MEDICAL RADIOLOGY
Diagnostic Imaging

Editors:
A. L. Baert, Leuven
K. Sartor, Heidelberg

Springer

Berlin
Heidelberg
New York
Hong Kong
London
Milan
Paris
Tokyo

Ali Guermazi (Ed.)

Radiological Imaging in Hematological Malignancies

With Contributions by

I. F. Abdelwahab · C. Adem · Y. Amano · T. Araki · J. Chiras · B. I. Choi · S. Choquet
K. B. M. Colquhoun · P. Costello · A. Coulon · K. Dan · M. A. Dimopoulos · E. Dion
P. J. DiPiro · G. D. Dodd III · E. K. Fishman · B. D. Fletcher · M. Furukawa · N. Furukawa
D. Galetta · A. Gangi · H. K. Genant · E. Gluckman · D. Gossot · A. Guermazi
R. P. Guillerman · S. Guth · J. K. Han · S. L. Hanna · G. Hermann M. C. Hull · A. Y. Kim
M. J. Klein · J. Kosiuk · T. Kumazaki · F. Lafitte F. E. Lecouvet · H. J. Lee · B. E. Maldague
J. Malghem · S. I. Marglin · T. Matsumoto · N. P. Mendenhall · B. Mesurolle · Y. Miaux
F. Mignon · S. Monzawa · L. A. Moulopoulos · C. G. C. Ooi · N. Oriuchi · B. R. Parker
I. M. Schmalfuss · S. Sheth · S. Sugai · K. Tajika · N. Tanaka · B. Taouli · O. Tokuda
H. Tonami · K. Tung · B. C. Vande Berg · E. Vázquez · I. Yamamoto

Series Editor's Foreword by

A. L. Baert

Foreword by

R. A. Castellino

With 584 Figures in 1268 Separate Illustrations, 96 in Color and 21 Tables

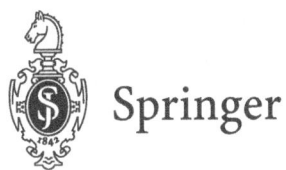 Springer

ALI GUERMAZI, MD
Visiting Associate Professor
Department of Radiology
Director, Radiographic Laboratory
Osteporosis & Arthritis Research Group
University of California, San Francisco
350 Pernassus Avenue, Suite 150
San Francisco, CA 94117
USA

MEDICAL RADIOLOGY · Diagnostic Imaging and Radiation Oncology
Series Editors: A. L. Baert · L. W. Brady · H.-P. Heilmann · M. Molls · K. Sartor

Continuation of Handbuch der medizinischen Radiologie
Encyclopedia of Medical Radiology

ISBN 978-3-540-43999-8   ISBN 978-3-642-18832-9 (eBook)
DOI 10.1007/978-3-642-18832-9

Library of Congress Cataloging-in-Publication Data

Radiological imaging in hematological malignancies / A. Guermazi, ed. ; with
    contributions by C. Adem ... [et al.] ; foreword by A. L. Baert.
        p. ; cm. -- (Medical radiology)
    Includes bibliographical references and index.
    ISBN 978-3-642-62313-4
        1. Lymphoproliferative disorders--Imaging. I. Guermazi, Ali. II. Series.
    [DNLM: 1. Hematologic Neoplasms--diagnosis. 2. Diagnostic Imaging--methods. WH
525 R1286 2003]
    RC646.2.R33 2003
    616.99'41807572--dc21   2003054384

http//www.springeronline.com
© Springer-Verlag Berlin Heidelberg 2004
Originally published by Springer-Verlag Berlin in 2004

The use of general descriptive names, trademarks, etc. in this publication does not imply, even in the absence of a specific
statement, that such names are exempt from the relevant protective laws and regulations and therefore free for general
use.

Product liability: The publishers cannot guarantee the accuracy of any information about dosage and application con-
tained in this book. In every case the user must check such information by consulting the relevant literature.

Cover-Design and Typesetting: Verlagsservice Teichmann, 69256 Mauer

21/3150xq – 5 4 3 2 1 0 – Printed on acid-free paper

Series Editor's Foreword

Due to the rapid development of chemotherapy and bone marrow transplantation, immense progress has been made over the past decade in the treatment concepts for hematological malignancies. At the same time, the new cross-sectional imaging modalities, in particular computed tomography (CT) and magnetic resonance (MR) imaging, have come to play a major role in the management of oncologic patients.

It is very important that radiologists should be familiar with modern imaging of the various hematological malignancies and with the changes that may be observed following treatment of these diseases.

This superbly illustrated volume covers all the relevant imaging features of the entire spectrum of hematological and bone marrow malignancies. The collaboration of many internationally well-known experts has resulted in first-rate, up-to-date, well written, and comprehensive chapters on all the main topics.

I would like to congratulate Dr. A. Guermazi and the authors most sincerely on producing this standard reference work on oncologic imaging. This outstanding book will certainly meet with great interest from radiologists with a special interest in oncology, but also from general and musculoskeletal radiologists. Hematologists and medical oncologists seeking to achieve better management of their patients will also greatly benefit from its contents. I am confident that it will meet with the same success with readers as previous volumes published in this series have done.

Leuven
ALBERT L. BAERT

Foreword

The malignant lymphomas (Hodgkin disease and the non-Hodgkin lymphomas) were the focus of intense investigation by clinicians and basic scientists for the latter half of the last century. As medical students 40 years ago, we were taught that Hodgkin disease was uniformly fatal. Remarkably, today the patients not only have an excellent likelihood of long-term survival, but the majority are cured of this disease. Only a few other malignancies – testicular cancer and some forms of childhood and adult leukemia come to mind – share this dramatic change in prognosis.

Not surprisingly, advances in the understanding of the basic biology of these diseases came largely from basic scientists and clinician–scientists. Development of novel – and often "aggressive" – therapeutic approaches was the result of insightful proposals by medical and radiation oncologists, often working in collaborative fashion. What is taken for granted today was, when first proposed and introduced in carefully constructed clinical trials, truly revolutionary and daring. Consider, for instance, megavoltage radiotherapy, a newly developed technology, to treat not only the site of known disease, but also adjacent lymph node groups that were clinically uninvolved! – and the simultaneous use of multiple, highly toxic, chemotherapeutic agents cycled over many months!

Medical imaging (not forgetting the assistance of our colleagues in surgical pathology) has provided important contributions to this team effort of clinical investigation. In the 1960s, lymphography demonstrated the relatively common occurrence of unsuspected retroperitoneal lymphadenopathy in patients otherwise felt to have disease limited to the neck or mediastinal lymph nodes. In the 1970s, CT provided additional information about involvement at other sites, such as the spleen, intra-abdominal lymph nodes, and gastrointestinal and genitourinary organs. The introduction of MR imaging in the 1980s and, more recently, the clinical acceptance of PET imaging has further expanded the ability to accurately display the tumor burden in patients with hematological malignancies. Importantly, comparison of serial imaging studies provides the most accurate and objective monitor of disease response, vital to guiding clinical trials and patient care.

In clinical practice, medical imaging studies are an integral component of the management of patients for most of the hematological malignancies discussed in this book. At the time of initial diagnosis, imaging studies provide information critical to appropriate staging, which guides therapeutic options. During treatment, imaging studies provide an objective measure of tumor response (or lack thereof). And, following completion of therapy, the patient enters a long period of clinical and imaging surveillance to monitor for possible tumor recurrence. Clearly central to these efforts is the careful performance and interpretation of these often-complex imaging studies. Importantly, the radiologist and nuclear medicine physician must provide strong guidance to the clinicians about which studies should – and which need not – be performed for optimal patient care. This is our responsibility, and we can best accomplish this by becoming active participants in the interdisciplinary management of these patients.

Dr. Ali Guermazi has undertaken the challenge of editing a comprehensive reference textbook addressing imaging studies in the hematological malignancies. To this end, he has enlisted the aid of an international group of clinician–investigators as contributors. They have shared their expertise in chapters that provide broad overviews of the basic biology and clinical manifestations of these disease entities, with appropriate emphasis on the varied imaging manifestations of these diseases and guidelines on appropriate utilization. The inclusion of chapters on the imaging manifestations of the effects of treatment adds to the value of this work.

Atherton, California

RONALD A. CASTELLINO

Professor of Radiology (emeritus) Stanford University School of Medicine
Chairman of Radiology (emeritus) Memorial Sloan-Kettering Cancer Center

Preface

The past 20 years have seen significant improvements in the diagnosis and treatment of patients with hematological malignancies. As new treatments have been developed, new side effects have appeared, and as patient life expectancy has increased, formerly unusual conditions have become more common. Rapid and accurate diagnosis is essential in these rapidly life-threatening conditions but is often difficult as clinical manifestations are rarely disease-specific. Imaging techniques, in combination with clinical and biological features, are essential for diagnosing many of these complications, as well as in differentiating between the manifestations of the underlying disease and complications of the treatment. These issues are directly addressed in this volume, which is one of the first books to deal specifically with imaging of the entire spectrum of hematological malignancies and to describe the use of the latest imaging modalities. Each of the 28 chapters was written by an expert internationally renowned in his or her field, making this the most complete volume currently available on this subject. This comprehensive treatise on radiological imaging in hematological malignancies combines a concise but, I hope, palatable text with a large number of carefully illustrated case presentations. All case diagnoses were verified, either histologically, where possible and/or appropriate, or by strong clinical or biological evidence.

After having spent more than 12 years as a radiologist at Saint-Louis Hospital in Paris, and after imaging and treating thousands of patients with hematological disorders, I believe that a book dedicated to the radiological aspects of these diseases will be of much use to radiologists and hematologists.

Many people have helped me to bring this project to fruition; without their assistance, which I gratefully acknowledge, this book would have never been published. I want especially to thank Professor Albert Baert, one of the leaders in radiology and the editor of European Radiology, who supported my idea and made its realization possible. Indeed, I approached him first about the appropriateness of such a book on radiology of hematological malignancies, and his positive answer was beyond my best expectations. Professor Baert was and is a mentor of my career. I am deeply grateful to him for his support. I would also like to thank Professor Ronald Castellino, who, during a meeting at his Californian retreat on a sunny day, gave me much encouragement and some very useful and practical advice. His support opened many doors and allowed me to secure the participation of internationally renowned radiologists, many of whom have worked with him and are leaders in their own right. I would like also to thank Professors Harry Genant, Klaus Sartor and Caroline Reinhold for their support and advice in writing this book.

During my radiologic training and fellowship, I had the pleasure to learn from Professors Jacques Chiras, Philippe Grenier, Gabriel Kalifa, Maurice Laval-Jeantet, and

Nicolas Sellier. Also during my time at Saint-Louis Hospital, I was fortunate to work with many talented physicians and radiologists. I would like to thank my many friends and colleagues from different departments at Saint-Louis Hospital, in particular those from the different departments of hematology. A special thank you to Doctor Yves Miaux, who gave me so much support during my years in France, and who is still "taking care" of me during my American experience.

I am grateful to the contributors, many of whom I now count among my friends, who have made this volume a reality. I am sure that their families suffered from their absence during the time they were working on their chapters. Thus, my thanks also go to their families, with my apologies.

I should not forget David Breazeale for his unconditional editorial assistance. He has reviewed every single sentence of the book. I also thank Ursula Davis of Springer-Verlag for always being there to answer my questions and for her endless patience.

Finally, I would like to thank my family, particularly my wife Noura and my daughter Dorra, for their support and love during all the time I spent working on the book. I also would like to thank all my friends in Tunisia, France and the United States for their support.

San Francisco   ALI GUERMAZI

"I will not permit considerations of religion, nationality, race, party politics, or social standing to intervene between my duty and my patient"

Hippocrates of Chios 470–410 BC

"In this manner, one passes up step by step until one reaches the very beginnings of all knowledge – namely, pure philosophy; to wit, metaphysics"

Abu Ali al-Husayn ibn Abd Allah ibn Sina (Avicenna) 980-1037

"Never allow the thought to arise in me that I have attained to sufficient knowledge, but vouchsafe to me the strength, the leisure and the ambition ever to extend my knowledge"

Abu Imran Musá ibn Ubayd Allah ibn Maymun al-Qurtubi (Maimonides) 1135–1204

Content

List of Abbreviations

AIDS: Acquired immunodeficiency syndrome
ALL: Acute lymphocytic leukemia
AML: Acute myeloid leukemia
BMT: Bone marrow transplantation
CLL: Chronic lymphocytic leukemia
CML: Chronic myeloid leukemia
CMV: Cytomegalovirus
CNS: Central nervous system
CSF: Cerebrospinal fluid
CT: Computed tomography
EBV: Epstein-Barr virus
FDG-PET: 2[(18)F]fluoro-2-deoxy-D-glucose-positron emission tomography
FLAIR: Fluid attenuated inversion-recovery
GVDH: Graft-versus-host disease
HD: Hodgkin disease
HIV: Human immunodeficiency virus
HRCT: High-resolution computed tomography
HSCT: Hematopoietic stem cell transplantation
HTLV: Human T lymphotropic virus
IGNB: Image-guided needle biopsy
IPI: International Prognostic Index
LDH: Lactate dehydrogenase
MALT: Mucosa-associated lymphoid tissue
MR: Magnetic resonance
NHL: Non-Hodgkin lymphoma
REAL: Revised European-American Lymphoma
STIR: Short tau inversion-recovery
US: Ultrasound
WHO: World Health Organization

1 MR Imaging of Bone Marrow

Bachir Taouli, Ali Guermazi, Elisabeth Dion, Harry K. Genant

CONTENTS

Bachir Taouli, MD
Assistant Professor, Department of Radiology, New York University Medical Center, 560 First Avenue, TCH-HW202, New York, NY 10016, USA
Ali Guermazi, MD
Visiting Associate Professor, Department of Radiology, University of California San Francisco, 350 Parnassus Avenue, Suite 150, San Francisco, CA 94117, USA
Elisabeth Dion, MD
Associate Professor, Department of Radiology, Pitié-Salpêtrière University Hospital, AP-HP, 83 Boulevard de l'Hôpital, F-75013 Paris, France
Harry K. Genant, MD
Professor of Radiology and Orthopaedics, Department of Radiology, University of California San Francisco, 350 Parnassus Avenue, Suite 150, San Francisco, CA 94117, USA

1.1 Introduction

In hematological malignancies, diagnosis and determination of disease stage, prognostic factors and response to treatment are important for adjusting the initial treatment to the spread and aggressiveness of the disease, for avoiding over or under-treatment during the course of the disease, and for comparing different therapies. Bone marrow imaging has advanced greatly with MR imaging, because MR presents a more global view of the bone marrow than biopsy material, and provides a better understanding of diffuse hematologic disease progression and resolution. Compared to other techniques, such as conventional radiography and CT, MR imaging is much sensitive to bone marrow disorders; however, it lacks specificity.

In this chapter, we will present the normal distribution and appearance of bone marrow at MR imaging, then discuss the different MR sequences that may be implemented for the imaging of bone marrow, and finally, describe the MR imaging patterns of marrow involvement in hematological malignancies at the time of diagnosis and after treatment, especially after radiation therapy.

1.2 Normal Bone Marrow Composition

Bone marrow occupies approximately 85% of the medullary bone cavity, the rest being occupied by a network of trabecular bone. It is constituted principally of fat and water, which makes assessment with MR imaging the modality of choice, particularly within the spine and pelvic girdle. MR imaging provides information about the bone marrow content rather than its mineral architecture, and alterations within the marrow signal can be easily seen using different MR imaging sequences. Normal bone marrow contains three components: trabecular bone, red (hematopoietic) marrow (Fig. 1.1a) and yellow (non hematopoietic) marrow (Fig. 1.1b). Red marrow is the active portion of bone marrow; it has a rich vascular supply, produces red cells, white cells and platelets, and contains about 40% fat, 40% water and 20% proteins in chemical composition, with a proportion of 60% hematopoietic cells to 40% fat cells (VANDE BERG et al. 1998a). Yellow marrow has a sparse vascular supply, contains mainly fat (80%) and a small proportion of water (15%); with 95% fat cells, its role is to provide nutritional support for red marrow (VOGLER and MURPHY 1988). The fraction of yellow marrow increases with age, as trabecular bone rarifies from osteoporosis, and is replaced by fat. Trabecular bone provides architectural support for red and yellow marrow. Accurate interpretation of signal intensity of bone marrow on MR imaging requires knowledge of the normal appearance and distribution of red and yellow marrow in the body.

1.2.1
Bone Marrow Conversion and Reconversion

Bone marrow is a dynamic organ that changes continuously through life, and therefore the MR appearance changes with age, in relation to the amount and distribution of red and yellow marrow (DOOMS et al. 1985; MOORE and DAWSON 1990; RICCI et al. 1990; DAWSON et al. 1992; KRICUN 1985). Conversion from red to yellow marrow is a physiologic process, occurs in a progressive manner, and is substantially completed by 25–30 years of age, proceeding in a centripetal direction from the extremities to the axial skeleton, starting in the distal bones of the extremities (feet and hands), and progressing finally to the proximal bones (humeri and femora) (Fig. 1.2). At birth and infancy, almost all marrow is red; by age 25, red marrow represents only half the marrow content, and is mostly restricted to the spine, sternum, ribs, pelvis, skull and proximal metaphyses of the humerus and femur, the remainder being fatty (Fig. 1.3).

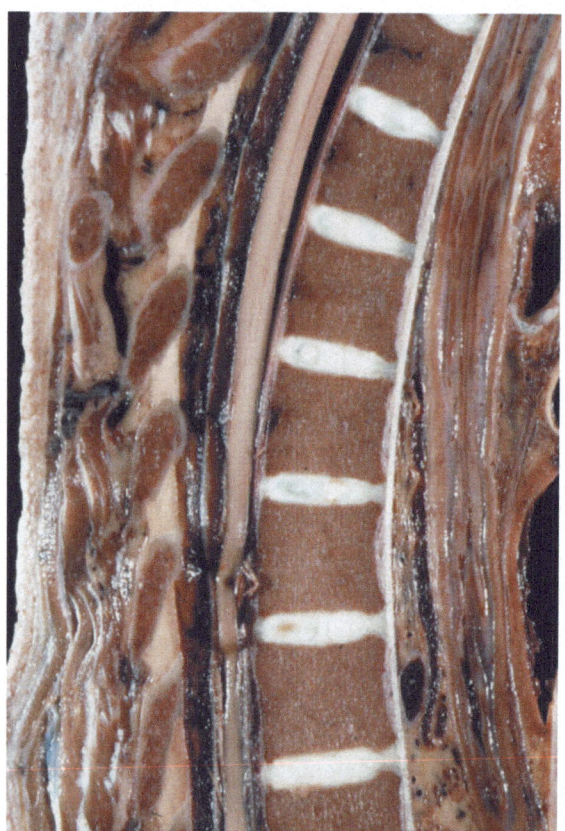 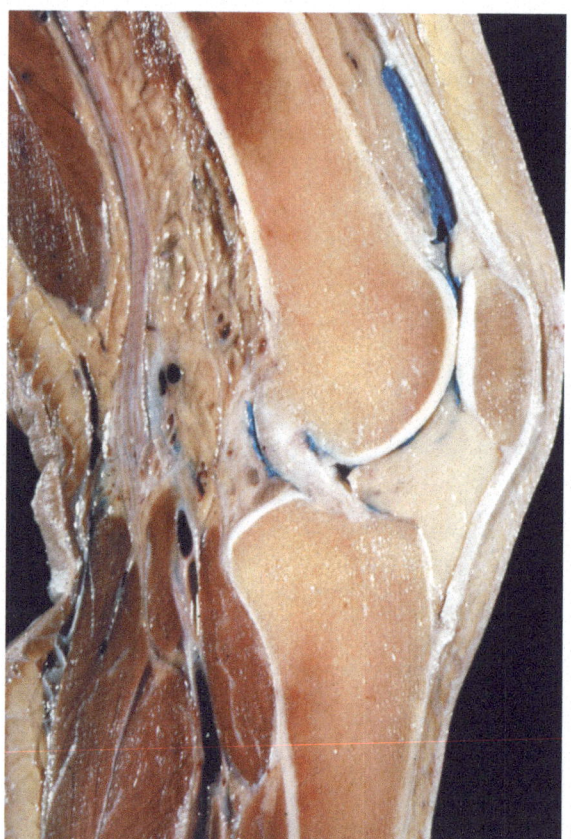

a   b

Fig. 1.1a,b. Anatomic specimens of normal red and yellow marrow in a 23-year-old man. **a** Sagittal anatomic specimen of the thoracic spine shows the normal appearance of red marrow. **b** Sagittal anatomic specimen of the knee shows normal appearance of yellow marrow in the knee, with some foci of red marrow in the distal femoral and proximal tibial metaphyses. *(Image courtesy of Dr. W. Rauschining)*

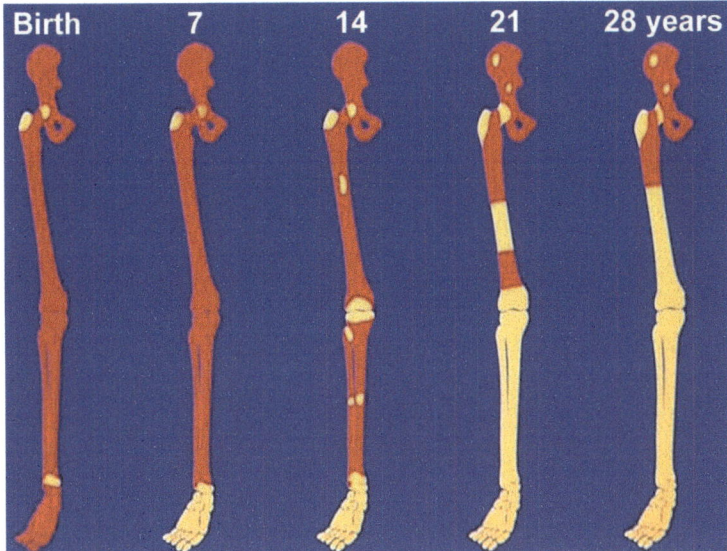

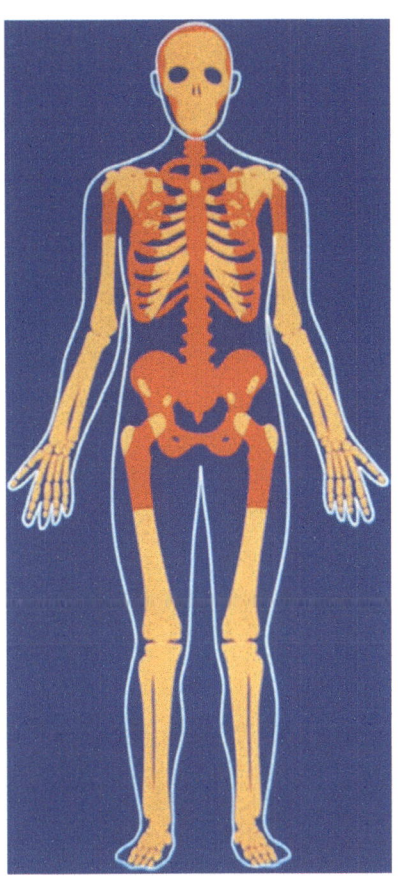

Fig. 1.2. Schematic of normal distribution of bone marrow in the lower limb with increasing age as seen in MR images. At birth, the majority of marrow is red. There is a physiologic progressive conversion from red to yellow marrow, completed by 25-30 years of age, proceeding in a centripetal direction from the extremities to the axial skeleton, occurring in the distal bones of the extremities (feet and hands) first, and progressing finally to the proximal bones (humeri and femora). *(Image courtesy of Drs. S. Moore and M. Kricun)*

Fig. 1.3. Schematic of normal distribution of young adult bone marrow. Macroscopic red marrow resides in the vertebral bodies, flat bones, and proximal metaphyses of the femora and humeri (red areas). The reminder of the skeleton (yellow areas) contains primarily yellow marrow. *(Image courtesy of Drs. S. Moore and M. Kricun)*

Benign hematopoietic marrow hyperplasia represents a normal variant of the marrow distribution in adults, and is recognized on MR imaging by the presence of low to intermediate signal on T1-weighted images in the distal metaphyses in asymptomatic young adults, especially in the distal femur (Fig. 1.4). Clues to normality also include absence of cortical destruction, poorly defined margins, and lack of epiphyseal involvement. It is associated with heavy smoking, long distance running, and with obesity in women. It is also seen in the menstruating age group (DEUTSCH et al. 1989; LANG et al. 1993; POULTON et al. 1993; SHELLOCK et al. 1992).

Red marrow reconversion is the reversal of normal physiological red marrow conversion to yellow marrow, in which yellow marrow progressively reconverts to red marrow. It proceeds from central to peripheral skeleton. It usually occurs in response to several disorders in which existing red marrow cannot meet the need for increased hematopoiesis such as chronic anemia, hypoxia (cyanotic heart disease), stress, and marrow infiltration or replacement. The reconversion occurs diffusely or as focal areas of red marrow in a background of yellow marrow.

1.3
MR Sequences Used to Image the Bone Marrow

MR signal of hematopoietic bone marrow depends on proton density and the T1 and T2 relaxation times. MR imaging sequences that show the fat and water differences are therefore useful. Using phased array coils, sagittal images of the spine and coronal images of the pelvis and proximal femurs can be obtained. Other sites can be imaged, depending on the location of clinical symptoms.

Conventional spin-echo sequences are helpful because of their great signal-to-noise ratio, and anatomic detail. Other sequences – such as STIR, fast spin-echo T2 sequences, diffusion-weighted imaging, and fat suppression techniques, as well as opposed-phase sequences – are also used to increase detection and characterization of bone marrow lesions (Table 1.1).

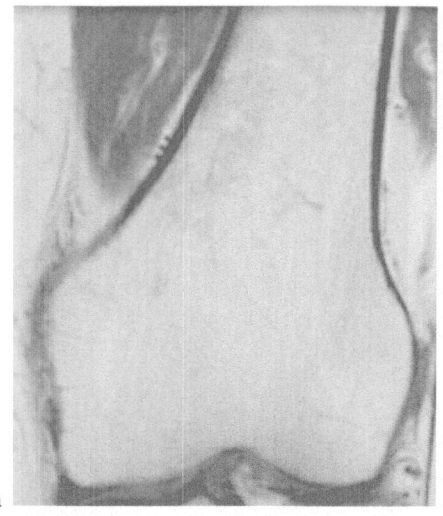

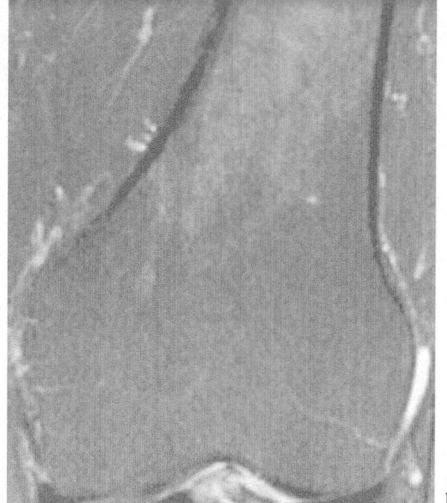

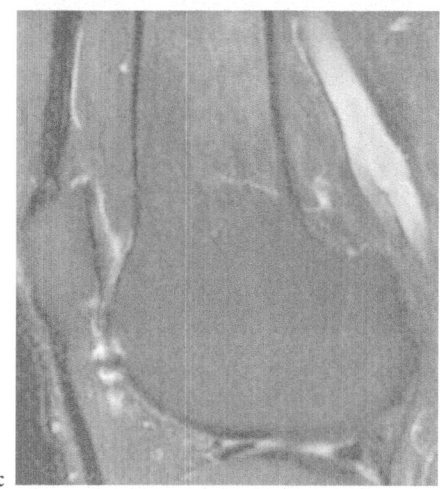

Fig. 1.4a–c. Normal red and yellow bone marrow in a 25-year-old woman. **a** Coronal spin-echo T1-weighted MR image of the knee shows red marrow with intermediate signal (higher than muscle), located in the distal femoral metaphysis. **b** Coronal and (**c**) sagittal fat-suppressed fast spin-echo T2-weighted MR images show fatty marrow which appears dark from fat suppression, and red marrow with intermediate signal, slightly higher than that of muscle.

Table 1.1. Characteristics of MR imaging sequences used to image the bone marrow

	T1-weighted sequence	Fast spin-echo T2-weighted sequence	STIR sequence	Opposed-phase sequence	Contrast-enhanced T1-weighted sequence
Fat suppression	No	Yes	No	No	Yes
Yellow marrow signal intensity	Bright	Dark	Dark	Dark	Dark with no or small enhancement
Red marrow signal intensity	Dark, but equal or higher than muscles and disks	Bright, equal or lower than muscle and disks	Bright, equal or lower than muscle and disks	Bright	Bright, with variable degree of enhancement
Marrow infiltration appearance	Dark, lower than muscles and disks	Bright, higher than muscle and disks*	Bright, higher than muscle and disks*	Bright	Bright, with strong enhancement
Advantages of the sequence	Very sensitive to marrow infiltration	Very sensitive to marrow infiltration	Very sensitive to marrow infiltration	Fast	Fast Possible differentiation of benign vs malignant vertebral fractures
Limitations of the sequence	None	Magnet field homogeneity for fat suppression	Lower signal to noise ratio than fast spin-echo T2-weighted sequence	Susceptibility artifacts	Still under evaluation Limited signal and resolution

*Exception: late stage myelofibrosis

1.3.1
T1-Weighted Spin-Echo Sequence

On T1-weighted images, tissue contrast is determined primarily by T1 characteristics. The use of spin-echo sequences is the most common approach to bone marrow imaging, and focal or diffuse lesions replacing fat will be easily detected on this sequence.

Fat has a short T1 relaxation time, and fatty marrow will appear hyperintense on T1-weighted images (Figs. 1.5–1.7). Red marrow, with lower fat content, will appear hypointense but remains iso or slightly hyperintense to muscles and intervertebral disks on the same images. On T1-weighted images, bone marrow signal intensity which is lower than muscle and discs in the spine is generally abnormal.

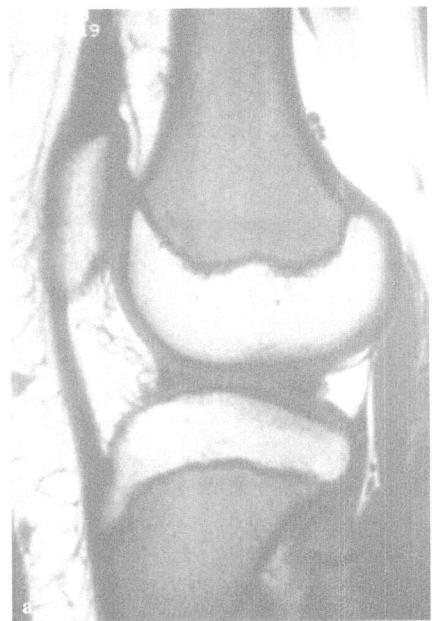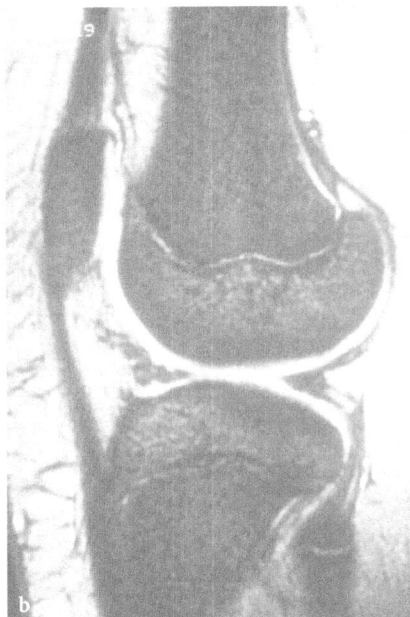

Fig. 1.5a,b. Normal red and yellow bone marrow in a 10-year-old boy. a Sagittal spin-echo T1-weighted MR image of the knee shows hyperintense fat marrow in the epiphyses and patella, and hypointense red marrow in the femoral and tibial metaphyses. b Sagittal gradient-echo T2-weighted MR image shows how the magnetic susceptibility effect from trabecular bone reduces bone marrow signal in both red and yellow marrow.

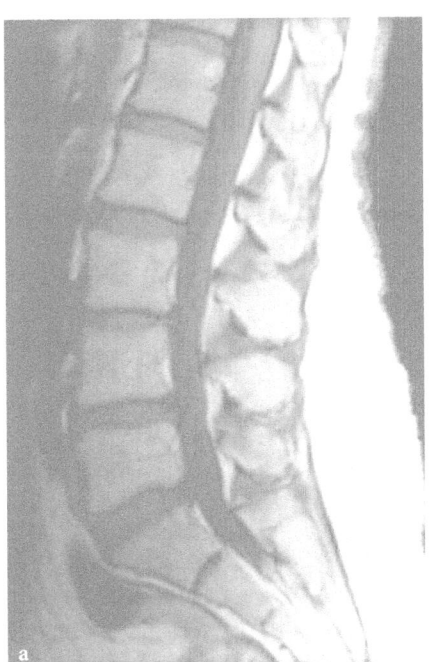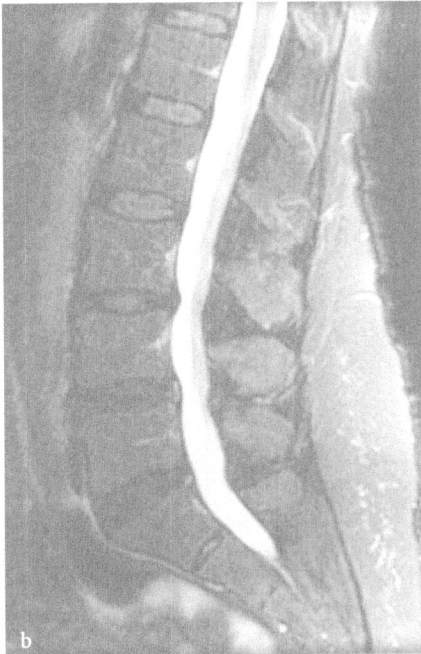

Fig. 1.6a,b. Normal appearance of the lumbar spine in a 57-year-old healthy woman. Sagittal (a) T1-weighted and (b) fat saturated fast spin-echo T2-weighted images show a normal signal pattern indicating a normal ratio of fatty and red marrow.

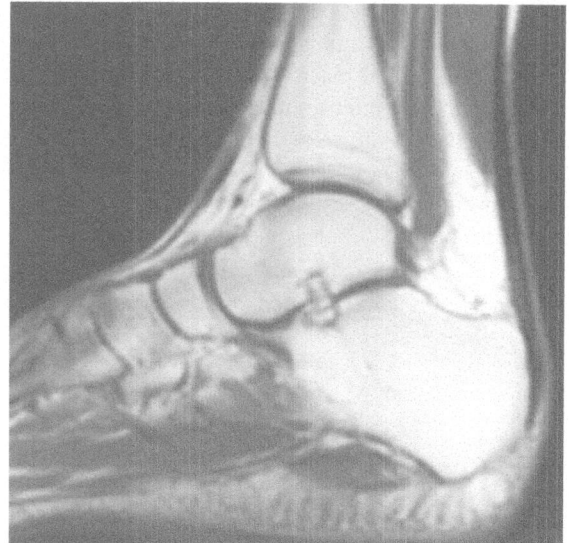
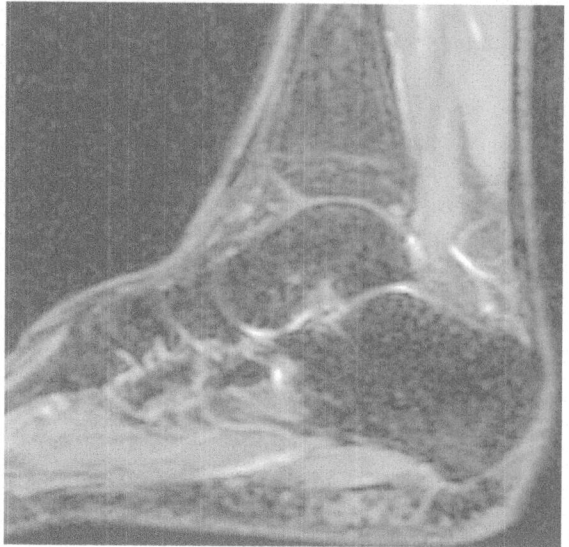

a
b

Fig. 1.7a,b. Normal yellow bone marrow in a 35-year-old woman. Sagittal MR images of the ankle show normal yellow marrow hyperintense on (a) T1-weighted and hypointense on (b) STIR images.

1.3.2
STIR Sequence

STIR sequence can be used to eliminate the signal from a selected tissue. It is a robust technique used to cancel the fat signal of the marrow by using an 180° inversion pulse. STIR images provide excellent conspicuity of cellular infiltration of the bone marrow, as good as fat-suppressed fast spin-echo T2-weighted images, but with less disturbance from field heterogeneity (MIROWITZ et al. 1994). This sequence is time consuming, and fast STIR (or turbo STIR) sequences can be used to decrease the imaging time.

Some recent studies have shown that whole-body MR imaging using turbo or fast-STIR can be used for the detection of metastases in patients with breast carcinoma and for patients with lymphoma (Fig. 1.8) or myeloma (Fig. 1.9) (WALKER and EUSTACE 2001; O'CONNELL et al. 2002; HARGADEN et al. 2003).

1.3.3
Fast Spin-Echo T2-Weighted Sequence

T2-weighted fast spin-echo (or turbo spin-echo) pulse sequences have replaced conventional spin-echo T2 sequences, offering the same image quality but with shorter acquisition times. For fat suppression, a saturation pulse with a narrow bandwidth is used; this

sequence needs a very homogeneous magnet field. On fast spin-echo images, red marrow generally demonstrates an intermediate signal intensity lower than that of yellow marrow. Indeed, the signal intensity of fat remains elevated and confusion between focal fat areas and lesions in red marrow may be difficult to resolve (CONSTABLE et al. 1992). Suppression of fat signal may be necessary to restore unequivocal distinction of fatty areas. On fat-suppressed fast spin-echo T2-weighted, and also STIR images, red marrow shows a signal intensity higher than that of yellow marrow (VANDE BERG et al. 1998a).

1.3.4
Gradient-Echo Sequences Using Chemical Shift Imaging

Most bone marrow pathology causes variations of the fat-to-water ratio, and the use of in-phase and out-of-phase MR sequences (Dixon technique) with different echo times that are sensitive to chemical shifts can be of high diagnostic sensitivity for imaging of bone marrow pathology. On in-phase images, the intra-voxel signal is proportional to the sum of water and fat protons, and normal yellow and red marrows appear hyperintense. On out-of-phase (opposed-phase) images, the contrast is related to the difference between the quantities of water and fat protons. With this technique, the red marrow will appear hypointense since it contains

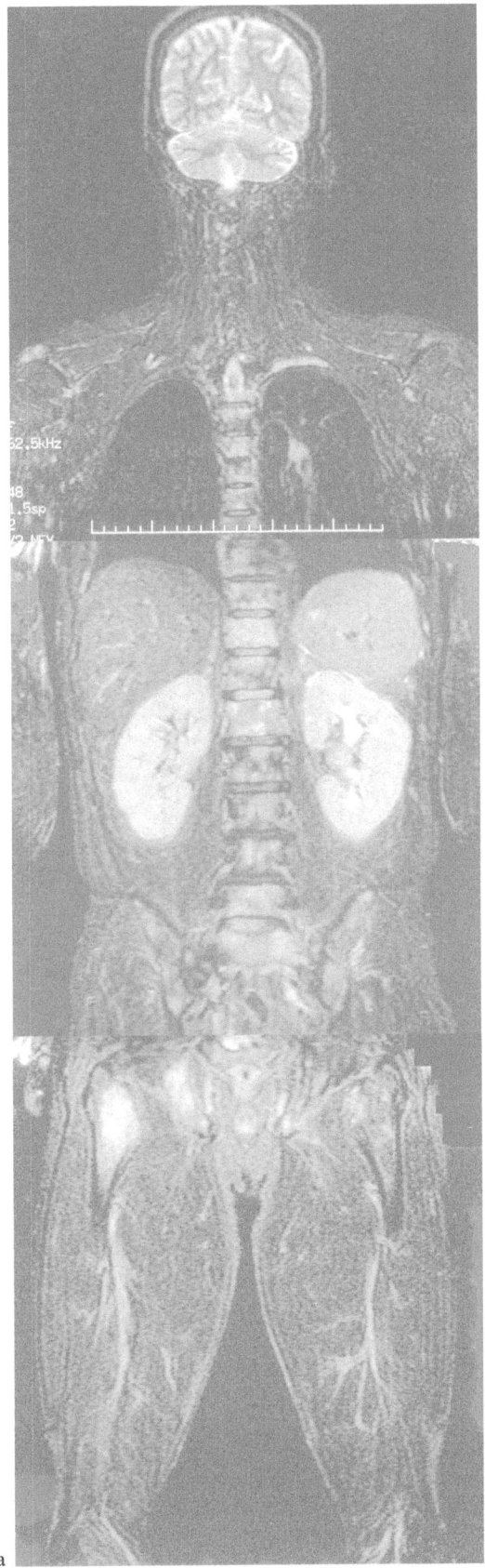

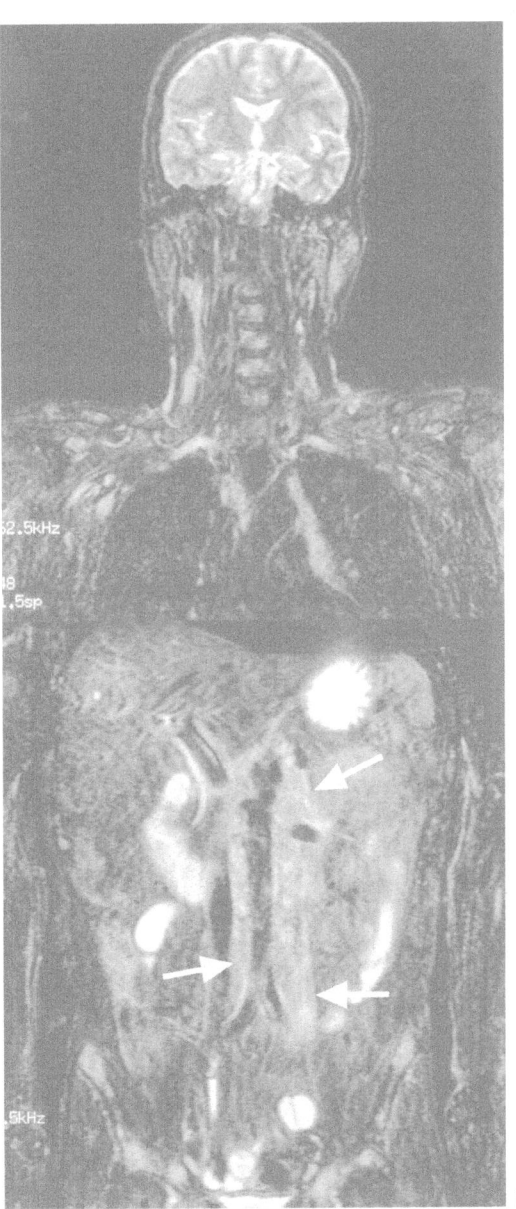

Fig. 1.8a,b. Diffuse involvement in a 51-year-old woman with Hodgkin disease. a, b Coronal whole-body fast STIR MR images show diffuse hyperintense areas in the cervical, thoracic and lumbar spine, ribs, ilia, and right femur. Large paraaortic lymph nodes (*arrows*) can be seen on (b). (*Image courtesy of Dr. M. Fukunaga*)

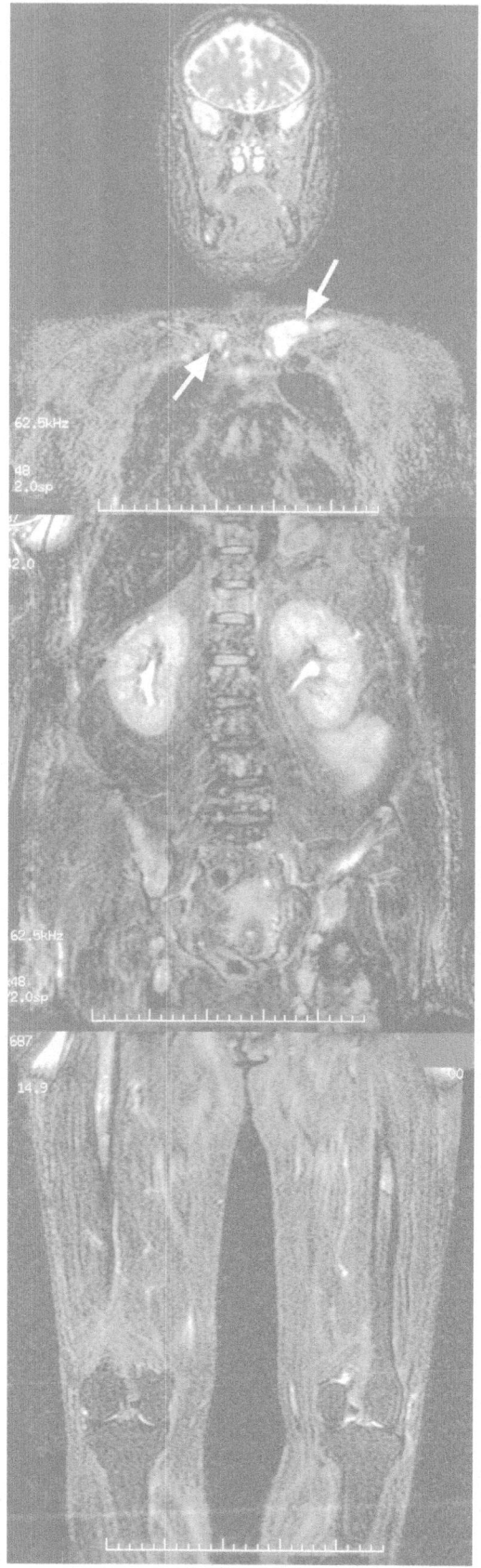

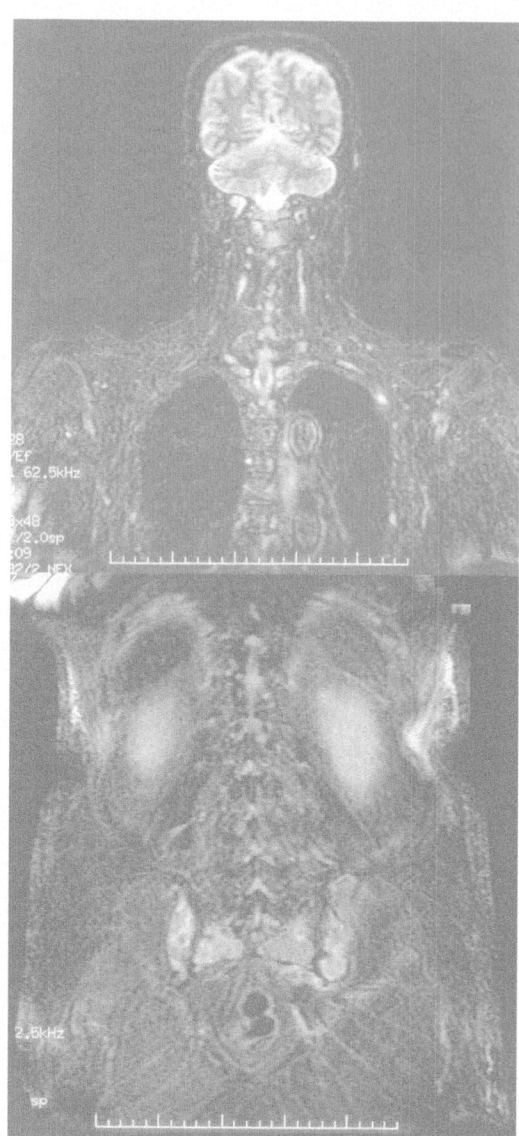

Fig. 1.9a,b. Diffuse involvement in a 61-year-old woman with multiple myeloma. **a, b** Coronal whole-body fast STIR MR images show hyperintense focal lesions in the clavicles (*arrows*), cervical, thoracic and lumbar spine, rib, ilia, sacrum, and femurs. *(Image courtesy of Dr. M. Fukunaga)*

approximately equivalent intra-voxel amounts of water and fat (Figs. 1.10, 1.11). Pathologic bone marrow as in inflammatory disease, edema and tumor infiltration will appear hyperintense on opposed-phase images, resulting in a high lesion-to-bone marrow contrast. Previous studies have shown that these sequences can help discriminate between neoplastic and nonneoplastic lesions of the bone marrow (DISLER et al. 1997; SEIDERER et al. 1999; ZAMPA et al. 2002).

1.3.5
Gadolinium Chelates Intravenous Injection

Intravenous contrast uptake is usually visualized on T1-weighted images, as unenhanced images are necessary for comparison. However, the changes visible on T1-weighted images are obscured by contrast enhancement without fat-suppression. Contrast-enhanced images can show abnormal soft tissue involvement, epidural (Fig. 1.12) and leptomenin-

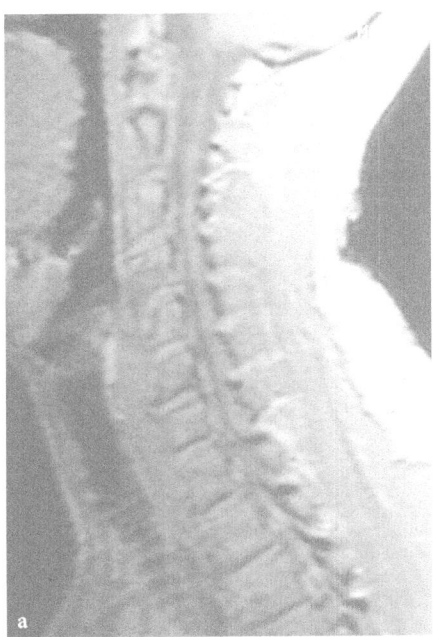
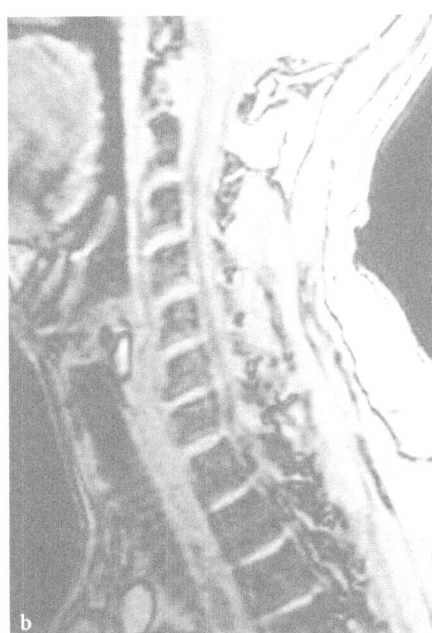

Fig. 1.10a,b. Chemical shift imaging of the cervical spine in a 38-year-old healthy man. Sagittal (a) in-phase and (b) opposed-phased MR images of the cervical spine show a normal signal drop on the out-of-phase image, related to the presence of microscopic fat in the vertebral bone marrow.

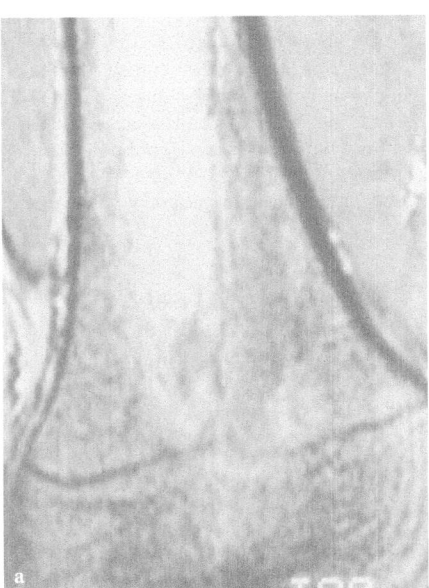
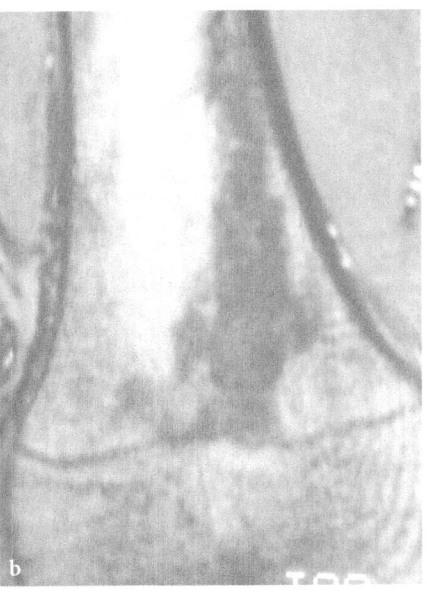

Fig. 1.11a,b. Normal appearance of yellow and red bone marrow in a 22-year-old woman. a Coronal in-phase gradient-echo MR image of the knee shows the red and yellow marrows have the same hyperintense signal. b On the out-of-phase gradient-echo MR image, the contrast between yellow and red marrow is more conspicuous, because of signal loss of the red marrow.

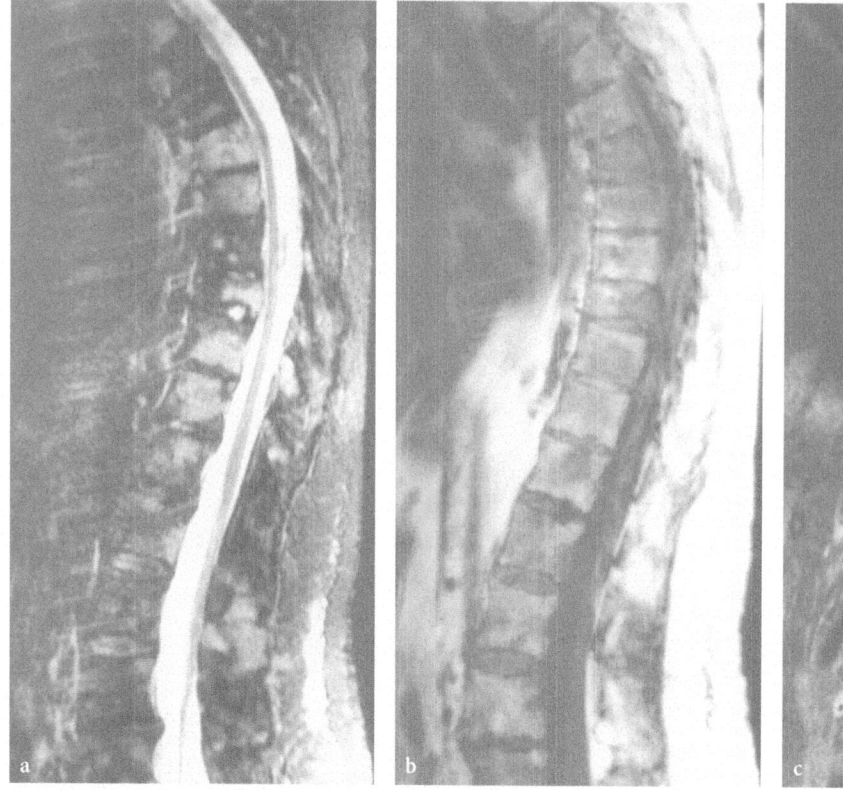

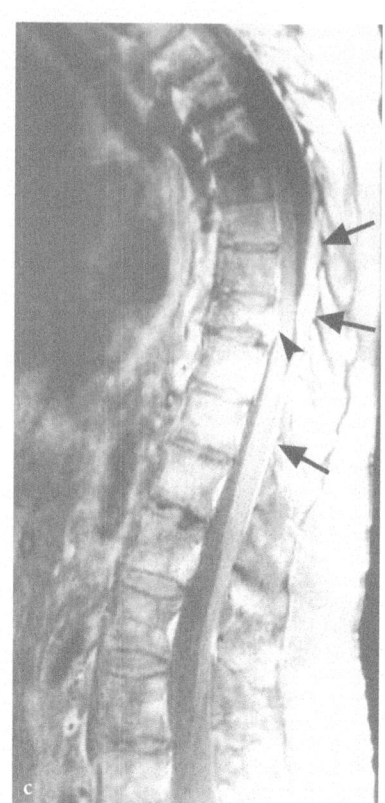

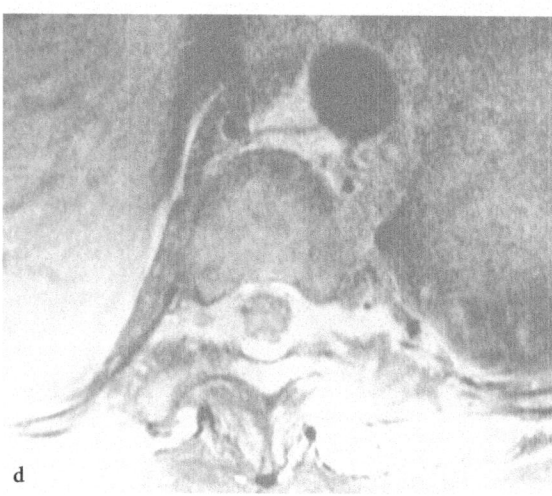

Fig. 1.12a–d. Epidural and spinal involvement in a 53-year-old woman with multiple myeloma. **a** Sagittal STIR MR image of the thoracolumbar spine shows diffuse hyperintense vertebral bone marrow infiltration and fracture of T8 vertebra. These lesions appear hypointense on (**b**) sagittal spin-echo T1-weighted MR image. **c** Sagittal contrast-enhanced fat-suppressed T1-weighted MR image shows diffuse and marked enhancement of abnormal marrow and also an anterior (*arrowhead*) and diffuse posterior (*arrows*) epidural enhancement. **d** Axial contrast-enhanced T1-weighted MR image at the level of T8 best demonstrates the epidural involvement.

geal enhancement. Contrast enhancement in healthy persons can vary greatly and is dependent on age. It is rarely conspicuous on visual inspection but can be detected by careful signal intensity measurements (SAIFUDDIN et al. 1994). In infants and to some extent children, diffuse marked enhancement of the vertebral (red) marrow can be seen (SZE et al. 1991). With increasing age, there is a significant decrease in contrast enhancement in normal bone marrow. In malignant bone marrow infiltration, the enhancement is usually higher than in normal bone marrow (BAUR et al. 1997), and the absence of contrast uptake almost certainly rules out involvement of bone marrow.

1.3.6
Diffusion-Weighted Imaging

Diffusion-weighted imaging allows for measurement of tissue microstructure and reflects the random motion

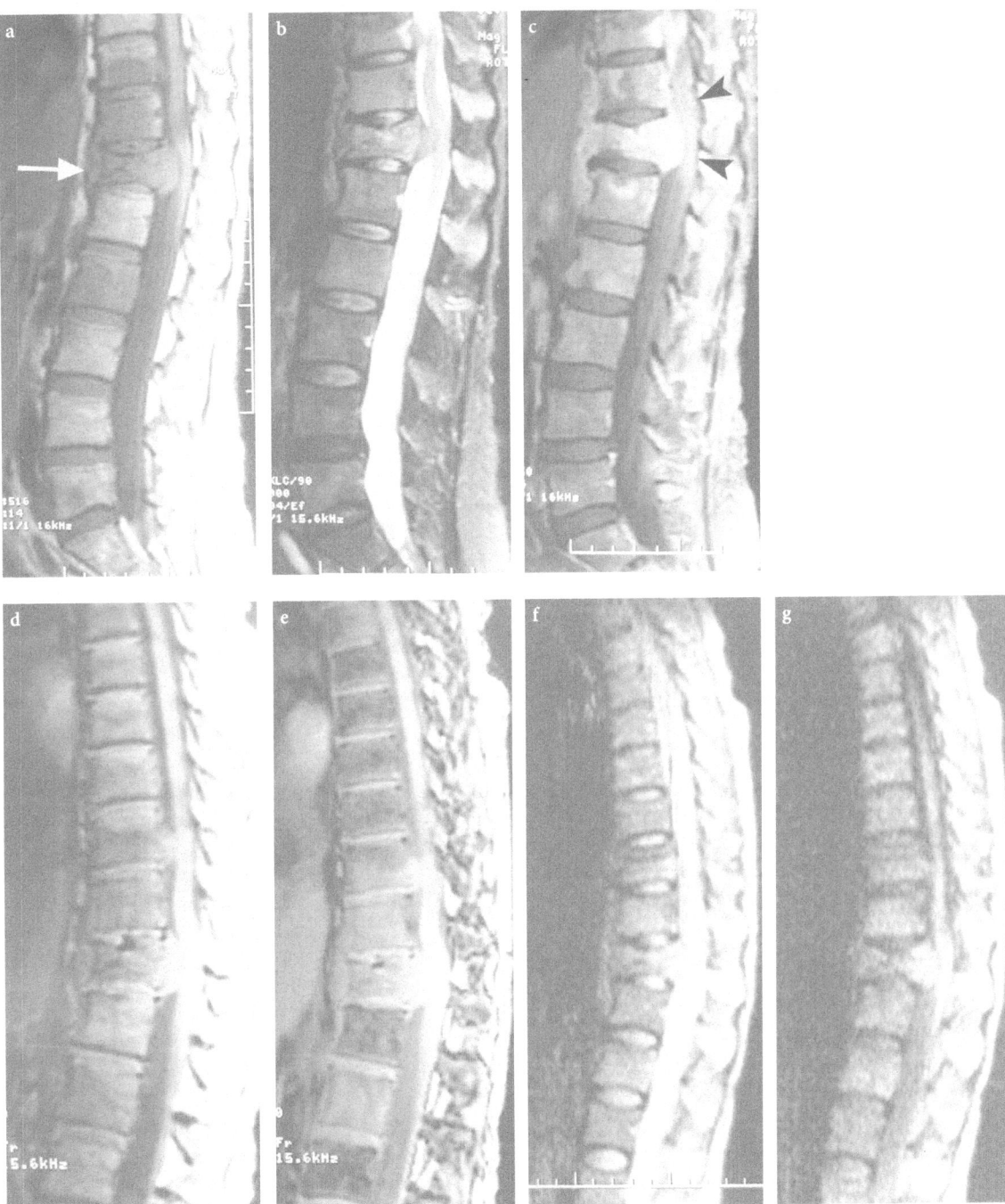

Fig. 1.13a–g. Multiple myeloma in a 53-year-old woman with multiple vertebral fractures. **a** Sagittal unenhanced spin-echo T1-weighted MR image of the thoracolumbar spine shows diffuse hypointense vertebral bone marrow infiltration at the levels of T10 to T12, L2 and L5, and vertebral fracture of T12 (*arrow*). These lesions appear mildly hyperintense on (**b**) sagittal fat-suppressed fast spin-echo T2-weighted image. **c** Sagittal contrast-enhanced T1-weighted MR image shows enhancement of abnormal marrow, particularly at the level of the vertebral fracture, with epidural enhancement and spinal cord compression (*arrowheads*). **d** In-phase and (**e**) out-of-phase MR images show signal attenuation of the red marrow, whereas the infiltrated bone marrow appears hyperintense on (**e**) due to the absence of fat content. Line scan diffusion-weighted images in which (**f**) b = 0 sec/mm² and (**g**) b = 750 sec/mm², show that vertebral fracture signal does not decrease after application of the diffusion gradient in relation to malignant infiltration. Note the complete attenuation of the cerebrospinal fluid and the decreased signal of the normally hydrated intervertebral disks.

of water protons. It provides a new method to study bone marrow alterations on the basis of altered water-proton mobility in various diseases (BAUR et al. 2003). In several recent studies, diffusion-weighted imaging was able to differentiate malignant from benign vertebral fractures, based on vertebral signal attenuation (BAUR et al. 1998; BAUR et al. 2001; SPUENTRUP et al. 2001). Using a steady state free precession sequence, BAUR et al. (1998, 2001) reported that pathologic compression fractures are hyperintense, whereas benign compression fractures are hypointense. They observed a decrease in the apparent diffusion coefficient (ADC), hypothesizing that hypercellularity by tumor cells reduced the extracellular space and mobility of water protons, resulting in increased signal on diffusion-weighted images (Fig. 1.13). In another study using diffusion-weighted imaging, the authors were able to differentiate benign vertebral fractures from malignant infiltration with 100% specificity, and the initial diagnosis was changed by the findings of diffusion-weighted imaging in 4 patients (SPUENTRUP et al. 2001).

1.3.7
MR Spectroscopy

The vertebral bone marrow fat/water ratios can be evaluated using MR spectroscopy, and this method can also quantify the reduction in fat fraction in infiltrative lesions (TRABER et al. 1996). MR spectroscopy has been also used to monitor hematopoietic reconstitution after bone marrow transplant (SCHICK et al. 1994).

1.4
MR imaging of Normal Bone Marrow

Yellow marrow
On T1-weighted images, yellow marrow has the same hyperintensity as subcutaneous fat. On non fat-suppressed T2-weighted images, yellow marrow will have an intermediate signal; on fat-suppressed T2-weighted and STIR images, it will be hypointense (Figs. 1.5–1.7). There is no significant signal intensity change in fatty marrow after contrast administration on spin-echo images, except on opposed-phase gradient-echo images.

Red marrow
Depending on the percentage of fat, red marrow will be relatively hypointense on T1-weighted images, but

always slightly hyperintense compared to muscle or intervertebral disks; and intermediate to hyperintense on STIR or fat-suppressed spin-echo and fast spin-echo T2-weighted images, where it appears similar to muscle (Figs. 1.14, 1.15). Because of the presence of fat – at least in adults – red marrow cannot be more hypointense than intervertebral disks or muscle on T1-weighted images. When the signal intensity of bone marrow appears lower than that of muscle or intervertebral disks, bone marrow infiltration should be highly suspected. After contrast intravenous injection, there is signal intensity enhancement of red marrow, but this appearance is rarely obvious on visual inspection.

Trabecular bone
Trabecular bone appears hypointense on both T1 and T2-weighted images, because of the low hydrogen content and magnetic susceptibility artifacts.

Marrow heterogeneity
On T1-weighted images, marrow heterogeneity can be caused by the presence of hyperintense areas due to focal yellow marrow which is a normal variant. Marrow heterogeneity can also be due to the presence of hypointense areas which can correspond to areas of red marrow, although it is sometimes difficult to distinguish from tumor infiltration. The features usually used to diagnose normal red heterogeneous marrow are: (1) symmetric distribution, (2) often parallel to subcortical bone, (3) with presence of central hyperintense areas corresponding to central fatty marrow. However, sometimes differentiating between the two entities can be extremely difficult (VANDE BERG et al. 1998b).

1.5
MR Imaging of Bone Marrow Infiltration in Hematological Malignancies

The thoracolumbar spine and the pelvic girdle contain 70% of the hematopoietic bone marrow in the body (CRISTY 1981) and are therefore the main sites of hematopoietic malignancies. The MR imaging appearance is completely nonspecific, showing hypointensity on T1 and hyperintensity on T2-weighted images, with replacement of normal yellow marrow. The only exception is advanced myelofibrosis, where the bone marrow appears hypointense on both T1 and T2-weighted sequences. Three patterns of involvement are described in malignant bone

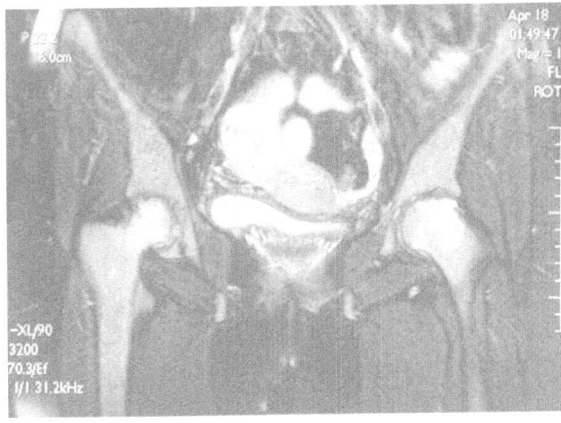
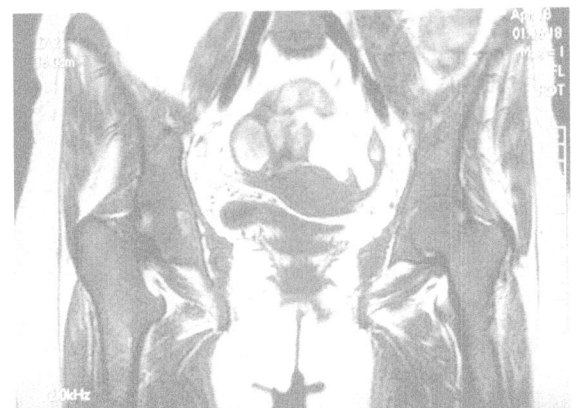
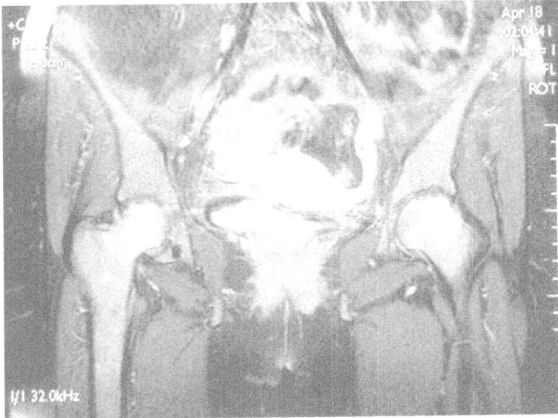

Fig. 1.14a–c. Normal bone marrow repopulation in a 55-year-old woman 2 months after bone marrow transplantation for multiple myeloma. Coronal MR images of the pelvis show the bone marrow is diffusely hyperintense on (a) fat-suppressed fast spin-echo T2-weighted, hypointense on (b) T1-weighted, and enhances (c) after contrast administration and fat suppression. These findings were found histologically to be related to normal red marrow repopulation. Bilateral femoral head osteonecrosis and edematous changes in the intertrochanteric are present.

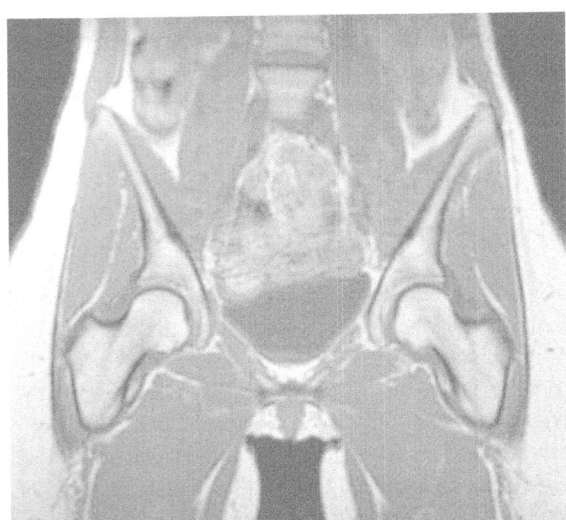
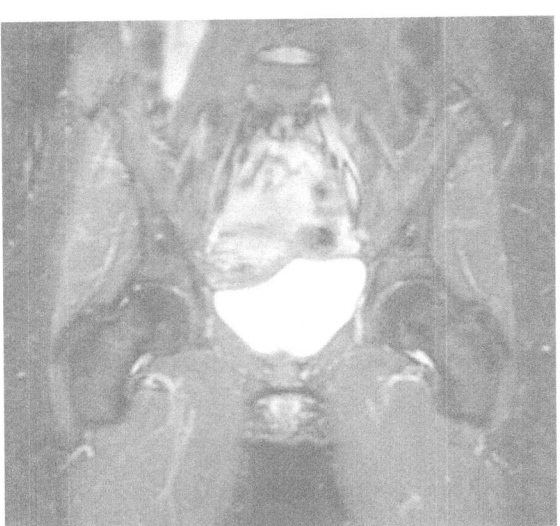

Fig. 1.15a,b. Normal red and yellow bone marrow in a 33-year-old woman. a Coronal spin-echo T1-weighted MR image of the pelvis and femora shows yellow marrow has the same hyperintensity as subcutaneous fat. The red marrow is intermediate in signal (higher than muscle) and is located in the proximal femoral metaphyses. b Coronal STIR MR image shows fatty marrow is hypointense, and red marrow with intermediate signal similar to muscle.

marrow infiltration: a focal pattern, consisting of focal lesions such as in metastatic disease; a diffuse pattern, typically seen in leukemia; and a variegated pattern, with multiple foci of infiltrative cells in a background of normal bone marrow.

1.5.1
Multiple Myeloma and Other Plasma Cell Dyscrasias

The diagnosis of solitary bone plasmacytoma requires histologic evidence of plasma cell infiltration at a single bony site, absence of clonal plasma cells at distant bone marrow sites, and a normal bone survey elsewhere. MR imaging should be used for staging of patients with solitary plasmocytoma to better assess the local extent of tumor (Fig. 1.16), to look for other foci of disease, and for follow-up, because some of these patients will eventually develop systemic disease (MOULOPOULOS et al. 1993a).

In multiple myeloma, MR imaging can show a focal or a diffuse pattern (Figs. 1.12, 1.17), or a salt-and-pepper (variegated) appearance of the bone marrow (STABLER et al. 1996), but it can also show a normal appearance. MR imaging can also depict epidural enhancement and vertebral fractures (Figs. 1.12, 1.17). Myelomatous lesions are usually hypointense on T1-weighted sequences, and hyperintense on fat-suppressed T2-weighted and STIR sequences (LIBS-HITZ et al. 1992; KUSUMOTO et al. 1997). MR imaging has been shown to be superior to bone radiographs for lesion detection in the spine and pelvis of patients with multiple myeloma (LECOUVET et al. 1999), and can be used for tumor mass assessment both at diagnosis and during follow-up in multiple myeloma (MOULOPOULOS et al. 1994; CARLSON et al. 1995). Quantitative contrast enhancement (RAHMOUNI et al. 1993a; STABLER et al. 1996) has been used for monitoring the response to treatment. Moreover, MR imaging is known to be of prognostic value in stage III patients (LECOUVET et al. 1998a) and has been shown to be more useful than radiographs in the follow-up of multiple myeloma patients with bone marrow transplants (AGREN et al. 1998).

1.5.2
Waldenström Macroglobulinemia

Waldenström macroglobulinemia is a rare, low-grade lymphoid malignancy infiltrating the bone marrow, lymph nodes and spleen with abnormal lymphoplasmocytoid cells. In one series, the bone marrow MR imaging involvement was diffuse (Fig. 1.18) or variegated, presenting the same appearance as in myeloma (MOULOPOULOS et al. 1993b). On the other hand, and in contrast to patients with multiple myeloma, no focal MR pattern was observed, and no normal MR imaging was found in any of the studied patients with macroglobulinemia (MOULOPOULOS and DIMOPOULOS 1997).

1.5.3
Lymphoproliferative Disorders

Bone marrow infiltration occurs in 5% to 15% of patients with HD, and 25% to 40% of patients with NHL (LINDEN et al. 1989). The presence of bone marrow infiltration classifies the patients in stage IV of disease. The diagnosis of marrow infiltration is obtained by bone biopsy, usually at the superior iliac crest, with a risk of sampling errors, even with bilateral iliac crest biopsies. MR imaging is known to be more sensitive than blind biopsy in detecting bone marrow invasion in lymphoma (SHIELDS et al. 1987; HOANE et al. 1991), and can show focal lesions distant from the iliac crests in patients with negative marrow biopsies, especially those with HD or intermediate to high-grade NHL. Therefore, MR imaging is used in conjunction with iliac crest biopsy in high-risk lymphoma patients. When present, bone marrow infiltration in lymphoma usually appears as diffuse (Figs. 1.19–1.21), and less frequently focal (OLSON et al. 1986; SHIELDS et al. 1987; HOANE et al. 1991). MR imaging can also depict soft tissue and epidural involvement, and also retroperitoneal lymphadenopathy. MR imaging is also useful to assess for post-treatment response.

1.5.4
Acute Leukemias

MR imaging is very sensitive in depicting bone marrow signal changes in patients with acute leukemia (Figs. 1.22, 1.23). Previous studies have reported that serial measurements of T1 relaxation time changes before and after treatment can differentiate responders from non responders (MOORE et al. 1986; THOMSEN et al. 1987; BENZ-BOHM et al. 1990; BOHNDORF et al. 1990). An increase in fat fraction (or decrease in T1 relaxation time) could be a good indicator of response to treatment (SCHICK et al. 1993), although this was not confirmed by another study (VANDE BERG et al. 1995). The changes in T1

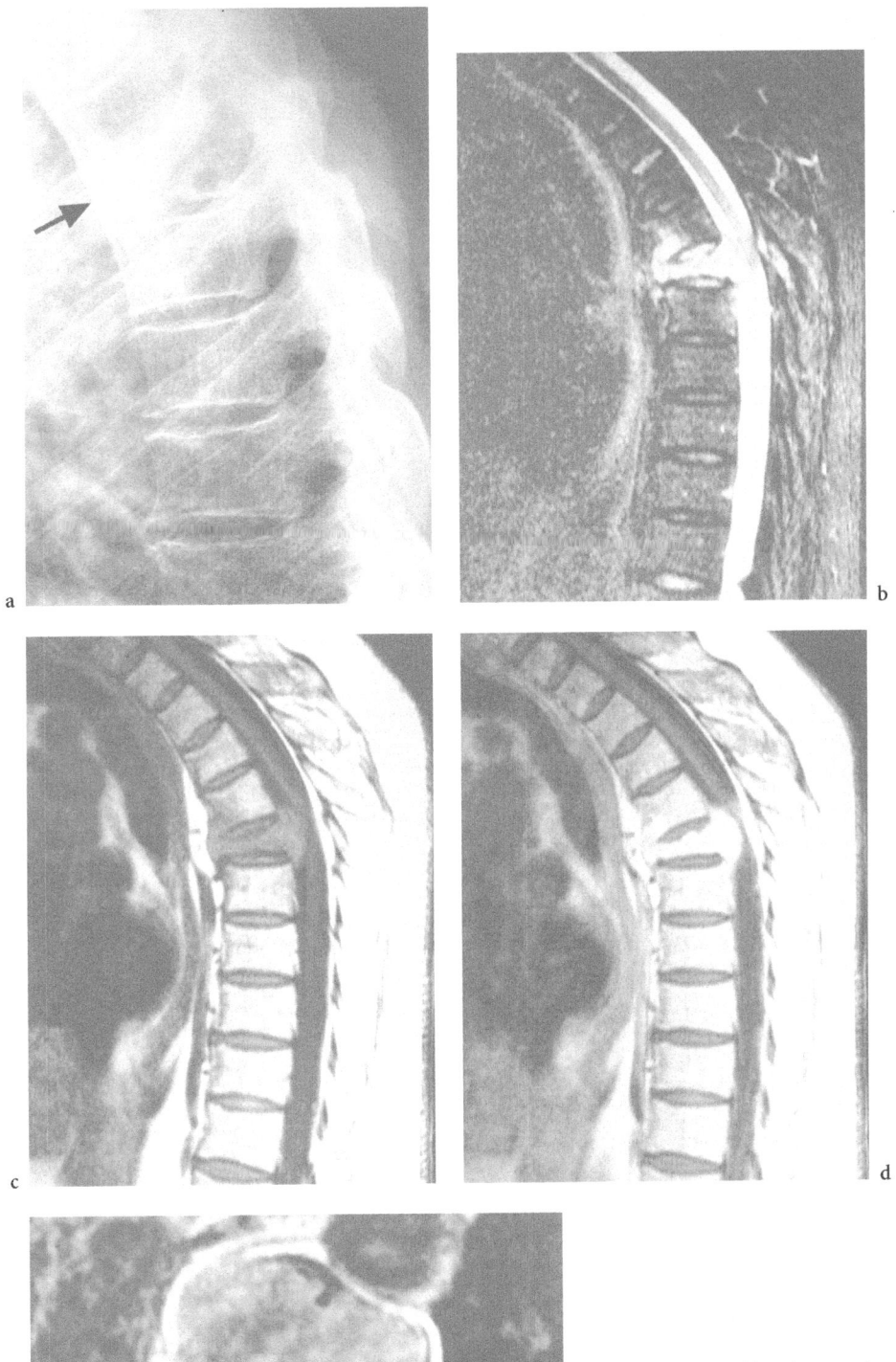

Fig. 1.16a–e. Focal involvement in a 62-year-old man with solitary plasmacytoma. **a** Lateral radiograph of the thoracic spine shows isolated fracture of the vertebral body of T5 (*arrow*). **b** Sagittal STIR MR image of the thoracic spine shows abnormal hyperintense signal of T5 with fracture, and also a contiguous involvement of T4. These lesions are hypointense on (**c**) sagittal spin-echo T1-weighted MR image and enhance strongly (**d**) after contrast administration. The T5 lesion extends posteriorly in the spinal canal with cord compression best seen on (**e**) axial contrast-enhanced T1-weighted MR image.

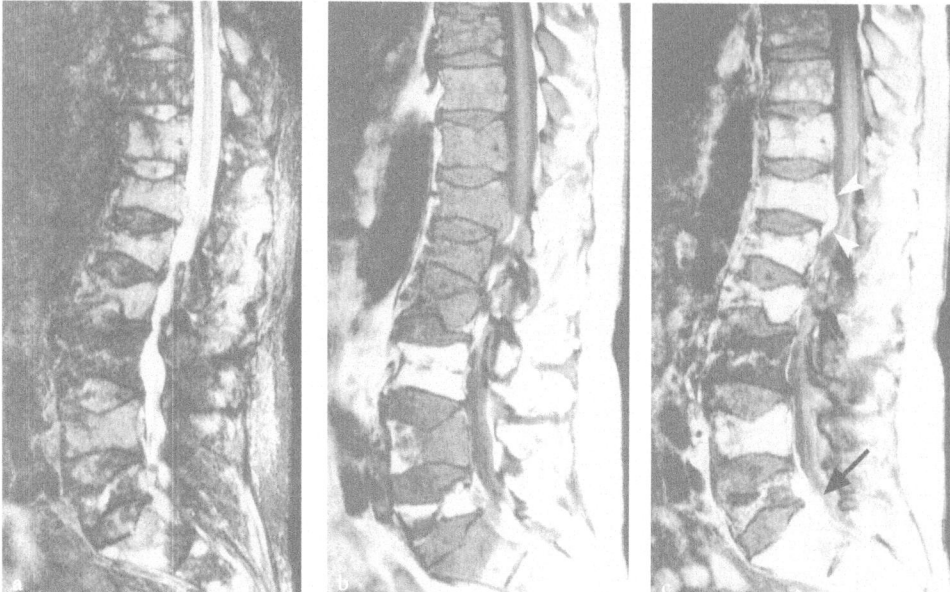

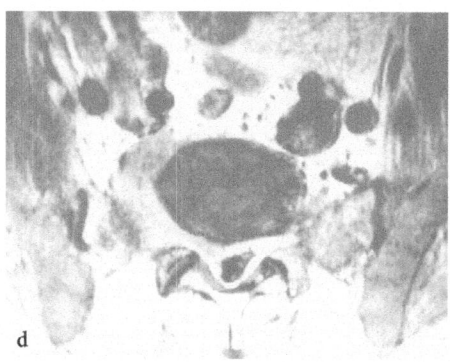

Fig. 1.17a–d. Diffuse involvement in a 58-year-old woman with multiple myeloma. a Sagittal STIR MR image of the thoracolumbar spine shows diffuse hyperintense vertebral bone marrow infiltration and multiple vertebral fractures. These lesions appear hypointense on (b) sagittal spin-echo T1-weighted MR image. c Sagittal contrast-enhanced T1-weighted MR image shows diffuse and marked enhancement of abnormal marrow and epidural enhancement at the level of T12-L1 (*arrowheads*). There is also a second foci of epidural enhancement at the level of L5-S1 (*arrow*) best seen on (d) axial contrast-enhanced T1-weighted MR image. The image (d) also demonstrates a heterogeneous involvement of iliac wings.

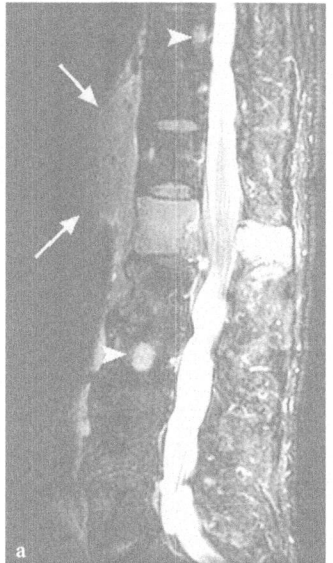

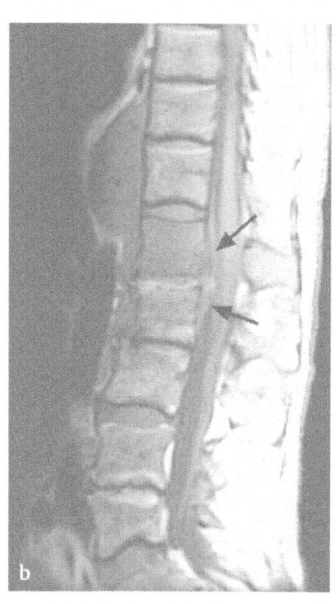

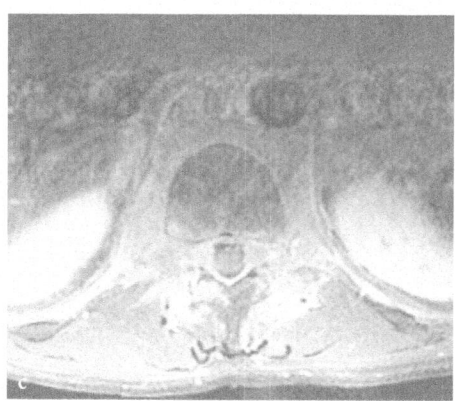

Fig. 1.18a–c. Epidural and spinal involvement in a 67-year-old man with Waldenström macroglobulinemia. a Sagittal STIR MR image of the thoracolumbar spine shows diffuse hyperintense vertebral bone marrow infiltration of L1 vertebra. This lesion appears hypointense on (b) sagittal spin-echo T1-weighted MR image. A large prevertebral mass (*white arrows*) is seen extending to the anterior epidural space (*black arrows*) with cord compression at the level of L1. There are also small marrow lesions (*arrowheads*) seen only on (a). c Axial contrast-enhanced fat-suppressed T1-weighted MR image at the level of L1 shows the prevertebral mass extending through the foramina with epidural involvement.

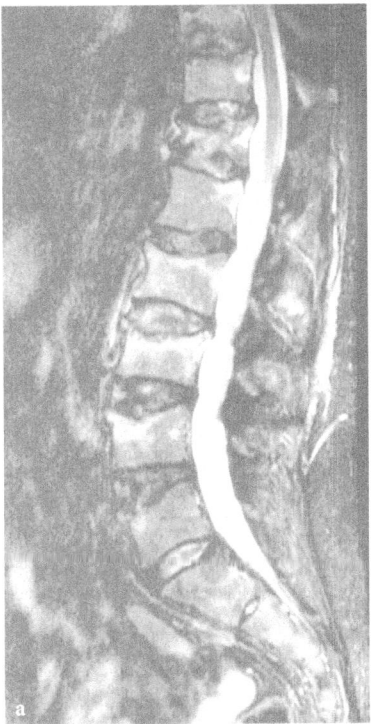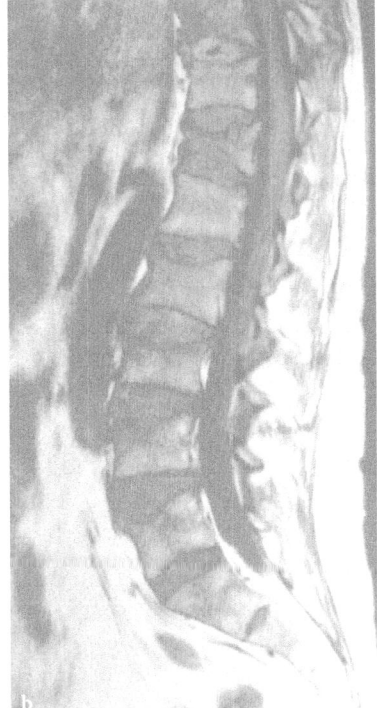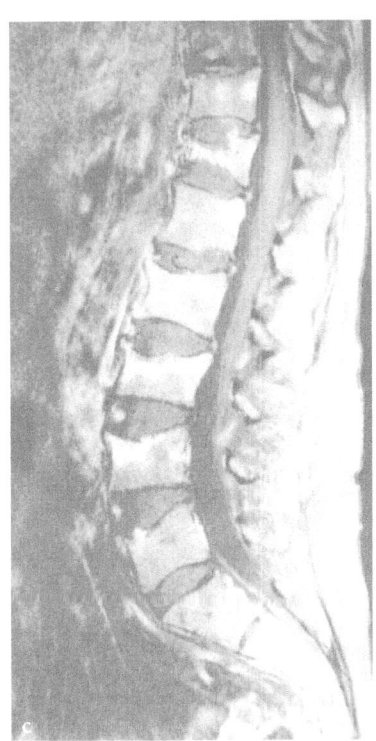

Fig. 1.19a–c. Diffuse involvement in a 42-year-old woman with non-Hodgkin lymphoma. **a** Sagittal STIR MR image of the thoracolumbar spine shows diffuse hyperintense vertebral bone marrow infiltration and multiple vertebral fractures. These lesions appear hypointense on sagittal (**b**) unenhanced spin-echo T1-weighted MR image and enhance markedly (**c**) after contrast administration and fat suppression.

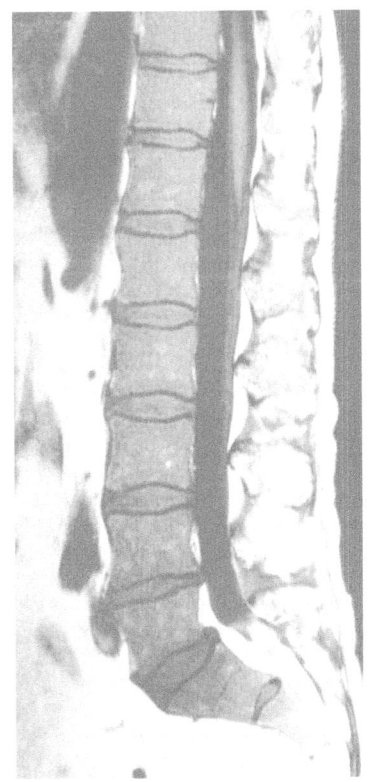

Fig. 1.20. Diffuse involvement in a 45-year-old woman with non-Hodgkin lymphoma. Sagittal spin-echo T1-weighted MR image of thoracolumbar spine shows diffusely hypointense bone marrow.

relaxation time may be affected by leukemic cell ablation and also by red marrow regeneration. VANDE BERG et al. (1995) concluded that post-treatment MR imaging lacks specificity to differentiate between active disease and red marrow regeneration in acute leukemia.

1.5.5
Myelofibrosis and Other Myeloproliferative Disorders

Bone marrow MR imaging in myeloproliferative disorders is an important tool for accurate diagnosis and monitoring and may be useful as an adjunct to bone marrow aspiration and biopsy (TAKAGI and TANAKA 1996).

Myelofibrosis is a chronic myeloproliferative disorder, which may be due to the proliferation of an abnormal clone of hematopoietic stem cells (idiopathic myelofibrosis), or secondary to several malignant and non malignant diseases (GUERMAZI et al. 1999). In idiopathic myelofibrosis, the normal fatty marrow is replaced by collagen, reticulin and cellular content, giving a typical hypointensity on T1 and T2-weighted

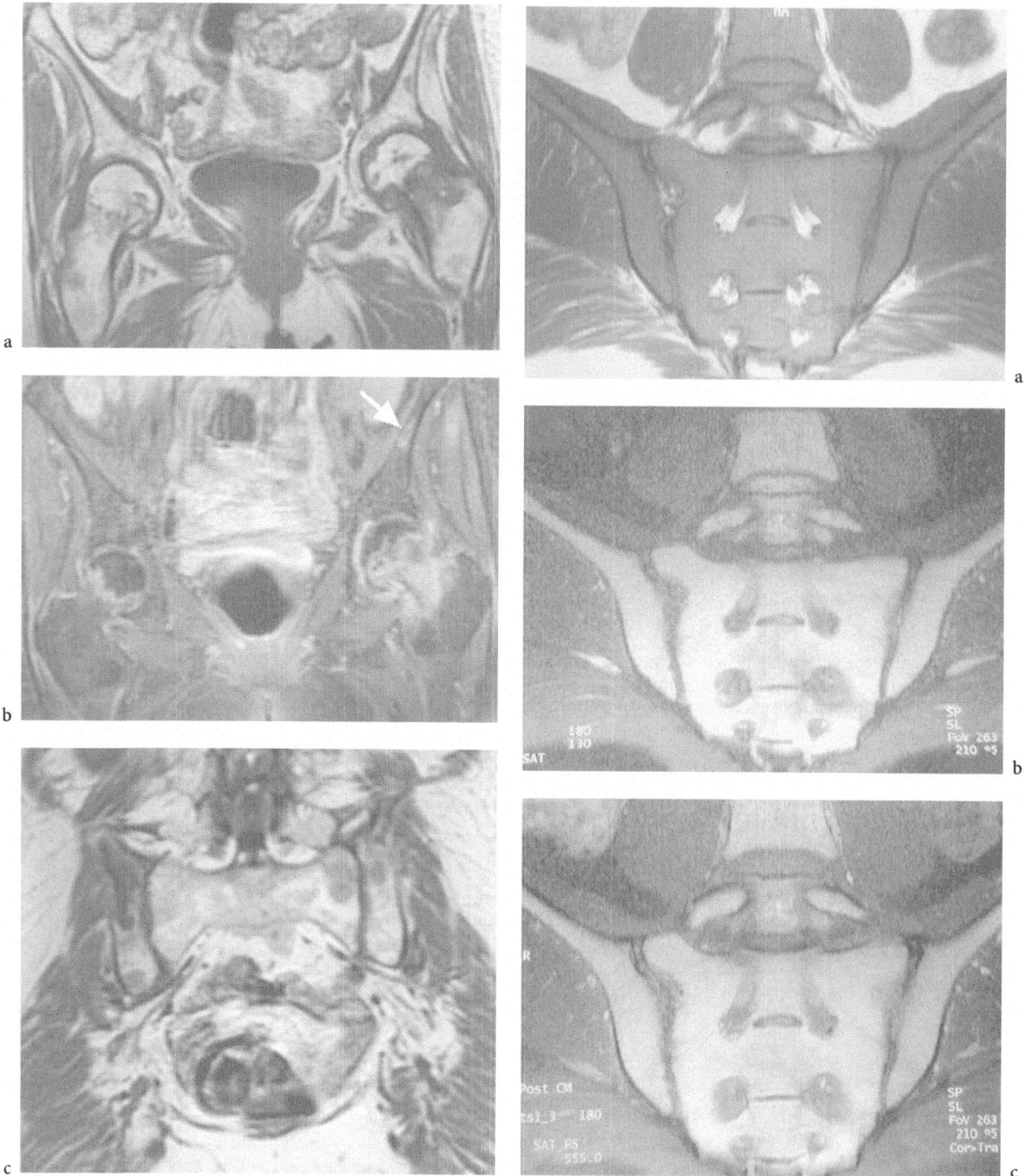

Fig. 1.21a–c. Diffuse involvement in a 70-year-old woman with non-Hodgkin lymphoma. Coronal MR images of the pelvis show heterogeneous lesion of the left femoral metaphysis appearing hypointense on (a) spin-echo T1-weighted and hyperintense on (b) fast spin-echo fat-suppressed T2-weighted images. A second lesion of the left iliac wing is also seen (*arrow*). c Coronal T1-weighted MR image posterior to (a) show additional hypointense lesions on iliac bones and sacrum. Bilateral femoral head osteonecrosis and left hip joint effusion are also present.

Fig. 1.22a–c. Bone marrow infiltration in a 12-year-old girl with acute myeloid leukemia. a Coronal fast spin-echo T1-weighted MR image of the pelvis shows a homogeneous hypointense replacement of the bone marrow. b The bone marrow appears hyperintense on coronal fat-suppressed fast spin-echo T2-weighted MR image. c Coronal contrast-enhanced fat-suppressed spin-echo T1-weighted MR image shows the homogeneous and marked enhancement of bone marrow. (*Image courtesy of Dr. S. Anderson*)

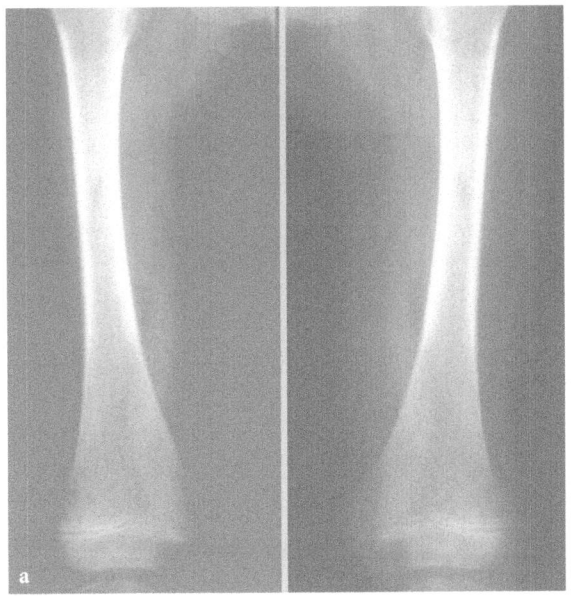

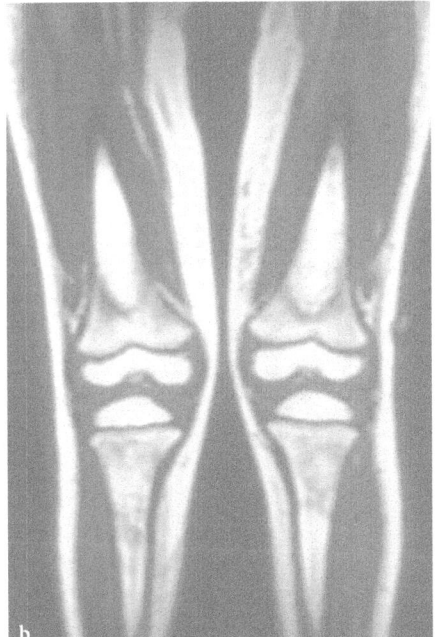

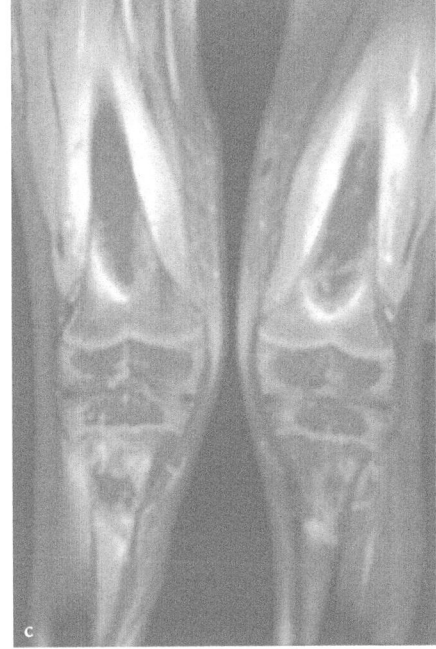

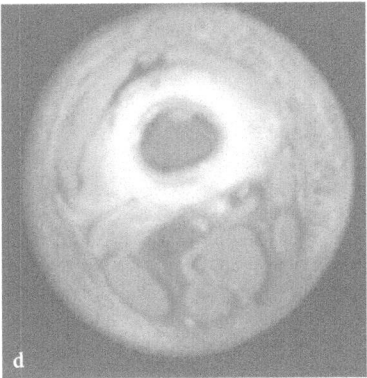

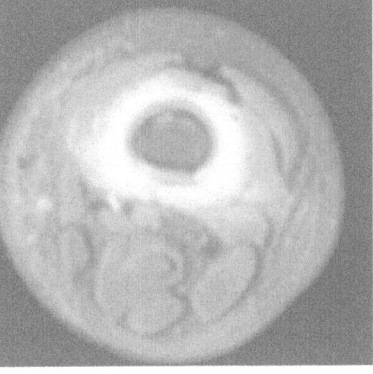

Fig. 1.23a–d. Periostitis in a 6-year-old boy with acute myeloid leukemia. a Anteroposterior radiographs of both femurs show subtle thickening of the cortical bone bilaterally. b Coronal spin-echo T1-weighted MR image of the lower limbs show diffuse bone marrow abnormalities corresponding to bone infarcts. There is no evidence of bone marrow infiltration. c Coronal and (d) axial fat-suppressed contrast-enhanced T1-weighted MR images confirm the bone infarcts and the absence of marrow infiltration but disclose a strong and bilateral soft-tissue enhancement surrounding the femoral diaphyses, corresponding to leukemic periostitis. *(Image courtesy of Dr. P. Kaplan)*

images in the late stage of fibrosis (Figs. 1.24, 1.25) (KAPLAN et al. 1992; GUERMAZI et al. 1999; ROZMAN et al. 1999; DIAMOND et al. 2002). This appearance can be also seen in patients with AIDS or iron overload (Fig. 1.26). However, in early stage myelofibrosis, the appearance is non specific, showing low signal on

T1-weighted images and high signal on STIR images (ALPDOGAN et al. 1998). KAPLAN et al. (1992) showed that patients with myelofibrosis and polycythemia vera and non fatty marrow in the proximal femur had significantly higher serum LDH and lower serum cholesterol levels than patients with fatty marrow.

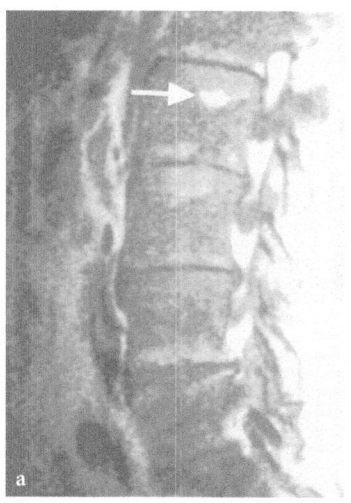
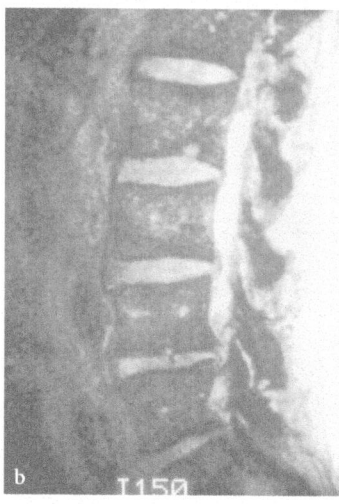

Fig. 1.24a,b. Stage III idiopathic myelofibrosis and secondary hemosiderosis in a 58-year-old woman. Sagittal (**a**) spin-echo T1-weighted and (**b**) gradient-echo T2-weighted MR images of lumbar spine show hypointensity of almost all marrow, with only a small focus of residual normal marrow in the L2 vertebral body (*arrow*). (*Image courtesy of Dr. P. Kaplan*)

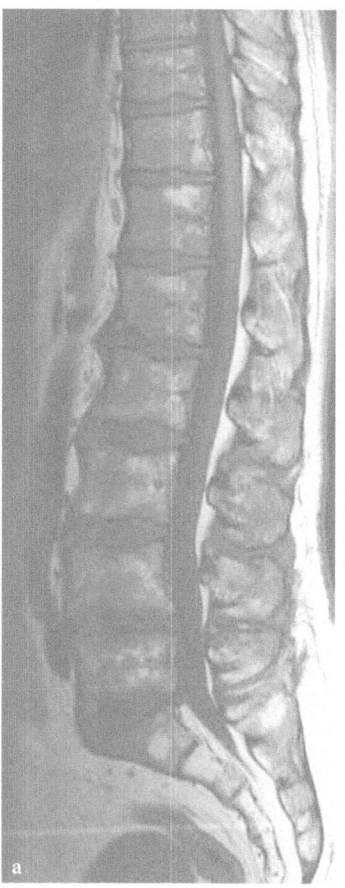
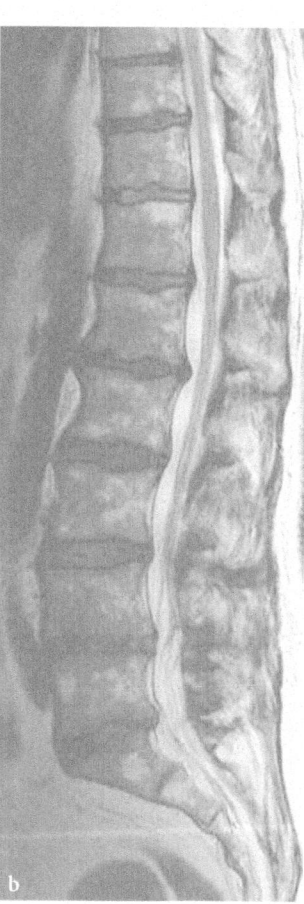

Fig. 1.25a,b. Stage III idiopathic myelofibrosis in a 61-year-old woman. Sagittal (**a**) spin-echo T1-weighted and (**b**) fast spin-echo T2-weighted MR images of thoracolumbar spine show hypointensity of almost all marrow, with small hyperintense foci of residual fatty marrow.

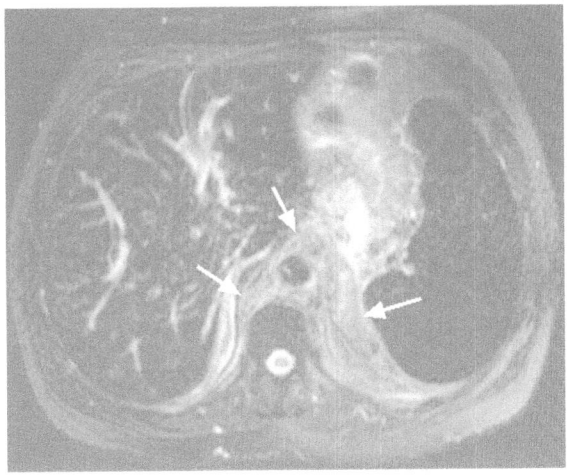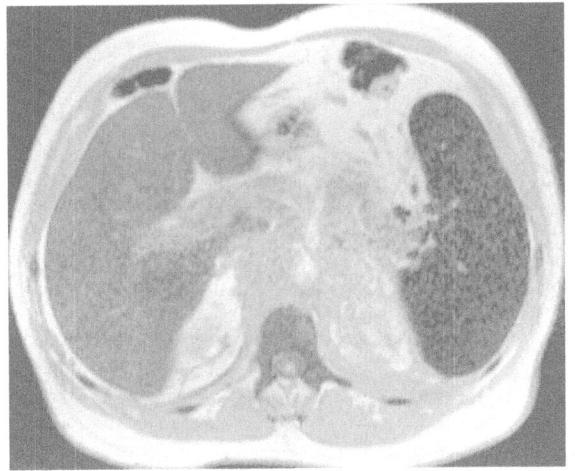

a
b

Fig. 1.26a,b. Hemosiderosis in a 58-year-old man with non-Hodgkin lymphoma and multiple prior blood transfusions. **a** Axial fast spin-echo fat-suppressed T2-weighted and (**b**) gradient-echo T1-weighted MR images of the abdomen show decreased liver and spleen signal, as well as a profound decreased signal of the vertebral bone marrow. A large non-Hodgkin lymphoma retroperitoneal nodal mass can be seen (*arrows*). Bone biopsy demonstrated increased iron content.

In polycythemia vera, the bone marrow of the axial skeleton appears diffusely and homogeneously hypointense on T1-weighted images (Fig. 1.27), indistinguishable from the appearance of myeloma or leukemia (MOULOPOULOS and DIMOPOULOS 1997).

In chronic leukemia, as in the other myeloproliferative disorders, the extent of marrow infiltration in the appendicular skeleton correlates with spleen size, which is a parameter indicative of disease extent. Bone marrow MR imaging findings in chronic leukemia do not differ from those of acute leukemia, and different studies have shown a significant prolongation of the T1 relaxation times compared with the normal range for hematopoietic bone marrow (Figs. 1.28, 1.29) (LECOUVET et al. 1998b; JENSEN 1990).

1.6
Post-Treatment Changes

During treatment, MR imaging is a valuable tool for the evaluation of response to treatment and for the diagnosis of benign bone marrow complications. Knowledge of post-therapeutic patterns is essential to avoid misinterpretation. However, the main drawback of MR imaging is its inability to differentiate residual lesions from fibrosis; needle guided-biopsy can be mandatory if treatment decision-making relies on the MR imaging result alone.

Initially after chemotherapy, the marrow is hypocellular with edema and necrosis, with corresponding diffuse hypointensity on T1-weighted images, and hyperintensity on T2-weighted images. After one week, the marrow is progressively colonized by fat cells, with a progressive hyperintensity T1. The administration of hematopoietic growth factors may delay the fatty infiltration or even cause marrow reconversion, simulating persistent disease or relapse.

Radiation therapy kills the hematopoietic cells as well as the malignant cells in the bone marrow. MR signal changes can be detected as early as 2 weeks after therapy begins (KAPLAN et al. 1992), showing initially edema and necrosis as diffuse low T1 signal and high signal on STIR (STEVENS et al. 1990a). About 2 weeks after the initiation of treatment, the signal of the bone marrow increases gradually on T1-weighted images and chemical shift imaging, and decreases on STIR images, in relation to fatty infiltration (Fig. 1.30) (STEVENS et al. 1990a; KAUCZOR et al. 1993), with possible areas of persistent red marrow surrounding the central marrow fat. The fatty infiltration is sharply limited to the radiation portals, and usually non reversible when the dose is equal to or higher than 50 Gy (CASAMASSIMA et al. 1989). Recurrent lesions will appear more conspicuous in a background of fatty marrow (Fig. 1.31). However, differentiation of regenerative red marrow and fibrosis from disease relapse can be difficult, and dynamic enhanced MR imaging has been used with success for that purpose in myeloma patients (RAHMOUNI et al. 1993b).

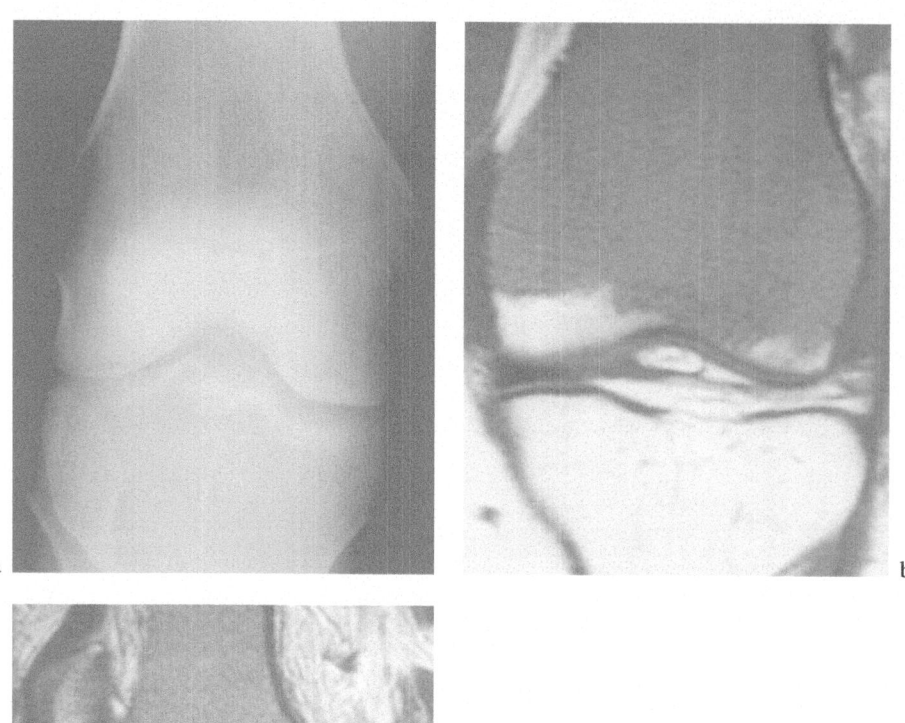

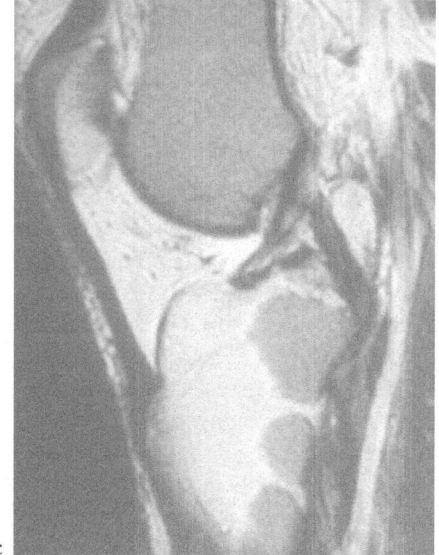

Fig. 1.27a–c. Bone marrow infiltration in a 60-year-old woman with poly-cythemia vera. a Anteroposterior radiograph of the knee shows no abnor-mality. b Coronal and (c) sagittal spin-echo T1-weighted MR images show heterogeneous bone marrow with hypointense areas of marrow replace-ment. *(Image courtesy of Dr. W. Palmer)*

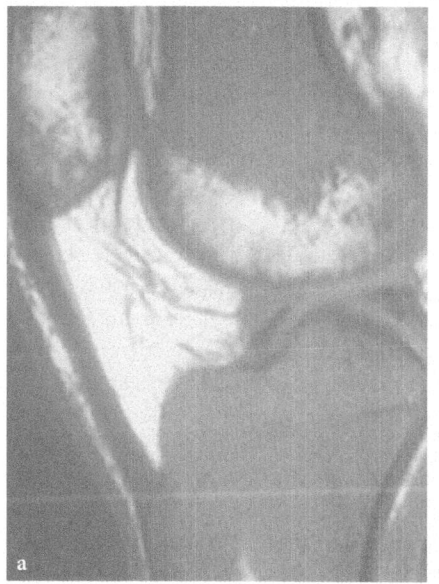

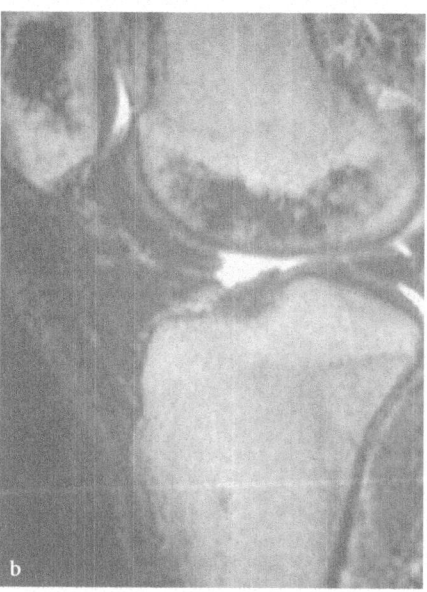

Fig. 1.28a,b. Bone marrow infiltration in a 21-year-old man with chronic myeloid leukemia. Sagittal (a) spin-echo T1-weighted MR image of the knee shows hypointense and heterogeneous bone marrow appearing hyper-intense on (b) fat-sup-pressed fast spin-echo T2-weighted MR image. These features correspond to the "Flip-Flop sign".

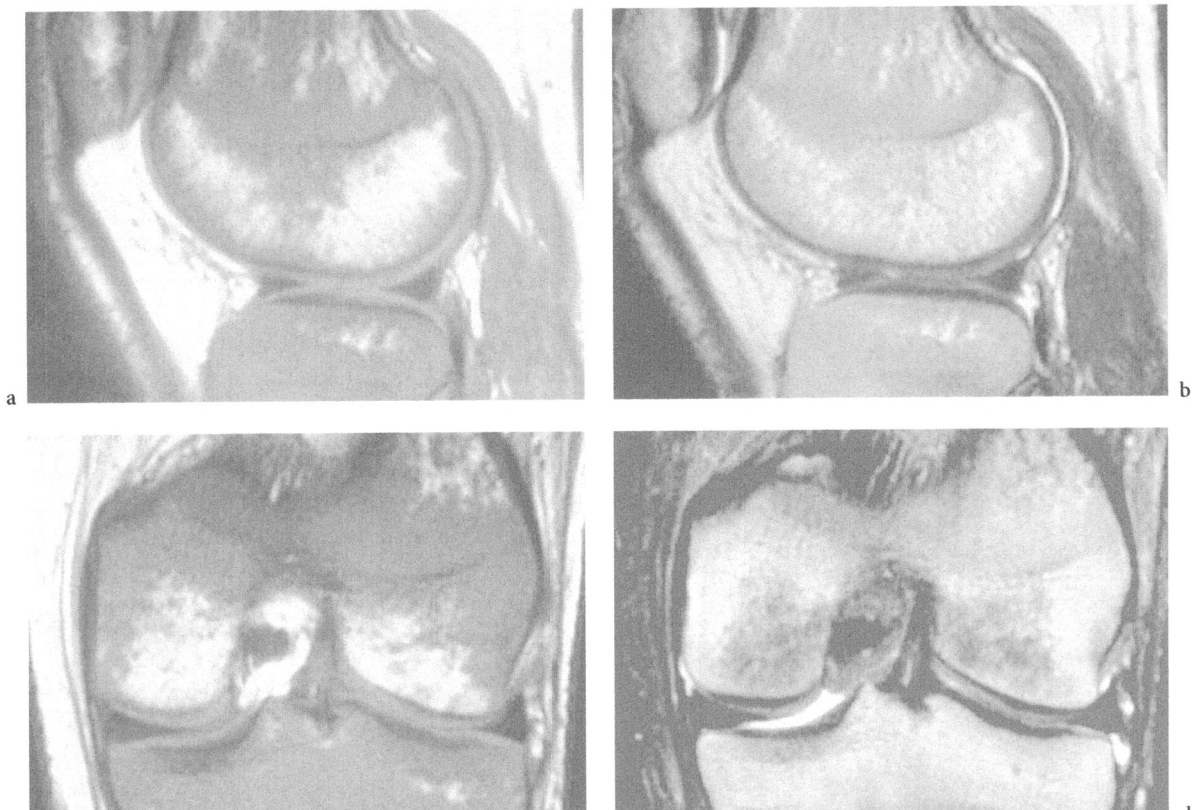

Fig. 1.29a–d. Bone marrow infiltration in a 21-year-old man with chronic myeloid leukemia. Sagittal (**a**) spin-echo T1-weighted and (**b**) fast spin-echo T2-weighted MR images of the knee show a heterogeneous replacement of the bone marrow, with the normal bone marrow appearing hyperintense. Coronal MR images clearly show the replacement of bone marrow with the remaining normal marrow appearing as hyperintense on (**c**) spin-echo T1-weighted and hypointense on (**d**) fat-suppressed fast spin-echo T2-weighted images.

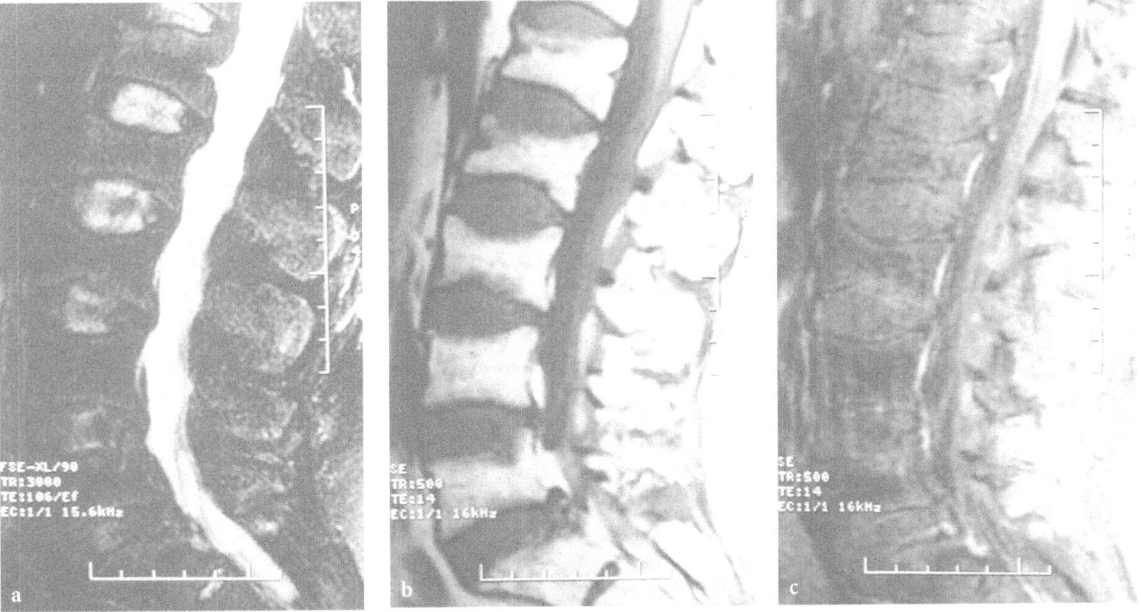

Fig.1.30a–c. Fatty replacement of the bone marrow in a 46-year-old man after radiation therapy for multiple myeloma. Sagittal (**a**) fat-suppressed fast spin-echo T2-weighted MR image of the lumbar spine shows diffuse homogeneous hypointensity that corresponds to homogeneous hyperintensity on (**b**) T1-weighted MR image. **c** Sagittal contrast-enhanced fat-suppressed T1-weighted MR image shows no abnormal enhancement.

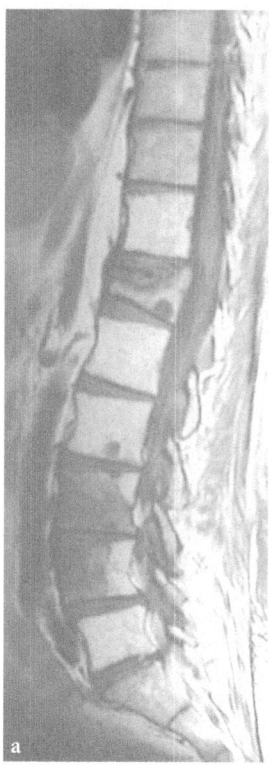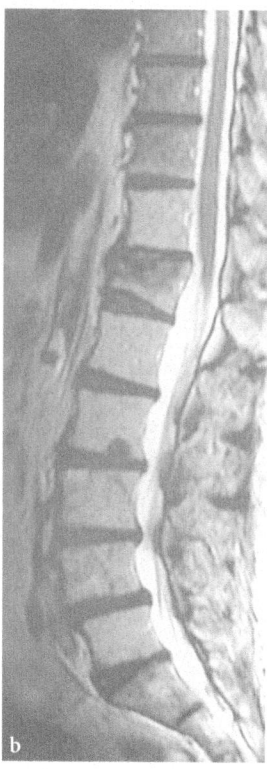

Fig. 1.31a,b. Marrow relapse in a 29-year-old man who underwent radiation therapy for non-Hodgkin lymphoma. Sagittal (**a**) T1-weighted and (**b**) fast spin-echo T2-weighted MR images show hyperintense marrow extending from T11 to L5, consistent with fatty replacement. There are several hypointense focal lesions in this area, better seen on (**a**) and corresponding to histologically proven recurrent marrow lesions, responsible for a pathologic fracture of T11. The vertebral marrow outside the radiation port has a red marrow appearance with intermediate signal intensity on (**a**) and hypointense on (**b**).

After bone marrow or stem cell transplantation, patients are followed with serial bone marrow aspirates and biopsies. MR imaging provides a noninvasive assessment of large volumes of bone marrow in these patients, and is a useful adjunct before and after BMT (Fig. 1.14). Immediately after the transplantation, marrow necrosis and edema is seen as low T1 signal and increased T2 signal. Within 3 months and up to 14 months after BMT, STEVENS et al. (1990b) observed in the majority of patients a characteristic band pattern consisting of a peripheral zone of intermediate signal intensity and a central zone of bright signal intensity on T1-weighted images. Histologically, the central zone corresponds to fatty marrow and the peripheral zone to regenerating hematopoietic marrow. MR imaging is also useful for selecting bone marrow harvest sites in patients who are candidates for autologous BMT.

1.7
Conclusion

Normal bone marrow has a variable appearance depending on the proportion of yellow and red marrow, which changes with age. Knowledge of these variations is mandatory for the interpretation of MR imaging of bone marrow. Despite its lack of specificity for bone marrow infiltration in hematological malignancies, MR imaging has become an important noninvasive method providing information on the diagnosis, staging, and monitoring of therapy in patients with hematological malignancies. In addition, MR imaging is unchallenged for the determination of the cause and level of spinal cord compression and vertebral fractures, and for the selection of patients for autologous bone marrow transplant.

References

Agren B, Rudberg U, Isberg B, Svensson L, Aspelin P (1998) MR imaging of multiple myeloma patients with bone-marrow transplants. Acta Radiol 39:36–42

Alpdogan O, Budak-Alpdogan T, Bayik M, Akoglu T, Kodalli N, Gurmen N (1998) Magnetic resonance imaging in myelofibrosis. Blood 92:2995–2997

Baur A, Dietrich O, Reiser M (2003) Diffusion-weighted imaging of bone marrow: current status. Eur Radiol 13: 1699–1708

Baur A, Huber A, Ertl-Wagner B, Durr R, Zysk S, Arbogast S, Deimling M, Reiser M (2001) Diagnostic value of increased diffusion weighting of a steady-state free precession sequence for differentiating acute benign osteoporotic fractures from pathologic vertebral compression fractures. AJNR Am J Neuroradiol 22:366–372

Baur A, Stabler A, Bartl R, Lamerz R, Scheidler J, Reiser M (1997) MRI gadolinium enhancement of bone marrow: age-related changes in normals and in diffuse neoplastic infiltration. Skeletal Radiol 26:414–418

Baur A, Stabler A, Bruning R, Bartl R, Krodel A, Reiser M, Deimling M (1998) Diffusion-weighted MR imaging of bone marrow: differentiation of benign versus pathologic compression fractures. Radiology 207:349–356

Benz-Bohm G, Gross-Fengels W, Bohndorf K, Guckel C, Berthold F (1990) MRI of the knee region in leukemic children. Part II. Follow up: responder, non-responder, relapse. Pediatr Radiol 20:272–276

Bohndorf K, Benz-Bohm G, Gross-Fengels W, Berthold F (1990) MRI of the knee region in leukemic children. Part I. Initial pattern in patients with untreated disease. Pediatr Radiol 20:179–183

Carlson K, Astrom G, Nyman R, Ahlstrom H, Simonsson B (1995) MR imaging of multiple myeloma in tumour mass measurement at diagnosis and during treatment. Acta Radiol 36:9–14

Casamassima F, Ruggiero C, Caramella D, Tinacci E, Villari N, Ruggiero M (1989) Hematopoietic bone marrow recovery after radiation therapy: MRI evaluation. Blood 73:1677–1681.

Constable RT, Anderson AW, Zhong J, Gore JC (1992) Factors influencing contrast in fast spin-echo MR imaging. Magn Reson Imaging 10:497–511

Cristy M (1981) Active bone marrow distribution as a function of age in humans. Phys Med Biol 26:389–400

Dawson KL, Moore SG, Rowland JM (1992) Age-related marrow changes in the pelvis: MR and anatomic findings. Radiology 183:47–51

Deutsch AL, Mink JH, Rosenfelt FP, Waxman AD (1989) Incidental detection of hematopoietic hyperplasia on routine knee MR imaging. AJR Am J Roentgenol 152:333–336

Diamond T, Smith A, Schnier R, Manoharan A (2002) Syndrome of myelofibrosis and osteosclerosis: a series of case reports and review of the literature. Bone 30:498–501

Disler DG, McCauley TR, Ratner LM, Kesack CD, Cooper JA (1997) In-phase and out-of-phase MR imaging of bone marrow: prediction of neoplasia based on the detection of coexistent fat and water. AJR Am J Roentgenol 169:1439–1447

Dooms GC, Fisher MR, Hricak H, Richardson M, Crooks LE, Genant HK (1985) Bone marrow imaging: magnetic resonance studies related to age and sex. Radiology 155:429–432

Guermazi A, de Kerviler E, Cazals-Hatem D, Zagdanski AM, Frija J (1999) Imaging findings in patients with myelofibrosis. Eur Radiol 9:1366–1375

Hargaden G, O'Connell M, Kavanagh E, Powell T, Ward R, Eustace S (2003) Current concepts in whole-body imaging using turbo short tau inversion recovery MR imaging. AJR Am J Roentgenol 180:247–252

Hoane BR, Shields AF, Porter BA, Shulman HM (1991) Detection of lymphomatous bone marrow involvement with magnetic resonance imaging. Blood 78:728–738

Jensen KE, Sorensen PG, Thomsen C, Christoffersen P, Henriksen O, Karle H (1990) Prolonged T1 relaxation of the hemopoietic bone marrow in patients with chronic leukemia. Acta Radiol 31:445–448

Kaplan KR, Mitchell DG, Steiner RM, Murphy S, Vinitski S, Rao VM, Burk DL, Rifkin MD (1992) Polycythemia vera and myelofibrosis: correlation of MR imaging, clinical, and laboratory findings. Radiology 183:329–334

Kauczor HU, Brix G, Dietl B, Jarosch K, Knopp MV, van Kaick G (1993) Bone marrow after autologous blood stem cell transplantation and total body irradiation: magnetic resonance and chemical shift imaging. Magn Reson Imaging 1993: 11:965–975

Kricun ME (1985) Red-yellow marrow conversion: its effect on the location of some solitary bone lesions. Skeletal Radiol 14:10–9

Kusumoto S, Jinnai I, Itoh K, Kawai N, Sakata T, Matsuda A, Tominaga K, Murohashi I, Bessho M, Harashima K, Heshiki A (1997) Magnetic resonance imaging patterns in patients with multiple myeloma. Br J Haematol 99:649–655

Lang P, Fritz R, Majumdar S, Vahlensieck M, Peterfy C, Genant HK (1993) Hematopoietic bone marrow in the adult knee: spin-echo and opposed-phase gradient-echo MR imaging. Skeletal Radiol 22:95–103

Lecouvet FE, Malghem J, Michaux L, Maldague B, Ferrant A, Michaux JL, Vande Berg BC (1999) Skeletal survey in advanced multiple myeloma: radiographic versus MR imaging survey. Br J Haematol 106:35–39

Lecouvet FE, Vande Berg BC, Michaux L, Malghem J, Maldague BE, Jamart J, Ferrant A, Michaux JL (1998a) Stage III multiple myeloma: clinical and prognostic value of spinal bone marrow MR imaging. Radiology 209:653–660

Lecouvet FE, Vande Berg BC, Michaux L, Scheiff JM, Malghem J, Jamart J, Maldague BE, Michaux JL, Ferrant A (1998b) Chronic lymphocytic leukemia: changes in bone marrow composition and distribution assessed with quantitative MRI. J Magn Reson Imaging 8:733–739

Libshitz HI, Malthouse SR, Cunningham D, MacVicar AD, Husband JE (1992) Multiple myeloma: appearance at MR imaging. Radiology 182:833–837

Linden A, Zankovich R, Theissen P, Diehl V, Schicha H (1989) Malignant lymphoma: bone marrow imaging versus biopsy. Radiology 173:335–339

Mirowitz SA, Apicella P, Reinus WR, Hammerman AM (1994) MR imaging of bone marrow lesions: relative conspicuousness on T1-weighted, fat-suppressed T2-weighted, and STIR images. AJR Am J Roentgenol 162:215–221

Moore SG, Bisset GS 3rd, Siegel MJ, Donaldson JS (1991) Pediatric musculoskeletal MR imaging. Radiology 179:345–360

Moore SG, Dawson KL (1990) Red and yellow marrow in the femur: age-related changes in appearance at MR imaging. Radiology 175:219–223

Moore SG, Gooding CA, Brasch RC, Ehman RL, Ringertz HG, Ablin AR, Matthay KK, Zoger S (1986) Bone marrow in children with acute lymphocytic leukemia: MR relaxation times. Radiology 160:237–240

Moulopoulos LA, Dimopoulos MA (1997) Magnetic resonance imaging of the bone marrow in hematologic malignancies. Blood 90:2127–2147

Moulopoulos LA, Dimopoulos MA, Alexanian R, Leeds NE, Libshitz HI (1994) Multiple myeloma: MR patterns of response to treatment. Radiology 193:441–446

Moulopoulos LA, Dimopoulos MA, Varma DG, Manning JT, Johnston DA, Leeds NE, Libshitz HI (1993b) Waldenstrom macroglobulinemia: MR imaging of the spine and CT of the abdomen and pelvis. Radiology 188:669–673

Moulopoulos LA, Dimopoulos MA, Weber D, Fuller L, Libshitz HI, Alexanian R (1993a) Magnetic resonance imaging in the staging of solitary plasmacytoma of bone. J Clin Oncol 11:1311–1315

O'Connell MJ, Hargaden G, Powell T, Eustace SJ (2002) Whole-body turbo short tau inversion recovery MR imaging using a moving tabletop. AJR Am J Roentgenol 179:866–868

Olson DO, Shields AF, Scheurich CJ, Porter BA, Moss AA (1986) Magnetic resonance imaging of the bone marrow in patients with leukemia, aplastic anemia, and lymphoma. Invest Radiol 21:540–546

Poulton TB, Murphy WD, Duerk JL, Chapek CC, Feiglin DH (1993) Bone marrow reconversion in adults who are smokers: MR Imaging findings. AJR Am J Roentgenol 161:1217–1221

Rahmouni A, Divine M, Mathieu D, Golli M, Dao TH, Jazaerli N, Anglade MC, Reyes F, Vasile N (1993a) Detection of multiple myeloma involving the spine: efficacy of fat-suppression and contrast-enhanced MR imaging. AJR Am J Roentgenol 160:1049–1052

Rahmouni A, Divine M, Mathieu D, Golli M, Haioun C, Dao T, Anglade MC, Reyes F, Vasile N (1993b) MR appearance of multiple myeloma of the spine before and after treatment. AJR Am J Roentgenol 160:1053–1057

Ricci C, Cova M, Kang YS, Yang A, Rahmouni A, Scott WW, Jr., Zerhouni EA (1990) Normal age-related patterns of cellular and fatty bone marrow distribution in the axial skeleton: MR imaging study. Radiology 177:83–88

Rozman C, Cervantes F, Rozman M, Mercader JM, Montserrat E (1999) Magnetic resonance imaging in myelofibrosis and essential thrombocythaemia: contribution to differential diagnosis. Br J Haematol 104:574–580

Saifuddin A, Bann K, Ridgway JP, Butt WP (1994) Bone marrow blood supply in gadolinium-enhanced magnetic resonance imaging. Skeletal Radiol 23:455–157

Schick F, Einsele H, Kost R, Duda S, Jung WI, Lutz O, Claussen CD (1994) Hematopoietic reconstitution after bone marrow transplantation: assessment with MR imaging and H-1 localized spectroscopy. J Magn Reson Imaging 4:71–78

Schick F, Einsele H, Bongers H, Jung WI, Skalej M, Duda S, Ehninger G, Lutz O (1993) Leukemic red bone marrow changes assessed by magnetic resonance imaging and localized 1H spectroscopy. Ann Hematol 66:3–13

Seiderer M, Staebler A, Wagner H (1999) MRI of bone marrow: opposed-phase gradient-echo sequences with long repetition time. Eur Radiol 9:652–661

Shellock FG, Morris E, Deutsch AL, Mink JH, Kerr R, Boden SD (1992) Hematopoietic bone marrow hyperplasia: high prevalence on MR images of the knee in asymptomatic marathon runners. AJR Am J Roentgenol 1992 158:335–338

Shields AF, Porter BA, Churchley S, Olson DO, Appelbaum FR, Thomas ED (1987) The detection of bone marrow involvement by lymphoma using magnetic resonance imaging. J Clin Oncol 5:225–230

Spuentrup E, Buecker A, Adam G, van Vaals JJ, Guenther RW (2001) Diffusion-weighted MR imaging for differentiation of benign fracture edema and tumor infiltration of the vertebral body. AJR Am J Roentgenol 176:351–358

Stabler A, Baur A, Bartl R, Munker R, Lamerz R, Reiser MF (1996) Contrast enhancement and quantitative signal analysis in MR imaging of multiple myeloma: assessment of focal and diffuse growth patterns in marrow correlated with biopsies and survival rates. AJR Am J Roentgenol 167: 1029–1036

Stevens SK, Moore SG, Kaplan ID (1990a) Early and late bone-marrow changes after irradiation: MR evaluation. AJR Am J Roentgenol 154:745–750

Stevens SK, Moore SG, Amylon MD (1990b) Repopulation of marrow after transplantation: MR imaging with pathologic correlation. Radiology 175:213–218

Sze G, Bravo S, Baierl P, Shimkin PM (1991) Developing spinal column: gadolinium-enhanced MR imaging. Radiology 180:497–502

Takagi S, Tanaka O (1996) The role of magnetic resonance imaging in the diagnosis and monitoring of myelodysplastic syndromes or leukemia. Leuk Lymphoma 23:443–450

Thomsen C, Sorensen PG, Karle H, Christoffersen P, Henriksen O (1987) Prolonged bone marrow T1-relaxation in acute leukaemia. In vivo tissue characterization by magnetic resonance imaging. Magn Reson Imaging 5:251–257

Traber F, Block W, Layer G, Braucker G, Gieseke J, Kretzer S, Hasan I, Schild HH (1996) Determination of 1H relaxation times of water in human bone marrow by fat-suppressed turbo spin echo in comparison to MR spectroscopic methods. J Magn Reson Imaging 6:541–548

Vande Berg BC, Malghem J, Lecouvet FE, Maldague B (1998a) Magnetic resonance imaging of normal bone marrow. Eur Radiol 8:1327–1334

Vande Berg BC, Malghem J, Lecouvet FE, Maldague B (1998b) Magnetic resonance imaging of the normal bone marrow. Skeletal Radiol 27:471–483

Vande Berg BC, Schmitz PJ, Scheiff JM, Filleul BJ, Michaux JL, Ferrant A, Jamart J, Malghem J, Maldague BE (1995) Acute myeloid leukemia: lack of predictive value of sequential quantitative MR imaging during treatment. Radiology 197:301–305

Vogler JB 3rd, Murphy WA (1988) Bone marrow imaging. Radiology 168:679–693

Walker RE, Eustace SJ (2001) Whole-body magnetic resonance imaging: techniques, clinical indications, and future applications. Semin Musculoskelet Radiol 5:5–20

Zampa V, Cosottini M, Michelassi C, Ortori S, Bruschini L, Bartolozzi C (2002) Value of opposed-phase gradient-echo technique in distinguishing between benign and malignant vertebral lesions. Eur Radiol 12:1811-1818

2 Nodal Involvement in Hodgkin Disease

Stephen I. Marglin

CONTENTS

2.1
Introduction

Hodgkin Disease (HD) is an uncommon disease, accounting for less than 1% of all neoplasms that occur yearly in the United States, and only 30% of all lymphomas. Despite this, it has been estimated that nearly 8,000 new cases of HD will be diagnosed in 2003, and that approximately 1,300 patients will die. These statistics, coupled with a appreciation for the remarkable advances that have been achieved in the understanding, diagnosis, staging, treatment, and prognosis of Hodgkin's, have caused HD to become a subject of fascination for oncologists and radiologists alike (Fig. 2.1).

In the past, considerable ambiguity existed concerning how best to evaluate newly diagnosed, previously untreated patients with HD. This lack of consensus was due, at least in part, to significant differences in the objectives that we, as physicians, were trying to achieve. These goals, i.e., maximum accuracy and scope of diagnostic information, utmost

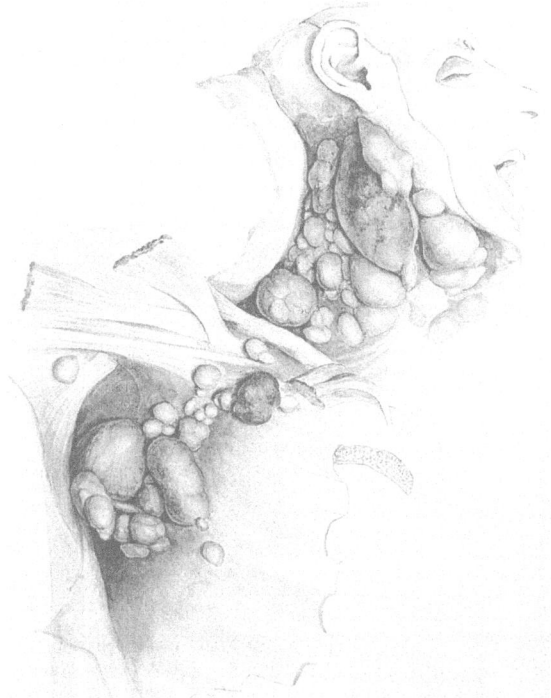

Fig. 2.1. A black and white reproduction of a water color painting by Robert Carswell (1793–1857). The patient, seen by Carswell at postmortem examination, was the seventh that Hodgkin described in his original manuscript.

Stephen I. Marglin, MD, FACR
Director of Radiology, Seattle Cancer Care Alliance, Associate Professor, Department of Radiology, University of Washington, 825 Eastlake Avenue, E., Seattle, WA 09109-1023, USA

economy in the utilization of limited resources, and minimization of patient discomfort, were often contradictory. These often incompatible goals, combined with the differing skills and preferences of the radiologists who perform the examinations, made it difficult to arrive at a consensus. However, in recent years, with the advent of newer imaging modalities, e.g., CT, MR imaging, and PET, this issue has, by and large, become moot. For that reason, a primary objective of this discussion will be to present an approach that is likely to be most applicable to the maximum number of patients. Because the impact of diagnostic imaging is greatest at the time of initial presentation, i.e., because this period coincides with the greatest opportunity for cure, this chapter will emphasize those issues that concern patients who are newly presenting and, as yet, untreated.

2.2
Principles of Oncologic Imaging

In deciding which examinations to obtain for the initial staging of patients with a new diagnosis of cancer, there are certain general principles that should be borne in mind. First and foremost, the information obtained should be worth the cost – the latter defined in both physical and monetary terms. If it is not anticipated that the information being sought is likely to alter a patient's stage or his/her treatment, the examination should probably not be performed. A second tenet, one that is only a little bit less axiomatic than the first, would hold that a test of limited accuracy should probably not be performed, even in instances where the prevalence of disease in a given location is known to be high. Third, although the "accuracy" of a screening test might be considerable, if the prevalence of disease in the location to be interrogated is low, the test should probably not be performed. As an illustration of this last point, consider the following quotation from 'The Fifth Discipline (SENGE 1990).

In a modern version of an ancient Sufi story, a passerby encounters a drunk on his hands and knees under a street lamp. He offers to help and finds out that the drunk is looking for his house keys. After several minutes, he asks 'Where did you drop them?' The drunk replies that he dropped them outside his front door. 'Then why look for them here?' asks the passerby. 'Because,' says the drunk, 'there is no light by my doorway.'

Although a test, like the street lamp above, might be extremely illuminating, it doesn't make sense to utilize it for the evaluation of sites where the prevalence of disease is low. An important qualification to the last two recommendations is related to situations in which the discovery of an abnormality would greatly affect therapy. If the "cost" of missing the presence of disease in a given location is regarded as critically high, the test may still be warranted.

Lastly, accurate interpretation of imaging examinations depends upon a comprehensive understanding of the anticipated behavior of a given neoplasm. In the case of HD, it has long been recognized that disease in newly presenting, untreated, patients, tends to spread by contiguity from one lymph node chain to others that are directly connected (ROSENBERG and KAPLAN 1966; ROTH et al. 1998). Contiguous in this context does not require physical proximity, but rather the presence of a direct communication via lymphatic channels. An example of this, initially noted by ROSENBERG and KAPLAN (1966), is the association between lower cervical and supraclavicular lymphadenopathy and upper abdominal lymphadenopathy and/or involvement of the spleen and splenic hilar nodes. This association is thought to occur via retrograde flow in the thoracic duct. Because the thoracic duct drains into the left subclavian vein, it is important to note that the association occurs more frequently with left-sided or bilateral supraclavicular involvement than it does with isolated right-sided lymphadenopathy. Knowledge of this behavior should make one reluctant to attribute lymphadenopathy in the iliac or inguinal lymph nodes to HD, if the patient presented with supraclavicular disease, particularly on the left, without evidence of disease in upper abdominal lymph nodes and/or the spleen. This presentation is sufficiently unusual as to call into question the diagnosis of HD.

2.3
Evaluating the Performance of an Imaging Modality

Current conventions call for reporting the 'performance' of an imaging modality in terms of the following parameters: sensitivity, specificity, positive predictive accuracy and negative predictive accuracy. These four descriptors are considerably more meaningful than the simple measure known as accuracy. Yet they also fail to provide a unique description of a test's diagnostic performance, because they only describe a single outcome achieved by a given investigator, based upon an arbitrary selection of a decision threshold. In doing so, they fall short of being able to tell us which test, among a number of competing possibilities, is the best. It is important to recognize that measurements such as these are actually "snapshots" of a dynamic process. If one wished to make a test more sensitive, one would only need to arbitrarily interpret a greater percentage of cases as positive; conversely, if one elected to interpret every examination as negative, the test results would, by definition, be 100% specific. Thus, the results that are presented in the literature actually represent those points along a continuum of possibilities, the so-called receiver operating characteristic (ROC) curve where an investigator or group of investigators have elected to establish their decision thresholds. The ROC curve is an experimentally derived description of the outcomes that result from intentionally varying the decision threshold, indicating all possible combinations of true positive and false positive interpretations (METZ 1978). Theory holds that measuring the area under a ROC curves provides a better estimate of a modality's performance than that which is provided by the static parameters

noted above. The advantage of this approach is that it explicitly takes into consideration not only the performance of the test, but also the performance of the of the individuals who are using it. While it works well for test results that do not overlap, when the curves intersect the incremental value of ROC area calculations is somewhat debatable. For a more detailed discussion of ROC methodology, the reader is encouraged to refer to references authored by Charles Metz (Fig. 2.2).

Of potentially greater clinical importance than the somewhat esoteric aspects of ROC analysis is an appreciation of the bias that may be inadvertently introduced by sub-specialists who practice at academic medical centers. The results achieved by these individuals do not necessarily translate into outcomes that one might expect from community radiologists, i.e., those who lack the luxury of sub-specialization. In many instances, it is more important to know what modalities your radiologist prefers and which ones he/she is most successful in performing, as opposed to the rarefied recommendations that the literature might suggest.

2.4
Background Information

The diagnosis of HD is based on the detection of large, multi-nucleated, giant cells, so-called Reed-Sternberg cells, embedded in a hyperplastic background of reactive lymphocytes, eosinophils, histiocytes, plasma cells, and neutrophils. It is notable that the number of malignant cells, i.e., the Reed-Sternberg cells, is remarkably low, relative to the number of reactive cells. The latter are not considered malignant, although, by size and weight, they account for almost the entire 'bulk' of the tumor. Rather, it is thought that the Reed-Sternberg cells elaborate cytokines that, in turn, attract inflammatory cells (POPPEMA et al. 1999). Cytokines may also be responsible for inducing fibrosis, mediating immune suppression, and causing systemic symptoms (KADIN 1994).

Because Reed-Sternberg cells are uncommon, it has been difficult to determine their cellular origin and/or their clonality. However, in recent years, techniques have been developed that permit the isolation of single cells, thereby permitting the application of standard molecular biological techniques. As a result, pathologists have successfully determined that Reed-Sternberg cells are clonal populations of B cells.

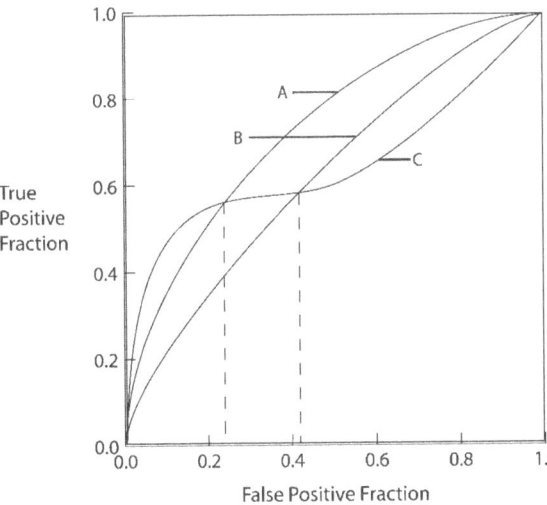

Fig. 2.2. Receiver operating characteristic curves for three 'competing' imaging modalities. The first, modality 'A' is superior to 'B' at all points, i.e., for any given true positive interpretation, the false positive fraction is less. Conclusions regarding modality 'C' are less certain. Before the first intersection, 'C' is superior to both 'A' and 'B'. After intersecting with 'B', it is inferior to both. Thus, much depends upon where on a given receiver operating characteristic curve an individual chooses to establish his/her threshold.

The majority of patients with HD present with painless cervical and/or supraclavicular adenopathy. Although this statement is accurate, it primarily reflects the fact that cervical and/or supraclavicular adenopathy is typical of patients with nodular sclerosing HD, a cell type that accounts for between 40% and 70% of patients.

Approximately 20–30% of newly presenting, untreated, patients with HD will have had so-called B symptoms during the six months preceding diagnosis, i.e., temperature higher than 38°C, drenching night sweats, and/or weight loss that exceeds 10% of baseline body weight. Usually the fever is low grade and irregular. However, in some patients it can be peculiarly repetitious. If the fever lasts approximately two weeks, and is followed by two weeks in which it is absent, only to return again, it is known as a Pel-Ebstein fever, and strongly suggests a diagnosis of HD.

The prevalence of HD has been noted to occur in a bimodal age distribution. Rates increase after age 10, peak in the third decade, and decline until age 45. The second peak begins after age 45, and tends to increase progressively over time. Patients who present with mediastinal disease tend to be younger than those who do not.

2.5
Epidemiology

The etiology of Hodgkin lymphoma remains unclear. In all likelihood, the 'cause' will ultimately be shown to be multifactorial, e.g., some combination of infectious, genetic, and immunologic factors. In favor of an infectious etiology, several reports have described outbreaks of HD among adults and children living in close proximity (GILMAN et al. 1999). In addition, siblings of children with HD have been shown to be at increased risk for developing the disease. There is also evidence that many patients with HD have been exposed to the EBV, and many have clinical histories of infectious mononucleosis (WEISS 2000; MACSWEEN and CRAWFORD 2003).

Other risk factors for the development of HD include male sex, higher social class, a family history of lymphoma, and infection with the human immunodeficiency virus. It has been suggested that delays or a decreased frequency of early infections may account for the increased prevalence that is associated with higher social class (PAFFENBARGER et al. 1977).

The argument for a genetic cause is based upon differences in HLA associations, and on observed differences in the prevalence of disease in different ethnic populations, independent of socioeconomic status (GLASER and JARRETT 1996; STILLER 1998; STARATSCHEK-JOX et al. 2002).

2.6
Classification

The history of pathology is notable for an ever changing, and usually expanding, system for the classification and characterization of disease. Without entering into a debate as to whether this is a good or a bad thing, the following quotation from Stan Kaufman of the Epimetrics Group (KAUFMAN 2002a; KAUFMAN 2002b), may be of interest.

"Regardless of the field of inquiry, taxonomists divide into "lumpers" and "splitters". The former consider the latter to be anal-retentive twonks who obsess over distinctions without differences, while the latter accuse the former of intellectual sloppiness or guile for conflating categories that should remain separate."

The classification schema for HD was relatively stable for the much of the past quarter century. It was accepted that HD consisted of four, separate, histologic types. These types could be distinguished morphologically, and more recently by immunohistochemical testing. The prevalence of the four histologies, and their clinical characteristics, are:

- Lymphocyte predominant   10%
- Nodular sclerosis   40% to 70%
- Mixed cellularity   30% to 50%
- Lymphocyte depletion   1%

During the past decade, advances in immunophenotypic testing have prompted a reassessment of this schema (HARRIS et al. 2000). A fifth histologic type, lymphocyte-rich classical Hodgkin lymphoma has been introduced, and a distinction has been drawn between the so-called classical forms of HD and a histologic type that bears the name nodular lymphocytic predominant Hodgkin lymphoma (Table 2.1).

It should be emphasized that nodular lymphocytic predominant Hodgkin lymphoma is not simply a variant, i.e., a different 'flavor', of lymphocyte rich classical HD. It is a distinct and separate entity, both morphologically and immunophenotypically (HARRIS et al. 1994). The fact that both have a small number of malignant cells in a background rich in lymphocytes is insufficient evidence to place them in the same category, or

Table 2.1. Histologic categorization of Hodgkin disease

Lymphocyte-rich classical Hodg-kin lymphoma (LRCHL)	Recently defined entity Male: Female = 2-4:1 Peak age of onset in 4th decade, i.e., older than NLPHL (DIEHL et al. 1999) Predominantly peripheral lymph nodes, e.g., neck Mediastinal and paraaortic disease is rare Stage I or II: 70–85% B symptoms: rare
Nodular sclerosis (NS)	Adolescents and young adults Female predominance Common presentation: localized disease, e.g., low cervical, supraclavicular and mediastinal
Mixed cellularity (MC)	Most prevalent in the young and the aged Advanced stage disease at presentation Somewhat poorer prognosis Strong association, in excess of 75%, with EBV infection
Lymphocyte depletion (LD)	Older age Extensive disease, usually symptomatic Abdominal adenopathy, spleen, liver and bone marrow involvement Peripheral adenopathy is unusual Association with HIV
Nodular lym-phocyte predom-inance (NLPHL)	Lack traditional Reed-Sternberg cells; Reed-Sternberg variants Male predominance Limited nodal disease at presentation, e.g., neck or inguinal Tendency to spare the mediastinum Stage I or II: 80% Indolent disease Tendency for late recurrence, i.e., lack of a plateau in failure-free survival (EKSTRAND and HORNING 2002)

even to view them as close relatives. Nodular lympho-cytic predominant Hodgkin lymphoma differs in that it lacks traditional Reed-Sternberg cells, and because it has a different immunophenotypic profile. Drawing attention to these differences, several pathologists have emphasized that the "Hodgkin lymphomas are two distinct diseases" (HARRIS 1999). Evolving acceptance of this position has led to a change in terminology, the more familiar term 'Hodgkin Disease' now gradually giving way to the term 'Hodgkin Lymphoma'.

2.7
Staging

The system by which HD is staged was originally promulgated in 1965 (LUKES and BUTLER 1966;

LUKES et al. 1966). Albeit modified, the primary features remains largely intact. In 1971, the system was amended to acknowledge that the prognosis for localized disease was essentially the same as for limited extranodal disease, when the latter occurs as a result of extracapsular extension (CARBONE et al. 1971). When it is possible to encompass the involved area within the confines of a conventional radiotherapy field, and when the area can reason-ably be treated with curative intent, no significant reduction in life expectancy is observed. This type of disease, i.e., limited extranodal spread, was given the designation 'E', in order to emphasize that its prognosis is significantly more favorable than is the case for stage IV disease (Table 2.2).

Table 2.2. Staging of Hodgkin disease

Stage I	One nodal site on either side of the diaphragm
Stage II	Two or more nodal sites on the same side of the diaphragm
Stage III	Lymph node disease on both sides of the dia-phragm. For purposes of this schema, the spleen is considered a lymph node
Stage IV	Disease that has disseminated beyond nodal sites

Prompted by the recognition that prognosis was adversely affected by 'bulky' disease (LISTER et al. 1989; CROWTHER and LISTER 1990), the system was further modified at the Cotswold meeting. Bulky, in this clinical context, was defined as tumor greater than 10 cm in maximum dimension, or tumor that measured more than one-third the widest transverse diameter of the chest.

As discussed above, stage of disease is further delineated by the presence or absence of constitu-tional, i.e., 'B' symptoms, by whether or not there is limited, extranodal, i.e., 'E' disease, and whether there is bulky, i.e., 'X' disease.

2.8
Prognostic Factors

Prognostic factors are parameters, often quantifi-able, that enable physicians to provide reasoned predictions of patient outcome. During the past decade, with improvements in disease assessment and, particularly, in treatment, a number of fac-tors that previously provided predictive value have lost their power. Thus, histological cell type, stage of disease, size of mediastinal masses, and the presence or absence of systemic symptoms, are all much less likely to prove helpful in predicting outcome. Newer information suggests that the parameters listed below are more important predictors of adverse outcome (HASENCLEVER and DIEHL 1998; HASENCLEVER 2002). Each is said to correlate with a decrease in survival rate of approximately 7–8% per year (HASENCLEVER and DIEHL 1998).

Age ≥ 45 years
Male sex
Stage IV
Hemoglobin < 10.5 g/dl
Albumin < 4 g/dl
Lymphocytes < 600/μl or < 8%
White blood count ≥ 15,000/μl

2.9
Sites of Disease

2.9.1
Peripheral Lymph Nodes

Although the majority of patients with HD present with axial adenopathy, i.e., enlarged lymph nodes in the chest or abdomen, other sites of nodal involvement are also possible. Examples of these include the preauricular, occipital, submaxillary and submental, anterior and posterior cervical (Fig. 2.3a), supraclavicular (Fig. 2.3b), infraclavicular, axillary (Fig. 2.4), epitrochlear, iliac, inguinal and femoral regions.

2.9.2
Neck

Of lymphomas that affect the head and neck, HD accounts for only 10–35%. In 70–80% of such cases, involvement is exclusively nodal (MALIS et al. 1998). In the remainder, the tumor involves extranodal lymphoid tissue in the palatine tonsils, nasopharyngeal tonsils (adenoids), lingual tonsils, tubal tonsils, and/or the lateral pharyngeal bands. This collection of lymphoid tissue is known collectively as Waldeyer's ring (HELLINGS et al. 2000). It is extremely uncommon for there to be isolated, i.e., stage I, involvement of Waldeyer's ring (Fig. 2.5) (KAPADIA et al. 1995; DUNPHY et al. 1996).

Approximately 25% of patients who present with involvement of Waldeyer's ring also have involvement of cervical/supraclavicular lymph nodes. Sixty-five percent will have coexistent mediastinal adenopathy, while 20% will have involvement of abdominal lymph nodes. Nearly 50% of cases will be of the mixed cellularity cell type, while 25% will be nodular sclerosis. When tissues from HD patients with involvement of Waldeyer's ring are compared to those obtained from patients with nodal tissue, the former demonstrate an increased prevalence of EBV (KAPADIA et al. 1995). Some have hypothesized that Waldeyer's ring may represent a reservoir for the virus.

The majority of patients with HD will have cervical and/or supraclavicular nodal involvement at the time they present. In Kaplan's analysis of 340 consecutive, untreated patients with HD, 55% had right side involvement, while 64% demonstrated involve-

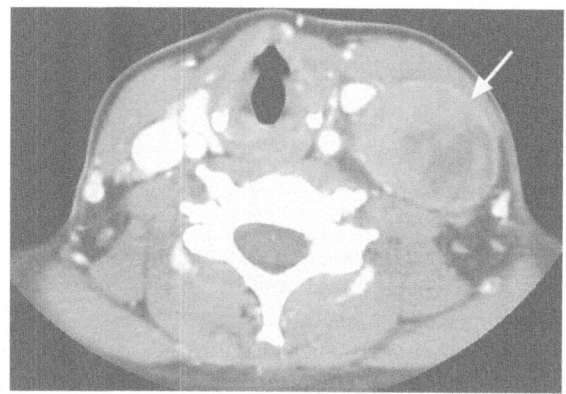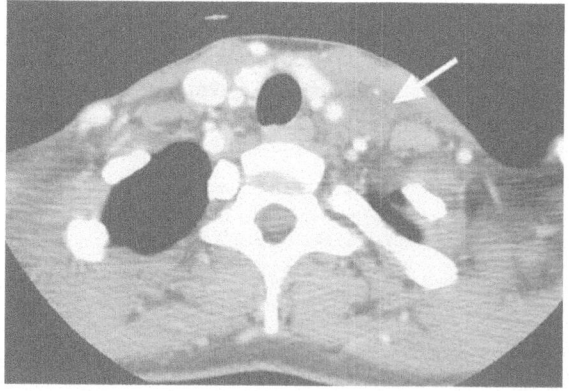

Fig. 2.3a,b. Nodular sclerosis Hodgkin disease in a 20-year-old woman with neck nodal involvement. **a** Axial contrast-enhanced CT scan of the neck demonstrates a markedly enlarged lymph node present at the base of the left side of the neck (*arrow*). **b** Axial contrast-enhanced CT scan of the upper thorax shows nodal disease extending into the left supraclavicular fossa (*arrow*).

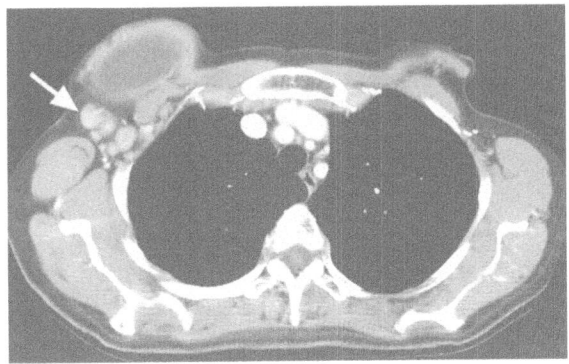

Fig. 2.4. Recent diagnosis of mixed cellularity Hodgkin disease in a 53-year-old woman with a prior history of breast carcinoma. Axial contrast-enhanced chest CT scan shows several markedly enlarged, albeit painless, right axillary lymph nodes (*arrow*).

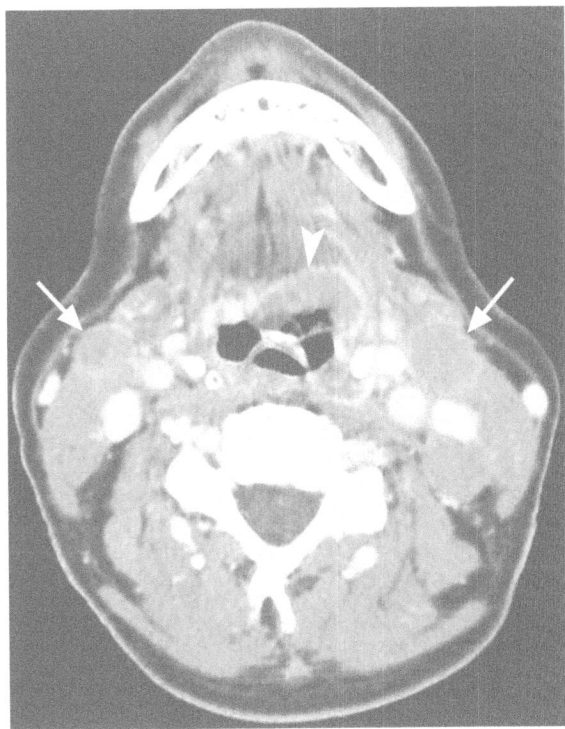

Fig. 2.5. Mixed cellularity Hodgkin disease in a 60-year-old man with involvement of extranodal tissue in Waldeyer's ring. Axial contrast-enhanced CT scan of the neck shows marked enhancement of the parapharyngeal soft tissue (*arrowhead*). In this instance, involvement is not isolated to Waldeyer's ring and several bilateral enhancing neck nodes (*arrows*) are also evident.

ment on the left (KAPLAN 1980). The mediastinum, left side of neck, and right side of neck were the most common locations of nodal disease in patients with nodular sclerosis or mixed cellularity cell types. Each of these sites was involved approximately 60% of the time. Prevalence in these locations was four or more times as common as in other nodal sites, either above or below the diaphragm. In contrast, the mediastinum was involved in only 8% of patients with the lymphocyte predominance cell type (MAUCH et al. 1993).

2.9.3
Thorax

Approximately 70% of patients with newly diagnosed HD present with evidence of intrathoracic disease (FILLY et al. 1976; KAPLAN 1980; CASTELLINO et al. 1986). Although mediastinal disease is common, isolated mediastinal involvement is not. It occurs in only 10% of patients. In most patients, if a diligent search is undertaken, lymphadenopathy will be detected in other sites. Only 15% of patients with intrathoracic HD will have adenopathy that is restricted to a single lymph node group, and only rarely are the nodes in the posterior mediastinum or cardiophrenic region involved (FILLY et al. 1976). Patients who present with mediastinal disease tend to be younger than those who do not.

Pulmonary parenchymal involvement occurs in up to 12% of newly diagnosed patients with HD (FILLY et al. 1976; STROLLO et al. 1997). In contrast to patients with NHL, pulmonary involvement in newly diagnosed patients with HD virtually never occurs without associated intrathoracic adenopathy. Fewer than 100 cases of this type of presentation have been reported. Lung involvement may be infiltrative or nodular, and the nodules may exhibit cavitation.

2.9.3.1
Plain Radiographs

Careful interpretation of chest radiographs in patients with HD has been shown to be capable of detecting most intrathoracic abnormalities (Figs. 2.6–2.8) (CASTELLINO et al. 1976). Furthermore, in almost every instance, these films serve as the initial portal through which patients with intrathoracic abnormalities pass. The relatively low cost of chest radiographs, combined with their ready availability and ease of performance, make them ideal for purposes of initial evaluation and periodic surveillance. Although

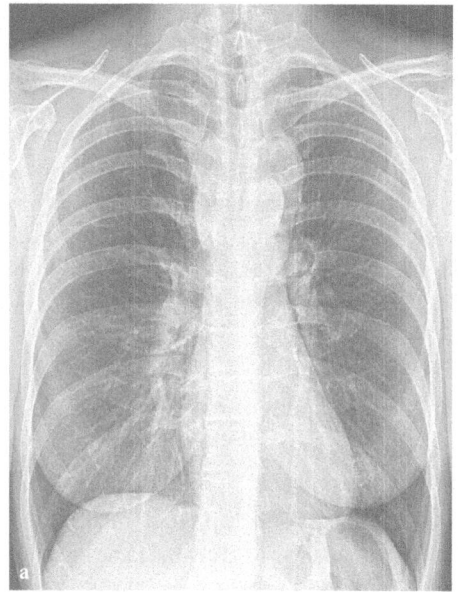

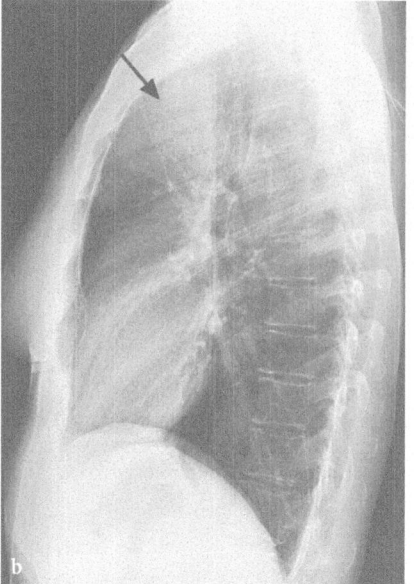

Fig. 2.6a,b. Nodular sclerosis Hodgkin disease in a 39-year-old woman with abnormal mediastinal contours. a Anteroposterior plain radiograph of the chest shows a double contour superimposed upon the aortic arch and right paratracheal regions. b Lateral plain radiograph of the chest shows a marked increase in opacity in the high retrosternal region (arrow). Lesser degrees of this abnormal opacity can be seen in patients whose frontal radiographs are either near-normal or entirely normal.

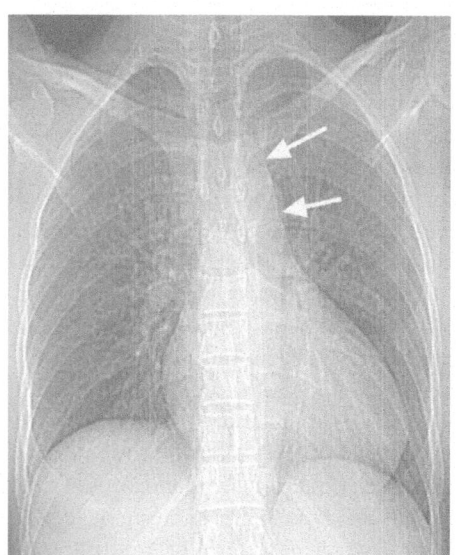

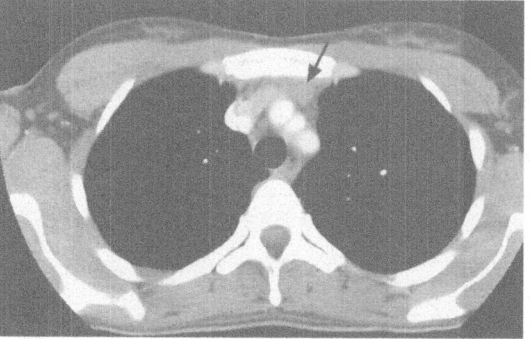

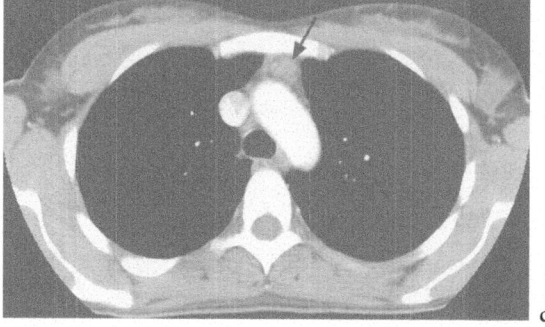

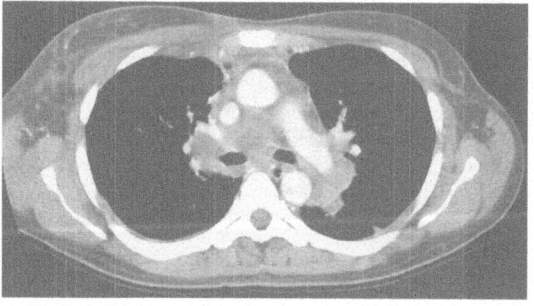

Fig. 2.7a–d. Nodular sclerosis Hodgkin disease in a 33-year-old man with mediastinal nodal involvement. a Anteroposterior plain radiograph of the chest demonstrates a double contour overlying and extending superiorly from the aortic arch (arrows). b Axial contrast-enhanced CT scan of the thorax shows abnormal nodal deposit posterior to the left side of the sternum, not to be confused with the left brachiocephalic vein (arrow). c Axial CT scan obtained 15 mm caudad to (b) shows the mass extending inferiorly, anterior to the aortic arch (arrow). Its rounded contours distinguish it from the normal thymus, which would be unlikely to be mass-like in the fourth-decade patient. d Axial CT scan at mid-thorax demonstrates extensive mediastinal and bilateral hilar lymphadenopathy.

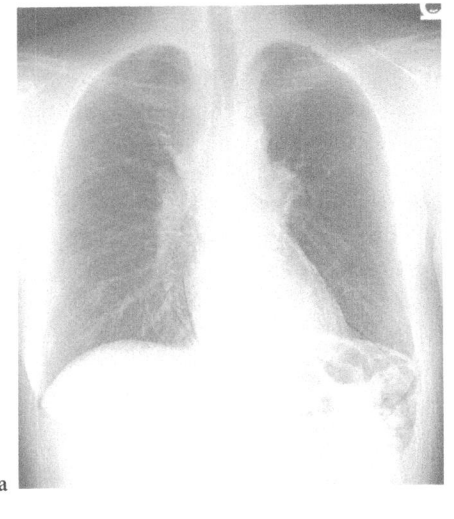

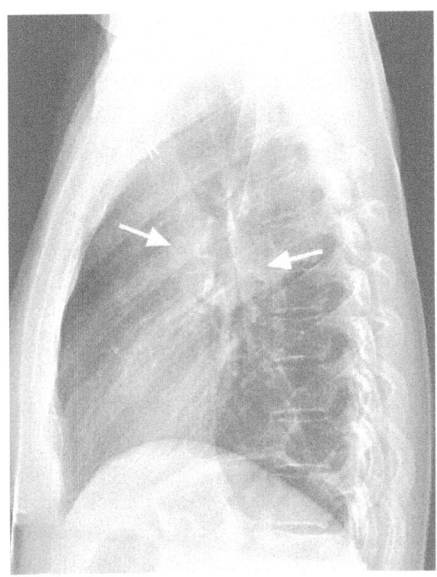

Fig. 2.8a,b. Nodular sclerosis Hodgkin disease in a 39-year-old woman with hilar nodal involvement. a Anteroposterior plain radiograph of the chest which is the product of a dual-energy subtraction of high density material, i.e., the ribs shows extensive bilateral hilar nodal involvement. b In the lateral radiograph, the enlarged lymph nodes (*arrows*) surround the central pulmonary arteries.

a

b

other examinations, e.g., CT or PET, are undeniably more sensitive and more specific, obtaining frontal and lateral chest radiographs is still recommended. They serve as an important baseline, and may provide information that will prove valuable during and after definitive therapy.

2.9.3.2
Computed Tomography

In 1976, investigators from Stanford reported on the additional information that could be obtained from the use of full-lung tomography versus that provided by routine chest radiographs (CASTELLINO et al. 1976). This analysis led, among other things, to the conclusion that tomography contributed relatively little when the results of the initial radiographs, carefully interpreted, were normal. When this form of analysis was extended to CT, a somewhat different conclusion was forthcoming. CT provided additional information in as many as 8% of patients whose chest radiographs were normal. In the aggregate, CT provided additional information in 15% of cases. Of note, in 9.4% (19/203) of the entire group of patients, and in 13.8% (9/65) of patients who were to be treated with radiotherapy alone, contemplated treatment was modified as a result of the new information (CASTELLINO et al. 1986). In 1988, HOPPER et al. performed a somewhat different, yet related, analysis in a group of 107 newly diagnosed patients with HD (HOPPER et al. 1988). When an analysis was performed on the effect that CT might have, relative to five possible treatment protocols, the authors

concluded that treatment would have been changed in between 6.5% and 62.7% of patients. On the basis of these two reports, it seems reasonable to obtain a chest CT in patients with newly diagnosed HD (Fig. 2.7).

Recently, a growing realization has emerged that the cure of HD has been obtained at a significant price. Second malignancies, both solid tumors and leukemia, have increased to a very significant degree (TUCKER et al. 1988; BITI et al. 1994; TRAVIS et al. 1994; METAYER et al. 2000; VAN LEEUWEN et al. 2000; DORES et al. 2002). Additionally, many patients suffer a severe degree of pulmonary impairment. Although multifactorial, many of the long-term complications appear to be related to the administration of radiotherapy. As a result, there is a tendency towards increased use of chemotherapeutic agents, and a corresponding decrease in the dose and frequency of radiation. It might therefore be argued that a chest CT need not be performed when the results of other tests have already led to a decision to treat with chemotherapy alone. If this option is chosen, a CT following treatment, i.e., for restaging, will likely be valuable as a baseline for subsequent surveillance.

2.9.3.3
Ultrasound

Ultrasound does not currently occupy a prominent position in the diagnostic armamentarium conventionally brought to bear on problems of mediastinal HD. In the early 1990s a group of European investigators reported upon the merits of sonography versus conventional chest radiographs and CT in the initial evaluation and post-treatment follow-up of patients with mediastinal lymphomas (WERNECKE et al. 1990a; WERNECKE et al. 1990b; WERNECKE and DIEDERICH 1994). Their data suggested that ultrasound might be more powerful than CT in evaluating response and in answering the important question of post-treatment residual tumor versus fibrosis. Perhaps because of training and technical requirements, mediastinal ultrasound has never garnered much enthusiasm in North America.

2.9.3.4
Magnetic Resonance Imaging

To date, a relative paucity of reports exist concerning the appropriate use of MR imaging in the pretreatment evaluation of newly presenting patients with HD (HOANE et al. 1994; DEVIZZI et al. 1997). Although small in number, these investigations suggest that MR imaging may be equally sensitive and possibly somewhat more specific than CT in the detection of mediastinal and hilar disease. However, the results would not appear to be statistically significant. Because pathological involvement of mediastinal and hilar nodes occurs in both HD and other thoracic neoplasms, e.g., carcinoma of the lung, a number of conclusions can plausibly be inferred from the literature on that subject. In 1991, the Radiology Diagnostic Oncology Group (RDOG) reported upon the results of a direct head-to-head comparison of CT and MR imaging in the staging of non-small cell bronchogenic carcinoma (WEBB et al. 1991). In this multi-institutional evaluation no significant difference was observed in the ability of the two modalities to detect significant pathologic abnormalities in mediastinal or hilar lymph nodes. The RDOG study also looked at the ability of MR imaging vs. CT to detect chest wall invasion and concluded that no significant difference existed. Recently, other authors have addressed this same question in patients with HD and NHL. These studies concluded that MR imaging appears to exceed the sensitivity and overall accuracy of CT in this one area. One of these manuscripts noted that the unique information obtained from performing MR imaging resulted in changes in radiation treatment planning in 3/15 (20%) patients (CARLSEN et al. 1993). Another potential value of MR imaging is in the detection of occult bone marrow involvement (BARBU et al. 1993; HOANE et al. 1994; VARAN et al. 1999). However, even with careful attention to detail, MR imaging is likely to be less accurate than CT in evaluating the lung parenchyma.

Could MR imaging function as an alternative to CT in the thorax? While the answer to this question is still open, the higher cost of MR imaging, its still somewhat limited availability, combined with the decreased sensitivity to the presence of lung involvement, tends to argue against its routine use. MR imaging is likely to be more useful as a tool for evaluating potentially important anatomical issues raised by CT, e.g., chest wall involvement, rather than as a modality to be regularly employed.

2.9.3.5
⁶⁷Gallium Scanning

For more than 30 years, ^{67}Gallium scanning has been utilized in the staging and reevaluation of patients with Hodgkin lymphoma (EDWARDS and HAYES 1970). After an initial period of optimism, the technique gradually declined in popularity, largely because of what were perceived to be an excessively large number of false negative diagnoses. It was not until the early 1980s that technical refinements, e.g., an increase in the administered dose, improved gamma camera resolution, and the introduction of tomographic techniques, provided the means for ^{67}Gallium to experience a resurgence (MCLAUGHLIN et al. 1990). Since 1980, a number of manuscripts have described ^{67}Gallium's ability to detect intrathoracic lymphadenopathy (ANDERSON et al. 1983; BLACKWELL et al. 1986; COHEN et al. 1986; RABY and INESON 1987; TUMEH et al. 1987). In general, the reported sensitivities and specificities are somewhat less than those obtained by CT. Given the prior recommendation, and given the fact that most centers routinely utilize CT for designing radiotherapy portals, the results would not appear to argue strongly for routine performance of ^{67}Gallium scanning.

Some have suggested that ^{67}Gallium can provide information that is sufficiently unique as to alter radiotherapy portals. In one study, the results of ^{67}Gallium scanning led to modifications in treatment planning in 3/26 newly presenting patients (12%) – primarily by extending coverage to the pericardium and the cardiophrenic lymph nodes, regions that would not have been adequately treated (JOCHELSON et al. 1988). ^{67}Gallium is also of value in determining whether a residual mass in a patient previously treated for HD contains viable tumor. The problem of the residual mass is both vexing and, unfortunately, quite common. Nearly 20% of all patients, and as many as 50% of children, will demonstrate a residual mass following treatment. ^{67}Gallium scanning has been utilized extensively as an adjunct in deciding whether such masses represent viable tumor or merely scarring/fibrosis. In adults, if a [67]Gallium scan is positive, the probability that tumor is present is high, approaching 100%. However in children, and at times in young adults, rebound thymic hyperplasia can cause abnormal gallium accumulation – accumulation that is visually indistinguishable from tumor. Some investigators have recommended that pediatric patients whose gallium scans remain or become positive following treatment should be further evaluated with Thallium-201. Thallium has been shown to have considerable affinity for certain tumors, without a corresponding propensity to accumulate in areas of inflammation or hyperplasia. At present, the cost-effectiveness and therefore the legitimacy of this recommendation remain uncertain. In both children and adults, if a [67]Gallium scan is negative, especially if the tumor previously demonstrated avidity for [67]Gallium, the results lend support to the impression that viable tumor no longer exists in that location. Unfortunately, as is the case with many tests, even these results are less than perfect. When the predictive accuracy of negative [67]Gallium scans was evaluated in patients who had been treated with chemotherapy, negative scans were found to be of limited value in predicting lymphoma sterilization and long-term prognosis. Suffice it to say that the subject of when, or whether, to utilize [67]Gallium scanning continues to remain ambiguous.

2.9.3.6
Positron Emission Tomography

While reports of the efficacy and prowess of [67]Gallium are intriguing, recent advances in PET imaging, for the most part, appear to have relegated [67]Gallium scanning to the status of a secondary modality. In routine clinical practice, PET scanning is performed using ^{18}F fluorodeoxyglucose. Malignant cells have been shown to have altered metabolism. As a result, they tend to rely upon glycolysis (WEBER 1983). The increased numbers of glucose transporters on the cell surface attract FDG which, when transported across the cell membrane, is converted to FDG-6 phosphate. The latter is not a suitable substrate for glycolysis, and the FDG-6 phosphate tends to accumulate. The degree of intracellular accumulation is therefore a reflection of the rate of glycolic metabolism (Fig. 2.9) (WEBER 1983).

In the past few years, a number of studies have become available that compare CT, [67]Gallium, and PET in the evaluation of patients with HD and NHL. While not all of these specifically deal with newly pre-

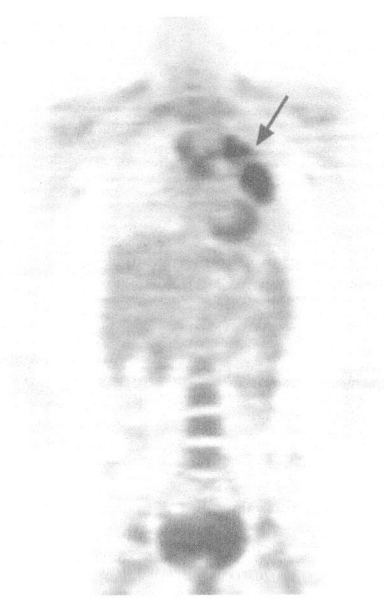

Fig. 2.9. Nodular sclerosis Hodgkin disease in a 25-year-old man with mediastinal nodal involvement. Coronal FDG-PET image shows extensive superior mediastinal lymphadenopathy, primarily on the left (*arrow*).

senting and previously untreated patients, the tenor of the findings suggest that PET is at least as effective as CT, and likely somewhat more so. This conclusion should come as no great surprise. CT relies almost upon the size of lymph nodes, and to a lesser degree their number, in assessing the likelihood of tumor involvement. Unfortunately, lymphoma can and often does exist in nodes that are normal in size. In addition, entities other than cancer can cause lymph nodes to enlarge, e.g., reactive hyperplasia. PET, on the other hand, evaluates metabolic activity, rather than size, in making these determinations (Fig. 2.10).

In a review of 28 consecutive, untreated patients with HD, PET and conventional imaging (primarily CT) were concordantly positive in 26% of the regions surveyed and negative in 68% (MENZEL et al. 2002). Where PET and CT disagreed, PET was positive in 5% when CT was negative, while CT was positive in 1% when PET was negative. Based upon the PET findings, the clinical stage for 4 patients was increased (14%), while in 2 it was decreased (7%). Subsequent follow-up served to validate the PET findings. In an additional five patients, PET detected more adenopathy than did CT, although this did not alter the stage of disease. An additional benefit of PET occurred in one patient who was thought to have stage II disease. PET detected stage bone marrow involvement, ren-

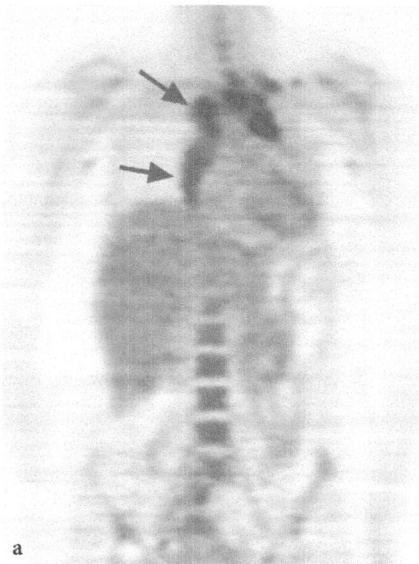
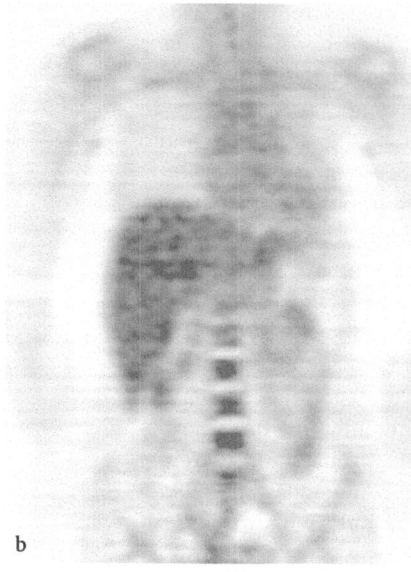

a   b

Fig. 2.10a,b. Nodular sclerosis Hodgkin disease in a 25-year-old woman with nodal involvement. **a** Coronal FDG-PET image obtained at presentation shows multiple abnormal nodal uptakes, primarily in the mediastinum (*arrows*). **b** Coronal FDG-PET image obtained following 4 months of chemotherapy demonstrates the complete resolution of the prior sites of abnormal nodal uptake.

dering the patient stage IV, a finding that was subsequently confirmed.

In a large interdisciplinary review, PET was approximately 10% more sensitive than CT while maintaining a specificity of approximately 85–90% (RESKE and KOTZERKE 2001).

Although PET scanning has obvious clinical appeal, there are numerous instances where issues such as infection, hemorrhage, and/or drug toxicity are aided by having a baseline CT examination. If economic considerations permit, obtaining both CT and PET at the outset is recommended (Fig. 2.11). Should this not be possible, PET would appear to be the examination of choice.

2.9.4
Abdomen and Pelvis

With some important exceptions, the approach that was taken to the evaluation of intrathoracic lymph nodes is mirrored in the approach employed for abdominal and pelvic lymph nodes.

2.9.4.1
Lymphography

In an earlier time, the assessment of abdominal/pelvic lymph nodes was indirect and markedly limited. Structures adjacent to lymph nodes, e.g., the inferior vena cava or the ureters, were opacified to see if, and to what degree, their course and position had been altered. In 1952, KINMONTH introduced a novel technique for can-

nulating lymphatics, thereby permitting the infusion of iodinated contrast. Initially, the contrast material was water soluble, and as a result it passed so rapidly through lymphatic channels as to preclude the acquisition of satisfactory nodal images. Approximately eight years later, when oily contrast was instilled into lymphatics on the dorsum of the feet, abdominal and pelvic nodes took up the contrast, thereby permitting assessment of internal architecture. The importance of this cannot be overestimated. Anatomic detail was of such a high degree that it was possible to detect lymphoma in nodes that were normal in size (Fig. 2.12), and to distinguish between tumor and conditions that might be confused with tumor, e.g., reactive hyperplasia, in enlarged nodes.

An extensive literature attests to the accuracy that can be obtained by lymphography in the evaluation of patients with HD. Numerous reports also attest to the contributions that this information can make to management decisions. In the largest series, one in which lymphography interpretations were compared with the results of staging laparotomies in 416 consecutive, untreated patients with HD, the following parameters of accuracy were obtained: sensitivity = 93%, specificity = 92%, positive predictive accuracy = 80%, negative predictive accuracy = 98%, overall accuracy = 92% (MARGLIN and CASTELLINO 1981). Few, if any, radiologic examinations have ever achieved this degree of pathologically confirmed performance (Fig. 2.13). Today, now that staging laparotomies are performed only rarely, the results of those examinations that follow must, necessarily, suffer from the lack of a reliable 'gold standard'.

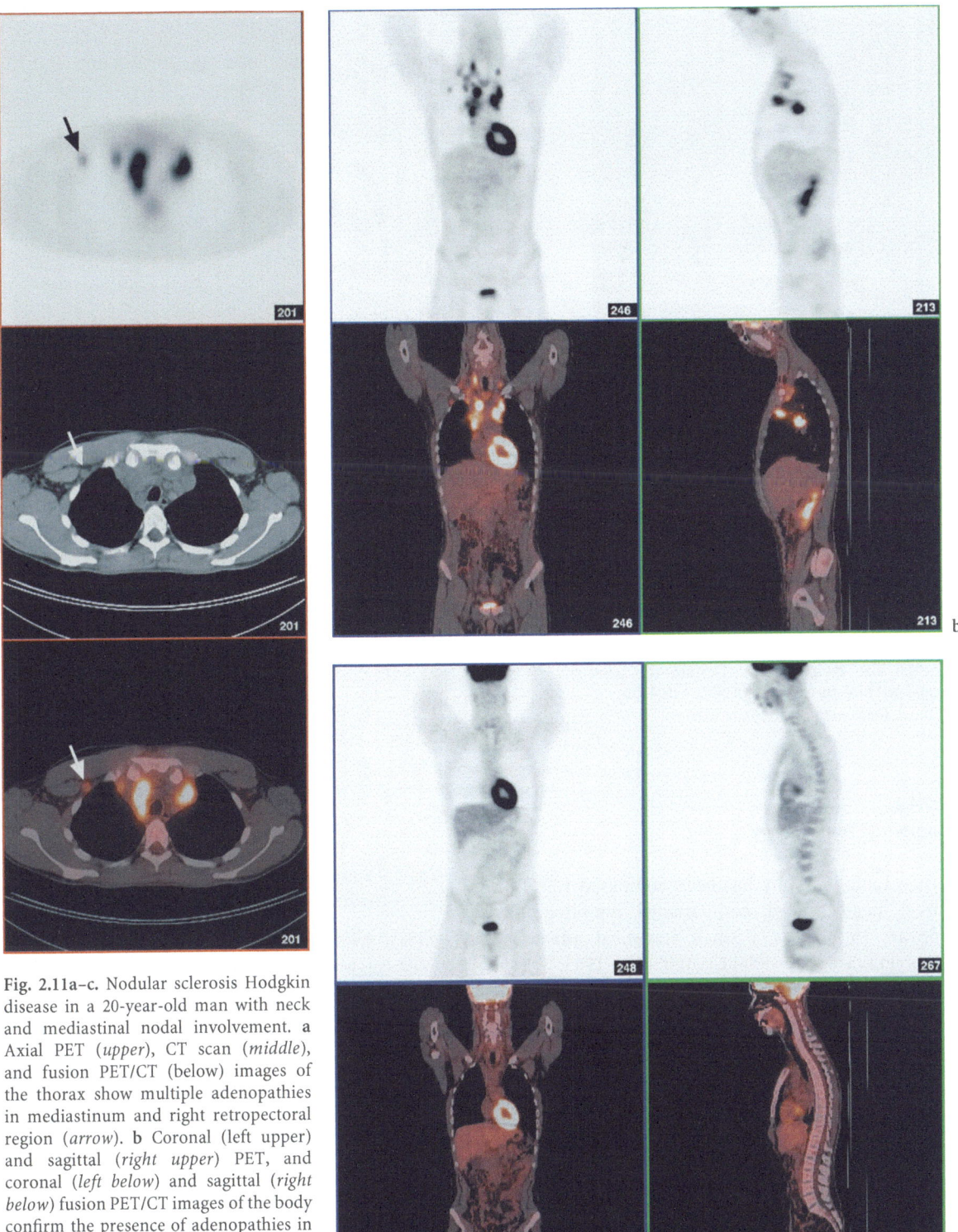

Fig. 2.11a–c. Nodular sclerosis Hodgkin disease in a 20-year-old man with neck and mediastinal nodal involvement. **a** Axial PET (*upper*), CT scan (*middle*), and fusion PET/CT (below) images of the thorax show multiple adenopathies in mediastinum and right retropectoral region (*arrow*). **b** Coronal (left upper) and sagittal (*right upper*) PET, and coronal (*left below*) and sagittal (*right below*) fusion PET/CT images of the body confirm the presence of adenopathies in the chest and also show adenopathies in supraclavicular areas and neck. The abdomen and pelvis are normal. About 2 months after chemotherapy, (**c**) repeated PET and fusion PET/CT images are negative. (*Image courtesy of Dr. C. Schiepers*)

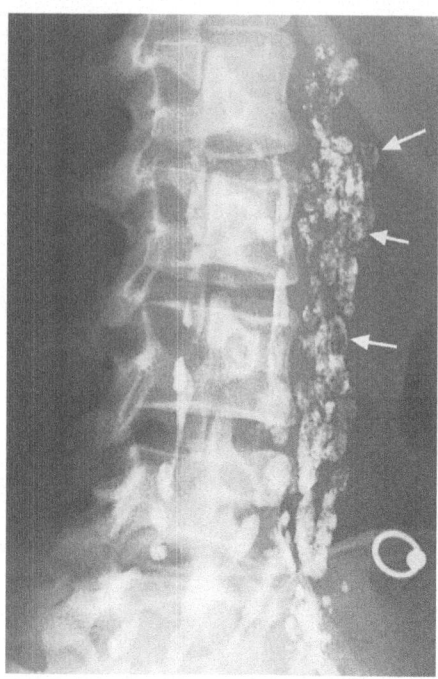

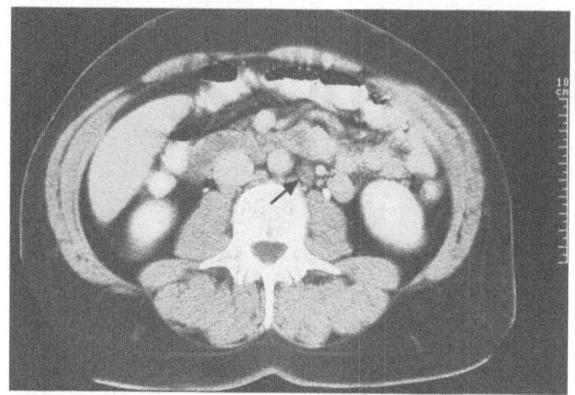

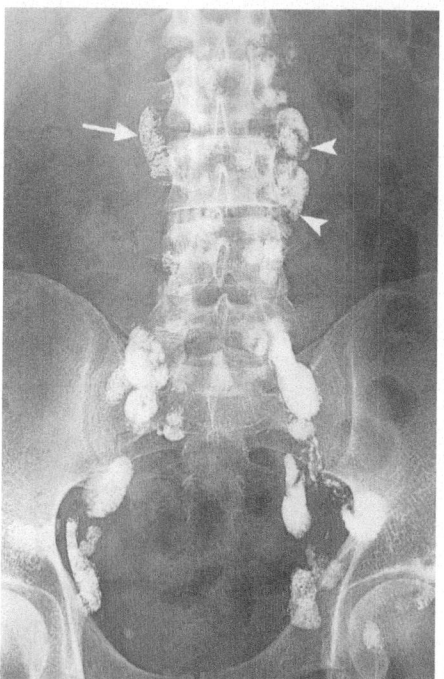

Fig. 2.12. Nodular sclerosis Hodgkin disease in an 18-year-old woman with subdiaphragmatic nodal involvement. Left posterior oblique view from a lymphogram demonstrates numerous normal size lymph nodes. Despite this, the nodal architecture is abnormal, exhibiting a diffuse, foamy appearance (*arrows*).

2.9.4.2
Computed Tomography

When lymphography has been compared to CT in direct, head-to-head, comparisons, lymphography appears to possess a small statistical advantage (CASTELLINO et al. 1984; CLOUSE et al. 1985; STRIJK et al. 1987; MANSFIELD et al. 1990). Proponents of CT have countered that CT should still be regarded as the examination of choice because of its broader purview, i.e., its ability to evaluate areas that are opaque to lymphography, e.g., the liver and spleen, as well as nodes in the upper abdomen, e.g. in the celiac axis, splenic hilus, porta hepatis, and mesentery. It is important to emphasize that when these benefits have been critically assessed, they have proven to be more theoretical than real. While it is true that CT can demonstrate foci of HD in the liver and spleen (Fig. 2.14), as a rule these deposits are so small as to prohibit reliable detection – especially at the time of initial presentation (OKAZAKI et al. 1985; MUNKER et al. 1995). In one study of 100 patients who underwent staging laparotomies, CT's sensitivity to the presence

Fig. 2.13a,b. Nodular sclerosis Hodgkin disease in a 48-year-old man with retroperitoneal nodal involvement. **a** Axial contrast-enhanced CT scan of the abdomen is interpreted as normal since the small size of the retroperitoneal lymph nodes (*arrow*) is inferior to 10 mm. **b** Anteroposterior radiograph from a lymphogram demonstrates multiple involved left paraaortic nodes. One of the nodes exhibits a focal filling defect (*arrowheads*), while others demonstrate the typical foamy architecture (*arrow*).

of splenic and/or hepatic involvement was only 37% (MUNKER et al. 1995). It is also important to note that the size of the spleen is a poor criterion for detecting splenic involvement. Thus, although a positive CT is quite accurate, i.e., one in which one or more focal lesions are detected, there are too many false negatives to place much reliance on the findings. Involvement of the liver occurs less frequently than splenic involvement and is almost invariably preceded by

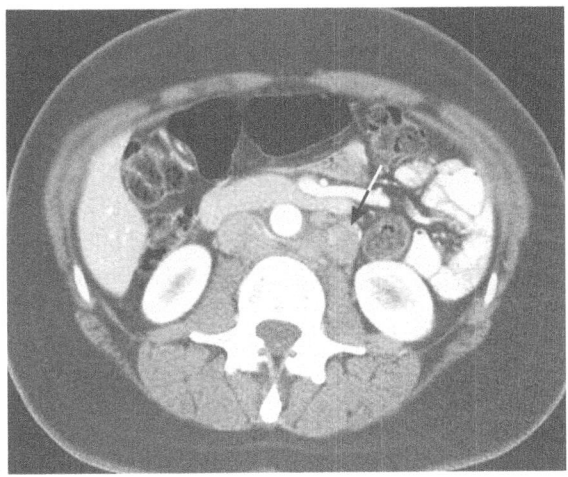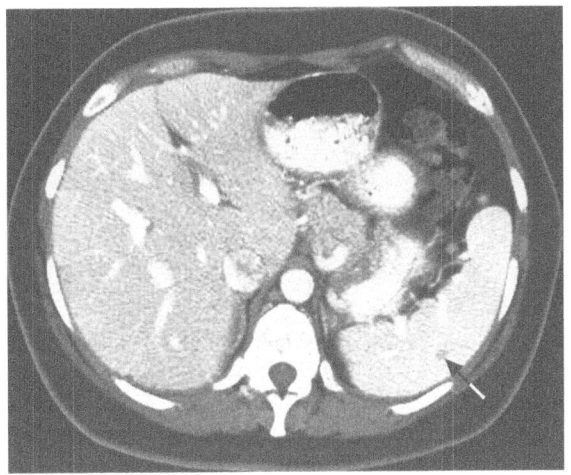

a
b

Fig. 2.14a,b. Nodular sclerosis Hodgkin disease in a 43-year-old woman with abdominal nodal and splenic involvement. **a** Axial contrast-enhanced CT scan of the abdomen shows conglomerate group of lymph nodes projecting to the left of the aorta (*arrow*). **b** Axial CT scan of the upper abdomen demonstrates a small focal filling defect in the spleen (*arrow*). It should be emphasized that the ability of CT to detect splenic involvement is limited.

the latter (KAPLAN 1980). When present, it usually manifests as infiltration of the periportal triad, making detection difficult. Although CT can visualize nodes in the celiac axis, splenic hilus, porta hepatis, and mesentery, CT relies almost exclusively upon increases in the size of the nodes as a criterion for pathological involvement, rather than upon alterations in nodal architecture. Staging laparotomies have revealed that when celiac axis or porta hepatis nodes contain tumor, in the absence of retroperitoneal involvement, the involved nodes are almost invariably normal in size and consequently would likely not have been detected by CT (Fig. 2.13).

Despite what many would regard as the superiority of lymphography over CT, during the past 10–15 years the former has inexorably given way to CT as the examination of choice – except in institutions with either a large cancer population and/or a specific interest in lymphography. This apparent paradox can be understood best in terms of the following two factors: (1) The reluctance of radiologists to champion an examination that they regard as tedious and difficult to perform and interpret; (2) the greater comfort that oncologists, as well as many radiologists, feel in reviewing CT.

At this juncture, it would probably be fair to say that neither lymphography nor CT can be regarded as satisfactorily sensitive to the presence of abdominal involvement in patients with HD. In one study, CT detected only 37% of cases with splenic and/or liver involvement (MUNKER et al. 1995). This is important since as many as 20–30% of patients with clinically staged IA–IIA lym-

phoma and 35% of patients with clinical stage IB–IIB lymphoma will have occult splenic or upper abdominal nodal involvement at the time of laparotomy.

2.9.4.3
[67]Gallium Scanning

In much the same way that [67]Gallium scanning has been advocated as a useful modality in the thorax, some enthusiasts have championed its use in the abdomen. Arguments against the routine performance of [67]Gallium scans are rooted in reports that such scans are insufficiently sensitive to confidently exclude abdominal organ and/or nodal involvement (FRONT et al. 1990; HAGEMEISTER et al. 1990; STOMPER et al. 1993). In one study, sensitivity for abdominal/pelvic disease was only 60% (BEKERMAN et al. 1984). While a positive scan can, and does, provide independent confirmation of involvement by lymphoma, as well as serving to confirm the results of other tests, a negative scan cannot be taken as strong evidence that lymphoma is not present. This is particularly true following treatment, when the accuracy of a negative interpretation is only 65%, in patients with advanced, i.e., stages III and IV, disease (SALLOUM et al. 1997; DELCAMBRE et al. 2000).

2.9.4.4
Magnetic Resonance Imaging

As in the thorax, the relatively small number of reports concerning the accuracy of MR imaging in assessing the abdomen in patients with HD precludes well-reasoned recommendations concerning its use. One report suggests that MR imaging can achieve the same degree of accuracy as does lymphography in evaluating retroperitoneal lymph nodes (TESORO-TESS et al. 1991). This conclusion is unexpected, if one extrapolates from earlier reports that compare CT and lymphography. Both MR imaging and CT utilize nodal enlargement, rather than alterations in internal architecture, to detect lymphadenopathy. MR imaging, however, possesses the additional advantage of being able to detect differences in signal characteristics between normal and pathologic tissue. However, since nodal involvement by HD is often minimal, it would seem unlikely that MR imaging will be able to detect adenopathy with an acceptably high degree of accuracy. It is possible, but as yet unproven, that MR imaging's ability to depict anatomy in more than one plane may translate into an increase in diagnostic accuracy. What would probably be the most reasonable conclusion is that MR imaging can be somewhat more sensitive than CT in identifying nodal involvement, but somewhat less specific (SKILLINGS et al. 1991).

In addition to surveying the retroperitoneum, MR imaging can also evaluate the spleen and liver. Limited information in this area suggests that MR imaging probably suffers from many of the same limitations that affect CT. However, in all likelihood, MR imaging is more sensitive to the presence of lymphoma than is CT (TESORO-TESS et al. 1991). An interesting and potentially valuable application of MR imaging is in the investigation of bone marrow involvement. In one report, MR imaging detected such involvement in 14 of 74 previously untreated patients with HD and NHL (TESORO-TESS et al. 1991). Because HD tends to infiltrate the bone marrow in a focal fashion, there is a considerable potential for sampling errors. The ability of MR imaging to survey large portions of the marrow would tend to facilitate image guided biopsies, as opposed to unguided sampling of the iliac crests.

2.9.4.5
Positron Emission Tomography

In recent years, there has been increasing enthusiasm for the use of FDG-PET in oncology. It is now generally conceded that PET is the single most accurate, examination for the evaluation of abdominal disease in patients with HD. The foundation on which this enthusiastic concession rests is somewhat less than rock-solid. The majority of the reports concern patients who were previously treated, thus

confounding the results. Of those reports that do deal with newly presenting, untreated patients, one might initially conclude that the advantage of PET is rather marginal. In one study of 28 sequential, newly presenting patients, PET and CT concurred in 163 assessments of organ and lymph node region involvement, and differed in only 5. However, upon closer inspection, PET contributed to a change in stage in 6 patients, i.e., 21% (MENZEL et al. 2002). In a series of 38 patients with HD, PET detected several sites of supradiaphragmatic disease that gallium did not, as well as splenic involvement that was also missed on gallium studies (VAN DEN ABBEELE et al. 2002). In another report, PET was said to have detected 92% of cases of splenic involvement. When interpreted as positive, the predictive accuracy of PET was 100%; a negative interpretation yielded a predictive accuracy of 95% (RINI et al. 2002). Although encouraging, given the frequency of microscopic involvement of the spleen, this degree of accuracy is puzzling. It is of obvious importance that efforts be made to replicate these results in larger series.

Although not the focus of this discussion, there is ample evidence that PET is very sensitive in the detection of residual disease, as well as in the assessment of possible disease recurrence. Another advantage of PET is its high prognostic predictive accuracy. When scanning of patients with HD and NHL was performed following treatment, 100% of those who were PET positive relapsed, while only 42% of those who were CT positive did so (JERUSALEM et al. 1999). PET performed early in the course of chemotherapy, on patients with NHL, has demonstrated the capacity to distinguish between those who will and those who will not respond to therapy. In one report, this determination could be made as early as seven days after the initiation of therapy, at which time the metabolic rates for responders were significantly lower than that of their counterparts (ROMER et al. 1998).

2.9.4.6
CT/PET Fusion

Thus far, I have described what might be called 'competing' modalities. Of these, PET provides important, often times crucial, metabolic information. CT, on the other hand, is the acknowledged leader in the provision of precise anatomic images. The fusion of metabolic and anatomic information has created what has come to be known as molecular imaging. Recent advances in instrumentation have resulted in the introduction of single machines that are capable of performing 'simultaneous' CT and PET examinations. In early reports,

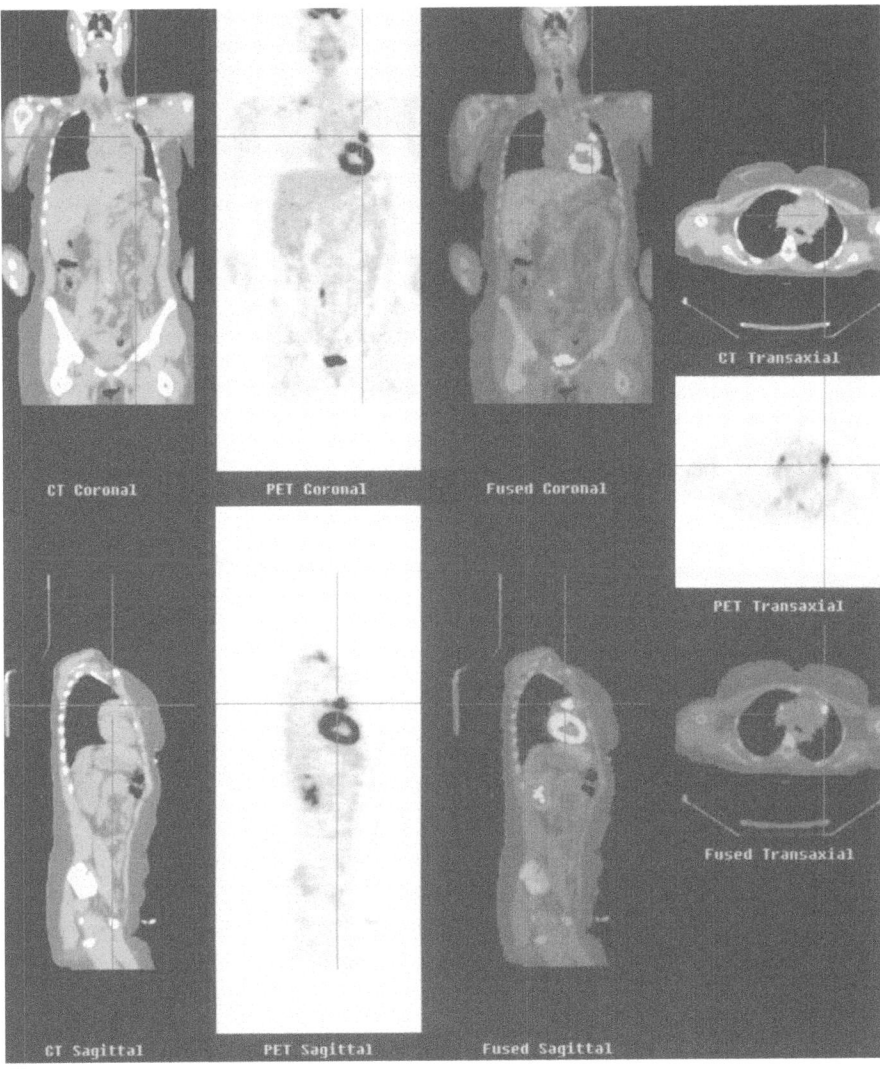

Fig. 2.15. Nodular sclerosis Hodgkin disease in a 25-year-old woman with diffuse supradiaphragmatic and subdiaphragmatic nodal involvement. The abnormalities are virtually impossible to detect with CT. Although visible with FDG-PET, the precise anatomic location is much more readily seen on the CT/PET fusion image.

integrated CT/PET scanners have proven to be both more sensitive and more specific than either modality alone or than the contemporaneous interpretation of two separate examinations (Fig. 2.15). The findings have resulted in a number of important changes in radiotherapy treatment planning.

An alternative to integrated CT/PET scanners is the use of fusion software. Such software currently costs between 1–5% of that of an integrated scanner. It is not restricted to PET images, but can also be utilized to fuse any pair of digital images in DICOM format, e.g., MR imaging. The images from both integrated scanners and those produced by fusion software suffer, to some degree, from problems of misregistration. Taking into consideration the fact that the briefest PET scanning time, to date, is 3 minutes, this is not surprising. The degree of misregistra-

tion of the two systems is likely comparable, between 2–6 mm., although this initial assessment has yet to be rigorously tested.

2.10
Conclusion

Much of the focus of this chapter has been on imaging that is performed at the time of initial presentation. This reflects a personal belief that the diagnostic challenge is usually greatest at that time, and that it coincides with the greatest opportunity to cure. Although salvage chemotherapy can be curative in a large number of patients with HD, it is likely that the physical, psychological, and monetary costs of the additional therapy are considerable. At this point in time, it seems reasonable to presume that the overall costs of care are likely to be lower if appropriate imaging is not avoided at the outset.

The issue of relevance is an important one. While extraordinary advances have been occurring in the field of diagnostic imaging, parallel improvements have been occurring in the systemic, i.e., chemotherapeutic, treatment of HD. These advances, coupled by a growing recognition that improvement in the outcome of HD has come at a high cost, have resulted in a shift away from radiotherapy, and a greater reliance upon chemotherapy. It legitimately could be argued that chemotherapeutic agents are less reliant upon accurate imaging than either radiotherapy or surgery.

It is difficult to prognosticate, but it seems likely that future advances in treatment will probably rely less upon imaging and more upon new areas of scientific investigation such as proteomics. Proteomics is defined as "a discipline in which the structure of proteins are determined with the aim of understanding their detailed functions, evolutionary relationships, and especially the structural changes in mutant proteins that make them unable to perform their function" (FARRAR 2002).

While we await the future, we need to practice in the present. At this juncture, my recommendations for the pre-treatment evaluation of patients with HD include the following:

- Chest x-ray
- CT of the chest abdomen and pelvis
- PET (or preferably some form of fusion imaging)

The added value of FDG-PET over CT still needs to be verified in large series of patients. This is particularly true given the current trend to administer chemotherapy even in early-stage disease (BAR-SHALOM et al. 2001).

A strong argument could also be made to refer newly presenting patients with HD to oncology centers that specialize in the evaluation and treatment of the disease. In such centers, lymphography would likely be available, and could be utilized, if clinical considerations warranted.

References

Anderson KC, Leonard RC, Canellos GP, Skarin AT, Kaplan WD (1983) High-dose gallium imaging in lymphoma. Am J Med 75:327–331

Barbu RR, Port JL, Elkowitz SS, Leonidas JC (1993) Marrow space imaging in Hodgkin's disease. MRI prior to biopsy for improved accuracy. Am J Pediatr Hematol Oncol 15:343–345

Bar-Shalom R, Mor M, Yefremov N, Goldsmith SJ (2001) The value of Ga-67 scintigraphy and F-18 fluorodeoxyglucose positron emission tomography in staging and monitoring the response of lymphoma to treatment. Semin Nucl Med 31:177–190

Bekerman C, Hoffer PB, Bitran JD (1984) The role of gallium-67 in the clinical evaluation of cancer. Semin Nucl Med 14:296–323

Biti G, Cellai E, Magrini SM, Papi MG, Ponticelli P, Boddi V (1994) Second solid tumors and leukemia after treatment for Hodgkin's disease: an analysis of 1121 patients from a single institution. Int J Radiat Oncol Biol Phys 29:25–31

Blackwell EA, Joshua DE, McLaughlin AF, Green D, Kronenberg H, May J (1986) Early supradiaphragmatic Hodgkin's disease. High-dose gallium scanning obviates the need for staging laparotomy. Cancer 58:883–885

Carbone PP, Kaplan HS, Musshoff K, Smithers DW, Tubiana M (1971) Report of the Committee on Hodgkin's Disease Staging Classification. Cancer Res 31:1860–1861

Carlsen SE, Bergin CJ, Hoppe RT (1993) MR imaging to detect chest wall and pleural involvement in patients with lymphoma: effect on radiation therapy planning. Am J Roentgenol AJR 160:1191–1195

Castellino RA, Filly R, Blank N (1976) Routine full-lung tomography in the initial staging and treatment planning of patients with Hodgkin's disease and non-Hodgkin's lymphoma. Cancer 38:1130–1136

Castellino RA, Hoppe RT, Blank N, Young SW, Neumann C, Rosenberg SA, Kaplan HS (1984) Computed tomography, lymphography, and staging laparotomy: correlations in initial staging of Hodgkin disease. Am J Roentgenol AJR 143:37–41

Castellino RA, Blank N, Hoppe RT, Cho C (1986) Hodgkin disease: contributions of chest CT in the initial staging evaluation. Radiology 160:603–605

Clouse ME, Harrison DA, Grassi CJ, Costello P, Edwards SA, Wheeler HG (1985) Lymphangiography, ultrasonography, and computed tomography in Hodgkin's disease and non-Hodgkin's lymphoma. J Comput Tomogr 9:1–8

Cohen MD, Siddiqui A, Weetman R, Provisor A, Coates T (1986) Hodgkin disease and non-Hodgkin lymphomas in children: utilization of radiological modalities. Radiology 158:499–505

Crowther D, Lister TA (1990) The Cotswolds report on the investigation and staging of Hodgkin's disease. Br J Cancer 62:551–552

Delcambre C, Reman O, Henry-Amar M, Peny AM, Macro M, Cheze S, Genot JY, Tanguy A, Switsers O, Van HL, Couette JE, Leporrier M, Bardet S (2000) Clinical relevance of gallium-67 scintigraphy in lymphoma before and after therapy. Eur J Nucl Med 27:176–184

Devizzi L, Maffioli L, Bonfante V, Viviani S, Balzarini L, Gasparini M, Valagussa P, Bombardieri E, Santoro A, Bonadonna G (1997) Comparison of gallium scan, computed tomography, and magnetic resonance in patients with mediastinal Hodgkin's disease. Ann Oncol 8:53–56

Diehl V, Sextro M, Franklin J, Hansmann ML, Harris N, Jaffe E, Poppema S, Harris M, Franssila K, van Krieken J, Marafioti T, Anagnostopoulos I, Stein H (1999) Clinical presentation, course, and prognostic factors in lymphocyte-predominant Hodgkin's disease and lymphocyte-rich classical Hodgkin's disease: report from the European Task Force on Lymphoma Project on Lymphocyte-Predominant Hodgkin's Disease. J Clin Oncol 17:776–783

Dores GM, Metayer C, Curtis RE, Lynch CF, Clarke EA, Glimelius B, Storm H, Pukkala E, van Leeuwen FE, Holowaty EJ, Andersson M, Wiklund T, Joensuu T, van't Veer MB, Stovall M, Gospodarowicz M, Travis LB (2002) Second malignant neoplasms among long-term survivors of Hodgkin's disease: a population-based evaluation over 25 years. J Clin Oncol 20:3484–3494

Dunphy CH, Saravia O, Varvares MA (1996) Hodgkin's disease primarily involving Waldeyer's ring. Case report and review of the literature. Arch Pathol Lab Med 120: 285–287

Edwards CL, Hayes RL (1970) Scanning malignant neoplasms with gallium 67. JAMA 212:1182–1191

Ekstrand BC, Horning SJ (2002) Lymphocyte predominant Hodgkin's disease. Curr Oncol Rep 4:424–433

Farrar WW (2002) Genomics, and the coming wave of proteomics and why the study of protein structure is important. In: www.biology.eku.edu/FARRAR/gen-prot.htm, Richmond

Filly R, Bland N, Castellino RA (1976) Radiographic distribution of intrathoracic disease in previously untreated patients with Hodgkin's disease and non-Hodgkin's lymphoma. Radiology 120:277–281

Front D, Israel O, Epelbaum R, Ben Haim S, Sapir EE, Jerushalmi J, Kolodny GM, Robinson E (1990) Ga-67 SPECT before and after treatment of lymphoma. Radiology 175: 515–519

Gilman EA, McNally RJ, Cartwright RA (1999) Space-time clustering of Hodgkin's Disease in parts of the UK, 1984–1993. Leuk Lymphoma 36:85–100

Glaser SL, Jarrett RF (1996) The epidemiology of Hodgkin's disease. Baillieres Clin Haematol 9:401–416

Hagemeister FB, Fesus SM, Lamki LM, Haynie TP (1990) Role of the gallium scan in Hodgkin's disease. Cancer 65: 1090–1096

Harris NL (1999) Hodgkin's lymphomas: classification, diagnosis, and grading. Semin Hematol 36:220–232

Harris NL, Jaffe ES, Diebold J, Flandrin G, Muller-Hermelink HK, Vardiman J (2000) Lymphoma classification – from controversy to consensus: the R.E.A.L. and WHO Classification of lymphoid neoplasms. Ann Oncol 11 Suppl 1:3–10

Harris NL, Jaffe ES, Stein H, Banks PM, Chan JK, Cleary ML, Delsol G, De Wolf-Peeters C, Falini B, Gatter KC (1994) A revised European-American classification of lymphoid neoplasms: a proposal from the International Lymphoma Study Group. Blood 84:1361–1392

Hasenclever D (2002) The disappearance of prognostic factors in Hodgkin's disease. Ann Oncol 13 Suppl 1:75–78

Hasenclever D, Diehl V (1998) A prognostic score for advanced Hodgkin's disease. International Prognostic Factors Project on Advanced Hodgkin's Disease. N Engl J Med 339:1506–1514

Hellings P, Jorissen M, Ceuppens JL (2000) The Waldeyer's ring. Acta Otorhinolaryngol Belg 54:237–241

Hoane BR, Shields AF, Porter BA, Borrow JW (1994) Comparison of initial lymphoma staging using computed tomography (CT) and magnetic resonance (MR) imaging. Am J Hematol 47:100–105

Hopper KD, Diehl LF, Lesar M, Barnes M, Granger E, Baumann J (1988) Hodgkin disease: clinical utility of CT in initial staging and treatment. Radiology 169:17–22

Jerusalem G, Beguin Y, Fassotte MF, Najjar F, Paulus P, Rigo P, Fillet G (1999) Whole-body positron emission tomography using 18F-fluorodeoxyglucose for posttreatment evaluation in Hodgkin's disease and non-Hodgkin's lymphoma has higher diagnostic and prognostic value than classical computed tomography scan imaging. Blood 94:429–433

Jochelson MS, Herman TS, Stomper PC, Mauch PM, Kaplan WD (1988) Planning mantle radiation therapy in patients with Hodgkin disease: role of gallium-67 scintigraphy. Am J Roentgenol AJR 151:1229–1231

Kadin ME (1994) Pathology of Hodgkin's disease. Curr Opin Oncol 6:456–463

Kapadia SB, Roman LN, Kingma DW, Jaffe ES, Frizzera G (1995) Hodgkin's disease of Waldeyer's ring. Clinical and histoimmunophenotypic findings and association with Epstein-Barr virus in 16 cases. Am J Surg Pathol 19: 1431–1439

Kaplan HS (1980) Hodgkin's disease. Harvard University Press, Cambridge

Kaufman SE (2002a) Lumpers and Splitters in Healthcare – I. In: http://www.epimetrics.com/topics/one-page?page_id= 196&topic=Commentary&page_topic_id=99. The Epimetrics Group, San Francisco

Kaufman SE (2002b) Lumpers and splitters in healthcare – II. In: www.epimetrics.com/topics/one-page?page_id=199& topic=Commentary&page_topic_id=99. The Epimetrics Group, San Francisco

Kinmonth JB (1952) Lymphangiography in Man. Clin Sci 11: 13–20.

Lister TA, Crowther D, Sutcliffe SB, Glatstein E, Canellos GP, Young RC, Rosenberg SA, Coltman CA, Tubiana M (1989) Report of a committee convened to discuss the evaluation and staging of patients with Hodgkin's disease: Cotswolds meeting. J Clin Oncol 7:1630–1636

Lukes RJ, Butler JJ (1966) The pathology and nomenclature of Hodgkin's disease. Cancer Res 26:1063–1083

Lukes RJ, Craver L, Hall T, Rappaport H, Ruber P (1966) Report of the Nomenclature Committee. Cancer Res 26:1311

Macsween KF, Crawford DH (2003) Epstein-Barr virus-recent advances. Lancet Infect Dis 3:131–140

Malis DD, Moffat D, McGarry GW (1998) Isolated nasopharyngeal Hodgkin's disease presenting as nasal obstruction. Int J Clin Pract 52:343–346

Mansfield CM, Fabian C, Jones S, Van SEJ, Grozea P, Morrison F, Miller TP, Seibert C, Ayyangar K (1990) Comparison of lymphangiography and computed tomography scanning in evaluating abdominal disease in stages III and IV Hodgkin's disease. A Southwest Oncology Group study. Cancer 66:2295–2299

Marglin S, Castellino R (1981) Lymphographic accuracy in 632 consecutive, previously untreated cases of Hodgkin disease and non-Hodgkin lymphoma. Radiology 140:351–353

Mauch PM, Kalish LA, Kadin M, Coleman CN, Osteen R, Hellman S (1993) Patterns of presentation of Hodgkin disease. Implications for etiology and pathogenesis. Cancer 71: 2062–2071

McLaughlin AF, Magee MA, Greenough R, Allman KC, Southee AE, Meikle SR, Hutton BF, Joshua DE, Bautovich GJ, Morris JG (1990) Current role of gallium scanning in the management of lymphoma. Eur J Nucl Med 16:755–771

Menzel C, Dobert N, Mitrou P, Mose S, Diehl M, Berner U, Grunwald F (2002) Positron emission tomography for the staging of Hodgkin's lymphoma – increasing the body of evidence in favor of the method. Acta Oncol 41:430–436

Metayer C, Lynch CF, Clarke EA, Glimelius B, Storm H, Pukkala E, Joensuu T, van Leeuwen FE, van't Veer MB, Curtis RE, Holowaty EJ, Andersson M, Wiklund T, Gospodarowicz M, Travis LB (2000) Second cancers among long-term survivors of Hodgkin's disease diagnosed in childhood and adolescence. J Clin Oncol 18:2435–2443

Metz CE (1978) Basic principles of ROC analysis. Semin Nucl Med 8:283–298

Munker R, Stengel A, Stabler A, Hiller E, Brehm G (1995) Diagnostic accuracy of ultrasound and computed tomography in the staging of Hodgkin's disease. Verification by laparotomy in 100 cases. Cancer 76:1460–1466

Okazaki A, Niibe H, Mitsuhashi N, Ito J, Nakajima N, Saito Y, Tamaki Y, Nagai T, Machinami R, Sakata N (1985) CT and pathologic studies on detecting hepatic involvement of malignant lymphoma. Gan No Rinsho 31:494–500

Paffenbarger RS Jr, Wing AL, Hyde RT (1977) Characteristics in youth indicative of adult-onset Hodgkin's disease. J Natl Cancer Inst 58:1489–1491

Poppema S, Potters M, Emmens R, Visser L, van den Berg A (1999) Immune reactions in classical Hodgkin's lymphoma. Semin Hematol 36:253–259

Raby N, Ineson N (1987) The role of gallium 67 scanning in the management of Hodgkin's disease. Br J Clin Pract 41: 553–556

Reske SN, Kotzerke J (2001) FDG-PET for clinical use. Results of the 3rd German Interdisciplinary Consensus Conference, "Onko-PET III," 21 July and 19 September 2000. Eur J Nucl Med 28:1707–1723

Rini JN, Manalili EY, Hoffman MA, Karayalcin G, Mehrotra B, Tomas MB, Palestro CJ (2002) F-18 FDG versus Ga-67 for detecting splenic involvement in Hodgkin's disease. Clin Nucl Med 27:572–577

Romer W, Hanauske AR, Ziegler S, Thodtmann R, Weber W, Fuchs C, Enne W, Herz M, Nerl C, Garbrecht M, Schwaiger M (1998) Positron emission tomography in non-Hodgkin's lymphoma: assessment of chemotherapy with fluorodeoxyglucose. Blood 91:4464–4471

Rosenberg SA, Kaplan HS (1966) Evidence for an orderly progression in the spread of Hodgkin's disease. Cancer Res 26:1225–1231

Roth SL, Sack H, Havemann K, Willers R, Kocsis B, Schumacher V (1998) Contiguous pattern spreading in patients with Hodgkin's disease. Radiother Oncol 47:7–16

Salloum E, Brandt DS, Caride VJ, Cornelius E, Zelterman D, Schubert W, Mannino T, Cooper DL (1997) Gallium scans in the management of patients with Hodgkin's disease: a study of 101 patients. J Clin Oncol 15:518–527

Senge PM (1990) The fifth discipline: the art and practice of the learning organization, 1st edn. Currency Doubleday, New York

Skillings JR, Bramwell V, Nicholson RL, Prato FS, Wells G (1991) A prospective study of magnetic resonance imaging in lymphoma staging. Cancer 67:1838–1843

Staratschek-Jox A, Shugart YY, Strom SS, Nagler A, Taylor GM (2002) Genetic susceptibility to Hodgkin's lymphoma and to secondary cancer: workshop report. Ann Oncol 13: 30–33

Stiller CA (1998) What causes Hodgkin's disease in children? Eur J Cancer 34:523–528

Stomper PC, Cholewinski SP, Park J, Bakshi SP, Barcos MP (1993) Abdominal staging of thoracic Hodgkin disease: CT-lymphangiography-Ga-67 scanning correlation. Radiology 187:381–386

Strijk SP, Boetes C, Rosenbusch G, Ruijs JH (1987) Lymphography and abdominal computed tomography in staging Hodgkin's disease. Rofo Fortschr Geb Rontgenstr Nuklearmed 146:312–318

Strollo DC, Rosado-de-Christenson ML, Jett JR (1997) Primary mediastinal tumors: part II. Tumors of the middle and posterior mediastinum. Chest 112:1344–1357

Tesoro-Tess JD, Balzarini L, Ceglia E, Petrillo R, Santoro A, Musumeci R (1991) Magnetic resonance imaging in the initial staging of Hodgkin's disease and non-Hodgkin lymphoma. Eur J Radiol 12:81–90

Travis LB, Curtis RE, Stovall M, Holowaty EJ, van Leeuwen FE, Glimelius B, Lynch CF, Hagenbeek A, Li CY, Banks PM, et al (1994) Risk of leukemia following treatment for non-Hodgkin's lymphoma. J Natl Cancer Inst 86:1450–1457

Tucker MA, Coleman CN, Cox RS, Varghese A, Rosenberg SA (1988) Risk of second cancers after treatment for Hodgkin's disease. N Engl J Med 318:76–81

Tumeh SS, Rosenthal DS, Kaplan WD, English RJ, Holman BL (1987) Lymphoma: evaluation with Ga-67 SPECT. Radiology 164:111–114

Van den Abbeele AD, Friedberg JW, Fischman A (2002) FDG-PET is superior to 67Ga scintigraphy in the staging and followup of patients with Hodgkin's lymphoma. J Nucl Med 43:30–31P

van Leeuwen FE, Klokman WJ, Veer MB, Hagenbeek A, Krol AD, Vetter UA, Schaapveld M, van Heerde P, Burgers JM, Somers R, Aleman BM (2000) Long-term risk of second malignancy in survivors of Hodgkin's disease treated during adolescence or young adulthood. J Clin Oncol 18: 487–497

Varan A, Cila A, Buyukpamukcu M (1999) Prognostic importance of magnetic resonance imaging in bone marrow involvement of Hodgkin disease. Med Pediatr Oncol 32: 267–271

Webb WR, Gatsonis C, Zerhouni EA, Heelan RT, Glazer GM, Francis IR, McNeil BJ (1991) CT and MR imaging in staging nonsmall cell bronchogenic carcinoma: report of the Radiologic Diagnostic Oncology Group. Radiology 178: 705–713

Weber G (1983) Biochemical strategy of cancer cells and the design of chemotherapy: G. H. A. Clowes Memorial Lecture. Cancer Res 43:3466–3492

Weiss LM (2000) Epstein-Barr virus and Hodgkin's disease. Curr Oncol Rep 2:199–204.

Wernecke K, Diederich S (1994) Sonographic features of mediastinal tumors. Am J Roentgenol AJR 163:1357–1364

Wernecke K, Vassallo P, Peters PE, Potter R, Luckener HG (1990a) Diagnostic imaging of mediastinal tumors. Sensitivity and specificity of sonography in comparison with computed tomography and conventional x-ray diagnosis. Radiologe 30:532–540

Wernecke K, Vassallo P, Potter R, Luckener HG, Peters PE (1990b) Mediastinal tumors: sensitivity of detection with sonography compared with CT and radiography. Radiology 175:137–143

3 Extranodal Hodgkin Disease

Ali Guermazi and Clara G.C. Ooi

CONTENTS

3.1
Introduction

Hodgkin disease (HD) is a lymphoid malignancy that has become, to a large extent, a curable disease. At presentation, HD is usually supradiaphragmatic,

Ali Guermazi, MD
Visiting Associate Professor, Department of Radiology, University of California, San Francisco, 350 Parnassus Avenue, Suite 150, San Francisco, CA 94117, USA
Clara G.C. Ooi, MD
Associate Professor and Honorary Consultant, Department of Radiology, University of Hong Kong, Room 405, Block K, Queen Mary Hospital, Pokfulam Road, Hong Kong SAR, China

with spread often occurring predictably from one nodal group contiguously to the next along the lymphatic pathways. HD is usually almost entirely confined to the lymph nodes. Although, at presentation or in the course of the disease, extranodal lesions may develop. Extranodal involvement in HD is very uncommon compared with non-Hodgkin lymphoma. Extranodal invasion of adjacent tissue is found in up to 15% of cases, and hematogenous spread in 5 to 10%. Even when dissemination occurs beyond the lymphoreticular system, certain patterns of associated spread are frequently evident. The extranodal disease, except spleen and thymus involvement, signifies stage IV HD. With the recent progress in therapy, the aim is currently to cure patients with HD and to limit long-term therapeutic toxicity. For these reasons, the therapeutic indications are tailored to the initial prognostic factors. All prognostic scores established for HD take account of either the presence of stage IV disease or the number of the extranodal sites. The initial staging is crucial for therapeutic decisions, demonstrating extranodal involvement or not. First, it must distinguish contiguous disease (E stage), which needs in addition local radiation therapy, from stage IV disease, which is treated with chemotherapy combined or not with general radiotherapy. Secondly, the number of extranodal involvement must be evaluated as it is considered prognostic. The purpose of this chapter is to present the various radiologic appearances of extranodal involvement in HD with emphasis on the pathophysiological mechanisms of tumoral spread. HD mainly spreads by means of lymphatic invasion or hematogenous dissemination. As a result, every organ system containing or not containing lymphoid tissue may be involved in HD. Extranodal involvement is more likely to occur at recurrence than at presentation. The differential diagnoses and diagnostic pitfalls will be discussed since extranodal HD may simulate other neoplastic or infectious diseases.

3.2
Thorax

Intrathoracic disease is more common in HD than in non-Hodgkin lymphoma (FILLY et al. 1976; NORTH et al. 1990). The presence and distribution of thoracic disease in patients with HD is important both in tumor staging and in treatment, especially when radiotherapy is planned (FILLY et al. 1976). There is currently a general agreement that CT is more sensitive and specific than plain radiographs in assessing chest disease (CASTELLINO et al. 1986; CARLSEN et al. 1993).

3.2.1
Lungs

Involvement of the lung parenchyma is rare (VAN DER SCHEE et al. 1990; SANDRASEGARAN et al. 1994) and accounts for 5.9–11.6% of cases (FILLY et al. 1976; NORTH et al. 1990; FISHMAN et al. 1991). It is bilateral in about 4.3% (FILLY et al. 1976). The lung is more frequently involved in secondary or recurrent disease than as a primary manifestation (NORTH et al. 1990; RADIN 1990; LEWIS et al. 1991; PINSON et al. 1992; CARTIER et al. 1999; DIEDERICH et al. 2001). At presentation, it is usually associated with hilar and/or mediastinal nodal disease (NORTH et al. 1990), but very few cases of primary pulmonary HD in the absence of mediastinal or hilar node disease have been reported (STRUM et al. 1985; RADIN 1990; PINSON et al. 1992; CARTIER et al. 1999). When the hilar adenopathy is unilateral, the parenchymal involvement, if present, is in the ipsilateral lung (FILLY et al. 1976; STRUM et al. 1985; NORTH et al. 1990). In treated patients, relapse in the chest is commonly seen in the lungs. In recurrent disease, pulmonary involvement without nodal disease is more common than it is at presentation (NORTH et al. 1990).

The most common feature is a direct extension from hilar nodes towards the lung. The second feature observed in HD is nodular lesions, often peripheral and showing poorly defined borders (Fig. 3.1). The nodules, with or without cavitation, tend to be single or few in number. There is a predilection for the upper lobes in primary pulmonary HD. Radiologic patterns also include masses (Fig. 3.2) or masslike consolidation and atelectasis of a lobe or segment. This may be due to bronchial compression by nodes or to endobronchial disease (Fig. 3.3). Bronchoscopy may be used to confirm endobronchial disease. The least common parenchymal manifestation is an interstitial infiltration representing disease along

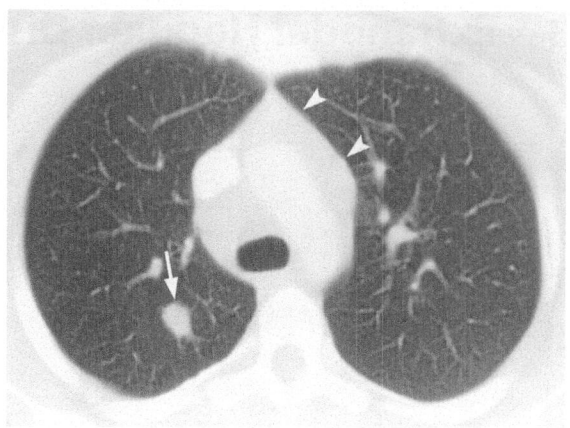

Fig. 3.1. Pulmonary involvement in a 19-year-old woman with nodular sclerosing Hodgkin disease. The patient had undergone treatment 18 months earlier and was in complete remission. Axial CT scan of the chest shows recurrent pulmonary disease with an ill-defined nodular lesion in the right lung (*arrow*). Mediastinal adenopathy is also seen (*arrowheads*). (With permission from [GUERMAZI et al. 2001])

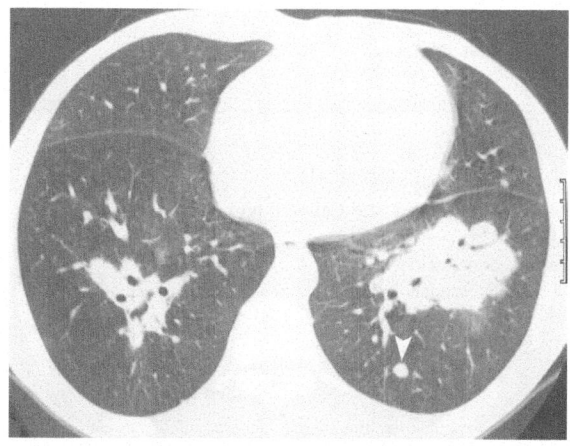

Fig. 3.2. Pulmonary involvement in a 38-year-old man with nodular sclerosing Hodgkin disease. The patient had undergone treatment 4 years and was in complete remission. Axial CT scan of the chest shows bilateral ill-defined lung masses with a nodular lesion in the left lung (*arrowhead*). There was no mediastinal adenopathy. (With permission from [GUERMAZI et al. 2001])

the lymphatic routes (FILLY et al. 1976; CASTELLINO et al. 1986; SHAHAR et al. 1987; NORTH et al. 1990; RADIN 1990; VAN DER SCHEE et al. 1990; FISHMAN et al. 1991; LEWIS et al. 1991; RICHARDSON and LONGO 1991; PINSON et al. 1992; SANDRASEGARAN et al. 1994; TREDANIEL et al. 1994). In general, primary pulmonary HD tends to have an upper lung zone and a relatively high incidence of cavitation (CARTIER et al. 1999). On the other hand, the typical appearance of

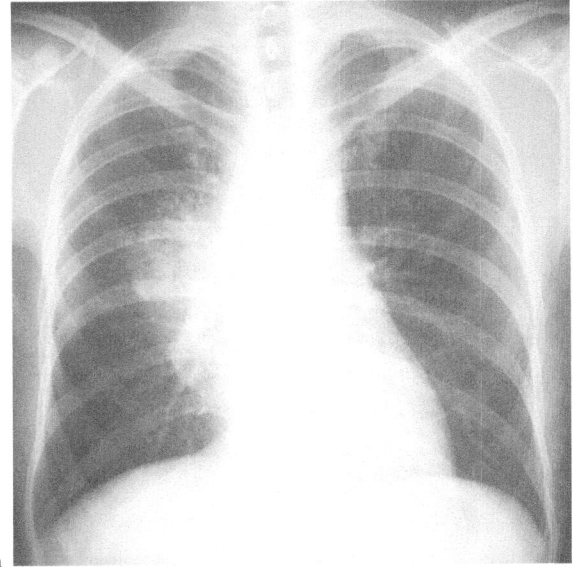
a

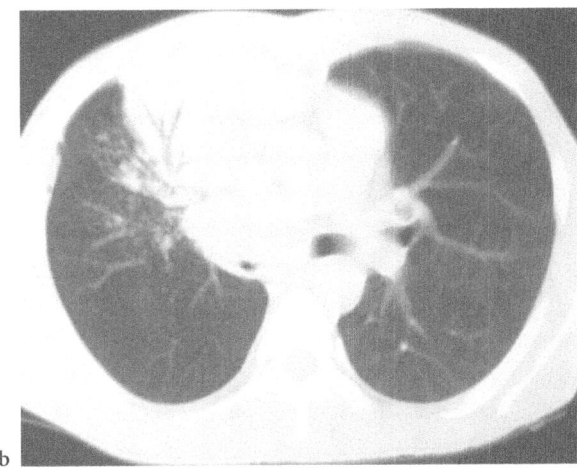
b

Fig. 3.3a,b. Endobronchial involvement in a 31-year-old man with nodular sclerosing Hodgkin disease who presented with respiratory symptoms. a Anteroposterior chest radiograph shows an ill-defined, right-sided hilar and mediastinal mass. b Axial CT scan of the chest demonstrates a pulmonary consolidation with an air bronchogram. There is a typical micronodulation along the bronchi. The patient underwent bronchoscopy, which demonstrated an endobronchial lesion due to Hodgkin disease. (With permission from [GUERMAZI et al. 2001])

secondary pulmonary HD consists of multiple, irregularly marginated pulmonary nodules (DIEDERICH et al. 2001).

When the above changes are seen in an untreated patient, pulmonary involvement can be diagnosed with confidence. In a treated patient, however, biopsy may be needed to differentiate relapse from infection, radiation pneumonitis, bronchoalveolar carcinoma, bronchiolitis obliterans, organizing pneumonia, Wegener granulomatosis, or drug-induced lung disease (Fig. 3.4) (LEWIS et al. 1991; SANDRASEGARAN et al. 1994; DIEDERICH et al. 2001; GUERMAZI et al. 2001).

CT is the method of choice for detecting lung anomalies, although most of the parenchymal involvement may be seen with chest radiographs (FILLY et al. 1976; CASTELLINO et al. 1986; NORTH et al. 1990; LEWIS et al. 1991; SANDRASEGARAN et al. 1994). Indeed, CT scans usually show more extensive parenchymal disease, or may demonstrate pulmonary involvement when the radiographs are normal, and may therefore change both the stage and the treatment of the disease (Fig. 3.5) (NORTH et al. 1990; LEWIS et al. 1991; DIEDERICH et al. 2001). Moreover, CT is used routinely in patients with lymphoma to assess response to therapy, evaluate recurrence, monitor patients before and after bone marrow transplantation, and diagnose complications such as pneumonia, radiation injury, and the occasional occurrence of secondary tumors (LEWIS et al. 1991).

3.2.2
Pleura

Pleural effusions are not uncommon at presentation (NORTH et al. 1990), and account for about 13% of cases (CASTELLINO et al. 1986). They are not of prognostic importance, unless associated with pleural mass, since they rarely contain malignant cells and

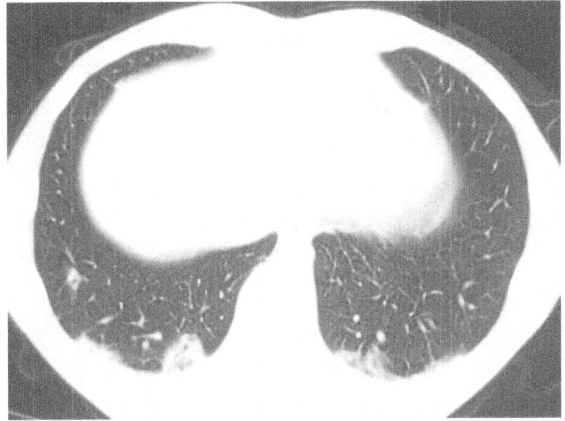

Fig. 3.4. Pulmonary toxicity in a 24-year-old man with nodular sclerosing Hodgkin disease. Axial CT scan of the chest 5 months after institution of C-MOPP-ABVD protocol chemotherapy demonstrates peripheral, ill-defined pulmonary consolidation bilaterally due to Bleomycin toxicity. (With permission from [GUERMAZI et al. 2001])

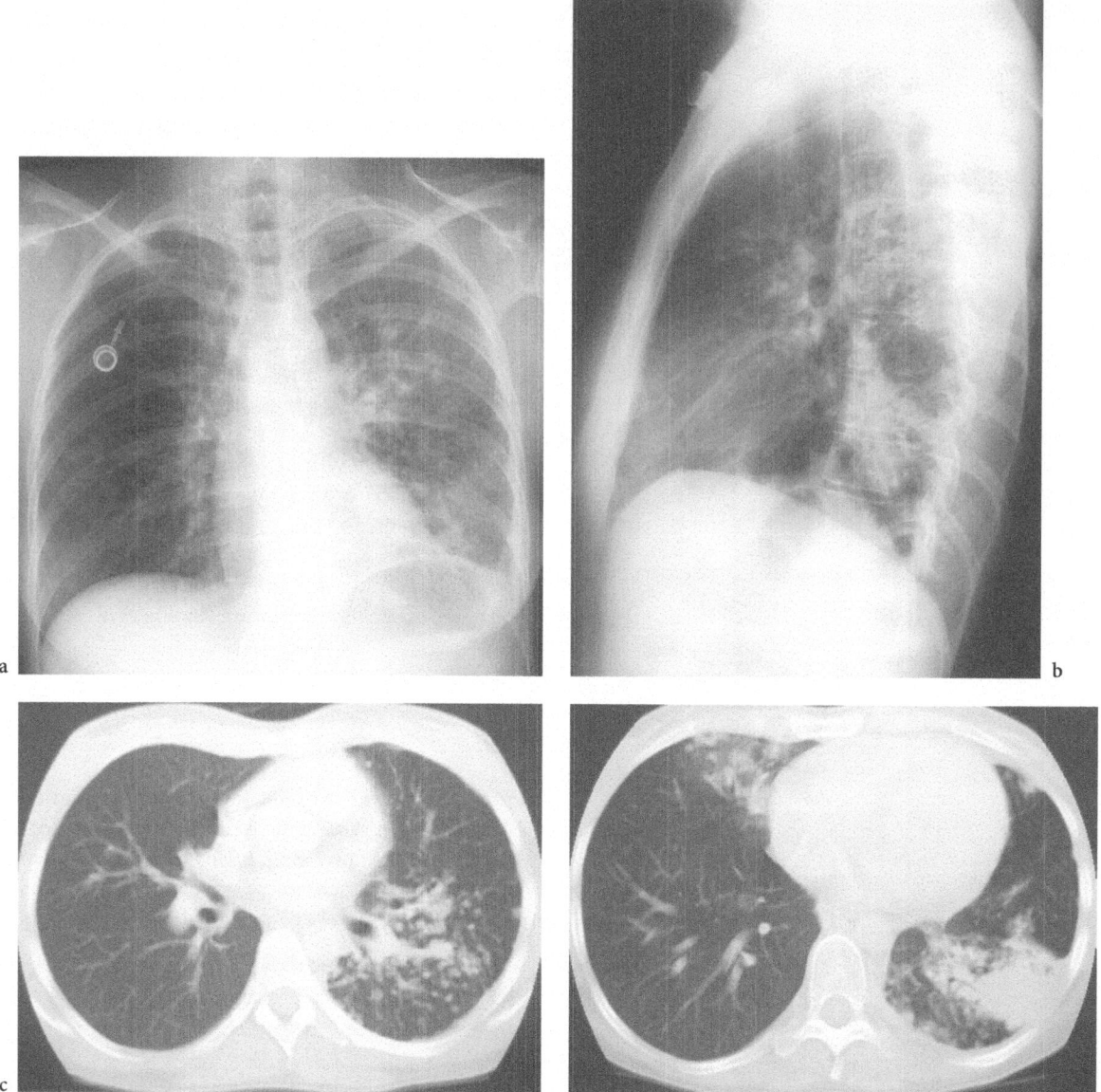

Fig 3.5a–d. Pulmonary involvement in a 25-year-old man with mixed-cellularity Hodgkin disease. The patient had undergone treatment 3 years earlier and was in complete remission. **a** Anteroposterior and (**b**) lateral chest radiographs demonstrate disseminated micronodular disease predominantly involving the left lung. A pulmonary consolidation in the left inferior lobe and a left pleural effusion are also seen. **c** Axial CT scan of the chest shows bilateral ill-defined peribronchial micronodular lesions less than 1 cm in diameter. **d** Axial CT scan obtained 4 cm caudad to (**c**) shows a shaggy left-sided mass with an air bronchogram, slight consolidation in the right middle lobe, and several peribronchial micronodular lesions. (With permission from [Guermazi et al. 2001])

resolve following treatment (Castellino et al. 1986; North et al. 1990; Sandrasegaran et al. 1994). Solid pleural masses, also called pleural-based masses, are less frequent (Fig. 3.6) (Aquino et al. 1999; Guermazi et al. 2001). They represent an underappreciated site of lymphoma (Shuman and Libshitz 1984). The pleural disease can occur as plaques, discrete nodules, or a combination of the two. Plaques may occur anywhere along the pleural surface and are frequently accompanied by fluid (Shuman and Libshitz 1984; North et al. 1990). A variety of other diseases can mimic the CT appearance of subpleural lymphoma. Thymoma, renal and testicular metastases are particularly confounding since they may have mediastinal nodes and pleural-based masses in combination. Pleural lipomas are relatively common and may be diagnosed with appropriate attenuation values (Shuman and Libshitz 1984).

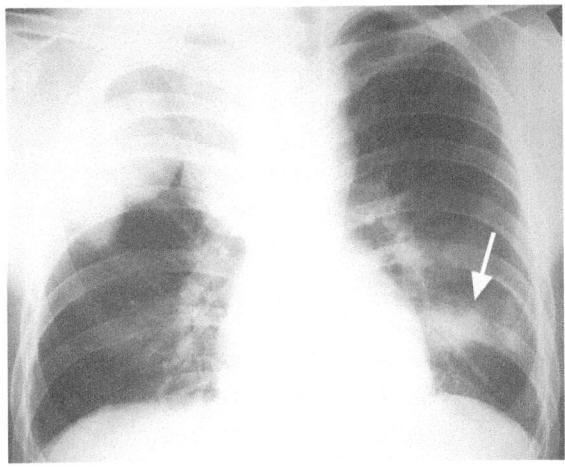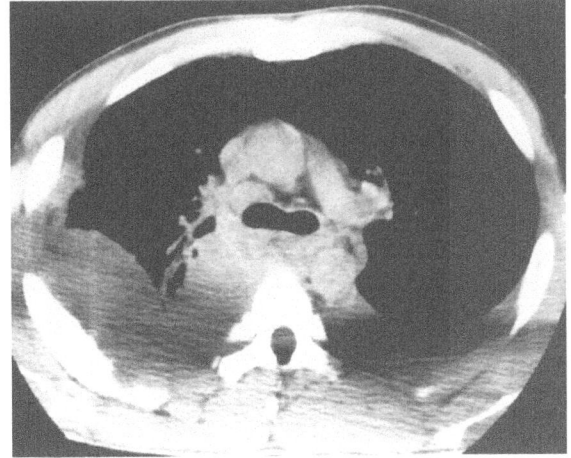

a   b

Fig. 3.6a,b. Pleural disease in a 26-year-old man with nodular sclerosing Hodgkin disease. The patient had undergone treatment 3 years earlier and was in complete remission. **a** Anterioposterior chest radiograph demonstrates pleural-based masses in the right apex. There is also a poorly defined left pulmonary consolidation (*arrow*). **b** Axial CT scan of the chest shows a right pleural mass and left pleural effusion. (With permission from [Guermazi et al. 2001])

3.2.3
Heart and Pericardium

Cardiac or pericardial disease apparently results from retrograde lymphatic spread, hematogenous spread, and direct extension from other intrathoracic tumor masses. The incidence of cardiac involvement by HD at autopsy is estimated at 7.5% (McDonnell et al. 1982).

Pericardial effusion may be seen in patients with large mediastinal masses (Castellino et al. 1986; North et al. 1990). It usually resolves in a short time following institution of chemotherapy. Invasion of the pericardium and superior vena cava by a right-sided hilar and mediastinal mass has been reported (Fig. 3.7) (North et al. 1990). A nodular mass in the pericardium was once noted in association with a large pericardial effusion (Castellino et al. 1986).

3.2.4
Thymus

Thymic enlargement is seen in 30–56% of patients who have intrathoracic involvement at first presentation (Castellino et al. 1986; North et al. 1990; Wong-You-Cheong and Radford 1995). However, HD involving only the thymus is rare (North et al. 1990; Wernecke et al. 1991) and may indicate a different disease (Heron et al. 1988). The clinical significance of thymic involvement in HD is as yet

unclear. With current staging and management, the thymus is considered a "lymph node" and, therefore, its involvement does not change the stage of the disease. The thymic origin of an anterior mediastinal mass in HD can frequently be diagnosed only on follow-up CT (Wernecke et al. 1991). The thymus remains enlarged in about one third of cases after treatment (Sandrasegaran et al. 1994). Following therapy, enlargement can be the result of recurrent disease, thymic rebound, or the development or persistence of thymic cysts (Heron et al. 1988; North et al. 1990; Wernecke et al. 1991; Wong-You-Cheong and Radford 1995). The timing of thymic enlargement in relation to therapy and the presence or absence of disease elsewhere may permit distinction between thymic relapse and rebound hyperplasia in most cases. When there is a doubt about the diagnosis, biopsy should be performed (Heron et al. 1988).

Distinguishing thymic enlargement is easier with CT than with conventional chest radiographs (North et al. 1990). The two morphologic criteria suggesting the presence of enlarged thymus are a triangular-shaped configuration of the mass (Fig. 3.8) or the presence of cysts (small areas of slightly reduced density) (Fig. 3.9) (Heron et al. 1988; Wernecke et al. 1991). Parasternal sonography has been suggested as an alternative technique for the diagnosis of thymic involvement but, since it does not eliminate the need for CT, its value is limited (Wernecke et al. 1991; Sandrasegaran et al. 1994).

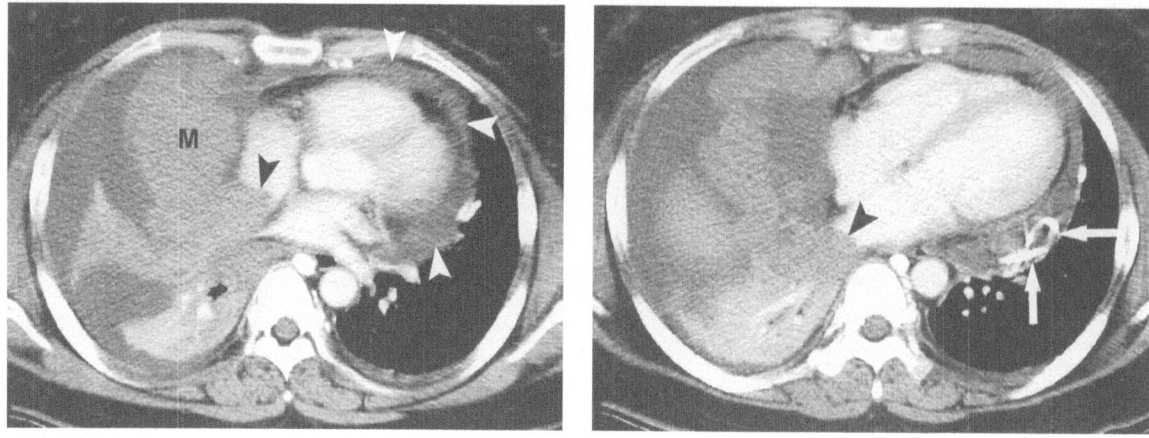

Fig. 3.7a,b. Pericardium involvement in a 30-year-old woman with nodular sclerosing Hodgkin disease. The patient presented with an anterior mediastinal mass a year earlier. **a** Axial contrast-enhanced CT scan of the chest shows a large anterior mediastinal mass (*M*) as well as an involvement of the right atrium (*black arrowhead*) and pericardium with pericardial effusion (*white arrowheads*). A right pleural effusion and collapse of the right lung are also seen. **b** The superior aspect of the left atrium is shown to be infiltrated (*arrowhead*). Note drainage catheter (*arrows*) within the pericardial effusion.

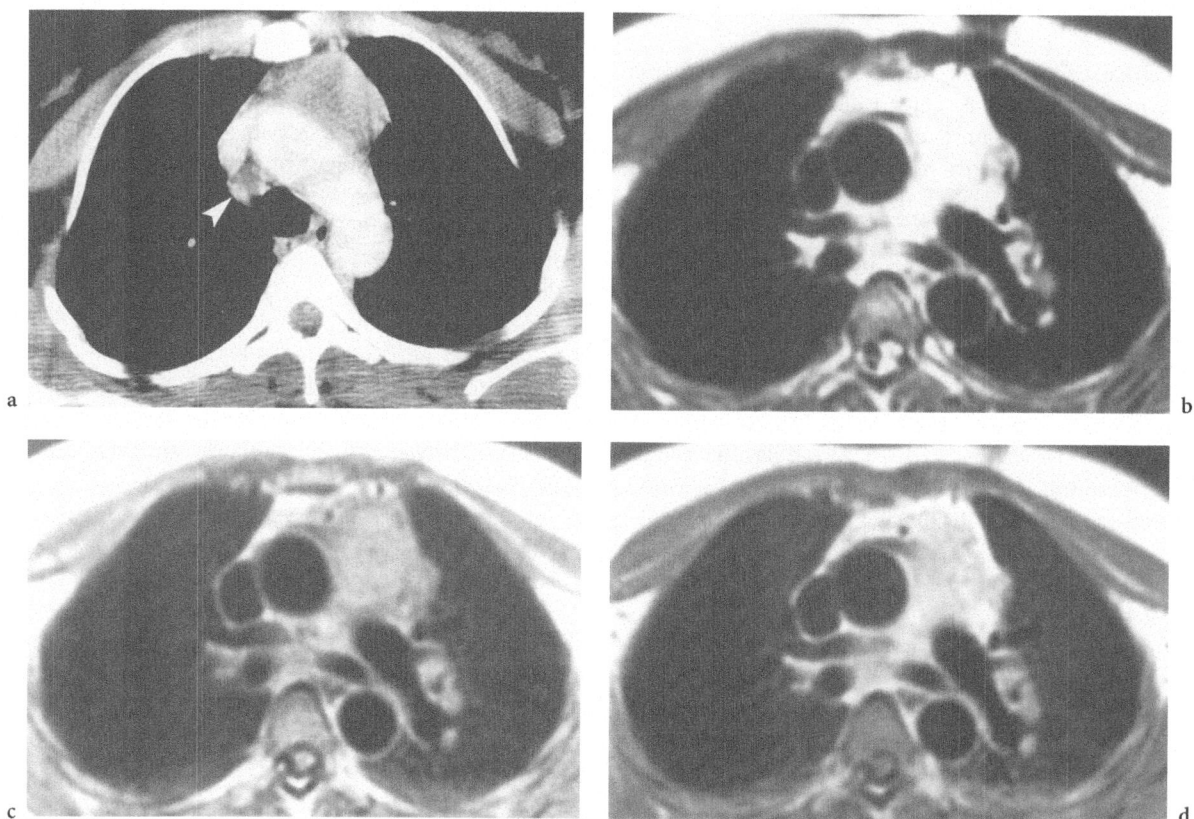

Fig. 3.8a–d. Thymic involvement in a 43-year-old man with nodular sclerosing Hodgkin disease. **a** Axial contrast-enhanced CT scan of the chest shows the thymus as a triangular prevascular lesion. Right laterotracheal adenopathy is also seen (*arrowhead*). The thymus appears hyperintense on (**b**) T2-weighted MR image and hypointense on (**c**) T1-weighted MR image. It enhances homogeneously (**d**) after contrast administration. (With permission from [Guermazi et al. 2001])

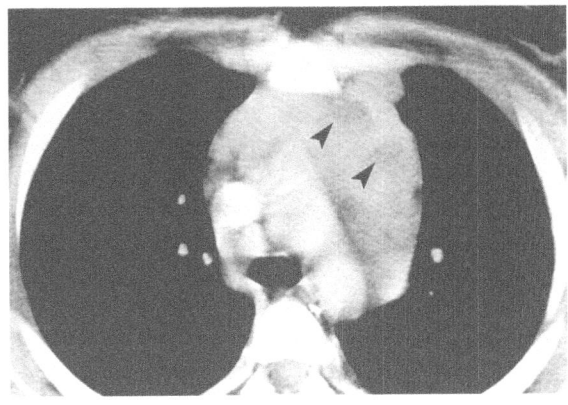

Fig. 3.9. Thymic involvement in a 24-year-old woman with nodular sclerosing Hodgkin disease. Axial contrast-enhanced CT scan of the chest shows an anterior prevascular mediastinal mass with small hypodense areas (*arrowheads*), findings that are suggestive of thymic involvement. Follow-up CT performed after radiation therapy (*not shown*) showed a triangular residual thymic gland. (With permission from [GUERMAZI et al. 2001])

3.2.5
Chest Wall

Chest wall involvement is not uncommon and occurs in about 6.4% of cases (CASTELLINO et al. 1986). It may be either an initial manifestation of the disease or a site of recurrence. If unrecognized, chest wall involvement increases the risk of treatment failure in patient with HD, since it changes the stage of disease and therefore needs more aggressive therapy (BERGIN et al. 1990; CARLSEN et al. 1993). The most common type of chest wall involvement is an infiltration of parasternal soft tissues by direct extension from anterior mediastinal nodes, mainly in cases of internal mammary node involvement. Occasionally, masses are seen beneath or between the pectoral muscles without contiguous mediastinal or axillary adenopathy (CHO et al. 1985; BERGIN et al. 1990; NORTH et al. 1990; CARLSEN et al. 1993). Thoracic spine involvement, when present, is frequently due to a direct spread from posterior mediastinal nodes (CHO et al. 1985; BERGIN et al. 1990; NORTH et al. 1990). Most patients with chest wall involvement have associated intrathoracic disease (NORTH et al. 1990; CARLSEN et al. 1993). However, occasionally chest wall masses may be seen without evidence of intrathoracic disease (CHO et al. 1985; NORTH et al. 1990).

CASTELLINO et al. (1986) showed that CT is the method of choice for detecting chest wall involvement since the disease was identified only on CT in 12 of 13 patients. More recently, it has been shown that MR imaging is more sensitive than CT (BERGIN et al. 1990; CARLSEN et al. 1993). Short tau inversion-recovery (STIR) and other fat saturation techniques are particularly sensitive in detecting chest wall invasion (BERGIN et al. 1990).

3.3
Abdomen and Pelvis

3.3.1
Spleen

The spleen is usually considered a "nodal organ" in HD, and an extranodal organ in non-Hodgkin lymphoma. We will however present the patterns of splenic involvement for a better understanding of progression in HD. The problem of detecting splenic involvement is still largely unsolved. Staging laparotomy has shown that the spleen is infiltrated in about 30–40% of patients at presentation (SHIRKHODA et al. 1990; SANDRASEGARAN et al. 1994). Splenic involvement is typically diffuse and only a small minority of cases present with nodules larger than 1 cm in size (Fig. 3.10). The size of the spleen is not of much help since diffuse infiltration may be present in spleens of normal size while mild to moderate reactive splenomegaly occurs in about 30% of patients in the absence of lymphoma deposits. Marked splenomegaly almost always indicates infiltration (CASTELLINO 1982; FISHMAN et al. 1991; SANDRASEGARAN et al. 1994).

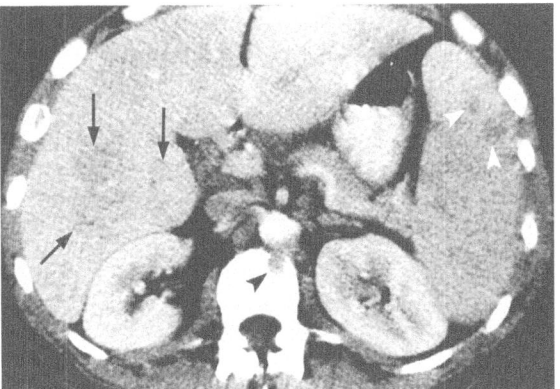

Fig. 3.10. Splenic and hepatic involvement in a 29-year-old man with nodular sclerosing Hodgkin disease. Axial contrast-enhanced CT scan of the abdomen shows marked enlargement of the spleen, which contains multiple areas of low attenuation (*white arrowheads*). There are also multiple, slightly hypodense lesions in the liver (*arrows*) and a small lytic bone lesion of the vertebral body (*black arrowhead*). (With permission from [GUERMAZI et al. 2001])

Nodules are characteristically hypoechoic on ultrasound and show low attenuation with reduced contrast enhancement compared with normal splenic tissue at CT (SHIRKHODA et al. 1990; FISHMAN et al. 1991; SANDRASEGARAN et al. 1994). Ultrasound may not detect very small deposits, and care must be exercised in interpreting CT images obtained during the early phase of a bolus contrast injection where the spleen may enhance very inhomogeneously mimicking tumor infiltration (SHIRKHODA et al. 1990). Detection of splenic lymphoma by MR imaging is not reliable because both the normal spleen and lymphomatous tissue may display similar signal intensity (SHIRKHODA et al. 1990). Nodules are hypo or isointense on T1-weighted images, hyperintense on T2-weighted images and show reduced enhancement after gadolinium compared with normal spleen (SANDRASEGARAN et al. 1994).

Diffuse involvement of the spleen in HD is non specific, and not detectable by US or CT (SHIRKHODA et al. 1990; SANDRASEGARAN et al. 1994; MUNKER et al. 1995). Indeed, it is generally accepted that in HD, the spleen may be enlarged but not involved, or of normal size yet infiltrated by tumor (SHIRKHODA et al. 1990).

3.3.2
Liver

Primary hepatic HD is very rare. However, secondary liver involvement is fairly common, usually associated with lymph node disease, and usually occurs late in the course of disease or with advanced stage disease (ZORNOZA and GINALDI 1981; SANDRASEGARAN et al.

1994; CHIM et al. 2000b). HD of the liver is almost invariably associated with disease of the spleen. Only one case of HD of the liver has been reported without splenic involvement. In fact, the more extensive the splenic disease, the greater the likelihood of liver involvement (SHIRKHODA et al. 1990). Liver involvement at the time of presentation is seen in 6–20% of patients (CASTELLINO 1982; FISHMAN et al. 1991; SANDRASEGARAN et al. 1994).

Liver involvement is usually diffuse, with discrete nodular lesions present in only 10% of cases (ZORNOZA and GINALDI 1981; SHIRKHODA et al. 1990; SANDRASEGARAN et al. 1994; CHIM et al. 2000b). The combination of diffuse and nodular types of lesions occurs in less than 3% of patients. The small number of positive findings, compared with the large number of studies reviewed, suggests that gross disease must be present before a pathological state can be detected by imaging modalities (ZORNOZA and GINALDI 1981). Indeed, HD occurs more often as miliary lesions (< 1 cm in diameter) (Fig. 3.11) than as masses (CASTELLINO 1982; FISHMAN et al. 1991; GUERMAZI et al. 2001). The diffuse or infiltrative form of the disease results in patchy and irregular infiltrates originating primarily in the portal areas.

Nodular disease in the liver shows the same characteristics as splenic disease on US, CT and MR images (SANDRASEGARAN et al. 1994). Despite imaging modalities advances, the sensitivity for detection of hepatic disease by US and CT is still low (MUNKER et al. 1995). Nevertheless, CT is currently the preferred imaging modality to evaluate lymphoma of the liver, with its sensitivity being increased with the use of dynamic liver scanning and the newer high resolution CT scanners (SHIRKHODA et al. 1990).

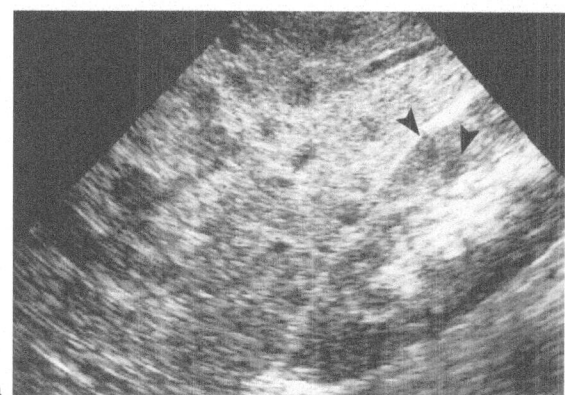
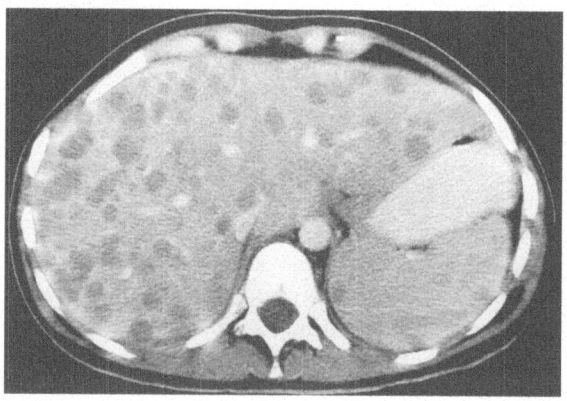

Fig. 3.11a,b. Hepatic and renal involvement in a 27-year-old woman with nodular sclerosing Hodgkin disease. The patient had undergone treatment 2 years earlier and was in complete remission. **a** Longitudinal US image shows hypoechoic nodular infiltration of the liver with involvement of the right kidney (*arrowheads*). **b** contrast-enhanced Axial CT scan of the abdomen shows multiple hypodense lesions within the liver and the spleen. (With permission from [GUERMAZI et al. 2001])

3.3.3
Pancreas

Pancreatic HD is extremely rare, and in almost all cases, it is secondary to contiguous lymph node disease (Fig. 3.12). Because the pancreas has no definable capsule, it may be difficult to distinguish adjacent lymph node disease from intrinsic pancreatic infiltration (SHIRKHODA et al. 1990).

3.3.4
Gastrointestinal Tract

HD rarely involves the gastrointestinal tract (CASTELLINO 1982; SANDRASEGARAN et al. 1994). Primary HD of the gastrointestinal tract usually involves a single site. Multiple sites are rarely involved in disseminated HD. Digestive HD has a lower 5-year survival rate than other forms (DODD 1990).

Primary HD of the esophagus seems to be extremely rare, especially in its isolated form (DODD 1990; TAAL et al. 1993; GELB et al. 1997; BOBICHON et al. 1998). Most cases of esophageal involvement are secondary (TAAL et al. 1993), and arise by extension from mediastinal lymph nodes (GELB et al. 1997). The radiologic appearances at barium swallow are always non specific, especially in early stages. A nodular aspect or irregular narrowing of the esophagus due to submucosal tumors represents the main pattern (TAAL et al. 1993). An unusual case of HD in a patient with AIDS who had esophageal perforation at presentation has been reported (GELB et al. 1997). Endoscopic ultrasonography is useful in the evaluation, staging, and follow-up of patients (BOBICHON et al. 1998).

The stomach is the most frequent site of malignant lymphoma of the gastrointestinal tract (LIBSON et al. 1994). Gastric HD accounts for about 9% of all gastric lymphomas (SODERSTROM and JOENSUU 1988; DODD 1990). However, primary gastric HD is extremely rare (SODERSTROM and JOENSUU 1988). Solitary lesions are usually antral in location but multifocal lesions may occur (LIBSON et al. 1994). The radiologic appearances of the gastric lymphomas generally reflect the gross pathology findings. Infiltrating form is the most frequent (Fig. 3.13), and may be difficult to differentiate from scirrhous carcinoma,

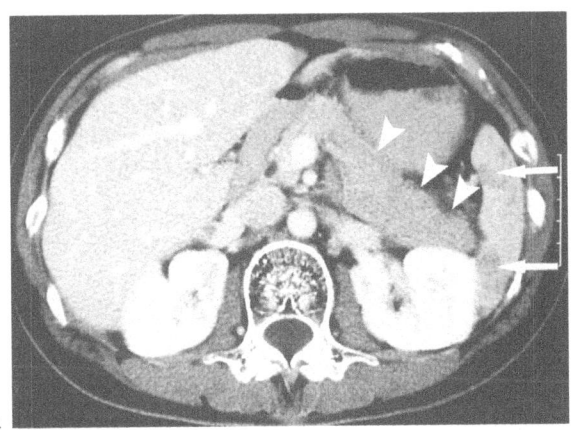

a

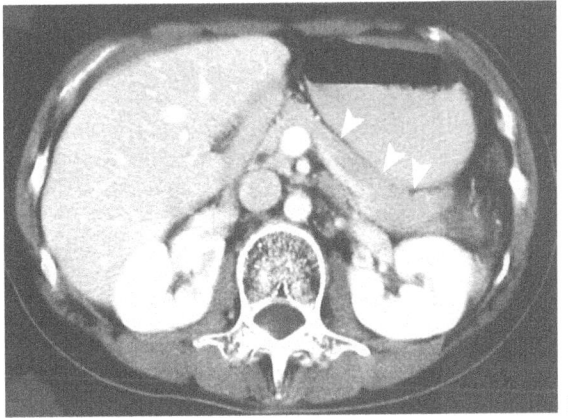

b

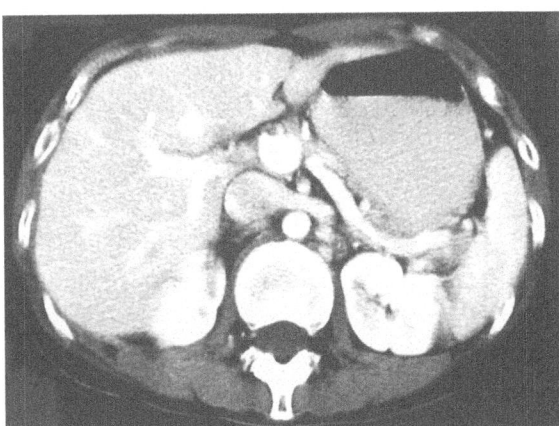

c

Fig. 3.12a–c. Pancreatic involvement in a 28-year-old woman with nodular sclerosing Hodgkin disease. The patient had undergone mantle field irradiation 3 years earlier with complete remission. a Axial CT scan shows diffusely enlarged body and tail of pancreas (*arrowheads*), which are slightly more hypodense than the head of the pancreas, and multiple hypodense lesions (*arrows*) in the spleen. Axial CT scans after 4 months of chemotherapy show normal (b) pancreas (*arrowheads*) and (c) spleen.

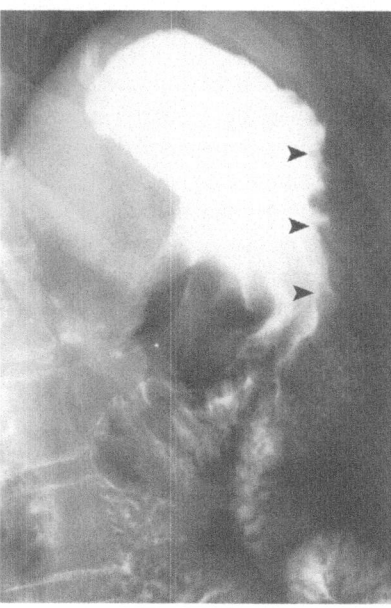

Fig. 3.13. Gastric involvement in a 19-year-old woman with mixed-cellularity Hodgkin disease. Image from a barium contrast study shows thickened folds in the body of the stomach (*arrowheads*). (With permission from [GUERMAZI et al. 2001])

particularly when HD with its associated fibrosis is involved. CT has proved particularly valuable in the diagnosis of gastric lymphoma, in demonstrating gastric wall thickening with a smoothly lobulated outer border (DODD 1990). Other radiologic appearances include large submucosal masses, and large ulcerating-masses (LIBSON et al. 1994).

HD involvement of the small intestine is the next most common site with jejunal, ileal and duodenal involvement in decreasing frequency (LIBSON et al. 1994). It may be associated with a sprue-like syndrome. Lymphomas associated with steatorrhea have a higher proportion of HD, and the tumors are often multiple (DODD 1990). Most lesions are focally stenotic, but other patterns include thick folds, effaced folds, and nodularity (Fig. 3.14) (LIBSON et al. 1994). A case of HD with intestinal perforation due to gut involvement was recently reported (GEETHA et al. 1999). Unlike non-Hodgkin lymphoma, excavation, fistulas, and aneurismal dilatation may occur but are uncharacteristic (LIBSON et al. 1994).

HD of the colon and rectum is uncommon (DODD 1990). The radiologic appearances reported include a solitary polypoid mass in transverse in one patient, and severe narrowing of the descending colon with adjacent mesenteric mass visible on CT in another patient (LIBSON et al. 1994).

3.3.5
Genitourinary System

The incidence of intrinsic involvement of genitourinary organ systems at presentation is rare (CASTELLINO 1982).

Renal involvement is extremely rare, HD being rather perirenal. Indeed, the radiologic appearance often consists of an invasion of the perirenal space by HD without renal parenchyma involvement. CT is the diagnostic modality of choice to detect renal and/or perirenal masses compared to urography or sonography (REZNEK et al. 1990).

Ureteral involvement is extremely rare. Only one recent case of HD presenting a ureteral origin has been reported. It was very particular due to its single growth in a ureteral situs and its early manifestation in comparison with the systemic disease. Urographic and CT features displayed a non specific thickening of the ureter wall which could not possibly be distinguished from involvement caused by urothelial heteroplastic lesions, metastasis via blood or lymph, distant tumors or isolated non-Hodgkin lymphomas (TOZZINI et al. 1999).

Bladder involvement is also extremely rare. The only two reported cases consisted of a nonspecific filling defect arising from the bladder wall (JONES 1989).

Very few cases of primary genital HD involving ovary or cervix have been reported, and only one case of primary HD of the vagina has been recently reported (PERIN et al. 2000).

3.4
Skeletal System

Although presenting symptoms due to bone involvement rarely occur in HD (GAUDIN et al. 1992), approximately 20% of patients with HD have radiographic bone involvement during the course of the disease. The poorer the prognosis by histologic type, the higher the incidence of bone destruction during the clinical course (EDEIKEN-MONROE et al. 1990).

3.4.1
Bone Marrow

Bone marrow involvement is rare at presentation so marrow biopsies are not systematically indicated as part of initial staging. During the course of illness,

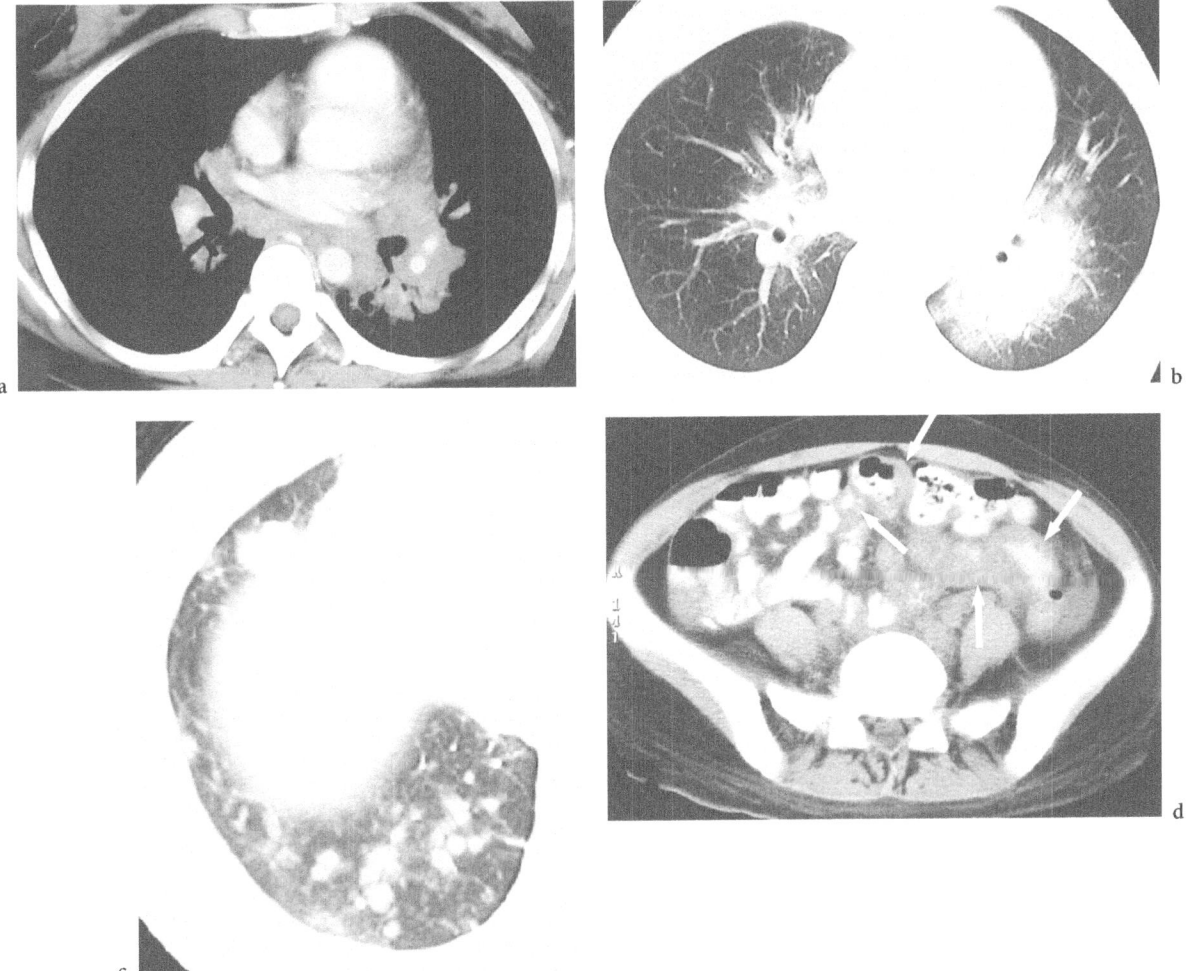

Fig. 3.14a–d. Small intestine involvement in a 21-year-old woman with nodular sclerosing Hodgkin disease. The patient had undergone bone marrow transplantation 4 years earlier. Axial contrast-enhanced CT scans of the chest at presentation show (**a**) mediastinal and bilateral hilar lymphadenopathy, as well as (**b**) perilymphatic infiltration of the surrounding lung parenchyma with consolidation, air bronchograms and ground glass opacification. The patient relapsed with disseminated disease 5 years later. Axial unenhanced CT scans show (**c**) multiple pulmonary nodules and (**d**) diffuse mural thickening of the proximal small bowel (*arrows*). There was also extensive involvement of the left lung, left pleural effusion and retroperitoneal lymphadenopathy (*not shown*).

5–32% of patients will develop marrow involvement (LINDEN et al. 1989; VARAN et al. 1999). When tumor infiltration is indicated with the imaging technique, clinical stage IV disease is presumed (LINDEN et al. 1989). HD is more likely to form focal lesions distant from the crests (Fig. 3.15) (HOANE et al. 1991).

MR imaging may be more sensitive than all other current imaging modalities in demonstrating bone marrow infiltration, and may be superior to blind bone marrow biopsies for detection of early disease (EDEIKEN-MONROE et al. 1990; GAUDIN et al. 1992; TOPRAK et al. 1997; VARAN et al. 1999). It may also be helpful in guiding the marrow biopsy (LINDEN et al. 1989; GAUDIN et al. 1992; TOPRAK et al. 1997). The STIR sequence is then very helpful, and generates images in which even small lesions are highly conspicuous (HOANE et al. 1991). A recent study demonstrates that MR imaging-positive patients had a higher relapse rate in the 24 month follow-up period than the MR imaging-negative patients (VARAN et al. 1999). Because of the often focal nature of bone marrow involvement, MR imaging and crest marrow sampling are complementary for improved marrow staging (HOANE et al. 1991).

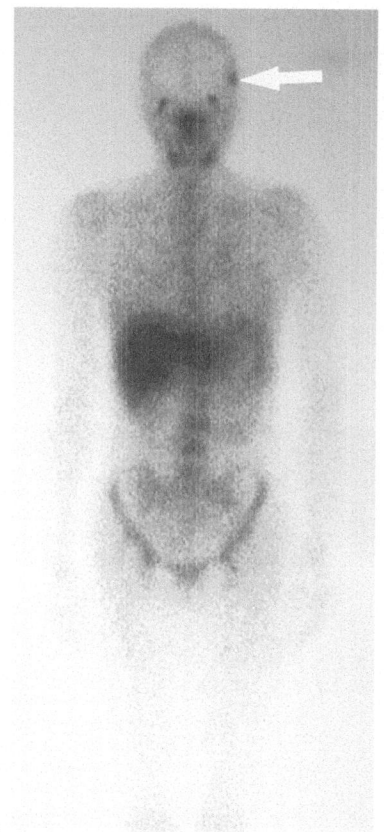

a

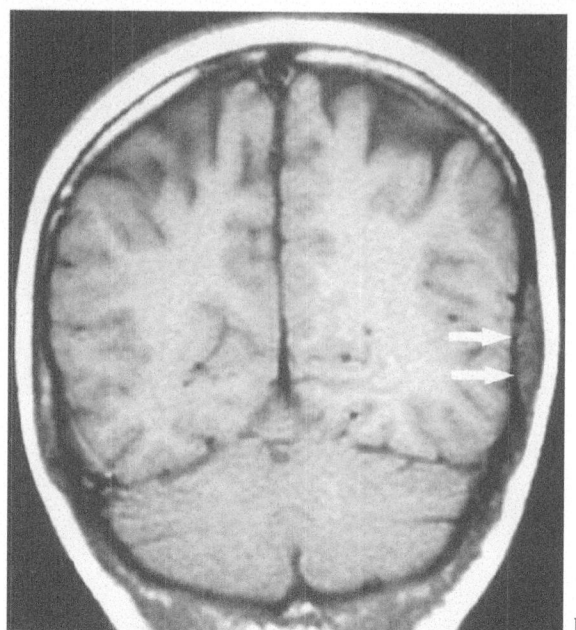

b

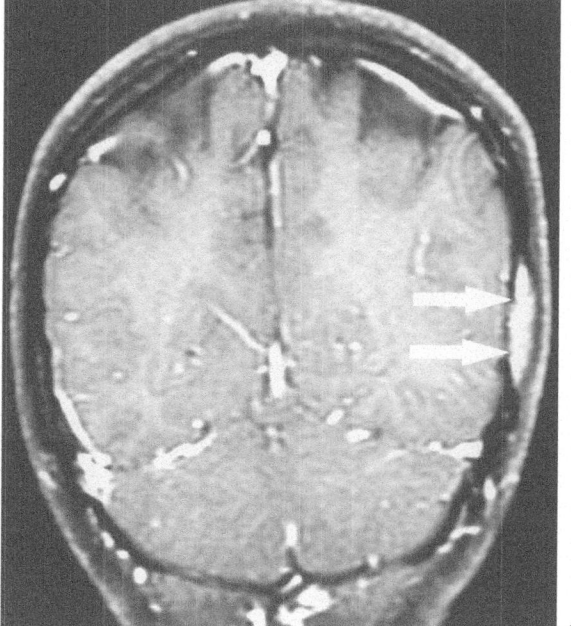

c

Fig. 3.15a–c. Skull vault involvement in a 30-year-old woman with Hodgkin disease. The patient had undergone chemotherapy for residual mediastinal disease. **a** Gallium-67 whole-body scan shows a hot spot in the left parietal bone (*arrow*). **b** Coronal T1-weighted MR image of the brain shows abnormal hypointense replacement of bone marrow in the diploic space of the left parietal bone (*arrows*). **c** Coronal contrast-enhanced T1-weighted MR image demonstrates marked enhancement of the lesion (*arrows*) consistent with bone marrow lymphomatous infiltration.

3.4.2
Bone

Osseous involvement occurs in 5–20% of patients during the course of HD, whereas it is seen in only 1–4% at the time of presentation (SULLI-VAN and SOLONICK 1987; EDEIKEN-MONROE et al. 1990; MIANO et al. 1990; GAUDIN et al. 1992; SANDRASEGARAN et al. 1994; GUERMAZI et al. 2001). It is indicative of a widespread and aggressive disease with poor prognosis (MIANO et al. 1990; GAUDIN et al. 1992), since it is usually associated with the most unfavorable histological subtypes (MIANO et al. 1990).

Primary bone HD probably does not exist (GAUDIN et al. 1992), in spite of the few cases reported as primary involvement without evidence of lymph node involvement (FRIED et al. 1995;

OSTROWSKI et al. 1999). Bone involvement may be either by contiguity or by a hematogenic process which is usually a late manifestation (GAUDIN et al. 1992; SANDRASEGARAN et al. 1994; GUERMAZI et al. 2001). The location of the bone lesions are, in decreasing order of frequency: dorsolumbar spine (Fig. 3.16), pelvis (Fig. 3.17), ribs (Fig. 3.18), femora, and sternum. Limb and cervical involvement are exceptional (SULLIVAN and SOLONICK 1987; PICCININI et al. 1991; GAUDIN et al. 1992; GUERMAZI et al. 2001). Focal extension from adjacent lymph nodes does not alter staging (SANDRASEGARAN et al. 1994).

Bone scintigraphy has a sensitivity and accuracy of 95% in detecting bone involvement but is not routinely indicated since most cases of bone HD are revealed on initial chest radiograph and CT scan (SANDRASEGARAN et al. 1994).

The radiographic features are nonspecific (GAUDIN et al. 1992). Lesions may be solitary (33%) or polyostotic (66%) (EDEIKEN-MONROE et al. 1990; OSTROWSKI et al. 1999; GUERMAZI et al. 2001). The edge is usually wide and ill-defined but may be marked by a sclerotic margin. A periosteal reaction, either lamellated (Fig. 3.19) or "sunburst", may occur with bone destruction. The lesions are predominantly osteolytic with blurred borders (Fig. 3.20), but rarely sclerotic or mixed (Fig. 3.21) (SULLIVAN and SOLONICK 1987; GAUDIN et al. 1992; GUERMAZI et al. 2001). Fractures are excep-

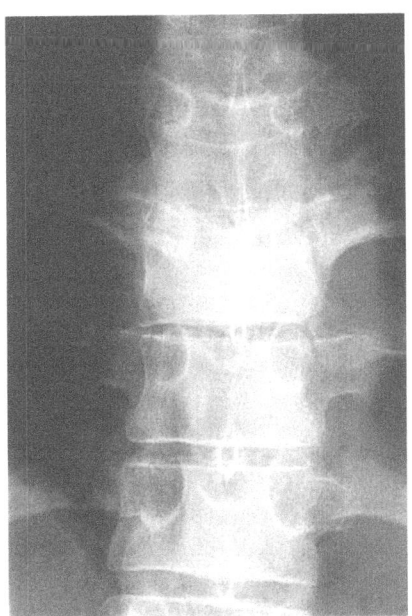

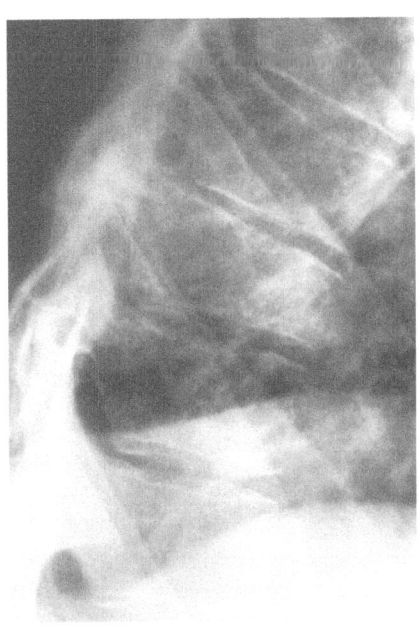

a

b

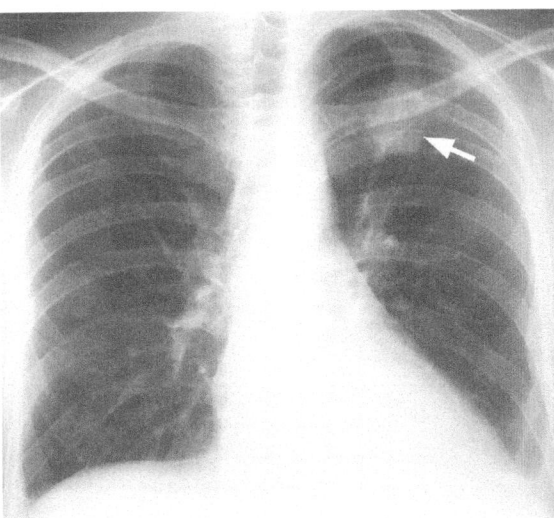

c

Fig. 3.16a–c. Dorsal spine involvement in a 29-year-old man with nodular sclerosing Hodgkin disease. a Anteroposterior and (b) lateral radiographs of the thoracic spine demonstrate an anterior collapse of the T9 body. c Anteroposterior chest radiograph shows a nodular lesion within the left lung (*arrow*), as well as a small left pleural effusion. (With permission from [GUERMAZI et al. 2001])

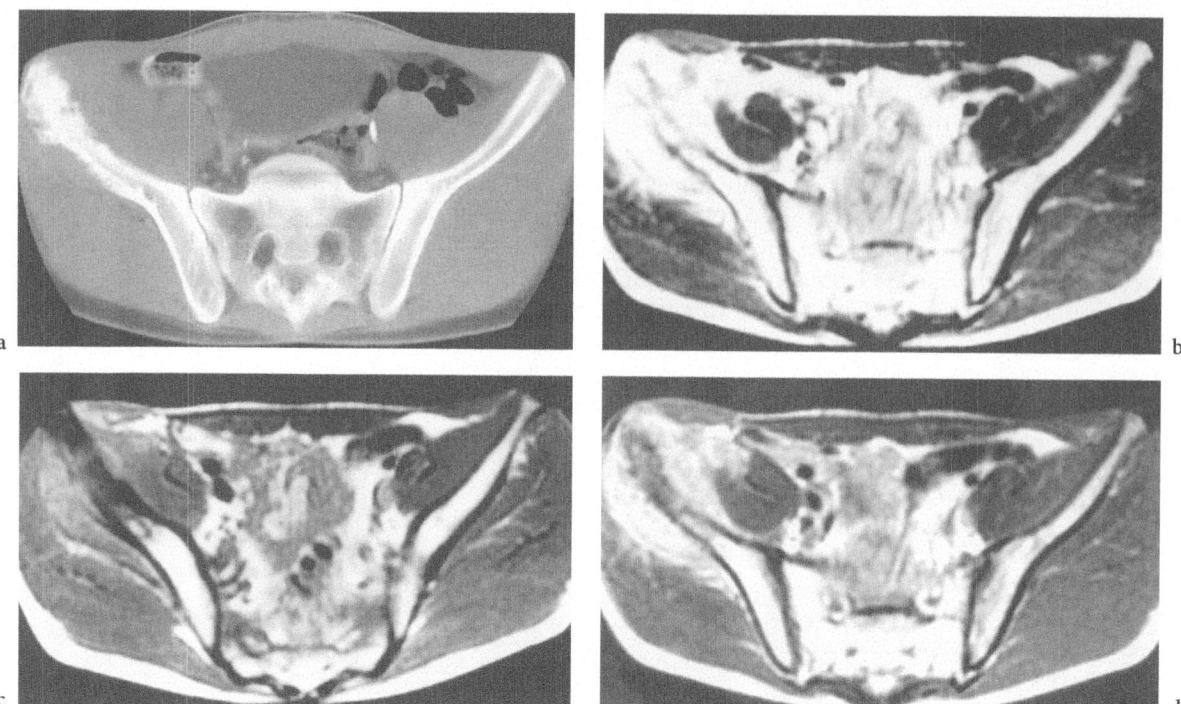

Fig. 3.17a–d. Iliac crest involvement in a 17-year-old man with mixed-cellularity Hodgkin disease. **a** Axial CT scan demonstrates a large soft tissue mass involving the right iliac crest and invading the surrounding muscles. The lesion appears hyperintense on (**b**) axial proton density-weighted MR image, isointense on (**c**) axial unenhanced T1-weighted MR image, and markedly enhances (**d**) after contrast administration. (With permission from [Guermazi et al. 2001])

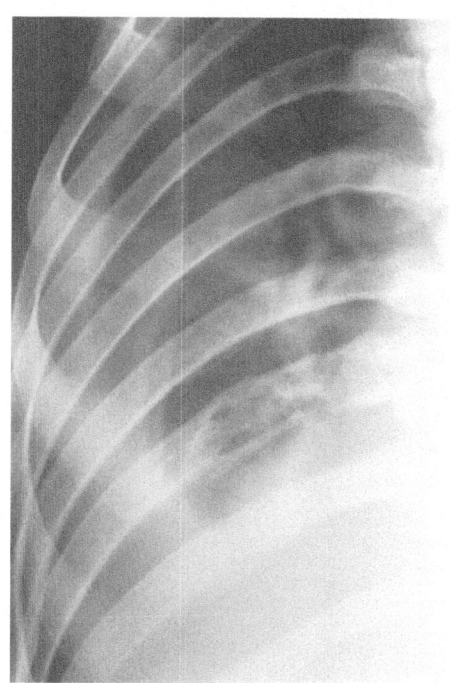

Fig. 3.18. Rib involvement in a 27-year-old man with nodular sclerosing Hodgkin disease. Anteroposterior radiograph demonstrates a mixed bone lesion in the posterior aspect of the right seventh rib. (With permission from [Guermazi et al. 2001])

tionally the first manifestations, although several observations of femoral and rib fractures have been reported (Gaudin et al. 1992). Soft-tissue tumors often appear adjacent to bone lesions (Edeiken-Monroe et al. 1990).

CT and MR imaging allow an upgraded assessment of bone texture and an accurate analysis of bone invasion by the tumoral process. CT may demonstrate bone lesions which are not visible on the radiographs (Gaudin et al. 1992).

The appearance of a bone mass in initial disease stages is rare, but the sternum is the most likely to be involved, perhaps due to its superficial location and its proximity to thoracic lymph ducts (Gaudin et al. 1992). The sternal mass is generally unique and develops over a variable time period, from several days to several months (Piccinini et al. 1991; Gaudin et al. 1992). Unlike other skeletal sites, it is often associated with good prognosis subtypes of HD, such as nodular sclerosing (Sullivan and Solonick 1987; Piccinini et al. 1991; Gaudin et al. 1992). The tumor is usually round or oval and of variable size (Fig. 3.22) (Stark and Jaramillo 1986; Gaudin et al. 1992).

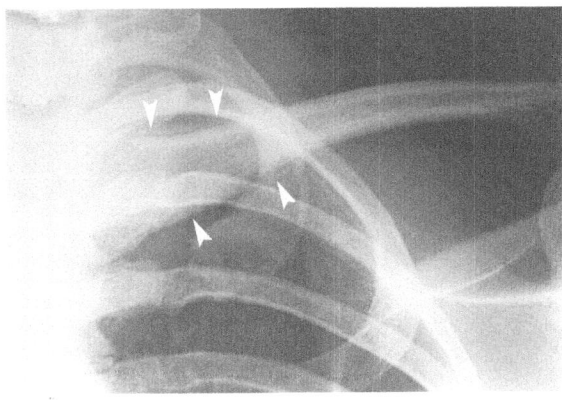
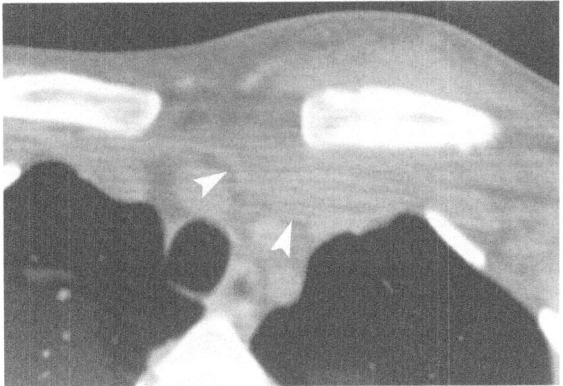

a   b

Fig. 3.19a,b. Clavicle involvement in a 25-year-old woman with nodular sclerosing Hodgkin disease. **a** Anteroposterior radiograph shows slight osteosclerosis of the proximal end of the right clavicle associated with lamellated periosteal reaction (*arrowheads*). **b** Axial CT scan demonstrates an associated soft-tissue mass with anterior mediastinal involvement (*arrowheads*), as well as the periosteal reaction. (With permission from [GUERMAZI et al. 2001])

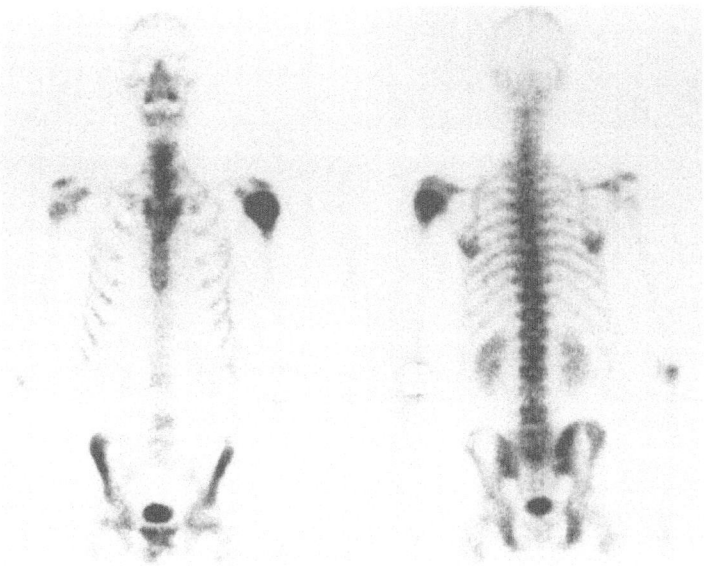
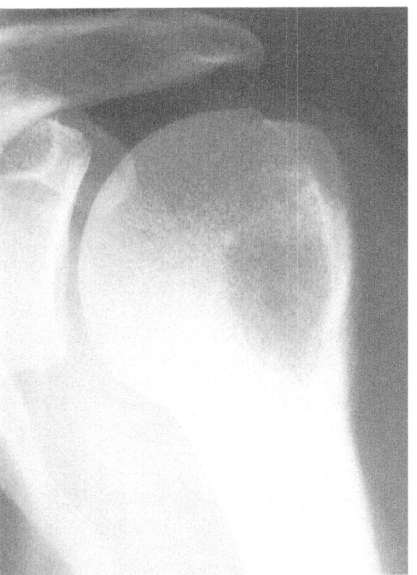

a   b

Fig. 3.20a,b. Humeral involvement in a 19-year-old man with nodular sclerosing Hodgkin disease. **a** Anterior (*left*) and posterior (*right*) bone scintigrams demonstrate markedly increased activity in the upper end of the left humerus. **b** Anteroposterior radiograph of the left humerus shows an ill-defined geographic area of bone destruction corresponding to the abnormality seen on scintigraphy. (With permission from [GUERMAZI et al. 2001])

Vertebral lesions occur most frequently in the dorsal and lumbar spine and least commonly in the cervical spine. Osteolysis is the rule (75%), but patchy sclerosis and "ivory vertebra" (20%) (Fig. 3.23), as well as mixed lytic and blastic lesions (5%), are frequent (EDEIKEN-MONROE et al. 1990; CAVALLI 1998; GUERMAZI et al. 2001). Vertebral collapse is also common (GAUDIN et al. 1992). Paravertebral soft-tissue masses occur consistently. Gouge defects of the anterior border of the vertebrae are frequently the result of erosion by lymph nodes (EDEIKEN-MONROE et al. 1990).

3.5
Head and Neck

Extranodal HD of the nasopharynx is manifested clinically in less than 1% of cases. However, about 20% of all cases have positive nasopharyngeal biopsies and some authors advocate nasopharyngeal biopsy as part of routine staging of HD (SANDRASEGARAN et al. 1994). The disease usually involves the rhinopharynx with or without laterocervical or jugulodigastric lymph nodes (Fig. 3.24). It

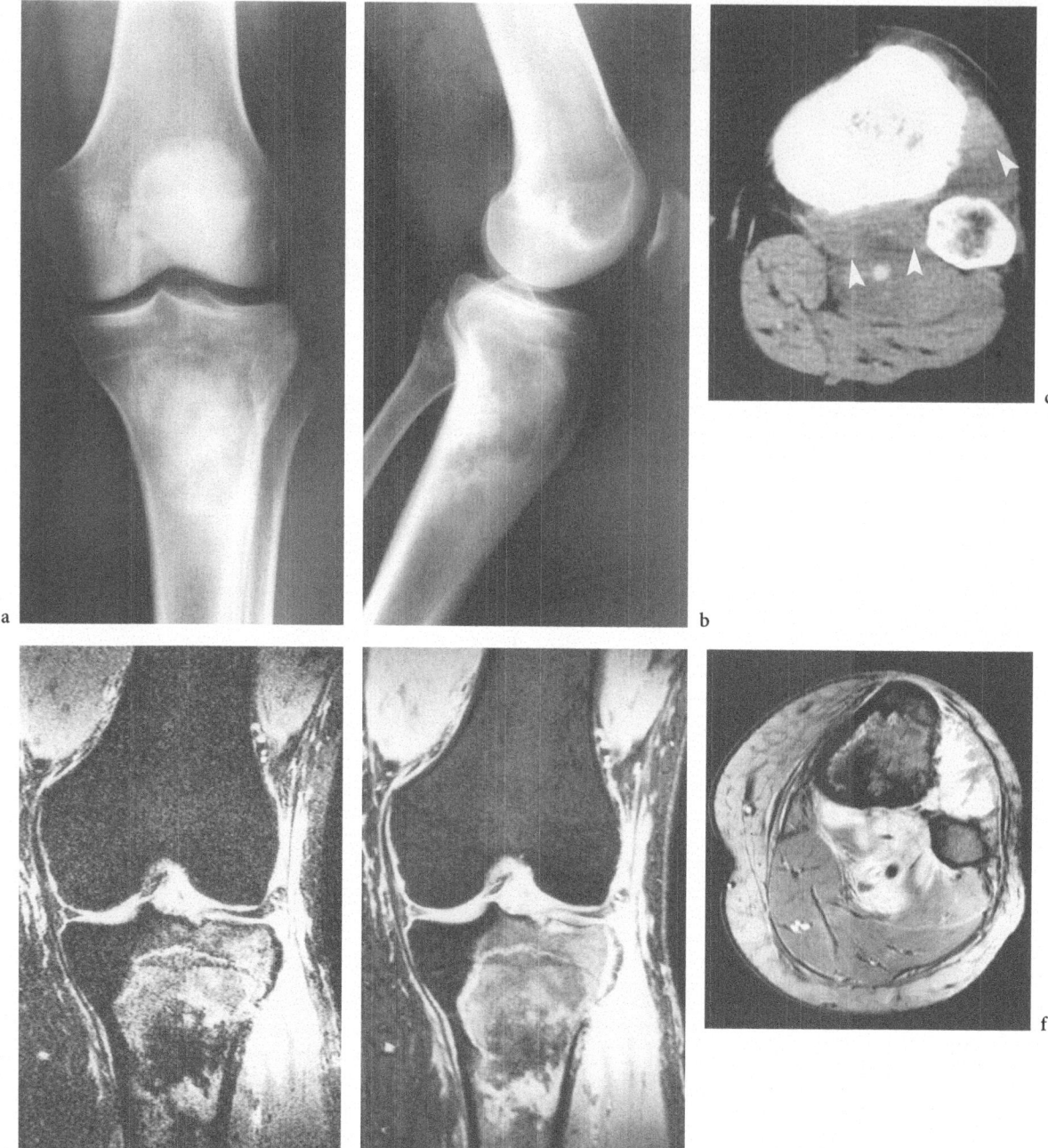

Fig. 3.21a–f. Tibial involvement in a 47-year-old man with nodular sclerosing Hodgkin disease. The patient had undergone treatment 5 years earlier and was in complete remission. **a** Anteroposterior and (**b**) lateral radiographs of the upper left knee demonstrate a large mixed lesion in the proximal tibia. No soft-tissue mass is identified. **c** Axial CT scan at the level of radiographic abnormality shows increased density in the medullary canal of the affected tibia. There is a slightly enhanced soft-tissue mass around the tibial metaphysis (*arrowheads*). **d** Coronal short tau inversion-recovery MR image shows a large lesion involving the entire proximal end of the tibia. **e** Coronal contrast-enhanced fat-suppressed T1-weighted MR image reveals striking heterogenous enhancement of the lesion with soft-tissue involvement. The hypointense area within the lesion corresponds to the osteosclerotic aspect. **f** Axial contrast-enhanced non fat-suppressed T1-weighted MR image better demonstrates the soft-tissue mass. (With permission from [GUERMAZI et al. 2001])

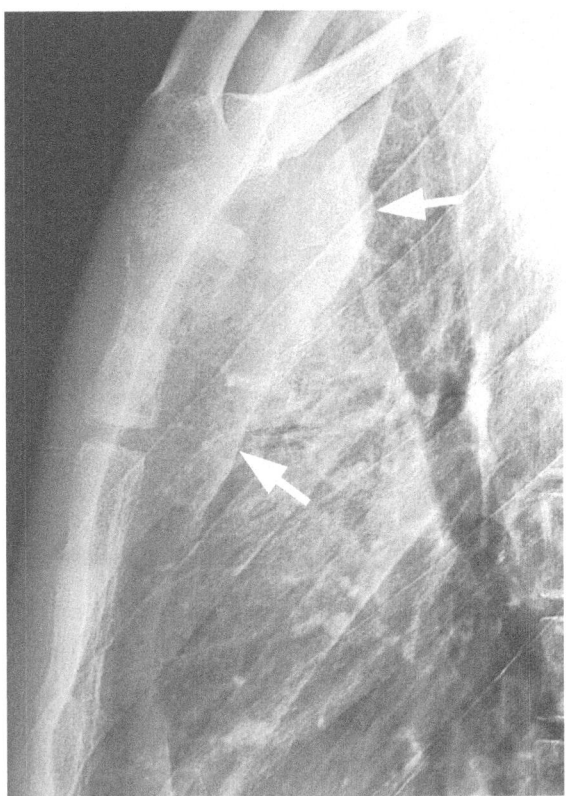
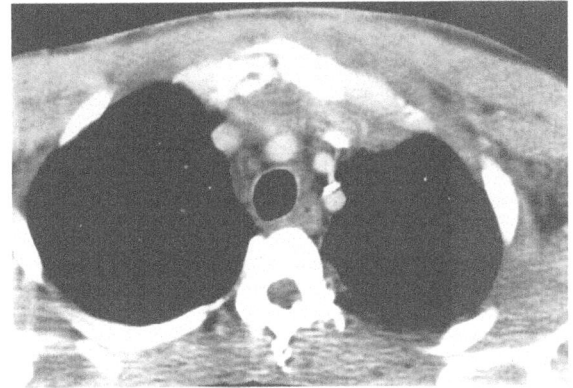
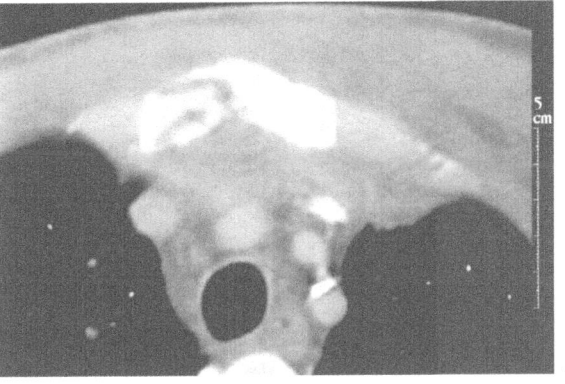

Fig. 3.22a–c. Sternal involvement in a 24-year-old man with nodular sclerosing Hodgkin disease. a Lateral radiograph demonstrates sternal involvement with an associated soft-tissue mass (*arrows*). b, c Axial contrast-enhanced CT scans show a manubrial lesion invading the anterior mediastinum and a mixed bone lesion of the sternum. (With permission from [GUERMAZI et al. 2001])

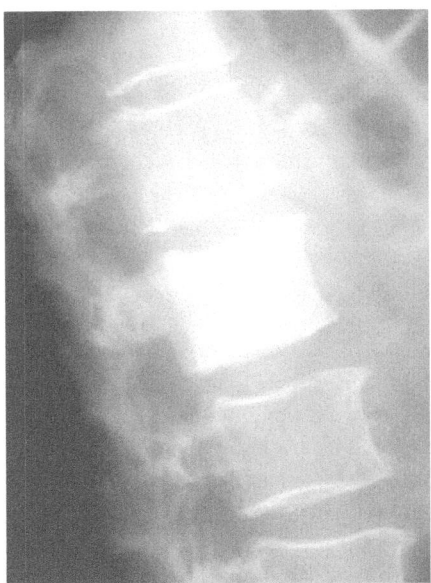

Fig. 3.23. Vertebral involvement in a 34-year-old woman with lymphocyte depletion Hodgkin disease. Lateral radiograph demonstrates an osteoblastic reaction in the second lumbar vertebra with "ivory vertebra" pattern. (With permission from [GUERMAZI et al. 2001])

generally involves young men, is localized and with good prognosis (ANSELMO et al. 2002).

A case was reported of a patient with a small focus of HD recurrence in the postnasal space associated with paraneoplastic cerebellar degeneration (TAPPIN and SATCHI 1995).

Primary thyroid HD is extremely rare. A few sporadic cases have been reported, while secondary involvement occurs in 2% of cases. HD of the thyroid occurs predominantly in elderly women. Involvement of only one lobe is common (VAILATI et al. 1991).

A case was reported of a patient with HD presenting as a cystic neck mass that most likely arose from a superiorly displaced thymic gland or thymic tissue remnants (BUTERA and FREEMAN 2000).

3.6
Central Nervous System

Central nervous system (CNS) involvement by HD is uncommon, with an overall incidence of 0.2% in

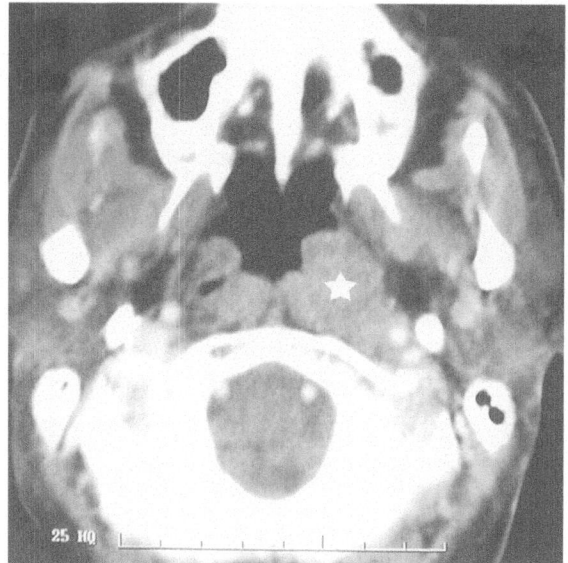
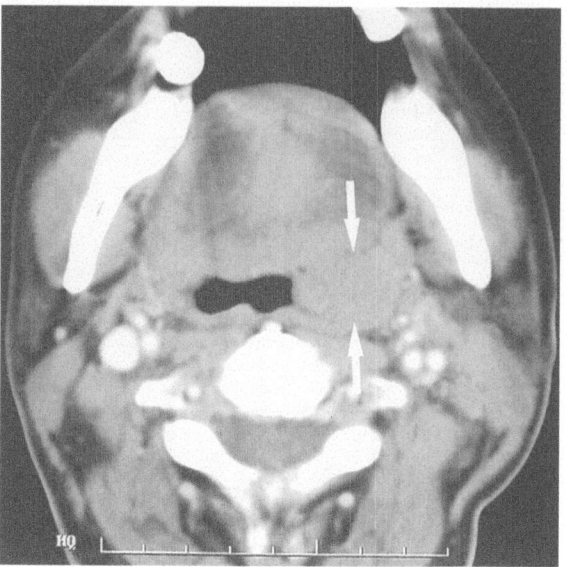

Fig. 3.24a,b. Nasopharyngeal involvement in a 53-year-old man with mixed-cellularity Hodgkin disease. The patient had multiple enlarged cervical and mediastinal lymph nodes. In addition, axial contrast-enhanced CT scans show (**a**) a soft-tissue lymphomatous mass in the left nasopharynx with filling in of the ipsilateral fossa of Rosenmuller (*star*), as well as (**b**) another soft-tissue lesion in the left pharyngeal tonsil (*arrows*).

the published series (HIGGINS and PESCHEL 1995; ANSELMO et al. 1996). Involvement of the brain or spinal cord by HD, whether primary or secondary, is generally a late manifestation. It constitutes a serious and potentially fatal threat to the patient (SCHEITHAUER 1979; ZIMMERMAN 1990). It is important to recognize that this complication may occur in patients who are apparently in remission (BLAKE et al. 1986). Lesions are more frequently intraspinal than intracranial (SCHEITHAUER 1979).

3.6.1
Brain

Brain HD involvement is so rare that a space-occupying lesion in the brain of a patient with known HD should prompt a second diagnosis (CUTTNER et al. 1979; BLAKE et al. 1986; SANDRASEGARAN et al. 1994). The existence of primary cerebral HD is still controversial. Rarely, HD may arise primarily in the dura, in the falx, and exceptionally in the brain parenchyma, meaning an isolated intracerebral manifestation (KLEIN et al. 1999). There is still doubt that histologic criteria for the diagnosis of HD of published cases are fulfilled because of limited immunohistochemical evidence. Actually, some former cases classified

as HD are considered B-cell lymphomas, encephalitis or reticulum cell sarcoma-microglioma after reevaluation (SCHEITHAUER 1979; KLEIN et al. 1999).

Secondary brain HD is an uncommon but wellknown complication of systemic HD, occurring in 0.2–0.5% of all cases in advanced stages (SAPOZINK and KAPLAN 1983; BLAKE et al. 1986; KLEIN et al. 1999). Various reports have suggested several mechanisms to explain intracranial involvement by HD (SAPOZINK and KAPLAN 1983). It was suggested that HD spreads to the dura, from which it extends into the subdural space, and from which it may penetrate through the arachnoid producing leptomeningeal dissemination within the subarachnoid space (BLAKE et al. 1986; ZIMMERMAN 1990). After analyzing concurrent sites of disease, it was concluded that this is not always the case, and that the hematogenous spread is probably the most common mechanism, since lesions may be unaccompanied by contiguous extraaxial deposits (SCHEITHAUER 1979; SAPOZINK and KAPLAN 1983). Risk factors for intracranial HD are still unclear. Since familial HD may be associated with immunodeficiency (SCHEITHAUER 1979; ASHIGBI et al. 1997), it was speculated that HD may be related to impaired immunologic status as is primary CNS lymphoma (ASHIGBI et al. 1997). Various intracerebral sites have been reported, with the major lesions being supratentorial (SCHEITHAUER 1979). The cerebral cortex and the meninges, particularly the inferior aspect of the brain, are most frequently involved but no area of the brain appears to be exempt (ASHIGBI et al. 1997; KLEIN et al. 1999). Anterior pituitary gland involvement has also been reported (ASHIGBI et al. 1997). Clinically, neurological signs or symptoms are usually absent although the brain cortex may be infiltrated (ANSELMO et al. 1996).

CT and MR imaging are equally effective in detecting brain HD (ZIMMERMAN 1990; SANDRASEGARAN et al. 1994). However, MR imaging provides direct multiplanar imaging in the coronal and sagittal planes in addition to the axial. Thus, it is ideal for detecting extracerebral tumor deposits in the subdural or epidural space (ZIMMERMAN 1990). The appearance of intracranial HD on CT can vary widely (CUTTNER et al. 1979; BLAKE et al. 1986). The common CT presentation is a hyperdense or isodense mass in the white matter, periventricular or basal ganglionic or cerebellar in location, with or without surrounding edema. The signal intensity of the tumor deposit remains hypo to isointense on all MR imaging sequences. Because of abnormally permeable tumor vessels, contrast-enhanced MR imaging makes these tumors more obvious (ZIMMERMAN 1990). HD most often involves the brain either as a mass or diffuse infiltrate of the meninges, with dural involvement much more common than parenchymal lesions. Intracranial involvement is usually the result of hematogenous metastasis or meningeal infiltration from systemic HD. Primary HD may involve parenchyma with or without dural attachment, leptomeninges, and the dura mater (CLARK et al. 1992). Two cases of intracerebral HD presenting as an isolated dural-based tumor were clinically and radiographically reported as indistinguishable from a meningioma (Fig. 3.25) (CHIM et al. 2000a; JOHNSON et al. 2000).

Paraneoplastic neurological syndromes rarely occur in HD. They may affect the brainstem, basal ganglia, and supratentorial brain cortex, but the cerebellum is the most frequent site involved. CT may be negative at presentation, and follow-up scans can show changes consistent with atrophy occurring as late as 7–25 months after the initial presentation with symptoms. Chemotherapy or radiotherapy of HD has improved symptoms and signs of paraneoplastic cerebellar degeneration in some instances. Spontaneous remission has also been described, but the findings may be progressive (KRISHNAN and BOCKENSTEDT 1994; TAPPIN and SATCHI 1995).

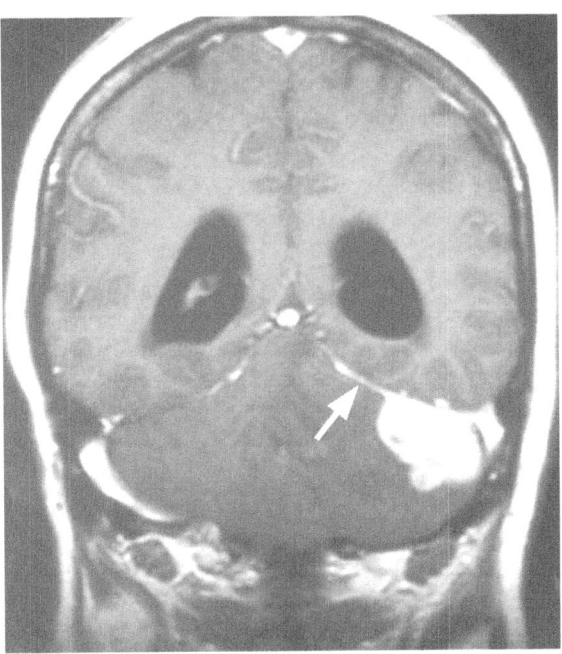

Fig. 3.25. Primary cerebral involvement in a 55-year-old woman with nodular sclerosing Hodgkin disease. Coronal contrast-enhanced T1-weighted MR image shows large enhancing mass with a dural tail sign (*arrow*) and arising from the inferior aspect of the tentorium cerbelli. (With permission from [JOHNSON et al. 2000])

3.6.2
Meninges

Hematogenous spread of HD to the leptomeninges and to the choroid plexus is another mechanism by which leptomeningeal tumor dissemination may be produced (SCHEITHAUER 1979; ZIMMERMAN 1990; SANDRASEGARAN et al. 1994). The meningeal deposits are best seen on coronal contrast-enhanced T1-weighted spin-echo MR images, which are considerably more sensitive than contrast-enhanced CT (ZIMMERMAN 1990; SANDRASEGARAN et al. 1994).

3.6.3
Spinal Cord and Cauda Equina

Intramedullary spinal cord metastases are uncommon in HD and have a poor prognosis. Only a few cases have been reported. CT may demonstrate an area of increased density in the substance of the cord. MR imaging, compared to CT, has a greater sensitivity and specificity for evaluation of the spinal cord. The T2-weighted MR images demonstrate increased signal within the spinal cord (LYDING et al. 1987).

HD very rarely presents initially with a paraspinal mass (TOPRAK et al. 1997; CITOW et al. 2001). The frequency of spinal cord compression, either at presentation or during the course of HD, is 3–7.6% (HIGGINS and PESCHEL 1995; TOPRAK et al. 1997). This involvement follows the distribution of paravertebral lymph nodes, which are more common in the upper-to-mid thoracic and mid-lower lumbar areas (Fig. 3.26) (ZIMMERMAN 1990; TOPRAK et al. 1997). Cases of cervical spine involvement have also been reported (Fig. 3.27) (HIGGINS and PESCHEL 1995). Although single epidural deposits are more frequent, multiple level involvement has been reported (TOPRAK et al. 1997). Tumor within the lymph node at these sites results in a paravertebral mass that extends through the intervertebral neural foramina to form an epidural mass that compresses the cord or cauda equina (ZIMMERMAN 1990; HIGGINS and PESCHEL 1995; MASCALCHI et al. 1995; TOPRAK et al. 1997). Concomitant vertebral bone involvement

has been observed in 32–42% of cases (MASCALCHI et al. 1995; TOPRAK et al. 1997). Spinal metastatic HD unaccompanied by contiguous meningeal or tumor deposits is extremely rare (SCHEITHAUER 1979). Furthermore, isolated primary extranodal HD involving the spine without lymphoma elsewhere is even more rare. Several authors have suggested that small elements in the epidural space may give rise to lymphoma (CITOW et al. 2001).

Detection of tumor in the paraspinal soft tissue and vessels is well shown by MR imaging (ZIMMERMAN 1990; SANDRASEGARAN et al. 1994; TOPRAK et al. 1997). No MR imaging feature can be regarded as pathognomonic. However, demonstration of a homogeneous isointense lesion which extends over more than one segment of the spine, which may have a paraspinal extension and is accompanied by diffuse vertebral marrow signal changes, should raise the suspicion of a primary or secondary spinal epidural lymphoma (HIGGINS and PESCHEL 1995; MASCALCHI et al. 1995). CT is superior in showing the extent of cortical bone destruction (Fig. 3.28) (ZIMMERMAN 1990; SANDRASEGARAN et al. 1994; Tet al. 2001).

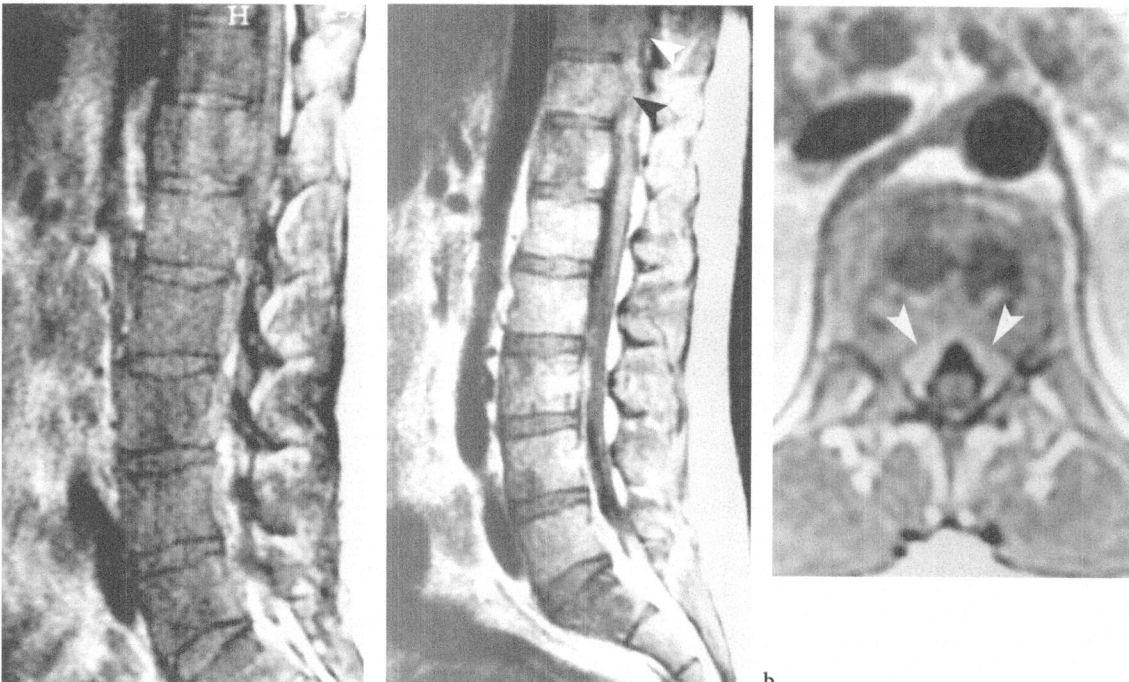

a   b
                                                                                                                                                      c

Fig. 3.26a–c. Spinal cord compression in a 34-year-old man with mixed-cellularity Hodgkin disease. The patient had undergone treatment 2 years earlier and was in complete remission. a Sagittal T1-weighted MR image shows subtle irregularities of the posterior margins extending from T10 to L1. The bone marrow is also heterogeneously involved and demonstrates decreased signal intensity. b Sagittal contrast-enhanced T1-weighted MR image demonstrates slight enhancement of the corresponding anterior epidural soft-tissue mass (*arrowheads*). Bone marrow enhancement is also seen. c Axial contrast-enhanced T1-weighted MR image obtained at the level of T12 shows impingement of the spinal cord by two anterolateral epidural masses (*arrowheads*). (With permission from [GUERMAZI et al. 2001])

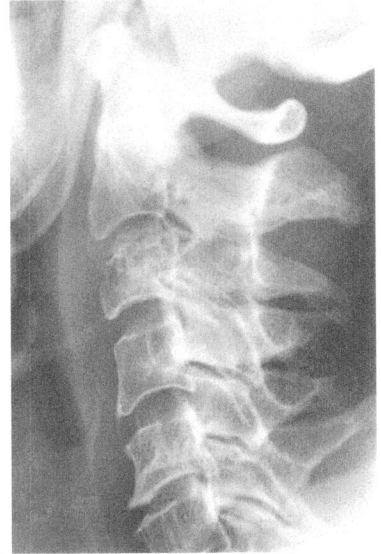
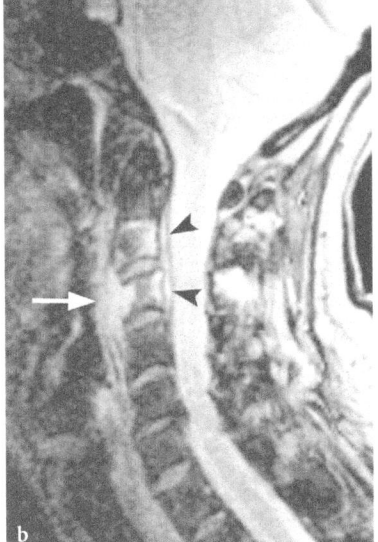
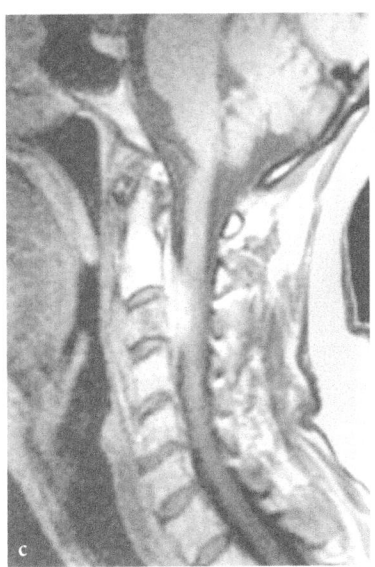
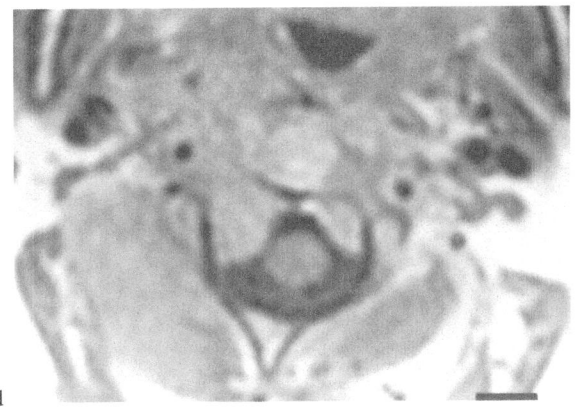

Fig. 3.27a–d. Cervical spine involvement in a 62-year-old woman with nodular sclerosing Hodgkin disease. **a** Lateral radiograph of the cervical spine demonstrates osteosclerosis of the posterior aspect of C2 and an osteolytic lesion of the C3 superior plate. **b** Sagittal T2-weighted MR image shows replacement of the anterior epidural space by a homogeneous lesion that extends from C2 to C3 and is slightly hyperintense relative to spinal cord (*arrowheads*). A soft-tissue mass is also seen anterior to the C3 vertebral body (*arrow*). The C1 and C2 bodies show hyperintense foci, findings that are consistent with replacement of the bone marrow. **c** Sagittal contrast-enhanced T1-weighted MR image demonstrates enhancement of the anterior epidural mass. **d** Axial contrast-enhanced T1-weighted MR image obtained at the level of C3 demonstrates impingement of the spinal cord by two anterolateral epidural masses that are connected with paravertebral soft-tissue masses through the intervertebral foramina. (With permission from [Guermazi et al. 2001])

3.7
Muscles

Muscles may occasionally be involved in HD. Most cases of paravertebral masses are invaded from retroperitoneal lymph nodes. A case of indolent course and late involvement of the striated gluteal muscle has been reported (Ariad et al. 1997).

3.8
Conclusion

Extranodal disease accounts for 15 to 30% of all HD cases. It is at the time of initial presentation that the therapeutic options are widest and the chance of cure is greatest. For this reason, when HD is diagnosed, extensive staging must be done to determine whether an extranodal involvement is a primary manifestation or dissemination of a systemic disease. The difference between these two conditions is important for prognosis, which is much less favorable in systemic HD. For this purpose, careful interpretation of CT is mandatory. In selected cases, ultrasonography and MR imaging may be useful depending on tumor location. In the future, metabolic positron emission tomography may provide more information about extranodal lymphoma than do the current imaging modalities.

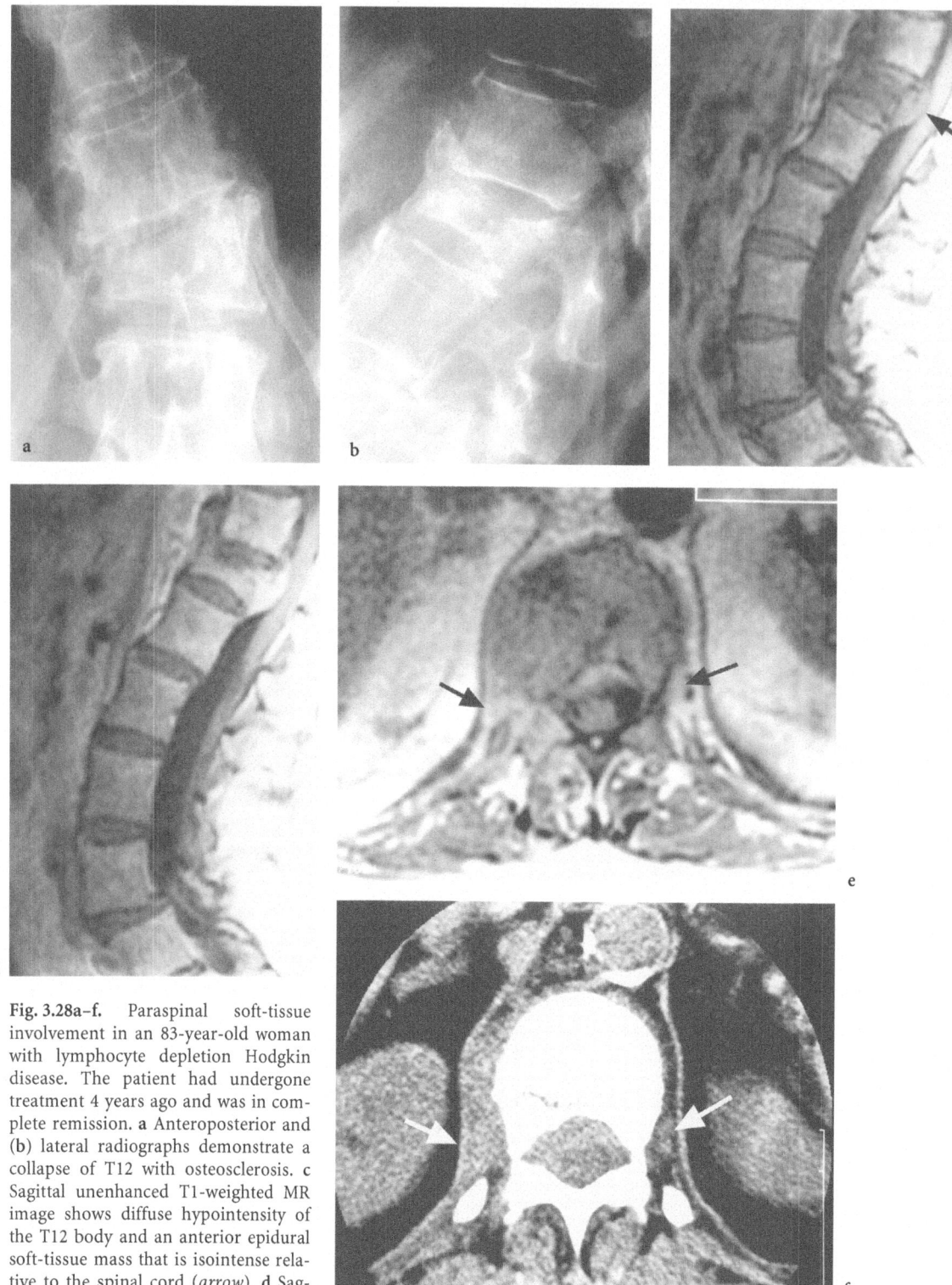

Fig. 3.28a–f. Paraspinal soft-tissue involvement in an 83-year-old woman with lymphocyte depletion Hodgkin disease. The patient had undergone treatment 4 years ago and was in complete remission. **a** Anteroposterior and (**b**) lateral radiographs demonstrate a collapse of T12 with osteosclerosis. **c** Sagittal unenhanced T1-weighted MR image shows diffuse hypointensity of the T12 body and an anterior epidural soft-tissue mass that is isointense relative to the spinal cord (*arrow*). **d** Sagittal contrast-enhanced T1-weighted MR image shows the mass with marked enhancement. Spinal cord compression is seen at this level. Axial contrast-enhanced (**e**) T1-weighted MR image and (**f**) CT scan show epidural extension of the soft-tissue lesion toward the spinal canal (*arrows*). The bone fracture is better demonstrated on the CT scan. (With permission from [Guermazi et al. 2001])

References

Anselmo AP, Proia A, Cartoni C, Baroni CD, Maurizi Enrici R, Delfini R, Avvisati G (1996) Meningeal localization in a patient with Hodgkin's disease. Description of a case and review of the literature. Ann Oncol 7:1071–1075

Anselmo AP, Cavalieri E, Cardarelli L, Gianfelici V, Osti FM, Pescarmona E, Maurizi Enrici R (2002) Hodgkin's disease of the nasopharynx: diagnostic and therapeutic approach with a review of the literature. Ann Hematol 81:514–516

Aquino SL, Chen MY, Kuo WT, Chiles C (1999) The CT appearance of pleural and extrapleural disease in lymphoma. Clin Radiol 54:647–650

Ariad S, Hatskelzon I., Benharroch D, Geffen DB (1997) Gluteal manifestation of advanced Hodgkin's disease. Skeletal Radiol 26:622–625

Ashigbi MY, Venkatraj U, Agarwal V, Bello J, Wiernik PH (1997) Intracranial Hodgkin's disease in two patients with familial Hodgkin's disease. Med Pediatr Oncol 28:255–258

Bergin CJ, Healy MV, Zincone GE, Castellino RA (1990) MR evaluation of chest wall involvement in malignant lymphoma. J Comput Assist Tomogr 14:928–932

Blake PR, Carr DH, Goolden AW (1986) Intracranial Hodgkin's disease. Br J Radiol 59:414–416

Bobichon R, Gaudin JL, Romand F, Pontette F, Thaunat JL, Souquet JC (1998) Esophageal involvement by Hodgkin's disease mimicking submucosal tumor. Endoscopy 30: S38–39

Butera J, Freeman NJ (2000) Case 1. Hodgkins's disease presenting as a cystic neck mass. J Clin Oncol 18:1150–1152

Carlsen SE, Bergin CJ, Hoppe RT (1993) MR imaging to detect chest wall and pleural involvement in patients with lymphoma: effect on radiation therapy planning. AJR Am J Roentgenol 160:1191–1195

Cartier Y, Johkoh T, Honda O, Muller NL (1999) Primary pulmonary Hodgkin's disease: CT findings in three patients. Clin Radiol 54:182–184

Castellino RA (1982) Imaging techniques for staging abdominal Hodgkin's disease. Cancer Treat Rep 66:697–700

Castellino RA, Blank N, Hoppe RT, Cho C (1986) Hodgkin disease: contributions of chest CT in the initial staging evaluation. Radiology 160:603–605

Cavalli F (1998) Rare syndromes in Hodgkin's disease. Ann Oncol 9:S109–113

Chim CS, Shek TW, Ooi GC, Liang R (2000a) Meningeal relapse in Hodgkin's disease. J Clin Oncol 18:1153–1155

Chim CS, Choy C, Ooi CG, Liang R (2000b) Hodgkin's disease with primary manifestation in the liver. Leuk Lymphoma 37:629–632

Cho CS, Blank N, Castellino RA (1985) Computerized tomography evaluation of chest wall involvement in lymphoma. Cancer 55:1892–1894

Citow JS, Rini B, Wollmann R, Macdonald RL (2001) Isolated, primary extranodal Hodgkin's disease of the spine: case report. Neurosurgery 49:453–456; discussion 456–457

Clark WC, Callihan T, Schwartzberg L, Fontanesi J (1992) Primary intracranial Hodgkin's lymphoma without dural attachment. Case report. J Neurosurg 76:692–695

Cuttner J, Meyer R, Huang YP (1979) Intracerebral involvement in Hodgkin's disease: a report of 6 cases and review of the literature. Cancer 43:1497–1506

Diederich S, Link TM, Zuhlsdorf H, Steinmeyer E, Wormanns D, Heindel W (2001) Pulmonary manifestations of Hodgkin's disease: radiographic and CT findings. Eur Radiol 11:2295–2305

Dodd GD (1990) Lymphoma of the hollow abdominal viscera. Radiol Clin North Am 28:771–783

Edeiken-Monroe B, Edeiken J, Kim EE (1990) Radiologic concepts of lymphoma of bone. Radiol Clin North Am 28:841–864

Filly R, Blank N, Castellino RA (1976) Radiographic distribution of intrathoracic disease in previously untreated patients with Hodgkin's disease and non-Hodgkin's lymphoma. Radiology 120:277–281

Fishman EK, Kuhlman JE, Jones RJ (1991) CT of lymphoma: spectrum of disease. Radiographics 11:647–669

Fried G, Ben Arieh Y, Haim N, Dale J, Stein M (1995) Primary Hodgkin's disease of the bone. Med Pediatr Oncol 24:204–207

Gaudin P, Juvin R, Rozand Y, Troussier B, Rose-Pittet L, Lebas JF, Pegourie B, Phelip X (1992) Skeletal involvement as the initial disease manifestation in Hodgkin's disease: a review of 6 cases. J Rheumatol 19:146–152

Geetha N, Thara S, Lali VS, Chitra S, Joseph F (1999) Intestinal involvement in Hodgkin's disease causing perforation. Am J Med 107:185–186

Gelb AB, Medeiros LJ, Chen YY, Weiss LM, Weidner N (1997) Hodgkin's disease of the esophagus. Am J Clin Pathol 108: 593–598

Guermazi A, Brice P, de Kerviler EE, Ferme C, Hennequin C, Meignin V, Frija J (2001) Extranodal Hodgkin disease: spectrum of disease. Radiographics 21:161–179

Heron CW, Husband JE, Williams MP (1988) Hodgkin disease: CT of the thymus. Radiology 167:647–651

Higgins SA, Peschel RE (1995) Hodgkin's disease with spinal cord compression. A case report and a review of the literature. Cancer 75:94–98

Hoane BR, Shields AF, Porter BA, Shulman HM (1991) Detection of lymphomatous bone marrow involvement with magnetic resonance imaging. Blood 78:728–738

Johnson MD, Kinney MC, Scheithauer BW, Briley RJ, Hamilton K, McPherson WF, Barton Jr JH (2000) Primary intracerebral Hodgkin's disease mimicking meningioma: case report. Neurosurgery 47:454–456; discussion 456–457

Jones MW (1989) Primary Hodgkin's disease of the urinary bladder. Br J Urol 63:438

Klein R, Mullges W, Bendszus M, Woydt M, Kreipe H, Roggendorf W (1999) Primary intracerebral Hodgkin's disease: report of a case with Epstein-Barr virus association and review of the literature. Am J Surg Pathol 23: 477–481

Krishnan K, Bockenstedt P (1994) Paraneoplastic cerebellar degeneration: a rare presentation of Hodgkin's disease. Clin Lab Haematol 16:359–362

Lewis ER, Caskey CI, Fishman EK (1991) Lymphoma of the lung: CT findings in 31 patients. AJR Am J Roentgenol 156:711–714

Libson E, Mapp E, Dachman AH (1994) Hodgkin's disease of the gastrointestinal tract. Clin Radiol 49:166–169

Linden A, Zankovich R, Theissen P, Diehl V, Schicha H (1989) Malignant lymphoma: bone marrow imaging versus biopsy. Radiology 173:335–339

Lyding JM, Tseng A, Newman A, Collins S, Shea W (1987) Intramedullary spinal cord metastasis in Hodgkin's disease. Rapid diagnosis and treatment resulting in neurologic recovery. Cancer 60:1741–1744

Mascalchi M, Torselli P, Falaschi F, Dal Pozzo G (1995) MRI of spinal epidural lymphoma. Neuroradiology 37:303–307

McDonnell PJ, Mann RB, Bulkley BH (1982) Involvement of the heart by malignant lymphoma: a clinicopathologic study. Cancer 49:944–951

Miano C, Donfrancesco A, Bonaldi U, Lombardi A, Baronci C, Rosati D (1990) Nodular sclerosing type of Hodgkin's disease: report of a case with unusual sternal localization at onset. Haematologica 75:95–96

Munker R, Stengel A, Stabler A, Hiller E, Brehm G (1995) Diagnostic accuracy of ultrasound and computed tomography in the staging of Hodgkin's disease. Verification by laparotomy in 100 cases. Cancer 76:1460–1466

North LB, Libshitz HI, Lorigan JG (1990) Thoracic lymphoma. Radiol Clin North Am 28:745–762

Ostrowski ML, Inwards CY, Strickler JG, Witzig TE, Wenger DE, Unni KK (1999) Osseous Hodgkin disease. Cancer 85:1166–1178

Perin T, Canzonieri V, Gloghini A, Volpe R, Scarabelli C, Carbone A (2000) Primary Hodgkin's disease of the vagina. Leuk Lymphoma 37:451–455

Piccinini L, Mauri C, Barbieri F, Luppi G (1991) With regard to a case of Hodgkin's disease with sternal involvement at onset. Haematologica 76:78–79

Pinson P, Joos G, Praet M, Pauwels R (1992) Primary pulmonary Hodgkin's disease. Respiration 59:314–316

Radin AI (1990) Primary pulmonary Hodgkin's disease. Cancer 65:550–563

Reznek RH, Mootoosamy I, Webb JA, Richards MA (1990) CT in renal and perirenal lymphoma: a further look. Clin Radiol 42:233–238

Richardson GE, Longo DL (1991) Multiple cavitating pulmonary nodules in Hodgkin's disease. Cancer 68:930–933

Sandrasegaran K, Robinson PJ, Selby P (1994) Staging of lymphoma in adults. Clin Radiol 49:149–161

Sapozink MD, Kaplan HS (1983) Intracranial Hodgkin's disease. A report of 12 cases and review of the literature. Cancer 52:1301–1307

Scheithauer BW (1979) Cerebral metastasis in Hodgkin's disease. Arch Pathol Lab Med 103:284–287

Shahar J, Angelillo VA, Katz D, Moore JA (1987) Recurrent cavitary nodules secondary to Hodgkin's disease. Chest 91:273–274

Shirkhoda A, Ros PR, Farah J, Staab EV (1990) Lymphoma of the solid abdominal viscera. Radiol Clin North Am 28:785–799

Shuman LS, Libshitz HI (1984) Solid pleural manifestations of lymphoma. AJR Am J Roentgenol 142:269–273

Soderstrom KO, Joensuu H (1988) Primary Hodgkin's disease of the stomach. Am J Clin Pathol 89:806–809

Stark P, Jaramillo D (1986) CT of the sternum. AJR Am J Roentgenol 147:72–77

Strum SB, Weiss A, McDermed JE, Rosen VJ (1985) Intrathoracic Hodgkin's disease. A case presentation with multiple pulmonary nodules in the absence of mediastinal or hilar node disease. Cancer 56:1953–1956

Sullivan WT, Solonick DM (1987) Case report 414: Nodular sclerosing Hodgkin disease involving sternum and chest wall. Skeletal Radiol 16:166–169

Taal BG, Van Heerde P, Somers R (1993) Isolated primary oesophageal involvement by lymphoma: a rare cause of dysphagia: two case histories and a review of other published data. Gut 34:994–998

Tappin JA, Satchi G (1995) Paraneoplastic cerebellar degeneration: a rare presentation of Hodgkin's disease. Clin Lab Haematol 17:206

Toprak A, Kodalli N, Alpdogan TB, Giral A, Celikel CA, Gurmen N, Bayik M (1997) Stage IV Hodgkin's disease presenting with spinal epidural involvement and cauda equina compression as the initial manifestation: case report. Spinal Cord 35:704–707

Tozzini A, Bulleri A, Orsitto E, Morelli G, Pieri L (1999) Hodgkin's lymphoma: an isolated case of involvement of the ureter. Eur Radiol 9:344–346

Tredaniel J, Peillon I, Ferme C, Brice P, Gisselbrecht C, Hirsch A (1994) Endobronchial presentation of Hodgkin's disease: a report of nine cases and review of the literature. Eur Respir J 7:1852–1855

Vailati A, Marena C, Aristia L, Nelva A, Cebrelli C, Ferrari E (1991) Primary Hodgkin's disease of the thyroid: report of a case and a review of the literature. Haematologica 76:69–71

van der Schee AC, Dinkla BA, van Knapen A (1990) Primary pulmonary manifestation of Hodgkin's disease. Respiration 57:127–128

Varan A, Cila A, Buyukpamukcu M (1999) Prognostic importance of magnetic resonance imaging in bone marrow involvement of Hodgkin disease. Med Pediatr Oncol 32:267–271

Wernecke K, Vassallo P, Rutsch F, Peters PE, Potter R (1991) Thymic involvement in Hodgkin disease: CT and sonographic findings. Radiology 181:375–383

Wong-You-Cheong J, Radford JA (1995) Case report: enlargement of a mediastinal mass during treatment for Hodgkin's disease may be due to accumulation of fluid within thymic cysts. Clin Radiol 50:61–62

Zimmerman RA (1990) Central nervous system lymphoma. Radiol Clin North Am 28:697–721

Zornoza J, Ginaldi S (1981) Computed tomography in hepatic lymphoma. Radiology 138:405–410

4 Nodal Involvement in Non-Hodgkin Lymphoma

Yasuo Amano, Kenji Tajika, Noboru Oriuchi, Kazuo Dan, Tatsuo Kumazaki

CONTENTS

Yasuo Amano, MD
Assistant Professor, Department of Radiology, Nippon Medical School, 1-1-5 Sendagi, Bunkyo-ku, Tokyo 113-8603, Japan
Kenji Tajika, MD
Assistant Professor, Division of Hematology, Department of the 3rd Internal Medicine, Nippon Medical School, 1-1-5 Sendagi, Bunkyo-ku, Tokyo 113-8603, Japan
Noboru Oriuchi, MD
Associate Professor, Department of Nuclear Medicine, Gumma University School of Medicine, 3-39-22 Showa-machi, Maebashi-shi, Gumma 371-8511, Japan
Kazuo Dan, MD
Professor, 3rd Department of Internal Medicine, Nippon Medical School, 1-1-5 Sendagi, Bunkyo-ku, Tokyo 113-8603, Japan
Tatsuo Kumazaki, MD
Professor, Department of Radiology, Nippon Medical School, 1-1-5 Sendagi, Bunkyo-ku, Tokyo 113-8603, Japan

4.1 Introduction

Malignant lymphoma is a hematological malignancy originating in the lymphocyte, lymphoid tissues, and immuno-related tissues. Because these tissues are so widely distributed, malignant lymphoma can occur not only in the lymph nodes but also in many extranodal organs such as the brain, salivary gland, thymus, stomach, and bone marrow.

Malignant lymphoma is classified into two types: Hodgkin disease and non-Hodgkin lymphoma (NHL). Hodgkin disease is a distinct pathological entity and usually involves the lymph nodes above the diaphragm, whereas the histopathological entity of NHL is very heterogeneous (Harris et al. 1999). Clinical features, treatment, and prognosis vary greatly in NHL, and accurate classification of this entity based on histological, immunological, and genetic features is required (Akasaka et al. 2000; Harris et al. 1999; Castellino 1991; Vallisa et al. 1999).

Because of the diverse nature of NHL and the recent emergence of several biological analyses for the condition, it is insufficient for clinical management to make the diagnosis of malignant lymphoma by diagnostic imaging only. One of the most important roles of diagnostic imaging for the management of malignant lymphoma is accurate determination of the clinical stage by depicting nodal and extranodal involvement (Cheson et al. 1999; Lister et al. 1989). The overall baseline before treatment of lymphoma can be obtained only with an imaging diagnosis. This contributes in part to the choice of therapy, and it is essential when comparing between the current regimen and a novel regimen or performing a multi-institutional study. In particular, NHL is often distributed in both nodal and extranodal tissues noncontiguously, and thus the combined use of several imaging techniques such as computed tomography (CT), magnetic resonance (MR) imaging, and positron emission tomography (PET) should be required. The other important role of diagnostic imaging is the assessment of the tumor response to chemotherapy and irradiation. Since diagnostic imaging can be repeated, visualizing the whole body with minimal invasiveness, and estimating the tumor location and volume, it is essential for follow-up of the primary lesion, observation of adverse effects associated with treatments, and early detection of local and distant recurrent tumors (CHESON et al. 1999).

In this chapter, we describe the clinical roles of diagnostic imaging for the management of NHL and its imaging features related to nodal involvement. The usefulness and limitations of each imaging modality are also discussed in detail.

4.2
Role of Diagnostic Imaging on Nodal Involvement in NHL

4.2.1
Practical Concepts of NHL

NHL is the group of malignant lymphoma other than Hodgkin disease. NHL occurs at all ages; the number of cases of NHL is gradually increasing in the world, partly because of the increase in acquired immunodeficiency syndrome (HOLFORD et al. 1992; SERRAINO et al. 1997). Although the main causes of NHL remain unknown, the association between NHL and some specific viruses and bacteria such as Epstein-Barr virus, hepatitis virus, and *Helicobacter pylori* has been indicated (JOSEPHS et al. 1988; SERRAINO et al. 1993; VALLISA et al. 1999). Human immunosuppressive virus (HIV) commonly leads to aggressive types of NHL involving both lymph nodes and extranodal organs (SERRAINO et al. 1993). Chronic thyroiditis (Hashimoto disease) and parotid adenitis (Sjögren disease) can lead to NHL in the endocrine system and salivary glands. Some epidemiologic tendencies have been suggested for NHL. Burkitt lymphoma is commonly found in Africa, and T-cell lymphoma and marginal zone B-cell lymphoma of mucosa-associated lymphoid tissues (MALT) lymphoma are more common in East Asia than in the West (MILLER 1996). On the other hand, follicular lymphoma is more common in Caucasians than in Asians and Africans (MILLER 1996; NAMBA 2000).

As the name of "non-Hodgkin" lymphoma indicates, this clinical entity is heterogeneous and includes a wide variety of histological disorders originating from lymphocytes, lymph nodes, and immune-related cells (e.g. natural killer cells). The World Health Organization Classification of Neo-

plastic Diseases of the Lymphoid Tissues demonstrates this wide variety of NHL (HARRIS et al. 1999). This neoplastic group consists of not only the "classical" non-Hodgkin lymphomas such as follicular lymphoma and diffuse large B-cell lymphoma, but also the re-categorized disorders including plasma cell myeloma, mantle cell lymphoma, hairy cell leukemia, mycosis fungoides, and peripheral T-cell lymphoma. This classification is largely based on the origins and locations of immune cells within the lymph nodes and immuno-related organs. Recently the importance of the immunophenotypic and genetic features of the neoplastic cells have been emphasized (AKASAKA et al. 2000).

Since NHL is the heterogeneous disorders of the lymph tissues, the clinical manifestations, therapeutic strategies, and prognosis largely depend on the histological, immunophenotypic, and genetic features of the neoplastic cells in the NHL. Although the Ann Arbor and Cotswolds classifications, which are adaptable to Hodgkin disease and largely determined by the diagnostic imaging, still have an important role in clinical treatment of NHL, these biological and histopathological analyses are now essential for classification and prediction of aggressiveness of NHL. Unlike Hodgkin disease, several types of NHL first involve the extranodal organs such as the skin and gastrointestinal tracts (Fig. 4.1) (HALLIDAY and BAXTER 2003). Follicular lymphoma is often indolent and "watch and wait" may be appropriate for some patients with this type of NHL (Fig. 4.2a,b). NHL often invades multiple lymph nodes non-contiguously (Fig. 4.3) (CASTELLINO 1991; HALLIDAY and BAXTER 2003). The International Prognostic

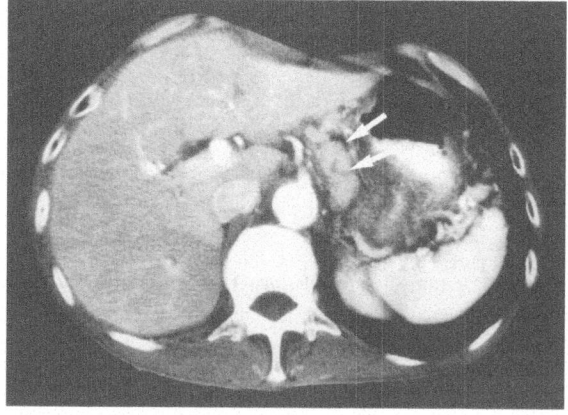

Fig. 4.1. MALT lymphoma in a 64-year-old man with involvement of lymph nodes close to the stomach. Axial contrast-enhanced CT shows the lymph nodes as homogeneously enhanced lesions (*arrows*).

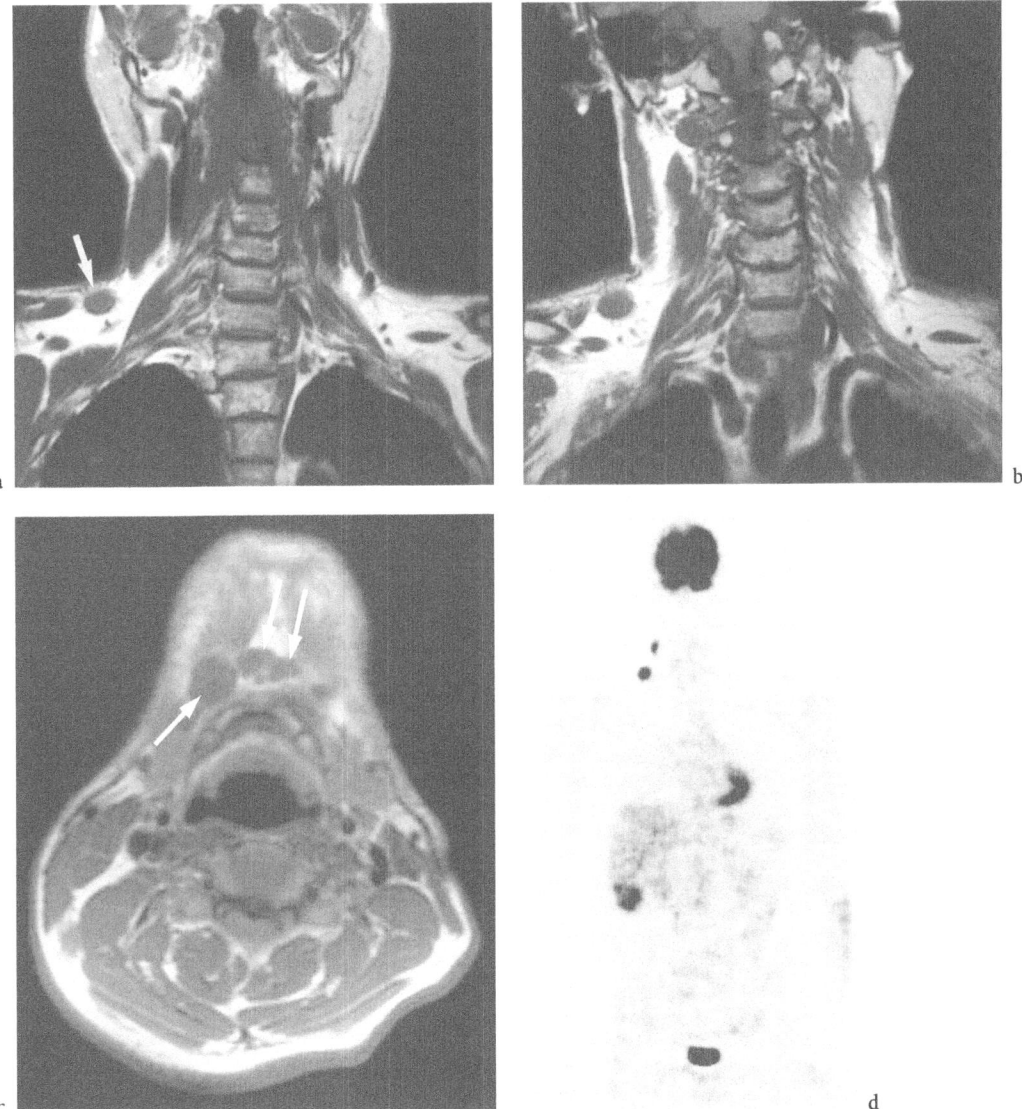

Fig. 4.2a–d. Follicular lymphoma in a 44-year-old man with cervical nodal involvement. **a** Coronal T1-weighted MR image shows right supraclavicular lymph node involvement (*arrow*). **b** Without treatment, this lymph node did not grow significantly for about six months after the first MR imaging examination. **c** Submental and anterior jugular lymph nodes are also found in axial T1-weighted MR image (*arrows*). **d** Although right supraclavicular and jugular lymph nodes lesions seem indolent in MR images, coronal FDG-PET indicates viability of this nodal involvement in non-Hodgkin lymphoma. Non-pathological uptake of FDG is found in brain, heart, colon, and urinary bladder.

Index shows that the prognosis of NHL depends on the status and age of patients and the lactate dehydrogenase values as well as the clinical staging (The International Non-Hodgkin's Lymphoma Prognostic Factor Project 1993). NHL is usually treated with CHOP-based regimen, but the lymphoma with high-intermediate risks based on age-adjusted international prognostic index or with aggressive clinical and histological manifestations should be treated with high-dose chemotherapy, monoclonal antibody

therapy, or other new agents possibly combined with peripheral blood stem cell transplant.

4.2.2
General Role of Diagnostic Imaging in Nodal Involvement in NHL

Although the clinical utility of genetic and histopathological analyses is emerging, there are still

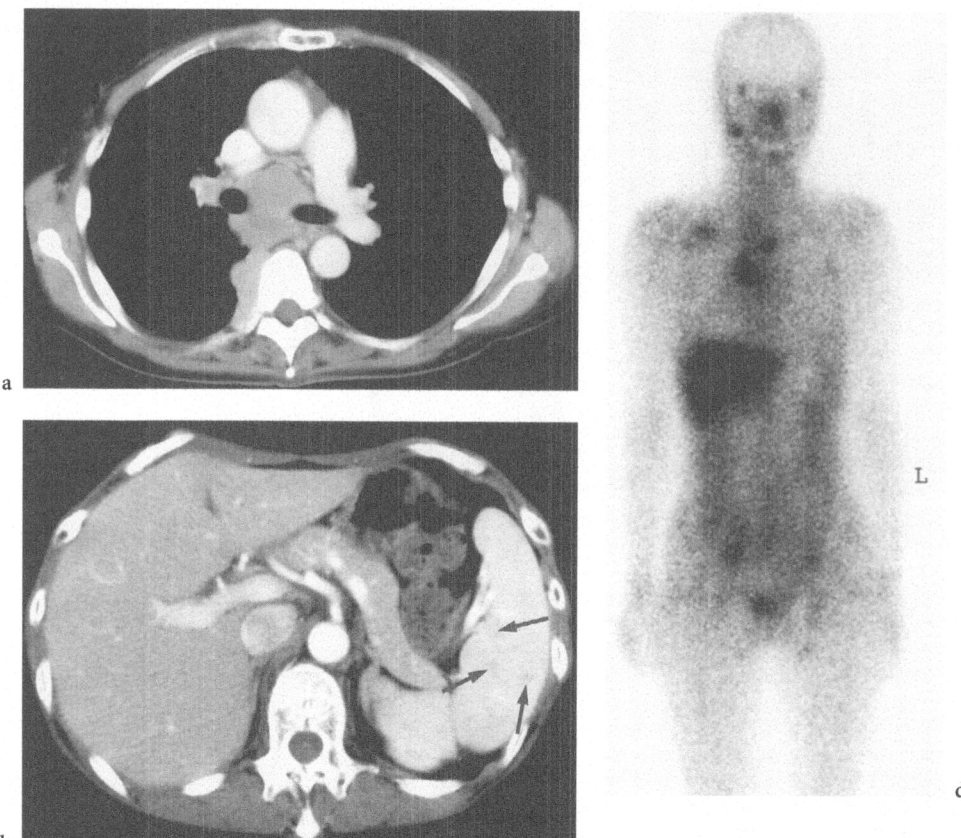

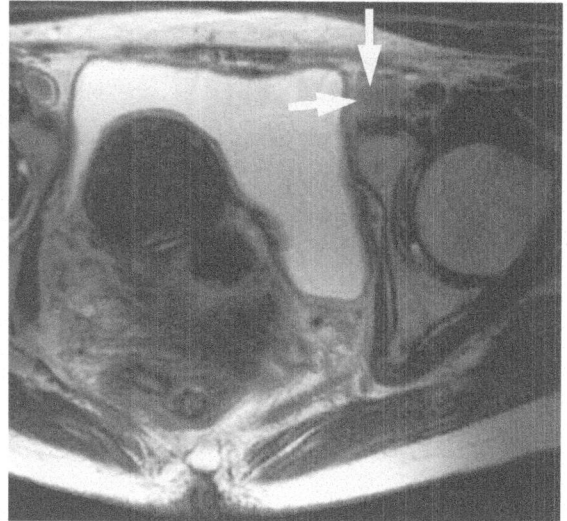

Fig. 4.3a–d. Diffuse large B-cell lymphoma in a 70-year-old woman with multiple lymph node involvement. **a** Axial contrast-enhanced CT of the chest shows subcarinal and right paraaortic lesions that enhance moderately. **b** Axial contrast-enhanced CT of the abdomen demonstrates small hypodense foci in the spleen (*arrows*), but does not depict any lymphadenopathy in the abdomen. **c** Axial T2-weighted MR image of the pelvis detects left inguinal lymphadenopathy with intermediate signal intensity between muscle and fat (*arrows*). **d** Gallium scintigraphy provides whole body imaging that shows right upper neck lymph nodes, mediastinal nodes, and bilateral inguinal nodes involved with non-Hodgkin lymphoma. Non-pathological accumulation of gallium is seen in the salivary gland, liver, bone marrow of vertebra, and colon.

three important roles for diagnostic imaging of NHL. First, diagnostic imaging can suggest the possibility of NHL when depicting single or multiple lymphadenopathy (Fig. 4.4). Enlarged lymph nodes showing homogeneous attenuation and contrast enhancement, conglomerates of lymph nodes, or multiple lymphadenopathy including superficial ones (i.e. axillary region and inguinal region) may suggest the possibility of NHL (CASTELLINO 1991; HALLIDAY and BAXTER 2003; ISHIKAWA and ANZAI 2002). When the vessels run through the enlarged lymph nodes (e.g. CT angiogram sign), the diagnosis of malignant lymphoma, both Hodgkin and non-Hodgkin, is possible (Fig. 4.5a,b). Especially

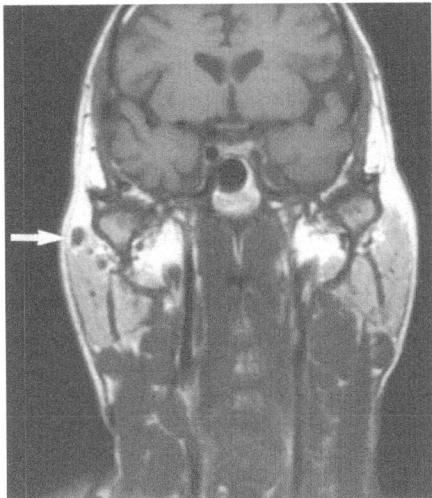

Fig. 4.4. Diffuse large B-cell lymphoma in a 57-year-old man with multiple cervical lymphadenopathy. Coronal T1-weighted MR image of the neck shows bilateral, multiple lymphadenopathy with isointensity to muscle. Right superficial pre-auricular lymph node is depicted (*arrow*), and this may be involved with non-Hodgkin lymphoma, although its diameter is below 1cm.

when the abnormal lymph nodes are distributed non-contiguously and superficially, the diagnosis of NHL should be considered rather than Hodgkin disease (Fig. 4.3). These imaging findings not only suggest NHL but also lead to the lymph nodes accessible for biopsy. For example, ultrasound, CT, and MR imaging clearly visualize lymphadenopathy in the supraclavicular, axillary, and inguinal regions that are easily accessible. Recently, CT guided biopsy has been used for lymphadenopathy in the trunk (Kono et al. 2000). Second, diagnostic imaging techniques are essential for the clinical staging and determination of the baseline before treatment of NHL (The International Non-Hodgkin's Lymphoma Prognostic Factor Project 1993; Lister et al. 1989). The International Prognostic Index recommends distinguishing between low-stage disease (i.e. stage I and II) and high-stage disease (i.e. stage III and IV). It is important to accurately determine the clinical staging for multi-institutional trials and to justify treatments. The overall baseline before treatment of NHL can be obtained only by the imaging

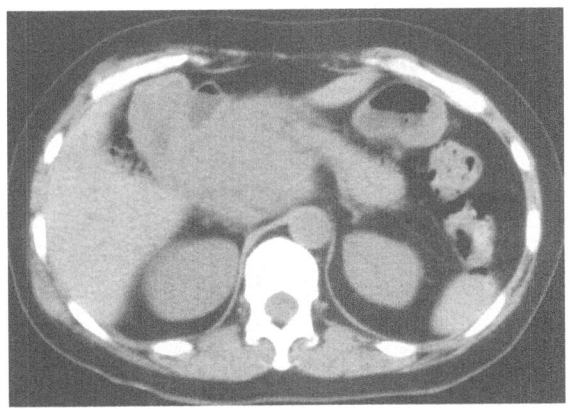

a

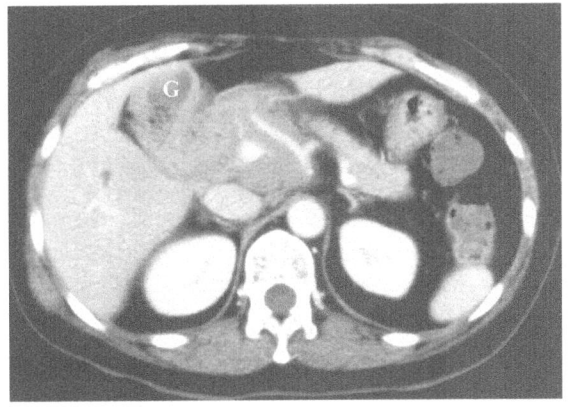

b

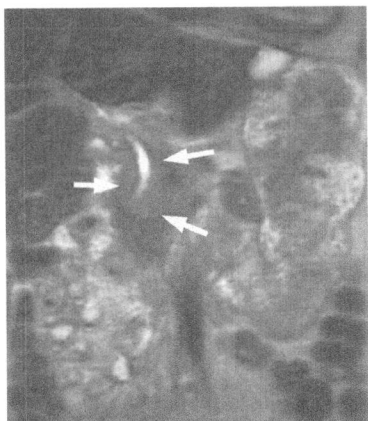

c

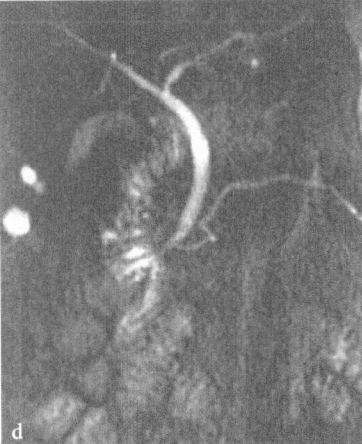

d

Fig. 4.5a–d. Diffuse large B-cell lymphoma in a 57-year-old woman with large abdominal lymph node involvement. a Axial unenhanced CT scan demonstrates a large mass with density identical to muscle in the right abdomen. b Axial contrast-enhanced CT scan shows that the mass enhances moderately and homogeneously. CT angiogram sign is observed, and the gallbladder (*G*) is surrounded by the tumor. c Coronal T2-weighted MR image shows that the common bile duct is also surrounded by lymphoma (*arrows*) but is not occluded. d Magnetic resonance cholangiopancreaticography (*MRCP*) image shows no abnormality in bile and pancreatic ducts, which indicates the involvement of non-Hodgkin lymphoma along the normal structures.

diagnosis. Third, the response to chemotherapy or radiation and the recurrent tumors after treatments are mainly evaluated with diagnostic imaging. Histopathological examination provides information on genetic abnormality, aggressiveness of the tumor, therapeutic strategies, possible response to treatment, and prognosis in each patient. Laboratory data such as lactate dehydrogenase, C-reactive protein, and some tumor markers may suggest recurrence of NHL. However, these examinations cannot quantify the tumor volume before and after treatment or recurrent tumors. Since the diagnostic imaging techniques are non-invasive, they can be performed repeatedly to measure the tumor volume after treatments (CHESON et al. 1999; LISTER et al. 1989). Because of the high spatial and contrast resolutions and unlimited view, diagnostic imaging has replaced surgical investigation in the clinical situations. In particular, CT and MR imaging are useful for accurate estimation of tumor bulk because of their high spatial resolution and multiplanar capability. Recently, PET has been reported to be valuable for assessment of tumor viability, which is often independent of the morphologic changes (HOANE et al. 1994; JERUSALEM et al. 1999; KOSTAKOGLU et al. 2000). Nodal involvement, in which fluorine-18-fluorodeoxyglucose (FDG) accumulates after treatments, is considered viable, even though the nodes decrease in size. Conversely, lesions that do not take up FDG should be scar tissue or non-viable nodes after treatment. The combined use of CT and FDG-PET is of great value for the determination of tumor response to treatments and is increasing the clinical utility of diagnostic imaging for NHL (HOANE et al. 1994).

4.3
Imaging Features and Assessment of Nodal Involvement in NHL

4.3.1
General Imaging Features of Nodal Involvement in NHL before Treatment

Although NHL includes a wide variety of histopathological entities, there are several imaging characteristics that are common to nodal involvement in NHL.

First, NHL tends to present with multiple lymphadenopathy as does Hodgkin disease. Unlike Hodgkin lymphoma, however, the nodal involvement in NHL is often non-contiguous in the whole body

(Fig. 4.3). Hodgkin disease usually involves supradiaphragmatic lymph nodes or thymus, while NHL often involves both supra- and infradiaphragmatic nodes (CASTELLINO 1991; Halliday and BAXTER 2003). NHL involves multiple lymph nodes in the thorax, while Hodgkin disease can involve a single superior mediastinal lymph node or thymus (HALLIDAY and BAXTER 2003). Therefore, NHL may be at a higher stage when it is identified (e.g. stage III or IV), and the whole body should be surveyed with combined imaging modalities so as not to miss small nodal involvement distant from the largest nodal group. Second, nodal involvement in NHL is often observed in the superficial regions such as the axillary, pre-auricular, and inguinal regions (Figs. 4.2c, 4.4). Regional lymphadenopathy close to extranodal involvements such as Waldeyer's ring, parotid gland, thyroid gland, stomach, and spleen is commonly investigated in NHL, but not in Hodgkin disease (Fig. 4.1) (HALLIDAY and BAXTER 2003). Diagnostic imaging can depict both extranodal and nodal involvement during a single examination. Third, the deep lymph node chains such as the spinal accessory lymph nodes and paraaortic lymph nodes are frequently involved in NHL (Figs. 4.3a, 4.6, 4.7) (ISHIKAWA and ANZAI 2002). Because these lesions cannot be palpated, diagnostic imaging, especially CT and MR imaging, are of great value for observation of deep lymph node chains in the head and neck and the trunk. Fourth, the lymph nodes involved in NHL are usually round and well-demarcated (Figs. 4.2a, 4.3c, 4.4, 4.7c). Even when the lymph nodes are small, the conglomerates of small round nodes strongly suggest nodal involvement in NHL. This imaging feature is often found in the upper neck, axillary region, and mediastinum in contrast-enhanced CT and MR imaging (Fig. 4.2c) (Halliday and Baxter 2003; Ishikawa and Anzai 2002). In both Hodgkin and non-Hodgkin lymphoma, extracapsular spread of tumor is rare prior to treatment. If extracapsular spread is observed in the neck and pelvis, metastasis from squamous cell carcinoma in these regions (e.g. nasopharynx, oropharynx, uterine cervix) should be considered rather than malignant lymphoma (ISHIKAWA and ANZAI 2002). Fifth, lymphadenopathy of NHL shows homogeneous density in non-contrast-enhanced CT and homogeneous signal intensity in MR imaging as does Hodgkin disease (Figs. 4.2a, 4.3c, 4.4, 4.5a). This lesion usually demonstrates homogeneous density similar to or slightly higher than muscle in CT, and homogeneously isointense to muscle in T1-weighted MR images and hyperintense to muscle in T2-weighted MR images (HAL-

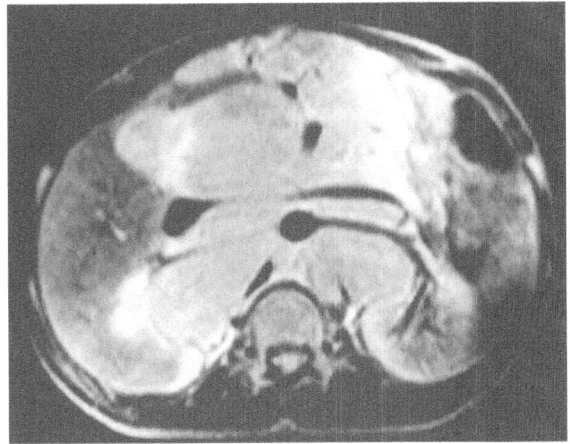

a

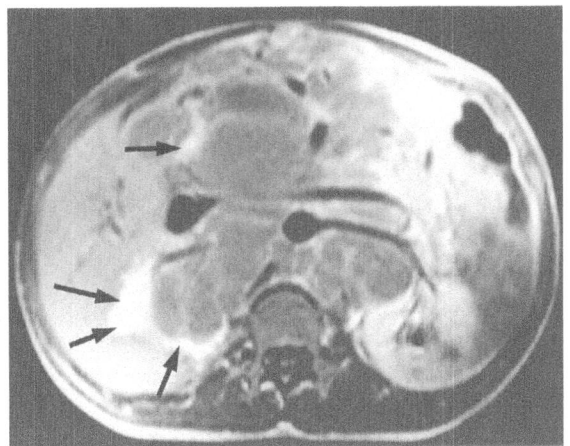

b

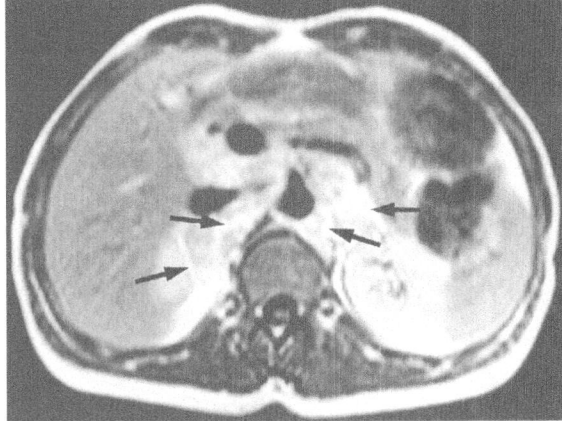

c

Fig. 4.6a–c. Follicular small B-cell lymphoma in a 40-year-old woman with large abdominal lymph node involvement. **a** Axial T2-weighted MR image shows a bulky lymphadenopathy in the abdomen. Extended visceral vessels are seen as flow voids in MR imaging. **b** Axial contrast-enhanced T1-weighted MR image demonstrates peripheral enhancement of this tumor (*arrows*). Central necrosis shows relatively hyperintensity in (**a**) T2-weighted MR image and does not enhance (**b**) after contrast administration. **c** Axial contrast-enhanced T1-weighted MR image after chemotherapy shows the tumor volume is significantly reduced, but enhancing lesions remain (*arrows*), indicating the viable lymphoma lesions. Additional course of chemotherapy is needed in this case.

LIDAY and BAXTER 2003; ISHIKAWA and ANZAI 2002; JUNG et al. 2000; URQUHART et al. 2002). When compared with adipose tissue, lymphadenopathy shows hypointensity in both T1 and T2-weighted MR images (Figs. 4.3c, 4.4). These features may suggest the high and compact cellularity of NHL. Contrast-enhanced CT and MR images demonstrate moderate and homogeneous contrast enhancement of the lymph nodes involved in malignant lymphoma, which indicates homogeneous tissue architecture and relatively low perfusion of the tumor (Figs. 4.3a, 4.5b) (RAHMOUNI et al. 2001). When non-enhancing regions are depicted in lymph nodes, this should reflect central necrosis or cystic changes in the tumors, and can lead to a diagnosis of lymphadenitis, reactive lymphadenopathy, and metastasis of squamous cell carcinoma rather than malignant lymphoma (ISHIKAWA and ANZAI 2002; URQUHART et al. 2002). However, in our experience, 10–15% of malignant lymphomas demonstrate central necrosis in the nodes (Fig. 4.6a,b) (AMANO et al. 1993).

Some reports have indicated that aggressive types of malignant lymphoma tend to show dystrophic changes such as central necrosis and calcification in the lymph nodes (APSTER et al. 2002; CLEARY et al. 1982; REHN et al. 1990). Therefore, when observing the central necrosis and cystic areas in cases of histologically proven NHL, more attention should be paid to evaluating the tumor response (Fig. 4.6). Sixth, lymphadenopathy associated with NHL can compress, but rarely invades vessels and normal structures such as the bile and pancreatic ducts, even when it is bulky (Fig. 4.6). Tumor growth along these normal structures without extracapsular spread is characteristic of both Hodgkin disease and NHL (Fig. 4.5). The so-called CT angiogram sign, which corresponds to the vessels penetrating enlarged lymph nodes, can lead to the diagnosis of malignant lymphoma rather than metastatic lymph nodes (Fig. 4.5b). This imaging feature is often observed in the mediastinum and abdomen which are not accessible by palpation and thus is useful for the diagnosis

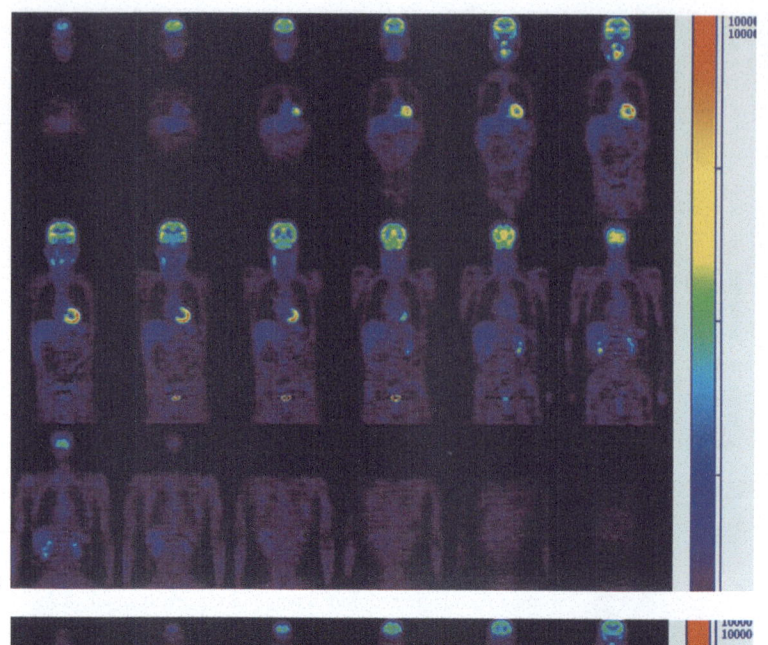

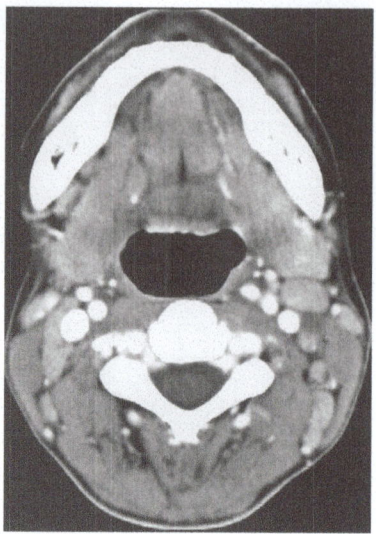

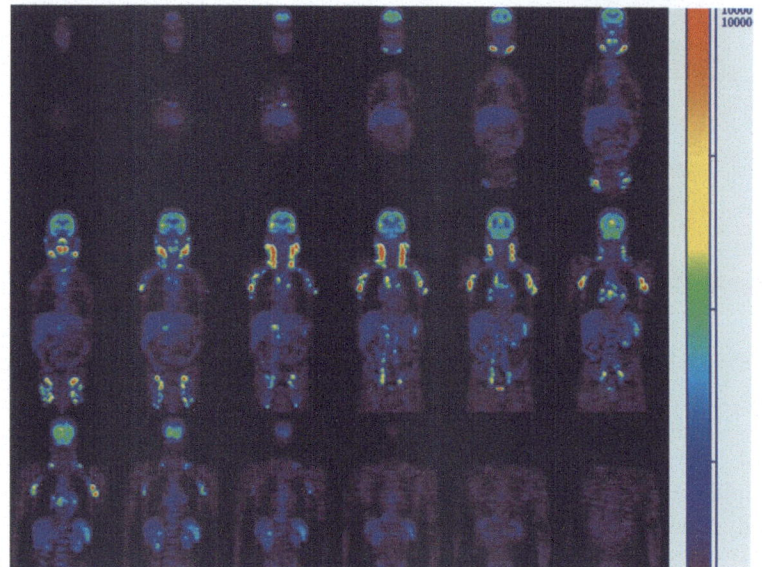

Fig. 4.7a–c. T-cell lymphoma in a 64-year-old man with recurrent lymph node involvement. **a** FDG-PET before treatment shows right cervical lymphadenopathy. **b** FDG-PET after treatment demonstrates recurrent nodal involvement with non-Hodgkin lymphoma in bilateral neck, axillary region, and pelvis. **c** Axial contrast-enhanced CT scan of the neck confirms multiple lymphadenopathy.

of malignant lymphoma. Seventh, gallium and FDG are usually absorbed into the viable tumor tissue of NHL (Figs. 4.2d, 4.3d, 4.7a,b). The attenuation of gallium in the nodes involved in malignant lymphoma is likely higher than other malignancies (FRONT et al. 1990). FDG is also taken up by NHL, and the sensitivity and specificity of the diagnosis of nodal and extranodal involvements from NHL is quite high (JERUSALEM et al. 1999; KOSTAKOGLU et al. 2000).

The imaging findings described above are common for many histological subtypes of NHL. Thus, we can recommend that hematologists should biopsy the lymph nodes when observing lymphadenopathy with these imaging features. CT and MR imaging demonstrate not only lymphadenopathy but also which lymph nodes are appropriate for biopsy. Biopsy guided by CT and MR imaging is now performed in some institutions (KONO et al. 2000). When these findings are not detected by tomographic images, the attenuation of gallium and FDG accumulation in the lymph nodes without apparent primary malignancies help make the diagnosis of malignant lymphoma. In addition, the imaging findings noted above must be the baseline findings for the assessment of tumor response to chemotherapy, irradiation, and bone marrow or stem cell transplantation.

4.3.2
Imaging Assessment of Response of NHL to Treatments

The response of NHL to treatment is determined by imaging diagnosis in addition to laboratory data such as lactate dehydrogenase. Because tomographic imaging modalities can estimate tumor volume and nuclear medicine can provide information on the tumor metabolism, they are of great value for the assessment of the tumor response to chemotherapy and irradiation (CASTELLINO 1991; CHESON et al. 1999; HOANE et al. 1994; JERUSALEM et al. 1999; KOSTAKOGLU et al. 2000; LISTER et al. 1989).

Tumor volume is still the most important, morphological indicator of the tumor response to treatments. Increased nodal size strongly indicates resistance of NHL to treatment, and the therapeutic strategy should be changed. Reduction of nodal volume indicates the tumor's response to the ongoing treatments and a favorable prognosis. NHL tends to decrease in size rapidly early in therapy, and continues shrinking for several weeks after treatment when the therapeutic regime is appropriate. Therefore, imaging diagnosis should be performed early in the therapeutic course to predict tumor response and resistance, late in the course to determine the degree of tumor response, and serially after the end of treatments to follow up the late effect of therapy on NHL and to detect recurrent tumors and to monitor adverse reactions. The follow-up imaging diagnosis is usually performed every 3–4 months during the first 2–3 years after the end of effective treatments. Thereafter, diagnostic imaging should be performed if clinical signs of recurrence are indicated by symptoms, laboratory tests or imaging examination. One disadvantage of this morphological assessment using tumor volume is that a decrease in tumor volume does not necessarily reflect reduced viability of NHL (JERUSALEM et al. 1999; LISTER et al. 1989). According to the Cotswolds classification, a lack of change in the residual masses may indicate nonviable lesions such as fibrosis and scar tissue after treatments (LISTER et al. 1989). However, when the necrotic or cystic area is reduced but the enhancing tumor remains, the tumor may be viable, and additional courses of chemotherapy and radiation therapy may be indicated (Fig. 4.6).

Unenhanced CT is useful for detecting calcification in the lymph nodes, which reflects the complete necrosis of tumor. However, this finding is very rare in NHL. Several MR imaging sequences have been reported to be useful for the assessment of viability of malignant lymphoma in the mediastinum and abdomen (NYMAN et al. 1989; RAHMOUNI et al. 2001). As described above, NHL usually shows intermediate intensity between muscle and fat in T2-weighted MR images prior to treatment. Decrease in signal intensity on T2-weighted MR images after treatments may indicate fibrosis, while a marked increase in signal intensity may reflect necrosis and cystic changes associated with treatment. Residual masses are often observed in mediastinal NHL after radiation therapy and thus T2-weighted MR imaging should be useful in differentiating between viable tumor and nonviable fibrosis as with Hodgkin disease (NYMAN et al. 1989). Contrast-enhanced CT and T1-weighted MR imaging demonstrate necrosis as a non-enhanced region in the tumor. When an enhanced region remains in the mass of NHL after treatment, the residual lesion should be considered viable even if the tumor volume decreases significantly (Fig. 4.6) (AMANO et al. 1993). In addition, one recent report suggests that the enhancement ratio can be an indicator of tumor recurrence in mediastinal lymphoma (RAHMOUNI et al. 2001).

Gallium scintigraphy and FDG-PET provide information on tumor viability after treatment, which is independent of the morphological changes in the tumor. Since NHL recurs both at the primary site and in lymph nodes distant from the primary nodes, the accumulation of these agents at the primary nodes should be carefully assessed both prior to and after treatments. Whole body scanning is also required to detect nodal involvement distant from the primary lesions (Fig. 4.7). Absence of gallium and FDG accumulation in the residual mass strongly indicates a nonviable lesion, even if the tumor volume does not decrease significantly. Conversely, the residual lesions with accumulations of these agents should be considered viable, although the lesion size decreases after chemotherapy and irradiation. A new uptake of gallium and FDG indicates wide spread of tumor and distant recurrence (Fig. 4.7b,c). Metabolic evaluation by nuclear medicine in combination with morphological evaluation of the tumor by CT and MR imaging enhances the clinical usefulness of diagnostic imaging for NHL.

4.4
Imaging Modalities for
Observation of Nodal Involvement in NHL

4.4.1
Computed Tomography

In clinical settings, CT is the most widely available imaging modality for the evaluation of nodal involvement in NHL. Because of its high spatial resolution, high reproducibility, unlimited view, and short examination time, CT should be first applied to the clinical assessment of NHL, as the Cotswolds classification recommends (LISTER et al. 1989). In particular, nodal involvement in the mediastinum, paraaortic region, retroperitoneal space, and inguinal region is shown most clearly with CT. In addition, CT is the only imaging technique to depict small pulmonary involvement in NHL. Unenhanced CT is very sensitive to nodal calcification in NHL, which is rare but a possible indicator of clinically aggressive lesions (APSTER et al. 2002). Contrast-enhanced CT visualizes lymphadenopathy adjacent to vessels, central necrosis of tumor, and the CT angiogram sign (Fig. 4.5b).

Recently developed multi-detector row CT (MDCT) can cover the whole body during a single examination (FOX et al. 1998). MDCT shows lymph node chains with reconstructed multiplanar images. The scan time of MDCT is so short that neither respiratory nor motion artifacts deteriorate image quality significantly. In addition, MDCT can reduce the dose of contrast agents and irradiation exposure. MDCT with four to 16 channels is the current version, and MDCT with flat panel detectors is being developed, which will be able to scan the whole body within 20–30 seconds with a thin slice thickness (1.25–2.5 mm), a subsecond gantry rotation (0.4–0.8 sec), and a higher scan pitch (> 13). MDCT is quite useful for assessment of nodal involvement in NHL, since NHL tends to invade lymph nodes non-contiguously, unlike Hodgkin disease.

The use of iodine contrast agents and irradiation are disadvantages of CT. Although unenhanced CT is often sufficient for the detection of lymphadenopathy associated with NHL, the CT angiogram sign and central necrosis in the tumor cannot be visualized without administration of an iodine contrast agent (Fig. 4.5a,b). Differentiation between pancreatic tumor and retroperitoneal lymph node involvement can be clarified only after rapid administration of contrast agents. However, iodine contrast agents sometimes induce minor and major adverse reactions such as vomiting, anaphylactoid reaction, and impairment of renal function. Irradiation exposure is basically hazardous for children and adolescents, although manufacturers are now developing automatic radiation dose-estimating systems that allow a reasonable reduction of radiation in MDCT. Soft tissue contrast is relatively poor in the head and neck region with CT. Tonsil and retropharyngeal lymph node enlargement in NHL is not easily distinguished from adjacent muscles with CT.

4.4.2
Magnetic Resonance Imaging

MR imaging, with its multiplanar capability, depicts the involved lymph node chains clearly, especially in the neck, paraaortic region, and pelvis (Fig. 4.4). The inherent high soft tissue contrast is also a big advantage over CT and ultrasound. T1 and T2-weighted MR images identify enlarged tonsil and retropharyngeal lymph nodes clearly. Unenhanced fat-suppressed T1-weighted MR imaging emphasizes the signal of the pancreas (SEMELKA and ASCHER 1993), which can be easily differentiated from retroperitoneal lymph nodes involved in NHL. The vessels running through the tumor can be seen as flow voids in unenhanced T1-weighted spin-echo (SE) and T2-weighted fast SE MR images (Fig. 4.5a) or as bright signals in gradient-echo MR angiography sequences.

T2-weighted MR imaging and contrast-enhanced T1-weighted MR imaging are reported to be available for assessing tumor viability (NYMAN et al. 1989; RAHMOUNI et al. 2001). T2-weighted MR imaging identifies central necrosis and cystic changes as a very hyperintense region and post-radiation fibrosis as hypointense (Fig. 4.5a). Contrast-enhanced T1-weighted MR imaging demonstrates the intratumoral necrosis and tumor perfusion clearly as does contrast-enhanced CT; the advantages of contrast-enhanced MR imaging are less nephrotoxicity and allergy of gadolinium-based agents. Some research centers are investigating ultrasmall superparamagnetic iron oxide as a lymph node-specific agent (WEISSLEDER et al. 1990). P-31 MR spectroscopy is also a non-invasive technique for measuring tumor viability and metabolism (NG et al. 1987).

Disadvantages of MR imaging are its lengthy examination time, low spatial resolution, and inability to detect pulmonary involvement of NHL. Fast MR imaging sequences can allow for breath-hold imaging and whole-body imaging (AMANO et al. 2003; SEMELKA and ASCHER 1993). However, when compared with spiral CT and MDCT, the scan time of MR imaging is much to long for a single screening tool. MR imaging can be recommended as such a tool with the histological types of NHL that tend to involve the central nervous system or the musculoskeletal system and which may be difficult to detect with CT. Lower spatial resolution associated with MR imaging may interfere with the depiction of small nodal involvement in NHL. In particular, motion artifacts and magnetic inhomogeneity in the periphery of the body (e.g. axillary region) in addition to the low spatial resolution can lead to underestimation of nodal involvement (AMANO et al. 2003).

4.4.3
Nuclear Medicine

Nuclear medicine is of great value for the assessment of tumor distribution and viability in NHL. An important advantage of nuclear medicine over CT and MR imaging is its ability to provide information on tumor viability independently of morphology. After treatment the residual mass is often observed at the primary site of NHL, and size and signal changes are indirect indicators of tumor viability in CT and MR imaging. However, nuclear medicine can assess viability directly. In addition, because NHL recurs both at the primary site and in lymph nodes distant from the primary nodes, the accumulation of these agents in the lymph nodes far from the primary lesion can be detected with this method. Nuclear medicine is much more clinically useful in NHL than in Hodgkin disease, and should be used for serial follow up of NHL after treatment.

4.4.3.1
Gallium Scintigraphy

Gallium scintigraphy was once the most commonly used method for detecting lymphoma lesions and assessing tumor viability before and after treatment (FRONT et al. 1990). Gallium citrate accumulates in active inflammatory and immune-related tissues 24–72 hours after its injection. Gallium scintigraphy covers the whole body during a single examination and is used to investigate the distribution and viability of NHL in the whole body (Fig. 4.3d). However, there are a couple of disadvantages. First, the spatial resolution of gallium scintigraphy is so low that it misses small nodal involvement in NHL even when lesions are viable. Second, there is some non-specific accumulation. Sarcoidosis, lymphadenitis, and reactive lymphadenopathy demonstrate the uptake of

gallium, which may make it difficult to differentiate between nodal involvement of NHL and other lymphadenopathies. In addition, pulmonary hilum lymph nodes commonly show non-pathological uptake of gallium. Gallium citrate accumulates in normal spleen and bone marrow, and these non-specific accumulations of gallium may lead to overestimation or underestimation of clinical staging and efficiency of treatment in NHL. Therefore, gallium scintigraphy is being replaced by PET, as PET is developed.

4.4.3.2
Fluorine-18-Fluorodeoxyglucose Positron Emission Tomography

FDG-PET is becoming the most powerful imaging modality for the assessment of nodal involvement in NHL (JERUSALEM et al. 1999; KOSTAKOGLU et al. 2000). FDG accumulates in tumor tissue with high glucose metabolism, and provides images with excellent sensitivity and high spatial resolution (Figs. 4.2d, 4.7a,b). Tumor viability can be assessed irrespective of tumor size and morphology with FDG-PET. Although lesion size is not accurate in this imaging, a combination of PET and CT provides information on both the metabolism and morphology of lymphoma lesions simultaneously. In addition, FDG-PET is useful for the detection of spleen and bone marrow infiltration by malignant lymphoma as well as nodal involvement. Because PET is performed shortly after the injection of FDG and covers the whole body during a single examination, this imaging method takes less time than other scintigraphic techniques.

There are a few disadvantages associated with FDG-PET: high cost, limited availability, and irradiation exposure. In addition, hyperglycemia may prevent the accumulation of FDG in the tumor tissue. FDG-PET is relatively insensitive to MALT lymphoma. However, new positron agents are now being developed to overcome these disadvantages (INOUE et al. 2001).

4.4.4
Lymphography and Other Imaging Techniques

Lymphography is the only imaging technique that can visualize the internal architecture of lymph nodes. It was formerly frequently used for clinical staging and for assessment of small lymph nodes possibly involved in malignant lymphoma. However, because of its limited view, complicated injection technique, use of lipid-soluble contrast agent, and the emergence of new imaging techniques, X-ray lymphography is rarely applied to nodal involvement in malignant lymphoma. Instead, MR lymphography using ultra-small iron oxide particles or gadolinium-based agents is being developed; it provides easy injection and tomographic images (TAUPITZ et al. 1993). However, its clinical utility remains undetermined.

Plain X-ray radiography can indicate lymphade-nopathy in the thorax, but does not visualize lymph nodes directly. Ultrasound is less expensive and is an easily accessible imaging technique for the depiction of nodal involvement in NHL. It detects enlarged lymph nodes, vessels in the nodes, and necrosis in the tumor tissues. The disadvantages are its inability to detect mediastinal lymph nodes, low reproducibility, and long examination time when covering the whole trunk. Imaging findings acquired by ultrasound in patients with known or suspicious NHL must be reconfirmed with CT or MR imaging.

4.5
Conclusion

Non-Hodgkin lymphoma includes a wide variety of histological entities. Nonetheless, NHL tends to dem-onstrate common imaging features and thus diagnos-tic imaging is clinically valuable. Diagnostic imaging can lead to the diagnosis of NHL and can identify the lymph nodes appropriate for biopsy. Because the nodal involvement in NHL is often noncontiguous in the whole body and extranodal involvement occurs simultaneously, diagnostic imaging covering the whole body is essential as the baseline before treatment. Since diagnostic imaging can visualize pathological lymph nodes non-invasively and repeatedly, it is essential for the assessment of tumor response to chemotherapy and radiation therapy and for the detection of recur-rent tumor near or far from the primary nodal involve-ment, which is more common in NHL than in Hodgkin disease. The combined use of PET and CT and/or MR imaging is becoming the standard for imaging diagno-sis of nodal involvement in NHL.

References

Akasaka T, Ueda C, Kurata M et al (2000) Nonimmnu-noglobulin (non-Ig)/BCL6 gene fusion in diffuse large B-cell lymphoma results in worse prognosis than Ig/BCL6. Blood 96:2907–2909

Amano Y, Tajika T, Uchiyama N et al (2003) Three-station black-blood fast short inversion time inversion-recovery magnetic resonance imaging for staging of malignant lymphoma: preliminary clinical results. Magn Reson Med Science 2:9–15

Amano Y, Takahama K, Hayashi H et al (1993) CT and MRI findings of malignant lymphoma with non-enhanced areas. Rinshou Houshasen 38:821–824

Apter S, Avigdor A, Gayer G et al (2002) Calcification in lym-phoma occurring before treatment. CT features and clini-cal correlation. AJR Am J Roentgenol 178:935–938

Castellino RA (1991) The non-Hodgkin lymphomas: practi-cal concepts for the diagnostic radiologist. Radiology 178: 315–321

Cheson BD, Horning SJ, Coiffier B et al (1999) Report of an international workshop to standardize response criteria for non-Hodgkin's lymphomas. J Clin Oncol 17:1244–1253

Cleary KR, Osborn BM, Butler JJ (1982) Lymph nodes infrac-tion foreshadowing malignant lymphoma. Am J Surg Pathol 6:435–442

Fox SH, Tanenbaum NL, Ackelsberg S et al (1998) Future direc-tions in Ct technology. Neuroimaging Clin N Am 8:497–513

Front D, Israel O, Epelbaum et al (1990) Ga-67 SPECT before and after treatment of lymphoma. Radiology 175:515–519

Halliday T, Baxter G (2003) Lymphoma: pictorial review I. Eur Radiol 13:1154–64

Harris NL, Jaffe ES, Diebold J et al (1999) World Health Organization classification of neoplastic diseases of the hematopoietic and lymphoid tissues: report of the clini-cal advisory committee meeting; Airlie House, Virginia, November 1997. J Clin Oncol 17:3835–3849

Hoane BR, Shields AF, Porter BA et al (1994) Comparison of initial lymphoma staging using computed tomography (CT) and magnetic resonance (MR) imaging. Am J Hema-tol 47:100–105

Holford TR, Zheng T, Mayne ST et al (1992) Time trends for non-Hodgkin's lymphoma: are they real? What do they mean? Cancer Res 52:5443s–5446s

Inoue T, Koyama K, Oriuchi N et al (2001) Detection of malignant tumors: whole-body PET with fluorine 18 alpha-methyl tyrosine versus FDG – preliminary study. Radiology 220:54–62

The International Non-Hodgkin's Lymphoma Prognostic Factor Project (1993). A predictive model for aggressive non-Hodgkin's lymphoma. N Engl J Med 329:987–994

Ishikawa M, Anzai Y (2002) MR imaging of lymph nodes in the head and neck. Magn Reson Imaging Clin N Am 10: 527–542

Jerusalem G, Beguin Y, Fassotte MF et al (1999) Whole-body positron emission tomography using 18F-fluorodeoxyglu-cose for posttreatment evaluation in Hodgkin's disease and non-Hodgkin's lymphoma has higher diagnostic and prognostic value than classical computed tomography scan imaging. Blood 94:429–433

Josephs SF, Buchbinder A, Streicher HZ et al (1988) Detection of human B-lymphotrophic virus (human herpes virus 6) sequences in B cell lymphoma tissues of three patients. Leukemia 2:132–135

Jung G, Heindel W, von Bergwelt-Baildon M et al (2000) Abdomi-nal lymphoma staging: is MR with T2-weighted turbo-spin-echo sequence a diagnostic alternative to contrast-enhanced spiral CT? J Comput Assist Tomogr 24:783–787

Kono Y, Kanazawa S, Hiraki Y (2000) CT-guided needle biopsy in malignant lymphoma: current techniques and its usefulness. Nippon Rinsho 58:110–114

Kostakoglu L, Goldsmith SJ (2000) Fluorine-18 fluorodeoxy-glucose positron emission tomography in the staging and follow-up of lymphoma: is it time to shift gears? Eur J Nucl Med 27:1564–1578

Lister TA, Crowther D, Sutcliffe SB et al (1989) Report of a committee convened to discuss the evaluation and staging of patients with Hodgkin's disease: Cotswolds meeting. J Clin Oncol 7:1630–1636

Miller RW (1996) Some US-Japanese differences in cancer occurrence-apparently inherent. GANN Monogr Cancer Res 44:13–28

Namba K (2000) Epidemiology and geo-pathology of malignant lymphoma with special emphasis on Japanese lymphomas. Nippon Rinsho 58:535–541

Ng TC, Vijayakumar S, Majors AW et al (1987) Response of non-Hodgkin lymphoma to ^{60}Co therapy monitored by ^{31}P-MRS in situ. Int J Radiat Oncol Bio Phys 13:1545–1551

Nyman RS, Rehn SM, Glimelius BL et al (1989) Residual mediastinal masses in Hodgkin disease; prediction of size with MR imaging. Radiology 170:435–440

Rahmouni A, Divine M, Lepage E et al (2001) Mediastinal lymphoma: quantitative changes in gadolinium enhancement at MR imaging after treatment. Radiology 219:621–628

Rehn SM, Nyman RS, Glimelius BL et al (1990) Non-Hodgkin lymphoma: predicting prognostic grade with MR imaging. Radiology 176:249–253

Semelka RC, Ascher SM (1993) MR imaging of the pancreas. Radiology 188:593–602

Serraino D, Pezzotti P, Dorrucci M et al (1997) Cancer incidence in a cohort of human immunodeficiency virus seroconverters. HIV Italian Seroconversion Study Group. Cancer 79:1004–1008

Taupitz M, Wagner S, Hamm B et al (1993) Interstitial MR lymphography with iron oxide particles: results in tumor-free and VX2 tumor-bearing rabbits. AJR Am J Roentgenol 161:193–200

Urquhart AC, Hutchins LG, Berg RL (2002) Distinguishing non-Hodgkin lymphoma from squamous cell carcinoma tumors of the head and neck by computed tomography parameters. Laryngoscope 112:1079–1083

Vallisa D, Berte R, Rocca A et al (1999) Association between hepatitis C virus and non-Hodgkin lymphoma, and effects of viral infection on histologic subtype and clinical course. Am J Med 106:556–560

Weissleder R, Elizondo G, Wittenberg J et al (1990) Ultrasmall superparamagnectic iron oxide: an intravenous contrast agent for assessing lymph nodes with MR imaging. Radiology 175:494–498

5 Central Nervous System Involvement in Non-Hodgkin Lymphoma

François Lafitte, Carmen Adem, Agnès Coulon, Jacques Chiras

CONTENTS

5.1 Introduction

Primary central nervous system (CNS) non-Hodgkin lymphoma (NHL) comprises 1 to 3% of primary brain tumors, 6% of all intracranial neoplasms and about 1% of all lymphomas (COULON et al. 2002). Onset is most common in the sixth and seventh decades. It usually presents as a brain tumor, but

FRANÇOIS LAFITTE, MD
Senior Radiologist, Department of Radiology, Adolphe de Rothschild Foundation, 25–29 Rue Manin, F-75019 Paris, France
CARMEN ADEM, MD
Senior Neuroradiologist, Department of Neuroradiology, Val de Grâce Military Hospital, 74 Boulevard du Port-Royal, F-75005 Paris, France
Agnès Coulon, MD
Clinical Fellow, Department of Radiology, Croix-Rousse Hospital, Grande Rue de la Croix-Rousse, F-69004 Lyon, France
Jacques Chiras, MD
Professor and Chairman, Department of Neuroradiology, La Salpêtrière University Hospital, 47–83 Boulevard de l'Hôpital, F-75013 Paris, France

may also involve the leptomeninges, eyes, and spinal cord. Its incidence has increased steadily in the last 20 years, in both immunocompromised and immunocompetent patients. Although the incidence is more frequent in immunodeficient states, especially AIDS, the pathogenesis remains unknown. The tumor develops initially in the periadventitial cells of the leptomeningeal vessels. It then invades the adjacent brain parenchyma and spreads into the perivascular spaces of the perforant vessels, before reaching the deep brain structures. This particular way of spreading is responsible for the diversity of the imaging patterns found in this condition.

The most common type of lymphoma affecting the brain is diffuse histiocytic lymphoma (GROSSMAN and YOUSEM 1994). Most primary CNS NHL are composed of diffuse large lymphomatous cells with a B phenotype, and cannot be histologically differentiated from systemic extra-nodal NHL. Secondary CNS involvement, less frequent than primary involvement, is more often observed in non-Hodgkin and in Burkitt lymphomas (MARSAULT et al. 1991).

In immunocompetent patients, primary NHL of the brain presents as solitary supratentorial lesions in about 80% of patients. The lesions involve mostly the supratentorial brain parenchyma, in deep or peripheral locations. The posterior fossa is involved in 10% of cases. Atypical forms with isolated ventricular or meningeal locations as well as multifocal or endovascular forms also occur. Ocular abnormalities such as uveitis or hyalitis are sometimes associated with brain involvement (ocular lymphoma). In immunocompromised patients, mostly those who are HIV positive, atypical forms are more frequent. NHL of the spinal cord involves mostly the leptomeningeal structure, but epidural or intramedullary locations may be encountered.

CT and MR imaging features are often suggestive, but atypical features and location are also common. Knowledge of these features, both typical and atypical, is important, since specific treatments are now available. The imaging patterns and differential diagnosis of lymphomas in immunocompromised patients differ from those in immunocompetent patients. Recent imaging techniques such as diffusion-perfusion imaging, MR spectroscopy and specific nuclear studies are useful in some specific cases, especially in helping to differentiate lymphoma from other cerebral lesions, such as toxoplasmosis.

5.2
Brain Involvement

5.2.1
Immunocompetent Patient

Most primary CNS NHL yield evocated features, yet atypical presentations are not uncommon. The classical features will be described first and then the atypical features, as well as particular forms such as multifocal lymphoma, endovascular lymphoma, cerebro-ocular lymphoma and secondary lymphoma. The main differential diagnoses are presented in each subchapter.

5.2.1.1
Classical Presentation

The classical presentation of primary CNS NHL is a solitary (80%) well demarcated intraparenchymatous lesion, with few edema or mass effects compared to the size of the lesion (KOELLER et al. 1997; SCHWAIGHOFER et al. 1989). The lesion can involve deep structures as well as peripheral white matter, but is often close to ventricular or meningeal structures. The corpus callosum is often involved, leading sometimes to a "butterfly pattern", as described in glioblastomas (Figs. 5.1, 5.2). Unlike secondary CNS lymphoma, bone and dural involvement are rare. The optic chiasm and pineal gland are rarely involved.

On CT, the lesion usually appears hyperdense or isodense before contrast administration (90%), probably due to the hypercellularity of the tumor (WATANABE et al. 1992). This feature is important for distinguishing primary CNS NHL from metastases or gliomas, which are more often hypodense (OSBORN 1994; PATCHELL 1995). Only a few cases of hypodense lymphomatous lesions have been described (GEOFFRAY et al. 1990).

On MR imaging, about 90% of the lesions are hypointense or isointense on T1-weighted images (COULON et al. 2002; KOELLER et al. 1997; SCHWAIG-HOFER et al. 1989; CANAPLE et al. 1996; JOHNSON et

al. 1997; BROWN et al. 1995; DE LA BLANCHARDIERE et al. 1997; FUROSAWA et al. 1998; GOLDSTEIN et al. 1991). The signal intensity on T2-weighted and fluid-attenuated inversion recovery (FLAIR) MR images is variable, but in most cases the tumor appears as an iso- or hypointense area surrounded by peripheral hyperintense edema (KOELLER et al. 1974; JOHNSON et al. 1997; JENKINS et al 1998). When presenting with iso or hypointense signal on T2-weighted MR images, primary CNS NHL can usually be distinguished from gliomas and demyelinating diseases, which are more commonly hyperintense. However, such T2 hypointensity can also be seen in gastrointestinal tract adenocarcinoma metastases and is related to the tumor hypercellularity and mucin hypersecretion. In primary CNS NHL, it probably reflects the increased nuclear-cytoplasmic ratio in these densely packed, highly cellular tumors (UEDA et al. 1995). After contrast administration, a strong and usually homogenous enhancement is observed on CT as well on MR imaging. Lack of enhancement of the lesions prior to treatment is very uncommon, but has been described in 10% of lesions in some series, which seems high (JOHNSON et al. 1997; CELLERIER et al. 1984; DEANGELIS 1995; NAMASI-VAYAM and TEASDALE 1992). Corticosteroids can also modify or negate the enhancement pattern, and therefore should not be administered prior to CT and MR imaging, unless there is significant intracranial hypertension.

Calcifications, cyst formation, and hemorrhage are uncommon features of primary CNS NHL prior to treatment. Calcifications occur most frequently after radiation therapy or chemotherapy or in primary glial tumors, particularly oligodendrogliomas. Hemorrhagic lymphomas are quite rare, but are described in the literature on MR imaging (UEDA et al. 1995). The differential diagnosis includes metastases such as melanoma, renal and lung cancers or choriocarcinoma, and glioblastoma that bleeds frequently. Necrotic lesions are also rare. They are preferentially found in metastases, or glioblastoma. Two to 6% of metastatic lesions yield necrotic or hemorrhagic components (OSBORN 1994). On MR imaging, there is a relation between necrosis and hyperintense signal on T2-weighted images and annular or heterogeneous enhancement (JOHNSON et al. 1997). Necrotic and hemorrhagic lesions are more frequent in patients with AIDS lymphomas (KOELLER et al. 1997; LANFERMANN et al. 1997; RUIZ et al. 1997; MARRELLE et al. 1994).

One of the most characteristic features of CNS lymphoma is a tendency to involve the ventricular

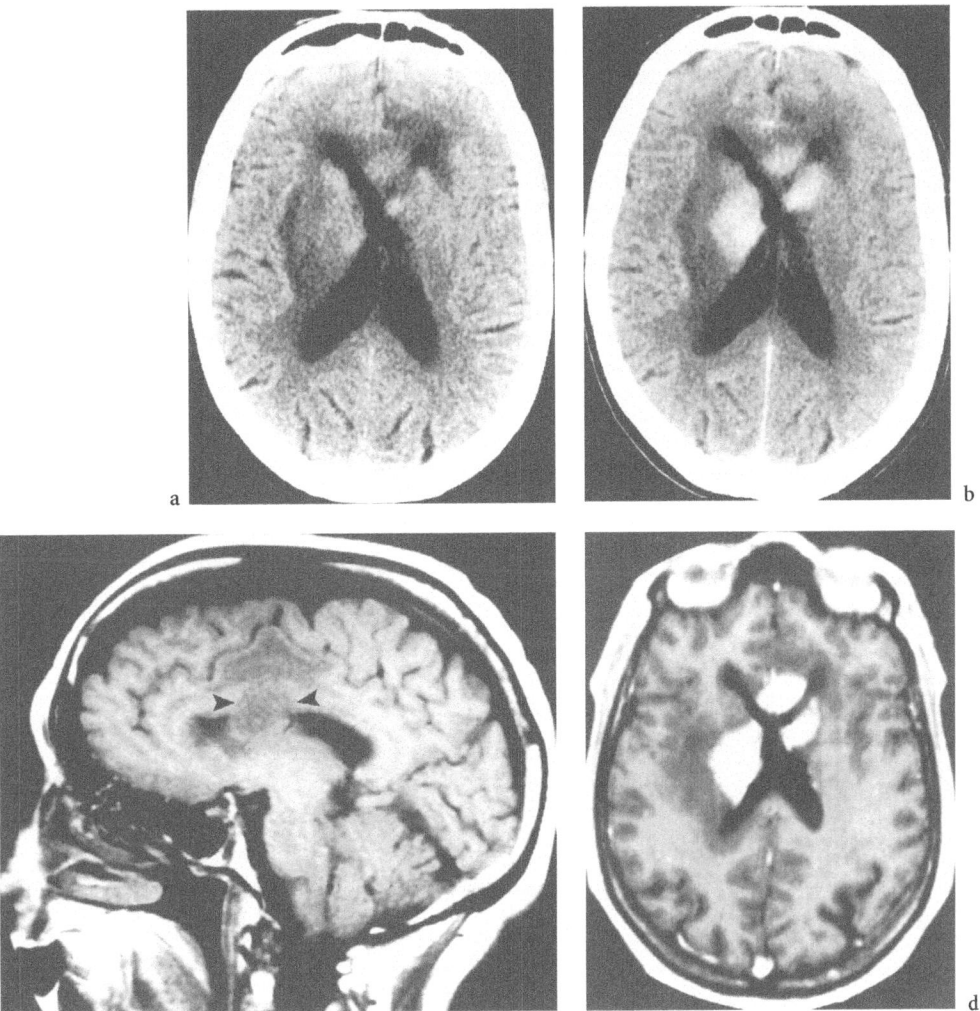

Fig. 5.1a–d. Cerebral non-Hodgkin lymphoma of the corpus callosum in a 63-year-old patient who presented with confusion. **a** Axial unenhanced CT scan shows a spontaneous hyperdense lesion of the corpus callosum and of the periventricular white matter. **b** Axial contrast-enhanced CT scan shows strong enhancement of the lesion. There is also a surrounding edema. **c** Sagittal unenhanced T1-weighted MR image demonstrates the hypointense corpus callosum lesion (*arrowheads*). **d** Axial contrast-enhanced T1-weighted MR image shows important and homogenous enhancement of the lesion.

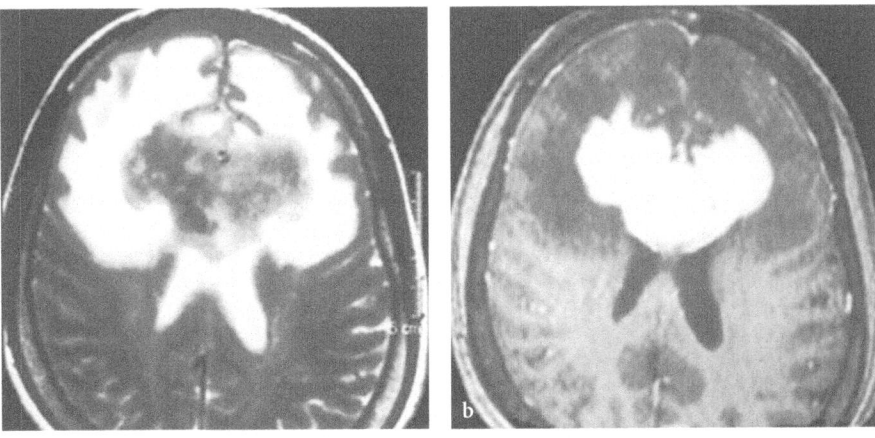

Fig. 5.2a,b. Cerebral non-Hodgkin Lymphoma in a 42-year-old woman with "butterfly pattern". **a** Axial T2-weighted MR image shows a hypointense lesion in the corpus callosum and both frontal lobes with important hyperintense surrounding edema. **b** Axial contrast-enhanced 3D spoiled gradient-echo (SPGR) T1-weighted MR image demonstrates strong enhancement of the lesion. (*Image courtesy of Dr. N. Martin-Duverneuil*)

ependyma, the meninges, or both. Such involvement is found in 60% to 80% of the cases on imaging, and in 100% at autopsy (GEOFFRAY et al. 1990; GOLDSTEIN et al. 1991; LANFERMANN et al. 1997; HOCHBERG and MILLER 1988). These findings support the theory that the lesion originates from the periadventitial cells of penetrating arterioles in the perivascular Virchow-Robin spaces (GUTMANN and KENDALL 1994). Local enhancement of the ventricular structures is found in about 20% of cases (COULON et al. 2002), most commonly in the lesions involving the deep brain matter (Fig. 5.3) (MURRAY et al. 1989; ARRUE et al. 1987). However, diffuse or localized meningeal enhancement is rare but often observed in CNS locations of non-CNS lymphoma or leukemia. Classically, meningeal and ventricular involvement is contiguous with a parenchymatous lesion, but a diffuse radiological meningitis or ventriculitis may exist, sometimes isolated (MURRAY et al. 1989; BALMACEDA et al. 1995). If CT and MR imaging demonstrate a good sensitivity for detecting diffuse meningeal involvement, cerebrospinal fluid (CSF) examinations are often negative in these cases (BALMACEDA et al. 1995). However, a positive CSF examination allows the diagnosis of primary CNS NHL and obviates the need for an invasive cerebral biopsy.

5.2.1.2
Main Atypical Patterns

In about 20% of immunocompetent patients, an atypical pattern is encountered, related to the type of enhancement, the location, or the number of the lesions.

5.2.1.2.1
Atypical Enhancement

The enhancement can be heterogeneous, mimicking glioma or sometimes encephalitis (Fig. 5.4). Rarely, a

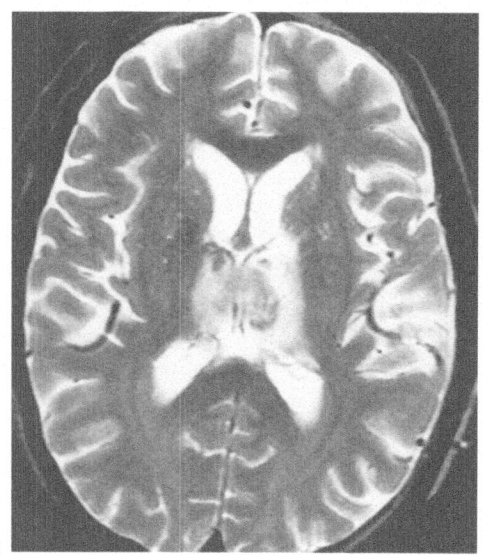

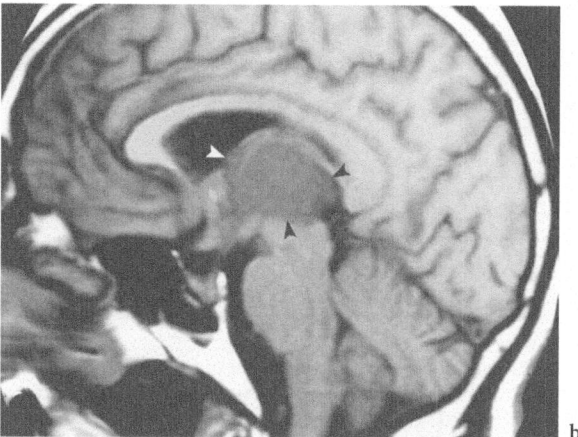

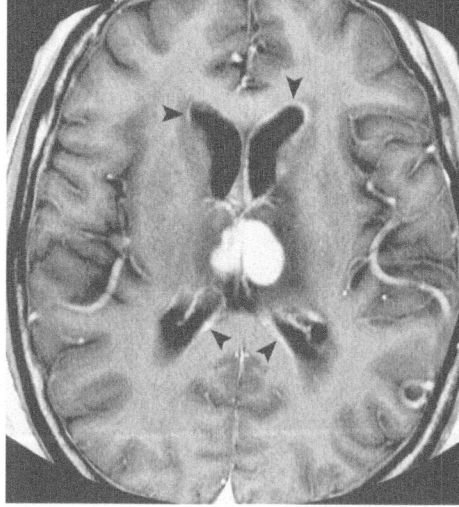

Fig. 5.3a–c. Cerebral non-Hodgkin lymphoma in a 58-year-old man who presented with intracranial hypertension. **a** Axial T2-weighted MR image demonstrates a lesion involving the parenchyma around the third ventricle. This lesion is isointense compared to the brain parenchyma and is surrounded by hyperintense edema. **b** Sagittal unenhanced T1-weighted MR image shows the mass is hypointense (*arrowheads*). **c** Axial contrast-enhanced T1-weighted MR image shows a strong enhancement of the lesion surrounding the third ventricle associated with ventriculitis (*arrowheads*). (With permission from [COULON et al. 2002])

ring enhancement as in cerebral abscesses or necrotic brain metastases is found. This pattern is more frequent in AIDS patients. Another presentation is a single lesion with nodular enhancement and important edema, as in brain metastases (Fig. 5.5). Gyral enhancement mimicking stroke is rarely observed.

Multiple patchy enhancement is sometimes seen in endovascular forms.

A lack of enhancement can be observed after corticosteroid administration, in some endovascular lymphomas, and in infiltrating forms where there is a diffuse involvement of the brain parenchyma with no mass

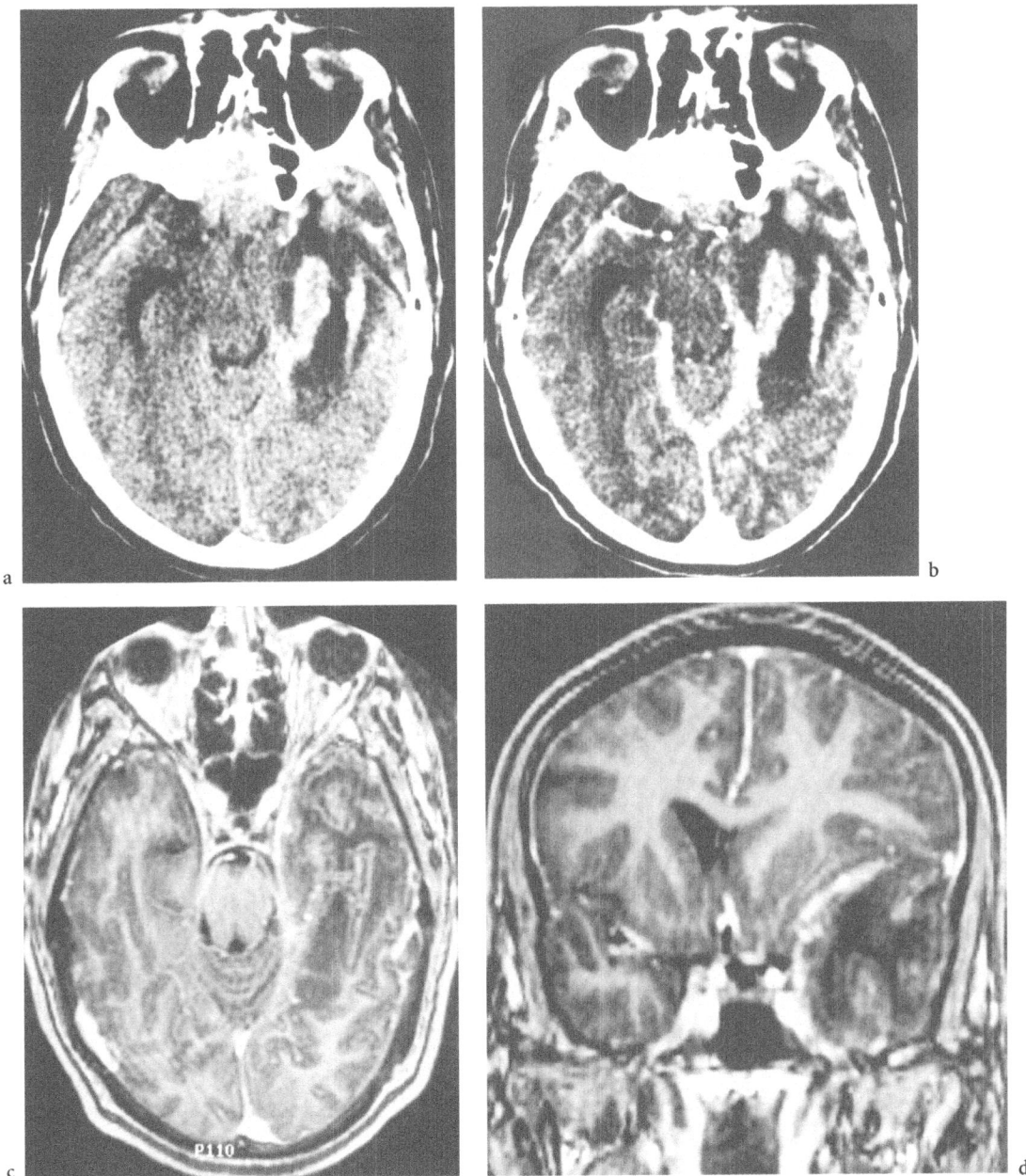

Fig. 5.4a–d. Cerebral non-Hodgkin lymphoma in a 38-year-old man who presented with intracerebral hemorrhage and aphasia. **a** Axial unenhanced CT scan demonstrates hemorrhagic left temporal lesion. **b** Axial contrast-enhanced CT scan shows a mild heterogeneous enhancement of the lesion. **c** Axial and (**d**) coronal contrast-enhanced 3D SPGR T1-weighted images show mild parenchymatous and meningeal enhancement. The radiological features are close to those observed in herpes meningoencephalitis, but clinical presentation is different. (With permission from [COULON et al. 2002])

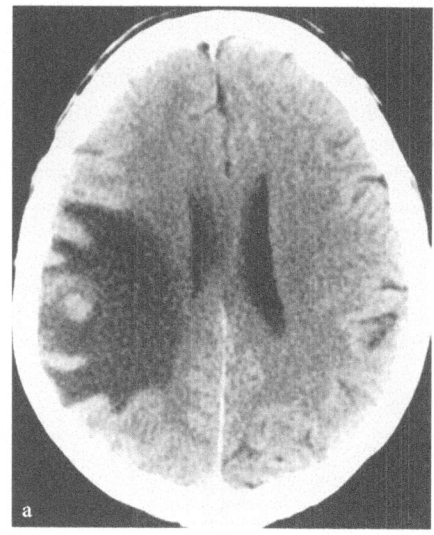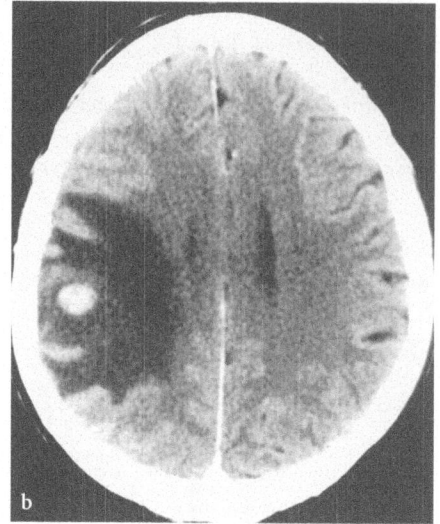

Fig. 5.5a,b. Cerebral non-Hodgkin lymphoma in a 45-year-old man who presented with left hemiplegia. **a** Axial unenhanced CT scan shows a spontaneous hyperdense nodular lesion of the right precentral gyrus with important peripheral edema. **b** There is strong nodular enhancement of the lesion after contrast injection, mimicking metastases.

formation (FURUSAWA et al. 1998; CELLERIER et al. 1984; MURRAY et al. 1989; DEANGELIS 1993; CARLSON 1996). These lesions appear as relatively symmetrical areas of hypodensity on CT and of hypointensity on T1-weighted MR images, with no or slight edema and mass effect. The diagnosis of lymphoma is difficult and often delayed. The differential diagnoses are demyelinating diseases, low-grade astrocytomas, gliomatosis cerebri, and progressive multifocal leukoencephalopathy in immunocompromised patients. In elderly patients, this feature may not be distinguished from leukoaraiosis. Involvement of the deep or superficial gray matter may help to exclude demyelinating diseases.

5.2.1.2.2
Atypical Location

1) *Isolated ventricular location.* In a few cases, only a pattern of ventriculitis is observed, with no associated parenchymal mass (Fig. 5.6). This ventricular enhancement can be diffuse or nodular, and most often concerns the periphery of the ventricular ependyma close to the deep white matter. The differential diagnoses are infectious disease, metastatic ventriculitis, or sarcoidosis, but the clinical presentations usually differ. A meningioma can also be considered in the case of an isolated intraventricular mass with strong homogeneous enhancement.

2) *Meningeal involvement.* A few cases of primary cerebral lymphoma presenting as meningeal masses are described in the literature (CARLSON 1996; ASHBY et al. 1988; ISLA et al. 1996; PAREKH et al. 1993; PETIOT et al. 1995). This meningeal involvement mimics meningioma on CT and MR

imaging (Figs. 5.7, 5.8). A dural tail can be observed, as with typical meningiomas. Osteocondensation close to the meningeal lesion, as well as calcifications, often observed in meningioma, are usually absent in cerebral lymphomas, although bony lyses can be observed, sometimes with an extension to the adjacent soft tissues (Fig. 5.9) (ISLA et al. 1996; PAREKH et al. 1993). This meningeal infiltration can be observed in the cerebral convexity, in the posterior fossa, as well as in unusual locations such as the cavernous sinus (Fig. 5.10) and jugum of sellae. It should be kept in mind when a meningeal mass is observed, that the differential diagnoses of meningioma include cerebral lymphoma as well as plasmocytoma, dural metastasis, Castleman disease, dural inflammatory disease and extraaxial cavernoma. Isolated leptomeningeal locations of primary cerebral lymphoma with enhancement of the cisterns and cranial nerves are rare and are more often seen in metastases of a systemic lymphoma (Fig. 5.11).

3) *Virchow-Robin spaces.* Rarely, multiple punctate foci of enhancement are seen, likely related to involvement of the perivascular spaces, also called Virchow-Robin spaces (Fig. 5.12).

4) *Skull base or convexity.* Involvement of the bony structure of the skull is mostly related to a meningeal lymphomatous mass (Fig. 5.9). The base as well as the top of the skull may be involved.

5) *Other locations.* Cerebral lymphoma can also involve the pituitary stalk (Fig. 5.13), the optic chiasm (Fig. 5.14), and the epiphyseal gland (Fig. 5.15), but these locations are rare. The differential diagnoses include the other tumoral conditions of the corresponding region.

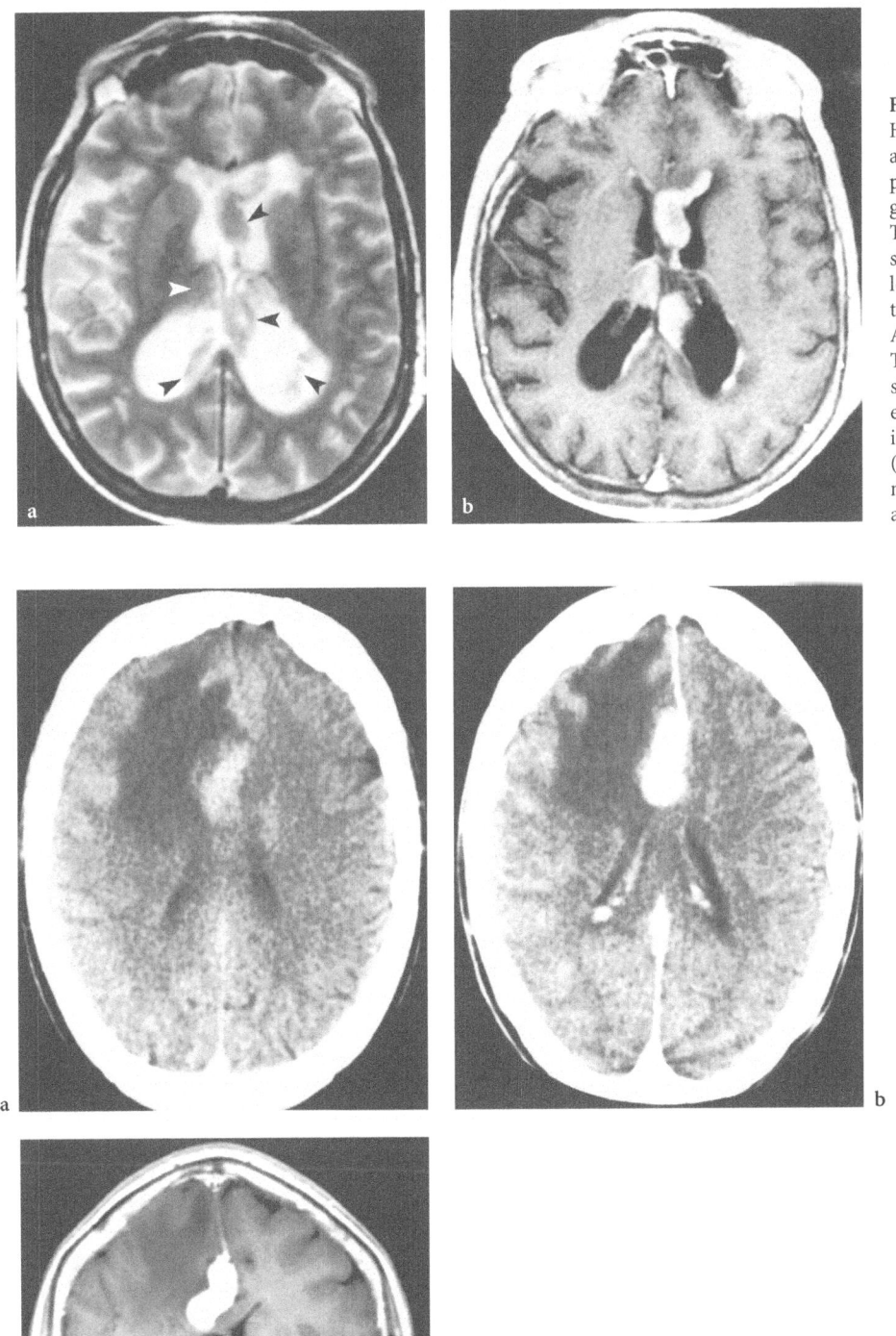

Fig. 5.6a,b. Cerebral non-Hodgkin lymphoma in a 79-year-old man who presented with meningeal syndrome. **a** Axial T2-weighted MR image shows multiple isointense lesions of the lateral ventricles (*arrowheads*). **b** Axial contrast-enhanced T1-weighted MR image shows multiple nodular enhancing lesions involving the lateral ventricles (ventriculitis). (With permission from [COULON et al. 2002])

Fig. 5.7a–c. Cerebral extra-axial non-Hodgkin lymphoma mimicking a falx meningioma in a 39-year-old woman. **a** Axial unenhanced CT scan shows a hyperdense extra-axial mass involving the cerebral falx, which strongly enhances (**b**) after contrast injection. Note the importance of associated edema. **c** Coronal contrast-enhanced T1-weighted MR image demonstrates a downwards displacement of the corpus callosum by the extra-axial mass. (With permission from [COULON et al. 2002])

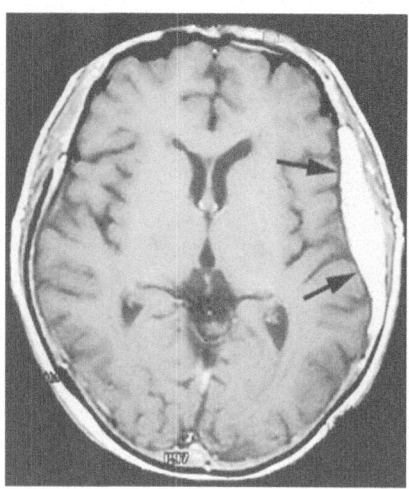

Fig. 5.8. Cerebral non-Hodgkin lymphoma of the meninges in a 42-year-old man. Axial contrast-enhanced T1-weighted MR image reveals an extra-axial atypical mass with linear meningeal enhancement, mimicking a left frontoparietal en-plaque meningioma (*arrows*). (*Image courtesy of Dr. N. Martin-Duverneuil*)

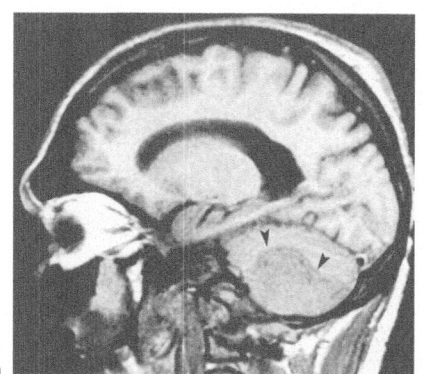

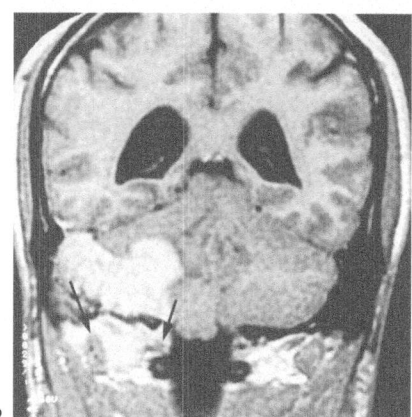

Fig. 5.9a,b. Cerebral non-Hodgkin lymphoma in a 26-year-old man who presented with intracranial hypertension. **a** Sagittal unenhanced T1-weighted MR image demonstrates a lesion of the posterior fossa, slightly hypointense compared to brain parenchyma (*arrowheads*). **b** Coronal contrast-enhanced T1-weighted MR image shows the important enhancement of the lesion, its extra-axial location, and the associated involvement of the adjacent skull base and soft tissues (*arrows*). (With permission from [COULON et al. 2002])

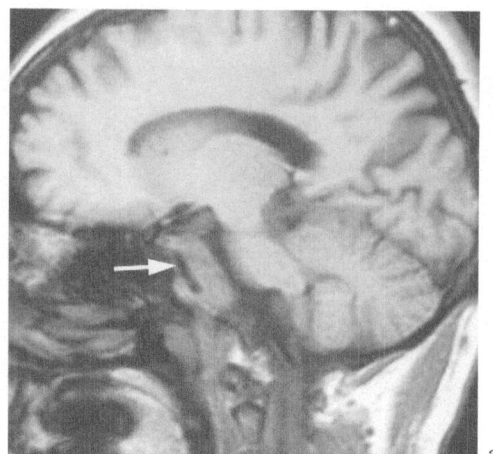

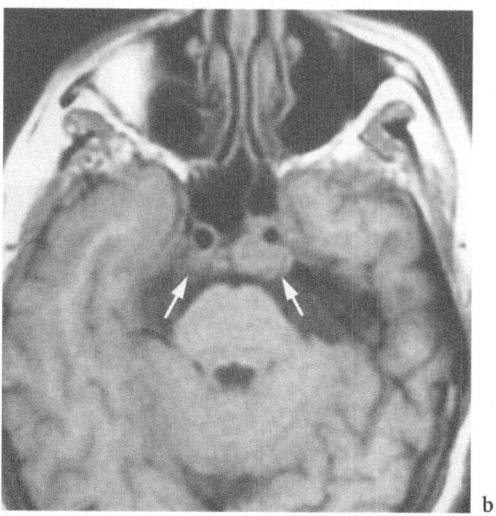

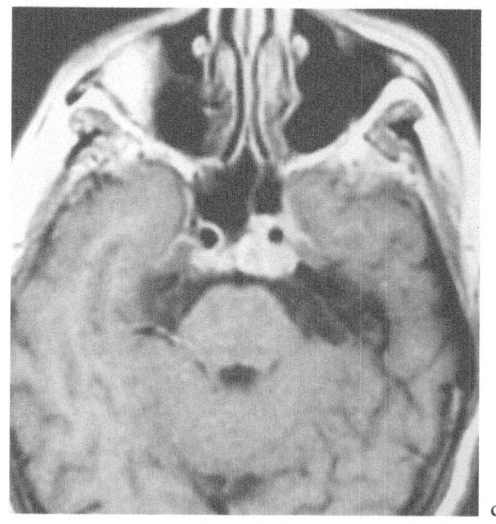

Fig. 5.10a–c. Cerebral extra-axial non-Hodgkin lymphoma in a 50-year-old man involving the cavernous sinuses. **a** Left parasagittal unenhanced T1-weighted MR image shows a mass involving the cavernous sinus and encasing the left internal carotid artery (*arrow*). **b** Axial unenhanced T1-weighted MR image shows the extra-axial lesion is bilateral and isointense to the cerebral parenchyma (*arrows*). **c** The lesion strongly enhances after contrast administration. (*Image courtesy of Dr. Y. Miaux*)

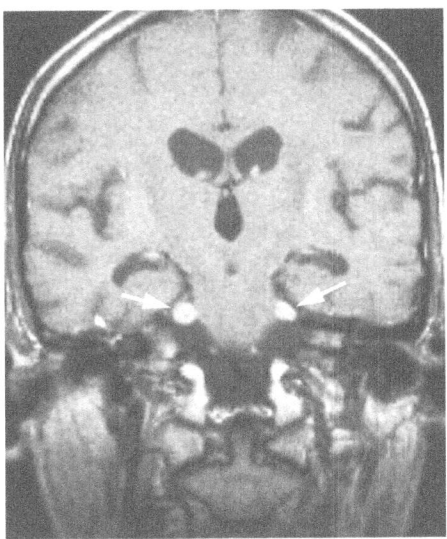

Fig. 5.11. Cerebral primary non-Hodgkin lymphoma in a 17-year-old boy involving the trigeminal nerves. Coronal contrast-enhanced T1-weighted MR image shows strong enhancement of the cisternal segments of bilaterally thickened trigeminal nerves (*arrows*). (*Image courtesy of Dr. Y. Miaux*)

5.2.1.2.3
Multifocal Forms

Multiple lesions occur in 11–47% cases of primary CNS NHL (Figs. 5.16, 5.17). They are more prevalent in immunocompromised patients. Isolated lobar involvement is frequent (70%), especially for the frontal and parietal lobes (COULON et al. 2002). Posterior fossa involvement is common (35%). Compared to monofocal primary CNS NHL, these lesions demonstrate a higher frequency of heterogeneous enhancement and areas of necrosis, but little edema and mass effect, unlike metastases. The differential diagnoses are metastases, even though often located at the white-gray matter junction, multifocal glioblastoma and abscess.

5.2.1.3
Specific Forms

5.2.1.3.1
Ocular and CNS Lymphoma

Ocular lymphoma is known to be associated with primary CNS NHL in 6 to 10% of cases, and to precede the disease in 10% (Fig. 5.18) (BLAY 1997). Furthermore, 10 to 20% of relapses occur in the eyeball (HOCHBERG and MILLER 1988; BLAY 1997). The

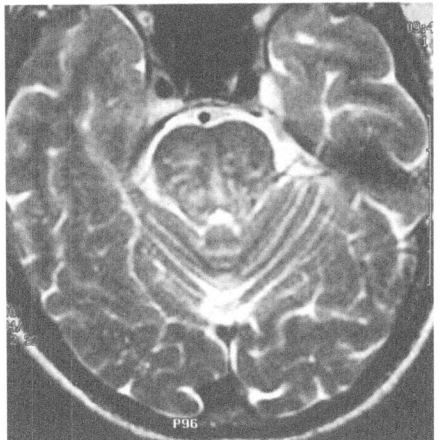

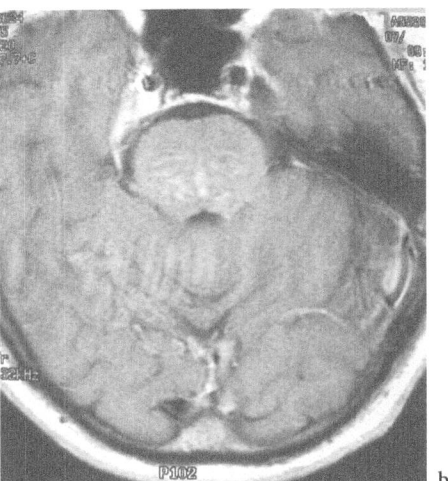

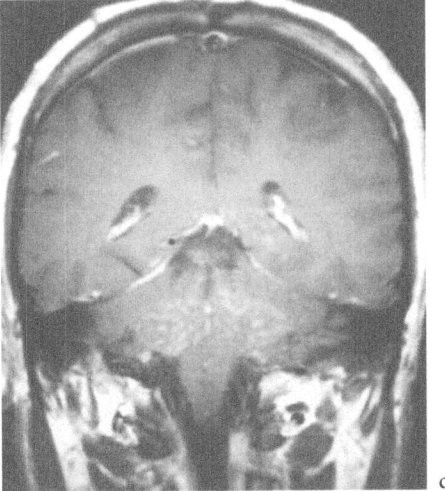

Fig. 5.12a–c. Cerebral non-Hodgkin lymphoma in a 60-year-old man who presented with ataxia and diplopia. **a** Axial T2-weighted MR image shows multiple bilateral hyperintense foci of the pons without mass effect. **b** Axial and (**c**) coronal contrast-enhanced T1-weighted MR images show multiple punctate enhancements, corresponding most likely to involvement of the Virchow-Robin spaces. (*Image courtesy of Dr. A. Guermazi*)

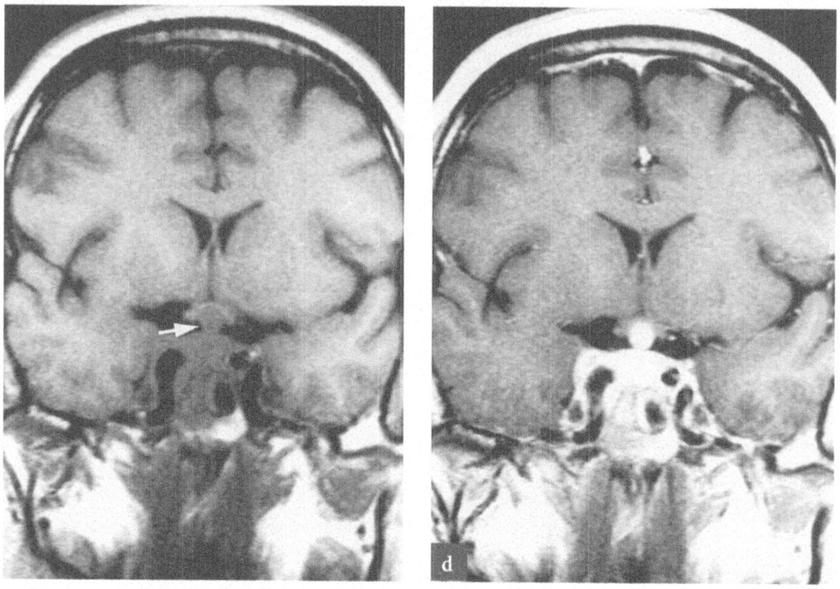

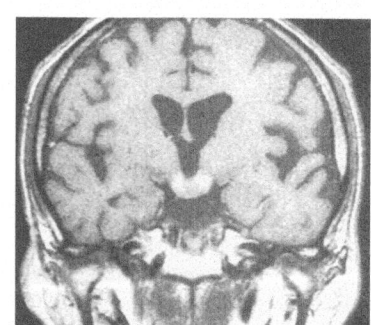

Fig. 5.13a–d. Cerebral primary non-Hodgkin lymphoma in a 28-year-old man involving the pituitary stalk. **a** Sagittal and (**b**) coronal unenhanced T1-weighted MR images demonstrate thickened, slightly hypointense pituitary stalk (*arrow*) which strongly and homogeneously enhances (**c, d**) after contrast administration.

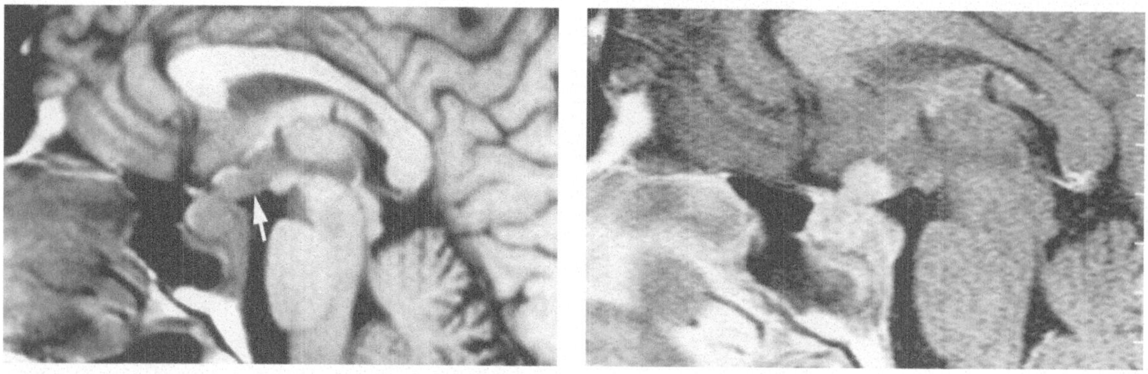

Fig. 5.14a–c. Cerebral primary non-Hodgkin lymphoma in a 59-year-old woman involving the opto-chiasmatic cistern. **a** Sagittal unenhanced T1-weighted MR image shows an extensive isointense supra-sellar mass involving the anterior optic pathways (*arrow*). **b** Sagittal and (**c**) coronal contrast-enhanced T1-weighted MR images show strong and homogenous enhancement of the lesion. *(Image courtesy of Dr. Y. Miaux)*

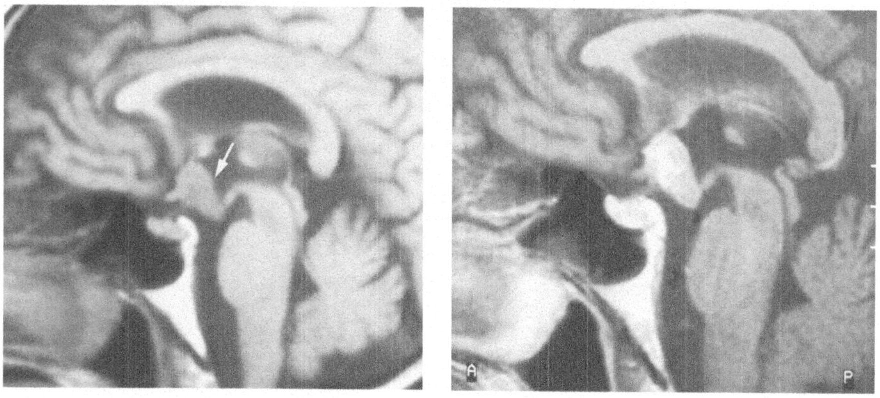

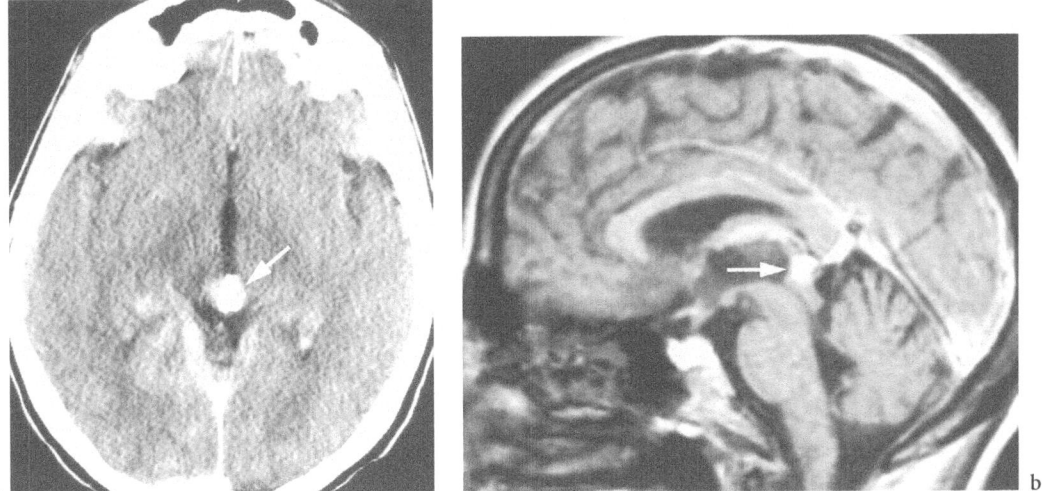

Fig. 5.15a,b. Cerebral primary non-Hodgkin lymphoma in a 38-year-old man involving the pineal gland. **a** Axial CT scan and (**b**) sagittal T1-weighted MR image after contrast administration show a focal lesion of the pineal gland (*arrow*) with significant enhancement. (*Image courtesy of Dr. Y. Miaux*)

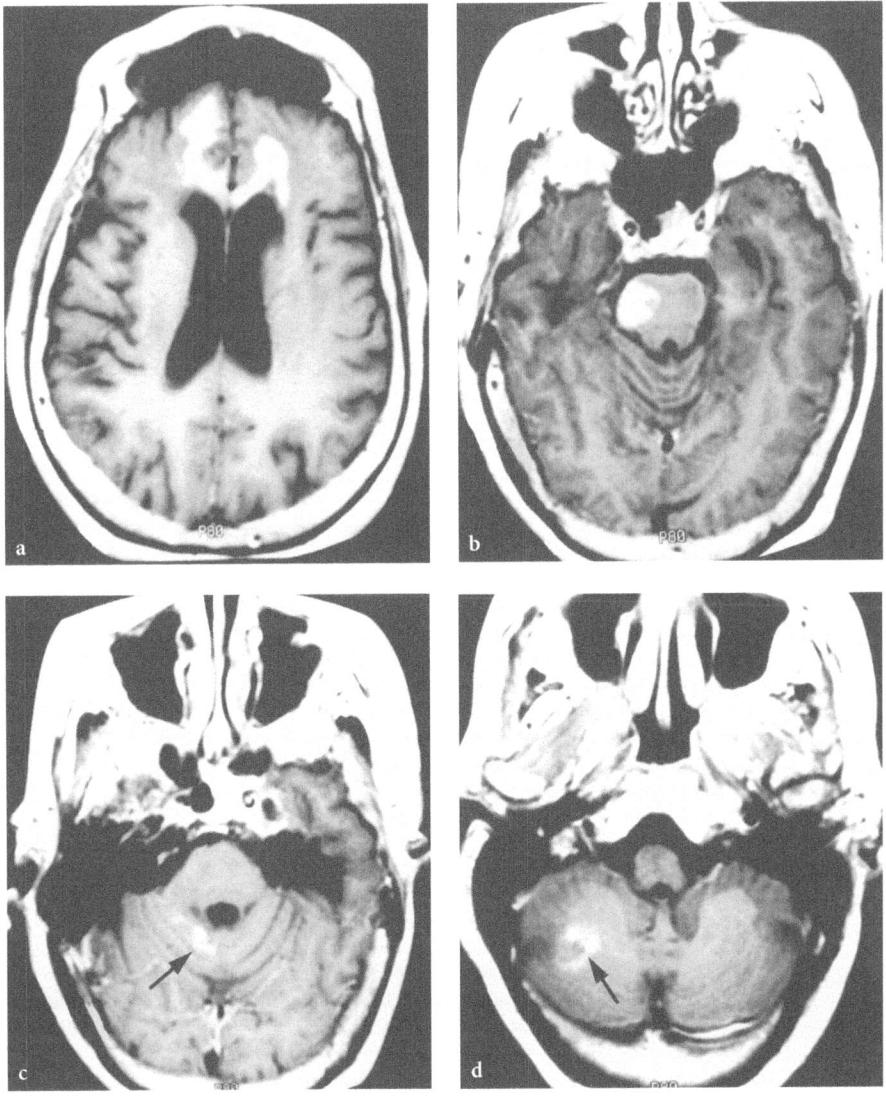

Fig. 5.16a–d. Multifocal cerebral non-Hodgkin lymphoma in an 80-year-old woman who presented with sensory loss. **a** Axial contrast-enhanced T1-weighted MR image shows a strong and homogenous enhancing area involving the frontal lobes and the genu of the corpus callosum. Several other contrast-enhanced lesions are visible involving (**b**) the pons, (**c**) the vermis (*arrow*) and (**d**) the inferior part of the right cerebellar hemisphere (*arrow*). (With permission from [Coulon et al. 2002])

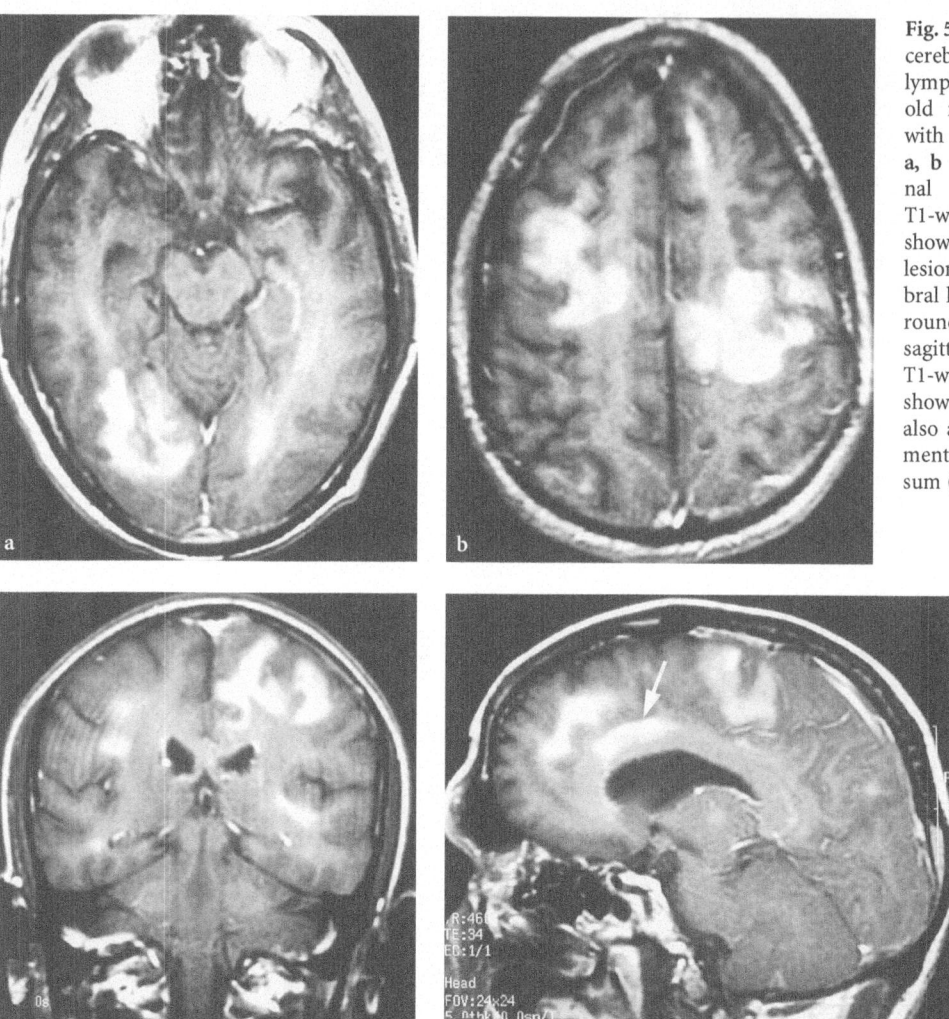

Fig. 5.17a–d. Multifocal cerebral non-Hodgkin lymphoma in a 49-year-old man who presented with brutal headache. **a, b** Axial and (**c**) coronal contrast-enhanced T1-weighted MR images show bilateral extensive lesions involving all cerebral lobes. Note mild surrounding edema. **d** Midsagittal contrast-enhanced T1-weighted MR image shows these lesions but also an extensive involvement of the corpus callosum (*arrow*).

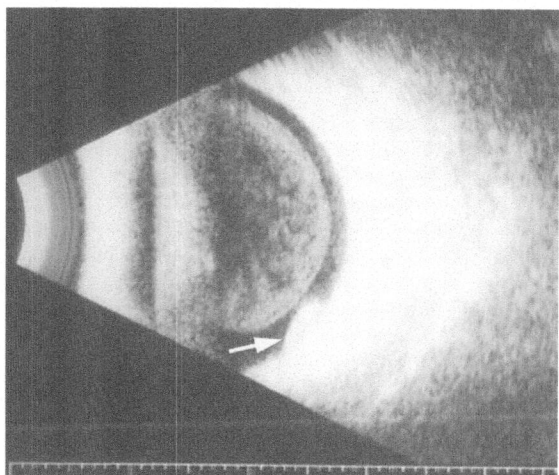

Fig. 5.18. Cerebral primary non-Hodgkin lymphoma in a 56-year-old man who presented with local recurrence, and abnormality of the posterior segment of the eye at the ophthalmologic exam. B-Mode US image of the eyeball demonstrates multiple thin echoes in the vitreous corresponding to lymphomatous cells, associated with a choroidal location of lymphoma (*arrow*).

lymphomatous cells can be found in the vitreous, choroid, retina, and optic nerve sheath. The presence of lymphomatous cells in the vitreous may be due to the direct propagation of tumoral cells from the brain to the eyeball via the subarachnoid spaces of the optic nerve sheath. In all cases of suspected primary CNS NHL, an ophthalmologic exam is mandatory to search for uveitis or hyalitis, since half of cases with ocular involvement are asymptomatic. With suggestive abnormalities such as uveitis or hyalitis, a vitreous biopsy may avoid an invasive brain biopsy, a concern especially in elderly patients (COULON et al. 2002; MAALOUF et al. 1997; ANGIOI-DUPREZ et al. 2002; HERAN et al. 2001).

5.2.1.3.2
Endovascular Lymphoma

In endovascular forms, also called intravascular malignant lymphomatosis, the histological findings are an extensive infiltration of small vascular structures of the brain by tumoral lymphocytes, leading to secondary vascular occlusion (MARTIN-DUVER-NEUIL et al. 2002). CNS involvement is frequent, but neurological symptoms as well as MR imaging findings are varied and nonspecific. Edema, infarct-like lesion of the cortex and basal ganglia related to vessel occlusion, or involvement of the white matter, are rarely found (Fig. 5.19). However, radial lesions of the white matter are suggestive. After contrast administration, enhancement is often moderate, but can be absent.

5.2.1.3.3
Brain metastases of a systemic lymphoma

Brain metastases usually involve the leptomeninges, leading to meningeal enhancement of basal cisterns, particularly affecting the cranial nerves, and sometimes meningeal structures of the convexity. Such patterns can also be observed in leukemias and leptomeningeal metastases, especially those from breast cancer, small-cell lung cancers, and in CSF dissemination of medulloblastomas and ependymomas (MARSAULT et al. 1991). However, lack of contrast enhancement also occurs, and hydrocephalus may be the only telltale sign (GROSSMAN and YOUSEM 1994). Dural invasion is very rare. Parenchymal locations are also rare: they are usually smaller than in primary CNS NHL and are more commonly multifocal.

5.2.1.4
New Imaging Techniques

5.2.1.4.1
Diffusion and perfusion imaging

Cerebral lymphomas often appear hyperintense in diffusion-weighted sequences (Fig. 5.20), with moderate decrease of the apparent diffusion coefficient (ADC). This may be related to the hypercellularity of this type of tumor. After bolus contrast injection, there is no peak of perfusion, and the relative cerebral blood volume (rCBV) value increases mildly in comparison to the adjacent normal brain, but less so

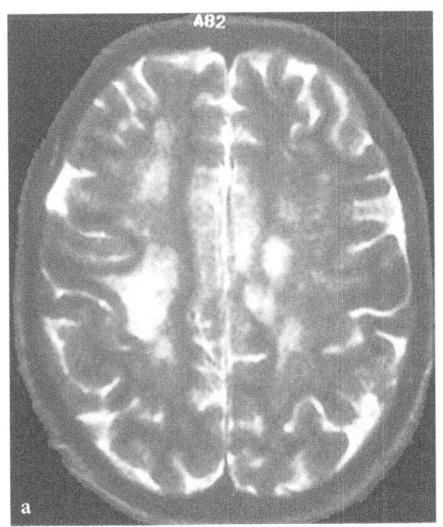 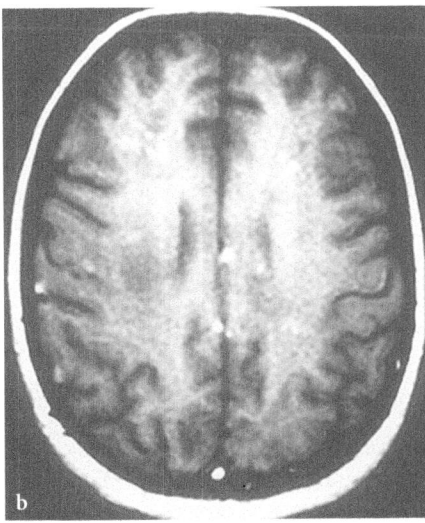

Fig. 5.19a,b. Cerebral intravascular malignant lymphomatosis in a 38-year-old man. **a** Axial T2-weighted MR image shows multiple hyperintense supratentorial lesions. **b** Axial contrast-enhanced T1-weighted MR image reveals numerous punctate cortical and subcortical enhancing spots. *(Image courtesy of Dr. N. Martin-Duverneuil)*

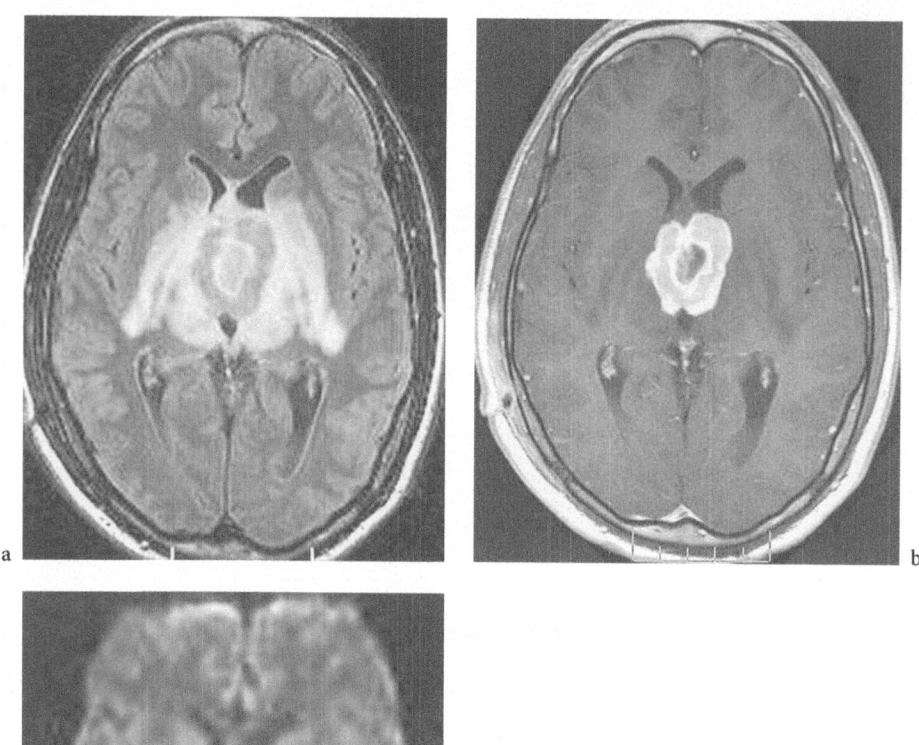

Fig. 5.20a–c. Cerebral non-Hodgkin lymphoma in a 20-year-old man who presented with headache and consciousness trouble. a Axial fluid-attenuated inversion recovery (FLAIR) MR image shows heterogeneous lesion around the third ventricle, isointense to brain parenchyma with central necrosis. b Axial contrast-enhanced T1-weighted MR image shows a strong rim enhancement of the lesion. c Axial echo-planar diffusion MR image shows the hyperintense periphery of the tissular part of the lymphoma, and the hypointense central necrosis.

than in high grade gliomas or metastases. The pattern observed in lymphomas is very different than in malignant gliomas, where a strong perfusion peak is usually observed (SUGAHARA et al. 1999).

5.2.1.4.2
Proton MR spectroscopy

Both primary and secondary lymphomas may involve the CNS. Marked elevation of the choline/creatine (Cho/Cr) ratio, significant reduction of the N-acetylaspartate (NAA)/Cr ratio, reduction of the Cr peak, and marked elevation of lipid/lactate resonances are common features of primary brain lymphoma, as are intra-axial masses. Activated macrophages within the lesion contain large amounts of mobile lipids, thus leading to an elevated lipid peak. Similar pattern spectra in gliomatosis and metastases can be encountered. Most secondary brain lymphomas are in leptomeningeal locations, allowing poor or no spectral characterization. As for other brain tumors, follow-up during therapy may be useful, showing a progressive reduction of Choline peak, increased NAA and Cr, and disappearance of lipid/lactate resonance, but without total recovery.

5.2.2
Immunodeficient Patient

5.2.2.1
General Considerations

Primary CNS lymphomas in immunodeficient patients, mostly with AIDS but also in other immunodepressive states, are related to chronic Epstein-Barr virus (EBV) infection, and present different patterns than lymphomas of immunocompetent patients. These lymphomas are often multifocal, ranging from 41% to 81% in clinical series (FINE and MAYER 1993; MIKOL et al. 1995) and from 80% to 100% in autopsy series (CHANG and ERNST 1997). They often grow rapidly, more than doubling in size within weeks. The rapid growth of the tumor is responsible for the preponderance of vascular supply at the edge of the tumor, leading to frequent

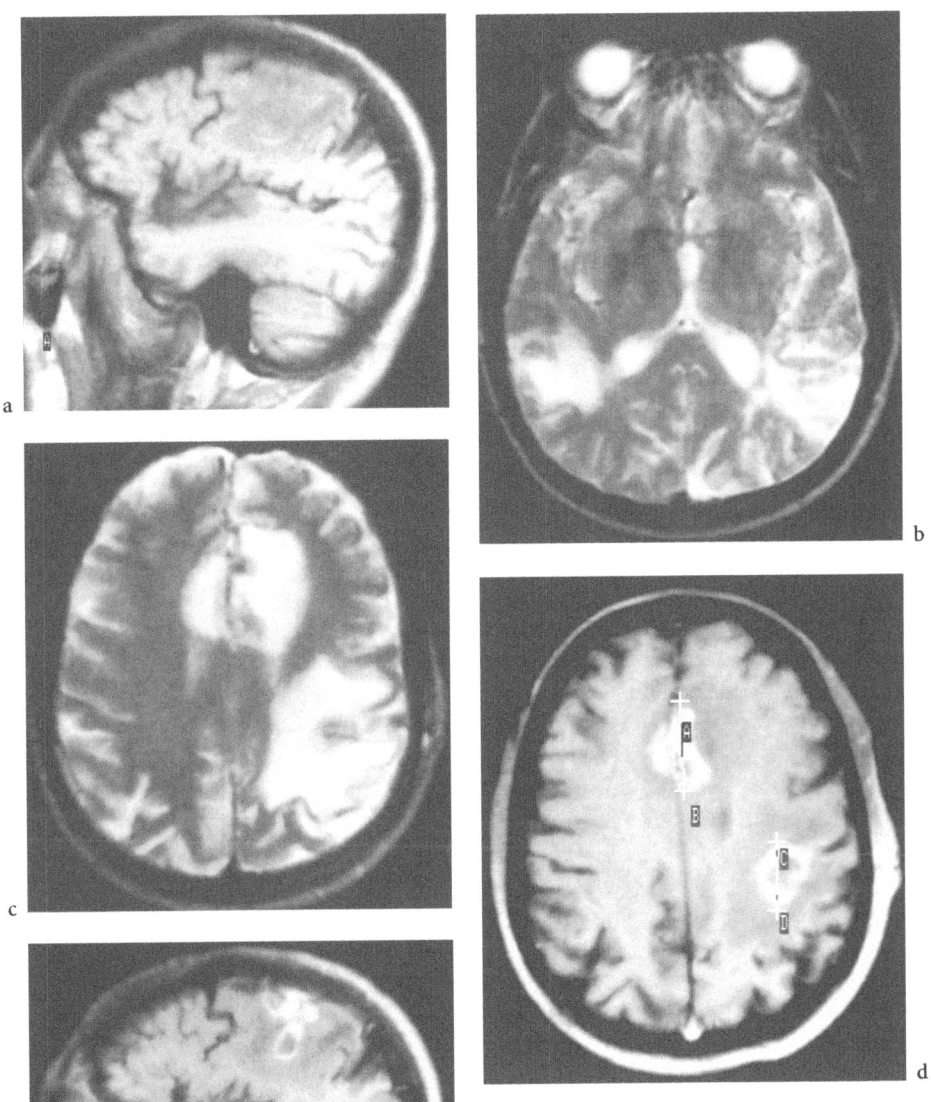

Fig. 5.21a–e. Cerebral multifocal non-Hodgkin lymphoma in a 52-year-old HIV positive man. **a** Sagittal unenhanced T1-weighted MR image shows hypointense parietal lesion. **b, c** Axial T2-weighted MR images demonstrate multiple ill-defined lesions involving both frontal and occipital lobes, surrounded by vasogenic edema. **d** Axial and (**e**) sagittal contrast-enhanced T1-weighted MR images show a heterogeneous enhancement of the different lesions, with central areas of necrosis. This pattern is often observed in lymphomas in AIDS patients, and makes the differential diagnosis with toxoplasmosis difficult.

areas of central necrosis, creating the ring pattern frequently observed after contrast administration (58% of cases), unlike the nodular enhancement usually observed in immunocompetent patients (Fig. 5.21). However, the other characteristics of the lesions do not differ from lymphoma in immunocompetent patients, with hyperdensity on CT, frequent iso or hypointensity on T2-weighted MR images, and mild or weak edema and mass effect. Spontaneous hemorrhage is uncommon but may occur after therapy with steroids or radiations (CHANG and ERNST 1997).

The main differential diagnoses are opportunist infections, especially toxoplasmosis. In toxoplasmosis, the lesions usually are smaller than in lymphoma, are located in the corticomedullary junction, thalamus or basal ganglia, are hyperintense on T2-weighted MR sequence, and are often multiple and sometimes hemorrhagic. The enhancement is usually annular and delayed compared to lymphoma. To distinguish lymphoma from toxoplasmosis, an antitoxoplasmic treatment is administered for eight days, before follow-up MR imaging. In lymphoma, there is a rapid increase in the size of the tumor (CORDOLIANI et al. 1992).

In AIDS related lymphoma, isolated ventriculitis can also be observed. An associated nodular enhancement is highly suggestive of lymphoma. In this context, a diffuse and thin enhancement is suggestive of a viral etiology such as cytomegalovirus (CMV) or varicella-zoster virus (VZV). A meningeal location with involvement of the cranial vault has also been described (THURNHER et al. 2001). Note that in AIDS patients, cerebral involvement of systemic lymphoma occurs in 25 to 40% of patients and is much more common than primary CNS lymphoma, which occurs in only about 5% of patients. As in immunocompetent patients, this secondary lymphoma usually involves the leptomeninges.

5.2.2.2
New Imaging Techniques

Since lymphoma in AIDS can display a large variety of patterns, and is often difficult to differentiate from toxoplasmosis, new imaging techniques have been developed to avoid brain biopsy in difficult cases.
1) *Dynamic MR imaging.* On dynamic contrast-enhanced MR imaging, lymphoma displays significantly greater enhancement than toxoplasmosis (LAISSY et al. 1994).
2) *Nuclear studies.* Thallium-201 single photon emission computed tomography (SPECT) scanning and 2-fluorine-18-fluoro-2-deoxy-D-glucose positron emission tomography (FDG-

PET) show promise for differentiating lymphoma from infectious lesions such as toxoplasmosis, with uptake of the isotope greater in lymphoma (JÄGER and RICH 2001; RUIZ et al. 1994). Sestamibi (MIBI) SPECT may also be helpful.
3) *Proton MR spectroscopy.* MR spectroscopy of lymphoma in AIDS shows a markedly elevated Choline peak, probably due to the increased cellularity and cell membrane turnover. There is a moderate elevation of lipids and lactate, with preservation of some normal metabolites. In a toxoplasmic lesion, lipids and lactate are markedly elevated, and other normal brain metabolites are virtually absent. However, these findings are not pathognomonic, and multiple pathologies are not uncommon in AIDS (CHANG and ERNST 1997; JÄGER and RICH 2001).
4) *Diffusion and perfusion imaging.* In lymphoma, the ADC is often decreased, and an increased rCBV is observed, in opposition to the toxoplasmosis abscess where the rCBV is reduced (MONJOUR et al. 1992).

5.3
Spinal Cord, Meninges and Roots

5.3.1
Primitive Lymphoma of the Spinal Cord

Primitive lymphoma of the spinal cord is rare (Fig. 5.22). It presents as a focal lesion surrounded by edema, with moderate mass effect. After contrast administration, enhancement of the lesion is strong and sometimes heterogeneous. Endovascular lymphoma of the spine is exceptional; it presents as a focal lesion of the spine, hyperintense on T2-weighted MR images, sometimes without enhancement.

5.3.2
Epidural Lymphoma

Primitive epidural lymphoma is also rare (Fig. 5.23). On MR imaging, the lesion presents as an epidural mass of linear shape, hypointense on T2-weighted sequences compared to CSF, with strong enhancement after contrast administration. Bony lyses are rare.

More frequent is epidural extension of a lymphoma involving the spine, or parameningeal masses extending from nodal locations of NHL. These lesions can grow through the intervertebral foramina (GROSSMAN and YOUSEM 1994).

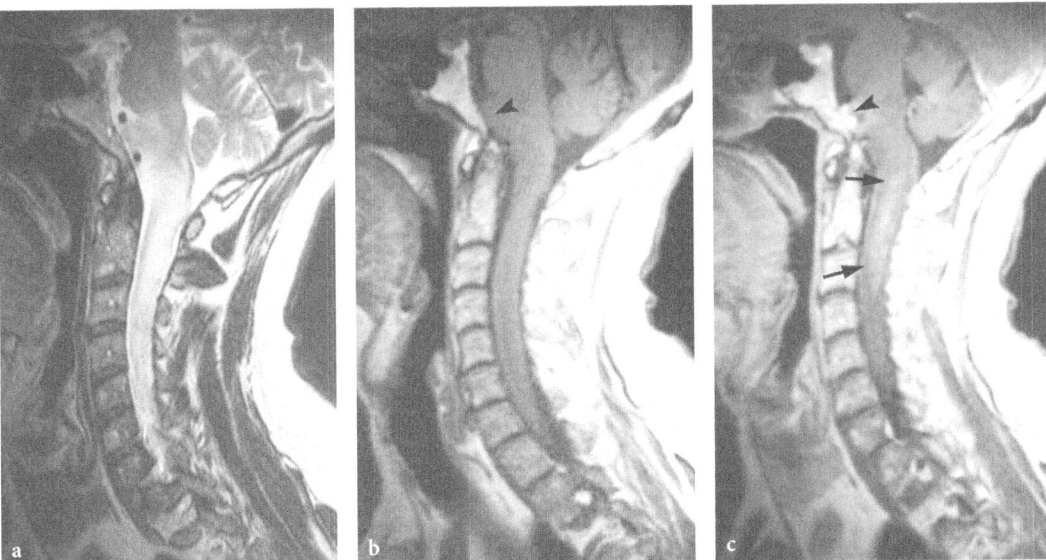

Fig. 5.22a–c. Intramedullary non-Hodgkin lymphoma in a 54-year-old man who presented with inferior limbs weakness. **a** Sagittal fast spin-echo T2-weighted MR image of the cervical spine shows an intramedullary hyperintense lesion extending from C1 to C3, involving also the inferior part of the medulla oblongata. **b** The lesion is isointense on sagittal unenhanced T1-weigthed MR image. **c** Sagittal contrast-enhanced T1-weighted MR image demonstrates enhancement of the lesion (*arrows*). Also note an isointense retroclival epidural mass (*arrowhead*) in (**b**) that strongly enhances in (**c**).

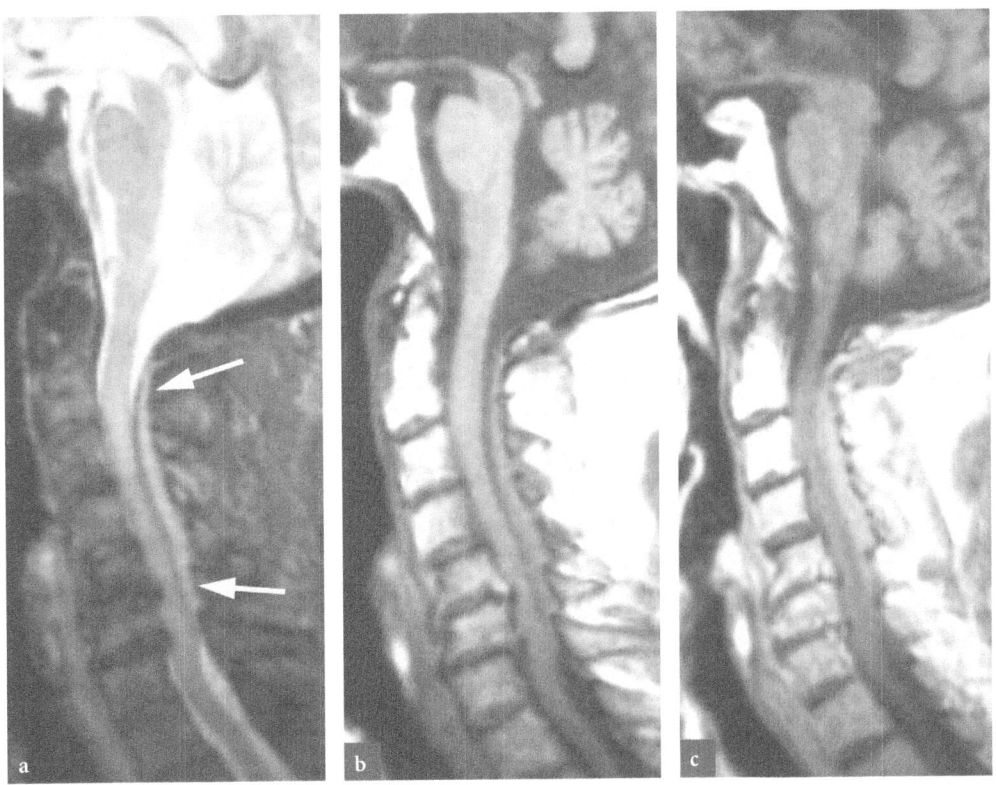

Fig. 5.23a–c. Spinal epidural non-Hodgkin lymphoma in a 47-year-old-man who presented with paraparesis. **a** Sagittal fat-suppressed T2-weighted MR image of the cervical spine shows a posterior epidural mass, isointense to the medulla, extending from the inferior part of C2 to C6 (*arrows*). Sagittal T1-weighted MR images show the lesion is isointense to the medulla (**b**) on unenhanced image, and enhances homogenously (**c**) after contrast administration.

5.3.3
Leptomeningeal Lymphoma

Leptomeningeal lymphomas are mostly a meningeal dissemination of a systemic lymphoma, especially at the late stage, or dissemination from a primitive brain lymphoma via the subarachnoid route (Fig. 5.24). Primitive leptomeningeal lymphomas are unusual (MONJOUR et al. 1992) and present the same pattern. In both cases, the lesions are difficult to see on plain T1 and T2-weighted MR sequences. Sometimes, the CSF signal is modified, and the conspicuity between CSF and cord may be diminished. They are much more obvious after contrast administration, which yields linear or nodular enhancement on nerve roots and/or in the cauda equina. In late stage disease, an enhancement of the entire subarachnoid space is found, called "sugar-coated appearance", as seen in metastatic infiltration (GROSSMAN and YOUSEM 1994). Sometimes, the lesions are less evident, with only a linear enhancement on the surface of the cord (pial metastases). The main differential diagnoses include subarachnoid metastases, mostly breast, lung and gastric carcinomas, dissemination of brain or spinal cord tumors such as medulloblastoma, ependymoma and glioblastoma, and inflammatory processes such as tuberculosis and sarcoidosis.

5.4
Conclusion

The frequency of cerebral lymphoma has increased steadily in the past 20 years, in both immunocompromised and immunocompetent patients. This diagnosis should not be overlooked, because it allows specific treatment. Although CT and MR imaging features are often evocative, atypical patterns are frequent and should be known, especially in AIDS patients. New imaging techniques like MR spectroscopy, diffusion-perfusion imaging and specific scintigraphies are useful in difficult cases, to avoid whenever possible an invasive brain biopsy, especially for deep brain lesions.

Acknowledgements
The authors thank Gilles Podevins for printing the images.

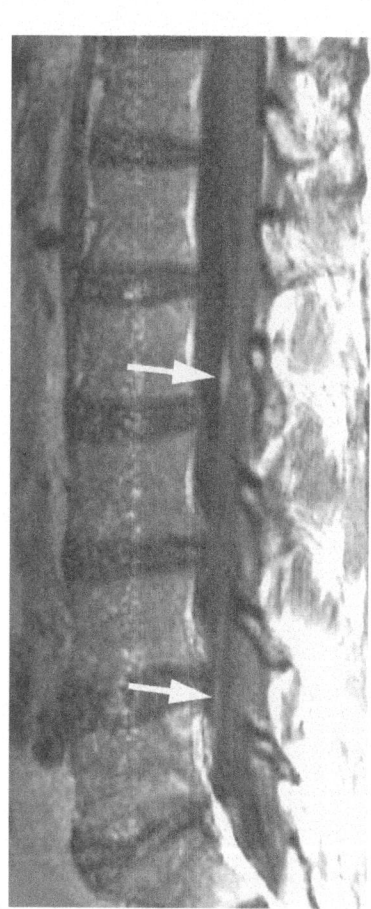 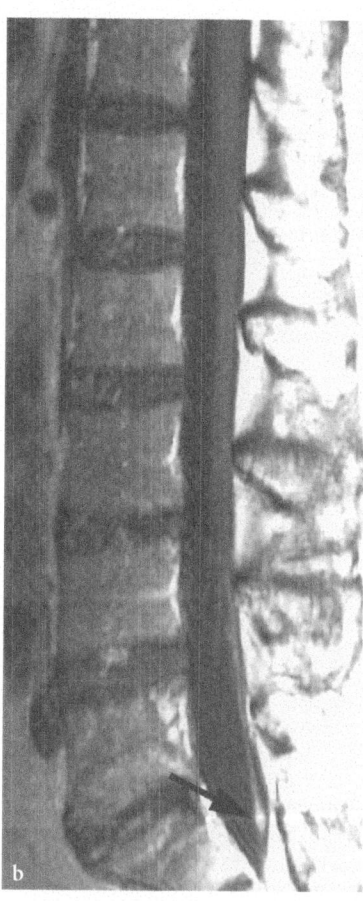

Fig. 5.24a,b. Leptomeningeal non-Hodgkin lymphoma in a 59-year-old-man who presented with a cerebral lymphoma and inferior limbs pain. **a, b** Sagittal contrast-enhanced fat-suppressed T1-weighted MR images of the lumbar spine show slight thickening of the lumbar arachnoid space with nodular enhancement of the cauda equina roots (*arrows*).

References

Angioi-Duprez K, Taillandier L, Gerin M, Berrod JP, George JL, Maalouf T (2002) Ocular involvement during primary central nervous system lymphoma. J Fr Ophtalmol 25: 147–153

Arrue P, Manelfe C, Delannes M, Prere J (1987) Cerebral localizations of non Hodgkin's malignant lymphomas. Contribution of X-ray computed tomography. J Radiol 68:777–784

Ashby MA, Bowen D, Bleehen NM, Barber PC, Freer CEL (1988) Primary lymphoma of the central nervous system: experience at Addenbrooke's hospital, Cambridge. Clin Radiol 39:173–181

Balmaceda C, Gaynor JJ, Sun M, Gluck JT, DeAngelis LM (1995) Leptomeningeal tumor in primary central nervous system lymphoma: recognition, significance, and implications. Ann Neurol 38:202–209

Blay JY (1997) Primary cerebral non-Hodgkin lymphoma in non-immunocompromised subjects. Bull Cancer 84: 976–980

Brown JH, Stallmeyer MJ, Lustrin ES, Chew FS (1995) Primary cerebral lymphoma. Am J Roentgenol 165:626

Canaple S, Rosa A, Deramond H, Desablens B, Legars D (1996) Clinico-radiological data of 48 cases of immunocompetent primary cerebral lymphoma. Rev Neurol 152:528–535

Carlson A (1996) Rapidly progressive dementia caused by nonenhancing primary lymphoma of the central nervous system. Am J Neuroradiol 17:1695–1697

Cellerier P, Chiras J, Gray F, Metzger J, Bories J (1984) Computed tomography in primary lymphoma of the brain. Neuroradiology 26:485–492

Chang L, Ernst T (1997) MR spectroscopy and diffusion-weighted imaging in focal brain lesions in AIDS. Neuroimaging Clin N Am 7:409–426

Cordoliani YS, Derosier C, Pharaboz C, Jeanbourquin D, Schill H, Cosnard G (1992) Primary brain lymphoma in AIDS. 17 cases studied by MRI before stereotaxic biopsies. J Radiol 6–7:367–376

Coulon A, Lafitte F, Hoang-Xuan K, Martin-Duverneuil N, Mokhtari K, Blustajn J, Chiras J (2002) Radiographic findings in 37 cases of primary CNS lymphoma in immunocompetent patients. Eur Radiol 12:329–340

DeAngelis LM (1993) Cerebral lymphoma presenting as a nonenhancing lesion on computed tomographic/magnetic resonance scan. Ann Neurol 33:308–311

DeAngelis M (1995) Current management of primary central nervous system lymphoma. Oncology 9:63–78

De la Blanchardiere A, Lesprit P, Molina JM, Zagdanski AM, Hennequin C, Garrait V, Decazes JM, Modai J (1997) Primary cerebral lymphoma in AIDS. Retrospective study of 20 patients. Presse Med 26:940–944

Ernst TM, Chang L, Witt MD, Aronow HA, Cornford ME, Walot I, Goldberg MA (1998) Cerebral toxoplasmis and lymphoma in AIDS: perfusion MR imaging experience in 13 patients. Radiology 208:663–669

Fine H, Mayer R (1993) Primary central nervous system lymphoma. Ann Intern Med 119:1093–1104

Furusawa T, Okamoto K, Ito J, Kojima N, Oyanagi K, Tokiguchi S, Sakai K (1998) Primary Central Nervous System Lymphoma presenting as diffuse cerebral infiltration. Radiat Med 16:137–140

Geoffray A, Laurent F, Drouillard J, Balu-Maestro C, Rogopoulos A, Bruneton JN (1990) Tomodensitometric aspects of brain lymphomas: apropos of 19 cases. Bull Cancer 77: 681–688

Goldstein D, Zeifer B, Chao C, Moser G, Dickson D, Hirschfeld D, Davis L (1991) CT appearance of primary CNS Lymphoma in patients with acquired immunodeficiency syndrome. J Comput Assist Tomogr 15:39–41

Grossman RI, Yousem DM (1994) Neuroradiology: the requisites, 1st edn. Mosby, St Louis

Gutmann J, Kendall B (1994) Unusual appearances of Primary Central Nervous System Non-Hodgkin's lymphoma. Clin Radiol 49:696–702

Heran F, Lafitte F, Berroir S, Blustajn J, Parrat E (2001) Atypical cerebral lymphoma with ocular onset: report of a case. J Neuroradiol 28:264–267

Hochberg FH, Miller DC (1988) Primary central nervous system lymphoma. J Neurosurg 68:835–853

Isla A, Alvarez F, Gutierrez M, Gamallo C, Garcia-Blazquez M, Vega A (1996) Primary cranial vault lymphoma mimicking meningioma. Neuroradiology 38:211–213

Jäger R, Rich P (2001) Cranial and intracranial pathology: intracranial tumours in adults. In: Grainger RG, Allisson DJ, Adam A, Dixon AK (eds) Diagnostic radiology: a textbook of medical imaging. Churchill-Livingstone, London, pp 2325–2350

Jenkins CN, Colquhoun IR (1998) Characterization of primary intracranial lymphoma by computed tomography: an analysis of 36 cases and a review of the literature with particular reference to calcification, haemorrhage and cyst formation. Clin Radiol 53:428–434

Johnson BA, Fram EK, Johnson PC, Jacobowitz RJ (1997) The variable MR appearance of primary lymphoma of the central nervous system: comparison with histopathologic features. Am J Neuroradiol 18:563–572

Koeller KK, Smirniotopoulos JG, Jones RV (1997) Primary central nervous system lymphoma: radiologic-pathologic correlation. Radiographics 17:1497–1526

Laissy JP, Soyer P, Tebboune J, Gay-Depassier P, Casalino E, Lariven S, Sibert A, Menu Y (1994) Contrast-enhanced fast MRI in differentiating brain toxoplasmosis and lymphomas in AIDS patients. J Comput Assist Tomogr 18: 714–718

Lanfermann H, Heindel W, Schaper J, Schröder R, Hansmann ML, Lehrke R, Ernestus RI (1997) CT and MRI imaging in primary cerebral non-hodgkin's lymphoma. Acta Radiologica 38:259–267

Maalouf T, Angioi-Duprez K, Guibaud I, Baty V, May T, Plenat F, Canton P, George JL (1997) Malignant non-Hodgkin lymphoma of the central nervous system with ocular site. Value of vitrectomy for diagnosis. J Fr Ophtalmol 20:693–696

Marelle L, Raphael M, Henin D, Vazeux R, Schuller E, Piette JC, Poisson M, Gentilini M, Hauw JJ (1994) Cerebral lymphoma in AIDS: clinical study and clinicopathological correlations. Rev Neurol 150:123–132

Marsault C, Le Bras F, Gaston A (1991) Imagerie du système nerveux, 2nd edn. Flammarion, Paris

Martin-Duverneuil N, Mokhtari K, Behin A, Lafitte F, Hoang-Xuan K, Chiras J (2002) Intravascular malignant lymphomatosis. Neuroradiology 44:749–754

Mikol J, Costagliola D, Polivka M, Thiebaut JB, Trotot P (1995) The epidemiology of cerebral lymphoma in AIDS. J Neuroradiol 22:204–206

Monjour A, Poisson M, Kujas M, Delattre JY (1992) Primary non-Hodgkin's malignant lymphoma of the central nervous system. Rev Neurol 148:589–600

Murray PA, Harnett AN, Thompson PI, Charlesworth M, Plowman PN (1989) Periventricular enhancement: a non-pathognomonic sign of intracerebral tumors. Br J Radiol 62:1075–1078

Namasivayam J, Teasdale E (1992) The prognostic importance of CT features in primary intracranial lymphoma. Br J Radiol 65:761–765

Osborn AG (1994) Brain tumors and tumorlike processes diagnostic. In: Osborn A (ed) Diagnostic neuroradiology. Mosby, St Louis, pp 620–622

Parekh H, Sharma RR, Keogh AJ, Prabhu SS (1993) Primary malignant non-Hodgkin's lymphoma of cranial vault: a case report. Surg Neurol 39:286–289

Patchell RA (1995) Metastatic brain tumors. Neurol Clin 13: 915–917

Petiot P, Croisile B, Bret P, Trillet M, Aimard G (1995) An aspect of intracerebral lymphoma in scanner X mimicking meningioma. Rev Neurol 151:580–582

Ruiz A, Ganz WI, Post MJ, Camp A, Landy H, Mallin W, Sfakianakis GN (1994) Use of Thallium-201 brain SPECT to differentiate cerebral lymphoma from toxoplasma encephalitis in AIDS patients. Am J Neuroradiol 15: 1885–1894

Ruiz A, Post MJ, Bundschu C, Ganz WI, Georgiou M (1997) Primary central nervous system lymphoma in patients with AIDS. Neuroimaging Clin N Am 7:281–296

Schwaighofer BW, Hesselink RJ, Press GA, Wolf RL, Healy ME, Berthoty DP (1989) Primary intracranial CNS lymphoma: MR manifestations. Am J Neuroradiol 10:725–729

Sugahara T, Korogi Y, Shigematsu Y, Hirai T, Ikushima I, Liang L, Ushio Y, Takahashi M (1999) Perfusion-sensitive MRI of cerebral lymphomas: a preliminary report. J Comput Assist Tomogr 23:232–237

Thurnher MM, Rieger A, Kleibl-Popov C, Schindler E (2001) Malignant lymphoma of the cranial vault in an HIV-positive patient: imaging findings. Eur Radiol 11:1506–1509

Ueda F, Takashima T, Suzuki M, Kadoya M, Yamashita J, Kida T (1995) MR Imaging of intracerebral malignant lymphoma. Radiat Med 13:51–57

Watanabe M, Tanaka R, Wakabayashi K, Takahashi H (1992) Correlation of computed tomography with the histopathology of primary malignant lymphoma of the brain. Neuroradiology 34:36–42

Zimmerman R (1990) Central nervous system lymphoma. Radiol Clin North Am 28:697–721

6 Head and Neck Involvement in Non-Hodgkin Lymphoma

MATTHEW C. HULL, ILONA M. SCHMALFUSS, NANCY PRICE MENDENHALL

CONTENTS

6.1 Introduction

Non-Hodgkin lymphomas are the most common hematological malignancies of the head and neck, comprising 5% of head and neck cancers (EVANS 1981). NHL often differs considerably from HD in presentation, behavior, treatment, and response. HD is characterized by contiguous disease sites with predictable responses to therapy, while NHL is a heterogeneous group of less predictable malignancies. The classification of NHL has evolved continually over the last 30 to 40 years. New techniques such as immunophenotyping, flow cytometry, and molecular genetic studies have revolutionized our understanding of NHL. Unique subclassifications have been identified that help predict the wide variations of behavior and response within what was previously classified as a single entity.

Treatment requires close cooperation among the surgeon, pathologist, radiologist, and medical and radiation oncologists. Surgery typically is restricted to obtaining tissue for diagnosis. Fine-needle aspiration may occasionally be sufficient, although excisional biopsy is generally preferred for assessment of the nodal architecture. Chemotherapy and radiation therapy both play major roles in treatment, often in combination. Low grade localized disease is often treated with radiation therapy alone. Advanced stage disease and intermediate to high-grade disease are typically treated with chemotherapy alone or sequentially with radiation therapy.

6.2 Epidemiology and Etiology

The American Cancer Society estimates that, in the United States in 2003, 53,400 people (28,300 men and 25,100 women) will be diagnosed with NHL and that 23,400 will die from this disease. This accounts for 4.5% of all cancer diagnoses. The median age at diagnosis is 65 years (GLASS et al. 1997).

There is a strong viral association with at least two types of NHL. The Epstein-Barr virus can be detected in lymphoma cells of 90% of children with African Burkitt lymphoma and HTLV-1 has been identified in the cells of an aggressive form of peripheral T-cell lymphoma (LINDAHL et al. 1974; POIESZ et al. 1980). There is an increased incidence of NHL in immune deficiency states such as post-transplant, acquired immune deficiency syndrome, and congenital disorders such as ataxia teleangiectasis and Wiscott-Aldrich syndrome.

MATTHEW C. HULL, MD
Radiation Oncologist, Department of Radiation Oncology, University of Florida College of Medicine, 2000 SW Archer Road, PO Box 100385, Gainesville, FL 32610-0385, USA
ILONA M. SCHMALFUSS, MD
Assistant Professor, Department of Radiology, University of Florida College of Medicine, Gainesville, FL 32610, USA
NANCY PRICE MENDENHALL, MD
Professor and Chairman, Department of Radiation Oncology, University of Florida College of Medicine, 2000 SW Archer Road, PO Box 100385, Gainesville, FL 32610-0385, USA

Non-Hodgkin lymphoma may be present in the lymph nodes or in extranodal sites. Forty to 60% of NHL present in extranodal sites and 1/3 to 2/3 of extranodal lymphomas occur in the head and neck area (MILLION et al. 1994). The head and neck region is second only to the stomach in number of localized extranodal NHL. The presenting symptoms depend on the site but patients are frequently asymptomatic. The most common extranodal locations within the head and neck are Waldeyer's ring (lymphoid tissue of the tonsil, nasopharynx, and base of tongue), salivary glands, thyroid, paranasal sinuses, and nasal cavity. Other sites, such as larynx, hypopharynx, and oral cavity are involved less frequently.

The most commonly involved lymph nodes are the internal jugular nodes; the occipital, preauricular, parotid, submaxillary, and submental lymph nodes are more commonly involved in NHL than in HD. The classic systemic B symptoms, (drenching night sweats, unexplained fever higher than 38°C, weight loss more than 10% over the preceding 6 months) common in HD, occur in only 10–15% of NHL patients at presentation.

6.3
Pathology

A series of classifications has been used for NHL since the mid 1960s. The Rappaport, Lukes-Collins, and Kiel Classifications were based primarily on cell morphology. The Working Formulation, proposed in 1982 based on morphology and biologic aggressiveness, and commonly used in the United States, classifies entities into low, intermediate, and high-grade. Immunologic and genetic techniques distinguishing between B and T-cell lineage and various molecular phenotypes led to the development of the REAL classification of lymphoid neoplasms and the subsequent REAL/WHO classification, which defined each entity by virtue of its morphologic, immunophenotype, genetic, and clinical features. One of the areas of greatest impact for this new classification is in the head and neck region. The majority of primary lymphomas in this region are extranodal, and include previously unclassified subtypes such as extranodal marginal zone B-cell lymphoma of MALT type, mantle cell, and NK/T-cell lymphomas. The identification and separation of these new subgroups with different natural histories, treatments, and prognoses may help to explain the heterogeneity in outcome of previous studies that combined these

newly distinguished subtypes. Until recently, studies have reported outcomes using the Kiel or Working Formulation classifications. Consistent reporting of studies using the REAL/WHO classification is necessary to define the optimal treatments for each subtype.

6.4
Imaging

Non-Hodgkin lymphoma is in the differential diagnosis of almost any radiographic imaging pattern. It is particularly difficult to distinguish between extranodal presentations of NHL and the more common epithelial primaries in this location, but there are some patterns of involvement that suggest NHL. As with epithelial malignancies, cross-sectional imaging (CT or MR imaging) is invaluable for the diagnosis, staging, and evaluation of treatment response evaluation, and post-therapy surveillance of NHL in the head and neck.

6.4.1
General Imaging Features

Location and Local Growth
NHL typically arises in the submucosa of structures with lymphatic tissue, such as tonsils, nasopharynx, base of tongue, and salivary glands. The mucosa is rarely invaded so ulceration is uncommon. NHL has a tendency to "sneak" along pathways of least resistance; typically displacing rather than invading anatomic structures. Diffuse infiltration of adjacent structures may rarely occur with low grade NHL. Frank invasion and obstruction of adjacent structures typically occurs only with intermediate or high-grade NHL such as Burkitt and NK/T-cell lymphomas (Fig. 6.1).

Internal Imaging Characteristics
Typically, NHL demonstrates homogenous attenuation on all imaging modalities (Figs. 6.1, 6.2). Classically, it is slightly hyperintense compared to adjacent muscles on T2-weighted MR images (Fig. 6.1b). Central necrosis is uncommon except in very aggressive NHL (Figs. 6.3–6.5) or in patients who are severely immunocompromised as in HIV (Fig. 6.3). Calcifications are rarely seen in lymphomas at diagnosis (< 1%), but may develop after treatment of aggressive subtypes (APTER et al. 2002).

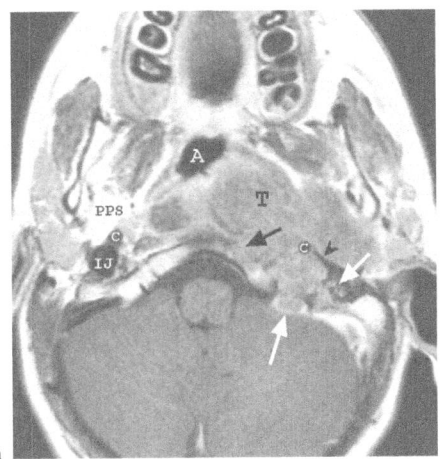
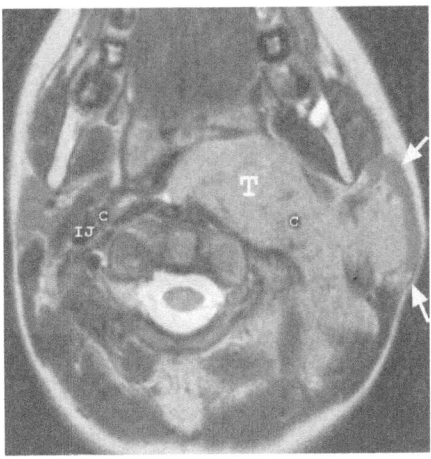

Fig. 6.1a,b. Parapharyngeal involvement in a 10-year-old boy with stage I Burkitt lymphoma. Axial MR images through the upper-neck demonstrate a large left parapharyngeal mass (*T*) with the classic imaging characteristics of lymphoma: homogenous enhancement on (**a**) contrast-enhanced T1-weighted image and slightly hyperintense compared to the adjacent muscles on (**b**) T2-weighted image. On (**a**), the tumor infiltrates the parapharyngeal fat planes on the left compared to the right (*PPS = parapharyngeal space*), compromises the upper airway (*A*), encases the internal carotid artery (*C*) posteriorly without luminal narrowing. The tumor also grows into the jugular foramen (*white arrows*) and completely compresses the internal jugular vein. Notice the normal appearance of the right internal jugular vein (*IJ*). In addition, the tumor wraps around the styloid process (*arrowhead*) without signs of erosion–a typical finding in lymphoma. However, there is disruption of the anterior cortex of the left inferior clivus (*black arrow*). This is a rather unusual finding in lymphoma but may happen in aggressive or large tumors. Notice also the hypointensity within the bone marrow just posterior to the cortical disruption. These findings are most consistent with additional bone marrow involvement. On (**b**), the mass infiltrates the deep and superficial lobes of the left parotid gland (*white arrows*).

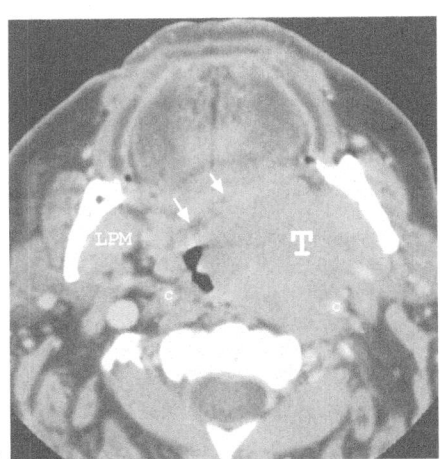
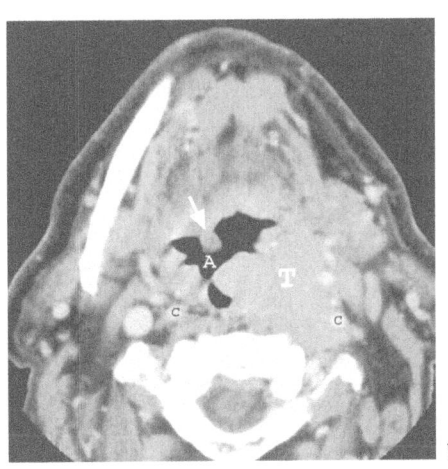

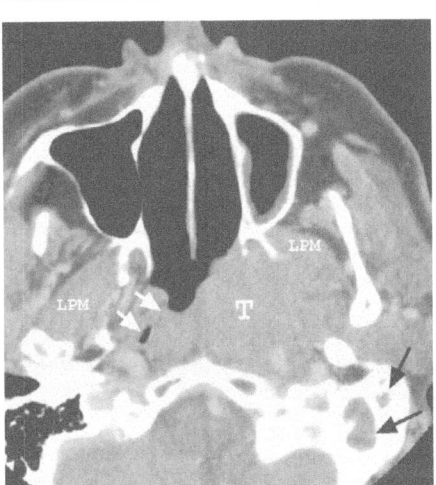

Fig. 6.2a–c. Tonsil involvement in a 68-year-old HIV positive man with stage II diffuse large B-cell lymphoma. **a, b** Axial contrast-enhanced CT scans demonstrate a large tumor (*T*) in the oropharynx involving the left lateral pharyngeal wall and pharyngeal space. The mass significantly compromises the upper airway (*A*). On (**a**), notice the complete obliteration of the left parapharyngeal fat planes. The left lateral pterygoid muscle (*LPM*) cannot be distinguished from the mass. This appearance could be due to infiltration and/or displacement of the lateral pterygoid muscle by the tumor. (The distinction could be made by MR imaging, see Fig. 6.1). The left internal carotid artery (*C*) is partially surrounded along its medial aspect by tumor without evidence of luminal narrowing. Notice also the marked anterior displacement of the uvula (*arrow*) on (**b**), and soft palate on the left, nicely indicated by the oblique position of the fat plane within the soft palate (*arrows*) on (**a**). **c** Axial contrast-enhanced CT scan cephalad to (**a, b**) shows the tumor (*T*) extending superiorly to involve the left nasopharyngeal soft tissues. The left lateral pterygoid muscle is displaced anteriorly. The left mastoid air cells (*black arrows*) are opacified secondary to obstruction of the eustachian tube by the tumor. Notice the normal appearance of the right eustachian tube opening (*white arrows*).

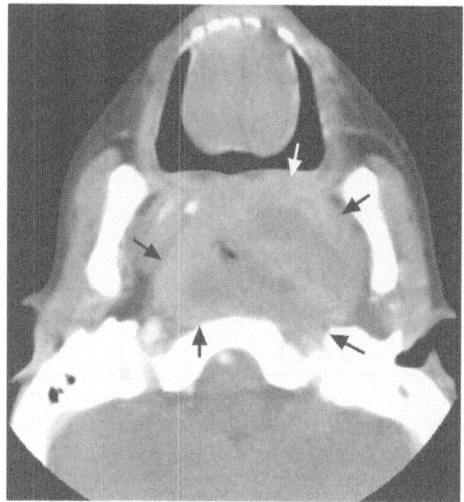
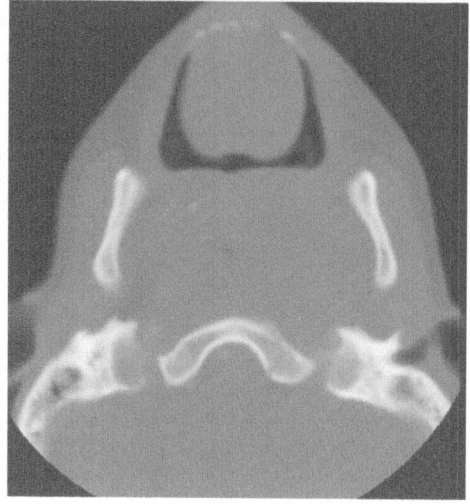

Fig. 6.3a,b. Nasopharyngeal involvement in an 8-year-old boy with AIDS and a diffuse large B-cell lymphoma. **a** Axial contrast-enhanced CT scan reveals a huge mass (*arrows*) in the nasopharynx bilaterally, worse on the left. The tumor shows an inhomogeneous enhancement pattern suggestive of focal necrosis typical of lymphoma in an immunocompromised patient. **b** The bone window image at the same level shows no signs of bone invasion despite the large tumor size, typical of lymphoma, in contrast to the more common squamous cell carcinoma which frequently invades bone.

Bone Involvement

Frank bone destruction is unusual for NHL even when associated with a large primary mass (Figs. 6.1, 6.3) (CHISIN et al. 1994). Sclerosis however, can be a manifestation of bone involvement in NHL. Occasionally, a localized area of bony destruction can represent a primary bone lymphoma. Bone erosion may be observed with low-grade lymphomas that have been present for a long time prior to diagnosis.

Neurotropic Spread

Rarely, lymphomas have a neurotropic pattern of spread. In particular, marginal zone lymphomas in the head and neck have been reported with extensive neurotropic spread (Fig. 6.6). Signs of neurotropic spread include enlargement of the involved nerve and/or nodular deposits of tumor in the vicinity of a nerve tract (GARCIA-SERRA et al. 2003).

Nodal Involvement

Lymph nodes involved by NHL typically show homogenous attenuation as described above under internal characteristics (Fig. 6.4). As noted previously, central necrosis is less common than with carcinoma and usually indicative of an intermediate or high-grade lymphoma, treatment effect, or immune compromise. The lymph nodes of the posterior triangle and upper mediastinum are more frequently involved than in squamous cell carcinomas (URQUHART et al. 2002; SOM et al. 1999).

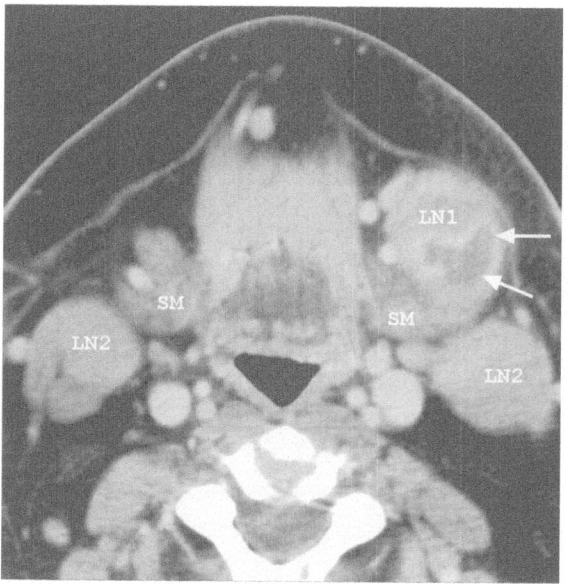

Fig. 6.4. Lymph node involvement in a 35-year-old man with stage II diffuse large B-cell lymphoma.. Axial contrast-enhanced CT scan demonstrates three enlarged lymph nodes (*LN1, LN2*) at the level of the submandibular glands (*SM*). The group 2A lymph nodes (*LN2* on each side) show homogenous attenuation typical of lymphoma. The group 1 lymph node (*LN1*) within the submandibular space on the left, however, shows a focal area of hypodensity (*arrows*) consistent with necrosis and suggestive of aggressive high-grade lymphoma in an immunocompromised patient, or of a treatment effect.

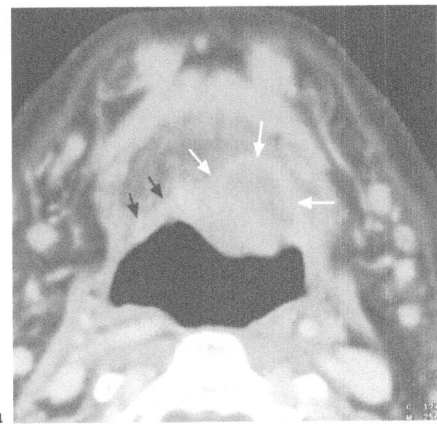
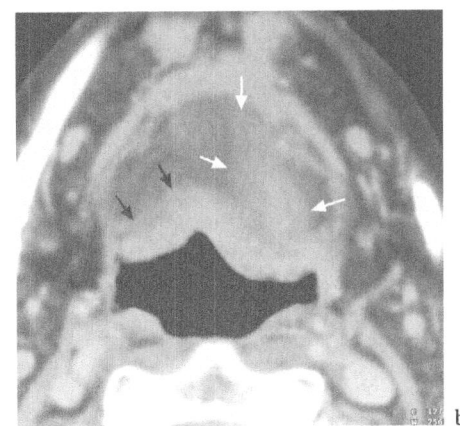
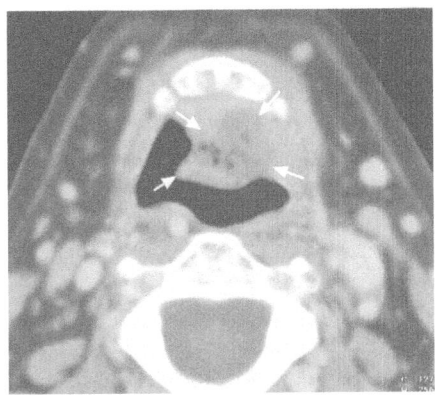

Fig. 6.5a–c. Tongue base involvement in a 68-year-old woman with stage II diffuse large B-cell lymphoma. a–c Axial contrast-enhanced CT images through the level of the base of the tongue demonstrate an infiltrating partially necrotic mass (*white arrows*) on the left extending slightly across midline to the right (a) and inferiorly to the level of the vallecula (c). The normal appearance of the lymphoid tissue (black arrows) at the tongue base level is demonstrated on the right.

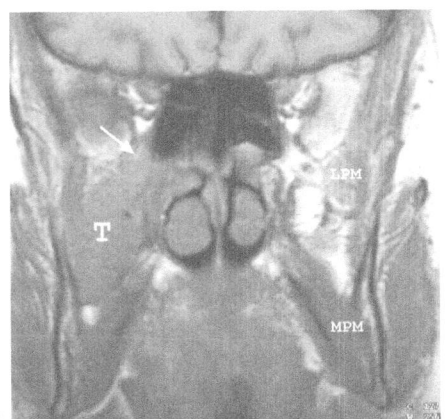
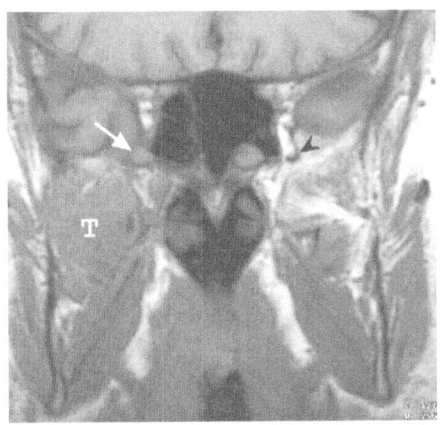
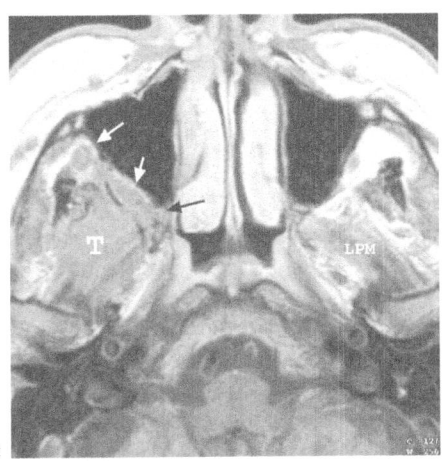

Fig. 6.6a–c. Masticator space involvement in a 65-year-old man with stage IE MALT lymphoma. a, b Coronal unenhanced T1-weighted MR images show a tumor mass (*T*) centered in the right masticator space. The tumor is partially infiltrating the right lateral pterygoid muscle (*LPM*) and shows no significant involvement of the right medial pterygoid muscle (*MPM*). On (a), the tumor continues superiorly via the right pterygopalatine fossa and inferior orbital fissure (*arrow*) into the foramen rotundum (*arrowhead*) to involve on (b), the second division of the right trigeminal nerve (*arrow*). c Axial contrast-enhanced T1-weighted MR image shows the mass also grows along the posterior wall of the maxillary sinus, indicated by loss of the right fat plane (*white arrows*), into the pterygopalatine fossa (*black arrow*).

6.4.2
Choice of Imaging Modalities

Computed Tomography
CT is usually the preferred modality for evaluation of NHL due to its widespread availability and relatively low cost. Its main disadvantages are radiation exposure and the use of iodinated contrast material. It is the method of choice for evaluation of cortical bone destruction.

Magnetic Resonance Imaging
The main strengths of MR imaging are excellent soft tissue resolution, improved visualization of perineural involvement, and delineation of bone marrow involvement. It can be helpful in evaluation of the low neck, as beam hardening artifacts compromise the evaluation of this area with CT. The multi-planar scanning capabilities of MR imaging have been a major advantage over CT in the past. The recent introduction of multi-slice helical CT scanners minimizes this advantage as the axial CT images can be reconstructed in any desirable plane, maintaining the image quality of the axial images.

Ultrasound
US is generally limited to evaluation of the salivary and thyroid glands. Nodal staging of lymphoma with ultrasound is a routine practice in Europe but is underutilized in the United States. The main disadvantages are operator dependence and reproducibility. US guidance is, however, very useful for localization and biopsy of suspicious lymph nodes.

Positron Emission Tomography
PET has the advantage of functional imaging. The avid uptake of FDG in follicular and aggressive subtypes of NHL make PET useful for staging, evaluation of treatment response, and post-treatment follow-up. For nodal staging, FDG-PET is approximately 10% more sensitive than MR imaging and/or CT and has a specificity of 85–90% (RESKE et al. 2001). PET is also able to identify more sites of involvement than a gallium-67 scan (WIRTH et al. 2002). While FDG-PET is suboptimal for MALT lymphomas of the head and neck, somatostatin-receptor scintigraphy using (111) In-labeled diethylenetriamine-pentaacetic acid (DTPA)-D-Phe (1)-octreotide is a promising approach. Somatostatin receptors are typically expressed in nongastric, MALT lymphomas. One study of 30 patients with extragastric MALT lymphoma reported that all sites of histologically documented involvement prior to treatment were PET-positive, whereas none of the scans were positive in patients with dissemination following gastric MALT lymphoma (RADERER et al. 2002).

6.5
Specific Sites of Involvement

6.5.1
Waldeyer's Ring

Waldeyer's ring is a circle of lymphatic tissue located in the tonsils, base of tongue, and nasopharynx. It remains controversial whether this should be considered nodal or extranodal tissue. The primarily IgG-secreting resident plasma cells and absence of a prominent marginal zone support a nodal origin, while its location along the aerodigestive tract and lack of afferent lymphatics is more consistent with extranodal lymphatic tissue.

Non-Hodgkin lymphoma, unlike HD, commonly involves Waldeyer's ring. Fifty to 60% of stage I and II extranodal NHL of the head and neck region are located in the Waldeyer's ring and 1/2 to 2/3 of these arise from the tonsils (GOSPADAROWICZ et al. 1995; SAUL et al. 1985; EZZAT et al. 2001). Patients with primary tonsillar lymphoma also have a 20–30% incidence of synchronous or metachronous gastrointestinal involvement (CHAN et al. 1990; HANNA et al. 1997). Diffuse large B-cell lymphomas comprise the majority of cases, followed by follicular, MALT, and Burkitt lymphomas (EZZAT et al. 2001). Potential signs and symptoms include sore throat, ear fullness or pain secondary to obstruction of the Eustachian tube, dysphagia, or airway obstruction.

Early-stage diffuse large B-cell lymphomas of Waldeyer's ring are commonly treated with CHOP (cyclophosphamide, doxorubicin, vincristine, and prednisone) chemotherapy and local–regional radiation therapy. Five-year survival for localized disease ranges from 60–90% (EZZAT et al. 2001; AVILES et al. 1996; LIANG et al. 1987). Patients older than 60 years have a somewhat poorer prognosis (EZZAT et al. 2001).

Radiographic Evaluation
Despite the fact that CT scans are the mainstay for evaluation of the Waldeyer's ring region, the appearance of extranodal NHL is not generally distinguishable from other malignancies in this area (HARNSBERGER et al. 1987). A large tumor mass with associated nonnecrotic adenopathy, without adjacent tissue or bone destruction is suggestive of NHL (Fig. 6.3). NHL

involving the tonsils (Fig. 6.7) frequently has a density and signal intensity similar to normal tonsillar tissue respectively on CT and MR imaging (KING et al. 2001). Hypertrophy of lymphoid tissue in Waldeyer's ring, occasionally seen in young adults or in HIV patients, can be indistinguishable from NHL. Only deep infiltration of the adjacent anatomic structures allows the radiologist to make the diagnosis of an underlying malignant lesion (Fig. 6.5).

6.5.2
Salivary Glands

Salivary gland NHL is uncommon, comprising approximately 5–10% of all NHL of the head and neck, and 2–5% of salivary gland neoplasms (JAEHNE et al. 2001). Lymphomas of the salivary glands are commonly associated with lymphoepithelial sialadenitis of Sjögren syndrome (LESA). Patients with lymphoepithelial sialadenitis have a 44 fold increased risk of developing salivary gland (Fig. 6.8) or extrasalivary lymphomas, up to 80% of which are marginal zone/MALT lymphoma (ZULMAN 1978; KASSAN et al. 1978; TALAL et al. 1967; ANDERSON et al. 1972). Major salivary gland NHL may have either an extranodal, or intraglandular/periglandular nodal presentation. The most common salivary gland nodal histology is follicular, whereas the most common extranodal

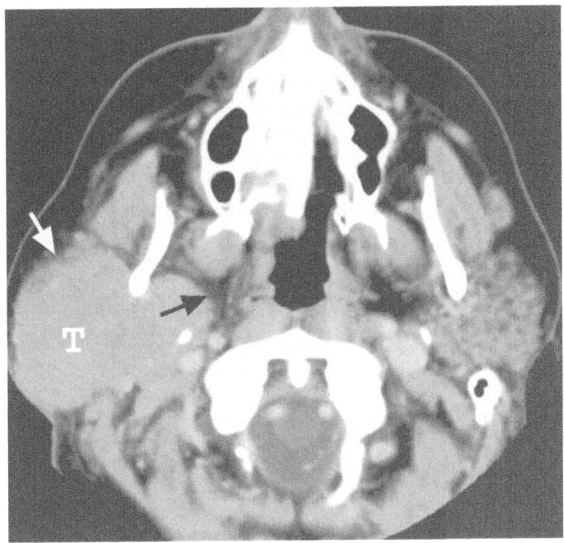

Fig. 6.8. Parotid gland involvement in a 30-year-old woman with stage IIE diffuse large B-cell lymphoma and Sjögren syndrome. Axial contrast-enhanced CT image through the parotid glands demonstrates a large mass (*T*) in the right parotid gland. Nearly the entire parotid gland has been infiltrated, with only a small portion of normal residual parotid gland parenchyma apparent along the anterior aspect (*white arrow*). The mass displaces and partially obliterates the fat pad within the parapharyngeal space on the right (*black arrow*). Notice the multinodular appearance of the left parotid gland reflecting the typical appearance of parotid gland in Sjögren syndrome.

histology is marginal zone lymphoma of the MALT type (JAEHNE et al. 2001). Nodal intraglandular presentations involve only the parotid gland since there are no lymph nodes within the submandibular gland. Other B-cell lymphomas arising from the salivary glands include diffuse large B-cell, mantle cell, lymphoplasmocytic, and small lymphocytic lymphomas. Primary salivary T-cell lymphoma is extremely rare with only three cases reported in the Western population (HEW et al. 2002).

The majority of patients present with painless swelling of the involved salivary gland. Clinically, most salivary gland lymphomas follow an indolent course, remaining localized and growing slowly over a prolonged period of time. Localized low-grade follicular and MALT lymphomas are typically treated with radiation therapy alone. Rapid progression raises concern for an intermediate or high-grade lymphoma, most commonly diffuse large B-cell lymphoma, arising either de novo, or as a transformation from a pre-existing MALT or follicular lymphoma. Upon completion of workup, if this more aggressive entity remains localized, treatment is with combined chemotherapy and radiation therapy.

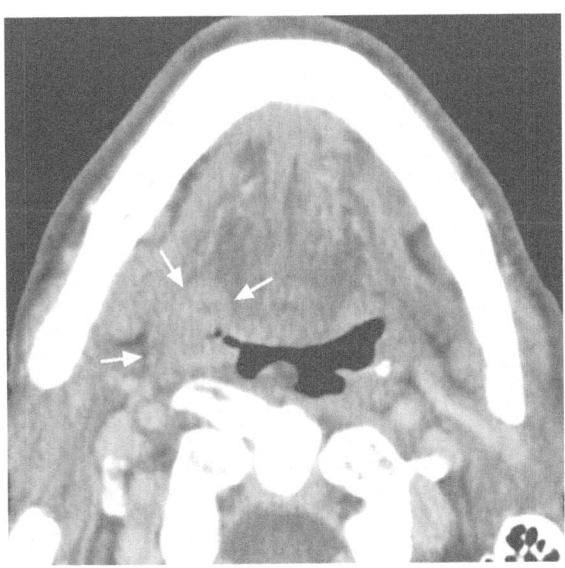

Fig. 6.7. Tonsil involvement in an 83-year-old man with stage II small lymphocytic lymphoma. Axial contrast-enhanced CT scan shows a mass (*arrows*) in the right tonsillar fossa with deep infiltration. The fat plane is preserved and no other areas of involvement were seen in this patient.

Radiographic Evaluation

The two types of lymphomatous involvement of the salivary gland, intraparenchymal and intraglandular nodal, can usually be identified by US. A heterogeneous internal echostructure is commonly noted in primary salivary gland lymphomas but is not specific, since similar ill-defined heterogeneous masses may be seen with carcinomas as well (YASUMOTO et al. 2001). Intraparenchymal involvement (Fig. 6.8) usually can be easily distinguished from the intraglandular nodal form of NHL on cross-sectional studies. The latter most often presents with multifocal and/or bilateral involvement of the parotid glands.

6.5.3
Ocular Adnexa

Lymphomas of the orbital tissues, conjunctiva, eyelid, lacrimal apparatus, and posterior orbit have been reported to comprise 10–55% of all orbital tumors with an increasing incidence over the last two decades (DUNBAR et al. 1990; WOTHERSPOON et al. 1993; TAKA-MAURA et al. 2001; MARGO et al. 1998; ESMAELI et al. 2002). These can occur as primary localized lesions or as a manifestation of systemic disease. The majority of primary lesions in both the anterior and posterior structures are MALT lymphomas, followed by diffuse large B-cell, and follicular lymphomas (AUW-HAED-RICH et al. 2001; COUPLAND et al. 1998; JENKINS et al. 2000; MANNAMI et al. 2001; NAKATA et al. 1999; WHITE et al. 1995; SASAI et al. 2001). Many orbital MALT lymphomas were previously classified as small lymphocytic lymphomas or pseudolymphomas. Diffuse large B-cell lymphomas are more likely to be located in the posterior structures of the orbit. Primary T-cell lymphomas represent approximately 1–3% of all ocular adnexal lymphomas (AUW-HAEDRICH et al. 2001; COUPLAND et al. 1999; HENDERSON et al. 1989; JENKINS et al. 2000). Secondary orbital lymphomas are more likely to be intermediate or high-grade (BESSELL et al. 1988). Primary intraocular lymphoma is a rare presentation, typically diffuse large B-cell lymphoma, which is associated with the development of subsequent central nervous system disease in 60–80% of cases (PETERSON et al. 1993; WHITCUP et al. 1993; AKPEK et al. 1999; GOLDEY et al. 1989).

Patients with orbital MALT lymphomas typically present with stage IE disease and painless unilateral orbital swelling. Between 10–20% of cases have bilateral involvement, 80% of which are synchronous (COUPLAND et al. 1998; WHITE et al. 1995; SASAI et al. 2001; KNOWLES et al. 1990; MCNALLY et al. 1987).

Conjunctival lymphomas develop bilateral disease approximately 45% of the time (SHIELDS et al. 2001). Reported rates of initial or subsequent systemic involvement are: conjunctiva, 20–31%; orbit, 35%; and eyelid involvement, 70%. A systemic workup is necessary for all cases (SHIELDS et al. 2001; KNOWLES et al. 1990). Ocular MALT lymphomas tend to remain localized until late in the course of the disease (ISAACSON et al. 1987, 1984). If the mass progresses it can cause proptosis, compromise vision, and cause ptosis. Conjunctival involvement usually presents with salmon-pink swelling and irritation.

Low grade localized orbital lymphoma is routinely treated with modest doses of radiation therapy in the range of 20–30 Gy with local control between 90–100% (BESSELL et al. 1988; FITZPATRICK et al. 1984; BOLEK et al. 1999). Patients with early stage intermediate or high-grade NHL are treated with combined chemotherapy and radiation therapy.

Radiographic Evaluation

US has been useful for the detection of intraconal and anterior lesions, although contrast-enhanced CT or MR imaging are the primary modalities for evaluation of the ocular adnexa (Fig. 6.9). CT is effective in evaluating the local extent of the primary lesion, regional adenopathy, and systemic disease. Orbital lymphoma masses are more likely to be hyperdense, mildly enhancing, and more sharply delineated on CT scan than benign lymphoid hyperplasia (FLANDERS et al. 1987). One study reported orbital lymphomas to be more homogeneous on CT compared to reactive lymphoid hyperplasia (75% vs. 23%) (WESTACOTT et al. 1991). Posterior tumors are usually located in the extraconal adipose tissue and conform to the orbital conus structures (Fig. 6.10). Actual invasion of the extraocular muscles is uncommon (Fig. 6.10). Bone destruction is rare and associated with high-grade histology (FLANDERS et al. 1987; WESTACOTT et al. 1991).

Orbital lymphomas are typically isointense to muscles on T1-weighted MR images. Most are hyperintense to fat and musculature on conventional or fat-suppressed T2-weighted MR images, and become slightly brighter relative to their appearance on proton density and T1-weighted MR images (VALVASSORI et al. 1999)

6.5.4
Thyroid Gland

Five to 10% of all thyroid nodules are malignant and approximately 5% of thyroid malignancies are

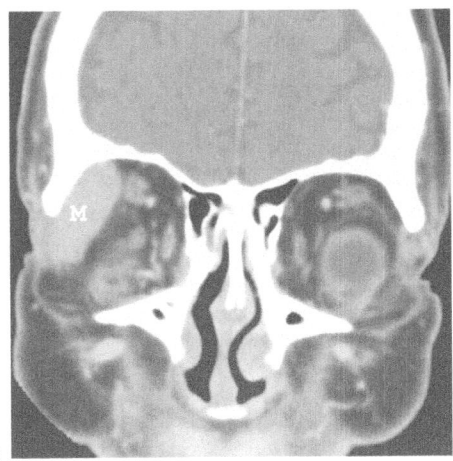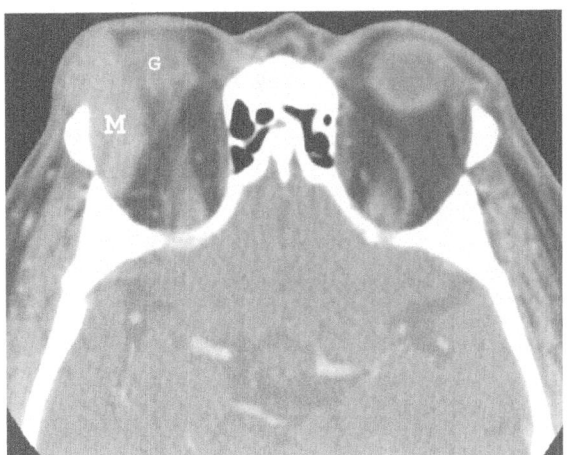

a   b

Fig. 6.9a,b. Lacrimal gland involvement in 64-year-old man with a stage IE MALT lymphoma. **a** Coronal and (**b**) axial contrast enhanced CT scans of the lacrimal gland show a mass (*M*) in the upper outer right orbit. The lacrimal gland could not be identified as a separate structure, suggesting lacrimal gland origin, which was confirmed by excisional biopsy. (*G = globe*)

primary thyroid lymphomas (MATSUZUKA et al. 1993; ROSAI et al. 1992). Patients with Hashimoto thyroiditis have a greater than 60 fold increased risk for developing NHL (PEDERSON et al. 1996; HYJEK et al. 1988; HOLM et al. 1985). The median age at diagnosis is 65 to 75 years with up to an 8:1 predominance of women (PEDERSON et al. 1996; JUNOR et al. 1992; PYKE et al. 1992; SKARSGARD et al. 1991; WOLF et al. 1992; LOGUE et al. 1992; COMPAGNO et al. 1980; BUTLER et al. 1990).

Primary thyroid NHL are a heterogeneous group of diseases. Diffuse large B-cell lymphoma, the most common histology, is more likely to present with or develop distant disease than MALT lymphoma. MALT lymphoma accounts for up to 25% of cases (GOSPODAROWICZ et al. 1995). Up to 75% of cases previously classified as anaplastic thyroid carcinoma have been reclassified retrospectively as thyroid lymphomas (WOLF et al. 1992; HOLTING et al. 1990). Primary T-cell lymphomas of the thyroid have been reported occasionally, more often in Asia, and appear to carry a worse prognosis than other thyroid lymphomas.

The majority of patients present with localized symptoms, most commonly a rapidly growing, non-tender mass. Thyroid lymphomas have a firm, rubbery consistency with a discrete nodule noted in 2/3 of patients. Dysphagia, hoarseness, or dyspnea may develop due to compression, or infiltration of local structures (MATSUZUKA et al. 1993; SIROTA et al. 1979). Regional lymph node involvement without distant disease is common. Approximately 50% of patients have abnormal laboratory thyroid function tests (HAMBERGER et al. 1983).

The role of surgery is primarily to obtain histologic diagnosis and for relief of acute symptoms. Stage I and II, low-grade lymphomas including the MALT subtype, are typically treated with radiation therapy alone to moderate doses of 30 to 45 Gy with local control greater than 95%, and overall survival rates of 90–100% (THIEBLEMONT et al. 2002; LAING et al. 1994; AOZASA et al. 1986). Diffuse large B-cell lymphoma is generally treated with CHOP-based chemotherapy and locoregional radiation therapy with local control. Overall survival rates exceed 70%. Adverse prognostic factors include high-grade histology, advanced stage, and older age (HA et al. 2001).

Radiographic Evaluation

A chest radiograph may demonstrate tracheal deviation due to an adjacent mass. Radionuclide scans typically demonstrate a cold nodule, however, patchy uptake, also typical of chronic thyroiditis, may make the diagnosis more difficult (ANSELL et al. 1999). Although US findings vary, three distinct patterns have been described: a solitary hypoechoic nodule with a few distal echos; a diffuse complex echo pattern due to intermixed uninvolved and lymphomatous tissue; and diffuse enlargement with a normal echo pattern (BRUNETON et al. 1986). US may be suboptimal for visualizing local invasion of surrounding structures (TAKASHIMA et al. 1995). US has been advocated for guidance of fine-needle aspiration and for follow-up on patients with a history of Hashimoto thyroiditis (TAKASHIMA et al. 1995; WIRTZFELD et al. 2001). CT is used to image the primary site and evaluate for regional and distant

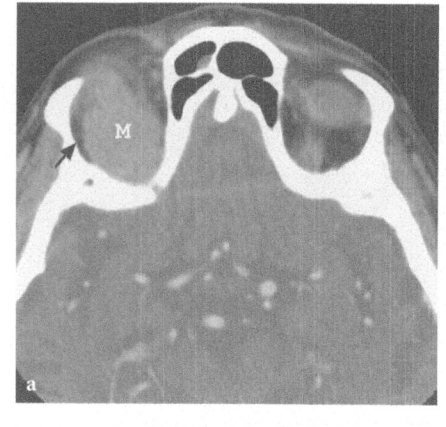
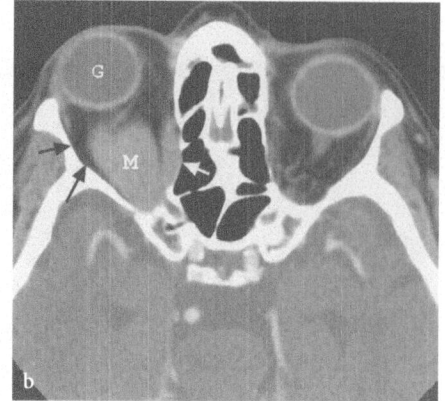
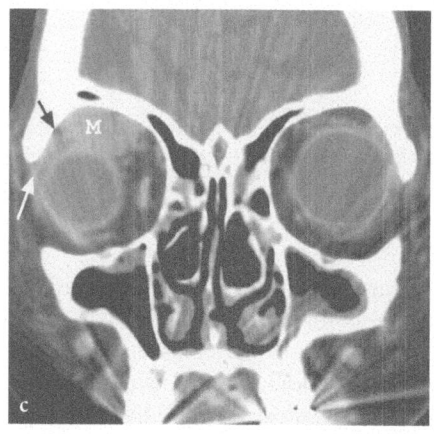
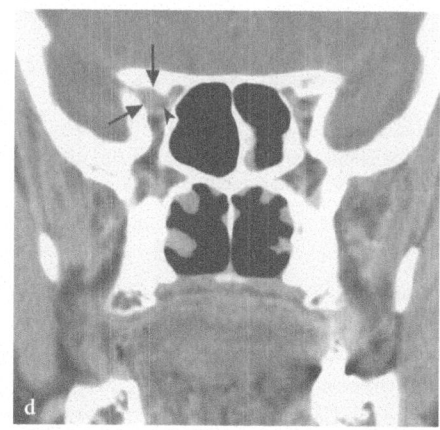

Fig. 6.10a–g. Orbital involvement in a 74-year-old woman with stage IE small lymphocytic lymphoma. **a, b** Axial contrast-enhanced CT scans through the orbit demonstrate a tumor mass (*M*) in the upper mid-orbit in an extraconal location, with preserved fat plane laterally (*black arrows*). There is significant enlargement of the right medial rectus muscle (*white arrow*). **c** Coronal contrast-enhanced CT scan through the orbit shows that the mass is separate from the lacrimal gland (*white arrow*) as seen by a thin preserved fat plane (*black arrow*) between the mass and the lacrimal gland. **d** Coronal contrast-enhanced CT scan posterior to (c) shows the mass extends posteriorly (*arrows*) to involve the superior orbital fissure evident from obliteration of the right fat plane in the superior aspect of the orbital apex (*arrowhead*). **e** Axial contrast-enhanced T1-weighted MR image exaggerates the posterior extension of the tumor since there is only a subtle difference between the tumor (*M*) and the bone marrow of the sphenoid wing (*arrows*). The enlargement of the medial rectus muscle (*arrowheads*) is suggestive of involvement of the muscle cone as well. Coronal (**f**) fat-suppressed T2-weighted and (**g**) contrast-enhanced T1-weighted MR images, however, confirm that the medial rectus muscle (*black arrow*) is not involved but rather inferiorly displaced by the medial lobulation of the tumor (*white arrows*). The mass causes significant compression of the right optic nerve sheath complex with complete obliteration of the CSF space around the optic nerve when compared to the uninvolved left side. The optic nerve (*arrowhead*) is also markedly displaced inferiorly as best appreciated on (**g**). Surgery confirmed that the lacrimal gland was not involved. (*G= globe*)

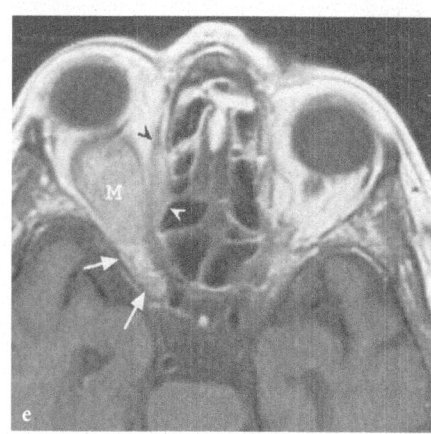
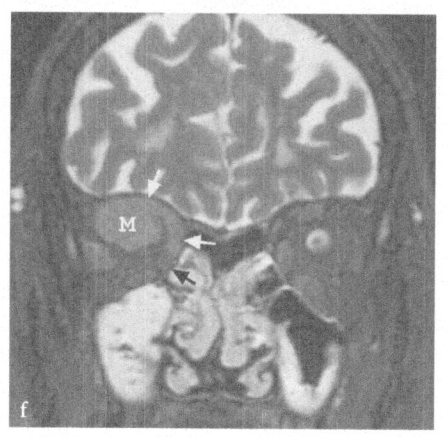
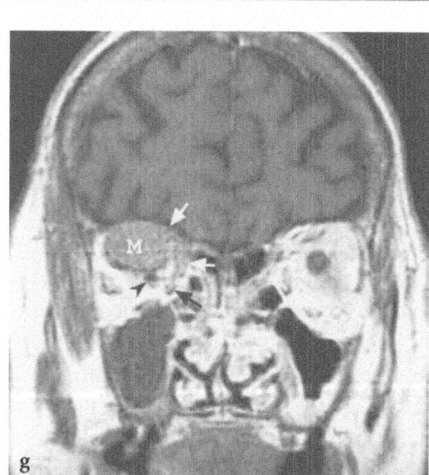

metastases. The primary tumor is hypodense on both unenhanced and contrast-enhanced CT scans. CT appearance has been classified into three types: solitary nodule (80%), multiple nodules (13%), and diffuse involvement (7%) (Fig. 6.11) (TAKASHIMA et al. 1988). Thyroid lymphoma is usually homogenously hypointense on both T1 and T2-weighted MR images. TAKASHIMA, et al. (1995) concluded that MR imaging is more accurate than CT or US in determining the extent of extrathyroidal spread, a factor that has been correlated with survival in some studies.

6.5.5
Sinonasal Cavities

Lymphoma is reported to account for approximately 10% of all sinonasal cancers (GRAU et al. 2001). Sinonasal lymphoma accounts for up to 2% of all NHL in the Western world and is primarily of B-cell origin (GRAU et al. 2001; ROBBINS et al. 1985; FRIERSON et al. 1984; FREEMAN et al. 1972). In Asia, these tumors are considerably more frequent comprising up to 7% of all NHL, and are predominantly of NK/T-cell origin (CHAN et al. 1987; Ho et al. 1984). These two types of lymphomas differ considerably in natural history and response to treatment despite their similar locations. The majority of B-cell neoplasms are diffuse large B-cell lymphomas and generally arise in the paranasal

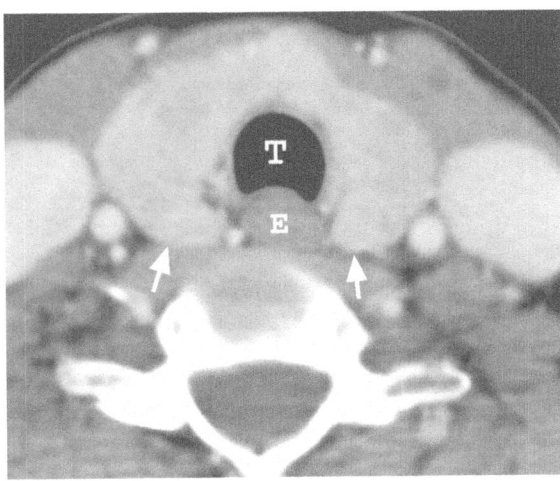

Fig. 6.11. Thyroid involvement in a 62-year-old woman initially diagnosed with an anaplastic thyroid cancer on fine needle aspiration, but later confirmed to have a stage IE diffuse large B-cell lymphoma. Axial contrast-enhanced CT scan through the lower neck demonstrates diffuse enlargement of the thyroid gland including the isthmus. The involved thyroid gland extends posteriorly into the trachea-esophageal groove bilaterally (*arrows*). (*T = trachea, E = esophagus*)

sinuses. The maxillary sinus is the most commonly involved paranasal sinus followed by the ethmoid, frontal, and sphenoid sinuses (BATSAKIS et al. 1979; YANG et al. 1986). The NK/T-cell lymphomas are more likely to be located centrally in the nasal cavity, arise in younger patients, and carry a poorer prognosis (QURAISHI et al. 2000; HATTA et al. 2001).

The clinical presentation correlates with histologic subtype. Low-grade lymphomas typically present with a mass and associated obstructive symptoms. High-grade lymphomas are more likely to present with aggressive signs and symptoms including ulceration, cranial nerve deficits, epistaxis, facial swelling, proptosis, and pain. NK/T-cell subtypes commonly present with nasal septal perforation and midline destruction (ABBONDANZO et al. 1995).

The majority of patients with diffuse large B-cell lymphoma are treated with combined chemotherapy and radiation therapy. The 5-year cause-specific survival for early stage disease is approximately 60% for B-cell lymphomas and approximately 30% for NK/T-cell lymphomas (QURAISHI et al. 2000; HATTA et al. 2001). There is some evidence that combined modality therapy employing up-front radiation therapy may be preferable for NK/T-cell lymphomas (RIBRAG et al. 2001).

Radiographic Evaluation
Non-Hodgkin lymphoma of the paranasal sinuses commonly presents as a soft tissue mass (Fig. 6.12) and is frequently associated with post-obstructive fluid. Maxillary sinus lymphomas usually present late with locally advanced tumors extending into adjacent sinonasal cavities, either eroding or permeating bone without evident bony destruction. CT is better for cortical bony changes, while MR imaging has superior delineation of soft tissue mass extension. Obstructive, inflammatory disease most often demonstrates hyperintensity on T2-weighted MR images differentiating it from most tumors, including lymphomas, which exhibit intermediate intensity (DEPENA et al. 1990). Dried out secretions and/or fungal colonization within the obstructed sinus reduces the hyperintensity of the inflammatory sinus disease on the T2-weighted MR images making it indistinguishable from NHL.

6.5.6
Larynx

Non-Hodgkin lymphoma of the larynx is rare, accounting for less than 1% of all laryngeal neo-

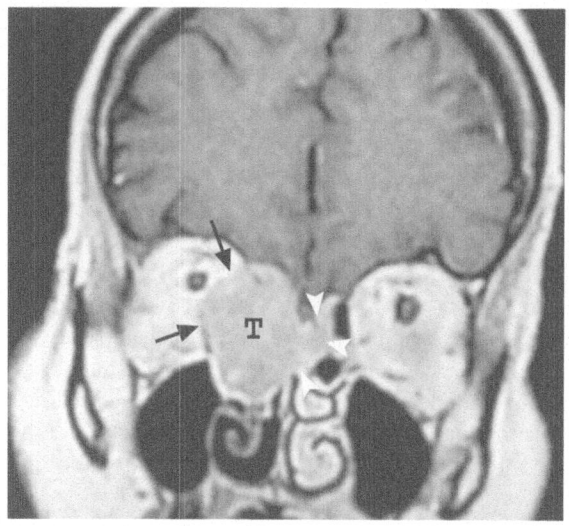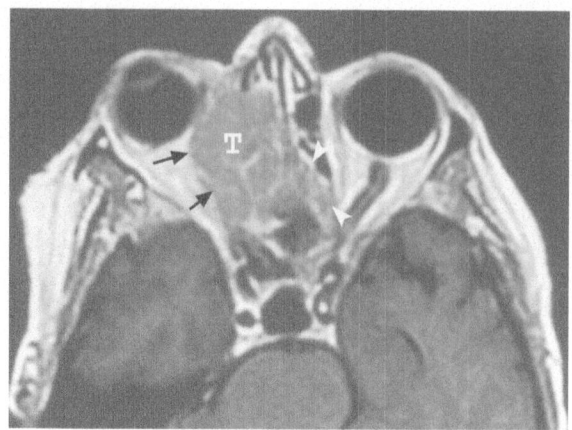

Fig. 6.12a,b. Ethmoid sinus involvement in a 70-year-old woman with stage IE diffuse large B-cell lymphoma. **a** Coronal and (**b**) axial contrast-enhanced T1 weighted MR images through the ethmoid sinuses demonstrate a tumor (*T*) centered in the right ethmoid air cells with extension (*arrowheads*) across the septum to the left. The tumor also grows laterally to involve the medial aspect of the orbit (*arrows*).

plasms (Ansell et al. 1997). The larynx may contain lymphatic tissue, primarily in the supraglottic region. The vast majority of reported cases are of B-cell origin, with diffuse large B-cell lymphoma the most common subtype. Follicular, small lymphocytic, and MALT subtypes have also been sporadically reported (Ansell et al. 1997; de Bree et al. 1998; Kato et al. 1997; Horny et al. 1996). Cases of T-cell and NK/T-cell lymphoma of the larynx are extremely rare, occurring primarily in the Asian population (Chan et al. 1997; Mok et al. 2001).

Most patients present with local complaints such as sore throat, hoarseness, dysphagia, or dyspnea. Examination usually reveals a bulky submucosal mass involving the supraglottis or aryepiglottic folds.

There is a paucity of information on the outcome of patients treated for primary NHL of the larynx. The Mayo Clinic reported local control in all 6 patients with stage IAE NHL of the larynx treated with radiation therapy alone. However, 4 patients had distant relapse, and 3 died from the lymphoma (Ansell et al. 1997). Excellent local and distant disease control of MALT lymphoma of the larynx can be achieved with radiation therapy alone at modest doses in the range of 30 Gy (de Bree et al. 1998).

Radiographic Evaluation
CT usually demonstrates a homogenous mass lesion arising from the supraglottic larynx without apparent

bone or cartilage destruction (Fig. 6.13). MR imaging also demonstrates a homogenous mass lesion arising from the submucosal region. The tumor may show intermediate signal intensity on both T1 and T2-weighted MR images. Marked enhancement of the mucosal layers on fat-suppressed T1-weighted MR images has also been noted (Takayama et al. 2001).

6.6
Conclusion

Non-Hodgkin lymphoma of the head and neck encompasses a group of diverse lymphoid malignancies with variable presentations, natural histories, and treatment responses. Localized low-grade NHL are typically treated with radiation therapy alone, with excellent local control. Localized intermediate and high-grade NHL are typically treated with combined chemotherapy and radiation therapy with results similar to other sites.

Understanding the radiologic patterns of presentation, natural history, and treatment response is essential for optimal management. Delineation of disease extent directs the treatment approach as well as design of the radiation therapy treatment fields. Functional imaging may also help in directing localized treatment and monitoring tumor response.

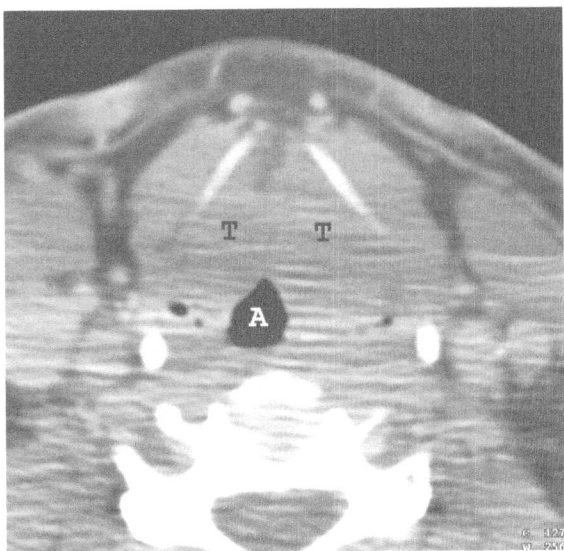 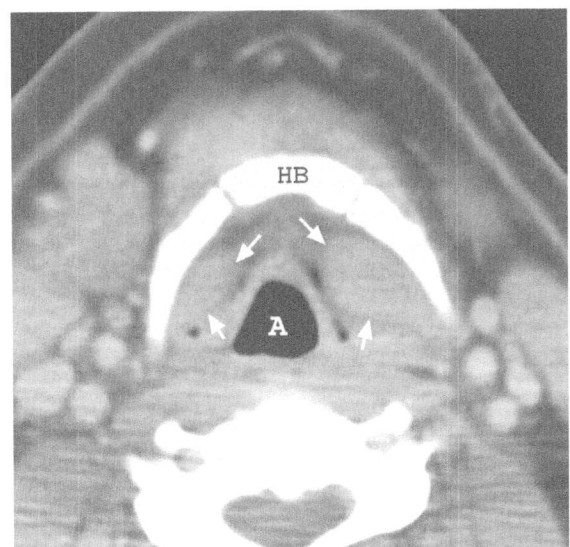

Fig. 6.13a,b. Laryngeal involvement in a 58-year-old man with stage IE MALT lymphoma. a Axial contrast-enhanced CT scan through the larynx demonstrates diffuse tumoral infiltration of the false vocal cords (*T*) bilaterally with significant thickening of the anterior commissure. b Axial contrast-enhanced CT scan cephalad to (a) shows the tumor extends superiorly to involve the aryepiglottic folds (*arrows*) bilaterally in a submucosal fashion. *(A = airway, HB = hyoid bone)*

References

Abbondanzo SL, Wenig BM (1995) Non-Hodgkin's lymphoma of the sinonasal tract. A clinicopathologic and immunophenotypic study of 120 cases. Cancer 75:1281–1291

Akpek EK, Ahmed I, Hochberg FH, et al. (1999) Intraocular-central nervous system lymphoma: clinical features diagnosis, and outcomes. Opthamol 106:1805–1810

Anderson LG, Talal N (1972) The spectrum of benign to malignant lymphoproliferation in Sjögren's syndrome. Clin Exp Immunol 10:199–221

Ansell SM, Habermann TM, Hoyer JD, et al. (1997) Primary laryngeal lymphoma. Laryngoscope 107:1502–1506

Ansell SM, Li CY, Lloyd RV, et al. (1999) Primary thyroid lymphoma. Semin Oncol 26:316–323

Aozasa K, Inoue A, Tajima K, et al. (1986) Malignant lymphomas of the thyroid gland. Analysis of 79 patients with emphasis on histologic prognostic factors. Cancer 58:100–104

Apter S, Avigdor A, Gayer G, et al. (2002) Calcification in lymphoma occurring before therapy: CT features and clinical correlation. AJR Am J Roentgenol 178:935–938

Auw-Haedrich C, Coupland SE, Kapp A., et al. (2001) Long term outcome of ocular adnexal lymphoma subtyped according to the REAL classification. Revised European and American Lymphoma. Br J Ophthalmol 85:63–69

Aviles A, Delgado S, Ruiz H, et al. (1996) Treatment of non-Hodgkin's lymphoma of Waldeyer's ring: Radiotherapy versus chemotherapy versus combined therapy. Eur J Cancer B Oral Oncol 32B:19–23

Batsakis JG (1979) Tumors of the head and neck: clinical and pathological considerations, 2nd edn. Williams and Wilkins, Baltimore

Bessell EM, Henk JM, Wright JE, et al. (1988) Orbital and conjunctival lymphoma treatment and prognosis. Radiother Oncol 13:237–244

Bolek TW, Moyses HM, Marcus RB, et al. (1999) Radiotherapy in the management of the orbital lymphoma. Int J Radiat Oncol Biol Phys 44:31–36

Bruneton JN, Schneider JN (1986) Radiology of lymphomas, 1st edn. Springer-Verlag, New York

Butler JS Jr, Brady LW, Amendola BE (1990) Lymphoma of the thyroid. Report of 5 cases and review. Am J Clin Oncol 13:64–69

Chan J, Ng CS, Isaacson PG (1990) Relationship between high-grade lymphoma and low-grade B-cell mucosa-associated lymphoid tissue lymphoma (MALToma) of the stomach. Am J Pathol 136:1153–1164

Chan JK, Ng CS, Lau WH, et al. (1987) Most nasal/nasopharyngeal lymphomas are peripheral T-cell neoplasms. Am J Surg Pathol 11:418–429

Chan JK, Sin VC, Wong KF, et al. (1997) Nonnasal lymphoma expressing the natural killer cell marker CD56: a clinicopathologic study of 49 cases of an uncommon aggressive neoplasm. Blood 89:4501–4513

Chisin R, Weber AL (1994) Imaging of lymphoma manifestations in the extracranial head and neck region. Leuk Lymphoma 12:177–189

Compagno J, Oertel JE (1980) Malignant lymphoma and other lymphoproliferative disorders of the thyroid gland. A clinicopathologic study of 245 cases. Am J Clin Pathol 74:1–11

Coupland SE, Krause L, Delecluse HJ, et al. (1998) Lymphoproliferative lesions of the ocular adnexa. Analysis of 112 cases. Ophthalmol 105:1430–1441

Coupland SE, Fossa HD, Assaf C, et al. (1999) T-cell and T/natural killer-cell lymphomas involving ocular and ocular adnexal tissues: A clinicopathologic, immunohistochemical, and molecular study of seven cases. Ophthalmol 106: 2109–2120

De Bree R, Mahieu HF, Ossen Koppelle GJ, et al. (1998) Malignant lymphoma of mucosa-associated lymphoid tissue in the larynx. Eur Arch Otorhinolaryngol 255:368–370

Depena CA, Van Tassel P, Lee YY (1990) Lymphoma of the head and neck. Radiol Clin North Am 28:723–743

Dunbar SF, Linggood RM, Doppke KP, et al. (1990) Conjunctival lymphoma: Results and treatment with a single anterior electron field. A lens sparing approach. Int J Radiat Oncol Biol Phys 19:249–257

Esmaeli B, Ahmadi MA, Manning J, et al. (2002) Clinical presentation and treatment of secondary orbital lymphoma. Ophthal Plast Resconstr Surg 18:247–253

Evans C (1981) A review of non-Hodgkin's lymphoma of the head and neck. Clin Oncol 7:23–31

Ezzat AA, Ibrahim EM, Weshi AN, et al. (2001) Localized non-Hodgkin's lymphoma of Waldeyer's ring: clinical features management, and prognosis of 130 adult patients. Head Neck 23:547–558

Fitzpatrick PJ, Macko S (1984) Lymphoreticular tumors of the orbit. Int J Radiat Oncol Biol Phys 10: 333–340

Flanders AE, Espinosa GA, Markiewicz DA, et al. (1987) Orbital lymphoma. Role of CT and MRI. Radiol Clin North Am 25:601–613

Freeman C, Berg JW, Cutter SJ (1972) Occurrence and prognosis of extranodal lymphomas. Cancer 29:252–260

Frierson HF Jr, Mills SE, Innes DJ Jr (1984) Non-Hodgkin's lymphoma of the sinonasal region: Histologic subtypes and their clinicopathologic features. Am J Clin Pathol 81:721–727

Garcia-Serra A, Mendenhall NP, Hinerman RW, et al. (2003) Management of neurotropic low-grade B-cell lymphoma: Report of two cases. Head Neck (in press)

Glass AG, Karnell LH, Menck HR (1997) The National Cancer Data Base report on non-Hodgkin's lymphoma. Cancer 80: 2311–2320

Goldey SH, Stern GA, Oblon DJ, et al. (1989) Immunophenotypic characterization of an unusual T-cell lymphoma presenting as anterior uveitis. A clinicopathologic case report. Arch Ophthamol 107:1349–1353

Gospodarowicz MK, Sutcliffe SB (1995) The extranodal lymphomas. Semin Radiat Oncol 5:281–300

Grau C, Jakobsen MH, Harbo G, et al. (2001) Sino-nasal cancer in Denmark 1982–1991–a nationwide survey. Acta Oncol 40:19–23

Ha CS, Shadle KM, Medeiros LJ, et al. (2001) Localized non-Hodgkin lymphoma involving the thyroid gland. Cancer 91:629–635

Hamberger JI, Miller JM, Kini SR (1983) Lymphoma of the thyroid. Ann Intern Med 99:685–693

Hanna E, Wanamaker J, Adelstein D, et al. (1997) Extranodal lymphomas of the head and neck. A 20 year experience. Arch Otolaryngol Head Neck Surg 123:1318–1323

Harnsberger HR, Bragg DG, Osborn AG, et al. (1987) Non-Hodgkin's lymphoma of the head and neck: CT evaluation of nodal and extranodal sites. AJR Am J Roentgenol 149:785–791

Hatta C, Ogasawara H, Okita J, et al. (2001) Non-Hodgkin's malignant lymphoma of the sinonasal tract–treatment outcome for 53 patients according to REAL classification. Auris Nasus Larynx 28:55–60

Henderson JW, Banks PM, Yeatts RP (1989) T-cell lymphoma of the orbit. Mayo Clin Proc 64:940–944

Hew WS, Carey FA, Kernohan NM, et al. (2002) Primary T-cell lymphoma of salivary gland: A report of a case and review of the literature. J Clin Pathol 55:61–63

Ho FC, Todd D, Loke SL, et al. (1984) Clinicopathologic features of malignant lymphomas in 294 Hong Kong Chinese patients, retrospective study covering eight-year period. Int J Cancer 34:143–148

Holm LE, Blomgren H, Lowhagen T (1985) Cancer risks in patients with chronic lymphocytic thyroiditis. New Eng J Med 312:601–604

Holting T, Moller P, Tschalargane C, et al. (1990) Immunohistochemical reclassification of anaplastic carcinoma reveals small and giant cell lymphoma. World J Surg 14:291–294, discussion 295

Horny HP, Ferlito A, Carbone A (1996) Laryngeal lymphoma derived from mucosa-associated lymphoid tissue. Ann Otol Rhinol Laryngol 105:577–583

Hyjek E, Isaacson PG (1988) Primary B-cell lymphoma of the thyroid and its relationship to Hashimoto's thyroiditis. Hum Pathol 19:1315–1326

Isaacson P, Wright DH (1984) Extranodal malignant lymphoma arising from mucosa-associated lymphoid tissue. Cancer 53:2515–2524

Isaacson PG, Spencer J (1987) Malignant lymphoma of mucosa-associated lymphoid tissue. Histopathol 11: 445–462

Jaehne M, Ussmuller J, Jakel KT, et al. (2001) The clinical presentation of non-Hodgkin's lymphoma of the major salivary glands. Acta Otolaryngol 121:647–651

Jenkins C, Rose GE, Bunce C, et al. (2000) Histologic features of ocular adnexal lymphoma (REAL classification) and their association with patient morbidity and survival. Br J Ophthalmol 84:907–913

Junor EJ, Paul J, Reed NS (1992) Primary non-Hodgkin's lymphoma of the thyroid. Eur J Surg Oncol 18:313–321

Kassan SS, Thomas TL (1978) Increased risk of lymphoma in sicca syndrome. Ann Intern Med 89:888–892

Kato S, Sakura M, Takooda S, et al. (1997) Primary non-Hodgkin's lymphoma of the larynx. J Laryngol Otol 111:571–574

King AD, Lei KI, Ahuja AT (2001) MRI of primary non-Hodgkin's lymphoma of the palatine tonsil. Br J Radiol 74: 226–229

Knowles DM, Jakobiec FA, McNally L, et al. (1990) Lymphoid hyperplasia and malignant lymphoma occurring in the ocular adnexa (orbit, conjunctiva, and eyelids): a prospective multiparametric analysis of 108 cases during 1977 and 1987. Hum Pathol 21:959–973

Laing RW, Hoskin P, Hudson BV, et al. (1994) The significance of MALT histology in thyroid lymphoma: a review of patients from the BNLI and Royal Marsden Hospital. Clin Oncol (R Coll Radiol) 6:300–304

Liang R, Ng RP, Todd D, et al. (1987) Management of stage I–II diffuse aggressive non-Hodgkin's lymphoma of the Waldeyer's ring: Combined modality therapy versus radiotherapy alone. Hematol Oncol 5:223–230

Lindahl T, Klein G, Reedman BM, et al. (1974) Relationship between Epstein-Barr virus (EBV) DNA and the EBV-determined nuclear antigen in Burkitt lymphoma biopsies and other lymphoproliferative malignancies. Int J Cancer 13:764–772

Logue JP, Hale RJ, Stewart AL, et al. (1992) Primary malignant lymphoma of the thyroid: A clinicopathological analysis. Int J Radiat Oncol Biol Phys 22:929–933

Mannami T, Yoshino T, Oshima K, et al. (2001) Clinical, histopathological, and immunogenetic analysis of ocular adnexal lymphoproliferative disorders: Characterization of malt lymphoma and reactive lymphoid hyperplasia. Mod Pathol 14:641–649

Margo CE, Mulla ZD (1998) Malignant tumors of the orbit. Analysis of the Florida Cancer Registry. Ophthalmol 105: 185–190

Matsuzuka F, Miyauchi A, Katayama S, et al. (1993) Clinical aspects of primary thyroid lymphoma: Diagnosis and treatment based on our experience of 119 cases. Thyroid 3:93–99

McNally L, Jakobiec FA, Knowles DM II (1987) Clinical, morphologic, immunophenotypic, and molecular genetic analysis of bilateral ocular adnexal lymphoid neoplasms in 17 patients. Am J Ophthalmol 103:555–568

Million RR, Cassisi NJ (1994) Management of head and neck cancer: a multidisciplinary approach, 2nd edn. JB Lippincott, Philadelphia

Mok JS, Pak MW, Chan KF, et al. (2001) Unusual T- and T/NK-cell non-Hodgkin's lymphoma of the larynx: a diagnostic challenge for clinicians and pathologists. Head Neck 23: 625–628

Nakata M, Matsuno Y, Katsumata N, et al. (1999) Histology according to the Revised European-American Lymphoma Classification significantly predicts the prognosis of ocular adnexal lymphoma. Leuk Lymphoma 32:533–543

Pederson RK, Pederson NT (1996) Primary non-Hodgkin's lymphoma of the thyroid gland: a population based study. Histopathol 28:25–32

Peterson K, Gordon KB, Heinemann MH, et al. (1993) The clinical spectrum of ocular lymphoma. Cancer 72: 843–849

Poiesz BJ, Ruscetti FW, Gazdar AF, et al. (1980) Detection and isolation of type C retrovirus particles from fresh and cultured lymphocytes of a patient with cutaneous T-cell lymphoma. Proc Natl Acad Sci USA 77:7415–7419

Pyke CM, Grant CS, Habermann TM, et al. (1992) Non-Hodgkin's lymphoma of the thyroid: is more than biopsy necessary? World J Surg 16:604–609

Quraishi MS, Bessell EM, Clark D, et al. (2000) Non-Hodgkin's lymphoma of the sinonasal tract. Laryngoscope 110: 1489–1492

Raderer M, Traub T, Formanek M, et al. (2002) Somatostatin-receptor scintigraphy for staging and follow-up of patients with extraintestinal marginal zone B-cell lymphoma of the mucosa associated lymphoid tissue (MALT)-type. Br J Cancer 85:1462–1466

Reske SN, Kotzerke J (2001) FDG-PET for clinical use. Results of the 3rd German Interdisciplinary Consensus Conference, "Onko-PET III" 21 July and 19 September 2000. Eur J Nucl Med 28:1707–1723

Ribrag V, Ell Hajj M, Janot F, et al. (2001) Early locoregional high-dose radiotherapy is associated with long-term disease control in localized primary angiocentric lymphoma of the nose and nasopharynx. Leukemia 15:1123–1126

Robbins KT, Fuller LM, Vlasak M, et al. (1985) Primary lymphomas of the nasal cavity and paranasal sinuses. Cancer 56:814–819

Rosai J (1992) Malignant lymphoma. In: Rosai J (ed) Atlas of tumor pathology, tumors of the thyroid gland. AFIP, Washington DC, pp 267–278.

Sasai K, Yamabe H, Dodo Y, et al. (2001) Non-Hodgkin's lymphoma of the ocular adnexa. Acta Oncol 40:485–490

Saul SH, Kapadia SB (1985) Primary lymphoma of Waldeyer's ring. Clinicopathologic study of 68 cases. Cancer 56: 157–166

Shields CL, Shields JA, Carvalho C, et al. (2001) Conjunctival lymphoid tumors: Clinical analysis of 117 cases and relationship to systemic lymphoma. Ophthalmol 108:979–984

Sirota DK, Degal RL (1979) Primary lymphomas of the thyroid. JAMA 242:1743–1746

Skarsgard ED, Connors JM, Robins RE (1991) A current analysis of primary lymphoma of the thyroid. Arch Surg 126: 1199–1203; discussion 1203–1204

Som PM, Curtin HD, Mancuso AA (1999) An imaging-based classification for the cervical nodes designed as an adjunct to recent clinically based nodal classifications. Arch Otolaryngol Head Neck Surg 125:388–396

Takamura H, Kanno M, Yamashita H, et al. (2001) A case of orbital solitary fibrous tumor. Ophthalmol 45:412–419

Takashima S, Ikezoe J, Morimoto S, et al. (1988) Primary thyroid lymphoma: evaluation with CT. Radiology 168: 765–768

Takashima S, Nomura N, Noguchi Y, et al. (1995) Primary thyroid lymphomas: evaluation with US, CT, and MRI. J Comput Assist Tomogr 19:282–288

Takayama F, Takashima S, Momose M, et al. (2001) MR imaging of primary malignant lymphoma in the larynx. Eur Radiol 11:1079–1082

Talal N, Sokoloff L, Barth WF (1967) Extrasalivary lymphoid abnormalities in Sjögren's syndrome (reticulum cell sarcoma, "pseudolymphomas" macroglobulinemia). Am J Med 43:50–65

Thiebelmont C, Mayer A, Dumontet C, et al. (2002) Primary thyroid lymphoma is a heterogeneous disease. J Clin Endocrinol Metab 87:105–111

Urquhart AC, Hutchins LG, Berg RL (2002) Distinguishing non-Hodgkin's lymphoma from squamous cell carcinoma tumors of the head and neck by computed tomography parameters. Laryngoscope 112:1079–1083

Valvassori GE, Sabris SS, Mafee RF, et al. (1999) Imaging of orbital lymphoproliferative disorders. Radiol Clin of North Am 37:135–150

Westacott S, Garner A, Moseley IF, et al. (1991) Orbital lymphoma versus reactive lymphoid hyperplasia: An analysis of the use of computed tomography in differential diagnosis. Br Ophthalmol 75:722–725

Whitcup SM, de Smet MD, Rubin BI, et al. (1993) Intraocular lymphoma. Clinical and histopathologic diagnosis. Opthamol 100:1399–1406

White WA, Ferry JA, Harris NL, et al. (1995) Ocular adnexal lymphoma. A clinicopathologic study with identification of lymphomas of mucosa-associated lymphoid tissue type. Ophthalmol 102:1994–2006

Wirth A, Seymour JF, Hicks RJ, et al. (2002) Flourine-18 fluorodeoxyglucose positron emission tomography, gallium-67 scintigraphy, and conventional staging for Hodgkin's disease and non-Hodgkin's lymphoma. Am J Med 112: 262–268

Wirtzfeld DA, Winston JS, Hicks WL Jr, et al. (2001) Clinical presentation and treatment of non-Hodgkin's lymphoma of the thyroid gland. Ann Surg Oncol 8:338–341

Wolf BC, Sheahan K, DeCoste D, et al. (1992) Immunohistochemical analysis of small cell tumors of the thyroid gland: an Eastern Cooperative Oncology Group study. Human Pathol 23:1252–1261

Wotherspoon AC, Diss TC, Pan LX, et al. (1993) Primary low-grade B-cell lymphoma of the conjunctiva: A mucosa-associated lymphoid tissue type of lymphoma. Histopathol 23:417–424

Yang PJ, Carmody RF, Seeger JF (1986) Computed tomography in hematologic malignancies of paranasal sinuses. J Comput Tomogr 10:1003–1005

Yasumoto M, Yoshimura R, Sunaba K, et al. (2001) Sonographic appearances of malignant lymphoma of the salivary glands. J Clin Ultrasound 29:491–498

Zulman J, Jaffe R, Talal N (1978) Evidence that the malignant lymphoma of Sjögren's syndrome is a monoclonal B-cell neoplasm. N Engl J Med 299:1215–1220

7 Thoracic Involvement in Non-Hodgkin Lymphoma

Pamela J. DiPiro, Philip Costello

CONTENTS

7.1 Introduction

Non-Hodgkin lymphoma (NHL) is known to involve multiple intra- and extrathoracic sites. Radiologic evidence of thoracic disease occurs in 45–48% of patients with NHL (CASTELLINO et al. 1996; ROMANO and LIBSHITZ 1998); the frequency at autopsy is 73% (VIETA and CRAVER 1941). Although the most common manifestation of thoracic lymphoma is intrathoracic nodal involvement, it can occur at multiple extranodal sites, including the thymus, thyroid, pulmonary parenchyma, pleura, pericardium, heart, chest wall, and breast. This chapter will review the various extranodal sites of thoracic involvement by NHL; the patterns of disease presentation; and the imaging evaluation at presentation, and in follow-up; as well as some points about recurrence.

7.2 Thymus

Thymic involvement by lymphoma has been more commonly described in Hodgkin disease (HD), with reported incidence of 30–56% at initial staging (HERON et al. 1988; KELLER and CASTELMAN 1974; WERNECKE et al. 1991b). To our knowledge, there are no large studies that have looked at the frequency of thymic involvement by NHL. However, lymphoblastic lymphoma, high-grade B-cell lymphoma and mucosa-associated lymphoid tissue (MALT) lymphoma of the thymus have all been described (Fig. 7.1) (STROLLO et al. 1999; YI et al. 1998). The radiologic findings of thymic lymphoma vary, and include thymic enlargement (generalized or with one or more focal masses); diffuse, mild contrast enhancement; and occasionally, cystic degeneration (at presentation or following therapy) (YI et al. 1998). Typically, there is associated nodal involvement, though isolated thymic lymphoma can occur. It is important to note that thymic enlargement following chemotherapy may be secondary to rebound hyperplasia.

Thymic involvement is most commonly evaluated with CT. Studies have shown the efficacy of ultrasound, though given the additional information provided with CT (regarding the remainder of the thorax, including pulmonary parenchyma), it is the test of choice (Fig. 7.2).

Pamela J. DiPiro, MD
Assistant Professor of Radiology, Harvard Medical School, Clinical Director of CT, Dana Farber Cancer Institute, 44 Binney Street, Boston, MA 02115, USA
Philip Costello, MD
Professor of Radiology, Harvard Medical School, Director of Thoracic Imaging, Brigham and Women's Hospital, 75 Francis Street, Boston, MA 02114, USA

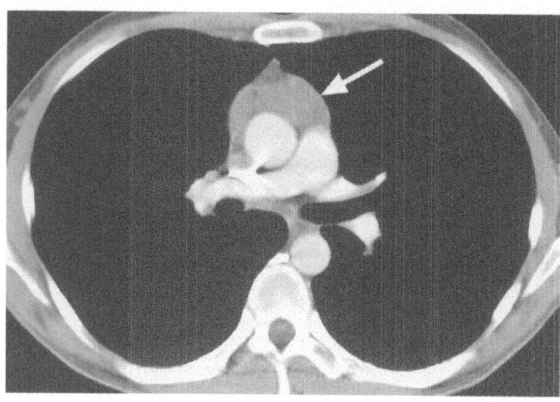

Fig. 7.1. Non-Hodgkin lymphoma of the thymus in a 41-year-old man. Axial contrast-enhanced CT scan reveals an anterior mediastinal mass (*arrow*) with no other sites of disease.

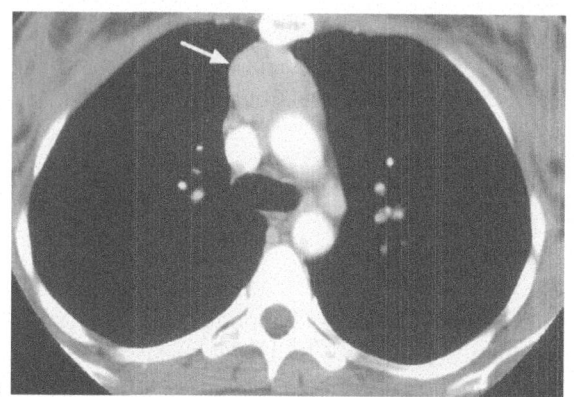

a

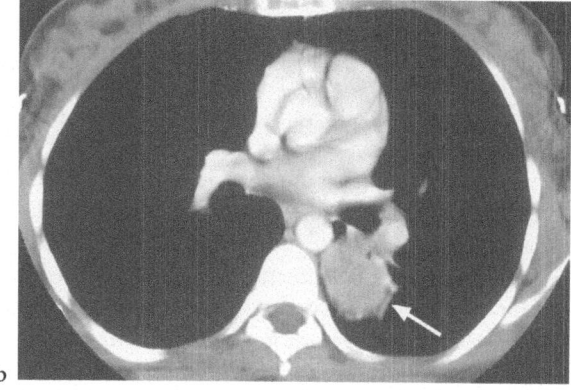

b

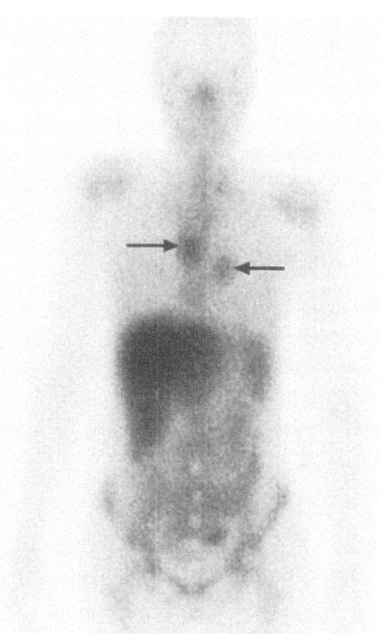

c

Fig. 7.2a–c. Non-Hodgkin lymphoma of the thymus and pulmonary parenchyma in a 23-year-old woman. a Axial contrast-enhanced CT scan reveals an anterior mediastinal mass (*arrow*). b More caudal CT image reveals a left lower lobe pulmonary mass (*arrow*). c Gallium scintigraphy reveals uptake at both sites (*arrows*), but is otherwise negative.

7.3
Thyroid

Primary thyroid lymphoma is rare, with a reported incidence of 1.8–8% of all thyroid malignancies, whereas secondary thyroid lymphoma reportedly occurs in upwards of 10% of cases (TAKASHIMA et al. 1988; COLTRERA 1999). In contrast to thymic involvement of NHL (where HD is much more common), thyroid involvement is nearly always secondary to NHL. Thyroid lymphoma is typically seen after the age of 50 (mean > 60 years), and more commonly affects women. The majority are seen in patients with a history of Hashimoto thyroiditis, and are typically B-cell lymphomas, though occasional MALT and T-cell lymphomas have been described (COLTRERA 1999).

Thyroid imaging can be accomplished by ultrasound, CT or MR imaging. Ultrasound typically depicts hypoechoic masses (TAKASHIMA et al. 1989a). The reported CT findings include solitary nodules, multiple nodules or diffuse goiter (TAKASHIMA et al. 1988; TAKASHIMA et al. 1989a). Lesions are typically

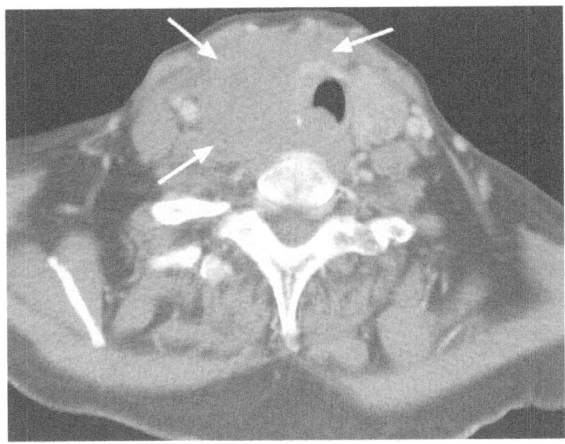

Fig. 7.3. Primary non-Hodgkin lymphoma of the thyroid in a 73-year-old woman presenting with a rapidly enlarging thyroid mass. Axial contrast-enhanced CT image reveals a homogeneous, non-calcified mass, predominantly involving the right thyroid lobe (*arrows*).

homogeneous, and the low frequency of calcification and necrosis are notable, possibly suggesting differentiation from anaplastic carcinoma (Fig. 7.3) (ISHIKAWA et al. 2002; TAKASHIMA et al. 1988). Earlier studies suggested that CT evaluation of thyroid lymphoma was superior to ultrasound (TAKASHIMA et al. 1989a). Although some more recent studies suggest that ultrasound with image-guided biopsy is the procedure of choice in differentiating Hashimoto thyroiditis from lymphoma (PODOLOFF 1996), there is some controversy as to whether or not an accurate diagnosis of thyroid lymphoma can be made with fine needle aspiration (COLTRERA 1999). Recently, immunohistochemical staining has improved diagnostic capabilities. MR imaging of thyroid lymphoma reveals a homogeneous mass with high intensity compared to Hashimoto thyroiditis on T2-weighted MR images. MR imaging also offers the ability to image in the coronal plane, which can be helpful for radiation therapy planning (TAKASHIMA et al. 1989b). Although thyroid lymphoma is hot on Ga-scintigraphy, it cannot be differentiated from Hashimoto thyroiditis, which is also Gallium-avid (COLTRERA 1999).

7.4
Pulmonary Parenchyma

The reported incidence of pulmonary parenchymal involvement by NHL at initial presentation is 13–24% (CASTELLINO et al. 1996; ROMANO AND LIBSHITZ 1998). However, in patients with AIDS-related lymphoma, its incidence is much higher, reported at 45–79% (SIDER et al. 1989; BLUNT and PADLEY 1995). Primary pulmonary NHL represents 0.4% of NHL and 3.6% of extranodal lymphomas (BERKMAN and BREUER 1993). Intraparenchymal pulmonary NHL may present without lymphadenopathy, (unlike HD, wherein pulmonary parenchymal involvement is nearly always associated with mediastinal or hilar lymphadenopathy at presentation). Pulmonary involvement is reportedly associated with hilar and/or mediastinal lymphadenopathy in 42–44% of NHL cases (BALIKIAN and HERMAN 1979; ROMANO and LIBSHITZ 1998). Three distinct radiological patterns of intraparenchymal pulmonary lymphoma have been described: nodular, bronchovascular (or lymphangitic) and pneumonic (or alveolar) (BRAGG 1978). More than one of these patterns is often noted simultaneously (BERKMAN and BREUER 1993; LEWIS et al. 1991).

The nodular form is the most common overall, typically measuring less than 3 cm, and often, possessing an ill-defined or shaggy border (Fig. 7.4) (BRAGG 1978; LEWIS et al. 1991; BERKMAN and BREUER 1993). Nodules may be unilateral or bilateral, solitary or multiple, frequently traverse lobar fissures, and have a predilection for the lower lobes and perihilar regions (Fig. 7.5) (TAKVORIAN and DIPIRO 2002). In addition, they may contain air bronchograms, and uncommonly, may cavitate.

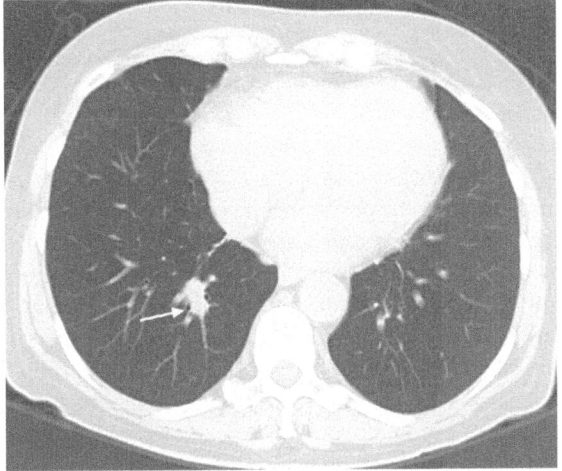

Fig. 7.4. Low-grade non-Hodgkin lymphoma in a 69-year-old woman presenting with a solitary pulmonary nodule. Axial CT image reveals an irregularly marginated, right lower lobe, solitary pulmonary nodule (*arrow*).

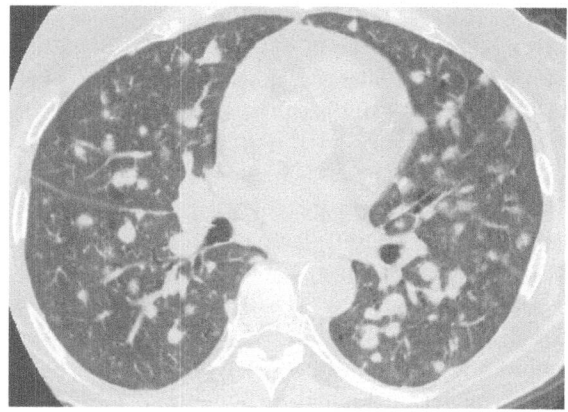

Fig. 7.5. Stage IV diffuse large cell non-Hodgkin lymphoma in a 61-year-old woman. Axial CT scan reveals multiple, bilateral, partially circumscribed pulmonary nodules.

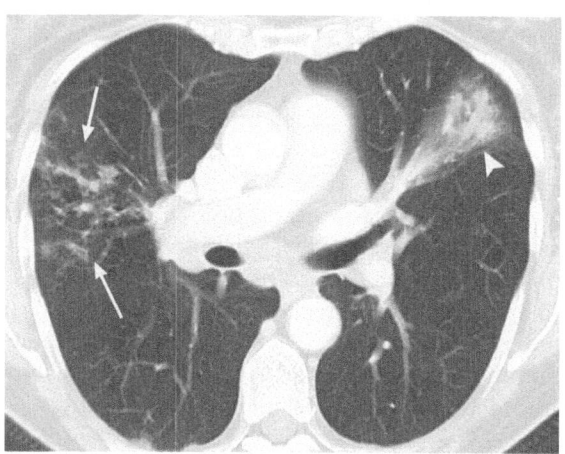

Fig. 7.6. Mantle cell non-Hodgkin lymphoma in a 65-year-old woman with bilateral lymphangitic extension. Axial CT image reveals reticular and nodular markings extending from the right hilum (*arrows*). Patchy opacity on the left is the result of more extensive involvement (*arrowhead*).

The bronchovascular or lymphangitic form spreads along the peribronchial or perivascular bundles. Infiltrates typically arise from direct spread from mediastinal lymph nodes. When located in the central or perihilar region, reticulonodular and coarse reticular markings radiate from the hilum into the adjacent lung (Fig. 7.6). When involvement is more extensive, a more focal patchy opacity may be seen. Radiographic findings may be due to direct tumor extension, causing parabronchial nodules delineating an air bronchogram, and/or due to obstruction of the central pulmonary lymphatics (more commonly seen with HD than NHL) (BERKMAN and BREUER 1993; BRAGG 1987; NORTH et al. 1990).

The pneumonic or alveolar form is the least common manifestation of pulmonary lymphoma, seen in 26% of patients with pulmonary NHL, and is radiographically indistinguishable from pneumonia (Fig. 7.7) (BERKMAN and BREUER 1993). Consolidation may be unilateral or bilateral, segmental or lobar, and is not associated with volume loss (Fig. 7.8).

Pulmonary MALT lymphoma, previously referred to as pseudolymphoma, is a relatively recently described subtype of B-cell lymphoma (ISAAKSON and WRIGHT 1983). It typically consists of aggregates of well-differentiated, extranodal B-cells (much less commonly, T-cells). MALT lymphomas are fairly indolent, remaining localized for a long time, and

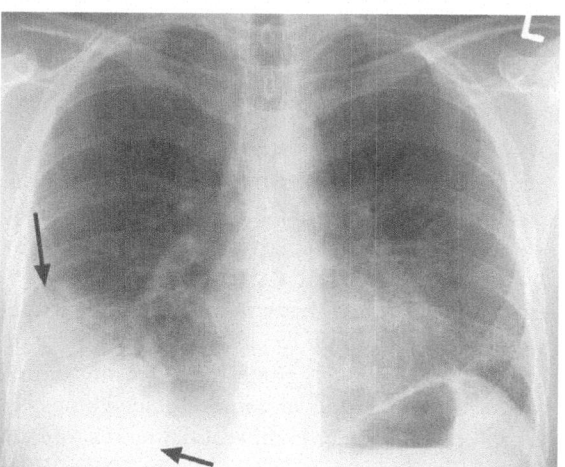

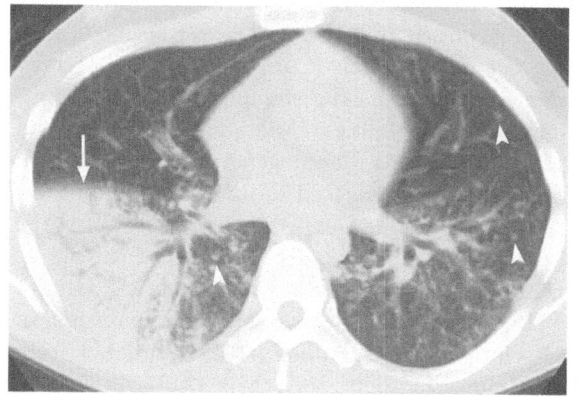

Fig. 7.7a,b. Primary pulmonary large cell non-Hodgkin lymphoma in a 25-year-old man who presented with dense right lower lobe consolidation that was refractory to antibiotics. **a** Posteroanterior chest radiograph shows dense right lower lobe opacity (*arrows*). **b** Axial CT image reveals dense consolidation with air bronchograms (*arrow*); small nodules are also present in both lower lobes (*arrowheads*). (With permission from [DiPiro PJ, Costello P (2000) Imaging of thoracic lymphoma. In: Contemporary diagnostic radiology. Lippincott Williams & Wilkins, Philadelphia])

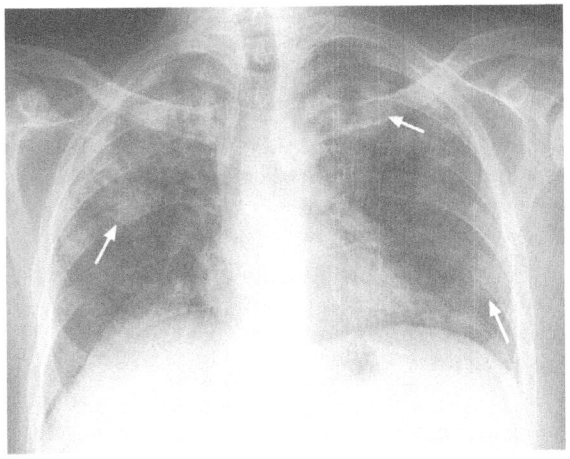

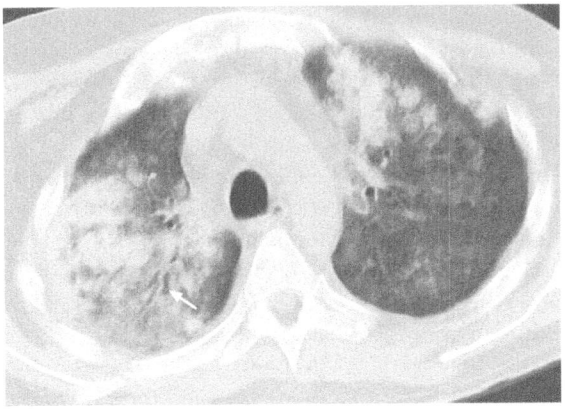

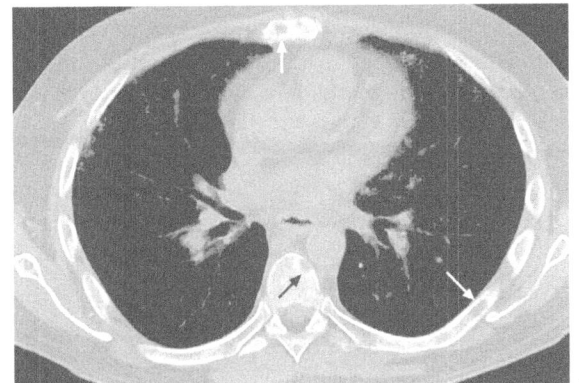

Fig. 7.8a–c. Recurrent B-cell non-Hodgkin lymphoma in a 50-year-old woman with both pulmonary and osseous involvement. **a** Posteroanterior chest radiograph reveals bilateral, patchy, alveolar opacities (*arrows*). **b** Axial CT image reveals patchy consolidation with right upper lobe air bronchograms (*arrow*). **c** Axial CT bone window reveals lytic bony lesions in the sternum, spine and ribs (*arrows*).

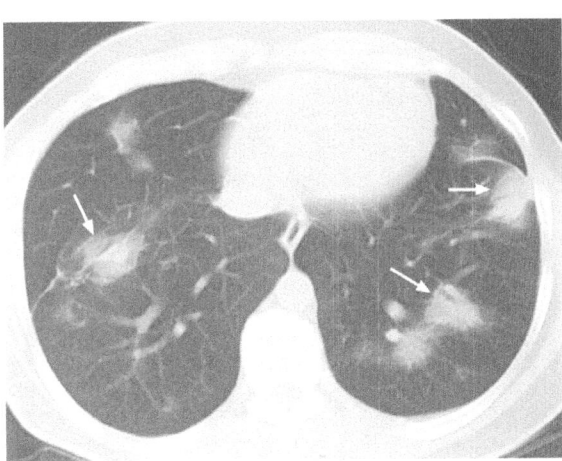

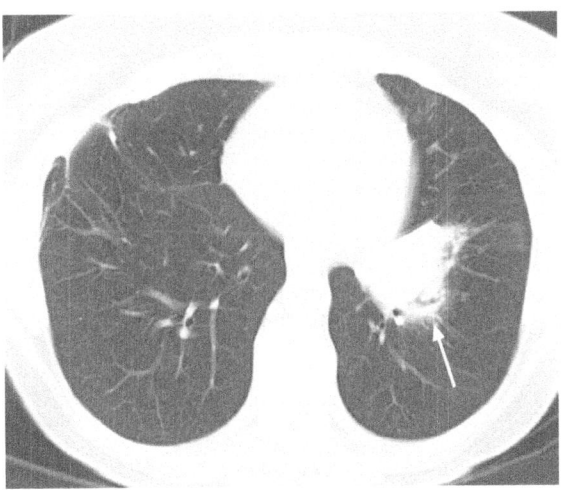

Fig. 7.9. Pulmonary MALT lymphoma in a 44-year-old man. Axial CT image reveals bilateral patchy areas of consolidation, some with air bronchograms (*arrows*), which have been generally stable since diagnosis was made, 10 years previously.

Fig. 7.10. Pulmonary MALT lymphoma in a 70-year-old woman. Axial CT image reveals focal area of dense consolidation with air bronchograms (*arrow*) in the left lower lobe.

are often clinically occult (Fig. 7.9). They are more commonly found in men, with a peak incidence in the sixth decade (BRAGG 1987; AU and LEUNG 1997). Radiographically, they most commonly present as areas of parenchymal consolidation with air bronchograms and/or ill-defined nodules, with or without air bronchograms (Fig. 7.10). More linear areas of attenuation and ground glass abnormalities have also been described (WISLEZ et al. 1999; KNISELY et al. 1999). They do not calcify, rarely cavitate, and are not commonly associated with pleural effusions or mediastinal lymphadenopathy (KNISELY et al. 1999; KING et al. 2000; LAZAR et al. 1996; MCCULLOCH et al. 1998). Prognosis is excellent, though treatment remains controversial, with therapeutic recommendations ranging from simple monitoring, to single agent chemotherapy, to surgical excision (CADRANEL et al. 2002).

Large cell lymphomas, which are more rare, and often present in patients with an underlying disorder such as immunodeficiency, most commonly manifest as diffuse lymphangitic infiltrates, and may progress rapidly (BERKMAN and BREUER 1993; CADRANEL et al. 2002). They may also present in the pneumonic/alveolar form, and be radiographically indistinguishable from pneumonia (Fig. 7.11) (BRAGG 1978). Prognosis is typically poor.

Although plain chest radiography often is the initial means of detection of pulmonary lymphoma, it is less sensitive than CT. In a retrospective study, plain chest radiography detected pulmonary parenchymal involvement in 13% of patients with NHL, while CT revealed disease in 24% of these patients (ROMANO and LIBSHITZ 1998). An earlier study suggested that despite the increased sensitivity of CT scans in the detection of thoracic lymphoma and accordant increase in disease stage, the increased sensitivity (over plain radiography) had no effect on the initial therapy of newly diagnosed patients with NHL (CASTELLINO et al. 1996). At many institutions, thoracic CT is performed at initial diagnosis to provide a more comprehensive evaluation, and to serve as a baseline for follow-up studies (MUSUMECI and TESORO-TESS 1994; SCUTELLARI et al. 2000; TAKVORIAN and DIPIRO 2002).

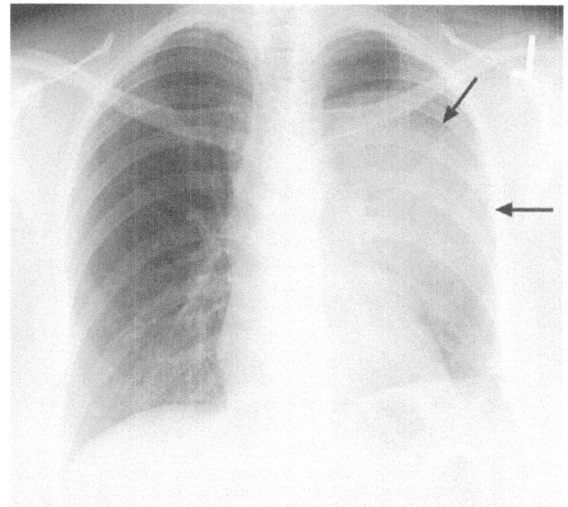

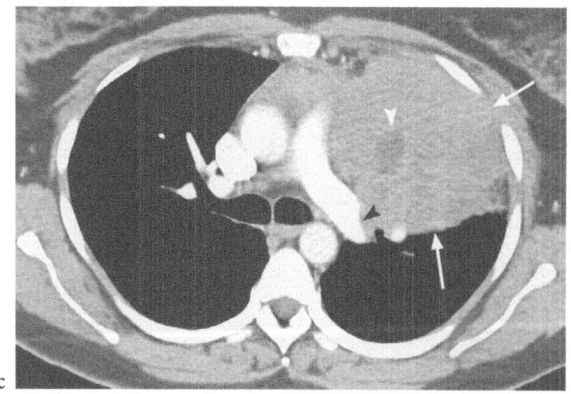

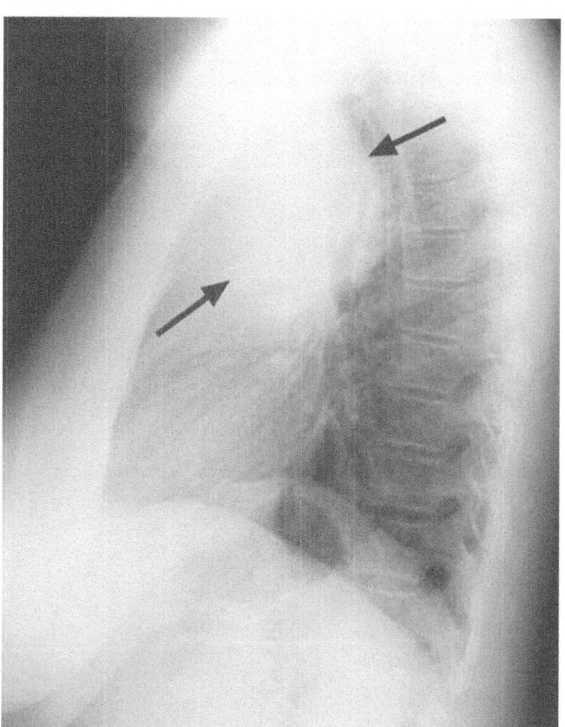

Fig. 7.11a–c. Pulmonary large cell non-Hodgkin lymphoma in a 40-year-old woman. **a** Posteroanterior and (**b**) lateral chest radiographs reveal a large, mass-like opacity in the left upper lobe (*arrows*). **c** Axial contrast-enhanced CT image shows large left upper lobe mass (*arrows*) with central necrosis (*white arrowhead*) extending into the mediastinum and compressing/invading the main left pulmonary artery (*black arrowhead*).

7.5
Pleura/Pericardium

Although pleural effusion may be the presenting manifestation of NHL, it is rarely the only site of disease. Twenty to seventy percent of patients with NHL and a pleural effusion have evidence of mediastinal disease, and 90% of these patients have disease elsewhere (Fig. 7.12) (BERKMAN and BREUER 1993). In a series of 181 patients, pleural effusions were detected radiographically in 20% of patients at initial presentation of NHL; 5% of patients also possessed focal soft tissue pleural masses (CASTELLINO et al. 1996). In another series, pleural disease was noted at presentation in 13% of patients with NHL, though no distinction between effusions and soft tissue masses was made (ROMANO and LIBSHITZ 1998). The latter, often presenting as small

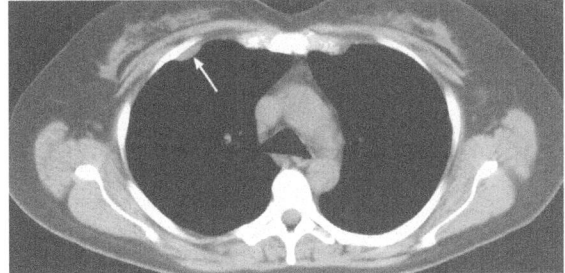

Fig. 7.13. Recurrent non-Hodgkin lymphoma in a 59-year-old woman. Axial CT image reveals a new right anterior pleural based mass (*arrow*).

pleural plaques or nodules, are typically due to tumor extension along the lymphatic channels (Fig. 7.13) (BRAGG 1978). SHUMAN and LIBSHITZ (1984), in a small series, noted solid pleural-based lymphoma in 8 of 24 (33%) patients with NHL, manifesting as subpleural nodules or plaques. These included both initial sites of presentation and recurrences. The authors noted that the patient population was skewed and the actual incidence is likely somewhat lower. Reportedly, 72% of patients with NHL have malignant pleural involvement at autopsy (BILLINGHAM et al. 1975). However, primary pleural lymphoma is rare.

Pleural effusions in patients with NHL may arise from different causes. They may result from direct extension of tumor to the pleura, a mechanism more commonly seen with carcinoma than lymphoma. Effusions may develop when lymphoma causes pulmonary lymphatic or venous obstruction. Finally, obstruction of the thoracic duct may result in chylothorax (BERKMAN and BREUER 1993; NORTH et al. 1990). When related to an obstructive process, pleural effusions will typically clear quite promptly with the institution of radiation or chemotherapy.

Pericardial disease (i.e., thickening and/or fluid) is described in 4–8% of patients presenting with NHL (CASTELLINO et al. 1996; ROMANO and LIBSHITZ 1998), particularly in patients with large mediastinal masses (Fig. 7.14). Pericardial effusions will typical resolve quickly with the onset of therapy. Soft tissue masses can also be seen involving the pericardium and infrequently, may invade the heart.

Although pleural and pericardial effusions may be detected on plain radiographs, they are better evaluated with cross sectional imaging – most commonly CT. CARLSEN et al. (1993) found that MR imaging is significantly more sensitive than CT in the detection of pleural disease, which may occur more frequently than previously recognized.

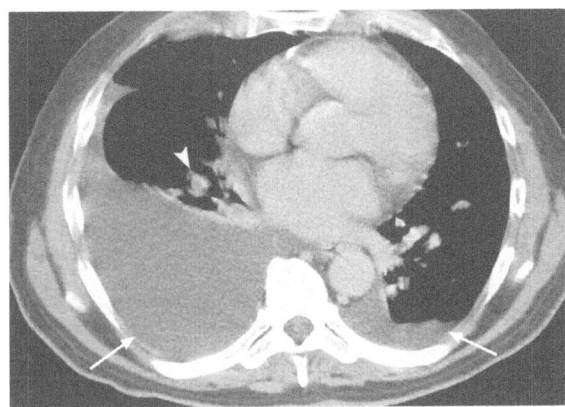

a

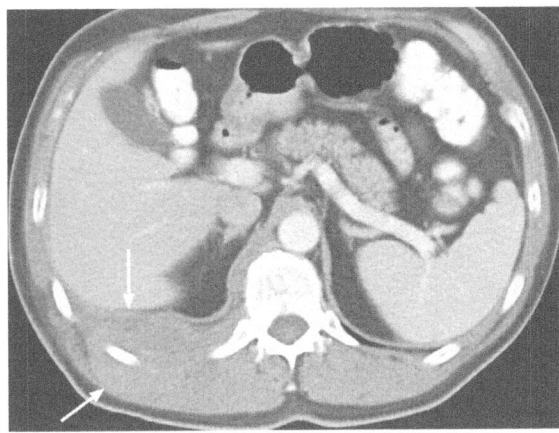

b

Fig. 7.12a,b. Recurrent non-Hodgkin lymphoma in a 57-year-old man presenting with bilateral pleural effusions; thoracentesis revealed no malignant cells. **a** Axial contrast-enhanced CT image reveals bilateral pleural effusions (*arrows*), right greater than left, with associated left lower lobe compressive atelectasis (*arrowhead*). **b** More caudal CT image shows a large, infiltrating, posterior chest wall mass, with attenuation value similar to that of muscle (*arrows*).

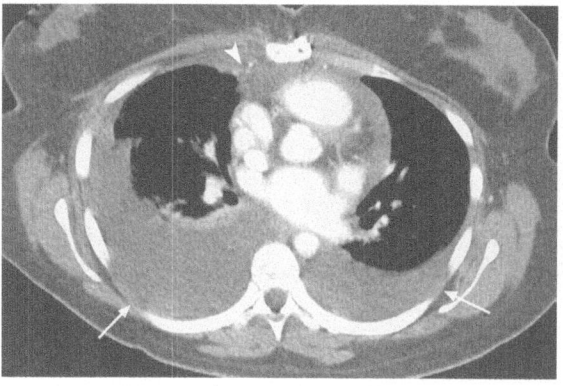

Fig. 7.14. Bilateral pleural and pericardial effusions in a 21-year-old woman with a large anterior mediastinal large cell non-Hodgkin lymphoma. Axial contrast-enhanced CT image reveals pleural (*arrows*) and pericardial (*arrowhead*) effusions that quickly resolved with chemotherapy.

7.6
Heart

Primary cardiac lymphoma is rare in immunocompetent people, reportedly accounting for 7 of 533 (1.3%) primary cardiac tumors and cysts in one series (McALLISTER and FENOGLIO 1978) and 0.5% of all extranodal lymphomas in another (ROLLA et al. 2002). The incidence of cardiac lymphoma in AIDS patients is higher. A review of the English language literature in 1992 revealed 22 patients with AIDS and cardiac lymphoma (HOLLADAY 1992). Metastases to the heart are more common; autopsy specimens reportedly revealed lymphomatous involvement in 20–24% of patients with disseminated NHL (ROBERTS et al. 1968; McDONNELL et al. 1982).

Historically, prognosis has been poor due to delayed diagnosis and critical site of disease. However, some more recent reports have suggested improved outcomes with earlier diagnosis and prompt treatment (CERESOLI et al. 1997). In a review of 50 cases (48 in literature and 2 additional cases), the most common presenting symptom was intractable congestive heart failure, with other reported symptoms of precordial pain, arrhythmias and cardiac tamponade (CERESOLI et al. 1997). Often, symptoms present late, with subsequent rapid decompensation.

Chest radiographs may reveal pericardial and or pleural effusions, from which cytologic diagnosis is sometimes derived. Transthoracic echocardiography and CT have been standard in the work-up of cardiac masses; however, transesophageal echocardiography and (MR imaging have revealed improved sensitivities of > 90% (Fig. 7.15) (CERESOLI et al. 1997).

7.7
Chest Wall

Thoracic wall involvement can be seen at initial presentation or at recurrence, either as a solitary site of disease or secondary to direct extension from mediastinal or parenchymal disease, in 4–5% of patients with NHL (CASTELLINO et al. 1996; PRESS et al. 1985). Thoracic wall masses commonly involve the pectoralis muscles, likely arising from the lateral thoracic and interpectoral lymph nodes (Fig. 7.16) (PRESS et al. 1985). Other sites of involvement include ribs (with lytic destruction and bony expan-

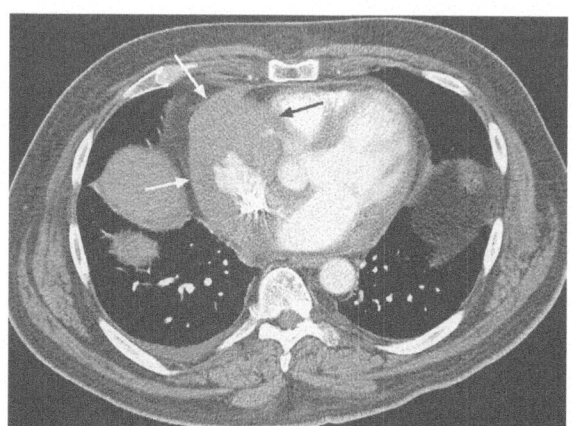

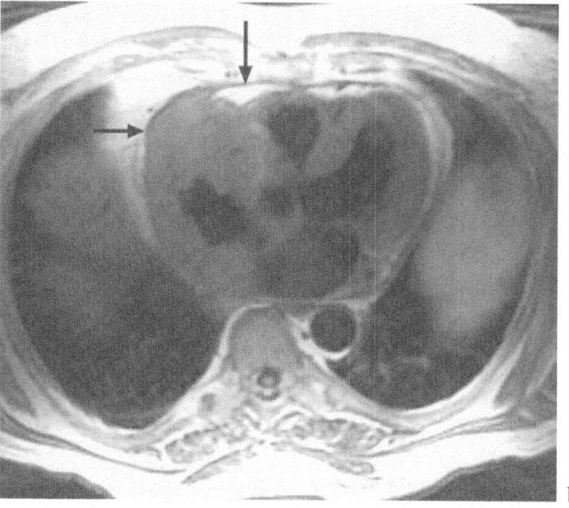

Fig. 7.15a,b. High-grade B-cell non-Hodgkin lymphoma in a 56-year-old woman presenting with cervical lymphadenopathy and a cardiac mass. **a** Axial contrast-enhanced CT image reveals a soft tissue mass that is inseparable from the pericardium, and surrounds the right atrium (*arrows*). **b** Axial T1-weighted MR image reveals encasement of the right atrium and a portion of the right ventricle, with invasion of the pericardial space and infiltration of the myocardium (*arrows*).

sion), vertebral bodies, chest wall that is contiguous with involved pleura or pulmonary parenchyma, and breast (BERGIN et al. 1990; PRESS et al. 1985).

Although CT is much more sensitive than plain films in the detection of chest wall disease, MR imaging has supplanted it as the modality of choice for the evaluation of chest wall lymphoma (Fig. 7.17) (BERGIN et al. 1990).

7.8
Breast

Mammary lymphoma is rare, with a reported incidence of primary breast lymphoma at 2.2% of all extranodal lymphomas (FREEMAN et al. 1972) and 0.05–0.53% of total breast malignancies (PETREK 1991). More commonly, breast involvement by lymphoma is secondary, presenting in conjunction with extramammary lymphomatous disease. Typically, patients present with a palpable mass, though some breast lymphoma is clinically occult, and detected on routine mammography (Fig. 7.18). Less commonly, a patient may present with a swollen, inflamed breast, often associated with ipsilateral axillary lymphadenopathy, an appearance indistinguishable from inflammatory breast carcinoma, and related to lymphatic obstruction (Fig. 7.19).

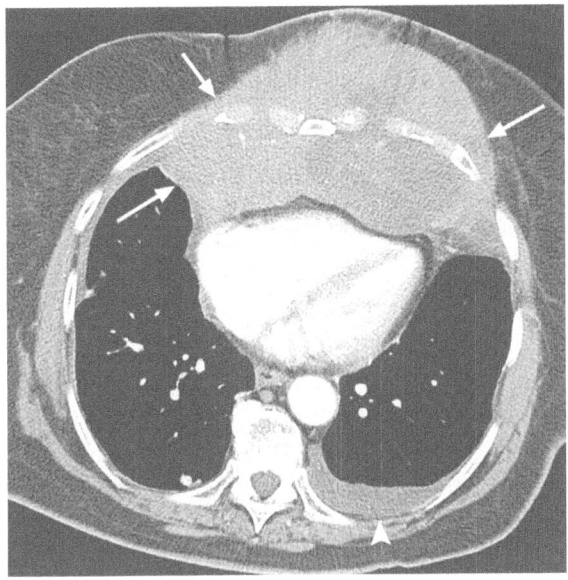

Fig. 7.16. Non-Hodgkin lymphoma in a 78-year-old woman. Axial contrast-enhanced CT scan shows left pleural effusion (*arrowhead*) and a large anterior chest wall mass (*arrows*).

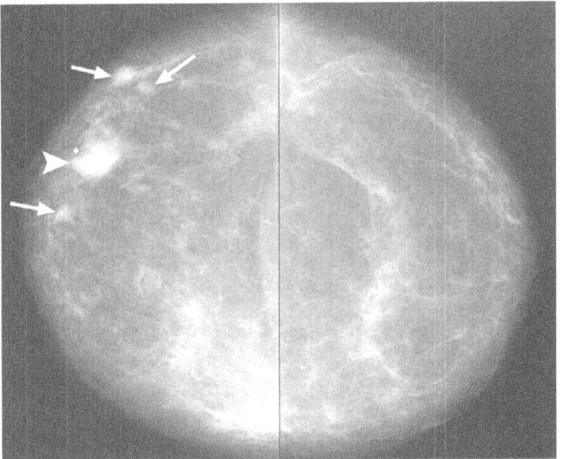

a

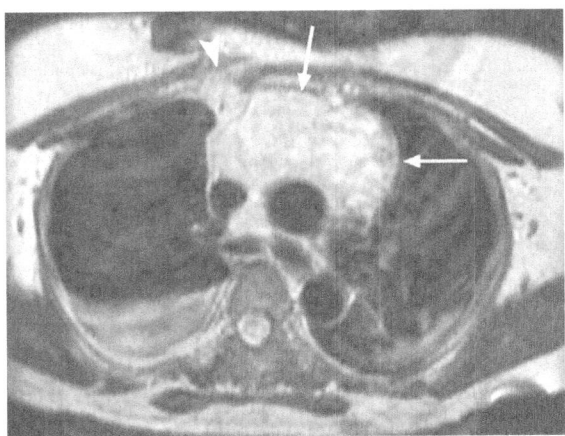

Fig. 7.17. Chest wall involvement by large B-cell non-Hodgkin lymphoma in a 54-year-old woman. Axial fast spin-echo T2-weighted MR image reveals subtle right anterior chest wall invasion (*arrowhead*) by a large anterior mediastinal mass (*arrows*). There is also a right pleural effusion. (With permission from [TAKVORIAN and DIPIRO 2002])

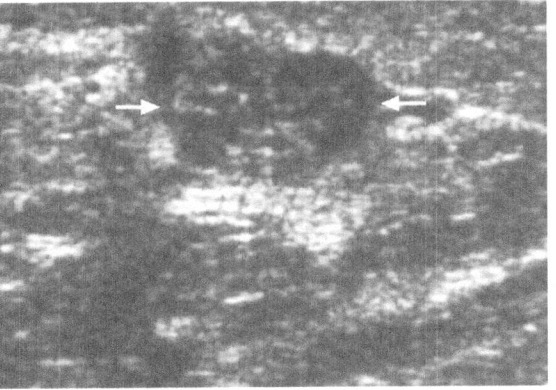

b

Fig. 7.18a,b. Primary non-Hodgkin lymphoma of the breast in a 66-year-old woman who presented with a palpable mass. a Craniocaudal mammographic view reveals three, small, non-calcified masses (*arrows*) in the left breast; a BB marks the largest, palpable lesion (*arrowhead*). b US image of the palpable area reveals an irregularly-marginated, hypoechoic mass (*arrows*).

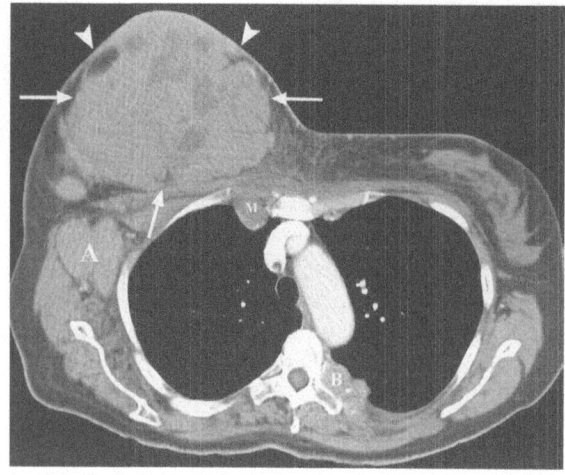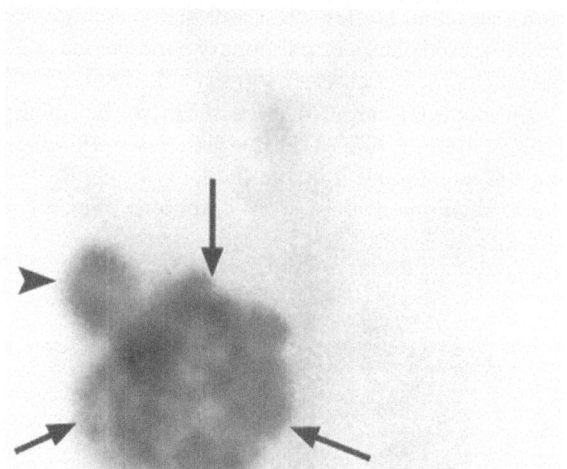

a   b

Fig.7.19a,b. Large cell non-Hodgkin lymphoma of the right breast in a 71-year-old woman who presented with redness and swelling of the breast, first noted after an automobile accident, when presumed contusion did not improve. **a** Axial contrast-enhanced CT image shows an 18 cm, necrotic right breast mass (*arrows*) with associated skin thickening (*arrowheads*) and extensive right axillary (*A*) and internal mammary (*M*) lymphadenopathy. Note a left costovertebral bone lesion (*B*). **b** Gallium scintigraphy shows marked uptake in the right breast (*arrows*) and axilla (*arrowhead*).

The mammographic appearance of breast lymphoma is non-specific, without pathognomonic or distinguishing features. The most common appearance is that of a solid, incompletely circumscribed or ill-defined, non-calcified mass. Sonographically, the masses are hypoechoic, predominantly homogeneous in echotexture, and often, possess posterior acoustic enhancement (DiPiro et al. 1996; Liberman et al. 1994).

7.9
AIDS-Related Lymphoma

AIDS-related lymphoma (ARL) is typically a high-grade, B-cell, Epstein-Barr virus (EBV)-positive, aggressive lymphoma, with a poor prognosis. ARLs tend to be extranodal, most commonly involving the central nervous system, bone marrow, bowel and mucocutaneous tissue, with less than 10% involving the thorax (Bazot et al. 1999). Earlier reports of ARL in the thorax described the most frequent findings as lung disease and pleural effusions (Sider et al. 1989; Blunt and Padley 1995). However, these studies included patients with documented disseminated disease, or made no distinction between disseminated and primary pulmonary disease. More recent studies have looked at primary pulmonary, AIDS-related lymphoma, and describe the most common findings as solitary or multiple, well-defined masses,

some with cavitation, but without associated lymphadenopathy or effusions (Figs. 7.20, 7.21) (Ray et al. 1998; Bazot et al. 1999). Findings are indistinguishable from infection, and require biopsy for diagnosis.

7.10
Posttransplantation Lymphoproliferative Disorder

Posttransplantation lymphoproliferative disorders (PTLD) comprise a spectrum from hyperplastic lesions to discrete NHL, and although rare, are a significant cause of mortality in allograft recipients (Muti et al. 2002). Onset of PTLD after solid organ transplantation varies widely from less than one month to several years. They are typically EBV-associated B-cell lymphoproliferative disorders that result from an immunocompromised patient's inability to fight neoplastic cellular activity. Fourteen percent of these lymphomas are of T-cell origin. The frequency of PTLD varies with the type of organ transplanted, being highest with heart-lung (9.4%), liver (2.2%), and heart (1.8%), likely related to more aggressive immunosuppression following these procedures (Dodd et al. 1992). Although PTLD has been noted with all immunosuppressive agents, specific agents have caused different organs to be affected (Trofe et al. 2002).

Seven percent of patients with PTLD manifest with thoracic tumors. The highest frequency (60%) has been reported following heart-lung transplanta-

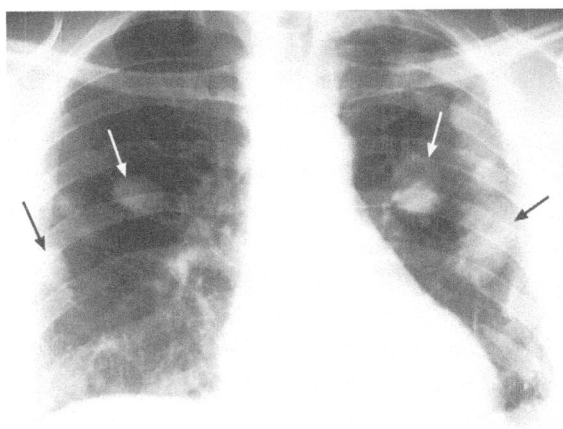

Fig. 7.20. High grade B-cell non-Hodgkin lymphoma in a 28-year-old HIV-positive man. Posteroanterior chest radiograph reveals multiple, bilateral pulmonary masses (*arrows*).

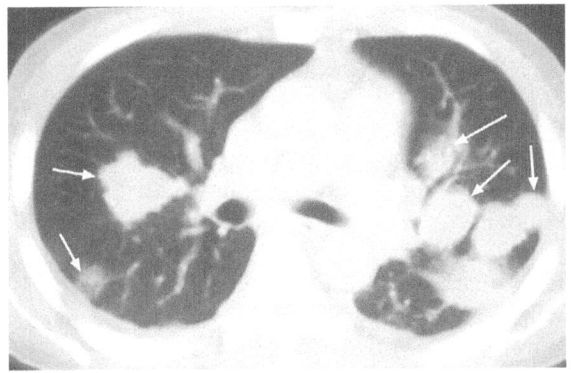

Fig. 7.21. Biopsy-proven non-Hodgkin lymphoma in a 35-year-old man with 18 month history of AIDS. Axial CT image reveals bilateral pulmonary masses (*arrows*).

tion. Thoracic sites of PTLD reported include the lungs, mediastinal lymph nodes, pleura and pericardium (Dodd et al. 1992). The most common pulmonary parenchymal presentation is multiple scattered nodules, ranging from 5 mm to 5 cm. They tend to be relatively well circumscribed and do not cavitate (Fig. 7.22). Other reported manifestations are alveolar opacities, or rarely, diffuse reticulonodular lesions. Pulmonary findings may be seen alone, or in combination with mediastinal or hilar lymphadenopathy. The latter is typically comprised of a few, nonconfluent, 2–4 cm nodes, though large masses have been described. Pleural effusions are often present, and pericardial effusions, with or without tumor invasion, have been described (Au and Leung 1997; Dodd et al. 1992; Lee et al. 1996). The appearance

is often non-specific, and may be radiographically inseparable from infection.

Treatment typically involves decrease in immunosuppression, which, early on, can reverse PTLD (Fig. 7.23). However, this also increases the risk of organ rejection. Surgical resection and chemotherapy may play roles in treatment, depending on the site and extent of tumor involvement. Although reversible if caught early, if diagnosis of PTLD is delayed, prognosis may be poor.

7.11
Staging and Follow-up Imaging Evaluation

7.11.1
CT

Although thoracic lymphoma is often first detected with plain chest radiography, several studies have documented increased sensitivity with CT (Castellino et al. 1996; Romano and Libshitz 1998). Despite this, the role of CT in the evaluation of thoracic NHL has been somewhat controversial. Khoury et al. (1986) concluded that CT was indicated in two specific groups of patients with NHL: those patients with stage I or II disease and questionable or normal chest radiographs (where CT would assist in staging), and those patients with definitely abnormal chest radiographs (where CT would help define radiation portals). Castellino et al. (1996), in a subsequent study of 181 patients with thoracic NHL, concluded that CT is not indicated in

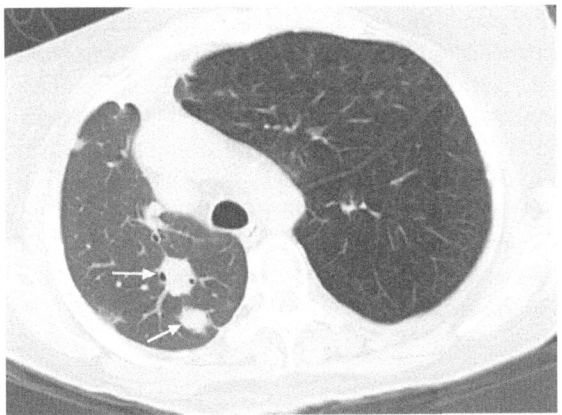

Fig. 7.22. Posttransplantation lymphoproliferative disorder in a 53-year-old woman, status post right lung transplant for severe chronic obstructive pulmonary disease. Axial CT image shows several right lung masses (*arrows*). Biopsy revealed large B-cell non-Hodgkin lymphoma.

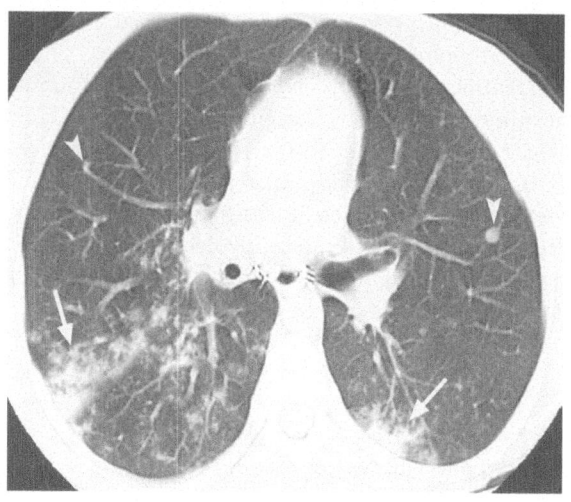
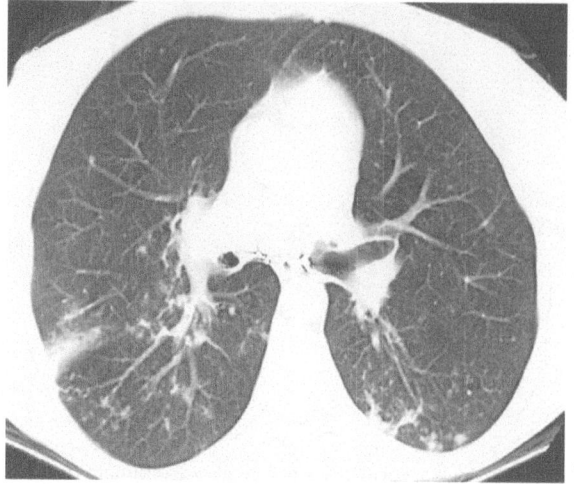

Fig. 7.23a,b. Posttransplantation lymphoproliferative disorder in a 21-year-old woman, 18 months post bilateral lung transplant for cystic fibrosis. The disorder regressed upon cessation of immunosuppression. **a** Axial CT image reveals bilateral ill-defined nodules (*arrowheads*) and alveolar opacities (*arrows*). Immunosuppressive agents were stopped. **b** Axial follow-up CT scan performed six days later, shows marked regression in nodules and alveolar opacities.

initial staging, despite its increased sensitivity, because the incremental information gained may increase disease stage, but has no effect on treatment decisions. Of late, CT is becoming the principal modality for initial staging of thoracic lymphoma, as it provides a more complete baseline staging evaluation and is useful for follow-up assessment of disease (MUSUMECI and TESORO-TESS 1994).

7.11.2
Ultrasound

Ultrasound, although noted to be comparable to CT in the evaluation of mediastinal lymphomas (WERNECKE et al. 1991a), is limited in application, and is not routinely used in initial staging of thoracic lymphoma. An exception is in those rare cases of cardiac lymphoma, where transthoracic and transesophageal echocardiography are utilized in cardiac evaluation. A second important role for ultrasound is in the evaluation of breast lymphoma, in the characterization of clinically palpable or mammographically detected breast masses.

7.11.3
MR imaging

Although MR imaging is at least equivalent to CT in the evaluation of mediastinal disease (HOANE et al. 1994), given its expense and time, as well as the

limited evaluation of the pulmonary parenchyma, it has not replaced CT in the initial staging evaluation of thoracic lymphoma. However, given its multiplanar, angiographic, and tissue differentiation capabilities, MR imaging is superior to CT in several specific situations. These include the evaluation of pericardial and cardiac involvement, suspected chest wall invasion and assessment of vascular patency/compromise (MUSUMECI and TESORO-TESS 1994; TAKVORIAN and DIPIRO 2002). A role for MR imaging in monitoring the effect of therapy and documenting tumor regression or predicting relapse has been described (RAHMOUNI et al. 1993; HILL et al. 1993; RAHMOUNI and ZERHOUNI 1990), but its use has not been widespread.

7.11.4
Radionuclide Imaging

7.11.4.1
Gallium-67 and Thallium-201 Scintigraphy

Gallium scintigraphy has been the gold standard for radionuclide imaging of lymphoma when performed using 10 mCi of gallium-67 citrate and acquiring both planar and single photon emission computed tomography (SPECT) images at 72 hours. The gallium-67 citrate binds to transferrin receptors in the tumor, making imaging possible. Gallium imaging has been used routinely for evaluation of high grade and intermediate grade lymphoma, both during and after therapy. Specifically, it has been used in prediction of prognosis (KAPLAN et al. 1990; FRONT et al. 2000), evaluation of a residual mass post-therapy, and in the diagnosis of recurrence (Fig. 7.24) (FRONT et al.

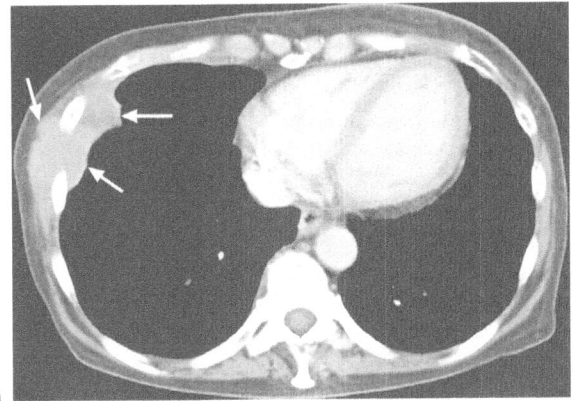

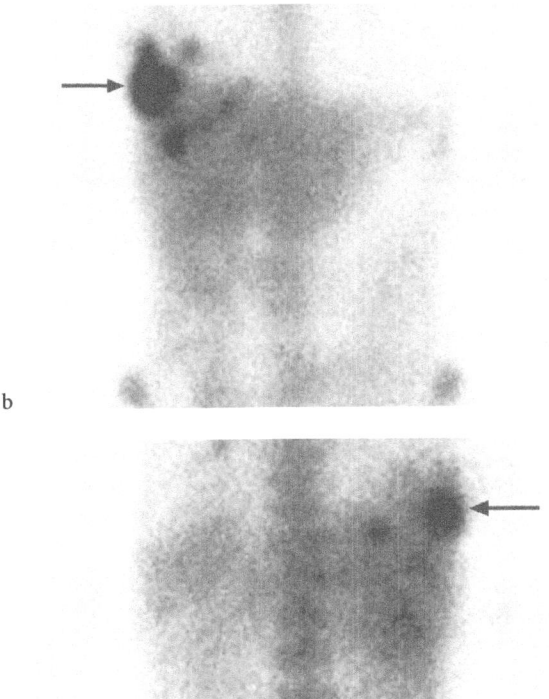

Fig. 7.24a–c. Recurrent non-Hodgkin lymphoma in a 56-year-old woman who presented one year previous with gastric lymphoma. a Axial contrast-enhanced CT image reveals a right anterolateral chest wall mass (arrows). b Anterior and (c) posterior gallium scintigraphic images reveal marked uptake in the chest wall (arrow), corresponding with the CT finding.

1997). Reported sensitivities and specificities for differentiating residual viable tumor from fibrosis are 76–100% and 75–96%, and for diagnosis of recurrence are 95% and 89%, respectively (FRONT et al. 1997). However, low-grade or follicular lymphomas are typically not of high gallium-avidity, and gallium scintigraphy is of low sensitivity. It is in the latter group of patients that Thallium-201 scintigraphy may be useful.

The mechanism of thallium uptake is not known, though several mechanisms may be involved, including blood flow, tumor viability, calcium channel mechanisms, the adenosine triphosphate sodium-potassium pump, and a co-transport system. In a small study comparing gallium and thallium, patient and site sensitivities in patients with low grade lymphoma for 67-Ga were only 56% and 32%, respectively, while for 201-Tl, they were both 100% (WAXMAN et al. 1996). Thallium use is not widespread, and is more typically used in following low grade, nodal lymphomas.

7.11.4.2
PET

Positron emission tomography (PET) is the newest and most promising radionuclide imaging modality. Using physiological, radioactively-labeled, tracer glucose (18-fluorine-2-fluorodeoxyglucose), the increased uptake and metabolism of tumor cells is identified and imaged. Studies of PET, thus far, have indicated high sensitivity and specificity for staging of lymphoma (KOSTAKOGLU et al. 2002b; WIRTH et al. 2002; STUMPE et al. 1998; BUCHMAN et al. 2001; MOOG et al. 1997; MOOG et al. 1998). In a recent study of patients with newly diagnosed or clinically recurrent aggressive lymphoma or HD, site and patient sensitivities were 100% for PET imaging, versus 71.5% and 80.3%, respectively, for gallium scintigraphy. Although varied results have been reported in assessment of residual masses and predicting relapse (MAISEY et al. 2000; MIKHAEEL 2000), more recent studies suggest that PET may play an important role in predicting prognosis, with resultant treatment implications and potential tailoring of treatment regimens (CREMERIUS et al. 2002; SPAEPEN et al. 2002; SPAEPEN et al. 2003; KOSTAKO-GLU et al. 2002a). Given the improved sensitivity, and specifically, the higher site positivity rate of PET over gallium scintigraphy, some people believe that PET should replace gallium scanning in the staging of patients with lymphoma. However, no large, prospective study comparing gallium scintigraphy and

PET imaging has yet been published. Despite PET's improved sensitivity over CT as well, it is generally agreed that PET is most useful for evaluating lymphoma patients when read in conjunction with CT imaging (Fig. 7.25). This relationship will be capitalized upon with the latest technology, possessing PET/CT fusion capabilities.

Some noted limitations of PET include the uptake of radioisotope within the neck musculature, which may be mistaken for disease, as well as the low sensitivity noted in low-grade lymphomas (with the exception of the follicular subtype) (JERUSALEM et al. 2001). False positive results are seen when reactive lymph nodes and thymic hyperplasia are interpreted as disease (BANGERTER et al. 1999). False negative scans have been described with MALT lymphomas. Although a case of increased FDG uptake with pulmonary MALT lymphoma was described (HARA et al. 2002), PET does not typically image extranodal B-cell MALT lymphomas (HOFFMANN et al. 1999; PAUL 1987).

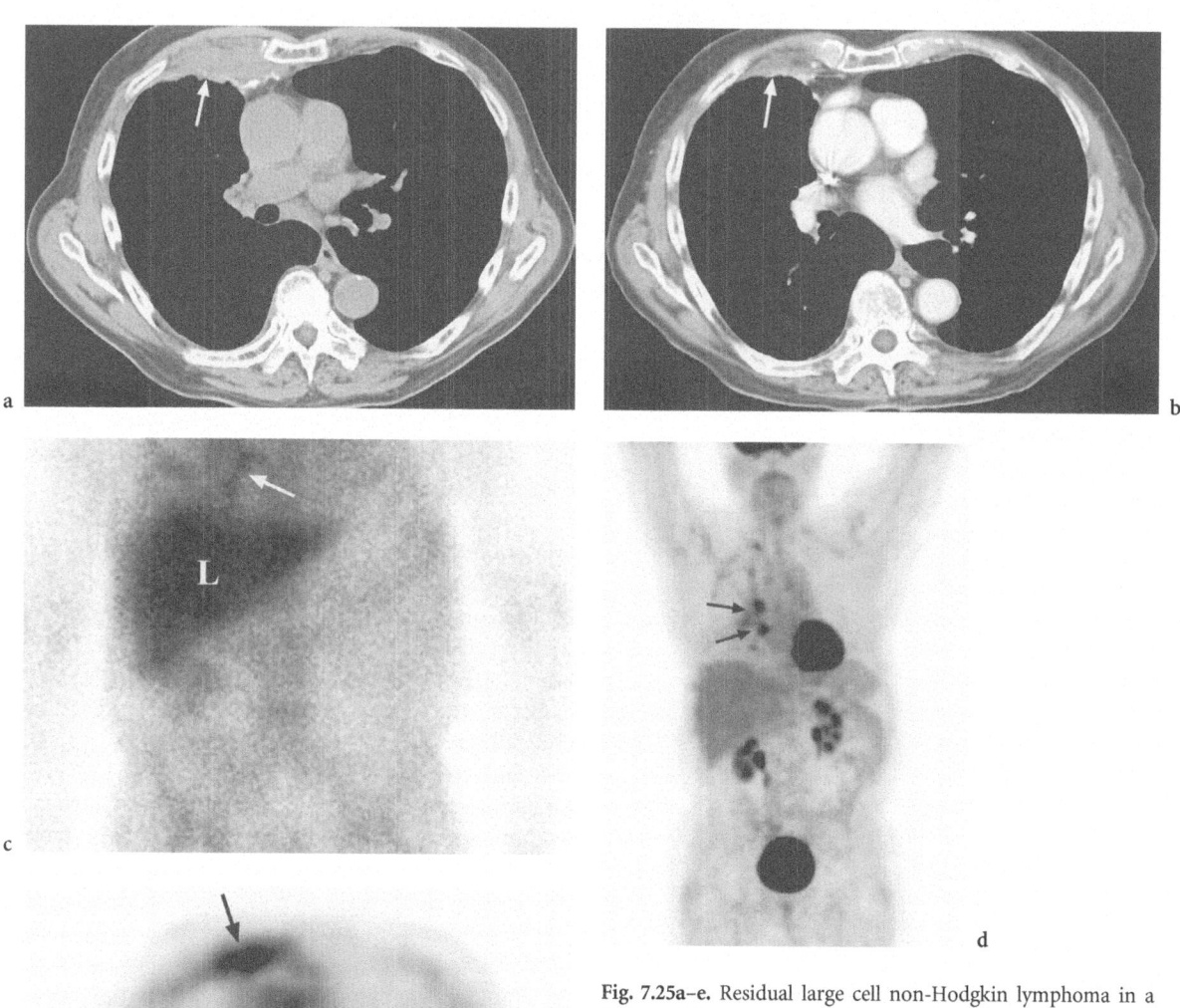

Fig. 7.25a–e. Residual large cell non-Hodgkin lymphoma in a 74-year-old woman, status post resection of anterior chest wall mass. **a** Pre-operative axial unenhanced CT image obtained following biopsy and talc pleurodesis, shows right parasternal chest wall mass (*arrow*). **b** Axial contrast-enhanced CT image obtained four months after surgical resection reveals minimal residual or recurrent soft tissue at the site of prior surgery (*arrow*). **c** Gallium scan reveals uptake in this region (*arrow*), cephalad to the liver (*L*). **d** Frontal maximum intensity projection (*MIP*) and (**e**) axial PET images reveal marked FDG uptake in the corresponding area (*arrows*). The mass regressed with chemotherapy.

7.12
Conclusion

Extranodal thoracic non-Hodgkin lymphoma can present at multiple sites and possess varied appearances. Over the last two decades, improvements in imaging technology have increased the sensitivity of detection of disease. With these advances in the detection of lymphoma and the improvements in predicting prognosis, trends toward more specific tailoring of therapies to each patient may be seen.

References

Au V, Leung AN (1997) Radiologic manifestations of lymphoma in the thorax. AJR Am J Roentgenol 168:93–98

Balikian JP, Herman PG (1979) Non-Hodgkin lymphoma of the lungs. Radiology 132:569–576

Bazot M, Cadranel J, Benayoun S, Tassart M, Bigot JM, Carette MF (1999) Primary pulmonary AIDS-related lymphoma: radiographic and CT findings. Chest 116:1282–1286

Bergin CJ, Healy MV, Zincone GE, et al (1990) MR evaluation of chest wall involvement in malignant lymphoma. J Comput Assist Tomogr 14:928–932

Berkman N, Breuer R (1993) Pulmonary involvement in lymphoma. Respir Med 87:85–92

Billingham ME, Rawlinson DG, Berry PF, Kempson RL (1975) The cytodiagnosis of malignant lymphomas and Hodgkin's disease in cerebrospinal, pleural and ascitic fluids. Acta Cytol 19:547–556

Blunt DM, Padley SPG (1995) Radiographic manifestations of AIDS related lymphoma in the thorax. Clin Radiol 50: 607–612

Bragg DG (1978) The clinical, pathologic and radiographic spectrum of the intrathoracic lymphomas. Invest Radiol 13:2–11

Bragg DG (1987) Radiology of the Lypmphomas. Curr Probl Diagn Radiol 16:183–206

Buchmann I, Reinhardt M, Elsner K et al (2001) 2-(fluorine-18)fluoro-2-deoxy-D-glucose positron emission tomography in the detection and staging of malignant lymphoma. A bicenter trial. Cancer 91:889–899

Cadranel J, Wislez M, Antoine M (2002) Primary pulmonary lymphoma. Eur Respir J 20:750–762

Carlsen SE, Bergin CJ, Hoppe RT (1993) MR Imaging to detect chest wall and pleural involvement in patients with lymphoma: effect on radiation therapy planning. AJR Am J Roentgenol 160:1191–1195

Castellino RA, Hilton SH, O'Brien JP, Portlock CS (1996) Non-Hodgkin Lymphoma: Contribution of Chest CT in the Initial Staging Evaluation. Radiology 199:129–132

Ceresoli GL, Ferreri AJM, Bucci E, et al (1997) Primary cardiac lymphoma in immunocompetent patients. Diagnostic and therapeutic management. Cancer 80:1497–1506

Coltrera MD (1999) Primary T-cell lymphoma of the thyroid. Head Neck 21:160–163

Cremerius U, Fabry U, Wildberger JE et al (2002) Pre-transplant positron emission tomography (PET) using

fluorine-18-fluoro-deoxyglucose (FDG) predicts outcome in patients treated with high-dose chemotherapy and autologous stem cell transplantation for non-Hodgkin's lymphoma. Bone Marrow Transplant 30:103–111

DiPiro PJ, Lester S, Meyer JE, et al (1996) Non-Hodgkin lymphoma of the breast: clinical and radiographic presentations. Breast J 2:380–384

Dodd GD 3rd, Greenler DP, Confer SR (1992) Thoracic and abdominal manifestations of lymphoma occurring in the immunocompromised patient. Radiol Clin North Am 30: 597–610

Freeman C, Berg JW, Cutler SJ (1972) Occurrence and prognosis of extranodal lymphomas. Cancer 29:252–260

Front D, Bar-Shalom R, Israel O (1997) The continuing clinical role of gallium 67 scintigraphy in the age of receptor imaging. Semin Nucl Med 27:68–74

Front D, Bar-Shalom R, Mor M et al (2000) Aggressive non-Hodgkin lymphoma: early prediction of outcome with 67Ga scintigraphy. Radiology 214:253–257

Hara M, Sugie C, Tohyama J et al (2002) Increased 18fluorodeoxyglucose accumulation in mucosa-associated lymphoid tissue type lymphoma of the lung. J Thorac Imaging 17: 160–162

Heron W, Husband JE, Williams MP (1988) Hodgkin Disease: CT of the Thymus. Radiology 167:647–651

Hill M, Cunningham D, MacVicar D et al (1993) Role of magnetic resonance imaging in predicting relapse in residual masses after treatment of lymphoma. J Clin Oncol 11: 2273–2278

Hoane BR, Shields AF, Porter BA, et al (1994) Comparison of initial lymphoma staging using computed tomography (CT) and magnetic resonance (MR) imaging. Am J Hematol 47:100–105

Hoffmann M, Kletter K, Diemling M et al (1999) Positron emission tomography with fluorine-18-2-fluoro-2-deoxy-D-glucose (F18-FDG) does not visualize extranodal B-cell lymphoma of the mucosa-associated lymphoid tissue (MALT)-type. Ann Oncol 10:1185–1189

Holladay AO, Siegel RJ, Schwartz DA (1992) Cardiac malignant lymphoma in acquired immune deficiency syndrome. Cancer 70:2203–2207

Isaacson PG, Wright DH (1983) Malignant lymphoma of mucosa associated lymphoid tissue: a distinctive B cell lymphoma. Cancer 52:1410–1416

Ishikawa H, Tamaki Y, Takahashi M et al (2002) Comparison of primary thyroid lymphoma with anaplastic thyroid carcinoma on computed tomographic imaging. Rad Med 20:9–15

Jerusalem G, Beguin Y, Najjar F et al (2001) Positron emission tomography (PET) with 18F-fluorodeoxyglucose (18F-FDG) for the staging of low-grade non-Hodgkin's lymphoma (NHL). Ann Oncol 12:825–830

Kaplan WD, Jochelson MS, Herman TS et al (1990) Gallium-67 imaging: a predictor of residual tumor viability and clinical outcome in patients with diffuse large-cell lymphoma. J Clin Oncol 8:1966–1970

Keller AR, Castleman B (1974) Hodgkin's disease of the thymus gland. Cancer 33:1615–1623

Khoury MB, Godwin JD, Halvorsen R, et al (1986) Role of chest CT in non-Hodgkin lymphoma. Radiology 158: 659–662

King LJ, Padley SPG, Wotherspoon AC, Nicholson AG (2000) Pulmonary MALT lymphoma: imaging findings in 24 cases. Eur Radiol 10:1932–1938

Knisely BL, Mastey LA, Mergo PJ, Voytovich MC, Zander D, Almasri NM, Collins J, Kuhlman JE (1999) Pulmonary Mucosa-Associated Lymphoid Tissue Lymphoma: CT and pathologic findings. AJR Am J Roentgenol 172:1321–1326

Kostakoglu L, Coleman M, Leonard JP et al (2002a) PET predicts prognosis after 1 cycle of chemotherapy in aggressive lymphoma and Hodgkin's disease. J Nucl Med 43: 1028–1030

Kostakoglu L, Leonard JP, Kuji I et al (2002b) Comparison of fluorine-18 fluorodeoxyglucose positron emission tomography and Ga-67 scintigraphy in evaluation of lymphoma. Cancer 94:879–888

Lazar EB, Whitman GJ, Chew FS (1996) Lymphoma of Bronchus-Associated Lymphoid Tissue. AJR Am J Roentgenol 167:116

Lee KS, Kim Y, Primack SL (1996) Imaging of pulmonary lymphomas. AJR Am J Roentgenol 168:339–345

Lewis ER, Caskey CI, Fishman EK (1991) Lymphoma of the lung: CT findings in 31 patients. AJR Am J Roentgenol 156:711–714

Liberman L, Giess CS, Dershaw DD, et al (1994) Non-Hodgkin lymphoma of the breast: imaging characteristics and correlation with histopathologic findings. Radiology 192: 157–160

Maisey NR, Hill ME, Webb A et al (2000) Are 18fluorodeoxyglucose positron emission tomography and magnetic resonance imaging useful in the prediction of relapse in lymphoma residual masses? Eur J Cancer 36:200–206

McAllister HA, Fenoglio JJ (1978) Tumors of the cardiovascular system. Armed Forces Institute of Pathology (ed) Atlas of tumor pathology. AFIP, Washington DC, pp 99–100

McCulloch GL, Sinnatamby R, Stewart S, Goddard M, Flower CDR (1998) High-resolution computed tomographic appearance of MALToma of the lung. Eur Radiol 8: 1669–1673

McDonnell PJ, Mann RB, Bulkley BH (1982) Involvement of the heart by malignant lymphoma: a clinicopathologic study. Cancer 49:944–51

Mikhaeel NG, Timothy AR, Hain SF et al (2000) 18-FDG-PET for the assessment of residual masses on CT following treatment of lymphomas. Ann Oncol 1:147–150

Moog F, Bangerter M, Diederichs CG et al (1997) Lymphoma: role of whole-body 2-deoxy-2-[F-18]fluoro-D-glucose (FDG) PET in nodal staging. Radiology 203:795–800

Moog F, Bangerter M, Diederichs CG et al (1998) Extranodal malignant lymphoma:detection with FDG PET versus CT. Radiology 206:475–481

Musumeci R, Tesoro-Tess JD (1994) New imaging techniques in staging lymphomas. Curr Opin Oncol 6:464–469

Muti G, Cantoni S, Oreste P, et al (2002) Post-transplant lymphoproliferative disorders: improved outcome after clinico-pathologically tailored treatment. Haematologica 87:67–77

North LB, Libshitz HI, Lorigan JG (1990) Thoracic lymphoma. Radiol Clin North Am 28:745–762

Paul R (1987) Comparison of fluorine-18 2-fluorodeoxyglucose and gallium-67 citrate imaging for detection of lymphoma. J Nucl Med 28:288–292

Petrek JA (1991) Breast diseases. In: Harris JR, Hellman S, Henderson IC, Kinne DW (eds) Lymphoma. Lippincott, Philadelphia, pp 806–807

Podoloff DA (1996) Is there a place for routine surveillance using sonography, CT, or MR imaging for early detection (notably lymphoma) of patients affected by Hashimoto's thyroiditis? AJR Am J Roentgenol 167:1337–1338

Press GA, Glazer HS, Wasserman TH et al (1985) Thoracic wall involvement by Hodgkin disease and Non-Hodgkin lymphoma: CT evaluation. Radiology 157:195–198

Rahmouni A, Tempany C, Jones R et al (1993) Lymphoma: monitoring tumor size and signal intensity with MR imaging. Radiology 188:445–451

Rahmouni AD, Zerhouni EA (1990) Role of MRI in the management of thoracic lymphoma. In: Zerhouni EA (ed) CT and MRI of the thorax. Churchill Livingstone, New York, pp 23–33

Ray P, Antoine M, Mary-Krause M, et al (1998) AIDS-related primary pulmonary lymphoma. Am J Respir Crit Care Med 158:1221–1229

Roberts WC, Glancy DL, DeVita VT Jr (1968) Heart in malignant lymphoma (Hodgkin's disease, lymphosarcoma, reticulum cell sarcoma and mycosis fungoides). A study of 196 autopsy cases. Am J Cardiol 22:85–107

Rolla G, Bertero MT, Pastena G, et al (2002) Primary lymphoma of the heart. A case report and review of the literature. Leuk Res 26:117–120

Romano M, Libshitz HI (1998) Hodgkin disease and non-Hodgkin lymphoma: plain chest radiographs and chest Computed Tomography of thoracic involvement in previously untreated patients. Radiol Med 95:49–53

Scutellari PN, Borgatti L, Spanedda R (2000) Non-Hodgkin's lymphomas of extranodal localization. Strategy for imaging diagnosis. Radiol Med 100:262–272

Shuman LS, Libshitz HI (1984) Solid pleural manifestations of lymphoma. AJR Am J Roentgenol 142:269–273

Sider LL, Weiss AJ, Smith MD, VonRoenn JH, Glassroth J (1989) Varied appearance of AIDS-related lymphoma in the chest. Radiology 171:629–632

Spaepen K, Stroobants S, Dupont P et al (2002) Early restaging positron emission tomography with (18)F-fluorodeoxyglucose predicts outcome in patients with aggressive non-Hodgkin's lymphoma. Ann Oncol 13:1356–1363

Spaepen K, Stroobants S, Dupont P et al (2003) Prognostic value of pretransplant positron emission tomography using fluorine 18-fluorodeoxyglucose in patients with aggressive lymphoma treated with high-dose chemotherapy and stem cell transplantation. Blood [epub ahead of print]

Strollo DC, Rosado-de-Christenson ML (1999) Tumors of the thymus. J Thorac Imaging14:152–171

Stumpe KD, Urbinelli M, Steinert HC et al (1998) Whole-body positron emission tomography using fluorodeoxyglucose for staging of lymphoma: effectiveness and comparison with computed tomography. Eur J Nucl Med 25:721–728

Takashima S, Ikezoe J, Morimoto S, Arisawa J, Hamada S, Ikeda H, Masaki N, Kozuka T (1988) Primary thyroid lymphoma: evaluation with CT. Radiology 168:765–768

Takashima S, Morimoto S, Ikezoe J, Arisawa J, Hamada S, Ikeda H, Masaki N, Kozuka T, Matsuzuka F (1989a) Primary thyroid lymphoma: comparison of CT and US assessment. Radiology 171:439–443

Takashima S, Ikezoe J, Morimoto S, Harada K, Kozuka T, Matsuzuka F (1989b) MR imaging of primary thyroid lymphoma. J Comput Assist Tomogr 13:517–518

Takvorian T, DiPiro PJ (2002) Staging of non-Hodgkin's lymphoma. In: Grossbard ML (ed) Malignant lymphomas. BC Decker Inc, Hamilton London, pp 67–83

Trofe J, Buell JF, First MR, et al (2002) The role of immu-nosuppression in lymphoma. Recent Results Cancer Res 159:55–66

Vieta JO, Craver LF (1941) Intrathoracic manifestations of the lymphomatoid diseases. Radiology 37:138–158

Waxman AD, Eller D, Ashook G et al (1996) Comparison of Gallium-67-citrate and Thallium-201 scintigraphy in peripheral and intrathoracic lymphoma. J Nucl Med 37: 46–50

Wernecke K, Vassallo P, Hoffmann G, et al (1991a) Value of sonography in monitoring the therapeutic response of mediastinal lymphoma: Comparison with chest radiogra-phy and CT. AJR Am J Roentgenol 156:265–72

Wernecke K, Vassallo P, Rutsch F, et al (1991b) Thymic Involvement in Hodgkin Disease: CT and Sonographic Findings. Radiology 181:375–383

Wirth A, Seymour JF, Hicks RJ et al (2002) Fluorine-18 fluo-rodeoxyglucose positron emission tomoography, gallium-67 scintigraphy, and conventional staging for Hodgkin's disease and non-Hodgkin's lymphoma. Am J Med 112: 320–321

Wislez M, Cadranel J, Antoine M, et al (1999). Lymphoma of pul-monary mucosa-associcted lymphoid tissue: CT scan findings and pathological correlations. Eur Respir J 14:423–429

Yi JG, Kim DH, Choi CS (1998) Malignant lymphoma of mucosa-associated lymphoid tissue (MALT lymphoma) arising in the thymus: radiologic findings. AJR Am J Roentgenol 171:899–900

8 Abdominal Involvement in Non-Hodgkin Lymphoma

Sheila Sheth, Elliot K. Fishman

CONTENTS

Sheila Sheth, MD
Associate Professor of Radiology, Johns Hopkins University
School of Medicine, Director of Biopsy Service, Department
of Radiology, Johns Hopkins Hospital, 600 N. Wolfe Street,
Baltimore, MD 21287, USA
Elliot K. Fishman, MD, FACR
Professor of Radiology and Oncology, Johns Hopkins Uni-
versity School of Medicine, Director, Diagnostic Radiology
and Body CT, Department of Radiology, Johns Hopkins
Hospital, 600 N. Caroline Street, JHOC 3254, Baltimore, MD
21287, USA

8.1 Introduction

Non-Hodgkin lymphomas (NHL) comprise a heterogeneous group of malignant tumors arising from B, T or natural killer lymphocytes or their precursors (Pileri et al. 1998). They represent the most common malignancy of the immune system, with approximately 50,000 new cases diagnosed every year in the United States (Armitage 1997). These lymphomas have been increasing at a rate of approximately 4% per year in the past few decades and are now the fifth most common cause of cancer death in the United States (Lionberger and Armitage 2001).

A detailed discussion of the various pathologic classifications of NHL is beyond the scope of this chapter. For the radiologist, suffice to know that several methods of categorizing NHL have been developed since the 1970s. In the 1980s, the old Rapaport classification based on morphologic appearance was abandoned in favor of the Working Formulation, which grouped NHL into low, intermediate and high grade tumors based on tumor growth patterns (follicular versus diffuse), cell size and patient survival (Armitage and Weisenburger 1998; Pileri et al. 1998). This new classification provided significant improvements in predicting clinical behavior and prognosis and helped select the most effective therapeutic options (Armitage and Weisenburger 1998). By the mid 1990s, progress in histologic diagnosis due to development of reproducible immunophenotyping techniques as well as advancement in therapeutic options had rendered the Working formulation obsolete. At the beginning of the 21st century, the most widely used classifications for NHL include the Revised European-American Lymphoma study group (REAL) classification that is being updated by the World Health Organization. This later method allows grouping NHL into clinically relevant categories based on demographic data, extent of disease, natural history and curability (Chan 2001).

The biologic behavior and prognosis of NHL are primarily determined by the histologic grade of the tumor and secondarily by clinical and/or anatomic stage (GLASS et al. 1997). The Ann Arbor staging classification, primarily designed for Hodgkin disease is also used for anatomic staging of NHL (CASTELLINO 1991). Over the past 2 decades, the development of effective treatment strategies has led to a significant improvement in the outcome of NHL. As accurate staging is an important prerequisite for planning therapy, imaging plays a vital role in the management of these patients.

8.2
Risk Factors for Non-Hodgkin Lymphoma

While the overall incidence of NHL is rising, particularly in the older population, individuals with an impaired immune system are at a much greater risk of developing NHL, as much as 40 to 100% higher, than the general population (CASTELLINO 1991).

8.2.1
Non-Hodgkin Lymphoma in HIV Patients

NHL is a common complication of HIV infection. The disruption of the immune system results in two main abnormalities predisposing these individuals to developing highly aggressive NHL. Loss of normal T-cell function leads to proliferation of B-cells infected with the Epstein Barr virus and development of immunoblastic lymphoma. In addition, chronic hyperactivation of B-cell lymphocytes is associated with Burkitt-like NHL and large cell non-cleaved NHL (MARTINEZ-MAZA and BREEN 2002).

HIV-related NHL are generally widespread at presentation. In the abdomen, lymphadenopathy is the most common manifestation of AIDS related NHL, followed by tumor involving the gastrointestinal tract (RADIN et al. 1993) and the liver (RIZZI et al. 2001). Aggressive tumors affecting multiple and unusual sites, including the heart and pericardium, epidural space, muscle groups, subcutaneous tissues and bone are characteristic features (Fig. 8.1).

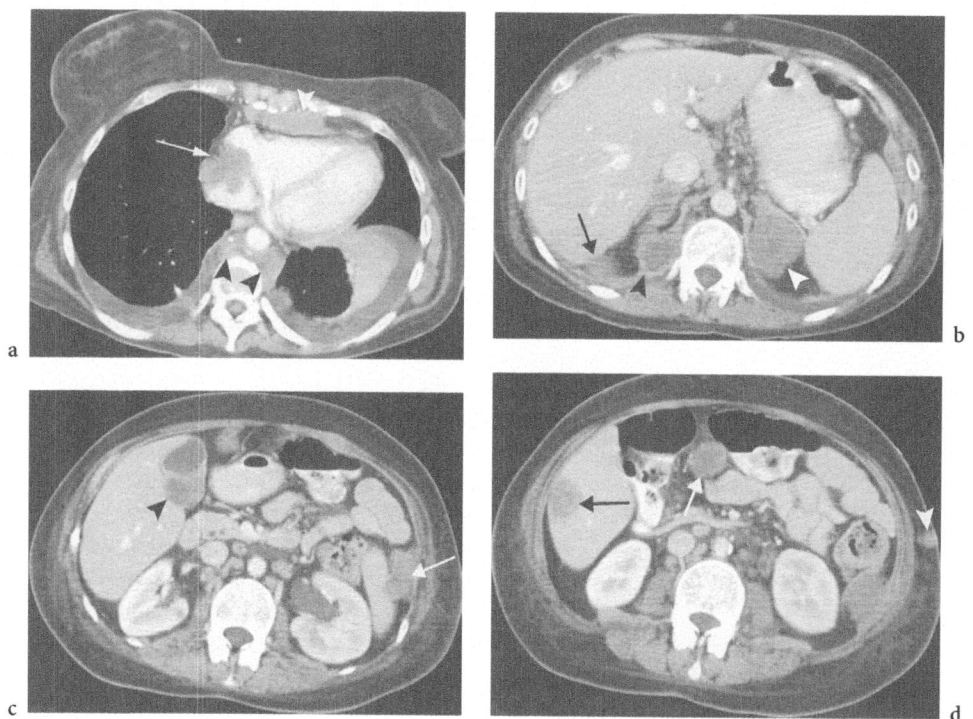

Fig. 8.1a–d. Extensive diffuse large B-cell lymphoma in a 36-year-old woman with HIV. **a** Axial contrast-enhanced CT scan of the lower thorax shows a soft tissue mass invading the right atrium (*arrow*). A large precardiac nodal mass is present (*white arrowhead*). Retrocrural lymphadenopathy and bilateral pleural effusions are seen (*black arrowheads*). **b** Axial contrast-enhanced CT scan of the upper abdomen shows bilateral adrenal masses (*arrowheads*), as well as soft tissue masses along the leaves of the diaphragm (*arrow*). **c** Axial contrast-enhanced CT scan at the level of the renal hila shows a hypoattenuating mass adjacent and invading the gallbladder (*arrowhead*), a peritoneal mass (*arrow*) and small retroperitoneal nodes. **d** Axial contrast-enhanced CT scan at the level of the lower pole of the kidneys shows a hypodense mass in the right hepatic lobe (*black arrow*) and soft tissue masses in the mesentery and posterior to the descending colon (*white arrow*). Note the subcutaneous nodule (*arrowhead*).

Histologic diagnosis, usually established by percutaneous image-guided biopsy, is essential for confirming the diagnosis and to exclude unusual infections and other malignancies such as Kaposi sarcoma and metastatic carcinoma (RIZZI et al. 2001).

8.2.2
Non-Hodgkin Lymphoma in
Solid Organ Transplant Recipients

Post transplant lymphoproliferative disorders (PTLD) develop in 1 to 10% of patients having received a solid organ transplant. The vast majority (close to 80%) of PTLD occurs within the first year after transplantation, with peak occurrence at 3 to 4 months, and are related to infection by the Epstein Barr virus caused by immunosuppression. Early onset PTLD regresses with adjustment of immunosuppressive therapy and is associated with a mortality rate of less then 40% (ARMITAGE et al. 1991). By contrast, approximately 20% of PTLD occur after the first year and resemble NHL occurring in immunocompetent patients. These lymphomas tend to be advanced stage with extranodal spread, require aggressive management and have a poor prognosis with a high mortality rate of at least 70% (Figs. 8.2, 8.3) (DOTTI et al. 2002; ARMITAGE et al. 1991).

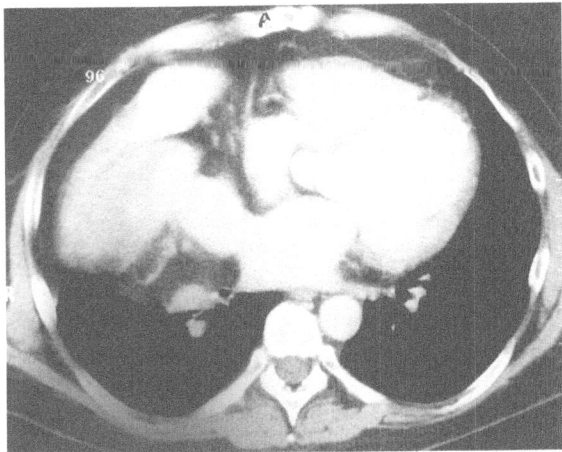
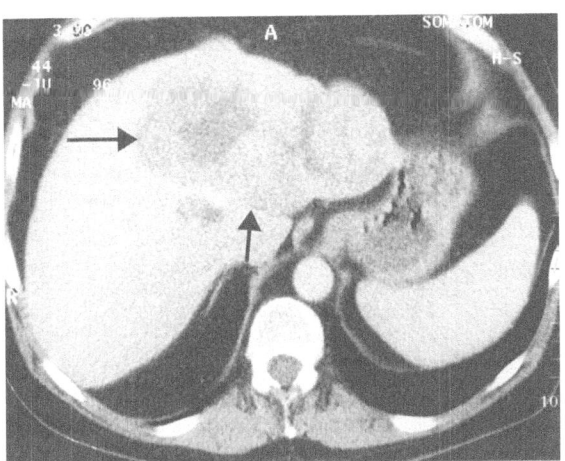

a   b

Fig. 8.2a,b. Hepatic lymphoma in a 52-year-old man with a history of heart transplant 8 years prior to current hospitalization. **a** Axial contrast-enhanced CT scan of the lower thorax shows the heart transplant. **b** Axial contrast-enhanced CT scan of the liver shows a large hypodense mass with central necrosis (*arrows*). The diagnosis of B-cell lymphoma was established by ultrasound guided biopsy of the hepatic mass.

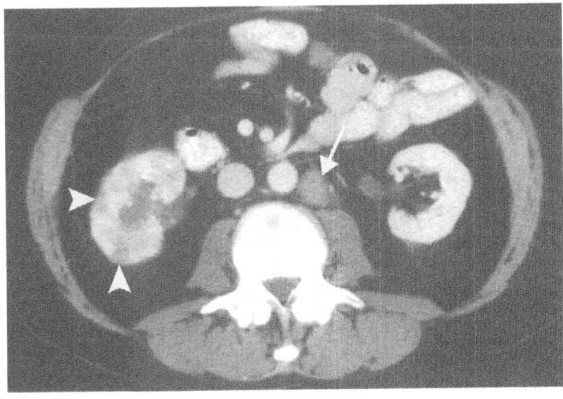
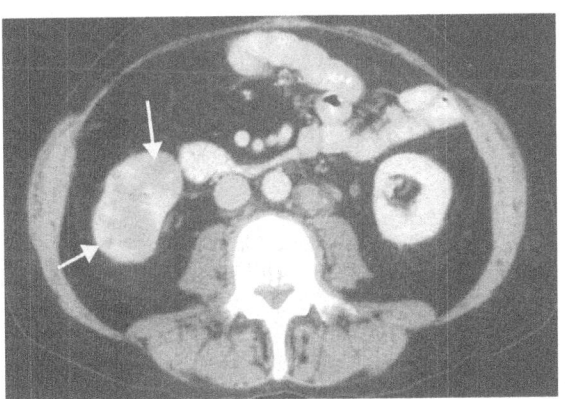

a   b

Fig. 8.3a,b. Renal lymphoma in a 60-year-old man with a history of liver transplant 10 years prior to presentation. **a** Axial contrast-enhanced CT scan at the level of the renal hila shows heterogeneous enhancement of the right renal cortex (*arrowheads*). There is mild hydronephrosis. Note the left paraaortic node (*arrow*). **b** Axial contrast-enhanced CT scan at the level of the lower poles of the kidneys shows that the lower pole of the right kidney is infiltrated by hypodense masses with poorly defined borders (*arrows*). The left paraaortic node is mildly enhancing.

8.3
Imaging Strategies for
Abdominal Non-Hodgkin Lymphoma

Anatomic staging is an essential component of treatment planning for NHL. Since the late 1970s, cross-sectional imaging modalities have almost entirely replaced staging laparotomy.

The appearance of NHL on cross-sectional imaging reflects their gross histologic morphology. Affected lymph nodes are diagnosed primarily based on abnormal size criteria. When lymphoma involves parenchymal organs, tumor cells may proliferate along the interstitium resulting in diffuse enlargement of the affected organ while preserving its overall shape. Alternatively, foci of lymphoma growing in a non-uniform fashion present as expansile masses with contour distortion (URBAN and FISHMAN 2000). Although one study suggested that high-grade lesions were associated with large nodular masses and low-grade NHL tended to be infiltrative (GORG et al. 1996), in general imaging characteristics do not predict the grade (high, intermediate or low) of the tumor.

8.3.1
Computed Tomography

Computed tomography (CT) remains the gold standard for the diagnosis, staging and post treatment monitoring of patients with suspected or known NHL (NEUMANN et al. 1983; SCUTELLARI et al. 2000). Heli-

cal technology, administration of intravenous contrast and image acquisition during the venous phase of enhancement are essential to reliably detect parenchymal organ infiltration. However, even if intravenous contrast cannot be utilized, CT is often adequate to detect large nodal disease often associated with NHL. Ingestion of oral contrast helps differentiate opacified bowel loops from mesenteric nodal disease.

Regardless of their location, lymphomatous foci usually appear as homogeneous masses of soft tissue attenuation with low or moderate enhancement after intravenous contrast administration (Fig. 8.4). Pronounced enhancement is unusual but does not exclude the diagnosis (POMBO et al. 1994). Bulky tumors tend to outgrow their blood supply and exhibit heterogeneous enhancement with areas of hypodense necrosis (Fig. 8.5).

8.3.2
Magnetic Resonance Imaging

Several studies in small series of patients have shown that magnetic resonance (MR) imaging with or without contrast enhancement can be as effective as helical CT in the evaluation of patients with NHL (Fig. 8.6) (JUNG et al. 2000; SKILLINGS et al. 1991). While at the present time MR imaging plays a secondary role in the diagnosis of NHL, its advantages over CT include depiction of marrow involvement (Fig. 8.7), spread to the uterus and ovaries and demonstration of infiltration of parenchymal organs in

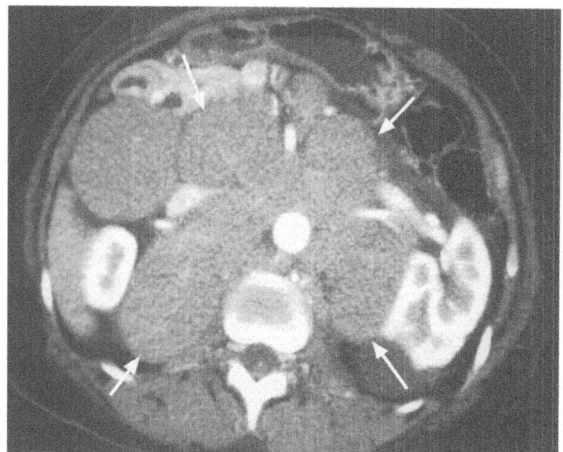

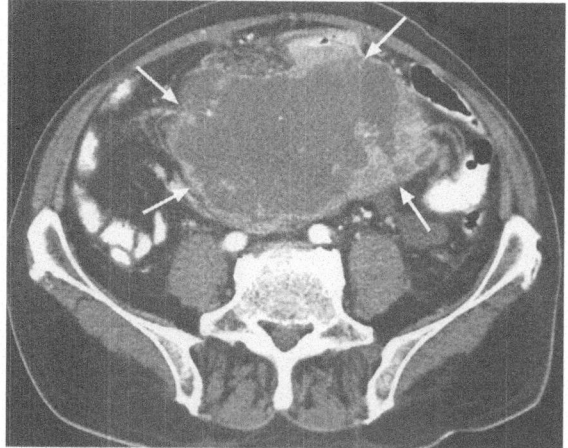

Fig. 8.4. Small cell lymphocytic lymphoma in a 72-year-old woman. Axial contrast-enhanced CT scan of the mid abdomen shows extensive mesenteric and retroperitoneal adenopathy (*arrows*). The nodes are homogeneous and mildly enhancing.

Fig. 8.5. Lymphoma of the mesentery in a 76-year-old man presenting with abdominal pain. Axial contrast-enhanced CT scan of the lower abdomen shows a very large mass in the mesentery (*arrows*). The center of the mass is of low attenuation suggesting necrosis.

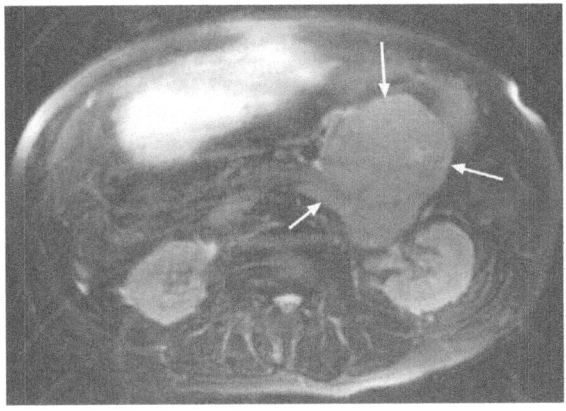
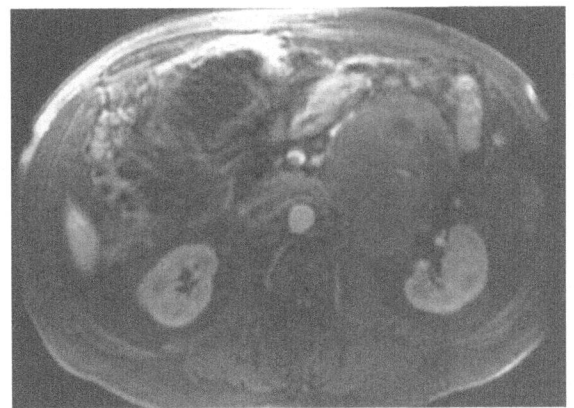

Fig. 8.6a,b. Non-Hodgkin lymphoma in a 66-year-old man with renal failure. a Axial fat-suppressed T2-weighted MR image of the mid abdomen shows a large left retroperitoneal mass with intermediate signal intensity (*arrows*). b Axial contrast-enhanced T1-weighted MR image with fat saturation of the mid abdomen shows some enhancement within the mass.

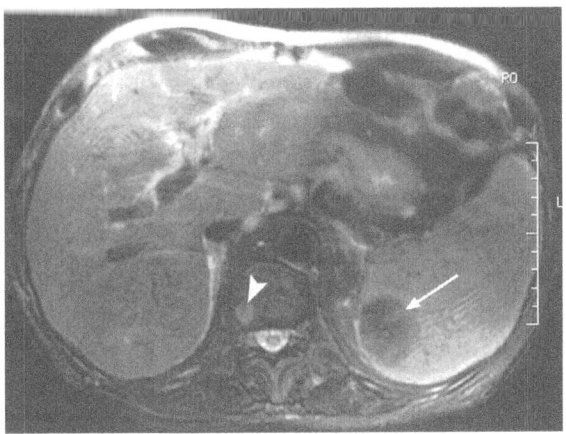
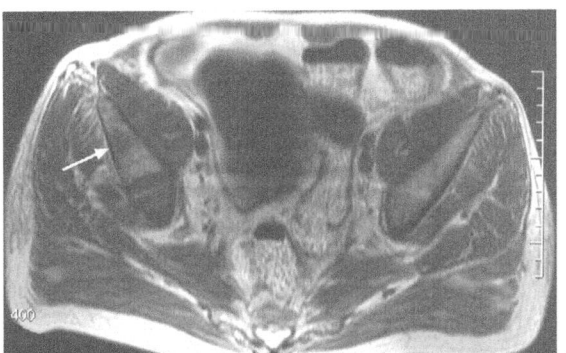
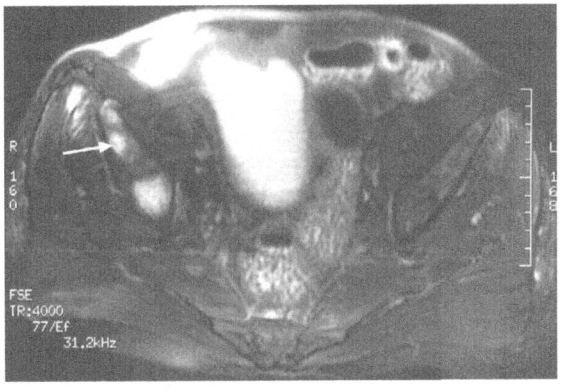

Fig. 8.7a–c. Staging MR in a 42-year-old man with peripheral T-cell lymphoma and chronic renal failure. a Axial fast spin-echo fat-suppressed T2-weighted MR image of the upper abdomen shows a lesion in the spleen (*arrow*). The lesion is of lower signal intensity than the normal parenchyma. Note the abnormal portocaval nodes and a hyperintense focus in the vertebral body indicating marrow involvement (*arrowhead*). Axial fast spin-echo (b) T1-weighted and (c) T2-weighted MR images of the mid pelvis show extensive marrow involvement in the right iliac wing (*arrow*). The lymphomatous foci are best seen as hyperintense lesions on the T2-weighted MR images.

cases where intravenous iodinated contrast administration is not desirable (JUNG et al. 2000)

8.3.3
Ultrasound

Ultrasound is not useful for the diagnosis because it routinely underestimates the extent of disease, particularly in the retroperitoneal and pelvic regions (NEUMANN et al. 1983). When they are visualized, lymphoma deposits appear as hypoechoic foci or masses and occasionally exhibit enough posterior sound enhancement to mimic cystic lesions (Fig. 8.8). Depiction of vascularity within the lesion on color Doppler ultrasound helps differentiate solid tumor from a fluid filled lesion (ISHIDA et al. 2001).

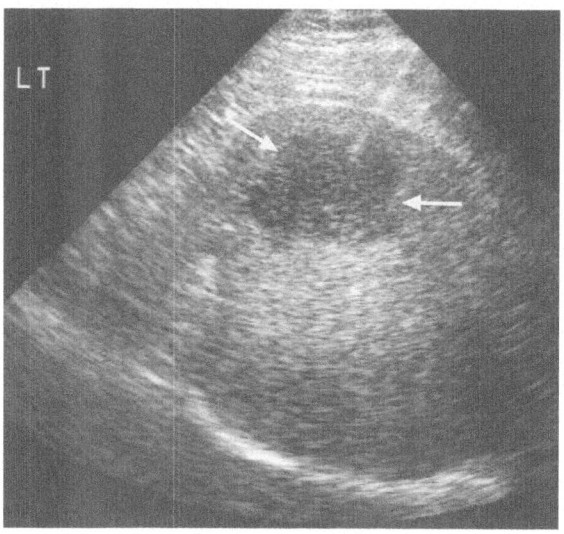

Fig. 8.8. Primary splenic lymphoma in a 38-year-old man. Transverse ultrasound of the spleen during fine needle aspiration shows a well-defined hypoechoic mass in the spleen (*arrows*). Note there is acoustic enhancement posterior to the lesion. The echogenic needle tip is easily seen within the mass.

While ultrasound is not used as a diagnostic test, it is the guidance modality of choice to perform percutaneous biopsy of abdominal lesions, regardless of their size and location, to obtain tissue sample for histologic analysis. The echogenic needle tip is easily depicted within hypoechoic NHL foci (Fig. 8.8) and the real time capability of ultrasound allows for faster procedure time and more accurate results compared with CT-guided procedure.

8.3.4
F-18 Fluorodeoxyglucose Positron Emission Tomography

F-18 fluorodeoxyglucose positron emission tomography (FDG PET) is a functional modality which images foci of accumulated FDG within malignant tumors (Fig. 8.9). Because it detects increased metabolic activity within lymphomatous deposits, FDG PET is likely to be more sensitive and specific then conventional anatomic imaging studies in detecting small additional tumor deposits, thereby refining initial staging. In a series of 81 newly diagnosed patients with lymphoma published by Moog and colleagues, FDG PET demonstrated 24 additional extranodal lesions not seen on CT, resulting in staging modification for 13 patients (MOOG et al. 1998). They found PET particularly valuable in detecting diffuse infiltration of the spleen with lymphoma and marrow involvement.

8.3.5
Prediction of Grade, Prognosis and Recurrence

Successful treatment of NHL requires effective assessment of disease response and early detection of recurrence. Attempts have been made with mixed results to correlate imaging features with disease outcome. Rodriguez and colleagues reviewed 63 patients with NHL and compared CT features with grade and prognosis. In untreated patients as well as patients treated with chemotherapy, marked inhomogeneity was associated with higher grade and worse prognosis (RODRIGUEZ et al. 1999). Dynamic CT allows measurement of the changes in attenuation values in tissue over time following a bolus of intravenous contrast. This technique estimates perfusion and capillary permeability in suspicious masses and may prove of value in assessing tumor activity (MILES and KELLEY 1997; DUGDALE et al. 1999).

Similarly, lack of enhancement after gadolinium injection on MR imaging appears to be a predictor for remission whereas contrast enhancement in residual masses after treatment may indicate residual or recurrent tumor (RAHMOUNI et al. 2001). Persistent residual soft tissue at the site of the original tumor after presumably successful therapy is a significant diagnostic dilemma. Cross-sectional imaging modalities such as CT rely almost entirely on change in tumor size overtime, and differentiation between inactive fibrous tissue and residual tumor may be challenging (Fig. 8.10). Because it presumably detects biologically active tissue, FDG PET appears to be most promising in identifying tumors that are likely to be refractory to standard therapeutic regimen as well as in differentiating active tumor from fibrous and scar tissue (Fig. 8.9). In a study by KOSTAKOGLU et al. (2002), patients with positive FDG PET findings after one cycle of treatment had shorter interval to recurrence compared to PET negative subjects. Other researchers have confirmed the value of interim PET during treatment: lack of uptake was associated with an 82% negative predictive value for treatment failure among 49 patients with aggressive NHL reported by MIKHAEEL et al. (2000).

8.4
Nodal and Splenic Non-Hodgkin Lymphoma

8.4.1
Lymphadenopathy

Enlargement of lymph nodes is the hallmark of abdominal NHL (Figs. 8.4, 8.11). Virtually any

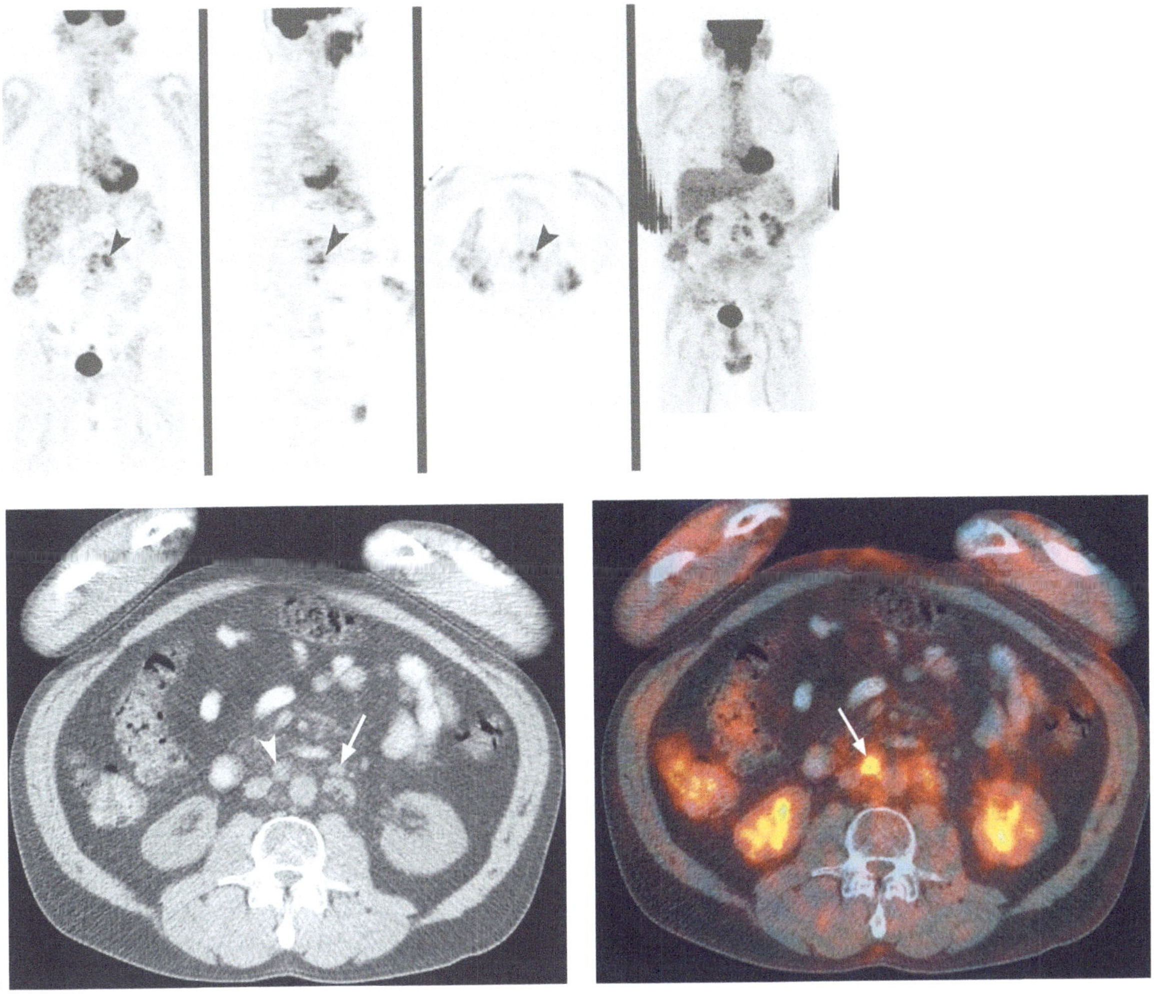

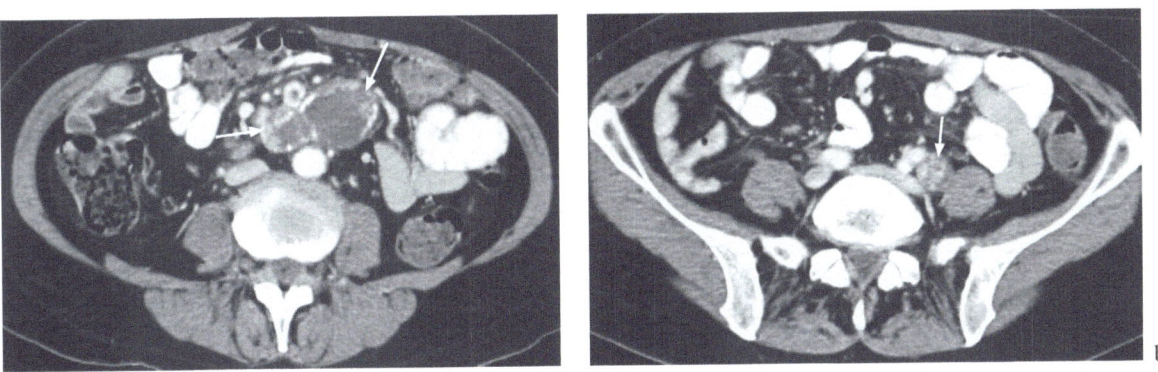

Fig. 8.9a–c. FDG-PET CT in a 52-year-old man with a history of low-grade lymphoma. **a** Coronal, sagittal and axial images acquired after intravenous injection of F-18FDG show discrete foci of increased metabolic activity in the aortocaval and left paraaortic regions (*arrowheads*) consistent with recurrent lymphoma in retroperitoneal lymph nodes. **b** Axial CT image from PET CT study shows small aortocaval (*arrowhead*) and paraaortic (*arrow*) nodes. **c** The fusion image shows intense metabolic activity in the aortocaval node (*arrow*), confirming recurrent lymphoma. (*Image courtesy of Drs R. Wahl and C. Cohade*)

Fig. 8.10a,b. Treated mesenteric lymphoma in a-53-year old man. **a** Axial contrast-enhanced CT scan of the mid abdomen shows a hypodense mass with rim calcifications in the mesentery (*arrows*). This mass had been stable for at least 1 year. **b** Axial contrast-enhanced CT scan of the lower abdomen shows a left common iliac node with punctate calcifications (*arrow*). Calcifications are more commonly seen after treatment.

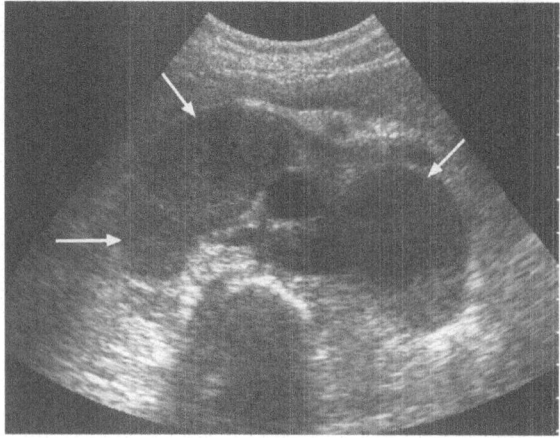

Fig. 8.11. Large B-cell lymphoma in retroperitoneal lymph nodes in a 55-year-old woman. Transverse ultrasound at the level of the mid abdomen shows large hypoechoic masses surrounding the aorta (*arrows*).

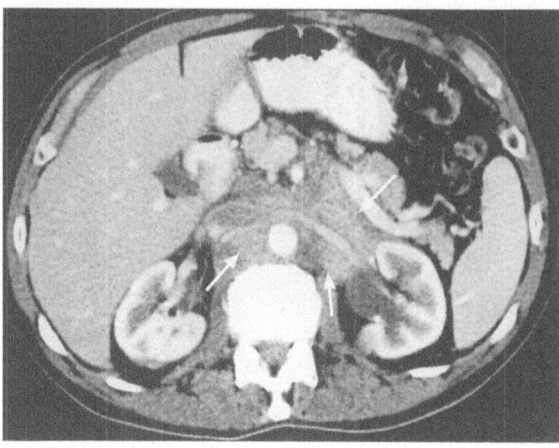

Fig. 8.13. Non-Hodgkin lymphoma in retroperitoneal nodes in a 66-year-old woman. Axial contrast-enhanced CT scan of the mid abdomen shows ill-defined mildly enhancing soft tissue in the retroperitoneum encasing the left renal vein and portion of the superior mesenteric artery (*arrows*).

nodal group can be affected including paraaortic and paracaval lymph nodes, iliac and obturator chains in the pelvis and nodes around the celiac axis, portocaval space and the peripancreatic region. Nodal NHL appears as well-defined, homogeneous, mildly enhancing masses on CT (Fig. 8.12) or displays an infiltrative pattern encasing but not occluding vessels (Fig. 8.13).

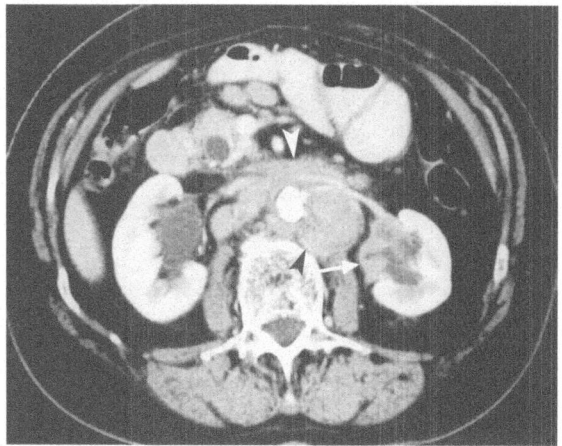

Fig. 8.12. Non-Hodgkin lymphoma in retroperitoneal nodes in a 77-year-old man. Axial contrast-enhanced CT scan of the mid abdomen shows discrete mildly enhancing enlarged nodes surrounding the aorta and inferior vena cava (*arrowheads*). They are encasing the left renal artery and vein. Note soft tissue thickening on the left renal pelvis (*arrow*) suggesting tumor spread and bilateral hydronephrosis.

8.4.2
Mesentery

NHL is the most common malignant neoplasm affecting the mesentery. Approximately 30 to 50% of patients with NHL harbor disease in the mesenteric lymph nodes. Imaging findings on contrast-enhanced CT or MR imaging include multiple rounded homogeneous masses (Fig. 8.14a), often encasing the mesenteric vessels and producing the "sandwich sign," a large lobulated "cake like" heterogeneous mass with hypodense areas of necrosis displacing small bowel loops (Fig. 8.5) or an ill defined infiltration of the mesenteric fat (MUELLER et al. 1980; MINDELZUN et al. 1996). Bulky retroperitoneal adenopathy commonly accompanies the mesenteric disease and should be a clue to the diagnosis (Fig. 8.4). Diffuse infiltration of the mesenteric fat has been described as "misty mesentery", (Fig. 8.14b) although this appearance is more commonly present after regression of pathologic nodes post treatment (MINDELZUN et al. 1996).

Occasionally, mesenteric lymphoma is accompanied by involvement of the omentum and peritoneum, an appearance indistinguishable from carcinomatosis (Fig. 8.15) (KIM et al. 1998).

Mesenteric lymphadenopathy caused by an infectious process needs to be differentiated from NHL, particularly in patients infected with HIV. Intra abdominal lymphadenopathy is the most common manifestation of abdominal tuberculosis and infection with Mycobacterium Avium Complex (MAC). CT

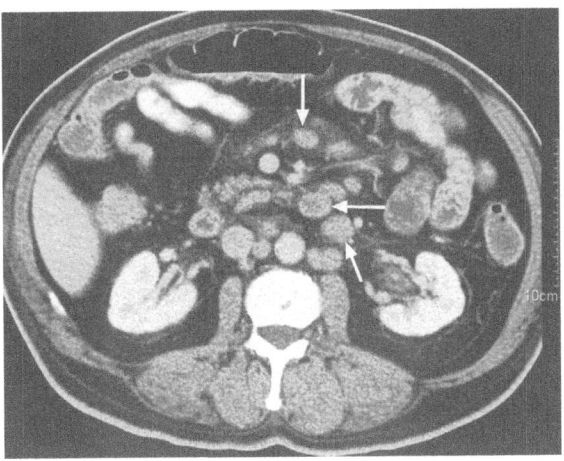
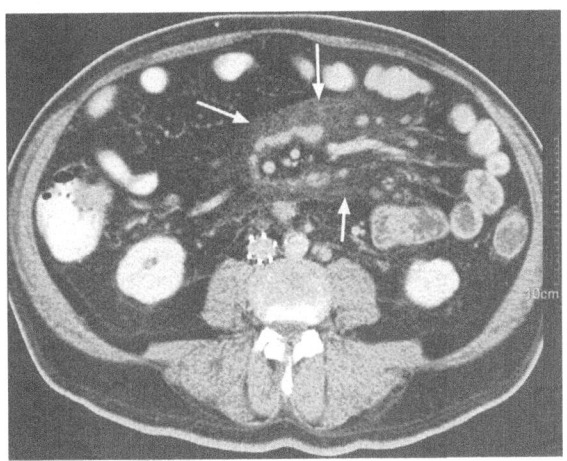

a   b

Fig. 8.14a,b. Non-Hodgkin lymphoma in the mesentery in a 52-year-old man presenting with abdominal pain and diarrhea. **a** Axial contrast-enhanced CT scan of the mid abdomen shows multiple small discrete nodes in the mesentery (*arrows*). Percutaneous biopsy of one of the nodes established the diagnosis. **b** Axial contrast-enhanced CT scan of the lower abdomen shows focal infiltration of the mesenteric fat, an appearance called "the misty mesentery" (*arrows*).

findings of predominant enlargement of mesenteric, peripancreatic and omental nodes, discrete adenopathy rather then confluent masses and the presence of central necrosis with rim enhancement (Fig. 8.16) or multilocular appearance of lymphadenopathy favors the diagnosis of atypical mycobacterial infection or tuberculosis (JADVAR et al. 1997; YANG et al. 1999).

Mesenteric NHL also needs to be distinguished from sclerosing mesenteritis (Fig. 8.17) and metastatic disease, particularly from carcinoid tumor. In the later case, the mesenteric mass often exhibits

strong enhancement after administration of intravenous contrast.

8.4.3
Spleen

Lymphoma is the most common malignant neoplasm affecting the spleen. Splenic involvement is present in up to 80% of cases and is usually associated with disease elsewhere in the thorax or abdomen. Isolated

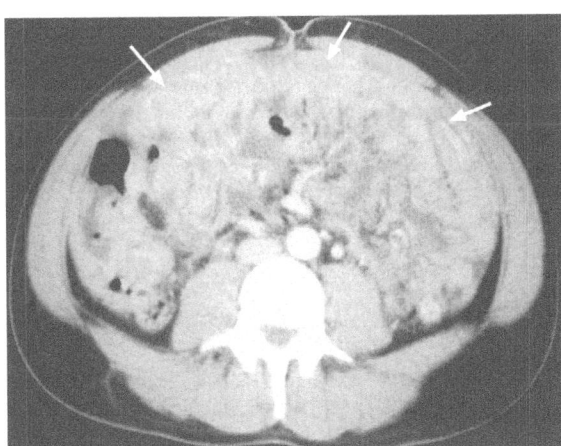
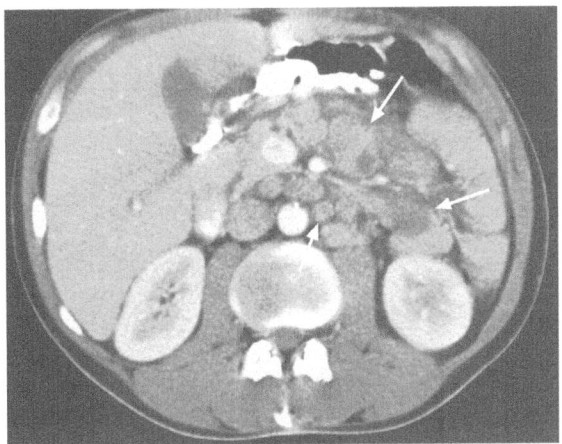

Fig. 8.15. Peritoneal lymphomatosis caused by Burkitt like NHL in a 41-year-old man. Axial contrast-enhanced CT scan of the mid abdomen shows diffuse infiltration of the mesentery and omentum by mildly enhancing soft tissue (*arrows*). The appearance cannot be distinguished from carcinomatosis.

Fig. 8.16. Mesenteric mycobacterial infection caused by MAI in a 38-year-old man with HIV. Axial contrast-enhanced CT scan of the abdomen shows multiple mesenteric and small retroperitoneal lymph nodes (*arrows*). Note that the nodes are not confluent and there are central hypodense areas in several of the nodes.

primary splenic lymphoma is much less common and requires splenectomy or image-guided biopsy for diagnosis (Fig. 8.18) (Brox and Shustik 1993).

Several patterns of splenic lymphoma can be recognized on imaging studies. Diffuse infiltration by malignant lymphocytes appears as diffuse splenomegaly, often with heterogeneous enhancement best seen in the portal venous phase of enhancement on contrast CT. Other appearances include a miliary pattern of multiple small masses or a few discrete larger lesions (Dachman et al. 1998). Regardless of their size, lymphomatous deposits are hypodense on

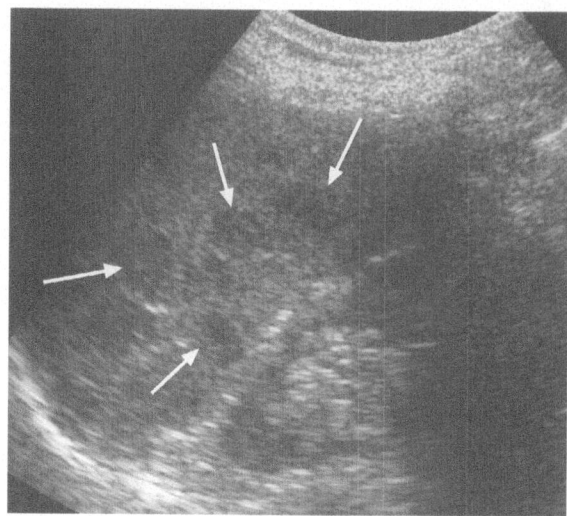

Fig. 8.19. Non-Hodgkin lymphoma involving the spleen in a 39-year-old man. Sagittal ultrasound of the spleen shows multiple hypoechoic lesions within a mildly enlarged spleen (*arrows*).

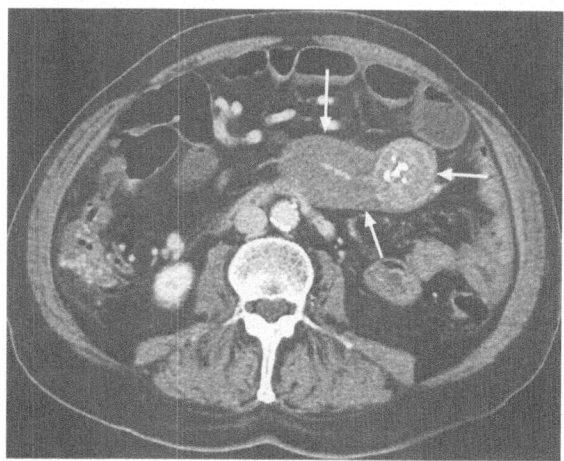

Fig. 8.17. Sclerosing mesenteritis in a 75-year-old man with abdominal pain. Axial contrast-enhanced CT scan of the abdomen shows a large mesenteric mass (*arrows*). Note the presence of coarse calcifications within portion of the mass. This would be unusual in untreated lymphoma.

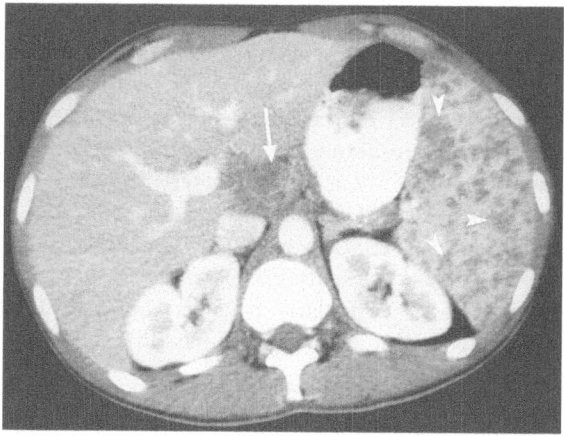

Fig. 8.20. Atypical mycobacterial infection involving the spleen and abdominal lymph nodes in a 40-year-old man with HIV. Axial contrast-enhanced CT scan of the upper abdomen shows innumerable small hypodense lesions within an enlarged spleen (*arrowheads*). Note the hypodense portocaval nodes (*arrow*). Fine needle aspiration of the lymph nodes demonstrated many acid fast bacilli within the aspirate.

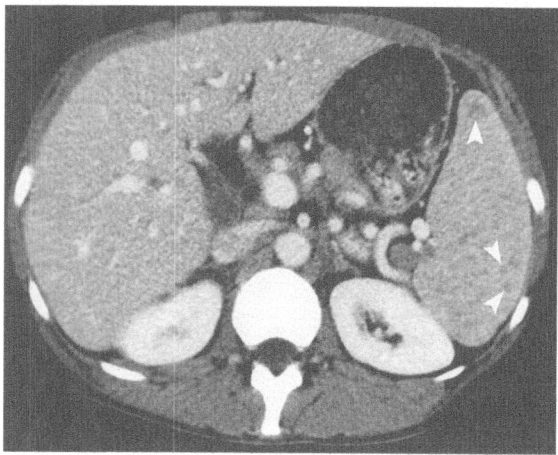

Fig. 8.18. B-cell lymphoma involving the spleen in a 44-year-old man. Axial contrast-enhanced CT scan of the spleen in the portal venous phase of enhancement shows multiple hypodense lesions within an enlarged spleen (*arrowheads*).

contrast CT (Fig. 8.18), hypoechoic on ultrasound (Figs. 8.8, 8.19) and appear hypointense on T1-wieghted and slightly hyperintense on T2-weighted MR images (fig. 8.7) (Urrutia et al. 1996).

Differential diagnosis of splenic lymphoma includes opportunistic infections (Fig. 8.20), particularly in immunocompromised patients, metastatic disease and sarcoidosis. Infectious nodules tend to be smaller and more uniform in size compared to lymphomatous foci (Warshauer et al. 1998).

8.5
Extranodal Non-Hodgkin Lymphoma

Extranodal NHL refers to disease affecting extranodal lymphoid tissue in the spleen and gastrointestinal tract or spread to organs that do not normally contain lymphatic tissue, such as the parenchymal abdominal organs. Extranodal disease is relatively common in certain subtypes of NHL, at initial diagnosis or during recurrence (CASTELLINO 1991).

8.5.1
Gastrointestinal Tract

The gastrointestinal tract (GI) is the most common site for extranodal NHL and is the primary location in 4–20% of cases (CRUMP et al. 1999; PANDEY et al. 1999). A variety of conditions predispose to the development of GI NHL. These include not only immunosuppression after solid organ transplantation and HIV infection but also Crohn disease, celiac disease and *Helicobacter pylori* infection (CRUMP et al. 1999).

The vast majority of these tumors affect the stomach, accounting for 74.8% of cases in one series of 371 patients with GI lymphoma (KOCH et al. 2001) In this series, small bowel lymphomas were a distant second (8.6% of cases), followed by the ileocecal valve (7% of patients). Multiple sites can occur, but isolated involvement of the duodenum, colon and rectum is rare (KOCH et al. 2001).

Most GI lymphomas originate in the mucosa-associated lymphoid tissue or MALT. With the exception of the stomach, where approximately 40% of tumors are low-grade, the majority of NHL is of an intermediate or aggressive subtype (HA et al. 1999).

8.5.1.1
Imaging Techniques

Single and double contrast techniques are traditionally used to image the GI. They provide unparalleled advantage for examination of mucosal abnormalities. However, CT is being utilized with increasing frequency in patients with non-specific abdominal complaints or suspected gastrointestinal pathology, particularly if the patient presents with an acute abdomen or signs of bowel obstruction (TAMM and FISHMAN 1996). Evaluation for abdominal adenopathy and involvement of other organs for staging purposes is best accomplished by CT. Administration of water rather than a positive oral contrast agent

and use of intravenous contrast material as well as multiplanar or three-dimensional reconstruction is helpful. While endoscopic ultrasound is increasingly being offered for the diagnosis and staging of gastric neoplasms, transabdominal ultrasound plays a minor role except to guide percutaneous biopsy of intestinal lesions that are difficult to reach endoscopically (CARSON et al. 1998). Similarly the role of MR imaging is still under investigation although a recent report boasts a higher sensitivity and specificity of MR imaging with half Fourier acquisition single shot (HASTE) sequence compared to single detector helical CT in a small series of 44 patients with suspected small bowel obstruction (BEALL et al. 2002).

8.5.1.2
Stomach

The stomach is the major site of GI lymphoma. A significant number of these tumors arise from MALT and are related to infection by *Helicobacter pylori* infection. Differentiation between low-grade and high-grade MALT lymphoma is critical for management and prognosis. Low-grade MALT lymphomas are superficially spreading lesions associated with a 90% 10-year survival rate (DE JONG et al. 1997) and usually respond to *H. pylori* eradication. By contrast, high-grade lymphomas require aggressive treatment and have poorer prognosis.

The radiographic manifestations of gastric lymphomas parallel their biological behavior and reflect the depth of invasion at histology. In a retrospective study comparing the radiographic findings in 29 patients with low-grade MALT gastric lymphoma and 28 patients with high-grade lesions, PARK et al. (2002) found significant differences between the 2 groups. Low-grade tumors typically appeared as a mucosal nodularity, shallow ulceration or mildly thickened folds on double contrast upper gastrointestinal series and depicted a normal appearance or minimal thickening of the gastric wall (1cm or less) on CT. In fact, CHOI et al. (2002) concluded that the absence of CT abnormality was a good predictor of a low-grade MALT lymphoma. The radiographic findings in high-grade lesions include bulky polypoid masses, markedly thickened folds (Fig. 8.21) and diffuse or focal gastric wall thickening (Figs. 8.22, 8.23) (often 4cm or more) on CT (MEGIBOW et al. 1983; BUY and MOSS 1982; FISHMAN et al. 1991; PARK et al. 2002; CHOI et al. 2002). Associated lymphadenopathy is seen in 67 to 75% of these patients (PARK et al. 2002; CHOI et al. 2002). Although it is often difficult to differentiate high-grade lymphoma from the

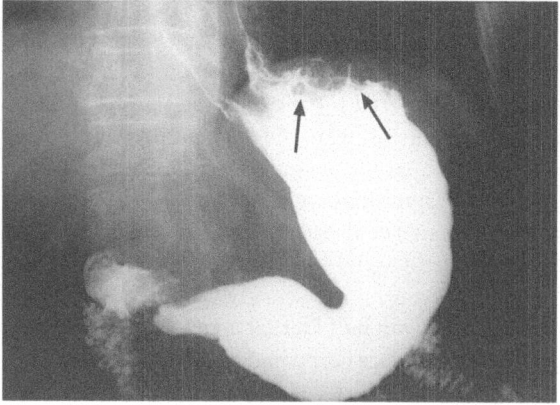

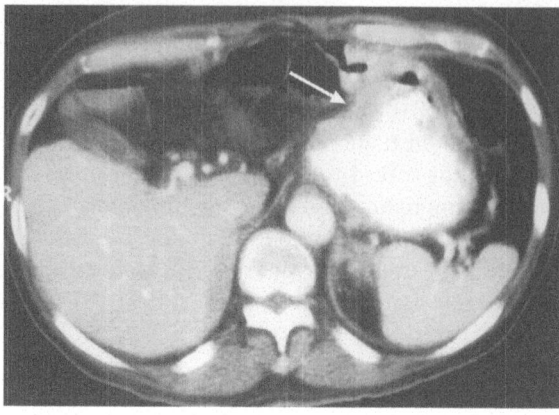

Fig. 8.21. Lymphoma of the gastric fundus in a 50-year-old woman. Image from a single contrast upper gastrointestinal examination shows a polypoid mass at the gastric fundus (*arrows*).

Fig. 8.22. Lymphoma of the stomach in a 62-year-old man. Axial contrast-enhanced CT scan of the stomach shows focal thickening of the gastric wall (*arrow*).

more common adenocarcinoma, severe gastric wall thickening of 5 cm or more as well as the presence of extensive adenopathy extending below the level of the renal hila favors the former diagnosis (FISHMAN et al. 1991).

8.5.1.3
Small Bowel

Small bowel lymphomas account for 20 to 50% of malignant tumors of the small bowel. Patients usually present with non-specific clinical symptoms of abdominal pain, weight loss or anemia. These tumors are more common in older men, with the exception of Burkitt lymphoma, which tends to affect adolescents or young adults. In a series of 119 cases of small bowel lymphomas, 66% were B-cell type and 34% were T-cell type. Nearly half of the patients with T-cell tumors had underlying enteropathy (DOMIZIO et al. 1993). Patients infected with HIV are at a particularly high risk of developing high-grade B-cell lesions.

BALTHAZAR et al. (1997) reviewed 42 patients with small bowel lymphoma and described two main CT patterns. The first pattern is that of homogeneous circumferential thickening of one or multiple segments of small bowel (Fig. 8.24). The second pattern is described as a focal mass causing aneurysmal dilatation of a small bowel loop (Fig. 8.25). Concomitant mesenteric or retroperitoneal adenopathy is often present. Cavitation or ulcerations can be seen within the mass. Lymphomatous masses sometimes cause small bowel obstruction or act as a lead point for intussusception (TAMM and FISHMAN 1996).

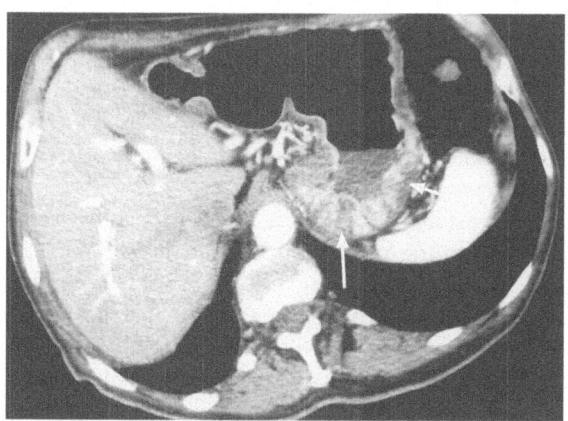

Fig. 8.23. T-cell lymphoma of the stomach in a 55-year-old man. Axial contrast-enhanced CT scan of the stomach shows subtle thickening and irregularities of the gastric folds near the fundus (*arrows*). Note how the use of water as oral contrast helps delineate the abnormality.

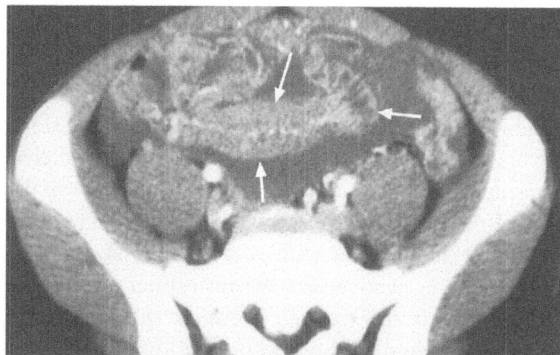

Fig. 8.24. Burkitt lymphoma of the small bowel in a 19-year-old man. Axial contrast-enhanced CT scan of the pelvis shows focal thickening of a small bowel loop (*arrows*). There is ascites present.

Primary lymphoma of the appendix is quite rare and typically presents with symptoms mimicking acute appendicitis. Marked thickening of the appendix with preservation of its vermiform shape or aneurysmal dilatation of the lumen should suggest the diagnosis, particularly in older patients (PICKHARDT et al. 2002).

Small bowel lymphoma is rarely diagnosed on ultrasound. Its appearance as hypoechoic thickening of a segment of bowel, the "pseudokidney sign", is non-specific and cannot be distinguished from inflammatory or other neoplastic diseases affecting the small bowel (SENER et al. 1989).

8.5.1.4
Colon

Colonic lymphoma comprises only about 6% of GI NHL (ZIGHELBOIM and LARSON 1994). The cecum followed by the rectum are the most common sites of involvement. Colonic NHL presents as a bulky polypoid mass or marked thickening of the affected segment (Figs. 8.26, 8.27) (LEVINE et al. 1997). As the tumor infiltrates the submucosa and may spare the mucosa, percutaneous biopsy may be preferable to the endoscopic approach.

8.5.2
Liver

Secondary spread to the liver occurs in 15 to 50% of patients with disseminated lymphoma and is more common at the time of recurrence (CIVARDI et al. 2002). In their series of over 400 patients with NHL, CIVARDI et al. (2002) found that hepatic lesions discovered during initial staging were incidental benign masses in nearly 60% of cases. By contrast, over half of the lesions newly detected during the course of the disease were malignant. Although most patients with hepatic NHL are asymptomatic, portal hypertension and hepatic insufficiency have rarely been associated with diffuse widespread infiltration by tumor (THOMPSON et al. 2001).

Primary hepatic lymphoma is quite rare, although immunocompromised patients and perhaps those infected with hepatitis C virus may be at increased risk (MAHER et al. 2001).

In the past, the sensitivity and specificity of CT to detect hepatic lymphoma was reportedly as low as 57% and 88% respectively (ZORNOZA and GINALDI 1981). With the advent of helical CT, both detection and characterization of all liver tumors, including lymphoma, has dramatically improved. Patterns of hepatic

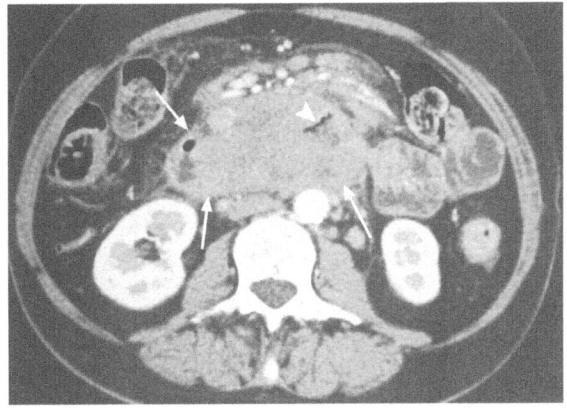

Fig. 8.25. B-cell lymphoma of the duodenum in a 44-year-old woman. Axial contrast-enhanced CT scan of the mid abdomen shows a lobulated mass in the expected location of the third portion of the duodenum (*arrows*). Note the ulceration within the mass (*arrowhead*). Percutaneous biopsy established the diagnosis.

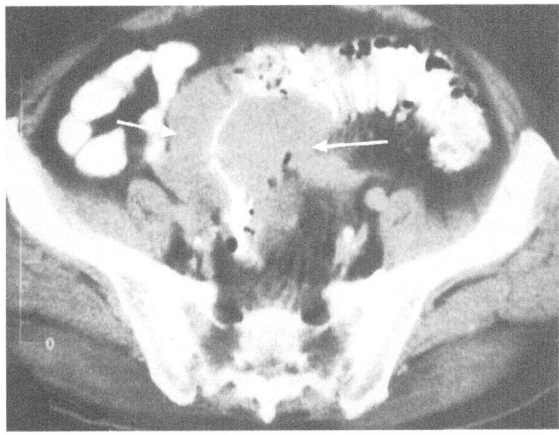

Fig. 8.26. Lymphoma of the sigmoid colon in a 65-year-old man with rectal bleeding. Axial contrast-enhanced CT scan of the pelvis shows marked thickening of a segment of the sigmoid colon with luminal narrowing (*arrows*).

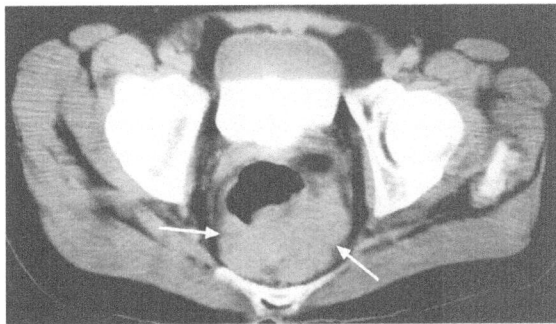

Fig. 8.27. Perirectal Burkitt lymphoma in a 63-year-old man. Axial contrast-enhanced CT of the pelvis shows an exophytic polypoid mass arising from the rectum (*arrows*).

lymphoma include hepatomegaly caused by diffuse infiltration of the liver, multiple masses or rarely a solitary lesion (MAHER et al. 2001). Foci of hepatic NHL typically have lower attenuation then the surrounding normal parenchyma at CT, with little enhancement post contrast or with a thin enhancing rim (Fig. 8.28) (MAHER et al. 2001; RIZZI et al. 2001). They are typically hypointense to the surrounding liver on T1-weighted MR sequence, and hyperintense on T2-weighted sequence (RIZZI et al. 2001) and hypoechoic compared to the normal liver on ultrasound (Fig. 8.29) (MAHER et al. 2001). Unfortunately, hepatic lymphoma cannot be definitively characterized by imaging, and requires percutaneous biopsy for definitive diagnosis.

8.5.3
Pancreas

As with other parenchymal organs, pancreatic NHL usually occurs in patients with extensive disease, either from infiltration of the organ by malignant lymphocytes or spread from adjacent lymph nodes. Primary pancreatic lymphoma is very rare, representing less then 0.5% of pancreatic tumors (BONI et al. 2002). The majority of primary pancreatic lymphoma presents as bulky lesions, which are located in the pancreatic head and are of B-cell type (NISHIMURA et al. 2001).

On imaging the task of the radiologist is to distinguish adenocarcinoma of the pancreas from pancre-atic and peripancreatic lymphoma. This distinction has important management implications, since surgery is generally not required for staging or treatment of pancreatic lymphoma and percutaneous biopsy generally yields enough tissue for diagnosis of the specific subtype of lymphoma (DI STASI et al. 1998). However pancreatic lymphoma has protean manifestations and cannot be reliably differentiated from adenocarcinoma in a significant number of cases.

Imaging features favoring the diagnosis of pancreatic lymphoma include the presence of a bulky mass with little or no biliary or pancreatic ductal obstruction (Fig. 8.30) and the presence of large peripancreatic lymph nodes or nodal enlargement below the level of the renal veins. In their review of the literature, FIDIAS et al. (1995) reported that obstructive jaundice is the presenting symptom of only 0.8% of patients with NHL. However, the presence of biliary tree dilatation should not exclude the diagnosis. Widespread infiltration of the pancreas can result in diffuse enlargement of the organ mimicking acute pancreatitis (Fig. 8.31) (MERKLE and GORICH 2002).

On gray scale ultrasound, both NHL and adenocarcinoma most often appear as irregularly shaped lobulated hypoechoic masses. In one small series, ISHIDA et al. (2002) found color Doppler ultrasound to be of some use: demonstration of peripancreatic vessels freely coursing through the masses without narrowing or turbulent blood flow would favor the diagnosis of NHL.

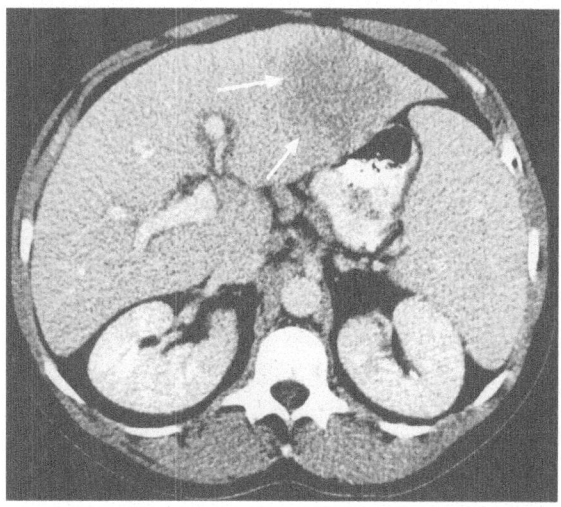

Fig. 8.28. Primary hepatic lymphoma in a 40-year-old man with HIV. Axial contrast-enhanced CT scan of the liver in the portal venous phase shows a low attenuation mass with ill defined borders in the left hepatic lobe (*arrows*).

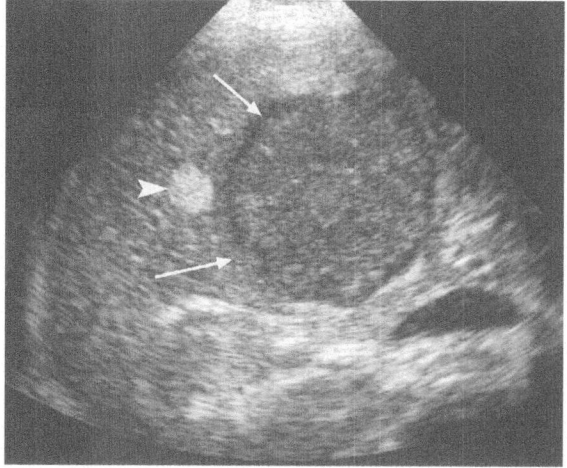

Fig. 8.29. Primary hepatic lymphoma in a 44-year-old man with HIV. Transverse ultrasound image of the right hepatic lobe shows a large hypoechoic mass (*arrows*). Note the adjacent well-defined echogenic lesion compatible with an incidental hemangioma (*arrowhead*).

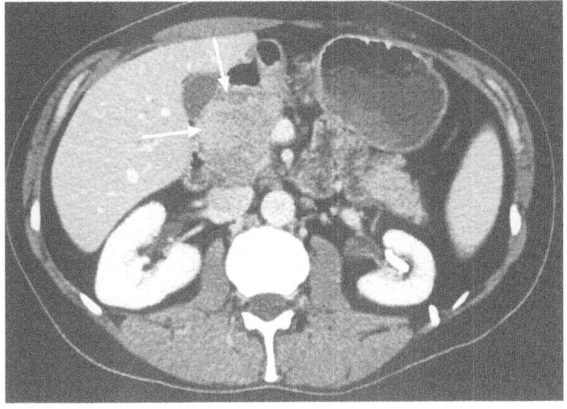

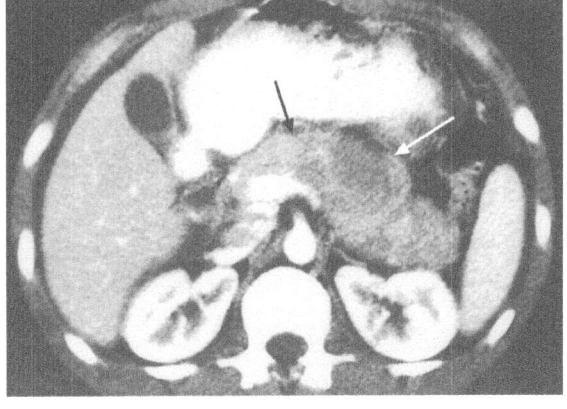

Fig. 8.30. Primary B-cell lymphoma of the pancreas in a 62-year-old man. Axial contrast-enhanced CT scan of the pancreas shows a bulky heterogeneous mass in the head of the pancreas (*arrows*). Note the absence of dilated biliary radicals in the liver.

Fig. 8.31. Recurrent B-cell lymphoma in a 42-year-old man with HIV. Axial contrast-enhanced CT scan of the pancreas shows diffuse enlargement of the pancreas (*arrows*). The parenchyma has low attenuation regions, an appearance mimicking pancreatitis.

8.5.4
Kidneys

Infiltration of the kidneys by NHL is common in patients with widespread disease. It is found in at least 50% of cases at autopsy and is increasingly being detected on cross sectional imaging studies. Most patients do not have any evidence of renal dysfunction. When present, renal failure is generally caused by ureteral obstruction or drug toxicity. Primary renal lymphoma is exceedingly rare and may present with acute renal failure caused by infiltration of the renal parenchyma by tumor cells (BROULAND et al. 1994).

Several patterns of renal lymphoma have been recognized on cross-sectional imaging studies (HEIKEN et al. 1983; COHAN et al. 1990; SHEERAN and SUSSMAN 1998; URBAN and FISHMAN 2000). The most common appearance, seen in at least 60% of patients, is that of bilateral multiple solid parenchymal masses (Figs. 8.32, 8.33). These lesions are hypoechoic on ultrasound and are homogeneous with lower attenuation than the normal renal parenchyma on contrast-enhanced CT. Invasion of the kidney by adjacent retroperitoneal lymph nodes is another common appearance (Fig. 8.34). These lymphomatous retroperitoneal masses often encase the renal vessels and invade or obstruct the ureter. Lymphoma can also infiltrate the renal parenchyma causing diffuse nephromegaly with preservation of the reniform shape of the kidney (Fig. 8.35). Atypical patterns include a solitary renal mass mimicking renal cell carcinoma (Fig. 8.36) and isolated perirenal

tumor resembling perirenal hematoma or extramedullary hematopoiesis (Fig. 8.37).

8.5.5
Adrenal Glands

Approximately 25% of patients with disseminated NHL are found to have adrenal involvement at autopsy. Disease confined to the adrenal glands (primary adrenal lymphoma) is very uncommon, with fewer than 100 case reports in the literature, often bilateral and associated with a poor prognosis, with many patients succumbing after just a few

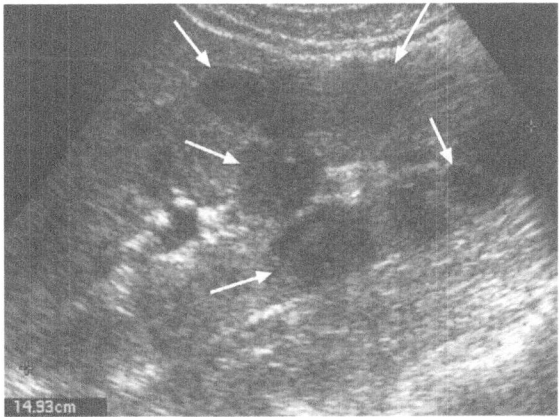

Fig. 8.32. Renal lymphoma in a 33-year-old man. Sagittal ultrasound of the right kidney shows multiple hypoechoic masses in the parenchyma (*arrows*). Note that the kidney is enlarged, but preserves its reniform shape.

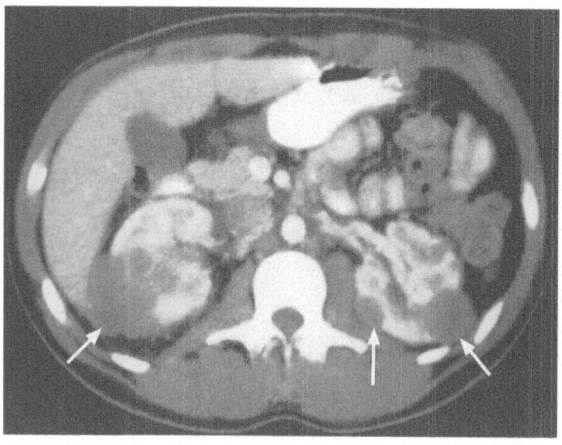

Fig. 8.33. Renal lymphoma in a 46-year-old woman. Axial contrast-enhanced CT scan of the kidneys shows multiple low attenuation masses in both kidneys (*arrows*).

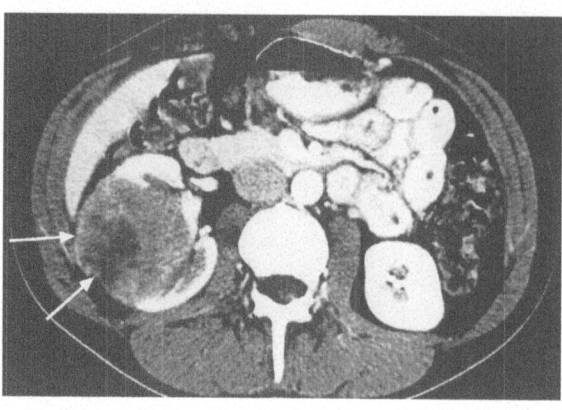

Fig. 8.36. Recurrent lymphoma in the right kidney mimicking a renal cell carcinoma in 41-year-old woman with history lymphoma. Axial contrast-enhanced CT scan of the kidneys shows a solitary heterogeneous mass in the right kidney (*arrows*). The diagnosis was established by percutaneous biopsy.

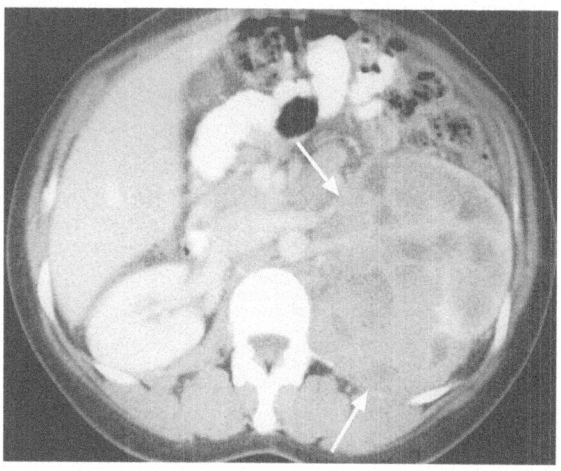

Fig. 8.34. Renal lymphoma in a 36-year-old woman. Axial contrast-enhanced CT scan of the abdomen shows a large heterogeneous left retroperitoneal mass extending into and infiltrating the left kidney (*arrows*).

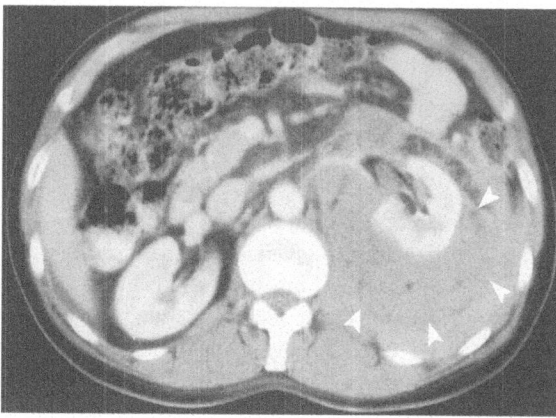

Fig. 8.37. Perirenal lymphoma in a 61-year-old man. Axial contrast-enhanced CT scan of the kidneys shows a large soft tissue mass in the perinephric space surrounding the left kidney (*arrowheads*). Note near normal enhancement of the renal parenchyma.

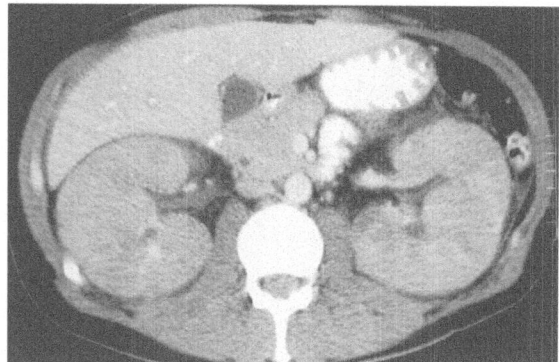

Fig. 8.35. Burkitt lymphoma involving both kidneys in a 22-year-old man. Axial contrast-enhanced CT scan of the kidneys in the nephrographic phase shows bilateral renal enlargement. There is heterogeneously decreased enhancement of the renal parenchyma.

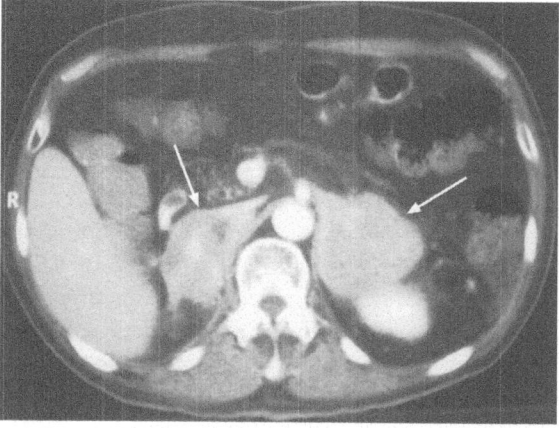

Fig. 8.38. Adrenal lymphoma in a 74-year-old man. Axial contrast-enhanced CT scan of the abdomen shows massive enlargement of both adrenal glands (*arrows*).

months (ELLIS and READ 2000). As many as two-thirds of patients with bilateral adrenal NHL experience clinical adrenal insufficiency (GAMELIN et al. 1992; KATO et al. 1996). This complication appears to be more common in patients with primary adrenal lymphoma. This diagnosis should be suspected in patients with adrenal insufficiency and bilateral adrenal masses and can be confirmed by percutaneous ultrasound or CT-guided biopsy (TAKAI et al. 1999).

On imaging, bilateral and often massive adrenal enlargement is seen. Typically the shape of the gland is preserved, a helpful distinguishing feature from adrenal metastases (Fig. 8.38). The masses are hypoechoic on ultrasound. On CT, homogeneous enlargement is seen with minimal enhancement after contrast administration. On MR imaging, adrenal lymphoma has been described as isointense to the kidney on T1 weighted images, hyperintense on T2-weighted sequence, and showing minimal enhancement following gadolinium administration (KATO et al. 1996).

8.5.6
Reproductive Organs

8.5.6.1
Testicles

NHL, usually diffuse large B-cell or Burkitt type, accounts for about 9% of testicular tumors and is one of the most common cause of testicular enlargement in men over the age of 60 (SHAHAB and DOLL 1999; MAZZU et al. 1995).

Two sonographic patterns have been described. In the diffuse infiltrative form the testicle is enlarged, maintains its ovoid shape and exhibits a diffusely heterogeneous echotexture. The testicle is diffusely hypervascular on color Doppler ultrasound, making differentiation with inflammatory or infectious orchitis difficult, although the clinical symptoms and the lack of epididymal enlargement should suggest the correct diagnosis (Fig. 8.39). The second pattern is that of single or multiple hypoechoic and hypervascular nodules (MAZZU et al. 1995). Bilateral involvement is common.

8.5.6.2
Ovaries and Uterus

Secondary infiltration of the female reproductive organ by NHL is more common then lymphoma primarily affecting the uterus or ovaries. If gynecological pathology is suspected, pelvic ultrasound or MR imaging are the imaging modalities of choice. Case reports describe the MR imaging findings in uterine lymphoma as diffuse enlargement of the uterus with a relatively homogeneous signal intensity and preservation of a normal junctional zone (KAWAKAMI et al. 1995; KIM et al. 1997). Primary lymphoma of the ovary is exceedingly uncommon, usually of the B-cell lineage. The possibility of ovarian lymphoma should be raised in the presence of bilateral solid ovarian masses on ultrasound (Fig. 8.40), homogeneously hypointense on T1-weighted MR imaging sequence, with mildly increased signal intensity on T2-weighted MR images and peripheral contrast enhancement after administration of gadolinium (FERROZZI et al. 2000).

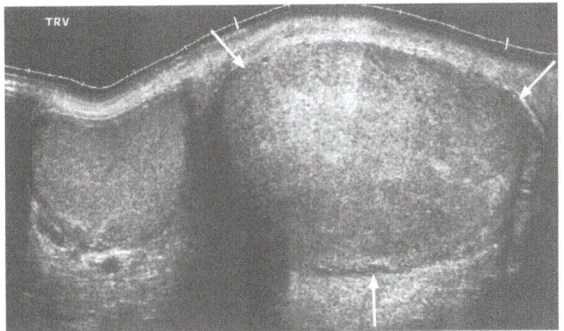

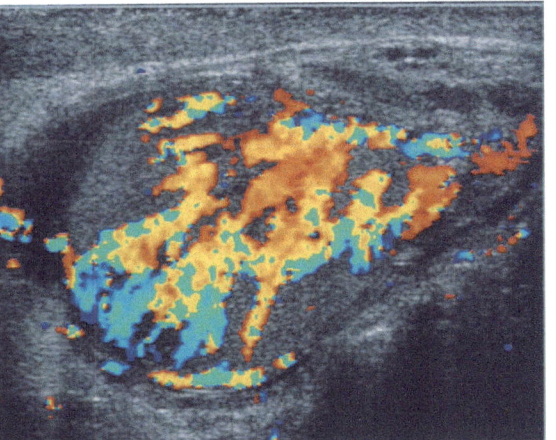

Fig. 8.39a,b. B-cell lymphoma of the testicle in a 68-year-old man. **a** Extended field of view ultrasound of the testicles shows an enlarged left testicle (*arrows*) diffusely infiltrated with multiple hypoechoic masses. Some of the lesions have ill defined borders. **b** Color Doppler image shows significant hypervascularity.

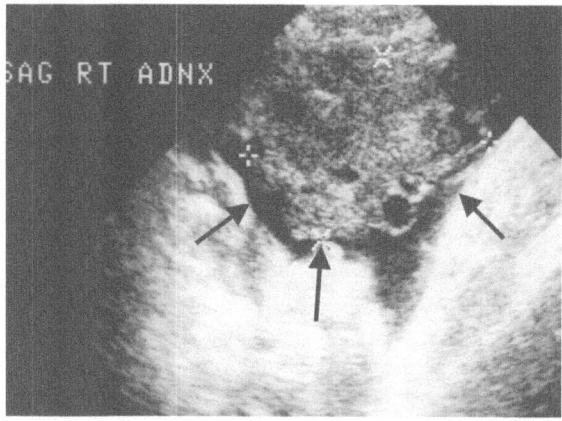

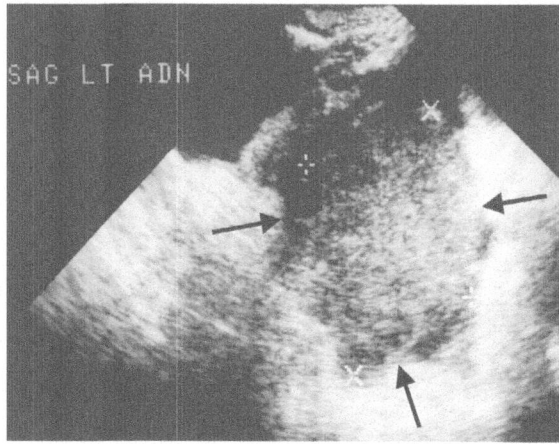

Fig. 8.40a,b. Lymphoma involving the ovaries in a 54-year-old woman. **a** Sagittal endovaginal ultrasound of the right ovary shows a heterogeneous predominantly solid mass replacing the right ovary (*arrows*). Ascites is present. **b** The left ovary has a similar appearance.

8.6
Conclusion

CT remains the modality of choice for the initial diagnosis, staging and monitoring of patients with non Hodgkin lymphoma. MR imaging is useful in selected cases, particularly in patients who are unable to receive intravenous iodinated contrast material. While ultrasound plays a limited role, except for evaluating spread to the reproductive organs, it is routinely used as a guidance modality for percutaneous biopsy.

References

Armitage JM, Kormos RL, Stuart RS et al (1991) Post-transplant lymphoproliferative disease in thoracic organ transplant patients: ten years of cyclosporine-based immunosuppression. J Heart Lung Transplant 10:877–886

Armitage JO (1997) The changing classification of non-Hodgkin's lymphomas. CA Cancer J Clin 47:323–325

Armitage JO, Weisenburger DD (1998) New approach to classifying non-Hodgkin's lymphomas: clinical features of the major histologic subtypes. Non-Hodgkin's Lymphoma Classification Project. J Clin Oncol 16:2780–2795

Balthazar EJ, Noordhoorn M, Megibow AJ et al (1997) CT of small-bowel lymphoma in immunocompetent patients and patients with AIDS: comparison of findings. AJR Am J Roentgenol 168:675–680

Beall DP, Fortman BJ, Lawler BC et al (2002) Imaging bowel obstruction: a comparison between fast magnetic resonance imaging and helical computed tomography. Clin Radiol 57:719–724

Boni L, Benevento A, Dionigi G et al (2002) Primary pancreatic lymphoma. Surg Endosc 16:1107–1108

Brouland JP, Meeus F, Rossert J et al (1994) Primary bilateral B-cell renal lymphoma: a case report and review of the literature. Am J Kidney Dis 24:586–589

Brox A, Shustik C (1993) Non-Hodgkin's lymphoma of the spleen. Leuk Lymphoma 11:165–171

Buy JN, Moss AA (1982) Computed tomography of gastric lymphoma. AJR Am J Roentgenol 138:859–865

Carson BW, Brown JA, Cooperberg PL (1998) Ultrasonographically guided percutaneous biopsy of gastric, small bowel, and colonic abnormalities: efficacy and safety. J Ultrasound Med 17:739–742

Castellino RA (1991) The non-Hodgkin lymphomas: practical concepts for the diagnostic radiologist. Radiology 178:315–321

Chan JK (2001) The new World Health Organization classification of lymphomas: the past, the present and the future. Hematol Oncol 19:129–150

Choi D, Lim HK, Lee SJ et al (2002) Gastric mucosa-associated lymphoid tissue lymphoma: helical CT findings and pathologic correlation. AJR Am J Roentgenol 178:1117–1122

Civardi G, Vallisa D, Berte R et al (2002) Focal liver lesions in non-Hodgkin's lymphoma: investigation of their prevalence, clinical significance and the role of Hepatitis C virus infection. Eur J Cancer 38:2382–2387

Cohan RH, Dunnick NR, Leder RA et al (1990) Computed tomography of renal lymphoma. J Comput Assist Tomogr 14:933–938

Crump M, Gospodarowicz M, Shepherd FA (1999) Lymphoma of the gastrointestinal tract. Semin Oncol 26:324–337

Dachman AH, Buck JL, Krishnan J et al (1998) Primary non-Hodgkin's splenic lymphoma. Clin Radiol 53:137–142

de Jong D, Boot H, van Heerde P et al (1997) Histological grading in gastric lymphoma: pretreatment criteria and clinical relevance. Gastroenterology 112:1466–1474

Di Stasi M, Lencioni R, Solmi L et al (1998) Ultrasound-guided fine needle biopsy of pancreatic masses: results of a multicenter study. Am J Gastroenterol 93:1329–1333

Domizio P, Owen RA, Shepherd NA et al (1993) Primary lymphoma of the small intestine. A clinicopathological study of 119 cases. Am J Surg Pathol 17:429–442

Dotti G, Fiocchi R, Motta T et al (2002) Lymphomas occurring late after solid-organ transplantation: influence of treatment on the clinical outcome. Transplantation 74: 1095–1102

Dugdale PE, Miles KA, Bunce I et al (1999) CT measurement of perfusion and permeability within lymphoma masses and its ability to assess grade, activity, and chemotherapeutic response. J Comput Assist Tomogr 23:540–547

Ellis RD, Read D (2000) Bilateral adrenal non-Hodgkin's lymphoma with adrenal insufficiency. Postgrad Med J 76: 508–509

Ferrozzi F, Tognini G, Bova D et al (2000) Non-Hodgkin lymphomas of the ovaries: MR findings. J Comput Assist Tomogr 24:416–420

Fidias P, Carey RW, Grossbard ML (1995) Non-Hodgkin's lymphoma presenting with biliary tract obstruction. A discussion of seven patients and a review of the literature. Cancer 75:1669–1677

Fishman EK, Kuhlman JE, Jones RJ (1991) CT of lymphoma: spectrum of disease. Radiographics 11:647–669

Gamelin E, Beldent V, Rousselet MC et al (1992) Non-Hodgkin's lymphoma presenting with primary adrenal insufficiency. A disease with an underestimated frequency? Cancer 69:2333–2336

Glass AG, Karnell LH, Menck HR (1997) The National Cancer Data Base report on non-Hodgkin's lymphoma. Cancer 80: 2311–2320

Gorg C, Weide R, Schwerk WB (1996) Sonographic patterns in extranodal abdominal lymphomas. Eur Radiol 6:855–864

Ha CS, Cho MJ, Allen PK et al (1999) Primary non-Hodgkin lymphoma of the small bowel. Radiology 211:183–187

Heiken JP, Gold RP, Schnur MJ et al (1983) Computed tomography of renal lymphoma with ultrasound correlation. J Comput Assist Tomogr 7:245–250

Ishida H, Konno K, Ishida J et al (2001) Splenic lymphoma: differentiation from splenic cyst with ultrasonography. Abdom Imaging 26:529–532

Ishida H, Konno K, Ishida J et al (2002) Abdominal lymphoma: differentiation from pancreatic carcinoma with Doppler US. Abdom Imaging 27:461–464

Jadvar H, Mindelzun RE, Olcott EW et al (1997) Still the great mimicker: abdominal tuberculosis. AJR Am J Roentgenol 168:1455–1460

Jung G, Heindel W, von-Bergwelt-Baildon M et al (2000) Abdominal lymphoma staging: is MR imaging with T2-weighted turbo-spin-echo sequence a diagnostic alternative to contrast-enhanced spiral CT? J Comput Assist Tomogr 24:783–787

Kato H, Itami J, Shiina T et al (1996) MR imaging of primary adrenal lymphoma. Clin Imaging 20:126–128

Kawakami S, Togashi K, Kojima N et al (1995) MR appearance of malignant lymphoma of the uterus. J Comput Assist Tomogr 19:238–242

Kim Y, Koh BH, Cho OK et al (1998) Peritoneal lymphomatosis: CT findings. Abdom Imaging 23:87–90

Kim YS, Cho O, Song S et al (1997) MR imaging of primary uterine lymphoma. Abdom Imaging 22:441–444

Koch P, del Valle F, Berdel WE et al (2001) Primary gastrointestinal non-Hodgkin's lymphoma: I. Anatomic and histologic distribution, clinical features, and survival data of 371 patients registered in the German Multicenter Study GIT NHL 01/92. J Clin Oncol 19:3861–3873

Kostakoglu L, Coleman M, Leonard JP et al (2002) PET predicts prognosis after 1 cycle of chemotherapy in aggressive lymphoma and Hodgkin's disease. J Nucl Med 43: 1018–1027

Levine MS, Rubesin SE, Patongrag-Brown L et al (1997) Non-Hodgkin's lymphoma of the gastrointestinal tract: radiographic findings. AJR Am J Roentgenol 168:165–172

Lionberger JM, Armitage JO (2001) Advances in the management of patients with non-Hodgkin's lymphoma. Expert Rev Anticancer Ther 1:43–52

Maher MM, McDermott SR, Fenlon HM et al (2001) Imaging of primary non-Hodgkin's lymphoma of the liver. Clin Radiol 56:295–301

Martinez-Maza O, Breen EC (2002) B-cell activation and lymphoma in patients with HIV. Curr Opin Oncol 14: 528–532

Mazzu D, Jeffrey RB Jr, Ralls PW et al (1995) Lymphoma and leukemia involving the testicles: findings on gray-scale and color Doppler sonography. AJR Am J Roentgenol 164: 645–647

Megibow AJ, Balthazar EJ, Naidich DP et al (1983) Computed tomography of gastrointestinal lymphoma. AJR Am J Roentgenol 141:541–547

Merkle EM, Gorich J (2002) Imaging of acute pancreatitis. Eur Radiol 12:1979–1992

Mikhaeel NG, Timothy AR, O'Doherty MJ et al (2000) 18-FDG-PET as a prognostic indicator in the treatment of aggressive non-Hodgkin's lymphoma-Comparison with CT. Leuk Lymphoma 39:543–553

Miles KA, Kelley BB (1997) CT measurements of capillary permeability within nodal masses: a potential technique for assessing the activity of lymphoma. Br J Radiol 70:74–79

Mindelzun RE, Jeffrey Jr RB, Lane MJ et al (1996) The misty mesentery on CT: differential diagnosis. AJR Am J Roentgenol 167:61–65

Moog F, Bangerter M, Diederichs CG et al (1998) Extranodal malignant lymphoma: detection with FDG PET versus CT. Radiology 206:475–481

Mueller PR, Ferrucci, Jr JT, Harbin WP et al (1980) Appearance of lymphomatous involvement of the mesentery by ultrasonography and body computed tomography: the "sandwich sign". Radiology 134:467–473

Neumann CH, Robert NJ, Canellos G et al (1983) Computed tomography of the abdomen and pelvis in non-Hodgkin lymphoma. J Comput Assist Tomogr 7:846–850

Neumann CH, Robert NJ, Rosenthal D et al (1983) Clinical value of ultrasonography for the management of non-Hodgkin lymphoma patients as compared with abdominal computed tomography. J Comput Assist Tomogr 7: 666–669

Nishimura R, Takakuwa T, Hoshida Y et al (2001) Primary pancreatic lymphoma: clinicopathological analysis of 19 cases from Japan and review of the literature. Oncology 60:322–329

Pandey M, Wadhwa MK, Patel HP et al (1999) Malignant lymphoma of the gastrointestinal tract. Eur J Surg Oncol 25:164–167

Park MS, Kim KW, Yu JS et al (2002) Radiographic findings of primary B-cell lymphoma of the stomach: low-grade versus high-grade malignancy in relation to the mucosa-associated lymphoid tissue concept. AJR Am J Roentgenol 179:1297–1304

Pickhardt PJ, Levy AD, Rohrmann Jr CA et al (2002) Non-Hodgkin's lymphoma of the appendix: clinical and CT findings with pathologic correlation. AJR Am J Roentgenol 178:1123–1127

Pileri SA, Milani M, Fraternali-Orcioni G et al (1998) From the REAL classification to the upcoming WHO scheme: a step toward universal categorization of lymphoma entities? Ann Oncol 9:607–612

Pombo F, Rodriguez E, Caruncho MV et al (1994) CT attenuation values and enhancing characteristics of thoracoabdominal lymphomatous adenopathies. J Comput Assist Tomogr 18:59–62

Radin DR, Esplin JA, Levine AM et al (1993) AIDS-related non-Hodgkin's lymphoma: abdominal CT findings in 112 patients. AJR Am J Roentgenol 160:1133–1139

Rahmouni A, Divine M, Lepage E et al (2001) Mediastinal lymphoma: quantitative changes in gadolinium enhancement at MR imaging after treatment. Radiology 219:621–628

Rizzi EB, Schinina V, Cristofaro M et al (2001) Non-Hodgkin's lymphoma of the liver in patients with AIDS: sonographic, CT, and MRI findings. J Clin Ultrasound 29:125–129

Rodriguez M, Rehn SM, Nyman RS et al (1999) CT in malignancy grading and prognostic prediction of non-Hodgkin's lymphoma." Acta Radiol 40:191–197

Scutellari PN, Borgatti L, Spanedda R (2000) Non-Hodgkin's lymphomas of extranodal localization. Strategies for imaging diagnosis. Radiol Med (Torino) 100:262–272

Sener RN, Alper H, Demirci A et al (1989) A different sonographic "pseudokidney" appearance detected with intestinal lymphoma: "hydronephrotic-pseudokidney". J Clin Ultrasound 17:209–212

Shahab N, Doll DC (1999) Testicular lymphoma. Semin Oncol 26:259–269

Sheeran SR, Sussman SK (1998) Renal lymphoma: spectrum of CT findings and potential mimics. AJR Am J Roentgenol 171:1067–1072

Skillings JR, Bramwell V, Nicholson RL et al (1991) A prospective study of magnetic resonance imaging in lymphoma staging. Cancer 67:1838–1843

Takai K, Hiragino T, Isoyama R et al (1999) A case of primary adrenal lymphoma diagnosed from percutaneous needle biopsy. Urol Int 62:31–33

Tamm EP, Fishman EK (1996) CT appearance of acute abdomen as initial presentation in lymphoma of the large and small bowel. Clin Imaging 20:21–25

Thompson DR, Faust TW, Stone MJ et al (2001) Hepatic failure as the presenting manifestation of malignant lymphoma. Clin Lymphoma 2:123–128

Urban BA, Fishman EK (2000) Renal lymphoma: CT patterns with emphasis on helical CT. Radiographics 20: 197–212

Urrutia M, Mergo PJ, Ros LH et al (1996) Cystic masses of the spleen: radiologic-pathologic correlation. Radiographics 16:107–129

Warshauer DM, Molina PL et al (1998) The spotted spleen: CT and clinical correlation in a tertiary care center. J Comput Assist Tomogr 22:694–702

Yang ZG, Min PO, Sone S et al (1999) Tuberculosis versus lymphomas in the abdominal lymph nodes: evaluation with contrast-enhanced CT. AJR Am J Roentgenol 172: 619–623

Zighelboim J, Larson MV (1994) Primary colonic lymphoma. Clinical presentation, histopathologic features, and outcome with combination chemotherapy. J Clin Gastroenterol 18:291–297

Zornoza J, Ginaldi S (1981) Computed tomography in hepatic lymphoma. Radiology 138:405–410

9 Musculoskeletal Involvement in Non-Hodgkin Lymphoma

George Hermann, Ibrahim Fikry Abdelwahab, Michael J. Klein

CONTENTS

9.1
Introduction

Lymphoreticular neoplasm of the reticulo-endothelial system is a well-known entity in which the tumor arises from lymphoid precursor cells. The disorders included in this group are NHL and HD, with a changing terminology. The old classification of primary NHL included lymphosarcoma and reticulum cell sarcoma. The cells of malignant lymphomas may exhibit various degrees of differentiation, which may be shown with immunohistochemistry (Resnick and Haghighi 1996; National Cancer Institute 1982).

George Hermann, MD, FACR
Professor of Radiology, Department of Radiology, Mount Sinai Medical Center, One Gustave L. Levy Place, New York, NY 10029-6574, USA
Ibrahim Fikry Abdelwahab, MD
Clinical Professor of Radiology, Weill Medical College, Cornell University of New York, Adjunct Clinical Professor of Pathology, Mount Sinai School of Medicine, 104-60 Queens Blvd #16A, Forest Hills, NY 11375, USA
Michael J. Klein, MD
Professor of Pathology, Head, Section of Surgical Pathology, Department of Pathology, University of Alabama at Birmingham School of Medicine, 1922 Seventh Avenue – Room 506, Birmingham, Alabama 35233, USA

Lymphomatous involvement of the skeleton may be the result of systemic lymphoma. Over 50,000 new cases of NHL were diagnosed in 1997 in the United States with a death rate predicted to be 50%. This puts the disease sixth in mortality among malignancies (Skarin and Dorfman 1997). Up to 20% of patients suffering from NHL show skeletal changes following the primary presentation. Not infrequently, however, skeletal changes may be part of the early manifestation of the disease (Resnick and Haghighi 1996). Skeletal involvement in HD is fairly common but is rarely seen at the time of onset of the disease.

Until the late 1920s, primary malignant bone lymphoma was not considered as a distinct entity in the literature. Oberling (1928) was the first to recognize that reticulum cell sarcoma may arise from the reticuloendothelial system of the bone and he identified it as a primary bone lymphoma. Accepting reticulum cell sarcoma as a distinct entity, Ewing (1939) added it to the Bone Sarcoma Registry of the American College of Surgeons. Parker and Jackson (1939) were the first to publish a complete study of 17 cases of reticulum cell sarcoma. However, Coley et al. (1950) published the first comprehensive report of 37 cases. They defined primary reticulum cell sarcoma of bone as a malignant tumor of bone that is histologically identical to reticulum cell sarcoma of other organs.

The majority of lymphomas presenting as primary lesions in the medullary cavities of single bones are NHL. Of these, the predominant phenotype is B-cell in origin (Boston et al. 1974; Pettit et al. 1990). The diagnosis of lymphomas may be made on a relatively small thin-needle biopsy, especially if the biopsy is CT or fluoroscopically directed and clinicopathologic correlation is made.

9.2
Histologic Presentation

Histologically, bone lymphoma is similar to lymph node disease. There is almost always a diffuse growth pattern with a mixture of large, atypical lymphocytes having grooved or polylobated nuclei (Fig. 9.1) and prominent nucleoli (FECHNER and MILLS 1993). The background small lymphocytes usually consist of reactive T-lymphocytes (PETTIT et al. 1990). Occasionally, there is an extensively fibroblastic background in which areas of the tumor appear hypocellular (Fig. 9.2). In these cases, the biopsy information may be confusing because the fibrous background can make the lymphoid cells appear spindled. In addition, biopsies of so dense a stroma in a confined osseous compartment may cause artifactual squeezing of the tumor cells, further confusing the diagnosis (Fig. 9.3).

The major tumor types to differentiate from malignant lymphoma histologically are Ewing sarcoma/primitive neuroectodermal tumor (PNET), metastatic neuroblastoma and small round cell tumors of soft tissue invading the bone. Of these, Ewing sarcoma/PNET causes the most histological confusion, not only because of its similarity to malignant lymphoma but because the age ranges of patients presenting with lymphoma and Ewing/PNET overlap significantly. In general, malignant lymphoma of bone shows more pleomorphism than Ewing sarcoma, which is more uniform and generally has smaller cells. In addition, lymphoma usually has considerable mitotic activity and its nuclei more often have prominent nucleoli than Ewing/PNET. Immunohistochemistry is normally used to ensure the differentiation of the tumor types. Lymphoma stains with leukocyte specific antigen while Ewing/PNET is negative since its cells do not arise from leukocyte precursors. Furthermore, B and T-lymphocyte-specific antigens can be applied to demonstrate tumor cell monoclonality, a certain and constant feature in malignant lymphomas. If there is any diagnostic confusion remaining, cytogenetic and molecular studies can demonstrate the reciprocal transformation or oncogene protein almost always found in Ewing/PNET.

Based on their experience, COLEY et al. (1950) set up three criteria for the diagnosis of primary reticulum cell sarcoma of bone: (a) A single bone is involved at first presentation; (b) Tumor is present in bone marrow; and (c) Primary tumor precedes metastasis by at least six months. If metastasis occurs, it must involve only the regional lymph nodes. Tumors with such criteria are usually associated with a relatively long survival, i.e., five-years in 50%, while in disseminated disease the survival rate is approximately 20% (EDEIKEN-MONROE et al. 1990).

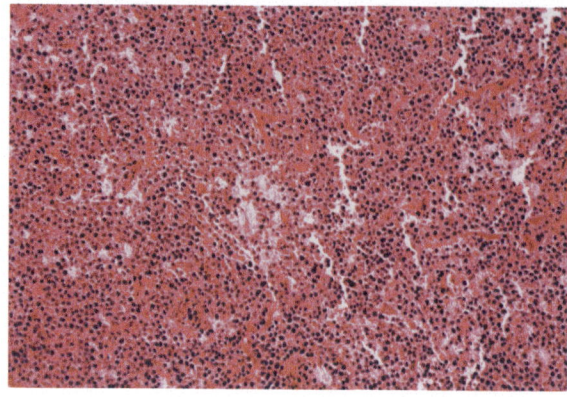

Fig. 9.1. Histopathological study with Hematoxylin eosin stain (original magnification, x250). This low magnification demonstrates replacement of bone marrow and fat by a uniform monomorphous lymphoid infiltrate.

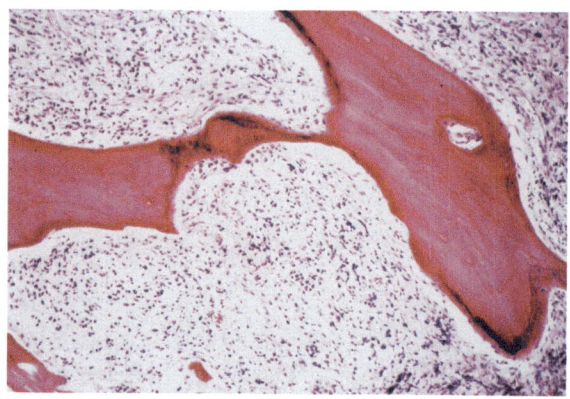

Fig. 9.2. Histopathological study with Hematoxylin eosin stain (original magnification, x100). Photomicrograph demonstrates replacement of the marrow by lymphoma in which the dominant feature is intercellular fibrosis and in which the lymphoid infiltrate appears paucicellular.

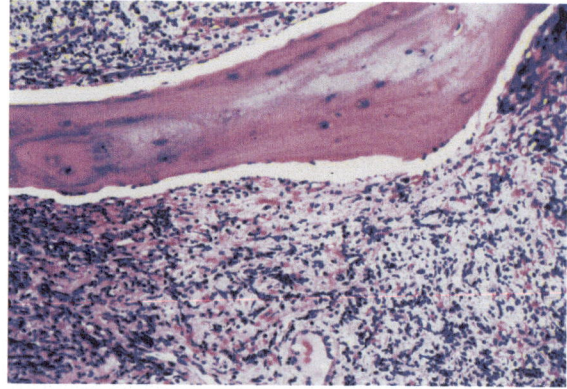

Fig. 9.3. Histopathological study with Hematoxylin eosin stain (original magnification, x250). This higher power magnification shows not only a paratrabecular infiltrate but also increased intercellular collagen.

IVINS and DAHLIN (1963) suggested a change in the name of reticulum cell sarcoma to malignant lymphoma. OSTROWSKI et al. (1986) revised the classification of COLEY et al. (1950) and described four groups of malignant lymphoma of bone. Group 1: primary solitary bone lymphoma. Group 2: primary multifocal bone lymphoma. In both groups neither distant nodal nor visceral involvement would be present at least 6 months following diagnosis. Group 3: patients develop distant nodal and/or visceral disease within 6 months. Group 4: patients have developed distant nodal and/or visceral disease at the time of the first diagnosis. The 5-year survival in group 1 was 58%, in group 2 was 42%, and in groups 3 and 4 was 22%.

Primary NHL of bone is one of the least common primary neoplasms, comprising lessthan 3% of primary bone tumors (WHITE et al. 1998; MULLIGAN et al. 1999) and approximately 5% of extranodal NHL (FREEMAN et al. 1972). In the majority of cases primary lymphoma of bone involves the appendicular skeleton. Over 50% of these tumors occur in the lower extremity, followed in frequency by the upper extremity and axial skeleton. There are very few detailed reports about primary lymphoma of bone in the literature. The old classification "reticulum cell sarcoma", described only the histology of the tumor.

9.3
Clinical Presentation

Skeletal involvement of systemic NHL is more common than primary bone lymphoma, and depends on the cellular maturity of the lesion. The more immature the lymphoma cells, the higher the incidence of skeletal involvement, which carries a poor prognosis. Also, when the lymphoma involves a single bone, the disease is considered Stage I, with a better prognosis. Regression of a solitary bone lesion has been reported (OHGI et al. 2002).

Primary NHL may occur in any age group. The age of patients at the onset of the disease is usually the fifth decade, with a male to female ratio of 1.8 to 1. BAAR et al. (1994) in their comprehensive study reviewed the clinicopathologic characteristics of 17 patients who were treated and followed-up between 1985–92. Using a combination of chemotherapy and/or radiotherapy the majority of patients remained alive and disease free at a median follow-up of 43 months.

Primary NHL can involve any bone. In most instances the primary site of involvement is the appendicular skeleton, predominantly the lower extremities, distal femur, proximal tibia. The humerus, pelvis, short tubular bones, irregular and flat bones, follow. Vertebral involvement is less common, occurring in about 4% of cases (PARKER and JACKSON 1939; MULLIGAN et al. 1999; CITOW et al. 2001).

Clinically, primary bone lymphoma may present with localized pain and swelling. The pain may be localized to the involved bone or referred to the neighboring joint. Mild to moderate pain may be responsible for the delay in diagnosis (PARKER and JACKSON 1939). The duration of symptoms in one series ranged from two months to four years. In the majority of cases symptoms have been present six months to one year before the patient seeks medical help. The patient's general condition is usually good. Weakness, weight loss and anemia are rare at presentation (SKARIN and DORFMAN 1997; PARKER and JACKSON 1939).

On physical examination the tumor may be palpable as a fusiform mass in about 2/3 of the patients. Occasionally, the mass may be ovoid or ill defined and its consistency varies.

9.4
Radiologic Presentation

The radiologic findings of bone lymphoma are widely discussed in the literature (SPAGNOLI et al. 1982; BEATTY et al. 1992; BRAUNSTEIN and WHITE 1980; VASSALLO et al. 1987; HAÜSSLER et al. 1999; COOK et al. 1996). The most common early feature is an osteolytic lesion with poorly defined margins (Fig. 9.4a). In most instances the lesion involves the metaphyseal, diaphyseal and occasionally the epiphyseal region of the long tubular bones. Sequester formation and pathologic fractures have been observed (RESNICK and HAGHIGHI 1996; WHITE et al. 1998; HICKS et al. 1995). The lesion shows a moth-eaten or permeative pattern and may be expansile (Figs. 9.4a, 9.5). While it is predominantly osteolytic, mixed sclerotic areas may be detected (Fig. 9.6a,b). The lytic nature of the lesion may be caused by the presence of an osteoclast-stimulating factor, a cytokine, which produces collagenase leading to bone resorption (GARRETT et al. 1987). In the normal person, cytokine is present and is considered as an osteoclast-activating factor. The cytokine activity depends on prostaglandin-E.

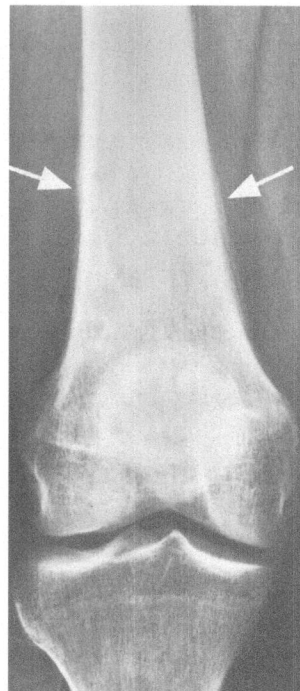

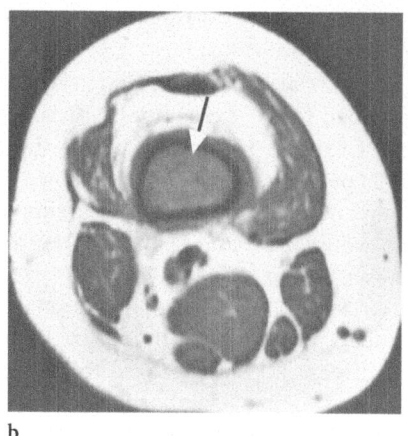

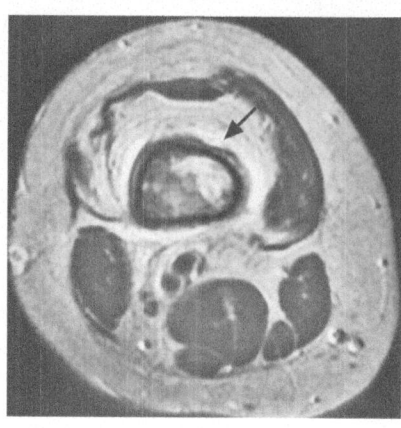

b   c

Fig. 9.4a–c. Primary non-Hodgkin lymphoma of the femur in a 53-year-old man. a Antero-posterior radiograph of the femur shows a permeative pattern involving the diametaphy-seal area. The cortex is thinned. Note the periosteal reaction (*arrows*). b Axial T1-weighted MR image reveals hypointensity replacing the fatty marrow and the periosseal tissue (*arrow*). c Axial T2-weighted MR image demonstrates a heterogeneous hyperintensity of the medullary cavity as well as the periosseal tissue (*arrow*).

a

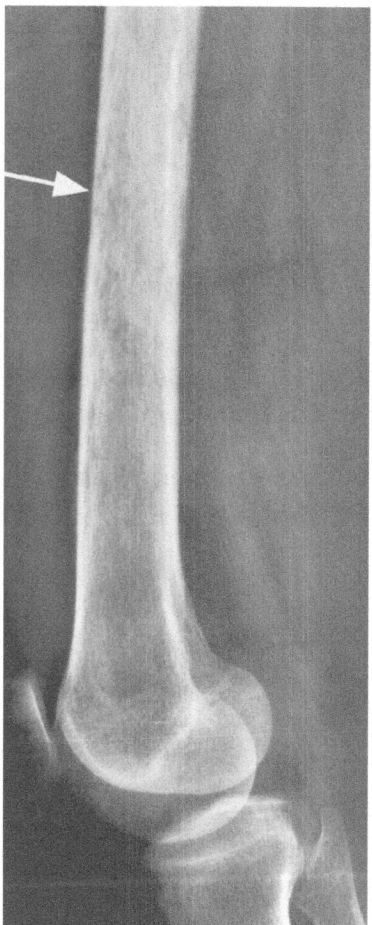

Fig. 9.5. Non-Hodgkin lymphoma of the femur in a 56-year-old woman. Lateral radiograph of the right femur shows moth eaten permeative pattern. The anterior cortex is thinned and eroded (*arrow*).

Therefore, prostaglandin inhibitors, like interferon, may limit or reduce the extent of the destructive process (MULLIGAN et al. 1999; GARRET et al. 1987).

As the lytic destructive process progresses, the cortex becomes thinned and is eventually destroyed (Fig. 9.7). Periosteal thickening may occur as a thin lamellated pattern (Fig. 9.7). The tumor may extend to the soft tissue, with the underlying cortex remaining relatively intact (HAÜSSLER et al. 1999; COOK et al. 1996). This may be explained by the fact that the tumor escapes from the medullary cavity through the minute vascular channels and is deposited in the surrounding soft tissue. This phenomenon may be demonstrated using new cross-sectional imaging modalities, such MR imaging (HICKS et al. 1995). Blastic forms of primary lymphoma of bone are extremely rare (Fig. 9.8a), less than 2% mentioned in the literature. MULLIGAN et al. (1999) recently reviewed over 200 pathologically proven cases and found

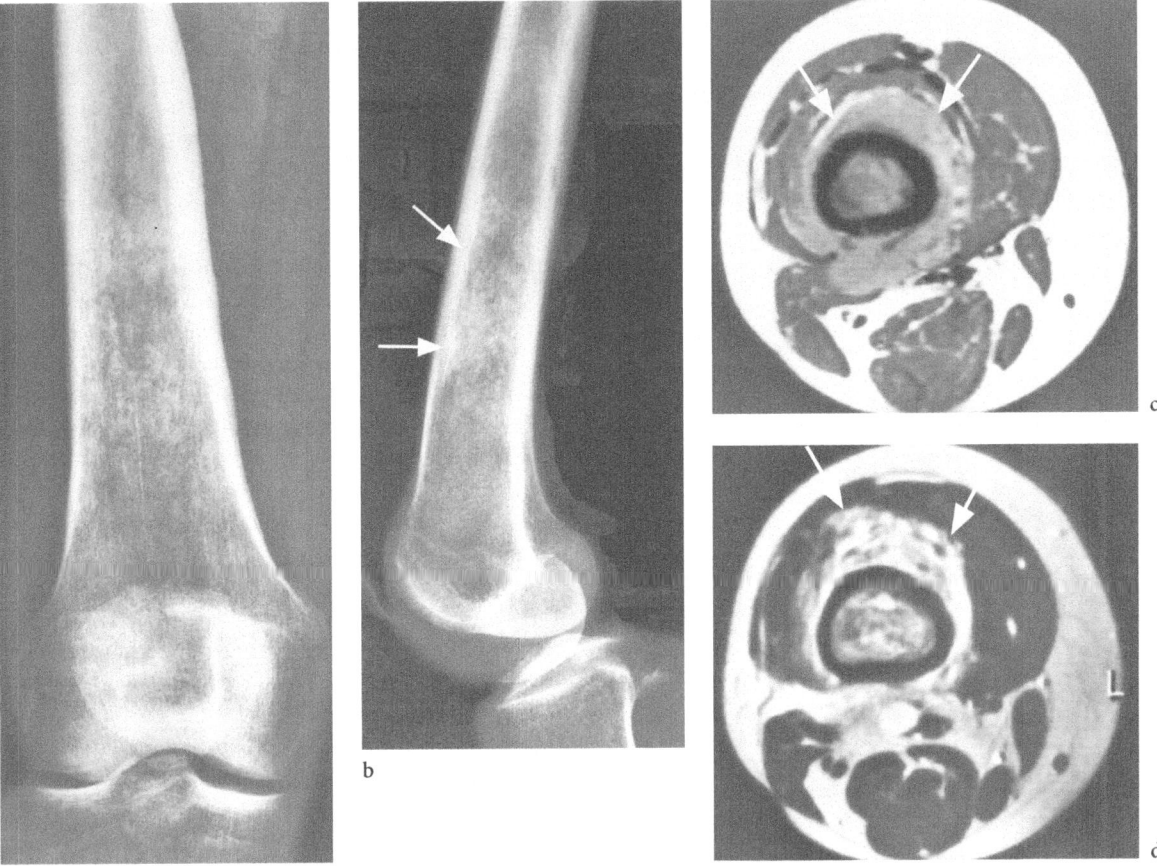

Fig. 9.6a–d. Non-Hodgkin lymphoma of the femur in a 46-year-old woman. **a** Anteroposterior and (**b**) lateral radiographs of the right femur show lytic lesion involving the middle third of the femoral shaft. Note the scattered sclerotic densities at the lower part of the shaft and linear endosteal sclerosis (*arrows*). There is slight periosteal reaction. **c** Axial T1-weighted MR image shows moderate hypointensity of the medullary cavity as well as the extraosseous soft tissue mass (*arrows*). **d** Axial T2-weighted MR image demonstrates a heterogeneous predominantly hypointense medullary cavity and the periosteal soft tissue mass (*arrows*).

only 2% in their series. On the other hand, primary soft tissue Hodgkin lymphomas often have blastic skeletal metastases (14%). A unique case of primary periosteal lymphoma has been published recently. The lesion arose from the periosteum and produced a moderate size soft tissue mass. The marrow remained uninvolved (CAMPBELL et al. 2003).

Many authors deny the existence of primary Hodgkin lymphoma of bone; a few cases have been documented in the literature (BOSTON et al. 1974; MIRRA 1980). LOVE et al. (1954) published 7 cases and CITOW et al. (2001) reported a case of isolated primary Hodgkin lymphoma in the spine. In this report, the fourth thoracic vertebra was replaced by an osteolytic lesion that extended to the epidural space as well as to the mediastinum.

Primary NHL may present as multifocal osseous lymphoma (Fig. 9.8). This is a multifocal primary tumor and not a hematogenous spread (VANEL et

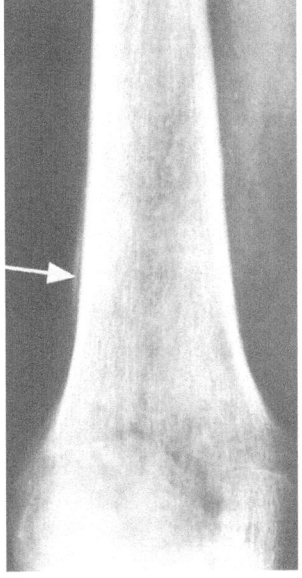

Fig. 9.7. Non-Hodgkin lymphoma of the femur in a 46-year-old woman. Anteroposterior radiograph of the femur shows lytic lesions of the femoral shaft. There is a minimal thinning of the cortex. Note the linear periosteal reaction (*arrow*).

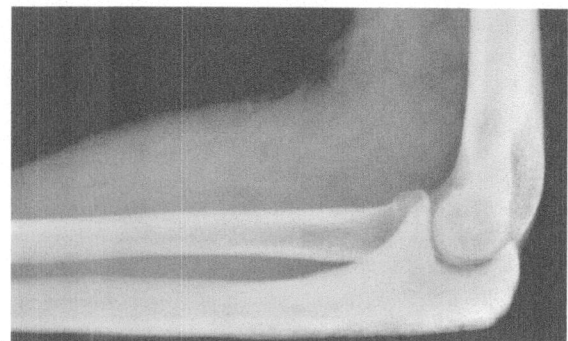

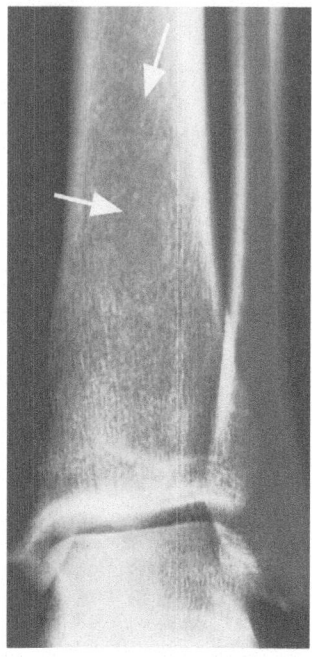

Fig. 9.8a,b. Multicentric non-Hodgkin lymphoma of the skeleton in a 16-year-old boy. **a** Lateral view of the forearm shows diffuse sclerotic changes involving the proximal radius. The cortex is uninvolved. **b** Anteroposterior radiograph of the distal leg shows a lytic lesion of the lower 1/3 of the tibia (*arrows*).

al. 1982; MELAMED et al. 1997). This interpretation is supported by the fact that patients in this group responded well to local therapy, promising a good prognosis (OSTROWSKI 1986). The clinical presentation of multifocal primary NHL is non-specific. Patients usually complain of vague pain but without constitutional symptoms. Plain radiographs therefore may underestimate bone lesions. Multiplicity of lesions may be overlooked unless scintigraphically evaluated. MELAMED et al. (1997) reported that only 25% of the lesions that were visualized on scintigraphy were detected by conventional radiograph in their cases. They did not describe any particular pattern in the uptake at the sites involved. LEESON et

al. (1989), on the other hand, described photopenia in the central portion of the lesion in their material. It is noteworthy that despite the fact that the first reported case of bone lymphoma represented primary multifocal bone disease, this entity gained little attention (WEILAND 1901). OSTROWSKI et al. (1986) reviewed the Mayo Clinic file and found 422 patients with malignant lymphoma of bone between 1907–82. In 179 patients lymphoma presented in one bone. In 82 patients lymphoma arose in multiple skeletal sites. Lymph nodes and inner organs were free of disease at the time of presentation and remained free at least 6 months following onset of the disease.

While conventional radiographs are the gold standard for detecting the primary bone lesions, newly applied cross-sectional imaging is extremely helpful in further evaluating the size and extent of the lesion. CT is essential to evaluate alteration in the bony cortex, and for detecting fine periosteal reaction (Fig. 9.9). MR imaging appears to be the most exact modality for detecting alterations in various marrow disorders. MR imaging can, in some instances, detect certain abnormalities in bone lesions that may direct our attention to a specific radiological diagnosis.

Normal bone marrow is constituted of fat, water and mineral, and each contributes to the signal intensities. Normal marrow has a different relaxation time than abnormal marrow. The portion of the mineral matrix of the marrow that represents the cortical trabecular bone produces essentially no signal since it lacks mobile protons. Fat is a major component of marrow that influences the signal from normal marrow resulting in a very short T1 relaxation time, compared to water. T2 relaxation time of fat, however, is relatively long.

Malignant processes such as lymphoma, leukemia, various metastases, and primary bone tumor infiltrate or replace the normal marrow with malignant tumor cells (Fig. 9.10) (VOGLER and MURPHY 1998). Some of these lesions (lymphoma, leukemia and myeloma) are considered primary marrow lesions originating in the red marrow. Others may be deposited in the bone marrow through hematogenous metastases. Tumorous lesions manifest as hypointense on T1 and are generally hyperintense on T2-weighted images. The signal intensity of the particular tissue on T2-weighted sequences, however, varies. It depends on cellularity, fluid content, fibrosis, necrosis, or inflammatory debris (VOGLER and MURPHY 1998). MR imaging is useful in defining accurately the extent of marrow infiltrate but it cannot characterize tissue histology. Consequently, it cannot, as a rule, differentiate benign from malignant lesions (HAÜSSLER et al. 1999; STIGLBAUER et al. 1992). Lesions, as noted above, which

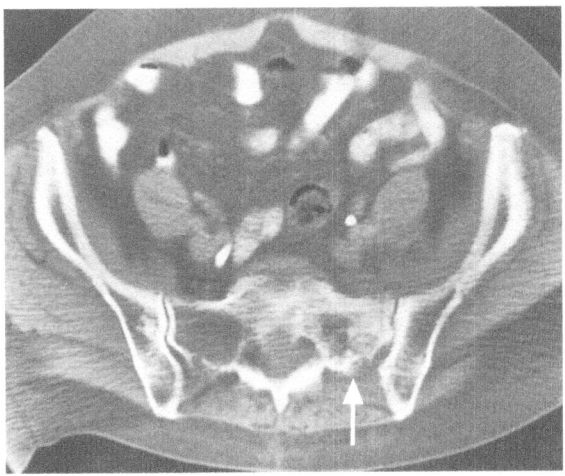

Fig. 9.9. Primary non-Hodgkin lymphoma of the sacrum in a 65-year-old woman. Axial CT scan of the pelvis shows a mixed lytic lesion alternating with sclerotic areas at the left side of the sacrum (*arrow*).

deposit in the medullary cavity, are hypointense on T1 and hyperintense on T2-weighted sequences (Figs. 9.10, 9.11). Recent studies, however, indicate that the marrow signal intensity of primary lymphoma of bone on T2-weighted images may show a variability that does not necessarily reflect the histologic findings such as avascularity and fibrosis (WHITE et al. 1998; STIGLBAUER et al. 1992; HERMANN et al. 1997; RAH-MOUNI et al. 1993).

VINCENT et al. (1992) observed primary bone lymphoma of the proximal tibia in a 35-year-old woman. MR imaging revealed hypointensity on T1, but also on T2-weighted images, which was predominantly low at the center of the lesion surrounded with hyperintensity. Open surgical biopsy revealed marked fibrosis. The peripheral hyperintense area that extended to the tibial plateau represented peritumoral edema. WHITE et al. (1998) reviewed 27 patients with primary NHL of bone. Nineteen were evaluated with MR imaging prior to surgery. On T1-weighted imaging, the signal intensity ranged from isointense to hypointense when compared with the surrounding muscle. T2-weighted imaging showed heterogeneity of signal intensity: hypointense, isointense and hyperintense compared with the subcutaneous fat. The majority of the lymphomas belonged to the isointense group. Only one of the T2-weighted images that showed hyperintensity had a significant amount of internal fibrosis. Histology showed moderate or only minimal fibrosis in the rest. It is questionable whether the degree of fibrosis and intralesional vascularity is responsible for the increased intensity on T2-weighted images (Fig. 9.4).

In a retrospective study, MULLIGAN et al. (1999) discussed the imaging features of 237 cases of primary lymphoma of bone. In the majority of cases the lesion involved the diametaphyseal site of the long bones of the femur, tibia, humerus, radius, ulna and fibula, in decreasing order. Of the 20 patients who underwent MR imaging, the authors discussed 15 in detail. The signal intensity on T1-weighted images appeared equal to the surrounding muscle (in 4 patients) or slightly hyperintense to the surrounding muscle (in 11 patients). On T2-weighted images, the signal intensity varied. Eight cases appeared isointense to subcutaneous fat, 1 hyperintense to fat, and 6 slightly less intense than fat.

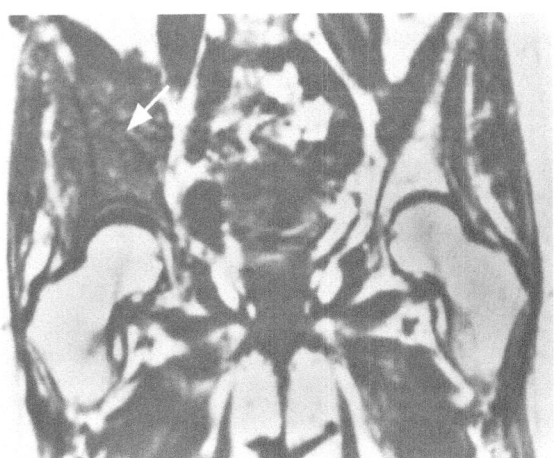
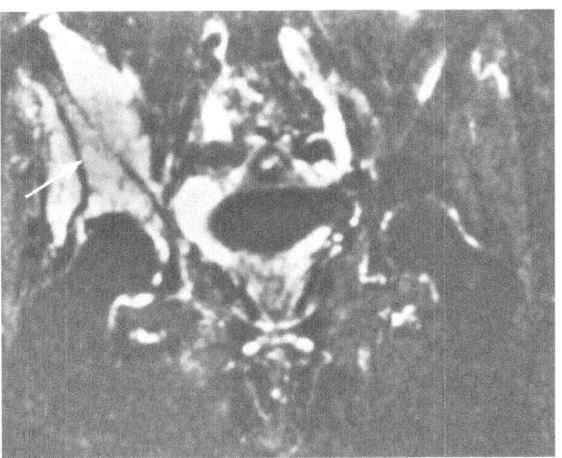

a   b

Fig. 9.10a,b. Primary non-Hodgkin lymphoma of the pelvis in an 82-year-old woman. **a** Coronal T1-weighted MR image of the pelvis shows homogenous hypointensity involving the right ileum (*arrow*) and surrounding muscles. The area becomes hyperintense on (**b**) coronal fat-supressed T2-weighted MR image (*arrows*). The inner cortex of the ileum is thinned. Note the large soft tissue mass around the ileum. (*Image courtesy of Dr. F. Feldman*)

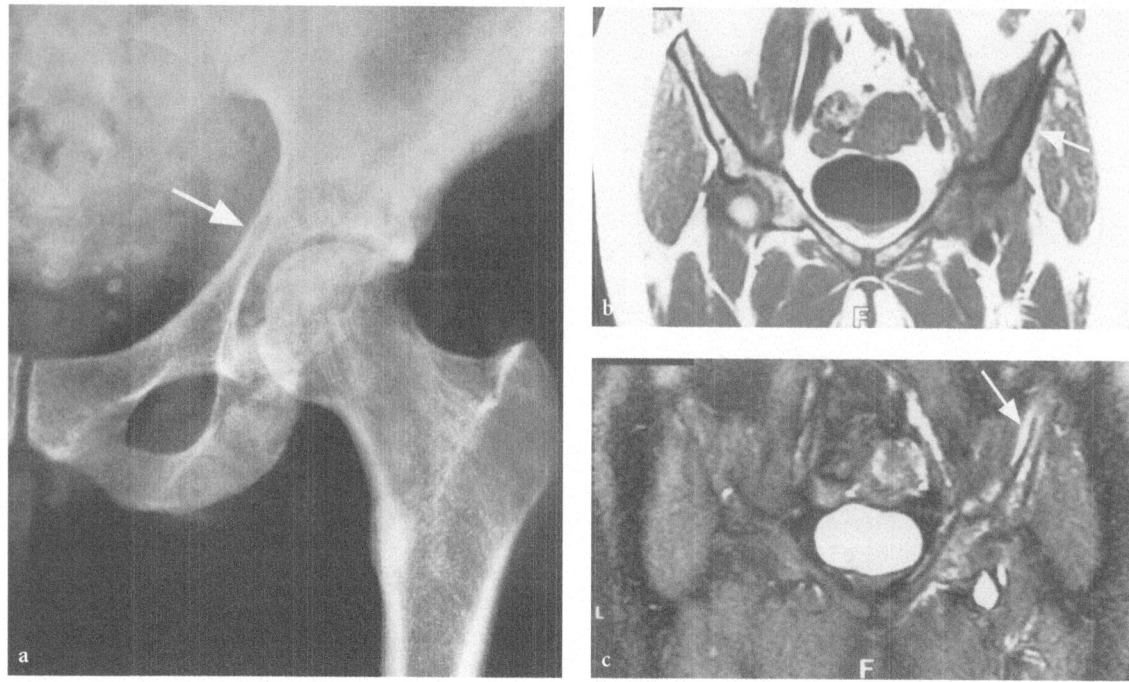

Fig. 9.11a–c. Non-Hodgkin lymphoma of the pelvis in a 45-year-old woman. **a** Anteroposterior radiograph of the left ileum demonstrates a mottled destruction of the left supra-acetabular area. Note the periosteal reaction along the inner aspect of the acetabulum (*arrow*). **b** Coronal T1-weighted MR image of the pelvis shows hypointensity of the left ileum (*arrow*). There is an involvement of the iliac muscle. **c** Coronal STIR MR image reveals a heterogeneous hyperintensity of the ileum. Note the hyperintensity along the inner aspect of the ileum (*arrow*).

STIGLBAUER et al. (1992) reported 7 patients with NHL of bone. They found that 6 of their 7 patients presented predominantly hypointensity relative to the surrounding fat on T2-weighted images. Histology revealed high content of fibrosis in all 6 cases. HERMANN et al. (1997) reviewing their own material, found hypointensity on T2-weighted images in 9 of their 10 cases. The histopathologic specimen showed high content of fibrosis suggesting an explanation for the characteristic signal pattern on MR images (Figs. 9.12, 9.13) (STIGLBAUER et al. 1992; HERMANN et al. 1997; VINCENT et al. 1992; NEGENDANK et al. 1990). The histologic sections of NHL are relatively homogeneous, uniformly cellular. On the other hand, in HD it is heterogeneous with large inflammatory cells.

9.5
Lymphoma of Skeletal Muscle

Lymphomatous involvement of the skeletal muscle is rare. It can occur in three forms: (a) Primary extranodal involvement; (b) Secondary involvement in disseminated form of the disease; and (c) Direct extension as a contiguous spread from regional bone or lymph node. In a large series, muscle involvement was observed in approximately 1.4% of patients. Primary involvement is extremely rare occurring in less than 0.2% in patients with lymphoma (HATEM et al. 1997; HOSONO et al. 1995). Muscle infiltration by lymphoma may manifest as a discrete mass, but more often as diffuse muscle enlargement. The most common site is the thigh, followed by the calf, psoas, deltoid, and paraspinal muscle (JEFFREY et al. 1991).

PILEPICH and CARTER (1997) reviewed CT scans of 5 patients with NHL. The CT density of the involved muscle was comparable to the normal muscle. Following contrast administration, lymphomatous muscle may appear hypodense or isodense to normal muscle (PANICEK et al. 1997). On the other hand, GRUNSHAW and CHALMERS (1992) observed significant enhancement of the lymphomatous muscle following contrast administration. Preservation of the inter-muscular fat planes has been described.

The appearance of soft tissue lymphoma on MR imaging is rarely discussed in the radiologic literature. METZLER et al. (1992) reported two patients, one with HD involving the psoas muscle as part of a disseminated disease, the second with NHL that involved the calf. The appearance of soft tissue neo-

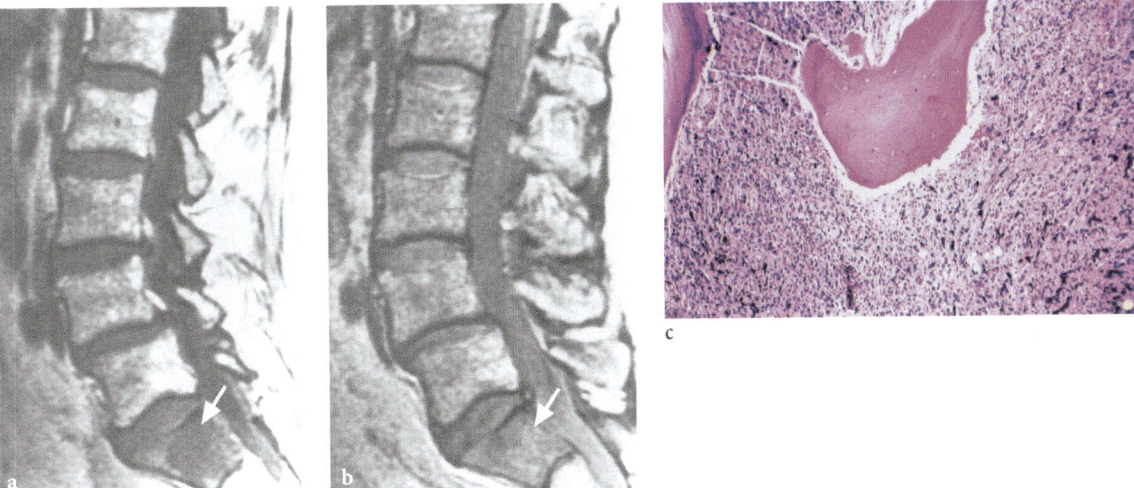

Fig. 9.12a–c. Non-Hodgkin lymphoma of the sacrum in a 65-year-old woman. **a** Sagittal T1-weighted MR image of the lumbosacral spine shows hypointensity of the upper segment of the sacrum (*arrow*). **b** Sagittal T2-weighted MR image shows the marrow remains hypointense (*arrow*). **c** Histological study shows a predominance of fibrous tissue. In addition, the lymphocytes are compressed and squeezed at the periphery of the photograph. The combination of fibrosis and squeeze artifact makes the lymphocytes appear spindled (original magnification, x100). (Reprinted with permission from [HERMANN et al. 1997])

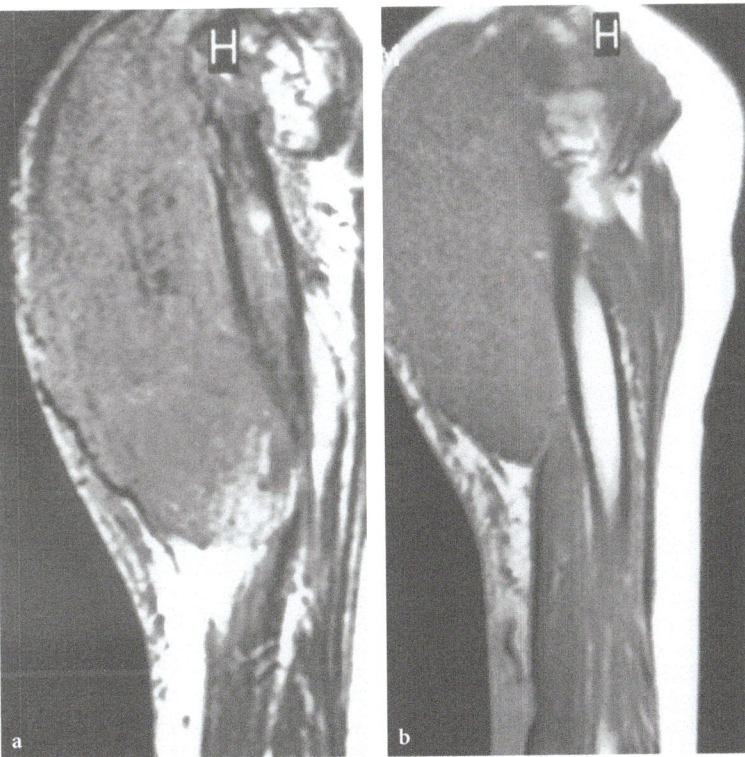

Fig. 9.13a,b. Non-Hodgkin lymphoma of the shoulder in a 35-year-old woman. **a** Sagittal T1-weighted MR image demonstrates a hypointense mass at the right shoulder region. **b** On sagittal T2-weighted MR image, the mass remains homogenously hypointense. (Reprinted with permission from [HERMANN et al. 1997])

plasms on MR imaging is typical but not specific. The majority of soft tissue lesions have a long T2 relaxation time that is hyperintense to fat on T2-weighted images and hypointense on T1-weighted images. Certain tumors such as fibromatosis, malignant fibrous histiocytoma, as well as scar tissue, mineralized masses, or tumors containing hemosiderin may show short T2 relaxation time. They are overall hypointense relative to fat on T2-weighted images (Lee and Glazer 1990). Metzler et al. (1992) observed decreased signal intensity on T2-weighted images in patients with NHL. The signal intensity on T1-weighted images appeared hypointense to fat and relatively hypointense on T2-weighted images. The lesion extends along the muscle fascicles while preserving the fat planes. The authors concluded that when a mass inside or around a muscle is hypointense or isointense to fat on T2-weighted images, lympho-proliferative disease should be included in the differential diagnosis (Fig. 9.14).

9.6
Skeletal Manifestation of Lymphoproliferative Disorders Following Organ Transplant

Lymphoproliferative disorder is a common complication of bone marrow and organ transplant and can be fatal if not recognized and treated properly (Hermann et al. 1999). The incidences range between 2–5% among patients receiving organ transplants. It is less common among kidney recipients and more common among liver, lung and heart recipients. Lymphoproliferative disorders may be manifested in various clinical forms. B-lymphocytes are found in organ transplant recipients receiving immunosuppressive therapy (Malatack et al. 1991; Newell et al. 1996; Penn et al. 1969). The EBV may stimulate B-lymphocyte proliferation. This virus that remains subclinical may infect large groups of patients in the pediatric population. When a patient is immunocompromised with EBV, the infection may be severe, even life threatening (Starzl et al. 1984; Morgan and Superina 1994; Ho et al. 1988; Breinig et al. 1987; Mulvihill et al. 1994).

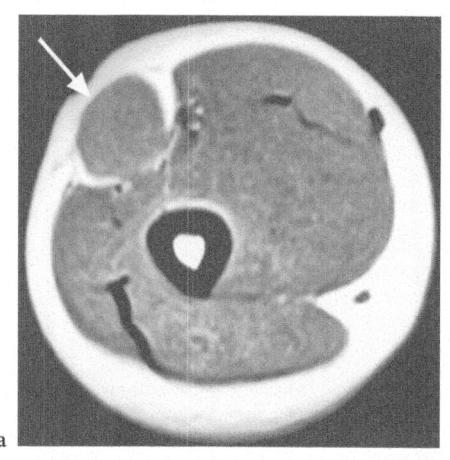

a

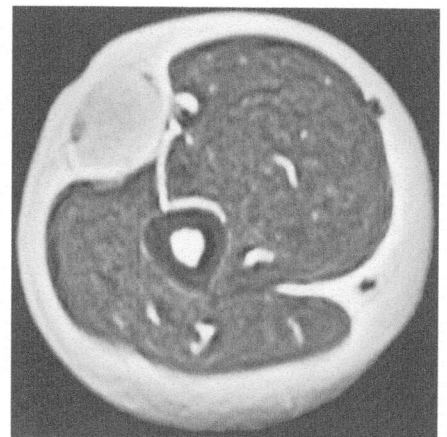

b

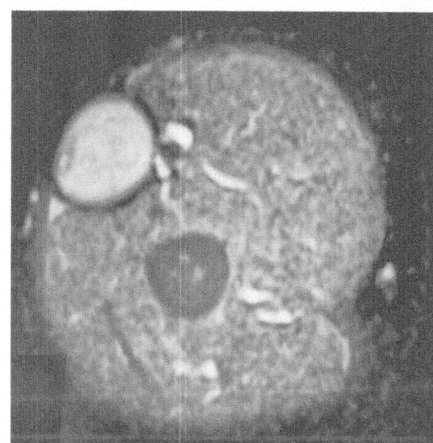

c

Fig. 9.14a–c. Non-Hodgkin lymphoma of the upper arm in a 39-year-old man. a Axial T1-weighted MR image demonstrates a discrete mass at the lateral aspect of the distal part of the upper arm. The mass is isointense to the muscles (*arrow*). b On axial T2-weighted MR image, the mass appears heterogeneously hyperintense. c On axial STIR MR image, the mass shows heterogeneous hyperintensity.

MATALACK et al. (1991) observed three different forms that may manifest in three clinical syndromes:

- Lymphadenopathy: patients may present with systemic lymphadenopathy with lymphatic tissue hyperplasia such as enlargement of the tonsils or axillary nodes. MATALACK et al. (1991) successfully treated his patients by removing the lymphoproliferative tissue and reducing the immunosuppressive cyclosporin. The patients remained symptom free up to 5 years following excision of the lymph nodes. None of these patients experienced organ rejection following reduction of the dose of immunosuppressive agents (STARZL et al. 1984).
- Systemic presentation: patients in this group presented with fever, vomiting, respiratory failure and progressive encephelopathy. Single or multiple organs may be involved. Immunosuppression in this group was completely withdrawn and reinstated only when graft rejection became severe. The patients remained free of symptoms 4 years following the onset of the disease.
- The third form consisted of patients who present with clinical signs and symptoms of lymphoma which is pathologically indistinguishable from NHL. This form of post-transplant lymphoproliferative disorder (PTLD) most often involves the gastrointestinal tract but any organ can be involved, including bone marrow (KAUSHIK et al. 2001). A recent report discussed a 67-year-old patient in whom the post transplant lymphoproliferative disorder manifested in a single bone only (Fig. 9.15) (HERMANN et al. 1999). The patient presented with thigh pain one year following orthotopic liver transplantation, while on immunosuppressive medication. Conventional radiographs showed destruction of the femur. MR imaging revealed hypointensity on T1-weighted images that remained relatively decreased on T2-weighted images. The results of an open biopsy were compatible with B-cell lymphoma. Histopathology revealed atypical lymphoid cells infiltrating the bone marrow and extending into the surrounding soft tissue. Treatment consisted of prophylactic fixation of the femur followed by radiation therapy. The medication tacrolimus (Prograf) was decreased and low-dose immunosuppressive therapy was continued.

9.7
Imaging of NHL by PET

During the past decade PET has become a useful imaging tool in evaluating tumor involvement in various organ systems (DALDRUP-LINK et al. 2001). FDG PET is useful for detecting nodal, extranodal and bone marrow infiltration by HD and NHL. The accumulation of FDG in tumor tissues depends on their metabolic rate of glucose use. The highest metabolizing tissues demonstrate the greatest accumulation. It is important to mention that low-grade lymphoma may be characterized by a low or undetectable level of accumulation of FDG as a result of reduced metabolic rate (Figs. 9.16, 9.17) (FELDMAN et al. 2003).

MOOG et al. (1998) compared PET scans with CT in evaluating extranodal malignant lymphoma. They concluded that PET scanning was at times able to detect diffuse bone marrow infiltration in a clinically occult stage. PET scanning could also direct bone marrow biopsy reducing the chance of sampling errors.

9.8
Conclusion

Musculoskeletal involvement by systemic NHL is more common than primary bone lymphoma. The more immature the lymphoma cells, the higher the incidence of skeletal involvement which carries a poor prognosis. Primary NHL of bone, on the other hand, is one of the most uncommon primary bone malignancies, accounting for less than 5% of all primary malignant bone tumors and approximately 1% of lymphomas cases. Primary NHL of soft tissue is even less common, with only scanty reports discussed in the literature. While conventional radiographic imaging is considered the gold standard in diagnosing primary NHL of bone, MR imaging is an excellent method of evaluation of the presence and extent of marrow infiltration. Recent observations indicate that primary NHL in bone marrow shows predominantly hypointensity on both T1 and T2-weighted images. The decreased signal intensity on T2-weighted images may be related to the prominent fibrosis that correlated well with the histopathologic features in our material. In recent years, PET scanning has become a promising method for detecting marrow infiltration by NHL as well as in following disease progression and regression during therapy.

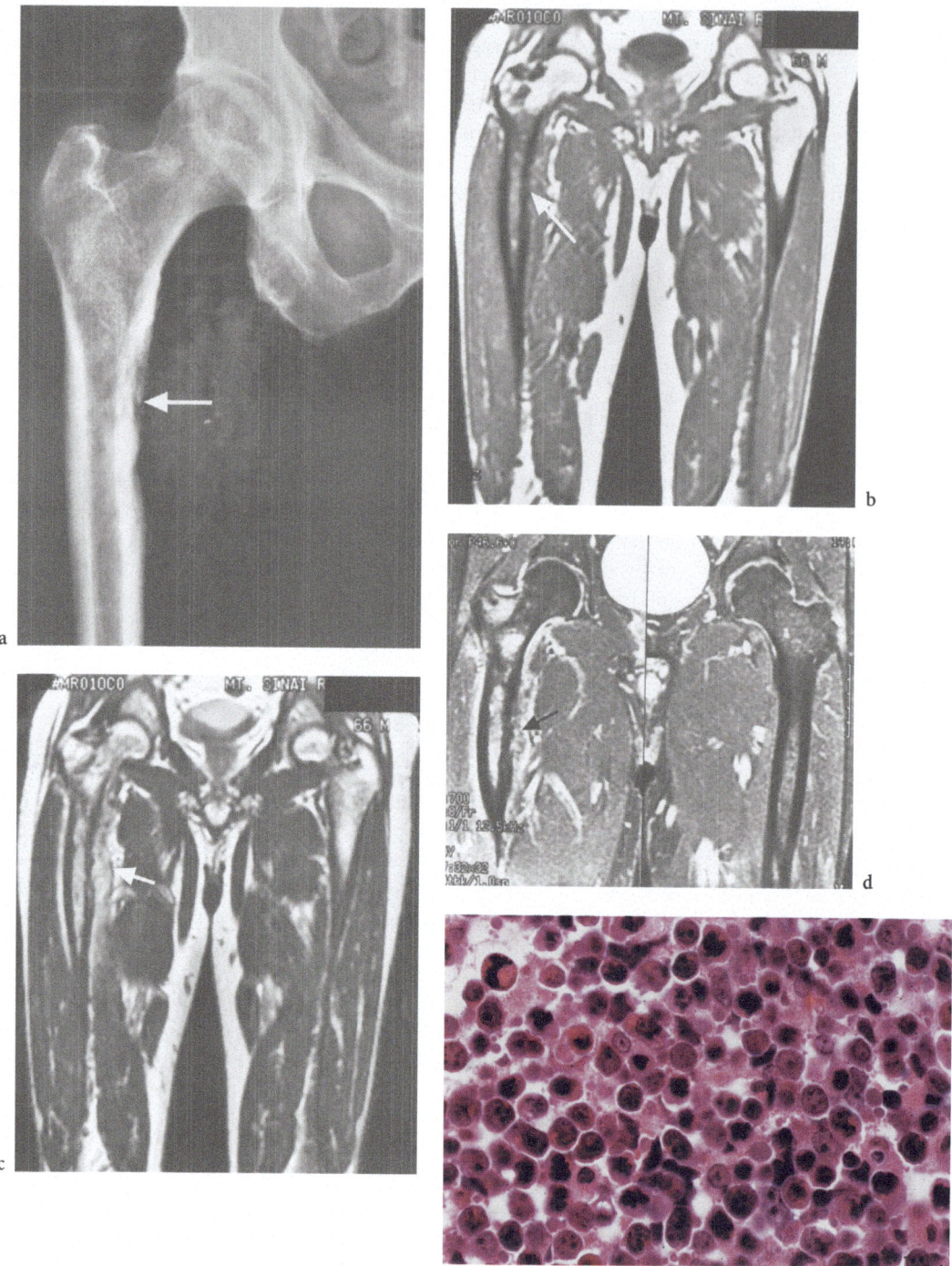

Fig. 9.15a–e. Primary non-Hodgkin lymphoma of the femur in a 66-year-old man after liver transplantation. **a** Anteroposterior radiograph of the right femur shows a lytic lesion of the upper 1/3 of the shaft. The inner cortex is destroyed (*arrow*). **b** Coronal T1-weighted MR images of both femurs reveals heterogeneous hypointensity of the medullary cavity of the right femur. Note the soft tissue mass adjacent to the medial aspect of the destroyed cortex (*arrow*). **c** Coronal T2-weighted MR image shows inhomogeneous marrow signal that is less intense than the subcutaneous fat. Scattered hyperintense foci are present. The soft tissue mass remains heterogeneously low in signal intensity (*arrow*). **d** Coronal contrast-enhanced T1-weighted MR image shows the abnormal marrow becomes heterogeneously hyperintense. The soft tissue also enhances (*arrow*). **e** Histological study shows detail of B-cell malignant lymphoma. Nuclear pleomorphism, prominent nucleoli, mitotic activity and even atypical mitotic activity (upper left and center) are easily discernible (Oil-immersion, original magnification, x787). (Reprinted with permission from [HERMANN et al. 1999])

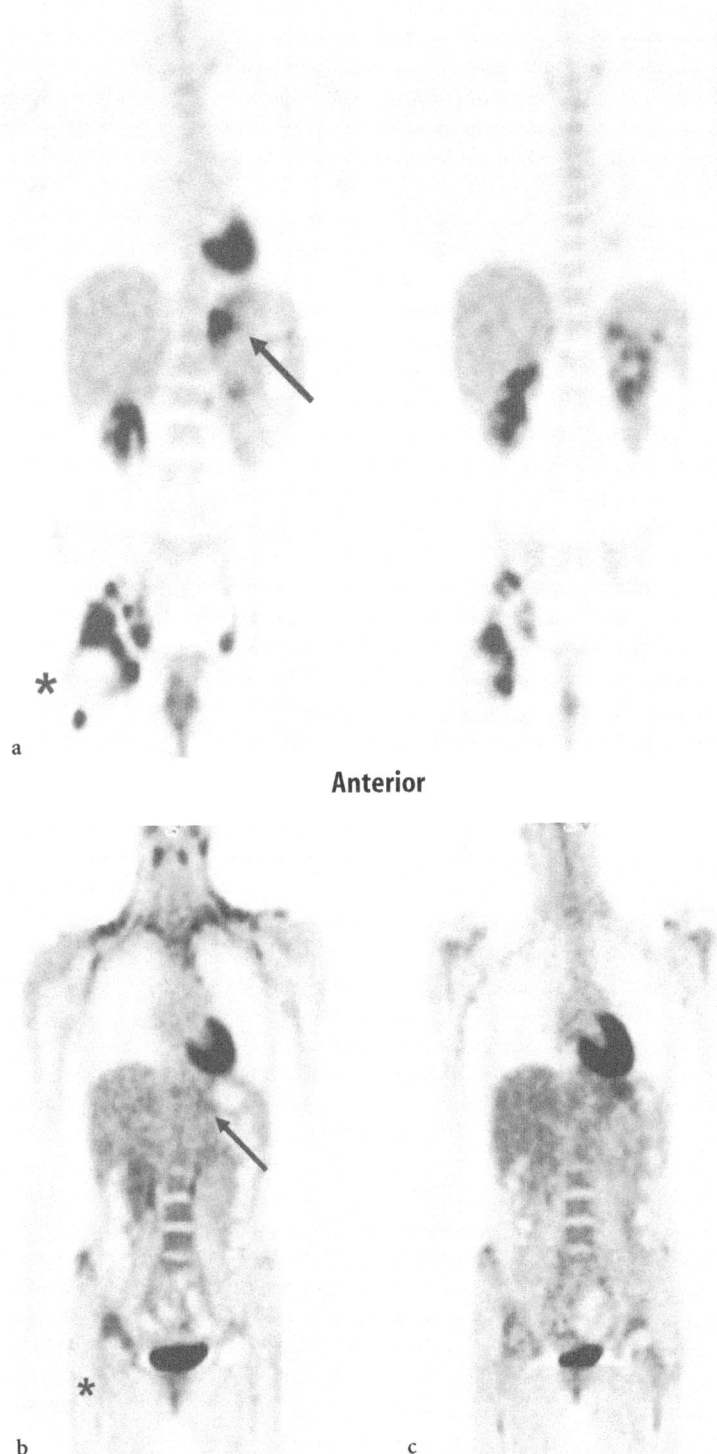

Fig. 9.16a–c. Non-Hodgkin lymphoma in a 52-year-old woman. **a** Pretreatment coronal FDG-PET scans reveal multiple uptakes in right hip/pelvis (*asterisk*) and left upper abdomen (*arrow*). **b** Immediate post therapy FDG-PET scan shows the resolution of the abdominal disease (*arrow*) but continued low level activity at the right side of the pelvis (*asterisk*). This could represent residual disease versus uptake in healing bone. **c** Follow-up FDG-PET scan shows generalized bone marrow stimulation from chemotherapy treatment effects and essentially complete resolution of the pelvic involvement. Often the apparent response of bone marrow and adjacent bone involved with disease appears to lag the response seen in soft tissues. This probably represents continued uptake due to repair of bone and marrow, and not necessarily disease. (*Image courtesy of Dr. B. Krynyckyi*)

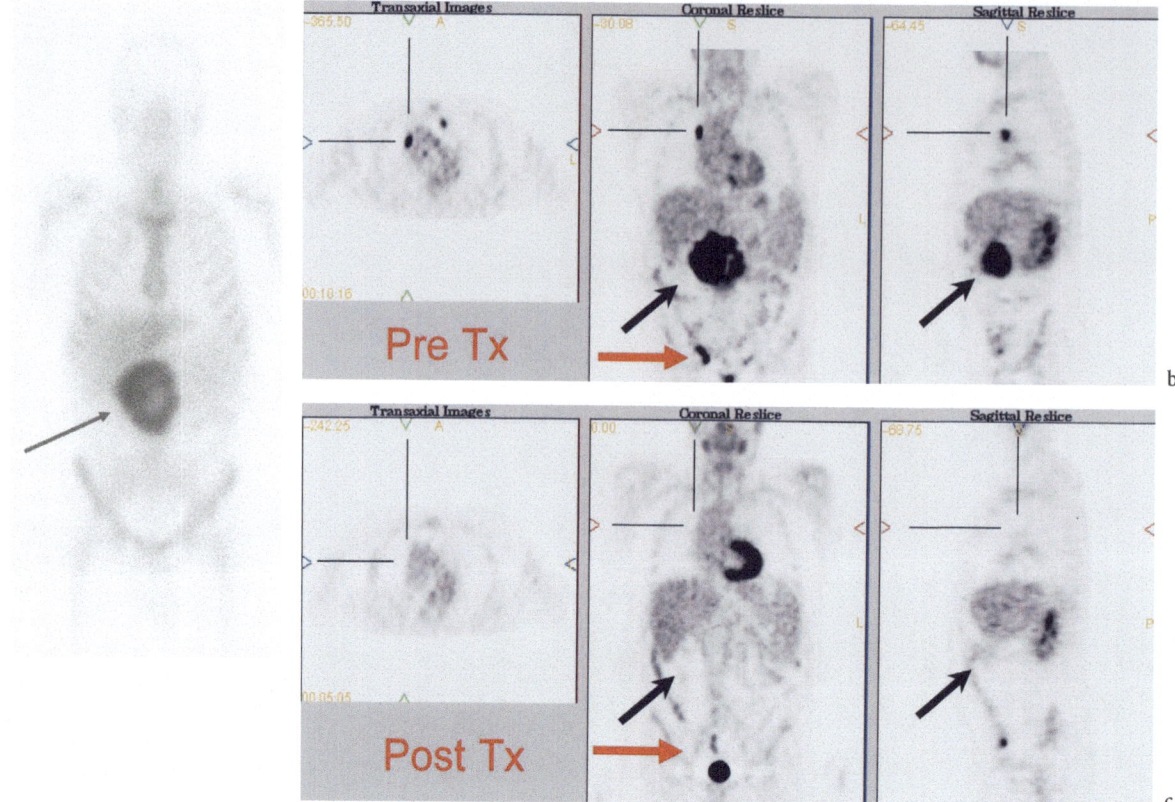

Fig. 9.17a–c. Non-Hodgkin lymphoma in a 57-year-old woman. **a** Initial Ga-67 scan shows only an abdominal lesion (*arrow*). **b** FDG-PET study performed at the same period than (**a**) shows same abdominal lesion (*black arrow*) and additional chest (*cross hairs*) and inguinal disease (*red arrow*) missed on the Ga-67 scan. **c** Follow-up FDG-PET study shows resolution of disease after treatment. (*Image courtesy of Dr. B. Krynyckyi*)

References

Baar J, Burkes RL, Bell R, Blackstein ME, Fernandes B, Langer F (1994) Primary non-Hodgkin's lymphoma of bone. Cancer 73:1194–1199

Beatty PT, Björkengren AG, Moore SG, Gelb AB, Gamble JG (1992) Case report 764. Primary lymphoma of bone, large cell, B-phenotype with articular involvement. Skeletal Radiol 21:559–561

Boston HC Jr, Dahlin DC, Ivins JC, Cupps RE (1974) Malignant lymphoma (so-called reticulum cell sarcoma) of bone. Cancer 34:1131–1137

Braunstein E, White S (1980) Non-Hodgkin lymphoma of bone. Radiology 135:59–63

Breinig MK, Zitelli B, Starzl T, Ho M (1987) Epstein-Barr virus cytomegalovirus and other viral infections in children after liver transplantation. J Infect Dis 156:273–279

Campbell SE, Filzen TW, Bezzant SM. Beall, DP, Burton MP, Sanders TG, Parsons TW (2003) Primary periosteal lymphoma: an unusual presentation of non-Hodgkin's lymphoma with radiographic, MR imaging, and pathologic correlation. Skeletal Radiol 32:231–235

Citow JS, Rini B, Wollmann R, Macdonald RL (2001) Isolated, primary extranodal Hodgkin's disease of the spine: case report. Neurosurgery 49:453–457

Cook, MA, Manfredi OL, Kasaw S, Murukutla S (1996) Primary skeletal lymphoma imaging and pathologic correlation. J Am Osteopath Assoc 10:610–612

Coley BL, Higinbotham NL, Groesbeck HP (1950) Primary reticulum-cell sarcoma of bone–summary of 37 cases. Radiology 55:641–658

Daldrup-Link HE, Franzius C, Link TM, Laukamp D, Sciuk J, Jürgens H, Schober O, Rummeny EJ (2001) Whole-body MR imaging for detection of bone metastases in children and young adults: Comparison with skeletal scintigraphy and FDG PET. AJR Am J Roentgenol 177:229–236

Edeiken-Monroe B, Edeiken J, Kim EE (1990) Radiologic concepts of lymphoma of bone. Radiol Clin North Am 28:841–864

Ewing J (1939) A review of the classification of bone tumors. Surg Gynec Obstet 68:971–976

Fechner RE, Mills SE (1993) Atlas of tumor pathology, 3rd edn, Armed Forces Institute of Pathology, Washington

Feldman F, van Heertum R, Manos C (2003) 18FDG PET scanning of benign and malignant musculoskeletal lesions. Skeletal Radiol 32:201–208

Freeman C, Berg JW, Cutler SJ (1972) Occurrence and prognosis of extranodal lymphomas. Cancer 29:252–260

Garrett IR, Durie BGM, Nedwin GE, Gillespie A, Bringman T, Sabatini M, Bertolini DR, Mundy GR (1987) Production of lymphotoxin, a bone-resorbing cytokine, by cultured human myeloma cells. N Engl J Med 317:526–532

Grunshaw ND, Chalmers AG (1992) Skeletal muscle lymphoma. Clin Radiol 43:399–400

Hatem SF, Petersilge CA, Park JK (1997) Musculoskeletal case of the day. Case 2. AJR Am J Roentgenol 169:288–289

Häussler MD, Fenstermacher MJ, Johnston DA, Harle TS (1999) MRI of primary lymphoma of bone: cortical disorder as a criterion for differential diagnosis. J Magn Res Img 9:93–100

Hermann G, Klein MJ, Abdelwahab IF, Kenan S (1997) MRI appearance of primary non-Hodgkin's lymphoma of bone. Skeletal Radiol 26:629–632

Hermann G, Abdelwahab IF, Capozzi J, Springfield D, Klein MJ (1999) Primary non-Hodgkin lymphoma of bone: unusual manifestation of lymphoproliferative disease following liver transplantation. Skeletal Radiol 28:175–177

Hicks DG, Gokan T, O'Keefe RJ, Totterman SMS, Fultz PJ, Judkins AR, Meyers SP, Rubens DJ, Sickel JZ, Rosier RN (1995) Primary lymphoma of bone–correlation of magnetic resonance imaging features with cytokine production by tumor cells. Cancer 75:973–980

Ho M, Jaffe R, Miller G, Breinig MK, Dummer JS, Makowka L, Atchison RW, Karrer FK, Nalesnik MA (1988) The frequency of Epstein-Barr virus infection and associated lymphoproliferative syndrome after transplantation and its manifestations in children. Transplantation 45:719–727

Hosono M, Kobayashi H, Kotoura Y, Tsuboyama T, Tsutsui K, Konishi J (1995) Involvement of muscle by malignant lymphoma. J Comput Assist Tomgr 19:455–459

Ivins JC, Dahlin DC (1963) Malignant lymphoma (reticulum cell sarcoma) of bone. Mayo Clin Proc 38:375–385

Jeffrey GM, Golding PF, Mead GM (1991) Non-Hodgkin's lymphoma arising in skeletal Muscle. Ann Oncol 1:501–504

Kaushik S, Fulcher AS, Frable WJ, May DA (2001) Posttransplantation lymphoproliferative disorder: osseous and hepatic involvement–Case Report. AJR Am J Roentgenol 177:1057–1059

Lee JKT, Glazer HS (1990) Controversy in the MR imaging appearance of fibrosis. Radiology 177:21–22

Leeson MC, Makely JT, Carter JR, Krupco T (1989) The use of radioisotope scans in the evaluation of primary lymphomas of bone. Orthop Rev 18:410–416

Love JG, Miller RH, Kernohan JW (1954) Lymphomas of spinal epidural space. Arch Surg 69:66–76

Malatack JF, Gartner JC Jr, Urbach AH, Zitelli BJ (1991) Orthotopic liver transplantation, Epstein-Barr virus, cyclosporine and lymphoproliferative disease: A growing concern. J Pediatr 118:667–675

Melamed JW, Martinez S, Hoffman CJ (1997) Imaging of primary multifocal osseous lymphoma. Skeletal Radiol 26:35–41

Metzler JP, Fleckenstein JL, Vuitch F, Frenkel EP (1992) Skeletal muscle lymphoma: MRI evaluation–Case Report. Magn Res Img 10:491–494

Mirra JM (1980) Lymphoma and lymphoma-like disorders. In: Mirra JM (ed) Bone tumors. Lea & Febiger Philadelphia, pp 1119–1185

Moog F, Bangerter M, Diederichs CG, Guhlmann A, Merkle E, Frickhofen N, Reske SN (1998) Extranodal malignant lymphoma: detection with FDG PET versus CT. Radiology 206:475–481

Morgan G, Superina RA (1994) Lymphoproliferative disease after pediatric liver transplantation. Pediatr Surg 29:1192–1196

Mulligan ME, Kransdorf MJ (1993) Sequestra in primary lymphoma of bone: prevalence and radiologic features. AJR Am J Roentgenol 160:1245–1248

Mulligan ME, McRae GA, Murphey MD (1999) Imaging features of primary lymphoma of bone. AJR Am J Roentgenol 173:1691–1697

Mulvihill DM, Munden MM, Edell D (1994) Lymphoproliferative disorder involving the liver following transplantation: CT appearance. J Comput Assist Tomogr 18:47–48

National Cancer Institute (1982) National Cancer Institute sponsored study of classifications of non-Hodgkin's lymphomas: summary and description of a working formulation for clinical usage. The non-Hodgkin's lymphoma pathologic classification project. Cancer 49:2112–2135

Negendank WG, Al-Katib AM, Karanes C, Smith MR (1990) Lymphomas: MR imaging contrast characteristics with clinical-pathologic correlations. Radiology 177:209–216

Newell KA, Alonso EM, Whitington PF, Bruce DS, Millis JM, Piper JB, Woodle ES, Kelly SM, Koeppen H, Hart J, Rubin CM, Thistlethwaite JR Jr (1996) Posttransplant lymphoproliferative disease in pediatric liver transplantation. Interplay between primary Epstein-Barr virus infection and immunosuppression. Transplantation 62:370–375

Oberling C (1928) Les réticulosarcomes et les réticuloendothéliosarcomes de la moelle osseuse (sarcomas d'Ewing). Bull Assoc Fr Etude Cancer (Paris) 17:259–296

Ohgi S, Ehara S, Satoh T, Kato S, Shimosegawa K, Ishida Y (2002) Spontaneous regression of malignant lymphoma of the lumbar spine. Skeletal Radiol 31:99–102

Ostrowski ML, Unni KK, Banks PM, Shives TC, Evans RG, O'Connell MJ, Taylor WF (1986) Malignant lymphoma of bone. Cancer 58:2646–2655

Panicek DM, Lautin JL, Schwartz LH, Castellino RA (1997) Non-Hodgkin lymphoma in skeletal muscle manifesting as homogeneous masses with CT attenuation similar to muscle. Skeletal Radiol 26:633–635

Parker F Jr, Jackson H Jr (1939) Primary reticulum cell sarcoma of bone. Surg Gynecol Obstet 68:45–53

Penn I, Hammond W, Brettschneider L, Starzl TE (1969) Malignant lymphomas in transplantation patients. Transplant Proc 1:106–112

Pettit CK, Zukerberg LR, Gray MH, Ferry JA, Rosenberg AE, Harmon DC, Harris NL (1990) Primary lymphoma of bone. A B-cell neoplasm with a high frequency of multilobated cells. Am J Surg Pathol 14:329–334

Pilepich MV, Carter BL (1980) Muscle enlargement in lymphoma patients. Radiology 134:521–523

Rahmouni A, Tempany C, Jones R, Mann R, Yang A, Zerhouni E (1993) Lymphoma: monitoring tumor size and signal intensity with MR imaging. Radiology 188:445–451

Resnick D, Haghighi P (1996) Myeloproliferative disorders. In: Resnick D (ed) Bone and joint imaging. W.B. Saunders, Philadelphia 1995; pp 625–638

Skarin AT, Dorfman DM (1997) Non-Hodgkin's lymphomas: current classification and management. CA Cancer J Clin 47:351–372

Spagnoli I, Gattoni F, Viganotti G (1982) Roentgenographic aspects of non-Hodgkin's lymphomas presenting with osseous lesions. Skeletal Radiol 8:39–41

Starzl TE, Nalesnik MA, Porter KA, Ho M, Iwatsuki S, Griffith BP, Rosenthal JT, Hakala TR, Shaw BW Jr, Hardesty RL, Atchison RW, Jaffe R, Bahnson HT (1984) Reversibility of lymphomas and lymphoproliferative lesions developing under cyclosporin-steroid therapy. Lancet 8377:583–587

Stiglbauer R, Augustin I, Kramer J, Schurawitzki H, Imhof H, Radaszkiewicz T (1992) MRI in the diagnosis of primary lymphoma of bone: correlation with histopathology. J Comput Assist Tomogr 16:248–253

Vanel D, Bayle C, Hartmann O, Rebibo G, Tamman S (1982) Radiological study of two disseminated malignant non-Hodgkin lymphomas affecting only the bones in children. Skeletal Radiol 9:83–87

Vassallo J, Roessner A, Vollmer E, Grundmann E (1987) Malignant lymphomas with primary bone manifestation. Pathol Res Pract 182:381–389

Vincent JM, Ng YY, Norton AJ, Armstrong P (1992) Case Report: primary lymphoma of bone – MRI appearances with pathologic correlation. Clin Radiol 45:406–409

Vogler JB III, Murphy WA (1998) Bone marrow imaging. Radiology 168:679–693

Weiland E (1901) Studien über das primär multiple auftretende lymphosarcom der knochen. Virchows Arch A 166:103–157

White LM, Schweitzer ME, Khalili K, Howarth DJC, Wunder JS, Bell RS (1998) MR imaging in primary lymphoma of bone: variability of T2-weighted signal intensity. AJR Am J Roentgenol 170:1243–1247

10 MALT Lymphoma

Ah Young Kim and Joon Koo Han

CONTENTS

10.1
Introduction

Mucosa-associated lymphoid tissue (MALT)-driven lymphoma, first described in 1983 by Isaacson and Wright, was only recognized in 1994 as a distinct entity of lymphoma in the revised European-American lymphoma (REAL) classification among the marginal zone B-cell lymphomas (HARRIS et al. 1994) as well as in the more recent classification proposed by the World Health Organization (WHO) (JAFFE et al. 1999).

Ah Young Kim, MD
Assistant Professor, Department of Radiology, Asan Medical Center, University of Ulsan College of Medicine, 388-1 Poongnapdong Songpagu, Seoul 138-736, Korea
Joon Koo Han, MD
Associate Professor, Department of Radioogy, Seoul National University Hospital, 28 Yongon-dong, Chongno-gu, Seoul 110-744, Korea

Histologically, MALT lymphoma is characterized by neoplastic marginal cells which display a variable combination of colonization of reactive germinal centers, plasmacytic differentiation, and destructive epithelial infiltration, forming lymphoepithelial lesions. MALT lymphomas are the most common subset of extranodal lymphoma and generally, arise from sites normally devoid of lymphoid tissue. Although it is well known that the stomach is the most common site of MALT lymphoma, it can also arise from various non-gastrointestinal sites, such as the salivary gland, conjunctiva, thyroid, orbit, lung, breast, kidney, skin, liver and prostate. The origin of MALT lymphoma is an accumulation of autoreactive lymphoid tissue generated by either chronic inflammatory disorders or autoimmune disease such as *Helicobacter pylori* infection in the stomach (WOTHERSPOON et al. 1991; WOTHERSPOON et al. 1993), follicular bronchiectasis in the lung (NICHOLSON et al. 1996), Sjögren disease in the salivary gland (ISAACSON 1990), Hashimoto thyroiditis (ISAACSON 1992), and reactive or inflammatory lesions of the orbit lymphoma (NERI et al. 1987). There are also literature reports of a correlation between hepatitis C virus infection and extranodal MALT lymphomas (ASCOLI et al. 1998; TKOUB et al. 1998).

This lymphoid tissue becomes genetically unstable with the acquisition of abnormalities such as translocations t11;18 and t1;14 trisomy 3, c-myc (8q24), and p53 (17p13) mutations leading to transformation into MALT lymphoma. MALT lymphomas are usually low-grade lymphomas. Histologic progression from a low-grade MALT lymphoma to a high-grade lymphoma is rare, occurring in less than 10% of the cases (THIEBLEMONT et al. 1997) and associated with other genetic events such as p16[Ink] or p53 inactivation.

Clinically, MALT lymphomas behave as an indolent disease with a prolonged clinical course. Unlike other lymphomas, these disorders tend to remain localized for prolonged periods and seldom involve the bone marrow at the time of presentation. Patients with MALT lymphomas show good outcome with a long disease-free survival and long overall survival and, consequently MALT lymphomas have been known as "pseudolymphomas". Although these lymphomas are believed not to disseminate as often as their nodal equivalents, MALT lymphoma presents as a disseminated disease in one-third of cases at diagnosis. However, this dissemination does not change the patient outcome (THIEBLEMONT et al. 2000).

Because of its distinctive clinical and pathologic characteristics comparable to other lymphomas, these MALT lymphomas provide new treatment insights. Hence, greater understanding of this new disease entity will be required for early detection and proper decision-making regarding treatment planning.

10.2
Clinicopathologic Consideration

The clinicopathologic features of malignant lymphoma traditionally have been discussed in the context of normal lymphoid tissue as exemplified by peripheral lymph nodes. However, between 25% and 40% of malignant non-Hodgkin lymphomas, the so-called primary extranodal lymphomas, arise outside the lymph nodes (FREEMAN et al. 1972; GREINER et al. 1995). These lymphomas can arise from extranodal lymphoid organs such as the spleen, from non-lymphoid organs containing a substantial amount of native lymphoid tissue such as the gastrointestinal tract, or from organs that are normally devoid of lymphoid tissue such as the brain. Studies of gastric lymphoma, the most common extranodal lymphoma, and certain other extranodal lymphomas, suggest that their clinicopathologic features are more closely related to the structure and function of so-called MALT than to those of peripheral lymph nodes (HALL and SMITH, 1970; HUSBAND 1982).

MALT is a term that describes lymphoid tissue under the epithelia of the gastrointestinal, respiratory, and urogenital tracts and their anlages. In contrast to peripheral lymph nodes which are adapted to deal with antigens carried to the nodes in afferent lymphatics, MALT appears to have evolved to protect mucosal tissue which is directly in contact with antigens in the external environment. MALT has been most thoroughly characterized in the gastrointestinal tract where it comprises four lymphoid compartments – Peyer patches, the lamina propria, the intraepithelial T lymphocytes, and the mesenteric lymph nodes. Among them, Peyer patches are most relevant to lymphomas. Unlike lymph nodes, Peyer patches are not encapsulated and lack afferent lymphatics. The B-

cell component is dominant and consists of a central follicle surrounded by a prominent marginal zone. This is surmounted by the dome epithelium containing clusters of intraepithelial B-cells; this constitutes the lymphoepithelium, a defining feature of MALT. These intraepithelial B-cells are different from the intraepithelial T cells that are present in the rest of the intestinal epithelium. Actually, MALT lymphomas show monoclonal B-cell proliferations and these B-cells have the same cytologic and immunophenotypic characteristics as the B-cells that are normally found around the mantle zones of Peyer patches (ISAACSON et al. 1986; MOORE and WRIGHT 1984; ABBONDANZO and SOBIN 1997). Therefore, these low-grade B-cell lymphomas which have the morphologic features of MALT with the high-grade lesions that may evolve from them are known as MALT lymphomas (ISAACSON and WRIGHT 1984; ISAACSON and SPENCER 1987; CHAN et al. 1990).

10.3
MALT Lymphoma of the Stomach

10.3.1
Background

The primary gastrointestinal lymphoma may be of B or T-cell origin (ISAACSON 1994). About 35% of gastrointestinal lymphomas are found in the stomach and are predominantly non-Hodgkin lymphoma of B-cell origin (ISAACSON 1994; LEWIN et al. 1978). Although the stomach is the most common primary site of extranodal lymphoma, primary gastric lymphoma is uncommon and constitutes only 2–5% of malignant gastric lesions because this organ is normally devoid of lymphoid tissue (AOZASA et al. 1985; FREEMAN et al. 1972). Most primary low-grade B-cell lymphomas of the stomach have been known as "pseudolymphoma" or "reactive lymphoreticular hyperplasia" because of their characteristic histopathologic features and favorable prognosis (TOKUNAGA et al. 1987). Recently, immunohistochemical methods have shown that most of these tumors are monoclonal B-cell proliferations and have emphasized the specificity of these B-cells, suggesting that they originate from MALT (BURKE et al. 1987; SPENCER et al. 1989; SIGAL et al. 1989; MOORE and WRIGHT 1984; ISAACSON et al. 1986; MYHRE and ISAACSON 1987). Therefore, these low-grade B-cell lymphomas, along with the high-grade B-cell lymphomas that evolve from them, are known as MALT lymphoma (ISAACSON and WRIGHT 1984; ISAACSON and SPENCER 1987; CHAN et al. 1990). This concept of MALT lymphoma has been incorporated into a new classification scheme, the REAL classification (HARRIS et al. 1994). Transformation to a large cell lymphoma is recognized in this new classification scheme. However, the criteria for distinguishing high-grade MALT type lymphomas from other large cell lymphomas have not been widely addressed (CHAN et al. 1990; MONTALBAN et al. 1995).

10.3.2
Clinical Considerations

Age

Low-grade gastric MALT lymphoma occurs predominantly in individuals over 50, but an increasing number of cases are being reported in younger patients. It is generally known that the mean age of MALT lymphoma patients is 50–60 years. CASTILLO et al. (1992) and HOSHIDA et al. (1997) reported no difference in the median ages between patients with high-grade and low-grade MALT lymphomas. However, KATH et al. (1995) and YOSHINO et al. (2000) reported a difference in the median ages between patients with low-grade (median, 58.5–59.9 years) and high-grade tumors (median, 66–68.5 years). According to the latter results, the mean age of patients with high-grade MALT lymphoma was 8.6 years more than that of patients with low-grade MALT lymphoma. Therefore, they suggest that it seems to take about one decade at least for high-grade transformation of low-grade MALT lymphoma. The number of men and women was nearly equal in the current study whereas a slight preponderance of men was found in the majority of previous studies (CHAN et al. 1990; AZAB et al. 1989; RUSKONE-FOURMESTRAUX et al. 1993).

Symptoms

The clinical presentation of gastric MALT lymphoma includes non-specific digestive symptoms, clinical indolence, and a slow course (MOORE and WRIGHT, 1984; ISAACSON et al. 1986). Persistent epigastric pain is the main presenting complaint and is often associated with acute bleeding, anemia or weight loss.

Frequency

The reported frequency of early stage disease in primary gastric lymphoma has increased since the acceptance of the MALT concept. In the current study, the percentage of stage I cases was 66%. The percentages of patients with stage I in previous reports adopting and not adopting the MALT concept, were approximately 50% and 26%, respectively. The frequency of low-grade, combined high- and low-grade, and high-grade types in the current study was 43%, 32%, and 18%, respectively, showing a lower frequency of high-grade MALT lymphomas and a higher frequency of combined high and low-grade MALT lymphomas than in previous reports (CASTRILLO et al. 1992; KATH et al. 1995; CHAN et al. 1990; NAKAMURA et al. 1995; RADASZKIEWICZ et al. 1992).

Clinical Behavior

In comparison to nodal low-grade B-cell lymphoma which, at the time of diagnosis, characteristically involves multiple lymph node sites and the bone marrow (stage IV), low-grade MALT lymphoma is usually confined to the site of origin (stage I_E or II_E) when diagnosed and is slow to disseminate. The highest reported incidence of bone marrow involvement is 10% (MONTALBAN et al. 1995). Splenic involvement has been described in some cases and interestingly, when this occurs the lymphomatous infiltrate is concentrated in the marginal zone (DU et al. 1997). The 10-year survival rate for patients with low-grade MALT lymphoma is approximately 80% compared to 40% to 50% for primary high-grade gastric lymphoma whether or not a minor low-grade component is present (COGLIATTI et al. 1991; DE JONG et al. 1997).

10.3.3
Helicobacter pylori and Gastric MALT lymphoma

It has recently been demonstrated that even though normal gastric mucosa contains no organized lymphoid tissue, the development of lymphoid follicles is a specific immunological response to chronic infection by *Helicobacter pylori* (STOLTE and EIDT 1989; HEILMANN and BORCHARD 1991). The association of high *H. pylori* infection rates (80–100%) with gastric lymphoma through a chronic gastritis has led to it being considered as a gastric carcinogen (ISAACSON and SPENCER 1993; WOTHERSPOON et al. 1991). This organism provokes an activation of cytotoxic and helper T-lymphocytes in the antral and fundic mucosa which stimulate the B-lymphocytes and plasma cells and induce the formation of lymphoid follicles, thus predisposing to the development of a MALT lymphoma (WOTHERSPOON et al. 1991; EIDT and STOLTE 1993; BAUERDORFER et al. 1997; CAMMAROTA et al. 1997). HUSSELL et al. (1993a,b) also found that the tumor B-cells themselves were not directly stimulated by *H. pylori*. This explains the observation that gastric MALT lymphomas, at least in the early phase of their growth, remain localized at the primary site as the lymphomas are dependent on activated T-cells which, while abundant in *H. pylori* gastritis, are unlikely to be present outside the gastric environment.

However, the prevalence of *H. pylori* infection varies worldwide between 20 and 100%, depending mostly on socioeconomic conditions (MEGRAUD et al. 1989; The EUROGAST Study Group 1993). Moreover, low positivity rates of *H. pylori* infection in gastric MALT lymphoma (42–59%) have also been reported in some recent Asian and Western studies, thus raising the question whether *H. pylori* infection is a universally crucial factor in the pathogenesis of gastric MALT lymphoma (XU et al. 1997; MIETTINEN et al. 1995; KARAT et al. 1995). NAKAMURA et al. (1997) and BOUZOURENE et al. (1999) reported the high relationship of *H. pylori* infection with low-grade MALT lymphomas (63–77%) in contrast to its relatively low correlation with high-grade MALT lymphoma (38–44%). According to their report, *H. pylori* infection was significantly correlated with the depth of invasion and the grade of the MALT lymphoma. It was also reported that the *H. pylori* density in patients with chronic gastritis who developed gastric MALT lymphoma, decreased significantly compared with that of similar patients who did not (NAKAMURA et al. 1998). These observations indicate that *H. pylori* infection tended to disappear with progression of the lymphoma, which suggests that *H. pylori* is more closely associated with the precursor or initial phase of gastric MALT lymphoma and might not be necessary for sustained lymphoma cell proliferation.

The notion that *H. pylori* infection and primary gastric lymphoma are related has been reinforced by the clinical and histological remission of some cases of low-grade lymphomas of the MALT type after *H. pylori* eradication by antibiotic therapy (WEBER et al. 1994; BAYERDORFFER et al. 1995; STOLTE and EIDT 1993). Recent studies reported that 70–80% of low-grade MALT lymphomas regress in response to eradication of *H. pylori* (WOTHERSPOON et al. 1993; BAYERDORFFER et al. 1997). However, antibiotic therapy for gastric MALT lymphoma appears to be effective only in low-grade disease restricted to the mucosa or submucosa.

10.3.4
Low-Grade Versus High-Grade MALT Lymphoma

Firstly, ISAACSON and WRIGHT (1983) classified primary B-cell MALT lymphoma into low-grade and high-grade lymphomas with or without evidence of a low-grade component. Pathologically, low-grade MALT lymphoma shows a diffuse infiltrate of small centrocyte-like cells that may invade the epithelial lining of gland of crypt and then form lymphoepithelial lesions (ISAACSON et al. 1986). In high-grade MALT lymphoma, large lymphoid cells transform from low-grade MALT lymphoma to form confluent clusters or sheets with or without areas of low-grade components (ISAACSON 1994). Glandular invasion is a rare event in high-grade MALT lymphoma, while in low-grade MALT lymphoma such event occurs quite often (CASTRILLO et al. 1992; CHAN et al. 1990). However, DE JONG et al. (1997) reclassified gastric MALT lymphoma into four categories, e.g. low-grade MALT lymphoma, mixed form, unequivocal high-grade transformation, and diffuse large B-cell lymphoma without reference to MALT, in order to determine the biological difference between gastric large B-cell lymphomas of MALT origin and those of putative non-MALT origin. They reported that no difference was seen in the clinical outcome of these high-grade categories and that the 10-year survival rate was approximately 45% for high-grade groups but 90% for classic low-grade MALT lymphoma. MONTALBAN et al. (1995) also reported that complete remission had been achieved in 91% of the patients in the low-grade group, but in substantially fewer patients (70%) in the high-grade group. These researchers suggested that the prognosis of gastric lymphoma depended primarily on the histologic grade and stage which are closely related. Histologic classification as low-grade and high-grade separates the distinctive groups of gastric MALT lymphoma which show striking clinical and prognostic differences.

Because of the role of *H. pylori* gastritis in the pathogenesis of gastric MALT lymphoma, considerable attention has been focused on the exciting possibility of treating these patients by eradicating *H. pylori* from the stomach without surgery, radiation or chemotherapy. However, as already indicated, untreated gastric MALT lymphomas may undergo blastic transformation, eventually leading to the development of more advanced, high-grade forms of gastric lymphoma. This pathologic sequence of events has major implications for patient prognosis; low-grade gastric MALT lymphomas are associated with 5-year survival rates of 75–91% (COGLIATTI et al. 1991; TAAL et al. 1996), whereas high-grade gastric lymphomas are associated with 5-year survival rates of less than 50% (TAAL et al. 1996).

A genetic change may be associated with the transition from gastritis to MALT lymphoma (CALVERT et al. 1995). It has further been proposed that MALT lymphoma may be a precursor of high-grade B-cell non-Hodgkin lymphoma in gastric tissue and that most high-grade lymphomas follow this evolutionary pathway (CHAN et al. 1990). High-grade B-cell gastric lymphoma may, however, arise de novo (PARSONNET et al. 1994; BROOKS and ENTERLINE 1983). Although the clinical symptoms of high-grade lymphoma and MALT lymphoma may be similar, they differ in several aspects. High-grade B-cell lymphoma has a relatively aggressive course as opposed to the more indolent and favorable outcome of MALT lymphoma. The endoscopic, microscopic, and histological appearance of the two entities also differ (TAAL et al. 1989; ISAACSON 1996). In high-grade gastric lymphoma, the extent of disease is usually greater at presentation, with involvement of adjacent organs and perigastric lymph nodes (COOPER et al. 1990). The diagnosis of high-grade gastric lymphoma can be established by endoscopic biopsy and spread outside the stomach can be assessed on CT and endoscopic ultrasound (TAAL et al. 1996; SUEKANE et al. 1993).

10.3.5
Radiologic Evaluation

10.3.5.1
Barium Examination

Gastric lymphomas are demonstrated on barium studies by a spectrum of findings, including thickened rugae, submucosal masses, centrally ulcerated (bull's eye or target) lesions, polypoid lesions, nodules, and ulcers. In particular, low-grade MALT lymphoma had a wider spectrum of appearance than high-grade MALT lymphoma. Many researchers have extensively investigated the radiographic features of gastric MALT lymphomas (KIM et al. 1999; PARK et al. 2002; THIEMBLEMONT et al. 2000). Although there are some differences in their results, most common findings of low-grade gastric MALT lymphomas are mucosal nodularity (30–52%) (Fig. 10.1) and ulcers of variable size, depth, and number (24-48%) (Figs. 10.2–10.4). The larger and deeper the gastric ulcers, the higher the grade of gastric MALT lymphomas. According to two

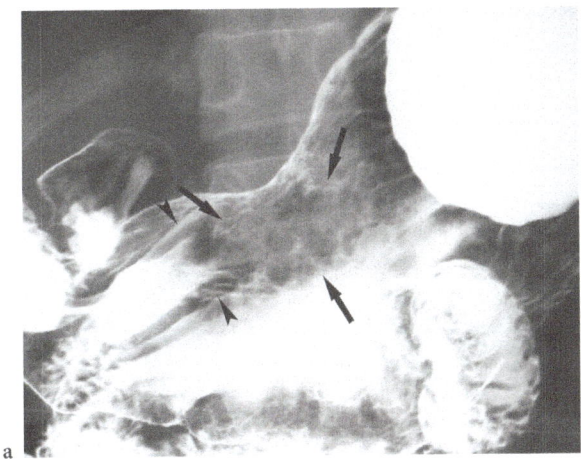

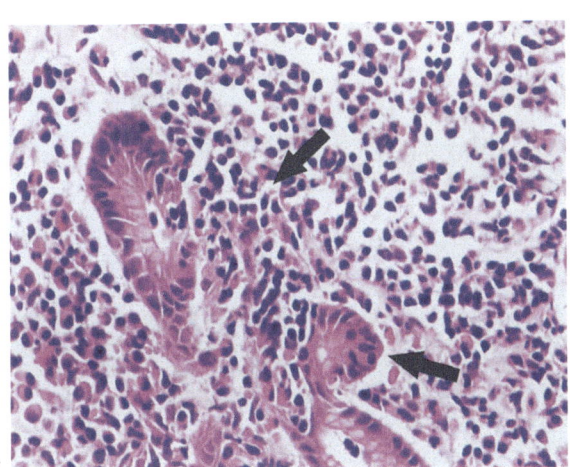

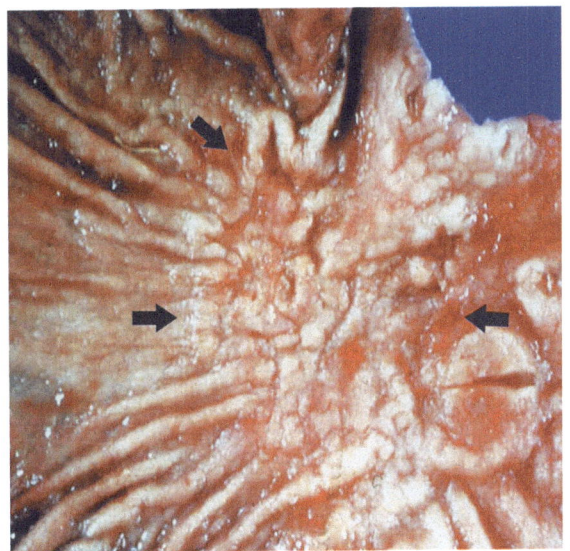

Fig. 10.1a–c. Low-grade gastric MALT lymphoma with mucosal nodularity in a 31-year-old woman. a Spot radiograph of upper gastrointestinal examination shows multiple nodules of variable sizes (*arrows*) with convergence of the surrounding rugae (*arrowheads*) in large areas of the gastric body and antrum. b Photograph of the resected specimen reveals mucosal nodularities (*arrows*) with disorganized rugal thickening. Note the convergent rugae that project to multiple points. c High-power photomicrograph (Hematoxylin-eosin stain; original magnification, ×400) shows lymphoproliferative lesion (*arrows*) composed of centrocyte-like lymphocytes and cells with plasmacytoid features and destruction of glandular structures.

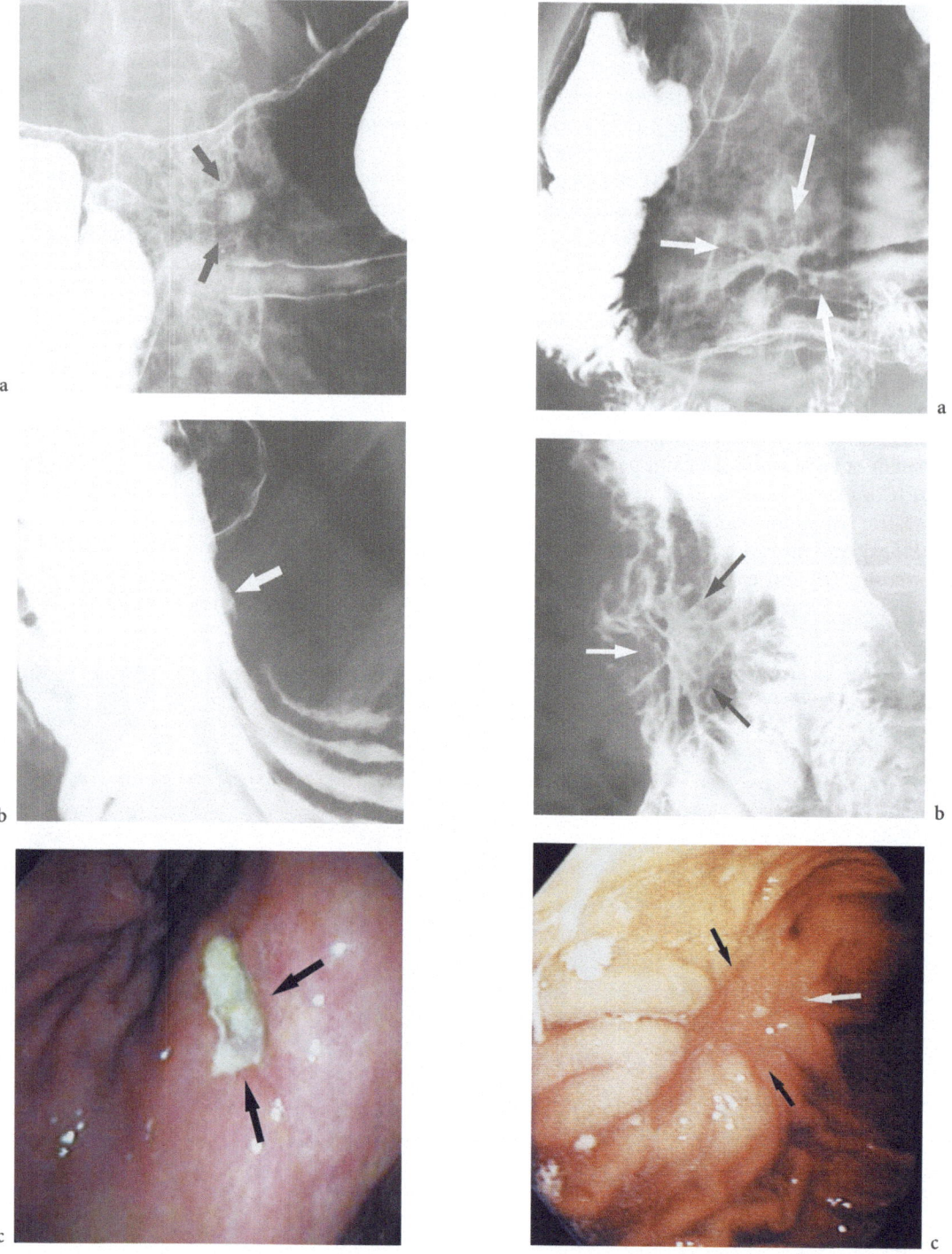

Fig.10.2a–c. Low-grade gastric MALT lymphoma with ulcer in a 55-year-old man. **a, b** Spot radiographs of upper gastrointestinal examination show a small depressed lesion with vague margins (*arrows*) on the lesser curvature side of the gastric body. **c** Endoscopic image reveals an ulcer (*arrows*) with hyperemic surrounding mucosa in gastric body.

Fig. 10.3a–c. Low-grade gastric MALT lymphomas with disorganized rugal thickening. **a** Spot radiograph of upper gastrointestinal examination shows a shallow irregular ulcer with convergent rugal thickening (*arrows*) in the posterior wall of the gastric body. **b** Spot radiograph of upper gastrointestinal examination and (**c**) endoscopic image of another patient demonstrate a large deep ulcer with vague ulcer margins (*arrows*) and marked rugal thickening that converges to a deep ulcer at the gastric high body.

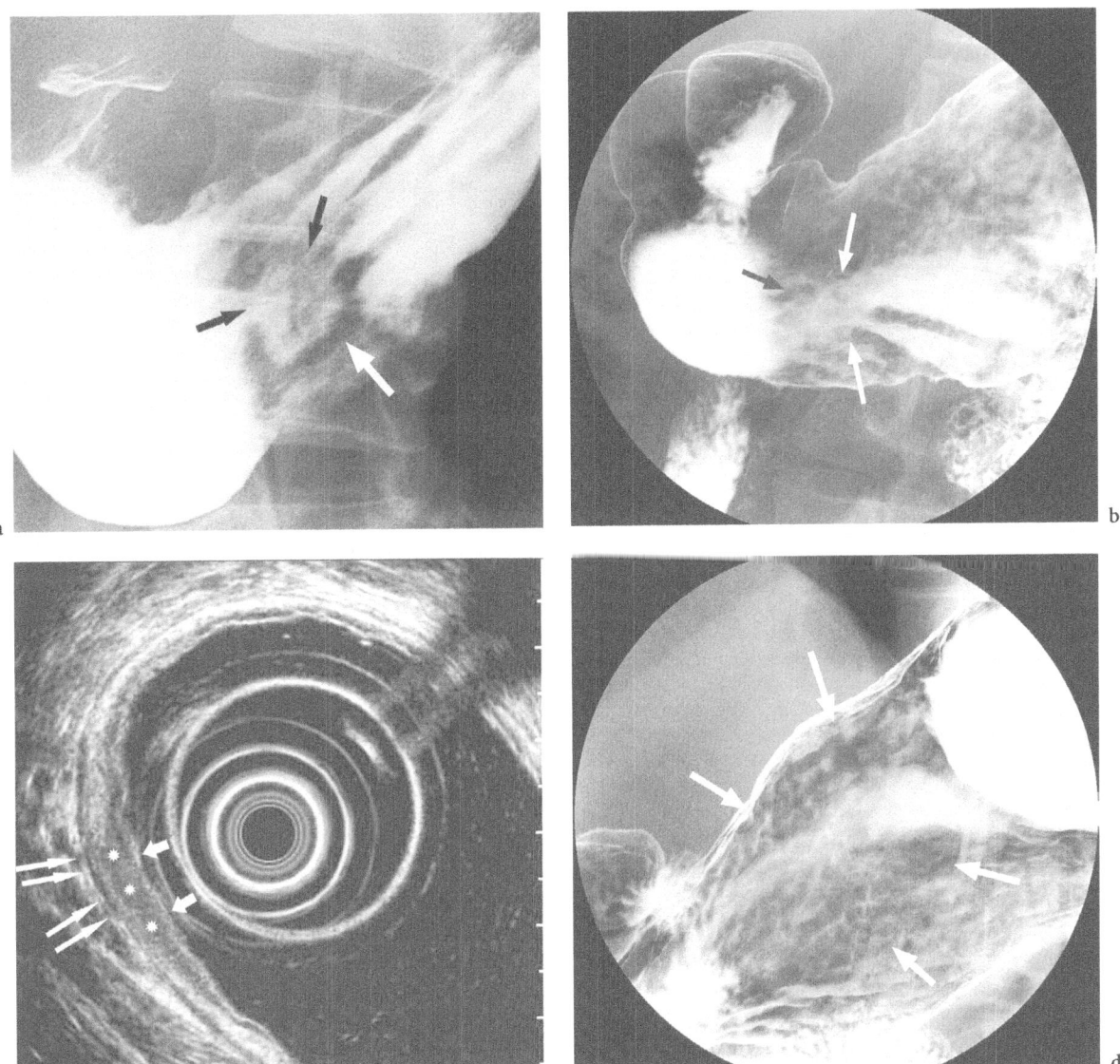

Fig. 10.4a–d. Low-grade gastric MALT lymphoma with multiple lesions in a 46-year-old woman. **a** Compression spot radiograph of the gastric body shows a shallow ulcer with convergent thick rugae (*arrows*) in the anterior wall. **b** Spot radiograph of upper gastrointestinal examination shows another shallow ulcer with vague margins (*arrows*) and disorganization of surrounding convergent folds in the posterior wall of the gastric body. **c** Endoscopic ultrasound image reveals an infiltrative hypoechoic lesion within submucosal layer (*asterisks*). Note the intact overlying mucosa (*thick arrows*) and underlying muscular layer (*double arrows*) in the posterior wall of the gastric body. **d** Coarse mucosal nodularities in large areas of the gastric high body (*arrows*) on barium examination were proved to be hypertrophic lymphoid follicles of *Helicobacter pylori* gastritis by endoscopic biopsy.

recent reports (PARK et al. 2002; THIEMBLEMONT et al. 2000), multiple erosions or shallow ulcers are frequently manifested in low-grade MALT lymphoma whereas deep ulcers are less frequently detected, while the most common findings of high-grade MALT lymphoma are a mass with or without ulcer (38–67%) (Fig. 10.5) and diffuse, very thick folds (28%) (Figs. 10.6, 10.7). The masses are larger in high-grade than in low-grade MALT lymphoma (AN et al. 2001).

These differences of radiologic manifestation between low-grade and high-grade gastric MALT lymphomas, which usually present as superficial spreading lesions of low-grade lymphoma and tumor-forming high-grade lymphoma, can be explained by the depth of tumor invasion. Endoscopic evaluation of gastric MALT lymphomas shows a similar observation (Fig. 10.4). TAAL et al. (1996) described the significant differences in

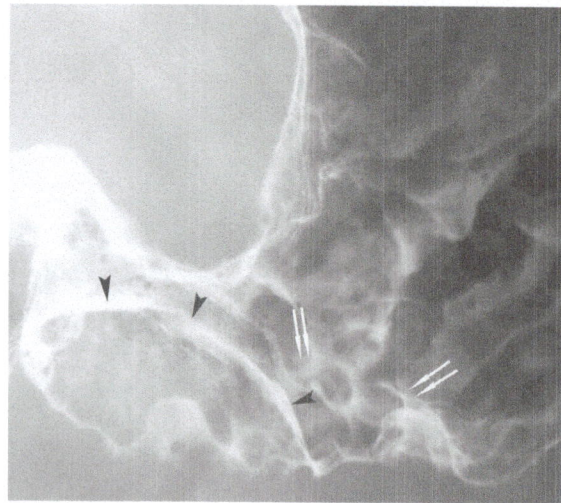

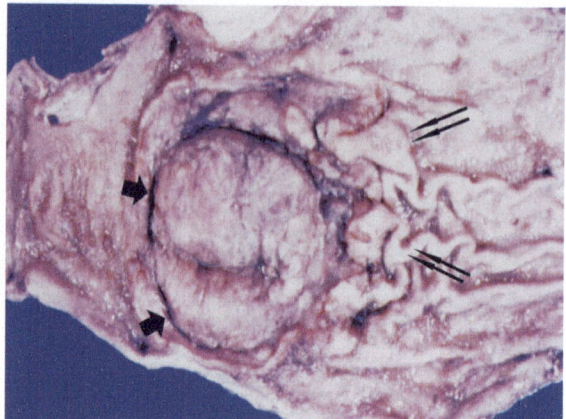

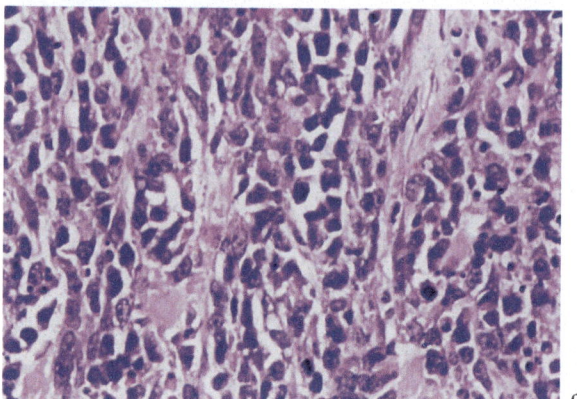

Fig. 10.5a–c. High-grade gastric MALT lymphoma with mass in a 64-year-old man. **a** Spot radiograph of upper gastrointestinal examination shows a well-demarcated mass (*arrowheads*) in the antrum and disorganized rugal thickening (*double arrows*). **b** Photograph of the resected specimen demonstrates marked disorganization of thick rugae (*double arrows*) proximal to the mass (*thick arrows*). **c** High-power photomicrograph (Hematoxylin-eosin stain; original magnification, ×400) reveals severe destruction of gastric glands by high-grade lymphoma cells. (With permission from [AN et al. 2001])

interpretation of the endoscopic findings, showing that the low-grade lymphomas were interpreted mainly as benign conditions such as benign ulcers (52% of cases), whereas the high-grade lymphomas were most often interpreted as malignancies such as advanced carcinoma (71% of cases).

Pitfalls

Most of the radiologic findings of barium examinations of gastric MALT lymphomas, i.e. mucosal nodularity, shallow or deep ulcer, rugal thickening, mass, and enlarged areae gastricae, are also demonstrated in gastric adenocarcinoma or lymphoma. In addition, the inadequate barium examination, shallow nature of the lesions, and nonspecific findings such as the mucosal nodularity and rugal thickening commonly seen in *H. pylori* gastritis, may contribute to the low detection rate of gastric MALT lymphoma on upper gastrointestinal barium examination.

Helicobacter pylori gastritis - On barium examination, *H. pylori* gastritis manifests as thickened, nodular rugae in the gastric antrum and enlarged areae gastricae (Fig. 10.8). Although all low-grade gastric MALT lymphomas do not have ulcers, the presence

of ulcers may be helpful in differentiating MALT lymphoma from *H. pylori* gastritis. However, some low-grade lymphomas manifesting as nodularity or thickened rugae alone are difficult to differentiate from *H. pylori* infection on the basis of findings on barium examination. Also, in contrast to the mucosal nodularities of MALT lymphoma, enlarged area gastricae of *H. pylori* gastritis tend to be more uniform in size and produce a sharply margined reticular network (SOHN et al. 1995). Usually, these lesions are less than 1 cm in diameter with clustered appearance and are most commonly seen in the distal antrum.

Intestinal metaplasia – Intestinal metaplasia consists of gastric mucosa resembling that of the intestine and considered as late stage of gastric carcinogenesis. On barium examination, radiologic findings of intestinal metaplasia include mucosal surface nodularity together with irregular thickening of the mucosal folds and enlarged areae gastricae. The nodular defects are usually even in size (mean, 6 mm) and diffuse in extent (Fig. 10.9). However, severity of intestinal metaplasia does not always correlate with the size of the nodules.

Gastric carcinoma – Differentiation from gastric carcinoma is the most frequent diagnostic problem

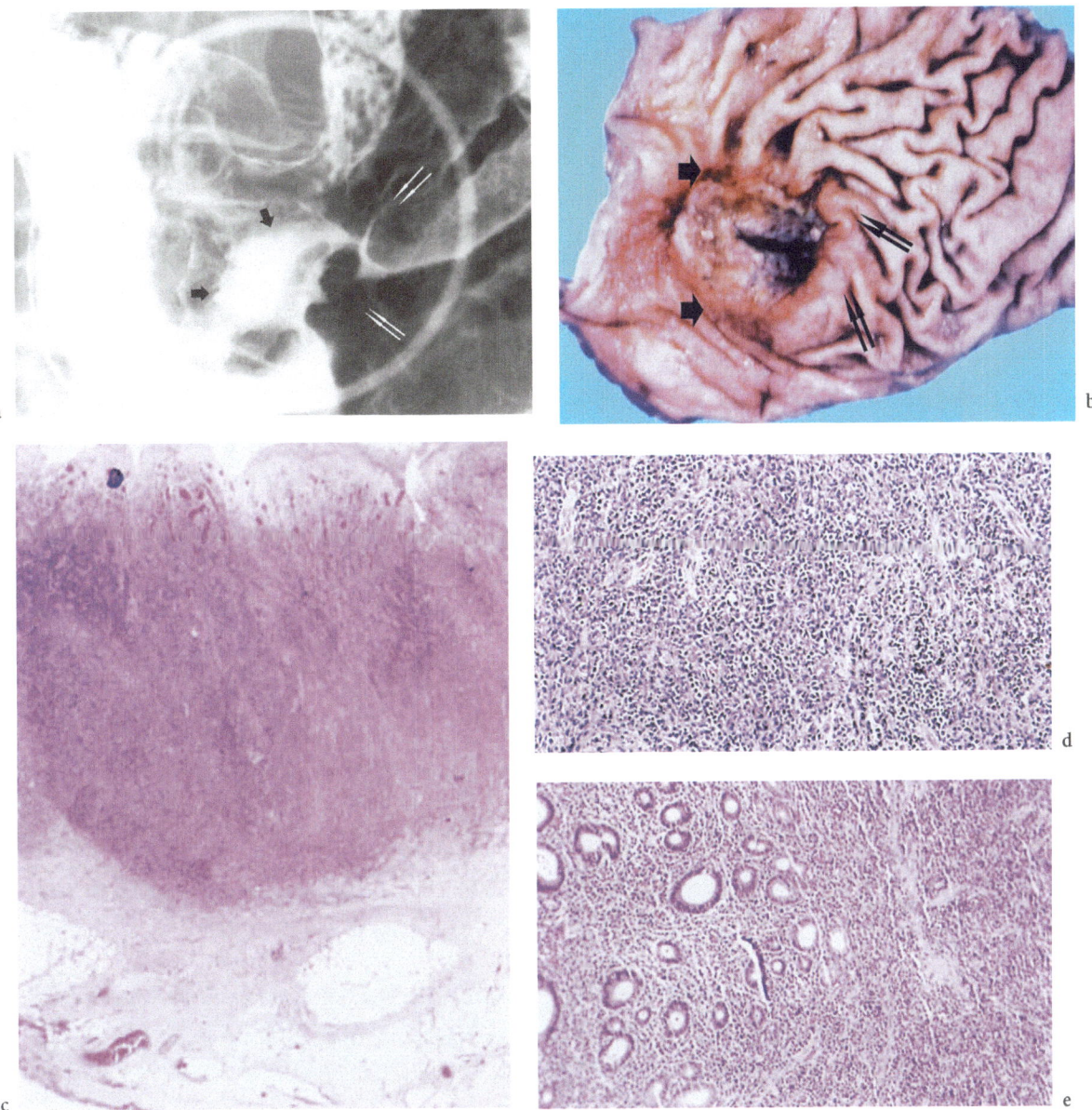

Fig. 10.6a–e. High-grade gastric MALT lymphoma with a large ulcer in a 45-year-old man. **a** Compression spot radiograph shows a large, deep ulcer (*solid arrows*) in the posterior wall of the antrum. Note prominent disorganization of the convergent thick rugae (*double arrows*). **b** Photograph of the resected specimen shows a large ulcer (*solid arrows*) and the disorganized rugal thickening (*double arrows*). **c** Low-power photomicrograph (Hematoxylin-eosin stain; original magnification, ×10) reveals expansile extension of tumor cells (blue stain) to the subserosa. This lymphoma is intermingled with (**d**) low-grade and (**e**) high-grade components (Hematoxylin-eosin stain; original magnification, ×100). (With permission from [AN et al. 2001])

because carcinoma also originates from mucosa and produces mucosal destruction and desmoplastic change in the submucosa (KITAMURA et al. 1996; SATO et al. 1986). In gastric carcinoma of the ulcerative type, these pathologic changes usually manifest as well-defined, irregular shallow ulcers with abrupt disruption of the normal mucosa; they often manifest

as a striking convergence of the rugae. In contrast, low-grade lymphoma arising from the lymphatic tissue in the deeper layer mainly produces submucosal tumor growth, and desmoplastic reaction is rare. Therefore, smooth enlarged rugae with slight convergence, indicating the submucosal nature of early lymphoma, and poorly defined ulceration,

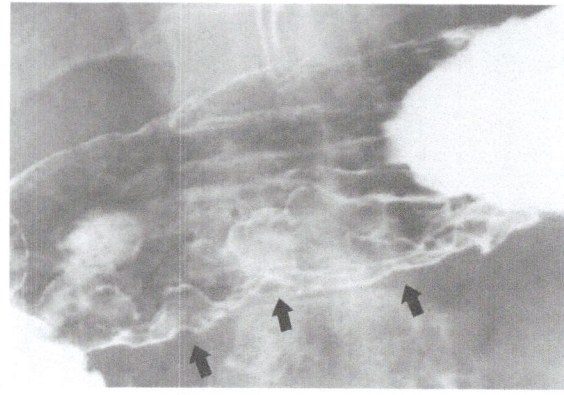

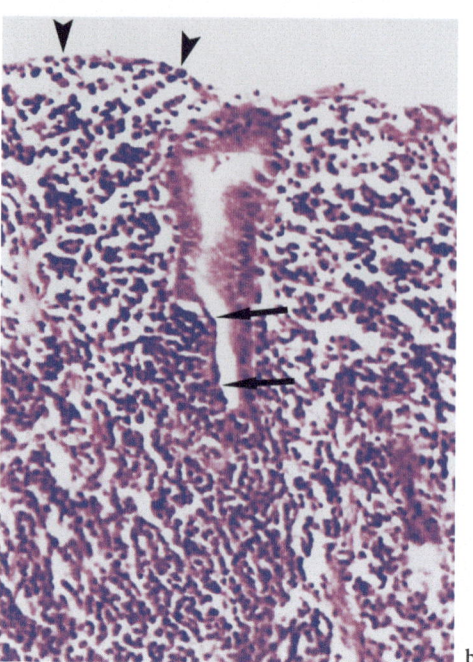

Fig. 10.7a,b. High-grade gastric MALT lymphoma with diffuse rugal thickening in a 45-year-old man. **a** Spot radiograph shows thickened nodular folds (*arrows*) in the greater curvature of the gastric body. **b** High-power photomicrograph (Hematoxylin-eosin stain; original magnification, ×200) shows the characteristic lymphoepithelial lesions formed by invasion of individual glands (*arrows*) or surface epithelium (*arrowheads*) by high-grade lymphoma cells that displace or destroy the glandular epithelium. (With permission from [AN et al. 2001])

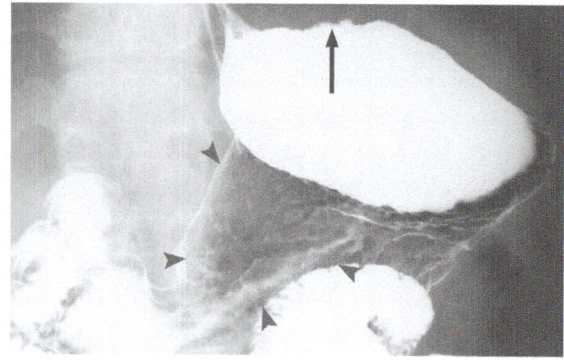

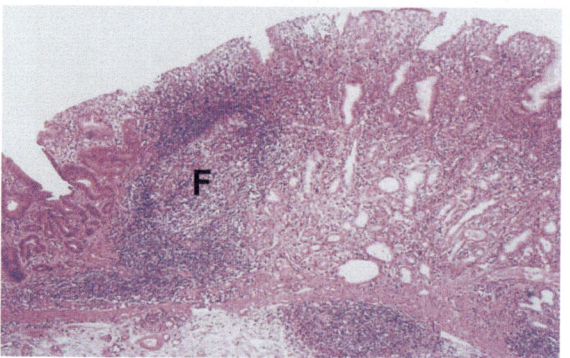

Fig. 10.8a,b. Helicobacter pylori gastritis in a 64-year-old man with advanced gastric cancer. **a** Spot radiograph of upper gastrointestinal examination shows clustered mucosal nodularities of uneven size (*arrowheads*) in the gastric body, along with gastric cancer (*arrow*) in the fundus. Note no visible fold convergence or ulceration. **b** Microphotograph (Hematoxylin-eosin stain; original magnification, ×100) of biopsy specimen obtained from the gastric body, where mucosal nodularity was seen on barium examination, discovers inflammation with formation of lymphoid follicles (*F*) within the gastric mucosa.

indicating poor desmoplastic reaction, are valuable findings favoring low-grade MALT lymphoma (SATO et al. 1986). Also, the higher prevalence of multiplicity (20–65%) of gastric MALT lymphoma can be helpful in its differential diagnosis from gastric carcinoma (KIM et al. 1999; THIEBLEMONT et al. 2000). In differentiating low-grade MALT lymphoma from early gastric carcinoma with ulceration, the presence of disorganized convergent rugae, vague ulcer margins, and multiple lesions may be useful findings (Fig. 10.4) (KIM et al. 1999).

10.3.5.2
Computed Tomography

Despite its questionable value for this use, computed tomography (CT) has been routinely used for the staging of primary gastric lymphomas and for monitoring treatment response (GRAU et al. 1996). Common CT findings of MALT lymphoma are gastric wall thickening and lymphadenopathy. Normally, gastric wall thickness should not exceed 4 mm on CT scanning, when the stomach

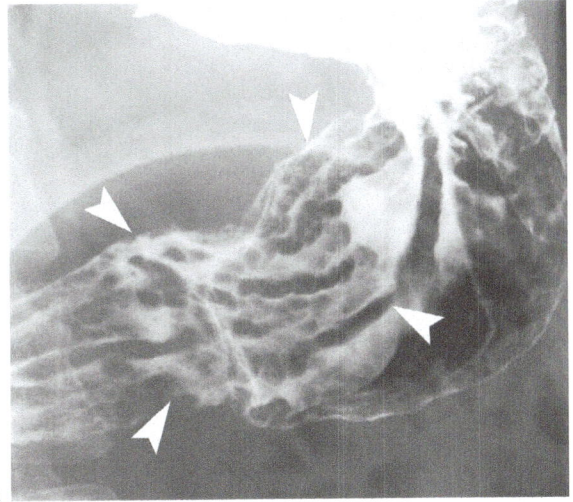

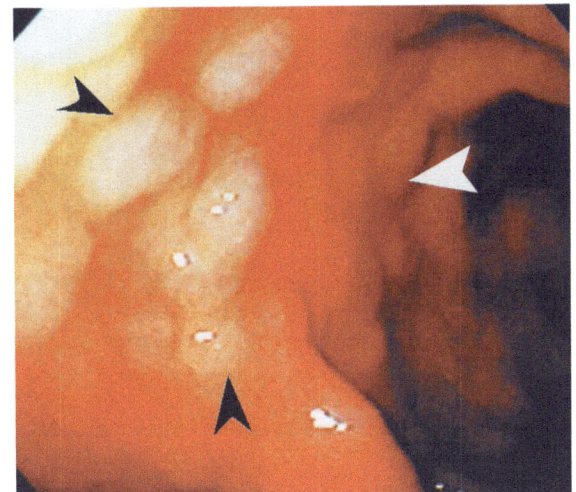

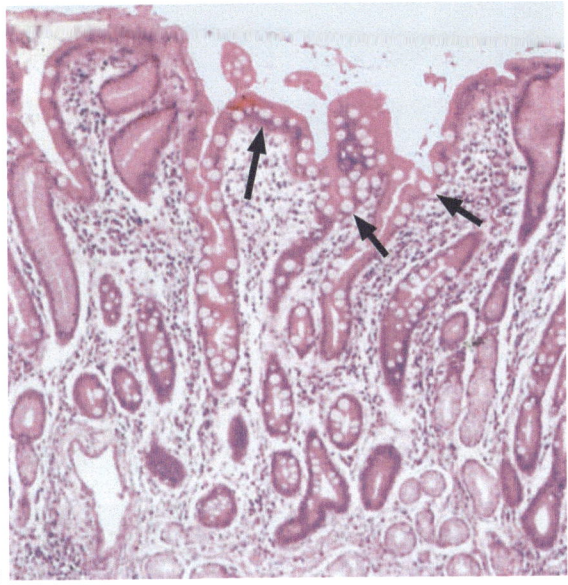

Fig. 10.9a–c. Intestinal metaplasia in a 57-year-old man. **a** Spot radiograph shows diffuse involvement of even-sized, sparse nodularity (*arrowheads*) in large area of gastric antrum. **b** Endoscopic image reveals diffuse even-sized nodules (*arrowheads*) with smooth mucosal surface in the gastric antrum. **c** Photomicrograph (Hematoxylin-eosin stain; original magnification, ×200) of biopsy specimen obtained from the antral lesions, mentioned above, shows the presence of intestinal metaplasia including goblet cells (*arrows*). Their outer surfaces appear to be nodular, causing nodularities on barium examination.

is adequately distended (WEGENER 1993). Usually there are no abnormal CT findings of low-grade MALT lymphoma (28–31%) or there may be minimal gastric wall thickening, 5–10 mm (Fig. 10.10) (KESSAR et al. 1999; GOLLUB et al. 1999; CHOI et al. 2002; PARK et al. 2002). In addition, there is rarely perigastric lymph node enlargement or involvement of adjacent organs. BLAZQUEZ et al. (1992) reported involvement of other mucosal sites, usually the lung, in some patients with gastric MALT lymphoma but there was no involvement of the spleen, lymph nodes or bone marrow.

This pattern of involvement as shown on CT of low-grade MALT lymphomas differs markedly from that of high-grade B-cell lymphomas. In the latter, the wall thickness is greater than that of the

low-grade type with a relatively wide range of 1.4 to 5 cm in mean thickness. Furthermore, adjacent organs were often involved and lymph nodes were invariably involved (67–75%) (Fig. 10.11) (CHOI et al. 2002; PARK et al. 2002). Bone marrow may also be infiltrated. High-grade B-cell lymphoma is overall a more aggressive disease.

According to recent studies (CHOI et al. 2002; PARK et al. 2002) comparing low and high-grade MALT lymphoma, there were significant differences in the thickness and extent of involvement of the gastric wall; both were thicker and wider in patients with high-grade histology. They stressed that diffuse gastric wall thickening to a severe or moderate degree, deep ulcer, and lymphadenopathy, were reliable findings of high-grade MALT lymphoma. Similarly,

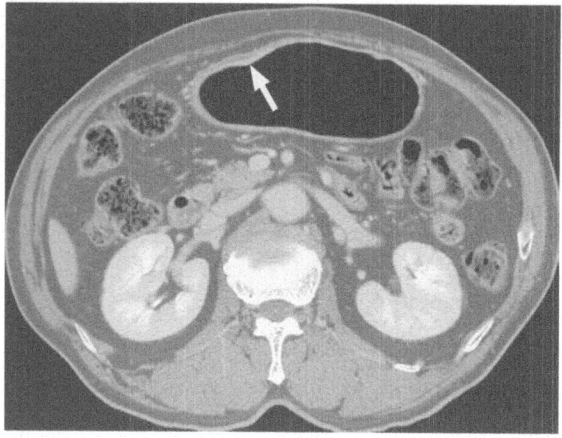

Fig. 10.10. CT of low-grade gastric MALT lymphoma in a 47-year-old man. Axial contrast-enhanced CT scan using effervescent oral agents shows minimal focal wall thickening (*arrow*) at anterior wall of gastric antrum. Perigastric lymphadenopathy is not visible.

KESSAR et al. (1999) suggested that the possibility of the lymphoma having been transformed into a high-grade form be considered if the lesion observed on follow-up CT appears to be more than mild gastric wall thickening. Alternatively, the absence of an abnormality on CT is highly predictive of low-grade MALT lymphoma. These different CT findings in low and high-grade lymphomas reflect the relationship between the gastric wall thickness and the depth of invasion of MALT lymphoma. Indeed, superficial spreading low-grade MALT lymphoma demonstrated the depth of invasion confined within the mucosa and submucosa (50–68%), and high-grade lymphoma showed the tumor extent beyond the muscularis propria (78–100%) on the histopathologic specimens (MONTALBAN et al. 1995; KESSAR et al. 1999).

10.3.6
Treatment Guidelines

Some preliminary data suggest that the rate of ongoing mutations gradually declines during disease progression and that the activity finally disappears in high-grade lesions. On the basis of that theory, it is suggested that in low-grade lymphoma, the eradication of *H. pylori* may abolish the antigenic drive of B-cell proliferation, leading to regression of the lymphoma (TAAL et al. 1996; ISAACSON 1999). In contrast to low-grade lymphoma, the proliferative process of high-grade lymphoma is probably fully autonomous and no longer dependent on antigenic drive and is

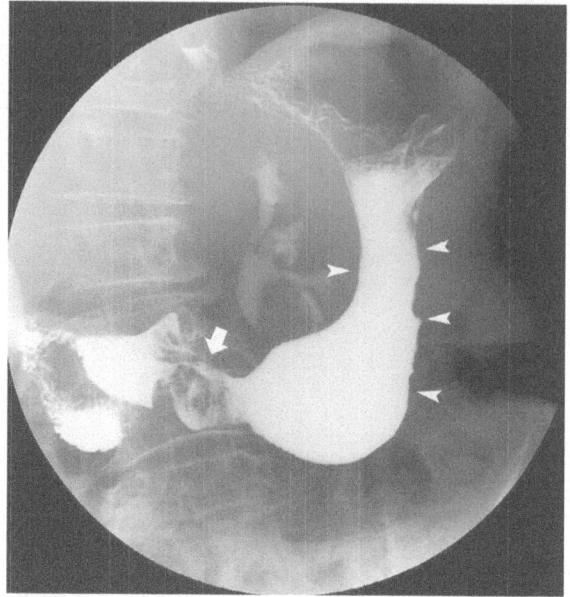

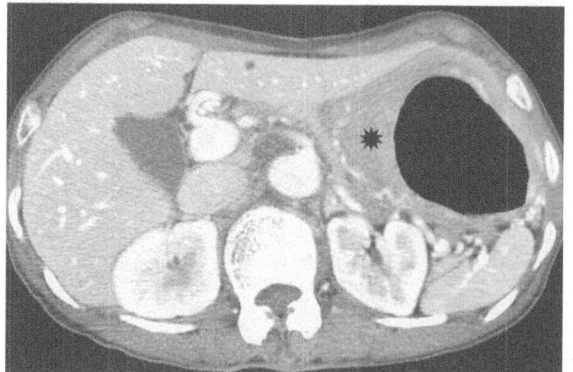

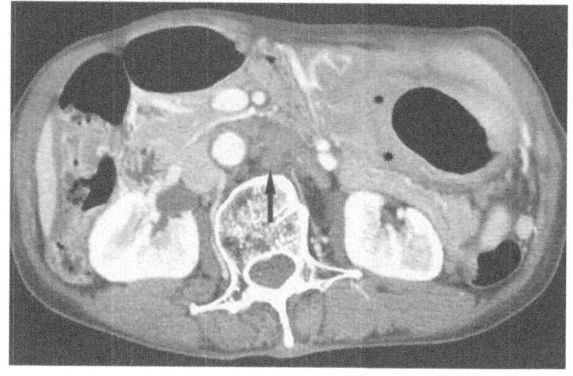

Fig. 10.11a–c. CT of high-grade gastric MALT lymphoma in a 47-year-old man. **a** Spot radiograph of barium examination in semierect position shows a large irregular shaped ulcer with fold convergence (*arrow*) in the gastric antrum and diffuse luminal narrowing with nodular thick rugae (*arrowheads*) along the gastric body. **b, c** Axial contrast-enhanced CT scans show marked and diffuse gastric wall thickening (*asterisks*) with perigastric lymphadenopathy, encasing perigastric vascular structures. Note conglomerated paraaortic lymphadenopathy (*arrow*).

therefore unresponsive to *H. pylori* eradication. This premise leads toward new therapies and augments the need to differentiate low-grade from high-grade MALT lymphoma before adopting a therapeutic approach. Hence, the therapeutic approach for gastric MALT lymphoma should be different according to the histologic grade, i.e. low or high-grade. Although treatment of low-grade MALT lymphoma remains controversial, medical treatment such as eradication of *H. pylori* or chemotherapy is usually the primary recommendation. Dual or triple therapy including antibiotics and a proton pump inhibitor seems very promising, resulting in 60–70% complete remission (BAYERDORFFER et al. 1995; ROGGERO et al. 1995). Many investigators supposed *H. pylori* eradication to be the first step of treatment, with surgery being reserved for those cases in which this treatment fails. On the other hand, high-grade MALT lymphoma is generally treated by radical gastrectomy and adjuvant chemotherapy with or without radiation therapy.

10.4
MALT Lymphomas of Other Sites

Although as many as 60% of all MALT lymphomas occur in the gastrointestinal tract, especially the stomach, the tumor often involves nonmucosal epithelia, e.g. salivary gland, thyroid, conjunctiva or breast, mucosal sites without a significant amount of normal lymphoid tissue, e.g. lung, or nonepithelial tissues, e.g. orbital soft tissue. The non-gastrointestinal sites more frequently involved by MALT lymphomas are the lung, orbital soft tissue, and head and neck (ZINZANI et al. 1999; THIEBLEMONT et al. 1997; KIM et al. 2001). These low-grade MALT lymphomas are also histologically remarkably homogeneous. Although none has been studied to the same depth as gastric lymphoma, there is no reason to believe that their biological or clinical behaviors are significantly different. In particular, a preceding chronic inflammatory disorder that results in "acquired MALT" is a common theme. Clearly, the causes of this chronic inflammation differ and their identification could provide new insights into treatment of these tumors comparable to the novel therapy for low-grade gastric MALT lymphoma.

10.4.1
Pulmonary MALT Lymphoma

MALT lymphoma of the lung, previously referred to as pseudolymphoma, also consists of aggregates of extranodal B-cells (T-cells in a small percentage of cases). MALT, sometimes known as bronchus-associated lymphoid tissue (BALT), has been shown to accumulate around bronchioles in neonates with pneumonia acquired in utero and in the fully developed lung as follicular bronchiolitis (GOULD and ISAACSON, 1993). It is assumed that pulmonary MALT lymphoma develops in the setting of this acquired MALT and this seems to be so in cases of pulmonary MALT lymphoma described in children with AIDS (TERUYA-FELDSTEIN et al. 1995). In a few cases, a temporal relationship between the respiratory infection and subsequent development of MALT lymphoma has been established (HOLLAND et al. 1991). MALT lymphoma may be seen in patients with dysgammaglobulinemia, Sjögren syndrome, various collagen vascular diseases, and HIV or AIDS (KRADIN and MARK 1983; McGUINNESS et al. 1995; TERUYA-FELDSTEIN et al. 1995). An autoimmune disease or other chronic antigenic stimulus may explain the nature of this tumor.

Most patients are asymptomatic, and the lesion of pulmonary MALT lymphoma is likely to be detected incidentally on chest radiographs (HOLLAND 1991). Despite the wide age range reported, i.e. from 11 to 80 years, middle-aged persons are most frequently involved (KINSELY et al. 1999; FEIGIN et al. 1977). According to a report reviewing 62 cases of primary pulmonary lymphomas (LI et al. 1990), patients with high-grade MALT lymphoma were older than those with low-grade MALT lymphoma, i.e. peak occurrence in the seventh versus the sixth decade.

Although radiographic presentation varies, with solitary or multiple nodules, alveolar or interstitial disease, and localized or diffuse involvement, common findings include a solitary or multifocal, round or segmental area of parenchymal consolidation (Figs. 10.12, 10.13) (HOLLAND et al. 1991; FEIGIN et al. 1977; JULSRUD et al. 1978). The consolidation may be central or peripheral, without a lobar predilection, and commonly shows a dense central lesion with an indistinct outer margin. Because these lesions are indolent, they may reach a large size before discovery. Air bronchograms commonly are present but cavitation, pleural effusions, and hilar or mediastinal lymphadenopathy are uncommon (KENNEDY et al. 1985). FEIGIN et al. (1977) reported that the most common radiographic finding in patients with pulmonary MALT lymphoma was the presence of sev-

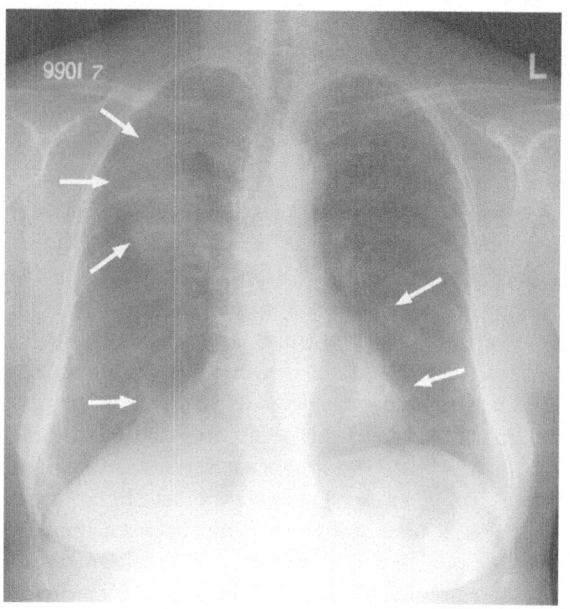

Fig. 10.12. Pulmonary MALT lymphoma in a 46-year-old man. Posteroanterior chest radiograph shows multifocal patchy consolidations (*arrows*), randomly scattered in both lungs. These lesions reveal indistinct outer margins but pleural effusion or hilar lymphadenoapathy is not seen.

eral, 2–5 cm sized masses scattered randomly in both lungs. They also found that there was neither pleural effusion nor lymphadenopathy.

On CT scans, the most common appearance of MALT lymphoma is an area of consolidation with air bronchograms (Figs. 10.12, 10.13), correlating histologically with a cellular lymphocytic infiltrate expanding the interstitium and compressing adjacent alveoli, producing air bronchograms. Nodules are the second most common CT finding in pulmonary MALT lymphoma, especially peribronchovascular nodules (KINSELY et al. 1999; McGUINNESS et al. 1995; CATTELANI et al. 1996). McGUINNESS et al. (1995) described numerous 2- to 4-mm diameter nodules superimposed on areas of ground-glass attenuation with associated bronchiectasis in their single case of pulmonary MALT lymphoma in a patient with AIDS.

However, it is still difficult to radiographically differentiate pulmonary MALT lymphoma from primary pulmonary lymphoma because the latter usually presents with localized areas of consolidation, with air bronchograms commonly present on chest radiographs and CT scans (BALIKIAN and HERMAN 1979). Therefore, diagnosis of MALT lymphoma requires

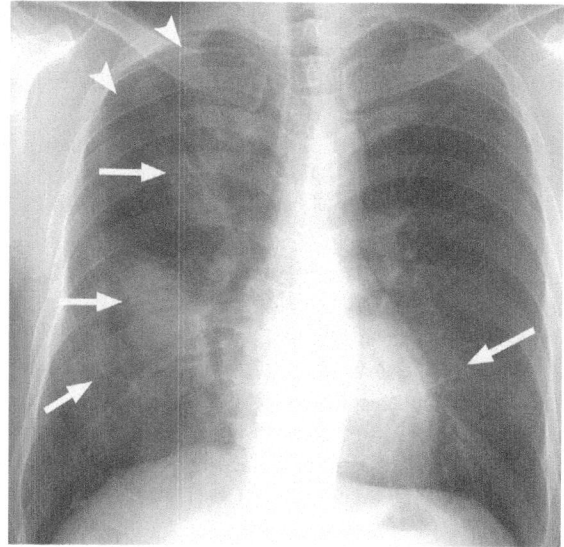

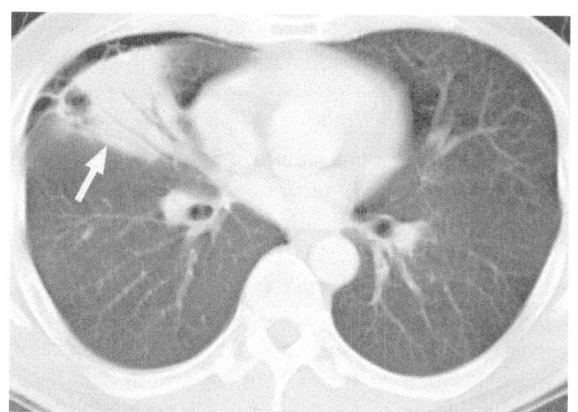

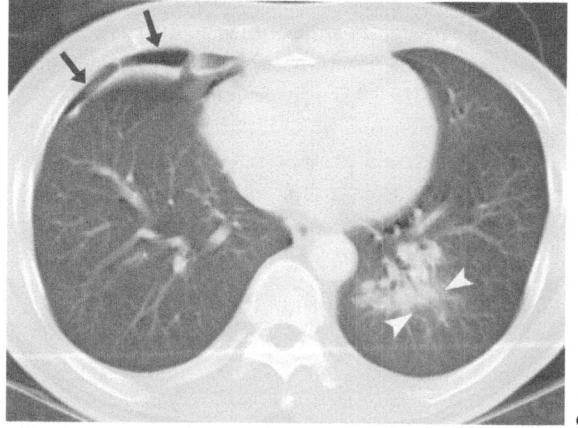

Fig. 10.13a–c. Pulmonary MALT lymphoma in a 57-year-old man. **a** Posteroanterior chest radiograph shows multifocal patchy consolidations (*arrows*) in both lungs. These mass-like lesions with indistinct borders contain air bronchograms. Right pneumothorax (*arrowheads*) and small pleural effusion after lung biopsy are also seen. **b** Axial CT scan reveals right middle lobe consolidation (*arrow*) with air bronchograms. **c** Axial CT scan of inferior lung level shows area of consolidation with air bronchogram superimposed on the area of ground-glass attenuation (*arrowheads*) in left lower lobe. Arrows remark extrapulmonary air, suggesting pneumothorax.

pathologic examination, including morphologic analysis, flow cytometry, and immunohistochemistry.

The preferred treatment of pulmonary MALT lymphoma is surgical resection, and the 5-year survival rate is greater than 80% after complete resection (COGLIATTI et al. 1991). However, in the review by LI et al. (1990) of 43 pulmonary MALT lymphomas, recurrences and metastases in the lung, stomach, lymph nodes, and salivary glands were seen in about 46% of the cases of low-grade MALT lymphoma of the lung. The median interval of relapse in this group was 30 months. From these results, they suggested that in pulmonary MALT lymphomas, local resection was the treatment of choice for limited disease with radiotherapy and chemotherapy reserved for locally advanced and disseminated disease, respectively. Because the presence of hilar or mediastinal adenopathy or chest wall invasion indicates unresectable, advanced disease with a poor prognosis, CT is needed for staging (MONTALBAN et al. 1995).

10.4.2
MALT Lymphoma of the Ocular Adnexa

Most orbital lymphomas are composed of monoclonal B-cells. Roughly 10% of non-Hodgkin lymphomas appear in the head and neck regions and lymphoid tumors account for 10% to 15% of orbital masses (PEYSTER and HOOVER 1984). True lymphoid tissue in the eye is found in the subconjunctiva and lacrimal gland. These two areas account for most of the lymphoreticuloses developing at these sites.

Similar to MALT lymphomas at other sites, low-grade MALT lymphomas of the orbit again arise in acquired MALT of the ocular adnexa (WOTHERSPOON et al. 1993; WOTHERSPOON et al. 1994). Low-grade B-cell lymphomas arising primarily in the orbit share all the clinical and histologic features of MALT lymphoma except for the absence of lymphoepithelial lesions, there being no epithelium in the orbit. This begs the question whether the designation "MALT" is entirely appropriate for this lymphoma. The same question arises with respect to low-grade B-cell lymphomas of the skin, dura mater, and even of the soft tissue, all of which have sometimes been characterized as MALT lymphomas.

Lymphoid neoplasms of the orbit span a large continuum of various classifications from malignant lymphomas to benign pseudolymphoma and pseudotumors (FLANDERS et al. 1987). Although there are no absolute imaging, clinical, or even laboratory tests to delineate all types of benign orbital lymphoid lesions

from malignant lymphomas, CT and MR imaging can be used to evaluate orbital lymphoid lesions. Despite there being no specific findings, the common finding is a solid homogeneous mass involving the lacrimal gland or other orbital adnexa. Such lesions have a tendency to present with bilateral involvement and mild enhancement. Of particular interest, in low-grade MALT lymphoma of conjunctiva, is their tendency to present as multifocal lesions possibly involving all four conjunctival quadrants. In addition, the shared feature of all orbital lymphoid tumors is their tendency to mold themselves around the orbital structures without evidence of bony erosion. In particular, a bulky lesion in the region of the lacrimal fossa not producing any bony erosion is most likely to be inflammatory or lymphoid (YEO et al. 1982).

MR imaging has proven to be as sensitive as CT for the diagnosis of orbital lymphoma and pseudotumors. It is well known that lymphomas may be more hypointense on T1-weighted MR images than pseudotumors, but lymphomatous lesions may be hyperintense on T2-weighted MR images. MONZEN (2001) reported that a solid homogeneous mass involving both the palpebral and orbital lobes of the lacrimal gland showed slight hyperintensity on T1-weighted MR images and hyperintensity on T2-weighted MR images with fat saturation (Fig. 10.14). They suggested that these MR imaging findings would be helpful in the diagnosis of MALT-type lymphoma.

Based on previous reports of patients with orbital low-grade lymphomas and pseudolymphomas, many of which will not be recognized as MALT lymphomas, surgical excision and radiotherapy show an excellent local control of MALT lymphomas and are recommended as the treatments of choice.

10.4.3
MALT Lymphoma of the Salivary Gland

Primary lymphoma of the salivary glands is an uncommon disease, representing only 1.7–3.1% of all neoplastic disorders of the salivary gland (SHARKEY 1977; GLEESON et al. 1986; SCHUSTERMAN et al. 1988). Among them, 21–50% of salivary gland lymphomas occur in patients affected by autoimmune diseases, particularly Sjögren syndrome (BARNES et al. 1998; MEHLE et al. 1993). MALT lymphoma can arise in any of the major or minor salivary glands. The parotid gland is most frequently involved, most likely because of the frequent presence of intraglandular lymph nodes and lymphoid tissue, which are usually absent in other

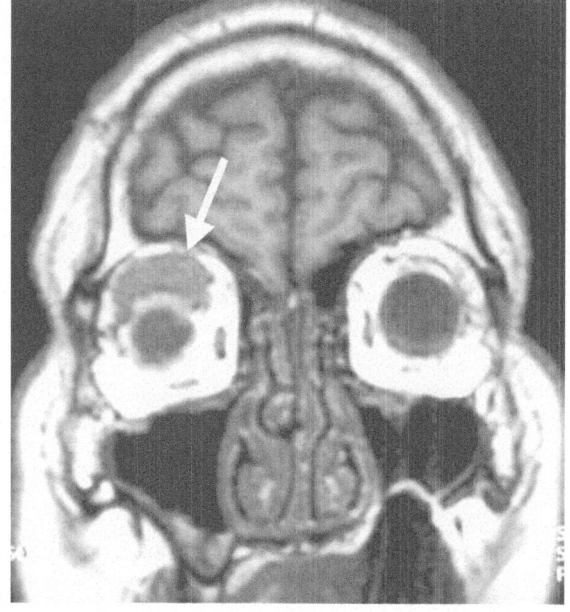

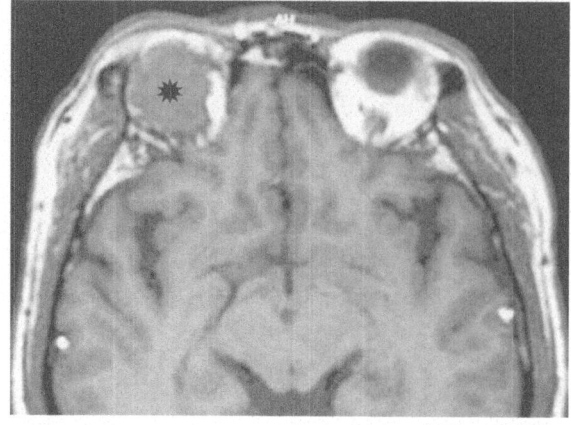

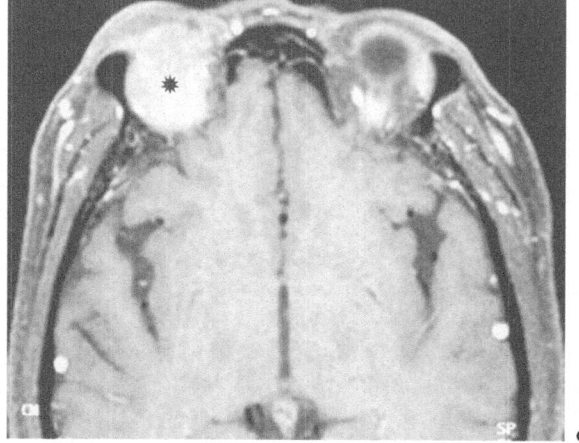

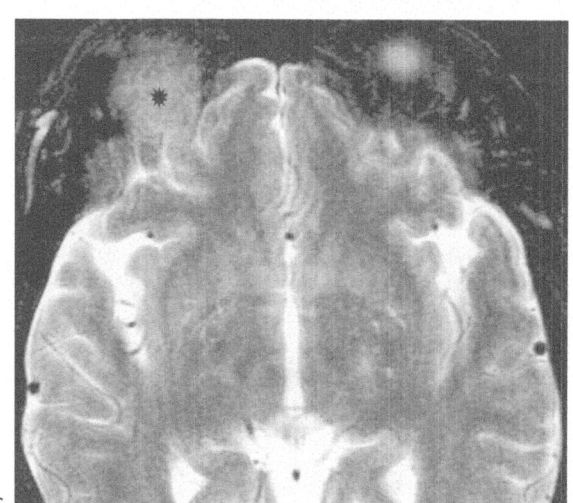

Fig. 10.14a–d. Low-grade MALT lymphoma involving ocular adnexa in a 63-year-old man. a The right superior rectus muscle is replaced by a solid homogenous mass (*arrow*). As compared with signal intensity of adjacent muscles, this mass (*asterisk*) is isointense on (b) T1-weighted MR image, slightly hyperintense on (c) T2-weighted MR image and enhances homogenously and intensely after (d) contrast administration. Note no evidence of tumor invasion into adjacent structures such as bone.

salivary glands (BATSAKIS 1986). Like the stomach, the salivary glands are normally devoid of lymphoid tissue. MALT accumulates in salivary gland tissue as a consequence of Sjögren syndrome and other as yet uncharacterized chronic inflammatory disorders. This lymphoid tissue at first accumulates as Peyer patch-like structures adjacent to dilated ducts. This progresses to the condition known as myoepithelial sialadenitis (MESA) (GENTA et al. 1993) where there is a diffuse lymphoid infiltrate of the salivary gland containing islands of coalescent ductal epithelium infiltrated by B-cells, so-called lymphoepithelial lesions.

Lymphomas of the salivary glands usually present with painless masses. Less frequent clinical mani-

festations are facial nerve paresis, painful mass and enlargement of cervical lymph nodes (BARNES et al. 1998). They rarely occur in patients younger than 50 years, and the sex distribution is roughly equal (GLEESON et al. 1986). Although there are few radiologic reports of MALT lymphoma of the salivary glands, the most common feature is a solid mass or mass-like enlargement of the involved salivary glands with a relatively homogeneous nature and mild, somewhat mixed enhancement (Fig. 10.15). Extensive lymphadenopathy is also frequently present. Typically, MALT lymphomas arising in the parotid gland tend to disseminate to other major and minor salivary glands, the lacrimal gland, stomach, and cervical lymph nodes. When salivary gland

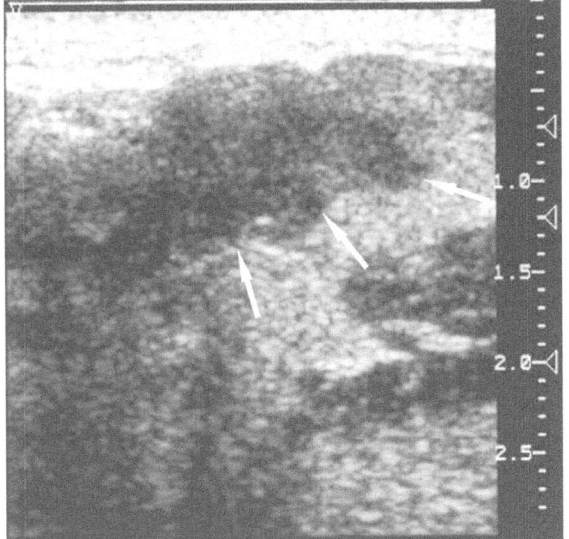

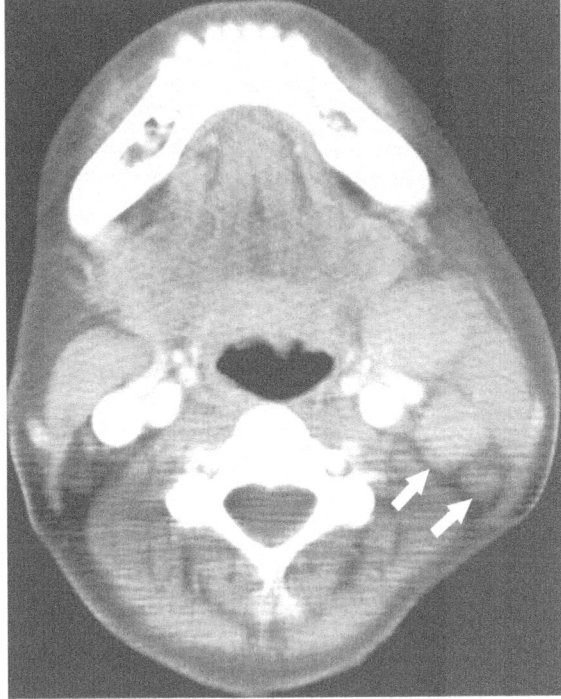

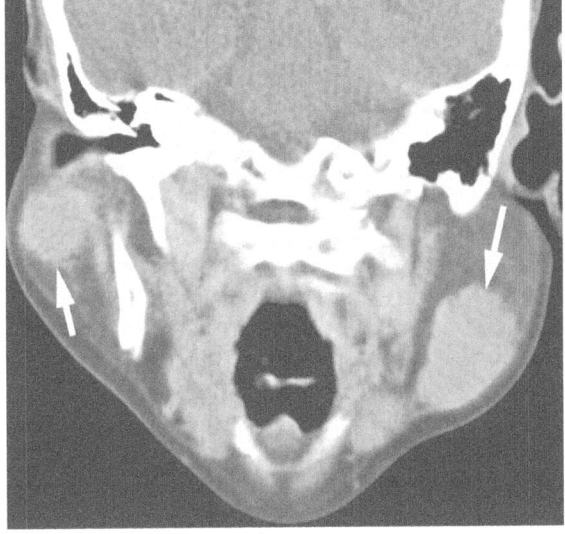

Fig. 10.15a–c. Low-grade MALT lymphoma involving salivary glands in a 56-year-old man. a Transaxial ultrasound image shows a well-defined low echoic mass (*arrows*) in the right submandibular gland. b Coronal reformatted image of contrast-enhanced CT scan shows well enhancing homogenous solid masses (*arrows*) within bilateral parotid glands. c At the lower level, axial CT scan reveals left cervical lymphadenopathy (*arrows*).

MALT lymphoma disseminates to lymph nodes, the lymph node histology is indistinguishable from so-called monocytic B-cell lymphoma. This may account for the reported tendency of monocytoid B-cell lymphoma to occur in association with Sjögren syndrome (NGAN et al. 1991). Whenever a diagnosis of nodal monocytoid B-cell lymphoma is considered, it is prudent to exclude primary salivary gland MALT lymphoma.

Although the best treatment of MALT lymphoma remains controversial, the tendency of this disorder not to disseminate for a long time suggests the choice of a local therapy – surgical treatment first. Radiotherapy or chemotherapy should be added in cases of partial removal, or of disseminated forms of this disease.

10.4.4
Proposals for Treatment

Currently, the largest reported series of non-gastrointestinal MALT lymphomas had a high complete remission (CR) rate of 79% and a high overall response rate of 100% (ZINZANI et al. 1999). With respect to the specific sites, all thyroid lymphoma patients obtained a CR (100%), whereas patients with involvement at other sites, e.g. lung, orbital soft tissue, skin, lacrimal gland, conjunctiva, or salivary gland, had CR rates ranging from 67% to 79%. A particularly poor response was noted among those patients with concomitant mucosal and bone marrow involvement who had a CR rate of only 34%

(GRAZIADEI et al. 1998). Therefore, the therapeutic approach should be modified according to which organs are involved.

Based on previous reports, chemotherapy was most effective for lung disease whereas surgical excision and radiotherapy or local IFNa2a were preferred for the orbital soft tissue and conjunctiva, respectively (ZINZANI et al. 1999). With regard to the specific therapeutic approaches, the effectiveness of combination therapy (chemotherapy plus radiation therapy) in the majority of sites, effectiveness of local treatment in particular sites where radiation therapy could be the cause of unpleasant and dangerous sequelae, and the role of chemotherapy (using CHOP or CHOP-like regimens) in the lung, should also be considered. Nevertheless, no firm conclusions can be drawn at this point regarding the most appropriate treatment with respect to the stage of the lymphoma.

The therapeutic approach to MALT lymphoma patients must be tailored to the specific site of the lymphoma, making it extremely difficult to stratify various early- and advanced-stage treatments. The demonstrated possibility of achieving successful results and long-lasting survival in all patients by means of differentiated therapeutic approaches in accordance with the particular extranodal site, underlines the importance of correctly identifying non-gastrointestinal MALT lymphoma.

10.5
Disseminated MALT Lymphoma

Low-grade gastric MALT lymphoma shows indolent tumor rarely involving adjacent organs and lymphadenopathy. However, these lymphomas can disseminate to other mucosal sites including primarily the lung, parotid gland, and small bowel, which occurs more frequently than has been previously reported (Fig. 10.16). BLAZQUEZ et al. (1992) found systemic manifestation in eight of 16 patients with low-grade gastric MALT lymphoma. Similarly, recent reports (THIEBLEMONT et al. 2000; ZINZANI et al. 1999) considering 76 to 158 cases of MALT lymphoma showed that about one-third of these patients presented with dissemination at the time of diagnosis. This contrasts with what has usually been reported in the literature (MONTALBAN et al. 1995) where MALT lymphoma presents as a localized disease in approximately 90% of the patients and remains confined to the site of origin for a prolonged period after diagno-

sis. However, this discrepancy seems to be explained by the site of origin presenting at the time of clinical manifestation. Because gastric discomfort or vague epigastric pain induces early clinical manifestation and the stomach is easily assessable to a diagnostic approach, gastric MALT lymphoma is likely to be detected at an early stage.

When dissemination has occurred, usually described as late in the course of the disease after many relapses (ZUCCA et al. 1998), its tendency is to metastasize to another site within the organ of origin or to another MALT-containing organ. This particular behavior, unique among lymphomas, has been described by ISAACSON (1995) as the MALT concept. Biologically, both dissemination inside the same organ of origin and inside MALT-containing organs, may be linked to the expression of special homing receptors or adhesion molecules at the surface of MALT normal cells and MALT lymphoma cells (DOGAN et al. 1997). THIEBLEMONT et al. (2000) reviewed 158 cases of MALT lymphoma, and found that one-third of these patients presented at diagnosis with dissemination. These multiple mucosal sites included not only the gastrointestinal tract, such as the stomach or intestines, but also non-gastrointestinal tract organs such as the lung. This is in keeping with the homing theory of neoplastic lymphocytes. However, in regard to another dissemination pattern observed in non-MALT sites such as the spleen or bone marrow, debate continues on whether or not dissemination is related to a preferential homing (HARRIS et al. 1996; DU et al. 1997).

Observations of some investigators who reported early dissemination of the MALT lymphoma led us to believe that at diagnosis, MALT lymphoma should be considered a multifocal disease with involvement in MALT or non-MALT-containing organs (DU et al. 1996). However, there has been no answer regarding the possible clinical impact and furthermore, the possible changes in diagnostic or therapeutic strategy as a result of this observation in patients presenting with MALT lymphoma. Indeed, THIEBLEMONT et al. (2000) observed the same outcome in patients with disseminated and localized MALT lymphoma, particularly with similar freedom-from-progression survivals. They concluded, despite the high percentage of dissemination, that MALT lymphoma is an indolent disease.

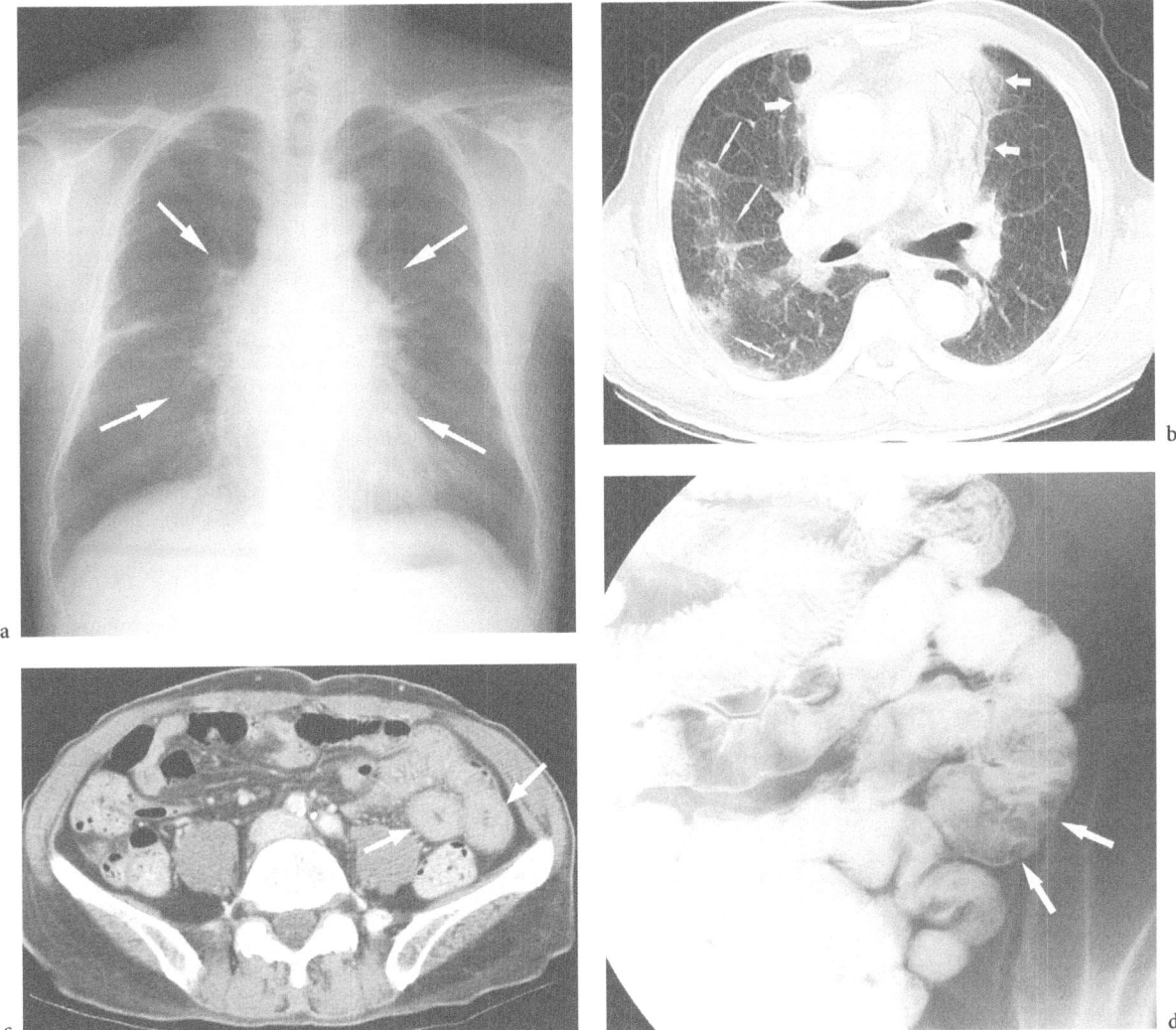

Fig. 10.16a–d. Disseminated MALT lymphoma in a 68-year-old man. **a** Posteroanterior chest radiograph shows indistinct bordered perihilar opacities (*arrows*) in both lungs. **b** Axial chest CT scan reveals poorly defined multifocal patchy consolidations (*thick arrows*) and ground-glass attenuations (*thin arrows*) in both lungs. **c** Axial image of abdominopelvic CT scan shows multifocal, concentric bowel wall thickening (*arrows*) in distal small bowel. **d** Spot radiograph of small bowel follow-through examination shows multiple mural nodules (*arrows*) and bowel wall thickening (*not seen*) in distal ileal loops. These lesions of lung and small bowel proved to be MALT lymphoma involvement on open biopsy and surgical resection.

10.6
Conclusion

MALT lymphomas behave as an indolent disease with a prolonged clinical course. Unlike other lymphomas, these disorders tend to remain localized for prolonged periods and show good outcome with a long overall survival. Because of the distinctive clinical and pathologic characteristics compared to other lymphomas, MALT lymphomas provide new treatment insights.

MALT lymphomas can arise not only from the gastrointestinal tract but also from various non gas-

trointestinal sites such as lung, salivary gland, conjunctiva, thyroid, and orbit. Among them, the stomach is the most common site for MALT lymphoma, resulting from lymphoid tissue acquired as the result of a *Helicobacter pylori* infection. Low-grade gastric MALT lymphoma is a curable disease by eradication of *H. pylori* and does not involve surgery, radiation therapy, or chemotherapy. Radiologists should be fully aware of the characteristic radiologic features of this disease, especially those findings found on barium and CT studies. Unfortunately, there is a low threshold for suggesting this diagnosis when suspicious findings are present, in particular on the barium study. An aggressive approach seems warranted for patients with possible radiographic findings of gastric MALT lymphoma because of the important ramifications of early diagnosis of this treatable form of malignant tumor.

Acknowledgements:
The authors are deeply grateful to Prof. Jin Seong Lee, Department of Radiology, University of Ulsan College of Medicine, Seoul, Korea, for invaluable advice and comments about pulmonary MALT lymphoma, and to Bonnie Hami, Department of Radiology, University Hospitals of Cleveland, OH, for her editorial assistance.

References

Abbondanzo SL, Sobin LH (1997) Gastric "pseudolymphoma": a retrospective morphologic and immunophenotypic study of 97 cases. Cancer 79:1656–1663

An SK, Han JK, Kim AY, et al (2001) Gastric mucosa-associated lymphoid tissue lymphoma: spectrum of findings at double contrast gastrointestinal examination with pathologic correlation. RadioGraphics 21:1491–1504

Aozasa K, Tsujimoto M, Inoue A et al (1985) Primary gastrointestinal lymphoma. A clinicopathologic study of 102 patients. Oncology 42:97–103

Ascoli V, Lo Coco F, Artini M et al (1998) Extranodal lymphomas associated with hepatitis C virus infection. Am J Clin Pathol 109:600–609

Azab MB, Henry-Amar M, Rougier P et al (1989) Prognostic factors in primary gastrointestinal non-Hodgkin's lymphoma. A multivariate analysis, report of 106 cases, and review of the literature. Cancer 64:1208–1217

Balikian JP, Herman PG (1979) Non-Hodgkin lymphoma of the lungs. Radiology 132:569–576

Barnes L, Myers EN, Prokopakis EP (1998) Primary malignant lymphoma of the parotid gland. Arch Otolaryngol Head Neck Surg 124:573–577

Batsakis JG (1986) Primary lymphomas of the major salivary glands. Ann Otol Rhinol Laryngol 95:107–108

Bayerdorffer E, Neubauer A, Rudolph B et al (1995) Regression of primary gastric lymphoma of mucosa-associated lymphoid tissue type after cure of Helicobacter pylori infection. MALT Lymphoma Study Group. Lancet 345:1591–1594

Bayerdorffer E, Miehlke S, Neubauer A, Stolte M (1997) Gastric MALT-lymphoma and Helicobacter pylori infection. Aliment Pharmacol Ther 11(Suppl 1):89–94

Blazquez M, Haioun C, Chaumette MT et al (1992) Low grade B cell mucosa associated lymphoid tissue lymphoma of the stomach: clinical and endoscopic features, treatment, and outcome. Gut 33:1621–1625

Bouzourene H, Haefliger T, Delacretaz F, Saraga E (1999) The role of Helicobacter pylori in primary gastric MALT lymphoma. Histopathology 34:118–123

Brooks JJ, Enterline HT (1983) Gastric pseudolymphoma. Its three subtypes and relation to lymphoma. Cancer 51:476–486

Burke JS, Sheibani K, Nathwani BN, Winberg CD, Rappaport H (1987) Monoclonal small (well-differentiated) lymphocytic proliferations of the gastrointestinal tract resembling lymphoid hyperplasia: a neoplasm of uncertain malignant potential. Hum Pathol 18:1238–1245

Calvert R, Randerson J, Evans P et al (1995) Genetic abnormalities during transition from Helicobacter-pylori-associated gastritis to low-grade MALToma. Lancet 345:26–27

Cammarota G, Tursi A, Papa A et al (1997) The growth of primary low-grade B-cell gastric lymphoma is sustained by Helicobacter pylori. Scand J Gastroenterol 32:285–287

Cattelani L, Solli P, Rusca M et al (1996) Primary pulmonary lymphoma: report of a case diagnosed by transbronchial biopsy. J Cardiovasc Surg 37:539–541

Castrillo JM, Montalban C, Obeso G, Piris MA, Rivas MC (1992) Gastric B-cell mucosa associated lymphoid tissue lymphoma: a clinicopathological study in 56 patients. Gut 33:1307–1311

Chan JK, Ng CS, Isaacson PG (1990) Relationship between high-grade lymphoma and low-grade B-cell mucosa-associated lymphoid tissue lymphoma (MALToma) of the stomach. Am J Pathol 136:1153–1164

Choi D, Lim HK, Lee SJ et al (2002) Gastric mucosa-associated lymphoid tissue lymphoma: helical CT findings and pathologic correlation. AJR Am J Roentgenol 178:1117–1122

Cogliatti SB, Schmid U, Schumacher U et al (1991) Primary B-cell gastric lymphoma: a clinicopathological study of 145 patients. Gastroenterology 101:1159–1170

Cooper DL, Doria R, Salloum E (1996) Primary gastrointestinal lymphomas. Gastroenterologist 4:54–64

de Jong D, Boot H, van Heerde P, Hart GA, Taal BG (1997) Histological grading in gastric lymphoma: pretreatment criteria and clinical relevance. Gastroenterology 112:1466–1474

Dogan A, Du M, Koulis A, Briskin MJ, Isaacson PG (1997) Expression of lymphocyte homing receptors and vascular addressins in low-grade gastric B-cell lymphomas of mucosa-associated lymphoid tissue. Am J Pathol 151:1361–1369

Du MQ, Xu CF, Diss TC et al (1996) Intestinal dissemination of gastric mucosa-associated lymphoid tissue lymphoma. Blood 88:4445–4451

Du MQ, Peng HZ, Dogan A et al (1997) Preferential dissemination of B-cell gastric mucosa-associated lymphoid tissue (MALT) lymphoma to the splenic marginal zone. Blood 90:4071–4077

Eidt S, Stolte M (1993) Prevalence of lymphoid follicles and aggregates in Helicobacter pylori gastritis in antral and body mucosa. J Clin Pathol 46:832–835

Feigin DS, Siegelman SS, Theros EG, King FM (1977) Nonmalignant lymphoid disorders of the chest. AJR Am J Roentgenol 129:221–228

Flanders AE, Espinosa GA, Markiewicz DA, Howell DD (1987) Orbital lymphoma. Role of CT and MRI. Radiol Clin North Am 25:601–613

Freeman C, Berg JW, Cutler SJ (1972) Occurrence and prognosis of extranodal lymphomas. Cancer 29:252–260

Genta RM, Hamner HW, Graham DY (1993) Gastric lymphoid follicles in Helicobacter pylori infection: frequency, distribution, and response to triple therapy. Hum Pathol 24:577–583

Gleeson MJ, Bennett MH, Cawson RA (1986) Lymphomas of salivary glands. Cancer 58:699–704

Gollub MJ, Latrenta L, Yahalom J et al (1999) Utility of abdominal CT in gastric MALT lymphoma (abstr). AJR Am J Roentgenol 172:56–57

Gould SJ, Isaacson PG (1993) Bronchus-associated lymphoid tissue (BALT) in human fetal and infant lung. J Pathol 169: 229–234

Grau E, Gomez A, Cunat A, Oltra C (1996) Computed tomography in staging of primary gastric lymphoma. Lancet 347:1261

Graziadei G, Pruneri G, Carboni N et al (1998) Low-grade MALT lymphoma involving multiple mucosal sites and bone marrow. Ann Hematol 76:81–83

Greiner TC, Medeiros LJ, Jaffe ES (1995) Non-Hodgkin's lymphoma. Cancer 75(Suppl 1):370–380

Hall JG, Smith ME (1970) Homing of lymph-borne immunoblasts to the gut. Nature 226:262–263

Harris NL, Jaffe ES, Stein H et al (1994) A revised European-American classification of lymphoid neoplasms: a proposal from the International Lymphoma Study Group. Blood. 84:1361–1392

Harris S, Wilkins BS, Jones DB (1996) Splenic marginal zone expansion in B-cell lymphomas of gastrointestinal mucosa-associated lymphoid tissue (MALT) is reactive and does not represent homing of neoplastic lymphocytes. J Pathol 179:49–53

Heilmann KL, Borchard F (1991) Gastritis due to spiral shaped bacteria other than Helicobacter pylori: clinical, histological, and ultrastructural findings. Gut 32:137–140

Holland EA, Ghahremani GG, Fry WA, Victor TA (1991) Evolution of pulmonary pseudolymphomas: clinical and radiologic manifestations. J Thorac Imaging 6:74–80

Hoshida Y, Kusakabe H, Furukawa H et al (1997) Reassessment of gastric lymphoma in light of the concept of mucosa-associated lymphoid tissue lymphoma: analysis of 53 patients. Cancer 80:1151–1159

Husband AJ (1982) Kinetics of extravasation and redistribution of IgA-specific antibody-containing cells in the intestine. J Immunol 128:1355–1359

Hussell T, Isaacson PG, Crabtree JE, Dogan A, Spencer J (1993a) Immunoglobulin specificity of low grade B cell gastrointestinal lymphoma of mucosa-associated lymphoid tissue (MALT) type. Am J Pathol 142:285–292

Hussell T, Isaacson PG, Crabtree JE, Spencer J (1993b) The response of cells from low-grade B-cell gastric lymphomas of mucosa-associated lymphoid tissue to Helicobacter pylori. Lancet 342:571–574

Isaacson PG (1990) Lymphomas of mucosa-associated lymphoid tissue (MALT). Histopathology 16:617–619

Isaacson PG (1992) Extranodal lymphomas: the MALT concept. Verh Dtsch Ges Pathol. 76:14–23

Isaacson PG (1994) Gastrointestinal lymphoma. Hum Pathol 25:1020–1029

Isaacson PG (1995) The MALT lymphoma concept updated. Ann Oncol 6:319–320

Isaacson PG (1996) Recent developments in our understanding of gastric lymphomas. Am J Surg Pathol 20(Suppl 1):S1–7

Isaacson PG (1999) Gastric MALT lymphoma: from concept to cure. Ann Oncol 10:637–645

Isaacson PG, Wright DH (1983) Malignant lymphoma of mucosa-associated lymphoid tissue. A distinctive type of B-cell lymphoma. Cancer 52:1410–1416

Isaacson PG, Wright DH (1984) Extranodal malignant lymphoma arising from mucosa-associated lymphoid tissue. Cancer 53:2515–2524

Isaacson PG, Spencer J, Finn T (1986) Primary B-cell gastric lymphoma. Hum Pathol 17:72–82

Isaacson PG, Spencer J (1987) Malignant lymphoma of mucosa-associated lymphoid tissue. Histopathology 11: 445–462

Isaacson PG, Spencer J (1993) Is gastric lymphoma an infectious disease? Hum Pathol 24:569–570

Jaffe ES, Harris NL, Diebold J, Muller-Hermelink HK (1999) World Health Organization classification of neoplastic diseases of the hematopoietic and lymphoid tissues. A progress report. Am J Clin Pathol 111(Suppl 1):S8–S12

Julsrud PR, Brown LR, Li CY, Rosenow EC 3rd, Crowe JK (1978) Pulmonary processes of mature-appearing lymphocytes: pseudolymphoma, well-differentiated lymphocytic lymphoma, and lymphocytic interstitial pneumonitis. Radiology 127:289–296

Karat D, O'Hanlon DM, Hayes N, Scott D, Raimes SA, Griffin SM (1995) Prospective study of Helicobacter pylori infection in primary gastric lymphoma. Br J Surg 82: 1369–1370

Kath R, Donhuijsen K, Hayungs J, Albrecht K, Seeber S, Hoffken K (1995) Primary gastric non-Hodgkin's lymphoma: a clinicopathological study of 41 patients. J Cancer Res Clin Oncol 121:51–56

Kennedy JL, Nathwani BN, Burke JS, Hill LR, Rappaport H (1985) Pulmonary lymphomas and other pulmonary lymphoid lesions. A clinicopathologic and immunologic study of 64 patients. Cancer 56:539–552

Kessar P, Norton A, Rohatiner AZ, Lister TA, Reznek RH (1999) CT appearances of mucosa-associated lymphoid tissue (MALT) lymphoma. Eur Radiol 9:693–696

Kim HJ, Kim AY, Kim TK et al (2001) Systemic manifestation of Mucosa-associated Lymphoid Tissue Lymphoma. Radiology 221:S685

Kim YH, Lim HK, Han JK et al (1999) Low-grade gastric mucosa-associated lymphoid tissue lymphoma: correlation of radiographic and pathologic findings. Radiology 212:241–248

Kinsely BL, Mastey LA, Mergo PJ et al (1999) Pulmonary mucosa-associated lymphoid tissue lymphoma: CT and pathologic findings. AJR Am J Roentgenol 172:1321–1326

Kitamura K, Yamaguchi T, Okamoto K et al (1996) Early gastric lymphoma: a clinicopathologic study of ten patients, literature review, and comparison with early gastric adenocarcinoma. Cancer 77:850–857

Kradin RL, Mark EJ (1983) Benign lymphoid disorders of the lung, with a theory regarding their development. Hum Pathol 14:857–867

Lewin KJ, Ranchod M, Dorfman RF (1978) Lymphomas of the gastrointestinal tract: a study of 117 cases presenting with gastrointestinal disease. Cancer 42:693–707

Li G, Hansmann ML, Zwingers T, Lennert K (1990) Primary lymphomas of the lung: morphological, immunohistochemical and clinical features. Histopathology 16:519–531

McGuinness G, Scholes JV, Jagirdar JS et al (1995) Unusual lymphoproliferative disorders in nine adults with HIV or AIDS: CT and pathologic findings. Radiology 197:59–65

Megraud F, Brassens-Rabbe MP, Denis F, Belbouri A, Hoa DQ (1989) Seroepidemiology of Campylobacter pylori infection in various populations. J Clin Microbiol 27:1870–1873

Mehle ME, Kraus DH, Wood BG, Tubbs R, Tucker HM, Lavertu P (1993) Facial nerve morbidity following parotid surgery for benign disease: the Cleveland Clinic Foundation experience. Laryngoscope 103:71–21

Miettinen A, Karttunen TJ, Alavaikko M (1995) Lymphocytic gastritis and Helicobacter pylori infection in gastric lymphoma. Gut 37:471–476

Montalban C, Castrillo JM, Abraira V et al (1995a) Gastric B-cell mucosa-associated lymphoid tissue (MALT) lymphoma. Clinicopathological study and evaluation of the prognostic factors in 143 patients. Ann Oncol 6:355–362

Montalban C, Manzanal A, Castrillo JM, Escribano L, Bellas C (1995b) Low grade gastric B-cell MALT lymphoma progressing into high grade lymphoma. Clonal identity of the two stages of the tumour, unusual bone involvement and leukemic dissemination. Histopathology 27:89–91

Monzen Y (2001) MALT-type lymphoma of the lacrimal gland: a case report. Nippon Igaku Hoshasen Gakkai Zasshi 61: 733–735

Moore I, Wright DH (1984) Primary gastric lymphoma-a tumour of mucosa-associated lymphoid tissue. A histological and immunohistochemical study of 36 cases. Histopathology 8:1025–1039

Myhre MJ, Isaacson PG (1987) Primary B-cell gastric lymphoma-a reassessment of its histogenesis. J Pathol 152:1–11

Nakamura S, Akazawa K, Yao T, Tsuneyoshi M (1995) A clinicopathologic study of 233 cases with special reference to evaluation with the MIB-1 index. Cancer 76:1313–1324

Nakamura S, Yao T, Aoyagi K, Iida M, Fujishima M, Tsuneyoshi M (1997) Helicobacter pylori and primary gastric lymphoma. A histopathologic and immunohistochemical analysis of 237 patients. Cancer 79:3–11

Nakamura S, Aoyagi K, Furuse M et al (1998) B-cell monoclonality precedes the development of gastric MALT lymphoma in Helicobacter pylori-associated chronic gastritis. Am J Pathol 152:1271–1279

Neri A, Jakobiec FA, Pelicci PG, Dalla-Favera R, Knowles DM 2nd (1987) Immunoglobulin and T cell receptor beta chain gene rearrangement analysis of ocular adnexal lymphoid neoplasms: clinical and biologic implications. Blood 70: 1519–1529

Ngan BY, Warnke RA, Wilson M, Takagi K, Cleary ML, Dorfman RF (1991) Monocytoid B-cell lymphoma: a study of 36 cases. Hum Pathol 22:409–421

Nicholson AG, Wotherspoon AC, Jones AL, Sheppard MN, Isaacson PG, Corrin B (1996) Pulmonary B-cell non-Hodgkin's lymphoma associated with autoimmune disorders: a clinicopathological review of six cases. Eur Respir J 9:2022–2025

Park MS, Kim KW, Yu JS (2002) Radiographic findings of primary B-cell lymphoma of the stomach: low-grade versus high-grade malignancy in relation to the mucosa-associated lymphoid tissue concept. AJR Am J Roentgenol 179: 1297–1304

Parsonnet J, Hansen S, Rodriguez L (1994) Helicobacter pylori infection and gastric lymphoma. N Engl J Med 330: 1267–1271

Peyster RG, Hoover ED (1984) Computerized tomography in orbital disease and neuro-ophthalomogy, 1st edn. Chicago Year Book Medical Publishers, Chicago

Radaszkiewicz T, Dragosics B, Bauer P (1992) Gastrointestinal malignant lymphomas of the mucosa-associated lymphoid tissue: factors relevant to prognosis. Gastroenterology 102: 1628–1638

Roggero E, Zucca E, Pinotti G (1995) Eradication of Helicobacter pylori infection in primary low-grade gastric lymphoma of mucosa-associated lymphoid tissue. Ann Intern Med 122:767–769

Ruskone-Fourmestraux A, Aegerter P, Delmer A, Brousse N, Galian A, Rambaud JC (1993) Primary digestive tract lymphoma: a prospective multicentric study of 91 patients. Groupe d'Etude des Lymphomes Digestifs. Gastroenterology 105:1662–1671

Sato T, Sakai Y, Ishiguro S, Furukawa H (1986) Radiologic manifestations of early gastric lymphoma. AJR Am J Roentgenol 146:513–517

Schusterman MA, Granick MS, Erickson ER, Newton ED, Hanna DC, Bragdon RW (1988) Lymphoma presenting as a salivary gland mass. Head Neck Surg 10:411–415

Sigal SH, Saul SH, Auerbach HE, Raffensperger E, Kant JA, Brooks JJ (1989) Gastric small lymphocytic proliferation with immunoglobulin gene rearrangement in pseudolymphoma versus lymphoma. Gastroenterology 97:195–201

Sharkey FE (1977) Systematic evaluation of the World Health Organization classification of salivary gland tumors: a clinicopathologic study of 366 cases. Am J Clin Pathol 67:272–278

Sohn J, Levine MS, Furth EE et al (1995) Helicobacter pylori gastritis: radiographic findings. Radiology 195:763–767

Spencer J, Diss TC, Isaacson PG (1989) Primary B cell gastric lymphoma. A genotypic analysis. Am J Pathol 135: 557–564

Stolte M, Eidt S (1989) Lymphoid follicles in antral mucosa: immune response to Campylobacter pylori? J Clin Pathol 42:1269–1271

Stolte M, Eidt S (1993) Healing gastric MALT lymphomas by eradicating H pylori? Lancet 342:568

Suekane H, Iida M, Yao T, Matsumoto T, Masuda Y, Fujishima M (1993) Endoscopic ultrasonography in primary gastric lymphoma: correlation with endoscopic and histologic findings. Gastrointest Endosc 39:139–145

Taal BG, den Hartog Jager FC, Burgers JM, van Heerde P, Tio TL (1989) Primary non-Hodgkin's lymphoma of the stomach: changing aspects and therapeutic choices. Eur J Cancer Clin Oncol 25:439–450

Taal BG, Boot H, van Heerde P, de Jong D, Hart AA, Burgers JM (1996) Primary non-Hodgkin lymphoma of the stomach: endoscopic pattern and prognosis in low versus high grade malignancy in relation to the MALT concept. Gut 39:556–561

Teruya-Feldstein J, Temeck BK, Sloas MM et al (1995) Pulmonary malignant lymphoma of mucosa-associated lymphoid tissue (MALT) arising in a pediatric HIV-positive patient. Am J Surg Pathol 19:357–363

The EUROGAST Study Group (1993) Epidemiology of, and risk factors for, Helicobacter pylori infection among 3194 asymptomatic subjects in 17 populations. Gut 34:1672–1676

Thieblemont C, Bastion Y, Berger F et al (1997) Mucosa-associated lymphoid tissue gastrointestinal and nongastrointestinal lymphoma behavior: analysis of 108 patients. J Clin Oncol 15:1624–1630

Thieblemont C, Berger F, Dumontet C et al (2000) Mucosa-associated lymphoid tissue lymphoma is a disseminated disease in one third of 158 patients analyzed. Blood 95: 802–806

Tkoub EM, Haioun C, Pawlotsky JM, Dhumeaux D, Delchier JC (1998) Chronic hepatitis C virus and gastric MALT lymphoma. Blood 91:360

Tokunaga O, Watanabe T, Morimatsu M (1987) Pseudolymphoma of the stomach. A clinicopathologic study of 15
cases. Cancer 59:1320–1327

Weber DM, Dimopoulos MA, Anandu DP, Pugh WC, Stein-
bach G (1994) Regression of gastric lymphoma of mucosa-
associated lymphoid tissue with antibiotic therapy for
Helicobacter pylori. Gastroenterology 107:1835–1838

Wegener OH (1993) Whole body computed tomography, 2nd
edn. Blackwell Scientific, Oxford

Wotherspoon AC, Ortiz-Hidalgo C, Falzon MR, Isaacson PG
(1991) Helicobacter pylori-associated gastritis and primary B-cell gastric lymphoma. Lancet 338:1175–1176

Wotherspoon AC, Doglioni C, Diss TC et al (1993) Regression
of primary low-grade B-cell gastric lymphoma of mucosa-
associated lymphoid tissue type after eradication of Helicobacter pylori. Lancet 342:575–577

Wotherspoon AC, Hardman-Lea S, Isaacson PG (1994)
Mucosa-associated lymphoid tissue (MALT) in the human
conjunctiva. J Pathol 174:33–37

Xu WS, Ho FC, Ho J, Chan AC, Srivastava G (1997) Pathogenesis of gastric lymphoma: the enigma in Hong Kong. Ann
Oncol 8(Suppl 2):41–44

Yeo JH, Jakobiec FA, Abbott GF, Trokel SL (1982) Combined
clinical and computed tomographic diagnosis of orbital
lymphoid tumors. Am J Ophthalmol 94:235–245

Yoshino T, Omonishi K, Kobayashi K et al (2000) Clinicopathological features of gastric mucosa associated lymphoid
tissue (MALT) lymphomas: high grade transformation and
comparison with diffuse large B cell lymphomas without
MALT lymphoma features. J Clin Pathol 53:187–190

Zinzani PL, Magagnoli M, Galieni P et al (1999) Nongastrointestinal low-grade mucosa-associated lymphoid
tissue lymphoma: analysis of 75 patients. J Clin Oncol 17:
1254–1258

Zucca E, Roggero E, Pileri S (1998) B-cell lymphoma of MALT
type: a review with special emphasis on diagnostic and
management problems of low-grade gastric tumours. Br
J Haematol 100:3–14

11 T-Cell Lymphoma

Hyun Ju Lee and Byung Ihn Choi

CONTENTS

Hyun Ju Lee, MD
Instructor of Diagnostic Radiology, Department of Radiology, Seoul National University College of Medicine, 28 Yongon-dong, Chongno-Gu, Seoul 110-744, Korea
Byung Ihn Choi, MD
Professor, Department of Radiology, Seoul National University College of Medicine, 28 Yongon-dong, Chongno-Gu, Seoul 110-744, Korea

11.1 Introduction

The T-cell lymphomas make up a heterogeneous group of aggressive neoplasms that share a T-cell immunophenotype. Although some of the diseases in T-cell lymphomas may have a protracted clinical course, the majority are the most aggressive hematopoietic and lymphoid neoplasms. In general, they have a poorer response to therapy and shorter survival times when compared to B-cell lymphomas and Hodgkin disease (Coiffier et al. 1990; Grogan et al. 1985; Kwak et al. 1991; Melnyk et al. 1997). Although uncommon, the incidence varies quite substantially in cohorts of aggressive non-Hodgkin lymphomas, depending on the series. T-cell lymphomas represent approximately 20–30% of all non-Hodgkin lymphomas in Far East countries and slightly less than 10% in Europe (Harris et al. 1994; Lee et al. 1999; Ko et al. 1998).

Most radiologists are unfamiliar with T-cell lymphomas because such lymphomas comprise a relatively small proportion of lymphoma and have a lower incidence in Western countries. The World Health Organization (WHO) classification of lymphoid neoplasm announced in 1999 aroused new interest in T-cell lymphoma (Harris et al. 1999a; Harris et al. 1999b; Harris et al. 2000a; Harris et al. 2000b). T-cell lymphomas involve various organs including the sinonasal cavity, intestinal tract, skin, lymph nodes, liver, airway, lung, and musculoskeletal system. The pattern of disease involvement is not random and specific clinicopathological entities of T-cell lymphoma have a particular primary location, clinical presentations, and pathological feature. Although the imaging features are often nonspecific, the radiologic features or location in several entities are quite different from those of lymphoma with B-cell phenotype (Lee et al. 2003). In this chapter, T-cell lymphomas will include "precursor T-cell lymphoblastic lymphoma/leukemia" and several clinicopathological entities of "peripheral T-cell lymphoma" based upon the WHO classification of lymphoid neoplasms. We will describe the clinical, pathologic, and radiologic features of each entity.

11.2
General Considerations

11.2.1
Classification and Diagnosis

The classification of lymphoid malignancy evolved steadily throughout the twentieth century. Non-Hodgkin lymphomas were separated from Hodgkin disease by recognition of the Reed-Sternberg cells early in the twentieth century. In the 1950s, Rappaport and colleagues recognized the importance of growth patterns for subdividing non-Hodgkin lymphomas. The Rappaport classification system, which was clinically relevant, was based on growth patterns in addition to cell size and shape. In the 1970s, it was recognized that non-Hodgkin lymphomas were derived from either T or B-cells. This led to immunologically based classifications of lymphomas such as the Lukes-Collins classification in the United States and the Kiel classification proposed by Lennert and associates in Europe. In an attempt to unify terminology and improve the effectiveness of communication between pathologists and clinicians, the Working Formulation was proposed in 1982. Over the next two decades the Kiel classification dominated clinical practice in Europe, whereas the Working Formulation became the main classification system in North America (FREEDMAN and NADLER 2001).

In the past two decades, increased understanding of the immune system and the genetic abnormalities associated with non-Hodgkin lymphoma have led to the identification of several previously unrecognized types of lymphoma. The recognition of these new and clinically relevant lymphomas led to proposals for a Revised European-American Lymphoma (REAL) classification of lymphoid neoplasms in 1994 (HARRIS et al. 1994). The new WHO classification was proposed in 1999 and is based on the REAL classification. In the new WHO classification, the most practical approach to lymphoma categorization was simply to define the diseases by taking into account the currently available morphologic, clinical, immunologic, and genetic information. In the WHO classification, there is no single gold standard and the importance of specific criteria for both definition and diagnosis differs among different diseases. Thus, lymphoma classification becomes simply a list of well-defined "real" clinical syndromes, that is, several clinicopathological entities that have clinical and therapeutic relevance. This system is presented in Table 11.1. Clinical studies have shown that this new system is clinically relevant and has a higher degree

Table 11.1. WHO classification of lymphoid malignancies

B-Cell Neoplasms

Precursor B-cell neoplasm

Precursor B-cell lymphoblastic lymphoma/Precursor B-cell acute lymphoblastic leukemia

Mature (peripheral) B-cell neoplasms

B-cell chronic lymphocytic leukemia/small lymphocytic lymphoma

B-cell prolymphocytic leukemia

Lymphoplasmacytic lymphoma

Splenic marginal zone B-cell lymphoma (± villous lymphocytes)

Hairy cell leukemia

Plasma cell myeloma/plasmacytoma

Extranodal marginal zone B-cell lymphoma of MALT type

Mantle cell lymphoma

Follicular lymphoma

Nodal marginal zone B-cell lymphoma (± monocytoid B-cells)

Diffuse large B-cell lymphoma

Burkitt lymphoma/Burkitt cell leukemia

T and NK-cell Neoplasms

Precursor T-cell neoplasm

Precursor T-cell lymphoblastic lymphoma/Precursor T-cell acute lymphoblastic leukemia

Mature (peripheral) T-cell neoplasms

T-cell prolymphocytic leukemia

T-cell granular lymphocytic leukemia

Aggressive NK cell leukemia

Adult T-cell lymphoma/leukemia (HTLV-1+)

Extranodal NK/T-cell lymphoma, nasal type

Enteropathy-type T-cell lymphoma

Hepatosplenic γδ T-cell lymphoma

Subcutaneous panniculitis-like T-cell lymphoma

Mycosis fungoides/Sézary syndrome

Anaplastic large cell lymphoma, primary cutaneous type

Peripheral T-cell lymphoma, not otherwise specified (NOS)

Angioimmunoblastic T-cell lymphoma

Anaplastic large cell lymphoma, primary systemic type

Hodgkin Disease

Nodular lymphocyte-predominant Hodgkin disease

Classical Hodgkin disease

Nodular sclerosis Hodgkin disease

Lymphocyte-rich classical Hodgkin disease

Mixed-cellularity Hodgkin disease

Lymphocyte-depletion Hodgkin disease

NOTE: HTLV, human T lymphotropic virus; MALT, mucosa-associated lymphoid tissue; NK, natural killer; WHO, World Health Organization.

of diagnostic accuracy than those used previously (Harris et al. 1999a; Harris et al. 1999b; Harris et al. 2000a; Harris et al. 2000b).

In the WHO classification, lymphoid malignancies are divided mainly into T-cell neoplasms, B-cell neoplasms, and Hodgkin disease. T-cell neoplasms are further divided into precursor T-cell neoplasms and peripheral T-cell neoplasms. B-cell neoplasms are divided in the same manner. The T-cell neoplasms are informally grouped according to their major clinical presentations: predominantly disseminated/ leukemic, primary extranodal, and predominantly nodal disease. Precursor T-cell neoplasms include an isolated entity called "precursor T-cell lymphoblastic lymphoma/leukemia". Among the peripheral T-cell neoplasms, primary extranodal and predominantly nodal diseases are called "peripheral T-cell lymphoma". A number of distinct clinicopathological entities are included in peripheral T-cell lymphoma (Table 11.2) (Harris et al. 1994; Harris et al. 1999a; Harris et al. 1999b; Harris et al. 2000a; Harris et al. 2000b).

Cytologic features and immunophenotypic markers have not been useful in the accurate pathologic diagnosis of T-cell lymphomas. Unlike B-cell lymphomas, immunophenotypic variation exists within specific disease entities, and many antigens are shared by different diseases. In addition, specific genetic abnormalities have not been identified for many of the T-cell lymphomas. Therefore, the diagnosis and classification of T-cell lymphomas proposed by the WHO emphasizes integrating clinical manifestations with morphologic, genetic, and immunologic features. The clinical syndromes and disease location (nodal versus extranodal) are important not only in diagnosis, but also in staging and prognosis (Harris et al. 1999a; Harris et al. 1999b; Harris et al. 2000a; Harris et al. 2000b).

11.2.2
Clinical Outcome

The prognosis of patients with non-Hodgkin lymphoma is best determined using the established prognostic factors. As an example, the International Prognostic Index (IPI) (Table 11.3) is a powerful predictor of outcome in all subtypes of non-Hodgkin lymphoma. Patients are assigned an IPI score based on the presence or absence of five adverse prognostic factors and may have none or all five of these adverse prognostic factors. Patients with T-cell lymphoma usually present with adverse prognostic factors, with 80% of patients having an IPI score of 2 and 30%

Table 11.2. T and NK-cell neoplasms: categorization according to major clinical presentation

Clinicopathological entities			Major clinical presentation
Precursor T-cell neoplasm		Precursor T lymphoblastic lymphoma/Precursor T-cell acute lymphoblastic leukemia	Predominantly disseminated disease
Peripheral T-cell neoplasm	Peripheral T-cell leukemia	T-cell prolymphocytic leukemia	Predominantly disseminated disease
		T-cell granular lymphocytic leukemia	
		Aggressive NK cell leukemia	
		Adult T-cell lymphoma/leukemia (HTLV1+)	
	Peripheral T-cell lymphoma	Extranodal NK/T-cell lymphoma, nasal type	Primary extranodal disease
		Enteropathy-type T-cell lymphoma	
		Subcutaneous panniculitis-like T-cell lymphoma	
		Mycosis fungoides/Sézary syndrome	
		Anaplastic large cell lymphoma, primary cutaneous type	
		Hepatosplenic γδ T-cell lymphoma	
		Anaplastic large cell lymphoma, primary systemic type	Predominantly nodal disease
		Angioimmunoblastic T-cell lymphoma	
		Peripheral T-cell lymphoma, not otherwise specified (NOS)	

Table 11.3. International Prognostic Index (IPI) for non-Hodgkin lymphoma

Five clinical risk factors	Age ≥ 60 years
	Serum lactate dehydrogenase levels elevated
	Performance status ≥ 2 (ECOG) or ≤ 70 (Karnofsky)
	Ann Arbor stage III or IV
	> 1 site of extranodal involvement
The meaning of IPI score	0,1 factor = low risk
	2 factors = low-intermediate risk
	3 factors = high-intermediate risk
	4,5 factors = high risk

(With permission from [Lee et al. 2003])

having an IPI score of 4. As this would predict, T-cell lymphomas are associated with a poor outcome, and less than 25% of patients survive 5 years after diagnosis. Treatment regimens are the same as those for diffuse large B-cell lymphoma, but patients with T-cell lymphoma have a poorer response to treatment (MELNYK et al. 1997; FREEDMAN and NADLER 2001).

Clinical relevance of immunophenotypes has been criticized since poor prognosis of T-cell lymphomas originates from either adverse prognostic factors or from the T-cell phenotype. However, comparison of B and T-cell lymphomas has not been stratified for differences in other established prognostic factors. Most studies have confirmed the findings that T-cell lymphomas occur more frequently in the elderly, with more advanced stage, frequent extranodal disease, and constitutional symptoms (ARMITAGE et al. 1989; CHOTT et al. 1990; COIFFIER et al. 1990; GROGAN et al. 1985; MONTALBAN et al. 1993; PINKUS et al. 1990; SU et al. 1988). These recognized poor prognostic factors thus may confound a meaningful comparison of these disorders. Recently, an attempt was made to correct for previous limitations in comparing T-cell lymphomas with aggressive B-cell non-Hodgkin lymphomas. Retrospective analysis assessed the prognostic value of immunophenotype in aggressive non-Hodgkin lymphomas with stratification for other prognostic factors using the IPI and M.D. Anderson prognostic tumor score (MDATS). This multivariate analysis showed that other prognostic factors and T-cell phenotype are the most significant predictors of failure-free survival and overall survival (JAGANNATH et al. 1986; MELNYK et al. 1997; RODRIGUEZ et al. 1992; The International Non-Hodgkin's Lymphoma Prognostic Factors Project 1993). Moreover, other prognostic factors and T-

cell phenotype were totally independent. This result means that T-cell phenotype is an independent and significant poor prognostic factor.

11.3
Peripheral T-Cell Neoplasms

11.3.1
Extranodal NK/T-Cell Lymphoma, Nasal Type

Clinical Features

Extranodal NK/T-cell lymphoma of nasal type was classified as "angiocentric lymphoma" in the REAL classification (HARRIS et al. 1994). It has been known by various names, including lethal midline granuloma, polymorphic reticulosis, and other more obscure terms such as progressive lethal granulomatous ulceration, malignant granuloma, nonhealing granuloma, and midline malignant reticulosis (EICHEL et al. 1996; STEWART 1993). All these diseases were destructive lesions involving the nasal cavity, oropharynx, upper palate, and larynx. However, with the advent of immunophenotyping, these lesions were found to be lymphoid in nature and so should now be regarded as an entity of peripheral T-cell lymphoma (JAFFE 1996b). Extranodal NK/T-cell lymphoma of nasal type is more common in Asia, South and Central America, and Mexico than in the United States and Europe. It accounts for approximately 12% of all non-Hodgkin lymphomas in Far East countries and approximately 2% in Europe (Ko et al. 1998; LEE et al. 1999; SALAR et al. 1997). Nearly half (45%) of all malignant lymphomas of the nasal cavity and nasopharynx are derived from NK/T-cells while 21% are derived from T-cells and 34% from B-cells (CHEUNG et al. 1998). B-cell lymphomas of the nose are rarely primary tumors and usually represent metastases from other lymph node sites (EICHEL et al. 1996). On the other hand, nasal T/NK-cell lymphomas are predominantly primary tumors (EICHEL et al. 1996; STEWART 1993).

Extranodal NK/T-cell lymphoma of nasal type presents clinically as a lethal midline granuloma or midfacial destructive lesion. The nose is the most frequently involved (Table 11.4). Palate and upper airway are other primary involved sites. Few cases occur in other extranodal sites such as the gastrointestinal tract and skin; therefore, nasal NK/T-cell lymphoma should be considered in the differential diagnosis for enteropathy-type T-cell lymphoma of the gastrointestinal tract, mycosis fungoides, and

Table 11.4. Clinicopathological entities of T-cell lymphomas and common primary involving organs

Clinicopathological Entity	Common Primary Involving Organ
Precursor T-cell lymphoma	
Precursor T lymphoblastic lymphoma/leukemia (precursor T-cell acute lympho-blastic leukemia)	Thymus
Peripheral T-cell lymphoma	
Extranodal NK/T-cell lymphoma, nasal type	Sinonasal cavity, upper airway
Enteropathy-type T-cell lym-phoma	Small bowel, colon
Subcutaneous panniculitis-like T-cell lymphoma	Subcutaneous fat
Mycosis fungoides	Skin
Anaplastic large cell lymphoma, primary cutaneous type	Skin
Anaplastic large cell lymphoma, primary systemic type	Lymph node, liver, spleen, lung
Angioimmunoblastic T-cell lym-phoma	Lymph node, liver, spleen, lung
Peripheral T-cell lymphoma, not otherwise specified	Lymph node, liver, spleen, lung
Hepatosplenic γδ T-cell lymphoma	Liver, spleen, bone marrow

(With permission from [Lee et al. 2003])

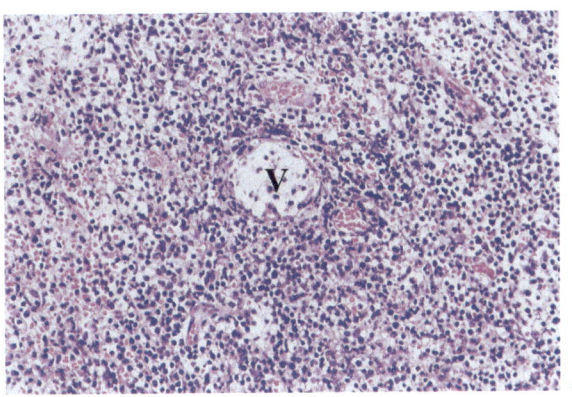

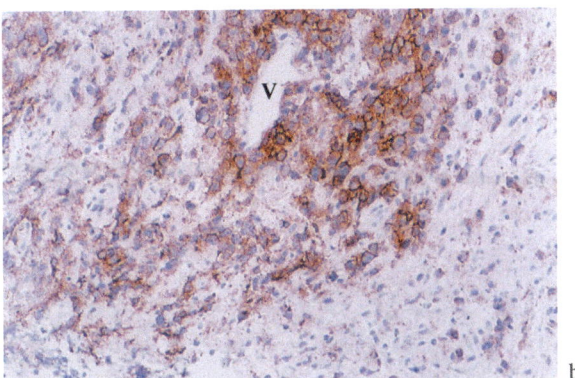

Fig. 11.1a,b. Nasal-type extranodal NK/T-cell lymphoma in a 36-year-old man with involvement of the nasal cavity. **a** Photomicrograph of a nasal mucosal biopsy specimen shows intense infiltration of atypical lymphoid cells into the perivascular area and vascular lumen (*arrow*). This is the appearance of "angiocentric invasion" in which atypical lymphoid cells obliterated the vascular lumen (*V*) (original magnification, ×200; hematoxylin-eosin stain). **b** Photomicrograph of NK-cell marker (CD56)-labeled tissue shows that atypical lymphoid cells react positively with the marker and appear brown. The atypical lymphoid cells are predominantly found in the perivascular area (original magnification, ×200; immunohistochemical stain on paraffin-embedded material) (*V= vascular lumen*).

cutaneous anaplastic large cell lymphoma (JAFFE et al. 1996b; KATOH et al. 2000). The course is highly aggressive and patients frequently have the hemophagocytic syndrome. When marrow and blood involvement occur, distinction between this disease and leukemia can be difficult. Some patients will respond to aggressive combination chemotherapy regimens, but the overall outlook is poor. (CHAN et al. 1987; FREEDMAN and NADLER 2001; JAFFE et al. 1996a; WEISS et al. 1994).

Pathological Features

"Angiocentric" invasion of lymphoid cells is a characteristic feature of this disorder (Fig. 11.1). Angiocentricity is seen in about half of all cases although it is occasionally found in other lymphoma subtypes. The tumor often shows polymorphic lymphoreticular infiltrates and necrosis (FERRY et al. 1991). Invasion of vascular walls by lymphoid cells causes occlusion of lumen. The vascular occlusion is usually associated with prominent ischemic necrosis of both tumor cells and normal tissue. Despite the characteristic pathologic features of nasal NK/T-cell lym-

phoma, difficulty in the diagnosis of this disorder, both clinically and pathologically, is well recognized. Pathological differentiation from chronic inflammation is difficult because atypical lymphoma cells and inflammatory lymphocytes mix at the site of ischemic necrosis. This lymphoma is highly associated with Epstein-Barr viral infection and immunophenotypic profile of tumor cells is CD2-positive, CD56-positive (natural killer cell marker) and CD3-negative (Fig. 11.1). Genotypically, the T-cell receptor gene in the germ line configuration allows classification (CHAN et al. 1987; FREEDMAN and NADLER 2001; JAFFE et al. 1996a; WEISS et al. 1994).

Radiologic Features

Little is known about the imaging features of extra-nodal NK/T-cell lymphoma of nasal type. Patients with nasal NK/T-cell lymphoma frequently present with symptoms confined to the nasal cavity. It shows a predilection for diffuse invasion of the nasal cavity, often involving both sides. In the smaller volume lymphomas, there is a tendency to spread as a diffuse thin sheet of tumor along the walls of the nasal cavity to envelop the nasal turbinates and nasal septum. In larger volume disease, a more discernible mass is seen with occasional spread to the nasopharynx or palate. Destruction of the midline structures – the nasal turbinates, nasal septum and palate – occur in half of the patients and tumor necrosis is frequently detected on CT or MR imaging (Fig. 11.2) (KING et al. 2000; LEE et al. 2003; OOI et al. 2000; TENG et al.

1990). Destruction of the lateral wall of the nasal cavity is rare. Invasion of the paranasal sinuses is less common compared with those invading the naso-pharynx and oropharynx (OOI et al. 2000). Regional nodal enlargement in nasal T/NK cell lymphoma is rare and more commonly associated with the B-cell lymphomas (CHEUNG et al. 1998). Interestingly, it is generally accepted that most lymphomas originating from maxillary sinus are B-cell lymphoma with good prognosis and those from nasal cavity or ethmoid sinus (Fig. 11.3) are peripheral T-cell lymphoma causing early death (NAKAMURA et al. 1997). There-fore, accurate definition of the primary site of sino-nasal lymphoma by imaging modality can confirm the correct diagnosis. Although it is very rare, the luminal narrowing and wall thickening in larynx and trachea on simple radiography and CT are pathologi-

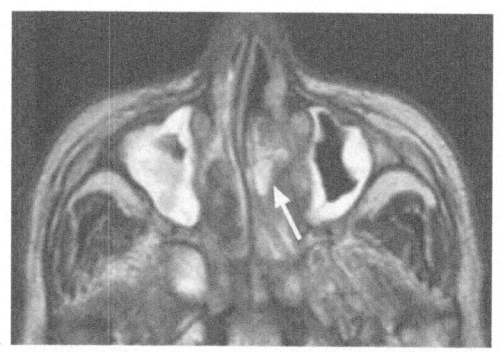
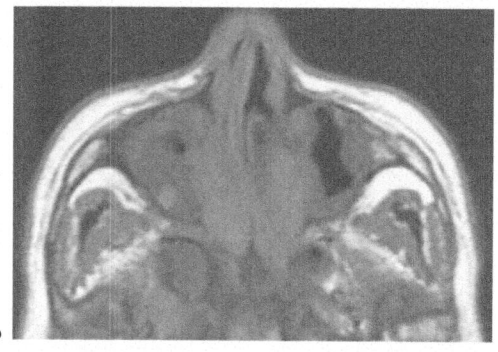
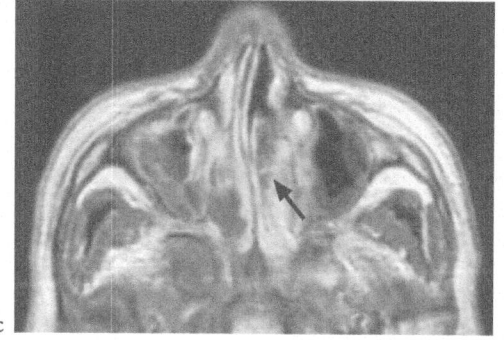
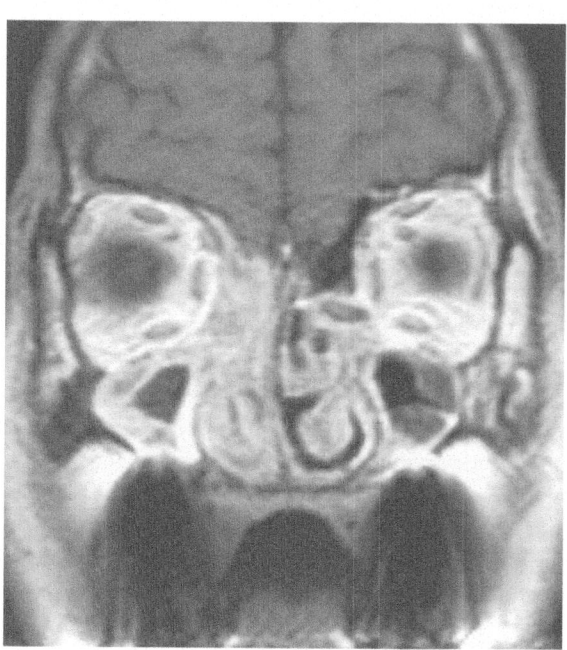

Fig.11.2a–d. Nasal-type extranodal NK/T-cell lymphoma in a 42-year-old man with involvement of the nasal cavity. He presented with nasal blockage. **a** Axial T2-weighted MR image shows a hypointense mass that fills the bilateral nasal cavity. Focal hyperintense area is found in the mass (*arrow*). Both maxillary antra are markedly hyperintense because of retained secretions. **b** The mass had intermediate signal intensity on axial T1-weighted MR image. **c** Axial contrast-enhanced T1-weighted MR image shows heterogeneous enhancement of the mass. Non-enhanced portion of the tumor (*arrow*) suggests necrosis. Note the thickening and enhancement of the wall of the bilateral maxillary sinus, an appearance suggestive of tumor infiltration. **d** Coronal contrast-enhanced T1-weighted MR image shows diffuse spread of the tumor along walls of nasal cavity to envelope nasal turbinates.

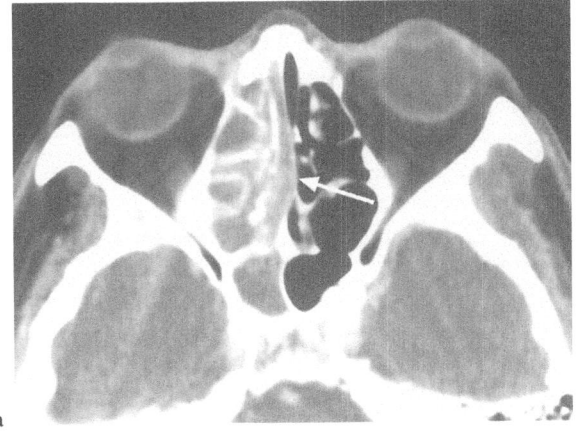

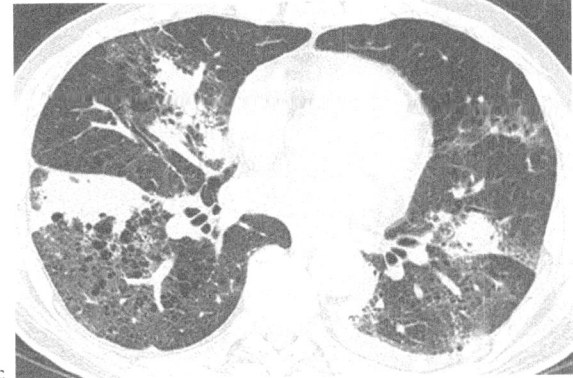

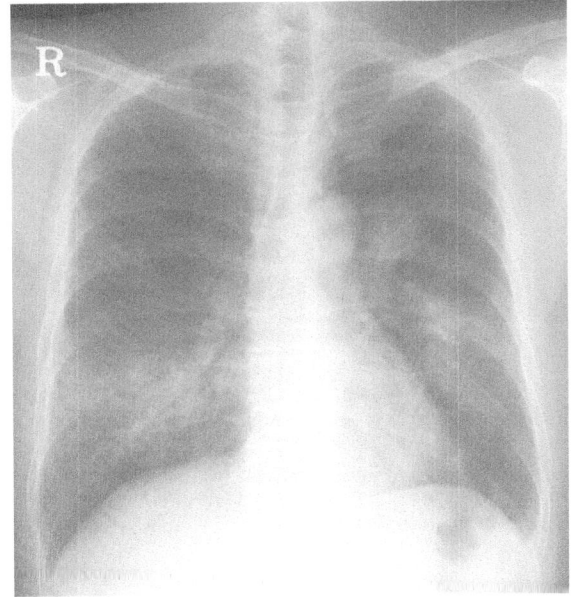

Fig. 11.3a–c. Nasal-type extranodal NK/T-cell lymphoma in a 63-year-old man. **a** Axial CT scan shows a mass filling the right ethmoid sinus (*arrow*). **b** Anteroposterior chest radiograph shows multifocal patchy infiltrations in both lungs. **c** Axial CT scan shows bilateral ill-defined peribronchovascular consolidations. Judging from the sinonasal and pulmonary manifestation, prospective radiologic diagnosis was Wegener granulomatosis. Open lung biopsy confirmed the diagnosis.

cally proved as NK/T-cell lymphoma of the nasal type (LEE et al. 2003).

The CT and MR imaging appearances are nonspecific and they cannot reliably distinguish this disease from other nasal cavity tumors such as squamous cell carcinoma, minor salivary gland tumors, rhabdomyosarcoma, and aggressive nonneoplastic lesions such as Wegener granulomatosis, sarcoidosis, cocaine abuse, fungal infection, leprosy, or syphilis (Fig. 11.3). The differential diagnosis relies more on clinical and histopathologic findings than radiologic findings (KING et al. 2000; LEE et al. 2003; OOI et al. 2000). However, it deserves mentioning that T2-weighted MR images may occasionally show slightly decreased or intermediate signal intensity of the tumor mass (Fig. 11.2). The intermediate signal is common for many malignant tumors of the head and neck and contrasts to the hyperintensity on T2-weighted images that is found almost exclusively in benign membrane and mucosal diseases. Therefore, this finding should raise suspicion of lymphoma (KING et al. 2000). Rare cases presented with soft tissue mass in the chest wall or extremities could not be distinguished from soft tissue sarcoma (Figs. 11.4, 11.5).

11.3.2
Enteropathy-Type T-Cell Lymphoma

Clinical Features

Enteropathy-type intestinal T-cell lymphoma was originally termed "malignant histiocytosis of the intestine", but has since been shown to be a peripheral T-cell lymphoma (ISAACSON et al. 1985). This disorder was classified as "intestinal T-cell lymphoma" in the REAL classification (HARRIS et al. 1994). Enteropathy-type intestinal T-cell lymphoma is a rare disorder and accounts for less than 1% of all non-Hodgkin lymphomas in Asia and Europe (KO et al. 1998; LEE et al. 1999; SALAR et al. 1997). It most frequently involves the small bowel (Table 11.4). The stomach or colon are affected less often. Patients present with abdominal pain, often associated with jejunal perforation. The course is aggressive and death usually occurs from multifocal intestinal perforation caused by refractory malignant ulcers. The prognosis is poor (HARRIS et al. 1994). Nasal NK/T-cell lymphoma and other clinicopathological entities of peripheral T-cell lymphoma may also occur in the gastrointestinal tract and should be considered in the

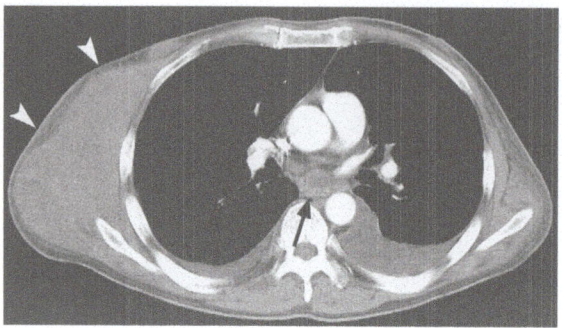

Fig. 11.4. Nasal-type extranodal NK/T-cell lymphoma in a 42-year-old man. Axial contrast-enhanced CT scan of the chest in mediastinal window setting shows soft tissue mass in right lateral chest wall (*arrowheads*). Bilateral pleural effusion and subcarinal lymph node enlargement (*arrow*) are also noted. In lung window setting, multiple nodules were seen in both lungs. This patient also had a sinonasal lymphoma.

differential diagnosis for enteropathy-type T-cell lymphoma of the gastrointestinal tract (JAFFE et al. 1996a; KATOH et al. 2000).

The relationship between enteropathy-type T-cell lymphoma and celiac disease or gluten-sensitive enteropathy is unclear, and the present consensus is that not all cases occur in the setting of enteropathy (ISAACSON 1994). Although it usually occurs in patients with untreated enteropathy, there are clearly cases in which there is neither history of celiac disease nor biopsy evidence of gluten sensitivity. Some have

suggested that these patients may have latent celiac disease in which the jejunal mucosa is histologically normal (LEVY and KOELLER 2003). However, this has not been firmly established.

Pathological Features

On gross examination, intestinal ulcers are present, often multiple, and often with perforation. A mass may or may not be present. Early lesions may show mucosal ulceration with only scattered atypical cells and numerous reactive histiocytes, without formation of masses. Adjacent mucosa may or may not show villous atrophy (CHOTT et al. 1992). Pathological differentiation from inflammatory bowel disease is difficult. Microscopically, atypical lymphoma cells and inflammatory lymphocytes are mixed at the site of mucosal ulceration (Figs. 11.6, 11.7). Therefore, if the biopsy is performed where inflammatory lymphocytes predominate, the pathologic diagnosis may be inflammatory bowel disease rather than lymphoma (LEE et al. 2001; LEE et al. 2002; TALLINI et al. 1993).

Radiologic Features

There are several reports of radiologic features of T-cell lymphoma involving the gastrointestinal tract. However, it is unclear whether these cases belong to enteropathy-type T-cell lymphoma. We think that most of the cases might be best classified into enteropathy-type T-cell lymphoma because they have clinical and histologic features in common

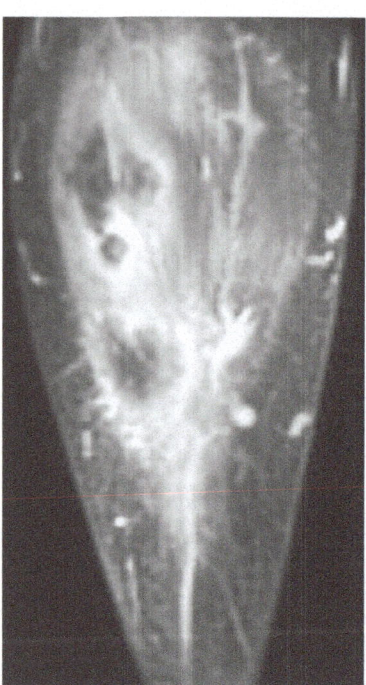
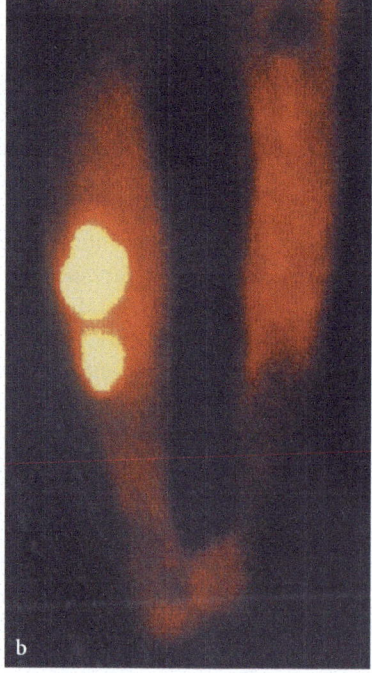

Fig. 11.5a,b. Nasal-type extranodal NK/T-cell lymphoma in a 66-year-old woman. **a** Coronal contrast-enhanced T1-weighted MR image shows predominantly peripherally enhanced tumor in the lower leg. Central hypointense area suggests central necrosis. The mass showed a heterogeneous hyperintensity on the axial T2-weighted spin-echo MR image and intermediate-signal-intensity on T1-weighted image. **b** Coronal FDG-PET demonstrates a corresponding increased uptake in the right lower leg. Normal increased uptake in heart and brain was also seen. In this patient, histopathologic findings were compatible with the nasal-type NK/T-cell lymphoma. However, there is no evidence of lymphoma in the sinonasal area.

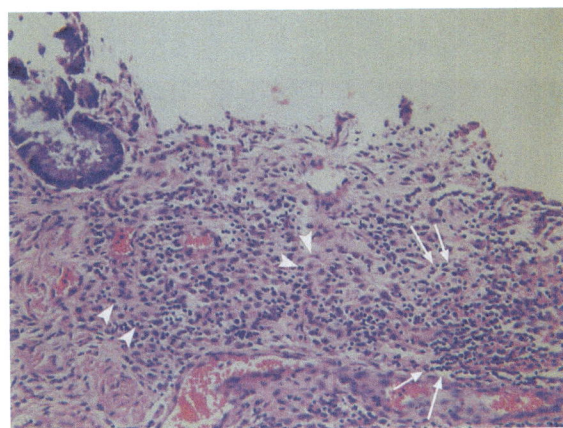

Fig. 11.6. Enteropathy-type T-cell lymphoma in a 44-year-old man with involvement of the colon. Photomicrograph of a colectomy specimen shows atypical lymphoid cells with abundant cytoplasm (*arrowheads*) and small inflammatory lymphocytes (*arrows*) mixed at the site of mucosal ulceration (original magnification, ×200; hematoxylin-eosin stain). The pathology report on the initial colonoscopic biopsy specimen concluded that the patient had chronic nonspecific colitis; the diagnosis was confirmed after colonic resection. (With permission from [LEE et al. 2003])

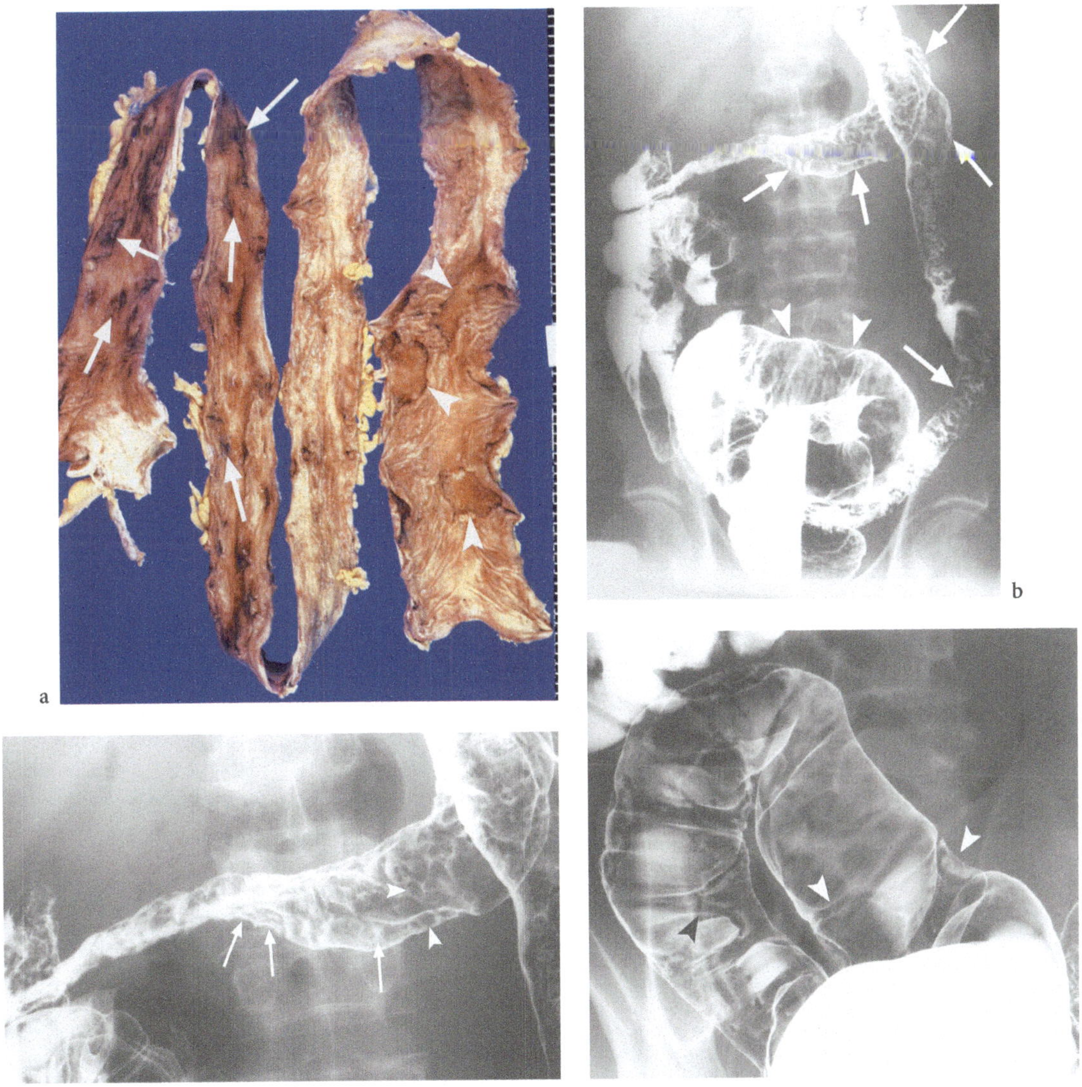

Fig. 11.7a–d. Peripheral T-cell lymphoma in a 44-year-old man with diffuse involvement of the colon. **a** Total colectomy specimen shows multiple small (*arrows*) and large (*arrowheads*) ulcerations of the entire colon. **b** Double-contrast barium enema image shows multiple geographic or aphthous ulcerations (*arrows*) in the entire colon and multiple pseudopolyps and unaffected areas between ulcerations. Deformity of the cecum and patent ileocecal valve were also noted at double-contrast barium enema examination (*not shown*). Large geographic ulceration (*arrowheads*) is depicted in the sigmoid colon. **c** Close-up view of the transverse colon demonstrates small aphthous ulcerations (*arrows*) and mucosal pseudopolyps (*arrowheads*). **d** Close-up view of the sigmoid colon shows multiple large geographic ulcerations (*arrowheads*). (With permission from [LEE et al. 2001])

with enteropathy-type T-cell lymphoma. Recent reports have described T-cell lymphoma of the colon manifested as either a diffuse or focal segmental lesion and showing extensive mucosal ulceration at double-contrast barium enema examination (Figs. 11.7, 11.8) (LEE et al. 2001; LEE et al. 2002; HSIAO et al. 1996). The T-cell lymphoma involving the small intestine also formed mucosal ulcers with short strictures (Fig. 11.9) and thick, nodular folds. Mesenteric adenopathy is typically identified at CT (LEVY and KOELLER 2003; LOBERANT et al. 1997; PERRET et al. 1998).

Unlike the more common B-cell lymphomas of the gastrointestinal tract, which may manifest as bulky annular masses or polypoid lesions in the distal small intestine, these radiologic findings of enteropathy-type T-cell lymphoma are similar to those of bowel ischemia or inflammatory bowel disease such as Crohn disease or tuberculous enterocolitis (Figs. 11.7–11.9). Because radiological and pathological diagnosis of enteropathy-type T-cell lymphoma is so difficult, clinical suspicion is very important. Enteropathy-type T-cell lymphoma should be suspected in patients with the radiologic features of inflammatory bowel disease with extensive ulcerations that are refractory to the treatment. Also, if there are shallow large geographic ulcerations in multiple locations, the diagnosis of enteropathy-type T-cell lymphoma might be considered (LEE et al. 2001). Moreover, ulcerative jejunoileitis, a rare complication of celiac disease is associated with thickened folds, multiple ulcers, strictures, and

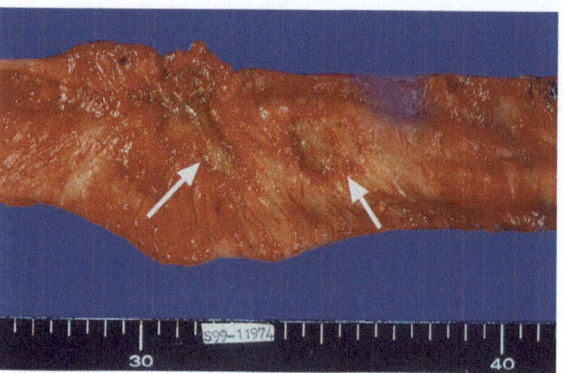

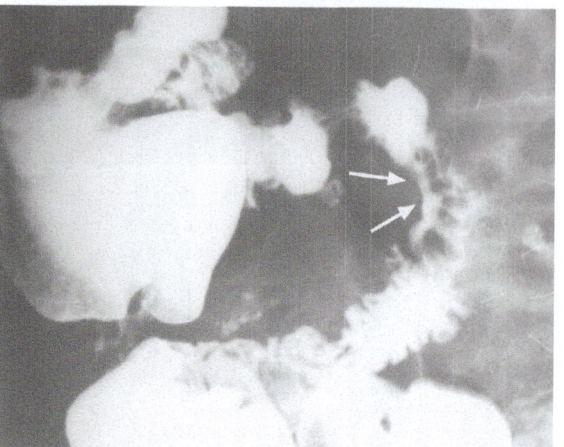

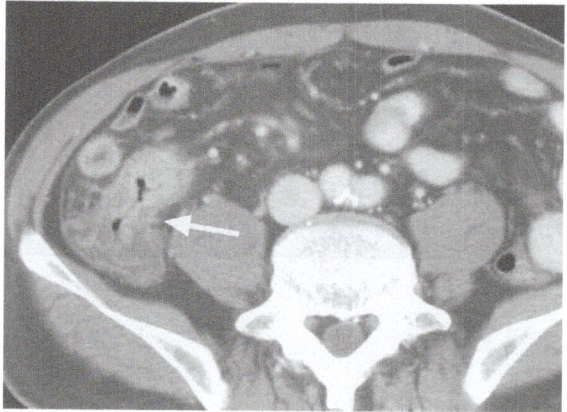

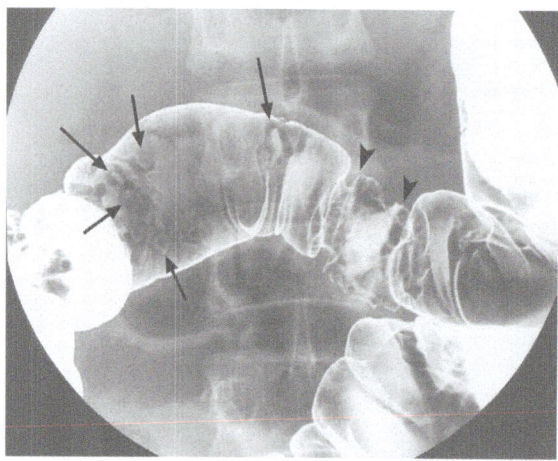

Fig. 11.8. Enteropathy-type T-cell lymphoma in a 37-year-old man with involvement of the colon. Image from a double-contrast barium enema study shows multiple aphthous ulcers (*arrows*) and segmental luminal narrowing (*arrowheads*) in the transverse colon. (With permission from [LEE et al. 2003])

Fig. 11.9a–c Enteropathy-type T-cell lymphoma in a 61-year-old man with involvement of the terminal ileum. **a** Photograph of the ileocecectomy specimen shows multiple irregular ulcers (*arrows*) in the terminal ileum. The prospective radiologic diagnosis was Crohn disease on the basis of the linear ulcers and pseudosacculation of the terminal ileum. Moreover, the pathologic diagnosis after the initial ileal biopsy was chronic nonspecific ileitis. The diagnosis was confirmed with surgical resection of the intestine. Scale is in 5-mm intervals. **b** Image from a barium study of the small intestine shows a linear ulcer (*arrows*) along the mesenteric border in the terminal ileum. **c** Axial contrast-enhanced CT scan shows wall thickening in the terminal ileum (*arrow*) and mesenteric fat infiltration around the ileum. (With permission from [LEE et al. 2003])

obstruction. Not only is its clinical and radiologic appearance identical to that of enteropathy-type T-cell lymphoma, but ulcerative jejunoileitis may coexist with lymphoma (ROBERTSON et al. 1983). Therefore, careful histopathologic examination and immunologic staining of tissue removed in patients with ulcerative jejunoileitis is recommended to identify occult lymphoma (ISAACSON 1994).

11.3.3
Mycosis Fungoides/Sézary Syndrome

Clinical Features

Mycosis fungoides and Sézary syndrome are the most common form of cutaneous T-cell lymphoma. This lymphoma is more often seen by dermatologists than radiologists. This disorder is more common in men and in blacks (FREEDMAN and NADLER 2001). It accounts for approximately 6% of all non-Hodgkin lymphomas in Europe but is very rare in Asian countries (KO et al. 1998; LEE et al. 1999; SALAR et al. 1997). Staging of cutaneous T-cell lymphoma was adapted from TNM criteria established in 1978 at the Mycosis Fungoides Cooperative Group-National Cancer Institute Workshop on cutaneous T-cell lymphoma (Tables 11.5, 11.6) (LAMBERG and BUNN 1979). As demonstrated in the Tables, staging is primarily determined by means of (a) the cutaneous manifestation of disease, (b) pathologically proved disease in lymph nodes, and (c) the presence of circulating Sézary cells. The disorder in which Sézary cells are found in the peripheral blood is called Sézary syndrome. Patients with Sézary syndrome present with generalized erythroderma and pruritus. Peripheral lymphadenopathy and hepatosplenomegaly are common (FREEDMAN and NADLER 2001).

Mycosis fungoides is an indolent lymphoma and typically has a long natural history. The patients often have several years of scattered plaque-like skin infiltrates before the diagnosis is finally established. This stage I disease, limited to the skin, may progress to involve large areas of the body surface with ulcers, nodules and cutaneous tumors. Extracutaneous disease including peripheral adenopathy is a late feature. Rare patients with localized early stage mycosis fungoides can be cured with radiotherapy, often total-skin electron beam irradiation. More advanced disease has been treated with topical glucocorticoids, topical nitrogen mustard, phototherapy, psoralen with ultraviolet A (PUVA), electron beam radiation, interferon, and systemic cytotoxic therapy. Unfortunately, these treatments are palliative. In its later

Table 11.5. TNM definitions in cutaneous T-cell lymphoma

Stage	Extent of cutaneous T-cell lymphoma
T1a	Limited patches < 10% total body surface area
T1b	Limited plaques < 10% total body surface area
T2a	Generalized patches > 10% total body surface area
T2b	Generalized plaques > 10% total body surface area
T3	Tumors ≥ 1
T4	Generalized erythroderma
N0	No clinically abnormal peripheral lymph nodes; pathologic findings negative for cutaneous T-cell lymphoma or no pathologic findings
N1	Clinically abnormal peripheral lymph nodes; pathologic findings negative for cutaneous T-cell lymphoma or no pathologic findings
N2	No clinically abnormal peripheral lymph nodes; pathologic findings positive for cutaneous T-cell lymphoma
N3	Clinically abnormal peripheral lymph nodes; pathologic findings positive for cutaneous T cell lymphoma
M0	No internal abnormalities or negative biopsy findings
M1	Internal organ abnormality (including thoracic, pelvic, or abdominal adenopathy) with positive biopsy findings or other confirmation
B0	No atypical lymphocytes; blood T-cell receptor gene is negative
B1	Atypical lymphocytes > 5% or blood T-cell receptor gene is positive

Table 11.6. Relation between clinical stage and TNM staging in cutaneous T-cell lymphoma

Clinical Stage	T	N	M	B
IA	1	0	0	0
IB	2	0	0	0
IIA	1, 2	1	0	0
IIB	3	0, 1	0	0
IIIA	4	0, 1	0	0
IIIB	4	0, 1	0	1
IVA	1–4	2, 3	0	0, 1
IVB	1–4	0–3	1	0, 1

stages, mycosis fungoides can cause peripheral lymphadenopathy, and finally progress to widespread extracutaneous visceral involvement. The extracutaneous involvement causes dramatic change in the 5-year survival rate (FREEDMAN and NADLER 2001). Those with limited disease have survival rates similar to the normal population. In contrast, Sézary syndrome has an aggressive course with a 5-year survival rate of 10% to 20% (KIM and HOPPE 1999).

Pathological Features

The abnormal lymphoid cells in mycosis fungoides resemble the membrane features of thymus-derived T lymphocytes and tend to infiltrate the skin and lymphoid tissue, sparing the marrow. Epidermotropism of solitary lymphocytes or small intraepidermal collections of lymphocytes (called Pautrier microabscess) can be seen in early patchy lesions of mycosis fungoides. Intraepidermal lymphocytes are usually neither strikingly atypical nor notably larger than those in the superficial dermis (Fig. 11.10) (Freedman and Nadler 2001; Harris et al. 1994). Early in the disease, biopsies are often difficult to interpret, and the diagnosis may only become apparent by observing the patient over time. In tumor stage, the normal structure of the skin is usually destroyed (Sander et al. 1997). Sézary syndrome involves the presence of characteristic abnormal lymphoid cells in the peripheral blood, the dermis, lymph nodes and visceral organs (Harris et al. 1994).

Radiologic Features

The cutaneous lesions of mycosis fungoides including patches, plaques, or erythroderma show no abnormalities on CT. In the stage with tumor formation, thickening or mass of the skin is seen on CT (Figs. 11.11, 11.12). The cutaneous lesions of mycosis fungoides are nonspecific and differentiation from other diseases including T-cell leukemia, and connective tissue disease is frequently not possible (Bass et al. 1993; Howlett et al. 1995; Miketic et al. 1993).

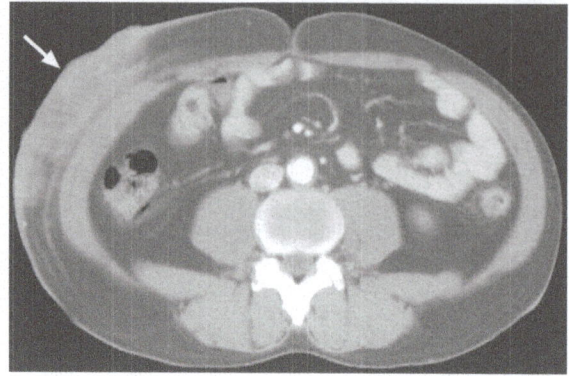

Fig. 11.11. Mycosis fungoides in a 51-year-old man. Axial contrast-enhanced CT scan shows a large tumor (*arrow*) in the anterior abdominal wall. The tumor involves the skin and subcutaneous fat.

Previous work has looked at the role of several modalities in the imaging of mycosis fungoides. Lymphangiography was able to demonstrate superficial involved nodes, but did not provide extra information to physical examination and biopsy (Castellino et al. 1979; Kulin et al. 1990). Gallium scintigraphy proved insufficiently sensitive or specific and was extensively degraded by bowel artifact in the abdomen and pelvis (Kulin et al. 1990). CT scanning for staging and follow-up is clearly indicated in patients with advanced mycosis fungoides (stage > I) and Sézary syndrome. The evaluation of the extracutaneous involvement, disease progression, and staging is the most important role of imaging in mycosis fungoides. For these reasons, CT demonstration of clinically unsuspected lymphadenopathy or abnormality in visceral organs such as hepatosplenomegaly is very important (Fig. 11.12). However, the literature is not clear on the use of CT during the initial staging of patients with clinical stage I mycosis fungoides. While some studies report no benefit from the routine use of CT in patients with early stage disease (Kulin et al. 1990; Rosen et al. 1986), others, in which CT raises the diagnostic stage of the patients and leads to a change in management, report clear benefit in staging, management, and prognosis (Bass et al. 1993; Howlett et al. 1995; Miketic et al. 1993).

11.3.4
Subcutaneous Panniculitis-Like T-cell Lymphoma

Clinical Features

Subcutaneous panniculitis-like T-cell lymphoma is a rare disorder. Clinically it is often confused

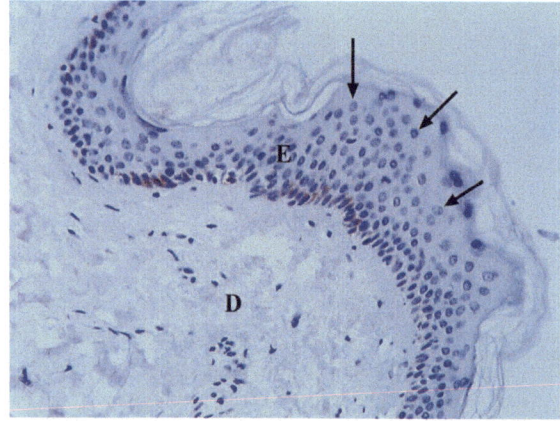

Fig. 11.10. Mycosis fungoides in a 63-year-old woman. Photomicrograph of a skin biopsy specimen shows small intraepidermal collection of lymphocytes (epidermotropism of lymphocytes) (*arrows*). Note the lack of striking nuclear atypia of the intraepidermal lymphocytes (original magnification, ×200; hematoxylin-eosin stain) (*D = dermis, E = epidermis*).

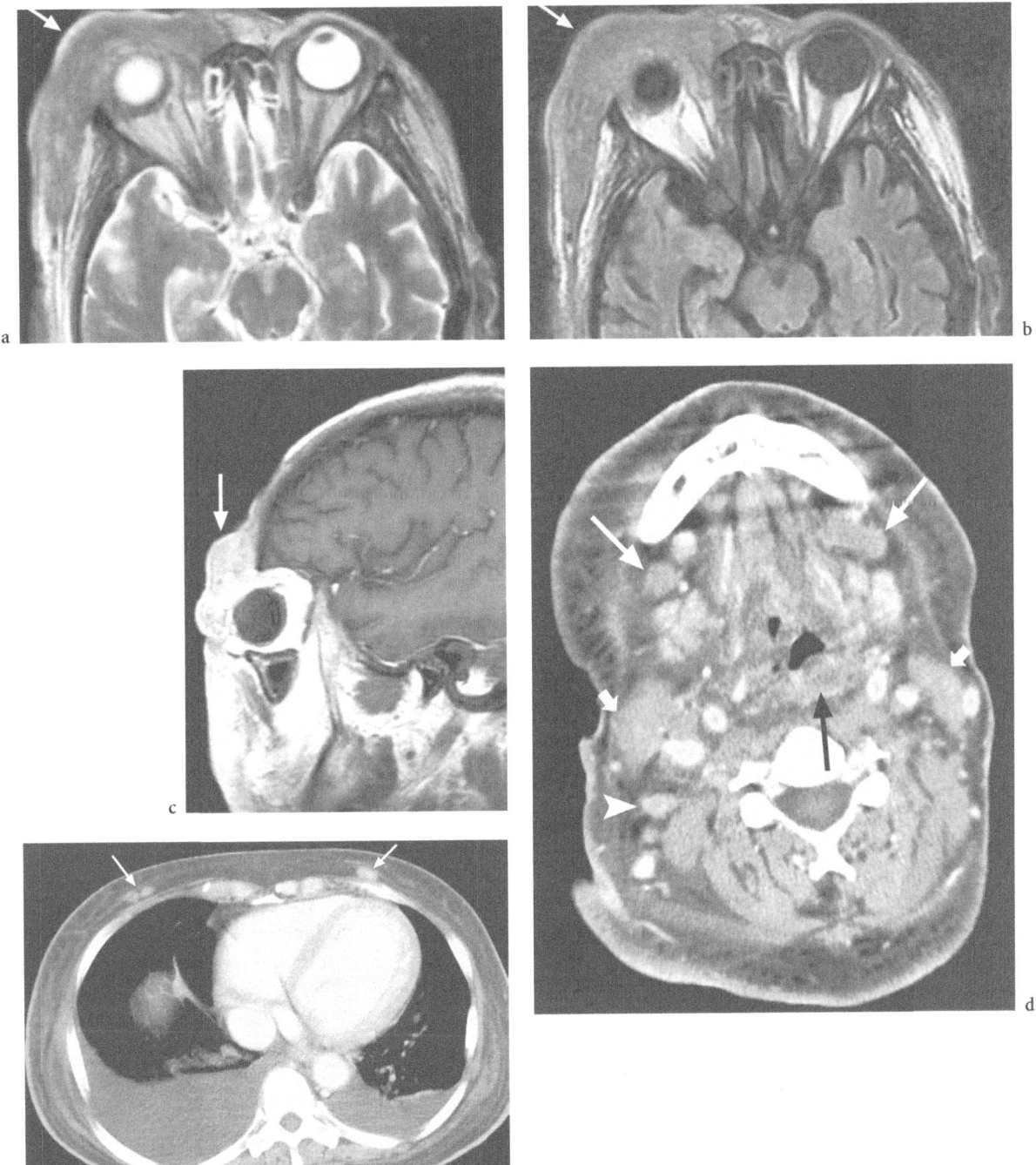

Fig. 11.12a–e. Mycosis fungoides in a 52-year-old woman. **a** Axial T2-weighted MR image shows a large tumor (*arrow*) involving the right upper eyelid. The tumor is hypointense and involves the skin and subcutaneous tissue. **b** Axial T1-weighted MR image shows that the mass has intermediate signal intensity (*arrow*). **c** Sagittal contrast-enhanced T1-weighted MR image shows a supraorbital mass with diffuse marked enhancement (*arrow*). **d** Axial contrast-enhanced CT scan obtained at the level of the hypopharynx shows enlarged lymph nodes in the submental area (*white arrows*), submandibular area (*thick short white arrows*), retropharyngeal area (*long black arrow*), and right spinal accessory chain (*arrowhead*). Laryngeal edema and edematous infiltration into the subcutaneous fat are also seen. Biopsy of the tumor and lymph nodes was performed. Pathologic analysis demonstrated mycosis fungoides involving the skin, subcutaneous tissue, and lymph nodes. Therefore, the patient had stage IV disease (T3 N3). **e** Axial contrast-enhanced chest CT scan shows multiple enhancing subcutaneous nodules (*arrows*) suggesting lymph nodes. Bilateral pleural effusion is also noted. (With permission from [Lee et al. 2003])

with inflammatory panniculitis associated with connective tissue disease. Patients present with multiple subcutaneous nodules, which progress and can ulcerate. Two clinical courses are observed: a prolonged course of recurrent panniculitis or a rapid clinical deterioration secondary to the hemophagocytic syndrome (profound anemia, ingestion of erythrocytes by monocytes and macrophages). The development of the hemophagocytic syndrome in this disorder is generally associated with a fatal outcome (Freedman and Nadler 2001; Harris et al. 1994; Lee et al. 2003).

Pathological Features

Histologically, this disorder characterized by a lymphohistiocytic infiltrate confined primarily to the fat lobules in subcutaneous tissue. Lymphoid cells commonly rim individual adipocytes (Fig. 11.13a). Karyorrhexis, fat necrosis, and cytophagocytosis are frequently seen (Lee et al. 2003; Sander et al. 1997).

Radiologic Features

Multiple subcutaneous nodules in patients with subcutaneous panniculitis-like T-cell lymphoma can be recognized on CT as multiple enhancing nodules (Fig. 11.13b). However, multiple subcutaneous nodules can be found in other diseases including inflammatory panniculitis associated with systemic lupus erythematosus or rheumatoid arthritis, cutaneous metastasis in malignant melanoma or breast cancer, or unusual subcutaneous nodules originating from bacterial, fungal, or parasitic infection. Radiologic differentiation is very difficult (Lee et al. 2003).

11.3.5
Anaplastic Large Cell Lymphoma, Primary Cutaneous Type

Clinical Features

Anaplastic large cell lymphoma (ALCL) can be further divided into two subgroups based on the initial location of anatomic presentation (Table 11.4). The first is systemic ALCL and the second is cutaneous Ki-1-positive ALCL. Cutaneous Ki-1-positive ALCL has a more indolent clinical course than systemic ALCL. Cutaneous lesions of Ki-1-positive ALCL typically present as solitary or multiple ulcerated nodules or plaques (Sander et al. 1997). Cutaneous ALCL occurs usually in older adults. Spontaneous regression is found occasionally (Freedman and Nadler 2001; Harris et al. 1999a; Harris et al. 1999b; Harris et al. 2000a; Harris et al. 2000b; Lee et al. 2003).

Pathological Features

Histologically, these lesions are typically composed of a diffuse dermal and subcutaneous infiltrate composed of large, bizarre, pleomorphic cells with Reed-Sternberg-like cells (Fig. 11.14a). These cells contain large irregular-shaped nuclei with prominent nucleoli and have abundant amphophilic to basophilic cytoplasm. The cells often preferentially cause perineural and perivascular invasion (Fig. 11.14b) (Lee et al. 2003; Sander et al. 1997).

Radiologic Features

There is virtually no radiologic literature on cutaneous ALCL. The radiologic features of cutaneous ALCL are described with the cases with mycosis fungoides in the reports about cutaneous T-cell lymphoma. Likewise in mycosis fungoides, the early

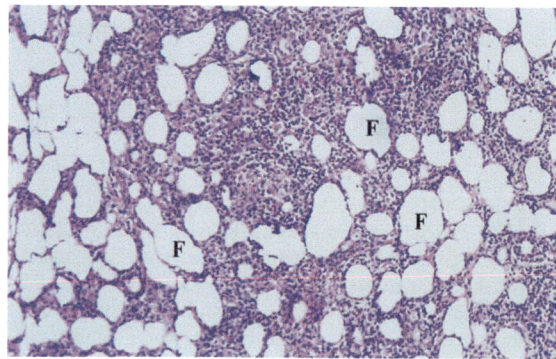
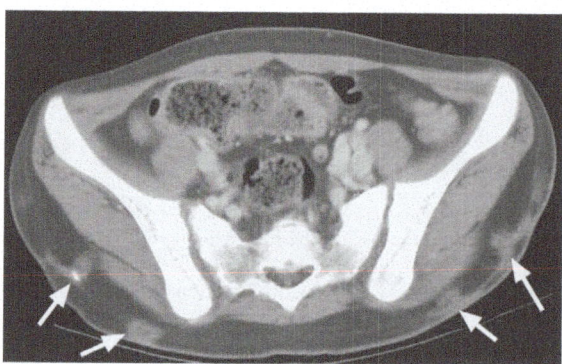

Fig. 11.13a,b. T-cell lymphoma in a 12-year-old girl with subcutaneous panniculitis-like. **a** Photomicrograph shows a lymphoid cell infiltrate in the subcutaneous fat layer. Lymphoid cells surround individual adipocytes (*F*) (original magnification, ×100; hematoxylin-eosin stain). **b** Axial contrast-enhanced CT scan of the abdomen shows multiple nodules (*arrows*) in the subcutaneous fat. At gross examination, the subcutaneous nodules gave rise to superficial elevated lesions on the skin.

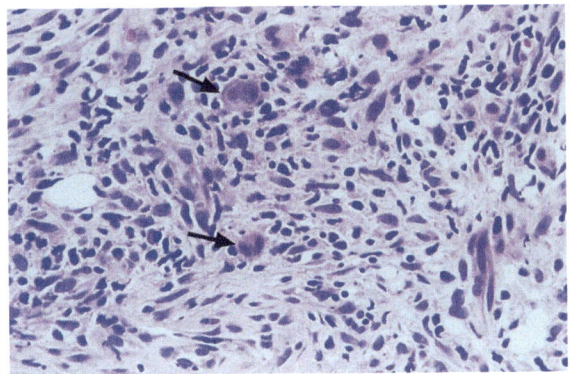
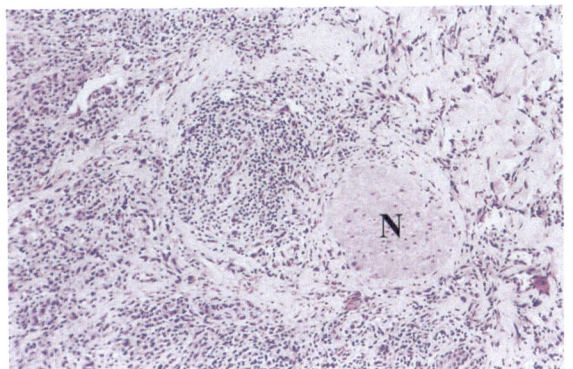

Fig. 11.14a,b. Primary cutaneous type ALCL in a 55-year-old man. a Photomicrograph shows scattered large lymphoid cells (i.e., anaplastic large cells) with pleomorphic nuclei, prominent nucleoli, and abundant cytoplasm (*arrows*) (original magnification, ×400; hematoxylin-eosin stain). b Photomicrograph of a skin biopsy specimen shows infiltration of atypical lymphoid cells with a perineural distribution (original magnification, ×100; hematoxylin-eosin stain) *(N = nerve)*.

lesions such as patches or plaques show no abnormalities on CT. In the stage with tumor formation, thickening or mass of the skin is seen on CT or MR imaging (Fig. 11.15) (Lee et al. 2003).

11.3.6
Anaplastic Large Cell Lymphoma, Primary Systemic Type

Clinical Features

This disorder is relatively rare, but may be diagnosed with increasing frequency as its features are more widely recognized. Systemic ALCL have a bimodal age distribution in children and adults. Common clinical presentation is generalized extensive lymph-

adenopathy. Patients most commonly present with disseminated stages. Extranodal sites including bone, soft tissue, skin, lung, pleura, and gastrointestinal tract are frequently involved. The bone marrow is also occasionally involved. The disorder presenting with a localized skin disease and a more indolent clinical course is a different disease than systemic ALCL and is termed "cutaneous ALCL" (Freedman and Nadler 2001; Harris et al. 1994).

Pathological Features

This disorder was previously diagnosed as undifferentiated carcinoma or malignant histiocytosis. The ALCL is a recently established category. Discovery of the Ki-1 antigen led to the identification of a new type

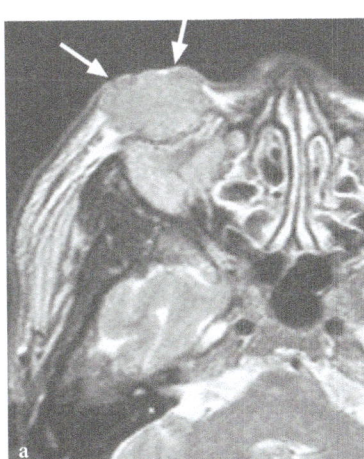
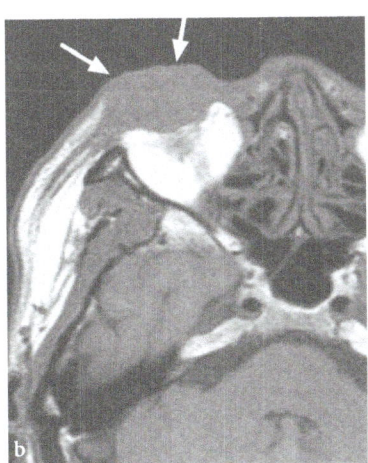
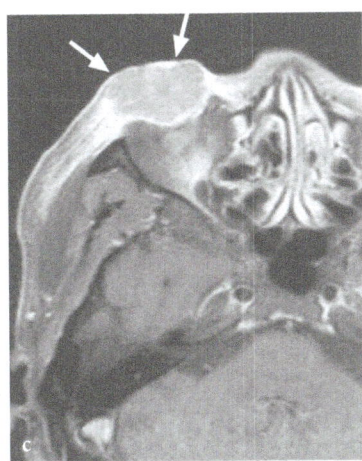

Fig. 11.15a–c. Primary cutaneous type ALCL in a 61-year-old man. a Axial T2-weighted MR image shows a mass (*arrows*) in the right eyelid. The mass has intermediate signal intensity. b Axial T1-weighted MR image shows that the mass has homogeneous hypointensity (*arrows*). c Axial contrast-enhanced T1-weighted MR image with fat saturation shows homogeneous enhancement of the mass (*arrows*). (With permission from [Lee et al. 2003])

of lymphoma. Some previously unclassified malignancies displayed this antigen. Subsequently, discovery of the chromosomal translocation t(2;5) and the resultant frequent overexpression of the anaplastic lymphoma kinase (alk) protein confirmed the existence of this entity (Harris et al. 1999a; Harris et al. 1999b; Harris et al. 2000a; Harris et al. 2000b; Lee et al. 2003; Sander et al. 1997). However, there is no single gold standard for the diagnosis of ALCL diagnosis requires both cellular morphology and immunophenotype. The diagnosis of ALCL is made when an expert hematopathologist recognizes the typical pleomorphic cells that contain irregular nuclei and prominent nucleoli. Documentation of the Ki-1 antigen positivity (Fig. 11.16), chromosomal translocation, and/or overexpression of alk protein confirm the diagnosis although they cannot be used as the defining criteria for ALCL (Freedman and Nadler 2001).

Radiologic Features

Because patients most commonly present with disseminated conditions, initial imaging work-up that covers the whole body is as important as the pathologic confirmation. Plain chest radiography, CT, radionuclear scintigraphy, and positron emission tomography (PET) are commonly used imaging modalities. In the thorax, mediastinal mass, mediastinal lymphadenopathy, multiple pulmonary nodules and pleural or pericardial effusion are seen frequently (Figs. 11.17, 11.18). Pleural or pericardial mass formation is common. Primary Ki-1-positive ALCL in a child that presented as a well-enhancing chest wall mass has been reported (Zaleski et al. 1997). In the abdomen, intraabdominal and retroperitoneal lymph node enlargement, mesenteric infiltration or mass,

diffuse intestinal wall thickening, and ascites are seen (Fig. 11.19). Peripheral lymph nodes in axillary, inguinal, and cervical area are diffusely enlarged in most of the patients. Brain, spinal cord, and muscles are rarely involved (Lee et al. 2003). In disseminated stage in other subtypes of peripheral T-cell lymphoma such as nasal type NK/T-cell lymphoma, enteropathy type T-cell lymphoma, and mycosis fungoides, the radiologic manifestations cannot be distinguished from those in this type of lymphoma.

11.3.7
Angioimmunoblastic T-Cell Lymphoma

Clinical Features

This is a relatively rare disorder, but is clinically distinctive. It accounts for less than 1% of all non-Hodgkin lymphomas in Asia and Europe (Ko et al. 1998; Lee et al. 1999; Salar et al. 1997). Although this disorder has been regarded as an abnormal immune reaction (angioimmunoblastic lymphadenopathy with dysproteinemia [AILD] or immunoblastic lymphadenopathy [IBL]), it is now generally accepted as an entity of peripheral T-cell lymphoma, because most cases show clonal rearrangements of T-cell receptor genes (Freedman and Nadler 2001; Harris et al. 1994). IBL-like T-cell lymphoma is another name for this disorder. Angioimmunoblastic T-cell lymphoma is characterized clinically by high fever, generalized lymphadenopathy, skin rash, hepatosplenomegaly, and hypergammaglobulinemia. The course is moderately aggressive, with occasional spontaneous remissions or protracted response to steroids, and infectious complications (Freedman and Nadler 2001).

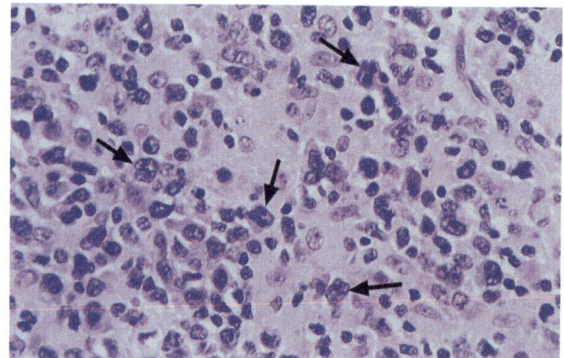
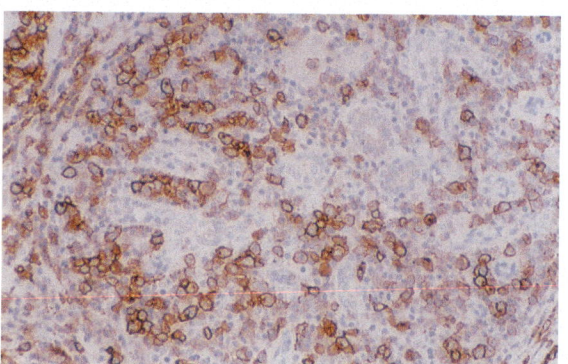

a   b

Fig. 11.16a,b. Primary systemic type ALCL in a 12-year-old girl. **a** Photomicrograph of a lymph node biopsy specimen shows diffuse proliferation of large lymphoid cells (i.e., anaplastic large cells) with pleomorphic nuclei, prominent nucleoli, and abundant cytoplasm (*arrows*) (original magnification, ×400; hematoxylin-eosin stain). **b** Photomicrograph of Ki-1 antigen-labeled tissue shows atypical lymphoid cells that react positively and appear brown (original magnification, ×200; immunohistochemical stain on paraffin-embedded material).

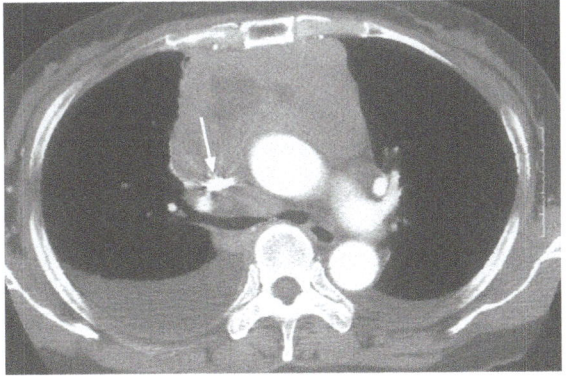

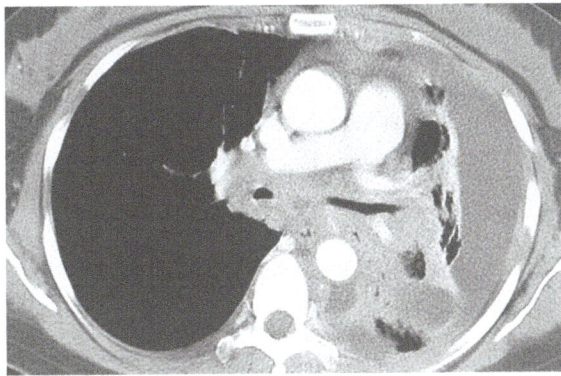

Fig. 11.17. Systemic anaplastic large cell lymphoma in a 49-year-old woman. Mediastinal window setting of axial contrast-enhanced chest CT shows bulky soft tissue mass in anterior mediastinum. The mass causes luminal narrowing of trachea as well as compression of superior vena cava (*arrow*). Bilateral pleural effusion is also noted.

Fig. 11.18. Systemic anaplastic large cell lymphoma in a 45-year-old woman. Axial contrast-enhanced chest CT shows soft tissue mass encasing the bronchi and pulmonary arteries. Pulmonary parenchymal invasion along the bronchovascular bundles and pleural effusion are noted.

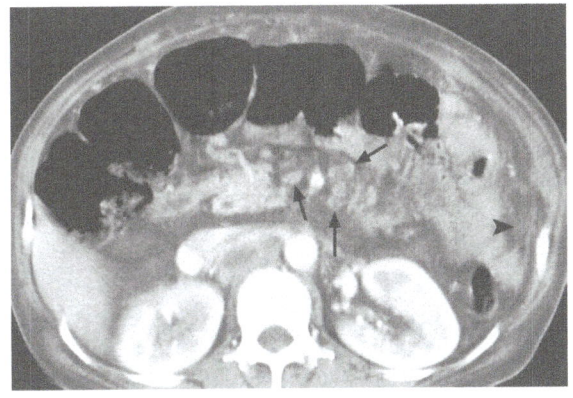

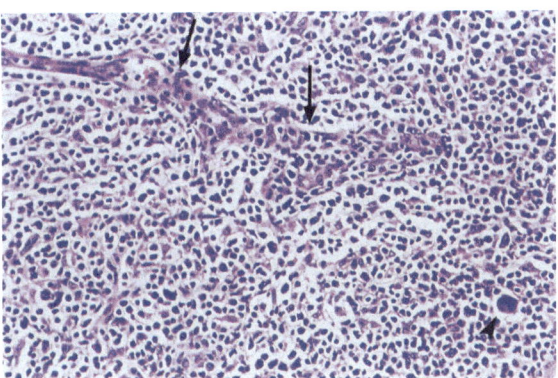

Fig. 11.19. Systemic anaplastic large cell lymphoma in a 56-year-old man. Axial contrast-enhanced CT scan of the abdomen shows multiple enlarged lymph nodes in the mesentery (*arrows*), dirty mesenteric infiltration, and peritoneal enhancement (*arrowhead*). These features suggest mesenteric lymphomatosis.

Fig. 11.20. Angioimmunoblastic T-cell lymphoma in an 18-year-old woman. Photomicrograph of a lymph node biopsy specimen shows diffuse proliferation of lymphoid cells and prominent vascular proliferation (*arrows*). The small lymphoid cells are admixed with immunoblasts (*arrowhead*) and plasma cells (original magnification, ×200; hematoxylin-eosin stain). The term angioimmunoblastic in the name of this condition is due to the vascular proliferation and admixed immunoblasts. (With permission from [LEE et al. 2003])

Pathological Features

Histologically, angioimmunoblastic T-cell lymphoma is characterized by prominent vascular proliferations. Affected lymph nodes show an effaced architecture caused by the proliferation of atypical lymphoid cells and arborizing endothelial venules. The infiltrate also contains eosinophils, plasma cells, and occasional immunoblasts (Fig. 11.20). The morphologic features are similar to those described for angioimmunoblastic lymphadenopathy (FREEDMAN and NADLER 2001; HARRIS et al. 1994; LEE et al. 2003).

Radiologic Features

Because patients most commonly present with disseminated conditions, the imaging features are not distinguished from those in other subtypes of lymphoma in disseminated state (Figs. 11.21–11.23). Radiographic manifestation of the thorax was reported. Paratracheal, anterior mediastinal, or hilar lymph node enlargement is the most common thoracic manifestation (Fig. 11.22a) (LIBSHITZ et al. 1977; LIMPERT et al. 1984). Widespread parenchymal infiltrates are infrequent, and a reticulonodular pat-

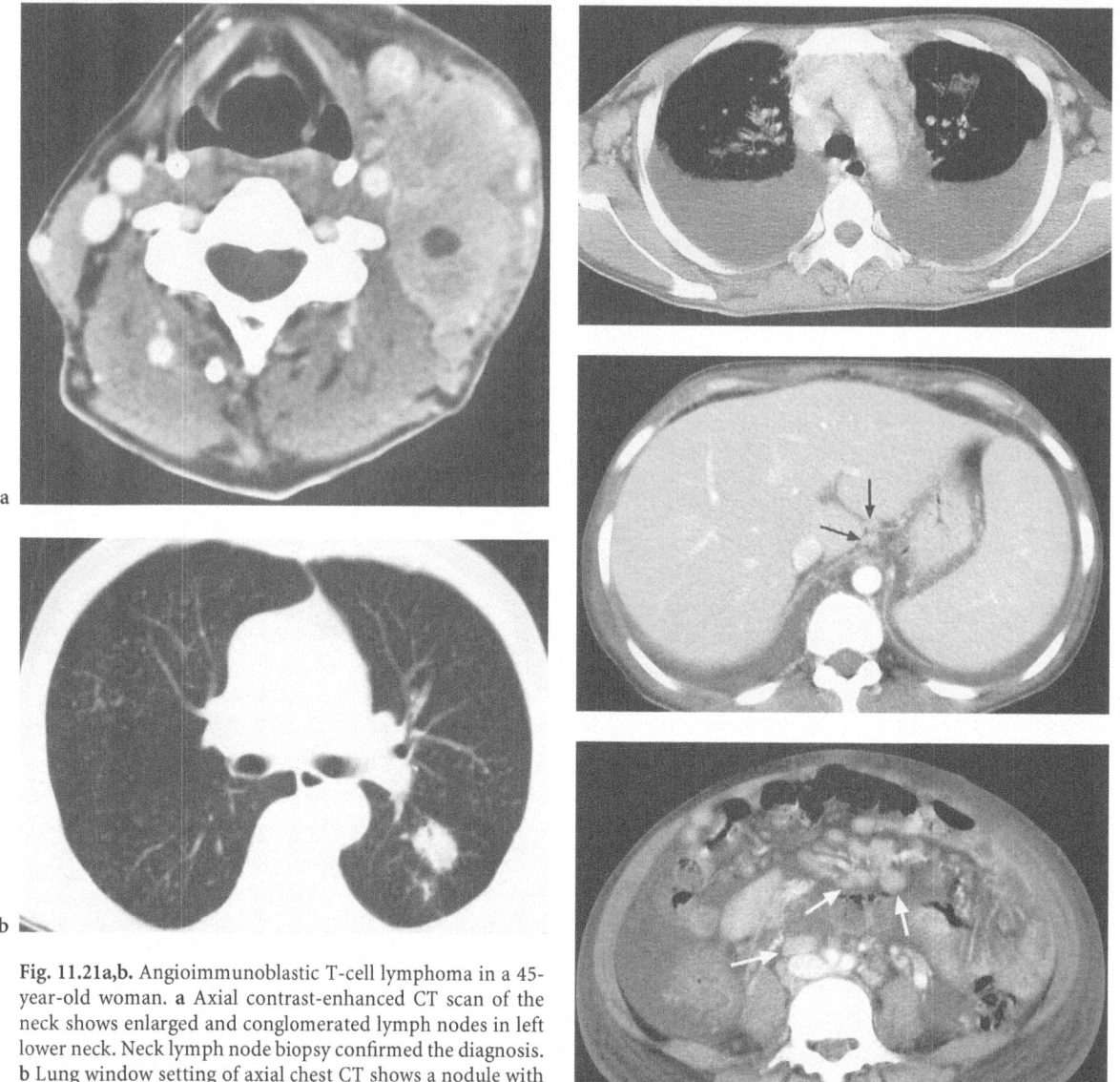

Fig. 11.21a,b. Angioimmunoblastic T-cell lymphoma in a 45-year-old woman. **a** Axial contrast-enhanced CT scan of the neck shows enlarged and conglomerated lymph nodes in left lower neck. Neck lymph node biopsy confirmed the diagnosis. **b** Lung window setting of axial chest CT shows a nodule with air-bronchogram in left lung. Disseminated small nodules in both lungs suggest underlying pneumoconiosis.

Fig. 11.22a–c. Angioimmunoblastic T-cell lymphoma in an 18-year-old woman. **a** Axial contrast-enhanced CT scan of the chest shows multiple enlarged lymph nodes in the prevascular, right lower paratracheal, and axillary areas. Bilateral pleural effusions are also noted. **b** Axial contrast-enhanced CT scan of the abdomen shows enlargement of the liver and spleen. Multiple lymph nodes are seen in the hepatic hilum (*arrows*). **c** Axial CT scan shows multiple enlarged lymph nodes in the mesentery and retroperitoneal area (*arrows*). Multiple enlarged mesenteric lymph nodes, mesenteric nodules, and ascites are suggestive of mesenteric lymphomatosis. (With permission from [LEE et al. 2003])

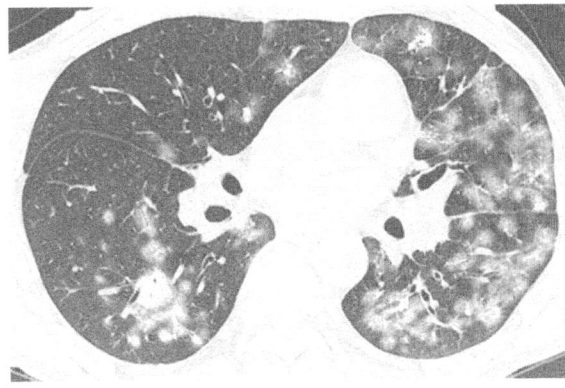

Fig. 11.23. Angioimmunoblastic T-cell lymphoma in a 42-year-old man. Lung window setting of axial high-resolution CT scan shows multiple variable-sized nodules in bilateral lungs. In this patient, multiple cervical lymph node enlargement and cutaneous lymphoma were also found. Nodal biopsy confirmed the diagnosis

tern with septal lines may be seen (ZYLAK et al. 1976). Pulmonary nodules are also encountered and pleural effusions are not uncommon (Figs. 11.21–11.23).

11.3.8
Hepatosplenic Gamma/Delta T-Cell Lymphoma

Clinical Features
Hepatosplenic gamma/delta (γδ) T-cell lymphoma is a rare, recently described subtype of peripheral T-cell lymphoma. It is characterized by hepatosplenomegaly without lymphadenopathy and significant cytopenia. This disorder has an aggressive clinical course and poor treatment outcome (FREEDMAN and NADLER 2001; LEE et al. 2003).

Pathological Features
Pathologically, lymphoma preferentially involves hepatic sinusoids, splenic red pulp and bone marrow. By definition, hepatosplenic γδ T-cell lymphoma must express the γδ T-cell receptor on cytogenetic study (FREEDMAN and NADLER 2001; HARRIS et al. 1994; LEE et al. 2003). Radiologic appearance is still unknown.

Radiologic Features
There is no radiologic literature about hepatosplenic γδ T-cell lymphoma. Hepatosplenomegaly may be detected on abdominal radiography, CT, or MR imaging (LEE et al. 2003).

11.3.9
Adult T-Cell Lymphoma/Leukemia

Clinical Features
Adult T-cell lymphoma/leukemia is one manifestation of infection by the human T lymphotropic virus-1 (HTLV1). The majority of patients are adults, who have antibodies to HTLV1. Most cases occur in Japan, but an endemic focus is found in the Caribbean, and sporadic cases are found in the United States (JAFFE et al. 1984; SWERDLOW et al. 1984; TOKUNAGA and SATO 1980; YAMADA 1983). Patients can be infected through transplacental transmission, blood transfusion, and by sexual transmission of the virus. Patients who acquire the virus from their mother through breast milk are most likely to develop lymphoma, but the risk is still only 2.5% and the latency averages 55 years (FREEDMAN and NADLER 2001; HARRIS et al. 1994).

Most common is the "acute form" in which the patient presents with an aggressive disease manifested by a high white blood cell count, lymphadenopathy, hepatosplenomegaly, hypercalcemia, lytic bone lesions, skin infiltration, and elevated LDH levels. The skin lesions can be papules, plaques, tumors, and ulcerations. True complete remissions are unusual and the median survival of patients is less than 1 year (FREEDMAN and NADLER 2001; HARRIS et al. 1994). Several clinical variants have been described (KIKUCHI et al. 1986). The rare "lymphomatous form" is characterized by isolated lymphadenopathy without leukemia. A "chronic form" with lower white blood cell count, without hypercalcemia or hepatosplenomegaly, has slightly longer survival. The rare "smoldering form" has mild lymphocytosis, which is demonstrably clonal, but a very indolent course (ABRAMS et al. 1985). Both chronic and smoldering forms often have skin rashes.

Pathological Features
The diagnosis of adult T-cell lymphoma/leukemia is made when an expert hematopathologist recognizes the typical morphologic picture. The pattern in lymph nodes is diffuse and usually there is a mixture of small and large atypical cells with pronounced polymorphism and nuclear pleomorphism. Marrow infiltration is diffuse, and ranges from sparse to marked. Examination of the peripheral blood will usually reveal characteristic, pleomorphic abnormal T-cell immunophenotypic (i.e., CD4-positive) cells with hyperlobated nuclei, which have been called "clover leaf" or "flower" cells. Clonally integrated HTLV1 genomes are found in all cases (FREEDMAN and NADLER 2001; HARRIS et al. 1994).

Radiologic Features

The reported radiologic features are mediastinal lymphadenopathy, omental lymphadenopathy causing a circumferential compression of portions of the duodenum and jejunum (Flores et al. 1998), and lymphomatous meningitis with steroid-induced epidural lipomatosis (Pennisi et al. 1985). Gallium-67 citrate scintigraphy shows a high uptake at the involved area (George et al. 1994). Radiological imaging could identify lytic bone lesions, hepatosplenomegaly, and cutaneous tumors.

11.3.10
Peripheral T-Cell Lymphoma, Not Otherwise Specified

Peripheral T-cell lymphoma can be difficult to understand and subclassify. Cases that do not fit into one of the defined entities of peripheral T-cell lymphoma are best left "Not otherwise specified (NOS)", reflecting the fact that we do not yet understand everything about lymphomas or the immune system. Problems include their rarity in Western patients, their apparent heterogeneity, and the difficulty of identifying the neoplastic cell population without a reliable immunophenotypic marker of T-cell malignancy (Harris et al. 1994). Peripheral T-cell lymphoma-NOS accounts for approximately 11% of all non-Hodgkin lymphomas in Korea and approximately 4% in Europe (Ko et al. 1998; Lee et al. 1999; Salar et al. 1997). This category includes heterogeneous diseases that require further definition.

Clinical Features

Patients are usually adults with generalized disease, occasionally with eosinophilia, pruritus or hemophagocytic syndromes. Lymph nodes, skin or subcutis, liver, spleen and other viscera may be involved. The clinical course is usually aggressive and relapses are more common than in B-cell lymphomas of similar histologic grades (Harris et al. 1994).

Pathological Features

The cases are stratified as medium-sized cell, mixed medium and large cell, large cell, and lymphoepithelioid cell types. For lack of definite criteria, these categories are imprecise and not reproducible (Harris et al. 1994, Harris et al. 1999a; Harris et al. 1999b; Harris et al. 2000a; Harris et al. 2000b).

Radiologic Features

Generalized lymphadenopathy is the most common finding. In patients presenting with disseminated conditions, the imaging features are not distinguished from those in other subtypes of lymphoma in disseminated state (Lee et al. 2003).

11.4
Precursor T-Cell Neoplasms

11.4.1
Precursor T-Cell Lymphoblastic Lymphoma/Leukemia

Clinical Features

Precursor T-cell malignancies can present either as acute lymphoblastic leukemia or as an aggressive lymphoma. These malignancies are more common in children and young adults, with men more frequently affected than women. It constitutes 40% of childhood lymphomas and 15% of acute lymphoblastic leukemias (Freedman and Nadler 2001; Harris et al. 1994). There is a consensus that precursor T-cell lymphoblastic lymphoma and precursor T-cell lymphoblastic leukemia are a single disease with different presentations. The precursor neoplasms presenting as solid tumors and those presenting with marrow and blood involvement are biologically the same disease, but with different clinical presentations. Precursor T-cell lymphoblastic lymphoma presents with a large mediastinal mass and pleural effusions. This disorder has a propensity to metastasize to the central nervous system, and central nervous system involvement is often present at diagnosis. Precursor T-cell acute lymphoblastic leukemia can present with bone marrow failure, and sometimes with very high white cell counts, a mediastinal mass, lymphadenopathy, and hepatosplenomegaly. Untreated, it is rapidly fatal; however, the majority of patients treated with chemotherapy can be cured. Patients who present with localized disease have an excellent prognosis. Advanced age is an adverse prognostic factor (Freedman and Nadler 2001; Harris et al. 1999a; Harris et al. 1999b; Harris et al. 2000a; Harris et al. 2000b).

Pathological Features

The tumor cells are morphologically identical to those of precursor B-cell lymphoblastic lymphoma/leukemia. The tumor cells are lymphoblasts, with round or convoluted nuclei, finely dispersed chromatin, inconspicuous nucleoli, and scant cytoplasm. The tumor cells are morphologically similar; therefore, immunophenotyping studies are necessary to distinguish this tumor from precursor B-cell lymphoblastic neoplasms (Freedman and Nadler 2001; Harris et al. 1994).

Radiologic Features

The radiographic presentations of several cases have been reported. There are isolated cases presenting with masses involving anterior mediastinum (KOITA et al. 1997; LEMAITRE et al. 1987; WILLEMSSEN et al. 2002), heart (WERNER et al. 2001), pleura (KARADENIZ et al. 2000), orbit (COOK and BARTLEY 1997; ESMAELI et al. 2001), pancreas (TAMURA et al. 1998), nasal cavity (KOITA et al. 1997), or breast (PAOLUCCI et al. 1981). A case presented with diffuse renal infiltration (JOSE et al. 1998) and a case with bulky lymphadenopathy in the oropharyngeal (Waldeyer's ring), submandibular, supraclavicular and inguinal nodal regions (GOLLARD et al. 1996) were also reported.

11.5
Conclusion

T-cell lymphoma can demonstrate a wide spectrum of disease in many organs. The specific clinicopathologic entities of T-cell lymphoma have particular primary locations and particular clinical and pathologic features. Most radiologic features of T-cell lymphoma are nonspecific and often simulate those of other neoplasms or inflammatory conditions. However, it is significant that the radiologic features of several entities including enteropathy-type T-cell lymphoma and nasal-type NK/T-cell lymphoma are quite different from those of lymphoma with the B-cell phenotype. Radiological demonstration of disease progression beyond the primary site is also clinically important because systemic dissemination in most of the entities leads to a dramatic change in the prognosis.

References

Abrams MB, Sidawy M, Novich M (1985) Smoldering HTLV-associated T-cell leukemia. Arch Intern Med 145: 2257–2258

Armitage JO, Greer JP, Levine AM, et al. (1989) Peripheral T-cell lymphoma. Cancer 63:158–163

Bass JC, Korobkin MT, Cooper KD, et al. (1993) Cutaneous T-cell lymphoma: CT in evaluation and staging. Radiology 186:273–278

Castellino RA, Hoppe RT, Blank N, et al. (1979) Experience with lymphography in patients with mycosis fungoides. Cancer Treat Rep 63:581–586

Chan JKC, Ng CS, Lau WH, et al. (1987) Most nasal/nasopharyngeal lymphomas are peripheral T-cell lymphomas. Am J Surg Pathol 11:418–429

Cheung MM, Chan JK, Lau WH, et al. (1998) Primary non-Hodgkin's lymphoma of the nose and nasopharynx: clinical features, tumor immunophenotype, and treatment outcome in 113 patients. J Clinical Oncol 16:70–77

Chott A, Augustin I, Wrba F, et al. (1990) Peripheral T-cell lymphomas: a clinicopathologic study of 75 cases. Hum Pathol 21:1117–1125

Chott A, Dragosics B, Radaszkiewicz T (1992) Peripheral T-cell lymphomas of the intestine. Am J Pathol 141:1361–1371

Coiffier B, Brousse N, Peuchmaur M, et al. (1990) Peripheral T-cell lymphomas have a worse prognosis than B-cell lymphomas: a prospective study of 361 immunophenotyped patients treated with the LNH-84 regimen. The GELA (Groupe d'Etude des Lymphomes Agressives). Ann Oncol 1:45–50

Cook BE Jr, Bartley GB (1997) Acute lymphoblastic leukemia manifesting in an adult as a conjunctival mass. Am J Ophthalmol 124:104–105

Eichel BS, Harrison EG, Devine KD, et al. (1996) Primary lymphoma of the nose including a relationship to lethal midline granuloma. Am J Surg 112:597–605

Esmaeli B, Medeiros LJ, Myers J, et al. (2001) Orbital mass secondary to precursor T-cell acute lymphoblastic leukemia: a rare presentation. Arch Ophthalmol 119:443–446

Ferry JA, Sklar J, Zukerberg LR, et al. (1991) Nasal lymphoma. A clinicopathologic study with immunophenotypic and genotypic analysis. Am J Surg Pathol 15:268–279

Flores LG 2nd, Nagamachi S, Nishii R, et al. (1998) Gallium-67 scintigraphy in the treatment and prognosis of acute adult T-cell lymphoma. Ann Nucl Med 12:105–108

Freedman AS, Nadler LM (2001) Malignancies of lymphoid cells. In: Fauci AS, Braunwald E, Isselbacher KJ (eds) Harrison's Online version 2.0. McGraw-Hill, New York, p 23

George CD, Wilson AG, Philpott NJ, et al. (1994) The radiological features of adult T-cell leukaemia/lymphoma. Clin Radiol 49:83–88

Gollard RP, Robbins BA, Piro L, et al. (1996) Acute myelogenous leukemia presenting with bulky lymphadenopathy. Case report and literature review. Acta Haematol 95: 129–134

Grogan TM, Fielder K, Rangel C, et al. (1985) Peripheral T-cell lymphoma: aggressive disease with heterogeneous immunotypes. Am J Clin Pathol 83:279–288

Harris NL, Jaffe ES, Stein H, et al. (1994) A revised European-American classification of lymphoid neoplasms: a proposal from the International Lymphoma Study Group. Blood 84:1361–1392

Harris NL, Jaffe ES, Diebold J, et al. (1999a) The World Health Organization classification of neoplastic diseases of the hematopoietic and lymphoid tissues. Report of the Clinical Advisory Committee meeting, Airlie House, Virginia, November, 1997. Ann Oncol 10:1419–1432

Harris NL, Jaffe ES, Diebold J, et al. (1999b) World Health Organization classification of neoplastic diseases of the hematopoietic and lymphoid tissues: report of the Clinical Advisory Committee meeting-Airlie House, Virginia, November 1997. J Clin Oncol 17:3835–3849

Harris NL, Jaffe ES, Diebold J, et al. (2000a) The World Health Organization classification of hematological malignancies report of the Clinical Advisory Committee Meeting, Airlie House, Virginia, November 1997. Mod Pathol 13:193–207

Harris NL, Jaffe ES, Diebold J, et al. (2000b) The World Health Organization classification of neoplastic diseases of the

haematopoietic and lymphoid tissues: Report of the Clinical Advisory Committee Meeting, Airlie House, Virginia,
November 1997. Histopathology 36:69–86

Howlett DC, Wong WL, Smith NP, et al. (1995) Computed
tomography in the evaluation of cutaneous T-cell lymphoma. Eur J Radiol 20:39–42

Hsiao CH, Lee WI, Chang SL, et al. (1996) Angiocentric T-cell
lymphoma of the intestine: a distinct etiology of ischemic
bowel disease. Gastroenterology 110:985–990

Isaacson PG (1994) Gastrointestinal lymphoma. Hum Pathol
25:1020–1029

Isaacson PG, O'Connor NT, Spencer J, et al. (1985) Malignant
histiocytosis of the intestine: a T-cell lymphoma. Lancet
2:688–691

Jaffe ES (1996) Classification of natural killer (NK) cell and
NK-like T-cell malignancies. Blood 87:1207–1210

Jaffe ES, Blattner WA, Blayney DW, et al. (1984) The pathologic
spectrum of adult T-cell leukemia/lymphoma in the United
States. Human T-cell leukemia/lymphoma virus-associated
lymphoid malignancies. Am J Surg Pathol 8:263–275

Jaffe ES, Chan JK, Su IJ, et al. (1996) Report of the workshop
on nasal and related extranodal angiocentric t/natural
killer cell lymphomas: definitions, differential diagnosis,
and epidemiology. Am J Surg Pathol 20:103–111

Jagannath S, Velasquez WS, Tucker SL, et al. (1986) Tumor
burden assessment and its implication for a prognostic
model in advanced diffuse large cell lymphoma. J Clin
Oncol 4:859–865

Jose MD, Bannister KM, Clarkson AR, et al. (1998) Diffuse
kidney infiltration with T-cell lymphoblastic lymphoma.
Nephrol Dial Transplant 13:1877–1878

Karadeniz C, Guven MA, Ruacan S, et al. (2000) Primary pleural lymphoma: an unusual presentation of childhood non-
Hodgkin lymphoma. Pediatr Hematol Oncol 17:695–699

Katoh A, Ohshima K, Kanda M, et al. (2000) Gastrointestinal
T cell lymphoma: predominant cytotoxic phenotypes,
including alpha/beta, gamma/delta T cell and natural killer
cells. Leuk Lymphoma 39:97–111

Kikuchi M, Mitsui T, Takeshita M, et al. (1986) Virus associated adult T-cell leukemia (ATL) in Japan: clinical,
histological and immunological studies. Hematol Oncol
4:67–81

Kim YH, Hoppe RT (1999) Mycosis fungoides and the Sezary
syndrome. Semin Oncol 26:276–289

King AD, Lei KI, Ahuja AT, et al. (2000) MR imaging of nasal
T-cell/natural killer cell lymphoma. AJR Am J Roentgenol
174:209–211

Ko YH, Kim CW, Park CS, et al. (1998) REAL classification of
malignant lymphomas in the Republic of Korea: incidence
of recently recognized entities and changes in clinicopathologic features. Hematolymphoreticular Study Group
of the Korean Society of Pathologists. Revised European-
American lymphoma. Cancer 83:806–812

Koita H, Suzumiya J, Ohshima K, et al. (1997) Lymphoblastic
lymphoma expressing natural killer cell phenotype with
involvement of the mediastinum and nasal cavity. Am J
Surg Pathol 21:242–248

Kulin PA, Marglin SI, Shuman WP, et al. (1990) Diagnostic
imaging in the initial staging of mycosis fungoides and
Sézary syndrome. Arch Dermatol 126:914–918

Kwak LW, Wilson M, Weiss LM, et al. (1991) Similar outcome of
treatment of B-cell and T-cell diffuse large-cell lymphomas:
the Stanford experience. J Clin Oncol 9:1426–1431

Lamberg SI, Bunn PA Jr (1979) Cutaneous T-cell lymphomas.
Summary of the Mycosis Fungoides Cooperative Group-
National Cancer Institute Workshop. Arch Dermatol 115:
1103–1105

Lee HJ, Han JK, Kim TK, et al. (2001) Peripheral T-cell lymphoma of the colon: double-contrast barium enema examination findings in six patients. Radiology 218:751–756

Lee HJ, Han JK, Kim TK, et al. (2002) Primary colorectal
lymphoma: spectrum of imaging findings with pathologic
correlation. Eur Radiol 12:2242–2249

Lee HJ, Im JG, Goo JM, et al. (2003) Peripheral T-cell lymphoma: spectrum of imaging findings with clinical and
pathologic features. Radiographics 23:7–26

Lee SS, Cho KJ, Kim CW, et al. (1999) Clinicopathological analysis of 501 non-Hodgkin's lymphomas in Korea
according to the revised European-American classification
of lymphoid neoplasms. Histopathology 35:345–354

Lemaitre L, Leclerc F, Marconi V, et al. (1987) Ultrasonographic findings in thymic lymphoma in children. Eur J
Radiol 7:125–129

Levy AD, Koeller KK (2003) Invited commentary. Radiographics 23:26–28

Libshitz HI, Clouser M, Zornoza J, et al. (1977) Radiographic
findings of immunoblastic lymphadenopathy and related
immunoblastic proliferations. AJR Am J Roentgenol 129:
875–878

Limpert J, MacMahon H, Variakojis D (1984) Angioimmunoblastic lymphadenopathy: clinical and radiological
features. Radiology 152:27–30

Loberant N, Cohen I, Noi I, et al. (1997) Enteropathy-associated
T-cell lymphoma: a case report with radiographic and computed tomography appearance. J Surg Oncol 65:50–54

Melnyk A, Rodriguez A, Pugh WC, et al. (1997) Evaluation of
the Revised European-American Lymphoma classification
confirms the clinical relevance of immunophenotype in
560 cases of aggressive non-Hodgkin's lymphoma. Blood
89:4514–4520

Miketic LM, Chambers TP, Lembersky BC (1993) Cutaneous
T-cell lymphoma: value of CT in staging and determining
prognosis. AJR Am J Roentgenol 160:1129–1132

Montalban C, Obeso G, Gallego A, et al. (1993) Peripheral T-
cell lymphoma: A clinicopathological study of 41 cases and
evaluation of the prognostic significance of the updated
Kiel classification. Histopathology 22:303–310

Nakamura K, Uehara S, Omagari J, et al. (1997) Primary non-
Hodgkin lymphoma of the sinonasal cavities: correlation of
CT evaluation with clinical outcome. Radiology 204:431–435

Ooi GC, Chim CS, Liang R, et al. (2000) Nasal T-cell/natural
killer cell lymphoma: CT and MR imaging features of a
new clinicopathologic entity. AJR Am J Roentgenol 174:
1141–1145

Paolucci R, Delledonne V, Bonati A (1981) T-lymphoblastic
lymphoma convoluted-cell type: mammographic picture.
Radiol Med (Torino) 67:453–455

Pennisi AK, Meisler WJ, Dina TS (1985) Lymphomatous
meningitis and steroid-induced epidural lipomatosis: CT
evaluation. J Comput Assist Tomogr 9:595–598

Perret RS, Borne J (1998) Case 3: T-cell lymphoma of the small
bowel developing in long-standing celiac disease (nontrop-
ical sprue). AJR Am J Roentgenol 171:858–860

Pinkus G, O'Hara CJ, Said JW (1990) Peripheral/post-thymic
T-cell lymphomas: a spectrum of disease. Cancer 65:
971–998

Robertson DA, Dixon MF, Scott BB, et al. (1983) Small intestinal ulceration: diagnostic difficulties in relation to coeliac disease. Gut 24:565–574

Rodriguez J, Cabanillas F, McLaughlin P, et al. (1992) A proposal for a simple staging system for intermediate grade lymphoma and immunoblastic lymphoma based on the "tumor score." Ann Oncol 3:711–717

Rosen ST, Gore R, Brennan J, et al. (1986) Evaluation of computed tomography and radionuclide scanning in the staging of cutaneous T-cell lymphoma. Arch Dermatol 122:884–886

Salar A, Fernandez de Sevilla A, et al. (1997) Distribution and incidence rates of lymphoid neoplasms according to the REAL classification in a single institution. A prospective study of 940 cases. Eur J Haematol 59:231–237

Sander CA, Kind P, Kaudewitz P, et al. (1997) The revised European-American classification of lymphoid neoplasms (REAL): a new perspective for the classification of cutaneous lymphomas. J Cutan Pathol 24:329–341

Stewart JP (1993) Progressive lethal granulomatous ulceration of the nose. J Laryngol Otol 48:657–701

Su IJ, Wang CH, Cheng AL, et al. (1988) Characterization of the spectrum of postthymic T-cell malignancies in Taiwan. A clinicopathologic study of HTLV-1-positive and HTLV-1-negative cases. Cancer 61:2060–2070

Swerdlow SH, Habeshaw JA, Rohatiner AZ, et al. (1984) Caribbean T-cell lymphoma/leukemia. Cancer 54:687–696

Tallini G, West AB, Buckley PJ (1993) Diagnosis of gastrointestinal T-cell lymphomas in routinely processed tissues. J Clin Gastroenterol 17:57–66

Tamura H, Ogata K, Mori S, et al. (1998) Lymphoblastic lymphoma of natural killer cell origin, presenting as pancreatic tumour. Histopathology 32:508–511

Teng MM, Chang CY, Guo WY, et al. (1990) CT evaluation of polymorphic reticulosis. Neuroradiology 31:498–501

The International Non-Hodgkin's Lymphoma Prognostic Factors Project (1993) A predictive model for aggressive non-Hodgkin's lymphoma. N Engl J Med 329:987–994

Tokunaga M, Sato E (1980) Non-Hodgkin's lymphomas in a southern prefecture in Japan: an analysis in 715 cases. Cancer 46:1231–1239

Weiss LM, Arber DA, Strickler JG (1994) Nasal T-cell lymphoma. Ann Oncol 10:39–42

Werner D, Schmeisser A, Daniel WG (2001) Images in cardiology: primary cardiac lymphoblastic T cell lymphoma. Heart 86:618

Willemssen F, Colla R, Vandevenne JE, et al. (2002) Mediastinal T-cell lymphoblastic lymphoma. JBR-BTR 85:172–173

Yamada Y (1983) Phenotypic and functional analysis of leukemic cells from 16 patients with adult T-cell leukemia/lymphoma. Blood 61:192–199

Zaleski CG, Abdenour GE (1997) Pediatric case of the day. Primary Ki-1-positive anaplastic large-cell lymphoma (ALCL) of the chest wall. Radiographics 17:227–231

Zylak CJ, Banerjee R, Galbraith PA, et al. (1976) Lung involvement in angioimmunoblastic lymphadenopathy (AIL). Radiology 121:513–519

12 Malignant Lymphoma in Sjögren Syndrome

Hisao Tonami, Itaru Yamamoto, Susumu Sugai

CONTENTS

12.1
Introduction

Sjögren syndrome is a chronic autoimmune disease associated with the production of autoantibodies and characterized by a progressive lymphocytic and plasma cell infiltration of the salivary and lacrimal glands leading to xerostomia and keratoconjunctivitis sicca (Fox et al. 1984). Sjögren syndrome may be primary or associated with another autoim-

Hisao Tonami, MD
Professor, Department of Radiology, Kanazawa Medical University, Daigaku 1-1, Uchinada, Kahoku, Ishikawa, Japan 920-0293
Itaru Yamamoto, MD
Professor, Department of Radiology, Kanazawa Medical University, Daigaku 1-1, Uchinada, Kahoku, Ishikawa, Japan 920-0293
Susumu Sugai, MD
Professor, Department of Internal Medicine, Division of Hematology and Immunology, Kanazawa Medical University, Daigaku 1-1, Uchinada, Kahoku, Ishikawa, Japan 920-0293

mune disease, most frequently rheumatoid arthritis (Anaya et al. 1996). An increased risk of malignant lymphoma in patients with Sjögren syndrome was first reported as early as 1963 (Bunim and Talal 1963). Subsequently, several case reports supported the association of lymphoma with Sjögren syndrome (Hornbaker et al. 1966; Talal et al. 1967) and recognized malignant lymphoma as the most serious complication in the progression of the disease (Kassan et al. 1978).

12.2
Etiology

In Sjögren syndrome, persistent antigenic challenge induces periductal lymphocytic aggregates that extend into and destroy the acinar parenchyma. The lymphoid infiltrate produces a localized parenchymal mass referred as a benign lymphoepithelial lesion (Cummings et al. 1971). The transformation from benign lymphoepithelial lesion characteristic of Sjögren syndrome to malignant lymphoma is probably a multi-step process (Fig. 12.1).

The benign lymphoepithelial lesion is generally composed of a mixture of polyclonal B-cell lymphocytes and T-cell lymphocytes. In contrast, malignant lymphoma represents neoplastic, monoclonal B-cell proliferations. Immunophenotypic analysis has been used in tissue samples from patients with Sjögren syndrome, showing oligoclonal or monoclonal B-cell expansion in 14–100% of cases (Fishleder et al. 1987). Some of these patients have developed overt malignant lymphoma, showing that Sjögren syndrome is a crossroad between autoimmunity and malignancy, and monoclonality may be a precursor for lymphoma development (Bhattacharyya et al. 1998). Morphologically benign and immunophenotypically oligoclonal lymphoid proliferations traditionally referred to as pseudolymphomas exhibit clonal immunoglobulin heavy or light chain gene rearrangements, indicating that most such lesions

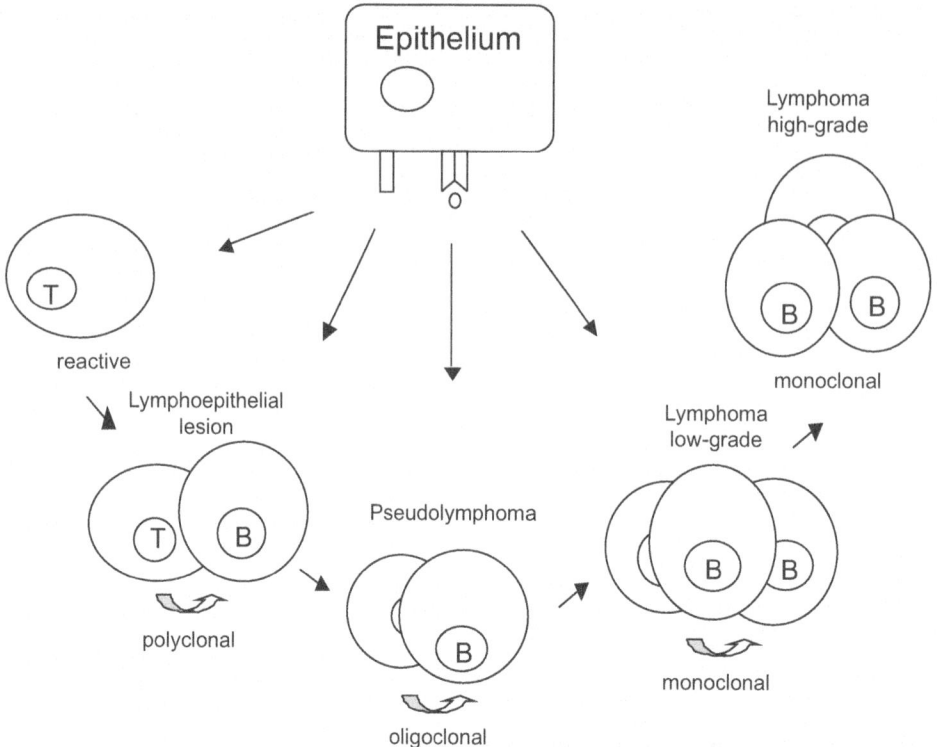

Fig. 12.1. Multi-step process to develop lymphoma in Sjögren syndrome. Benign lymphoepithelial lesion characteristic of Sjögren syndrome is composed of a mixture of T-cells and B-cells which is polyclonal. On the other hand, pseudolymphoma is composed of oligoclonal and MALT lymphoma is composed of monoclonal B-cell expansion.

represent early forms of low-grade B-cell lymphoma. Factors associated with monoclonal or malignant transformation during the course of disease are not fully understood. However, dysregulation in the mechanisms leading to apoptosis, hyperstimulation of B-cells, or infectious agent may contribute to malignant lymphoproliferation in Sjögren syndrome (MARIETTE 1999).

12.3
Incidence

The risk of lymphoma in patients with Sjögren syndrome reached 6.4 cases per 1000 per year (44 times greater than in a normal healthy population) in 136 women with Sjögren syndrome followed for an average of 8.1 years (KASSAN et al. 1978). Comparable results (10–15% of patients with Sjögren syndrome developed malignant lymphoma during follow-up of more than 15 years) were obtained in several reports (PISA et al. 1991; PARIENTE et al. 1992; KRUIZE et al. 1996; SUTCLIFFE et al. 1998).

12.4
Histology

The majority of malignant lymphomas associated with Sjögren syndrome are B-cell non-Hodgkin lymphomas (MARIETTE 1999). Both T-cell non-Hodgkin lymphomas and Hodgkin lymphomas are very rare. To date, various histologic subtypes of B-cell non-Hodgkin lymphomas have been described in patients with Sjögren syndrome, including follicular lymphomas (PAVLIDIS et al. 1992), diffuse large cell lymphomas (ZULMAN et al. 1978), and especially marginal zone B-cell lymphomas (ISAACSON and SPENCER 1987). The term marginal zone B-cell lymphoma includes low-grade B-cell mucosa-associated lymphoid tissue (MALT) lymphomas and monocytoid B-cell lymphomas. MALT lymphomas commonly present with localized extranodal disease involving glandular epithelial tissues and monocytoid B-cell lymphomas represent the nodal counterpart of MALT lymphomas (SHIN et al. 1991; HARRIS et al. 1994). It has been reported that MALT lymphoma accounts for 46–56% of the malignant lymphomas that develop in patients with Sjögren syndrome (ROYER et al. 1997). Previous studies have established that MALT lymphomas arise from the physiological MALT, like in the small intestine or, more frequently, from the acquired MALT occurring following different chronic inflammatory disorders (Isaacson and Wright 1984). The commonest examples of acquired MALT are represented by *Helicobacter pylori* induced chronic gastritis, lymphoid interstitial pneumonitis, Hashimoto thyroiditis, and Sjögren syndrome (Wotherspoon et al. 1991). Recently, it has been shown that marginal zone B-cell lymphomas, especially MALT lymphomas can progress to high-grade diffuse large cell lymphomas (Chan et al. 1990; Zucca et al. 1998). In the light of these data, a large number of malignant lymphomas occurring in patients with Sjögren syndrome reported in the literature can be reclassified as marginal zone B-cell lymphomas either of low-grade or of low-grade transformed into high-grade lymphomas.

12.5
Imaging Features

12.5.1
Initial Imaging Features

Initial imaging features of malignant lymphomas in patients with Sjögren syndrome are not substantially different from those reported in the other lymphomas occurring in patients without an underlying Sjögren syndrome (Tonami et al. 2002a). Although both extranodal and nodal involvements are observed, extranodal manifestation is more common in Sjögren syndrome (Royer et al. 1997). The extranodal site is often the salivary gland, but other extranodal sites including the lacrimal gland, the thyroid gland, Waldeyer's ring, the lung, and the stomach are also involved (Voulgarelis et al. 1999).

12.5.1.1
Salivary Gland

The salivary gland is one of the major targets of Sjögren syndrome. Approximately 55% of all extranodal lymphomas associated with Sjögren syndrome affect the salivary gland (Biasi et al. 2001). Most reported lymphomas of the salivary gland have been found in the parotid gland (Grevers et al. 1994; Tagnon et al. 2002). There are only isolated reports of lymphoma in the submandibular gland (Tonami et al. 2002a). The majority of lymphomas of the salivary gland are MALT lymphomas arising

from benign lymphoepithelial lesions characterizing Sjögren syndrome (Stewart et al. 1994; Sato et al. 2002). The imaging appearance of malignant lymphomas of the salivary gland varies with the pathologic distribution of the disease. Most commonly, the lymphoma is confined to the gland, and one to several benign appearing masses are identified within the gland (Som and Brandwein 2002). Usually, each mass is homogenously hypodense on unenhanced CT scans (Fig. 12.2). The lymphoma tends to show hypointense to native gland tissue on T1-weighted MR images, iso- to hyperintense on T2-weighted MR images, and may enhance moderately on contrast-enhanced T1-weighted MR images (Fig. 12.3) (Vogl et al. 1996). If the gland is diffusely infiltrated, the lesion will be seen either with poorly defined margins or involving the entire gland (Fig. 12.4).

In some cases, multiple cystic lesions may be observed within the gland, corresponding to lymphoepithelial cysts which have been described as a common finding in Sjögren syndrome or human immunodeficiency virus positivity (Som et al. 1995).

12.5.1.2
Lacrimal Gland

The lacrimal gland is also one of the chief organs targeted by Sjögren syndrome (Bloch et al. 1965). The lymphomas originating from the lacrimal gland are

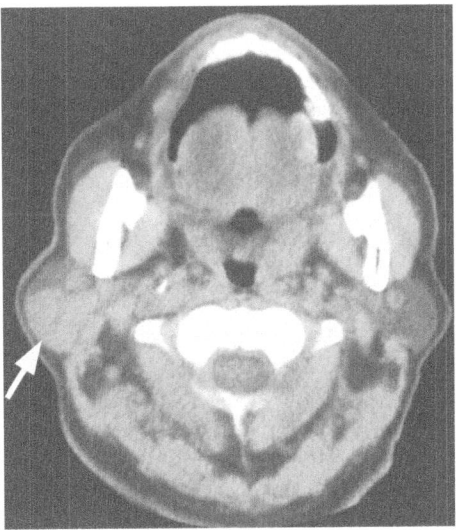

Fig. 12.2. Diffuse medium cell lymphoma of the parotid gland in a 67-year old man. He was simultaneously diagnosed as having Sjögren syndrome and malignant lymphoma. Axial unenhanced CT scan shows a lobulated mass (*arrow*) in the right parotid gland. The mass is homogenous and hypodense to the native parotid tissue.

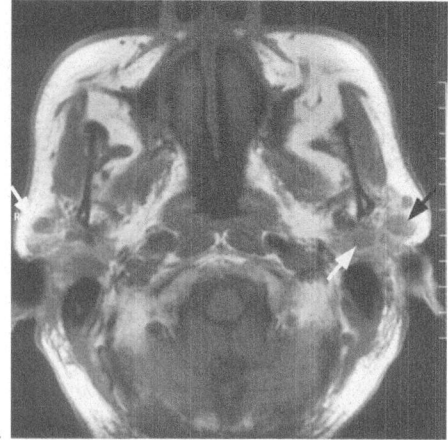

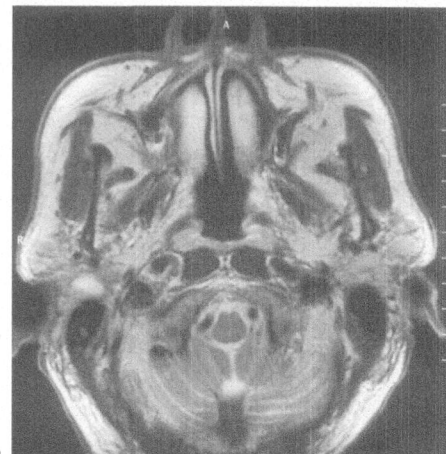

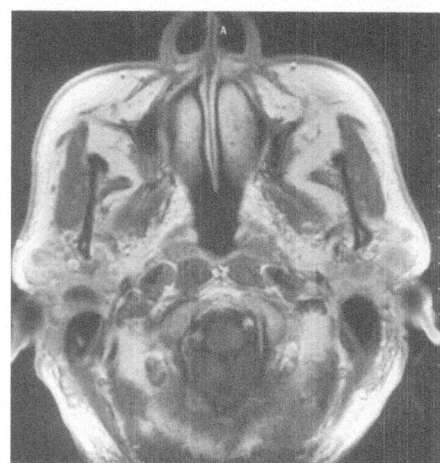

Fig. 12.3a–c. MALT lymphoma of the parotid glands in a 72-year-old man. The disease duration of Sjögren syndrome prior to the onset of malignant lymphoma was 8 years. **a** Axial spin-echo T1-weighted MR image shows multiple hypointense masses (*arrows*) in the bilateral parotid glands. **b** Axial fast spin-echo T2-weighted MR image shows the masses to be isointense to the native parotid tissue. **c** Axial contrast-enhanced spin-echo T1-weighted MR image shows the masses show moderate enhancement.

usually low-grade, with an indolent course (KIRATLI et al. 1999). CT or MR imaging show unilateral or bilateral, lobulated or round mass, molding adjacent structures without causing indentation (TONAMI et al. 2002b). In addition, a wedge shaped enlargement of the lacrimal gland which molds and drapes onto the globe, with more frequent evidence of anterior or posterior extension, is seen (Fig. 12.5). On T1-weighted MR images, the lymphomas exhibit iso- to hyperintensity in comparison with the extraocular muscles, and moderate to marked enhancement on contrast-enhanced MR images. Since these imaging features are relatively nonspecific, it may be difficult to differentiate malignant lymphomas from benign lymphoid hyperplasia or pseudolymphomas, especially in the context of an underlying Sjögren syndrome (Figs. 12.5, 12.6) (POLIO et al. 1996).

12.5.1.3
Waldeyer's Ring

The occurrence of malignant lymphoma in Waldeyer's ring in patients with Sjögren syndrome is less common. The most common sites are the palatine and lingual tonsils, followed by nasopharynx (RODALLEC et al. 2002). The imaging finding of these lesions is an asymmetric thickening of the pharyngeal mucosa, or a solitary mass (Fig. 12.7). The signal intensity of adenoid is similar to that of lymphoma, and distinction of between normal lymphoid tissue and lymphoma may be difficult on CT and MR imaging.

12.5.1.4
Thyroid Gland

Most of the lymphomas originating from the thyroid gland in Sjögren syndrome are MALT lymphomas (NAKANO et al. 1999). Although the thyroid gland is devoid of native lymphoid tissue, lymphoid tissue is acquired during the course of Sjögren syndrome. The relationship of Hashimoto thyroiditis and malignant lymphoma is well established, suggesting that lymphocytes infiltrating the tissue of Hashimoto thyroiditis undergo blastic change due to persistent antigenetic challenge (SCHOLEFIELD et al. 1992). In the same way, lymphoma of the thyroid gland is developed as a result of autoimmune reactions in Sjögren syndrome. Lymphoma of the thyroid gland may present as a diffuse enlargement of the gland, or as multiple nodules, but more commonly it presents as a solitary mass. Usually it is hypoechoic on ultrasound and hypodense on unenhanced CT scans (Fig. 12.8) (RODALLEC et al. 2002). The lymphoma is usually hypo to isointense to

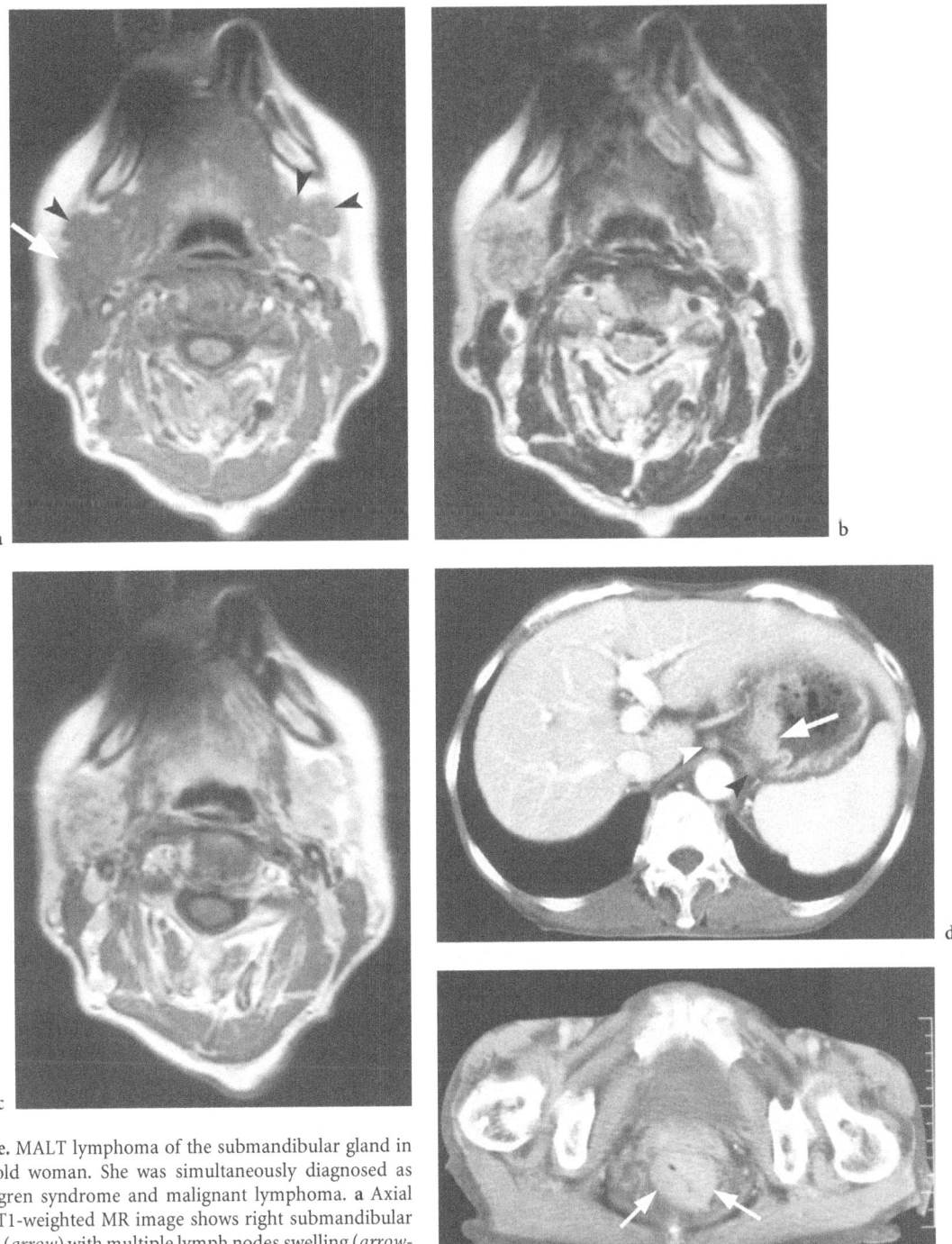

Fig. 12.4a–e. MALT lymphoma of the submandibular gland in a 64-year-old woman. She was simultaneously diagnosed as having Sjögren syndrome and malignant lymphoma. **a** Axial spin-echo T1-weighted MR image shows right submandibular gland mass (*arrow*) with multiple lymph nodes swelling (*arrowheads*). The mass is isointense to muscles. **b** Axial fast spin-echo T2-weighted MR image shows mass to be hypointense to subcutaneous fat. **c** Axial contrast-enhanced spin-echo T1-weighted MR image shows diffuse enhancement. She was treated with radiation therapy followed by chemotherapy, achieving complete remission. Axial contrast-enhanced CT scans obtained 1 year later show abnormal wall thickening (*arrows*) suggestive of disease spread to stomach (**d**) and rectum (**e**). Note few enlarged lymph nodes in perigastric regions (*arrowheads*). (With permission from [TONAMI et al. 2002a])

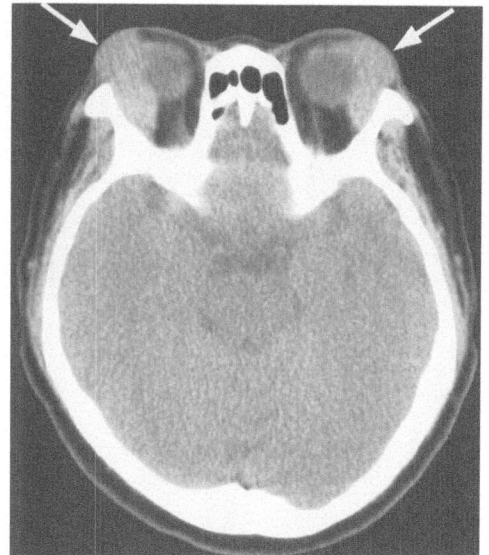

a

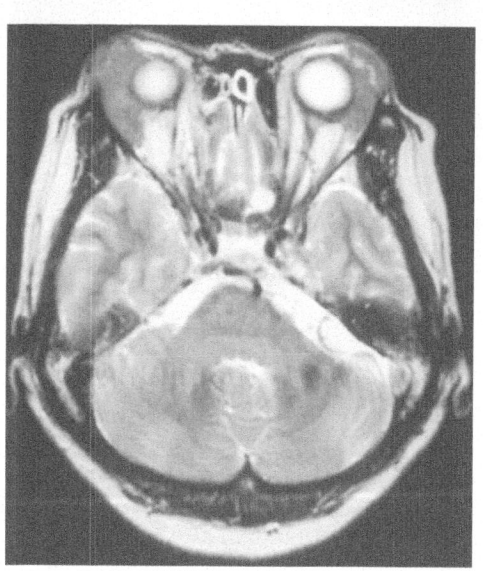

b

c

native thyroid tissue on T1-weighted MR images and hyperintense on T2-weighted MR images.

12.5.1.5
Lung

The majority of lymphomas of the lung in patients with Sjögren syndrome arise from bronchus-associated lymphoid tissue, which is a component of the much larger and more extensive MALT (LIAO et al. 2000). The most common CT findings are air-space consolidation or nodules with prominent air bronchograms (Fig. 12.9) (LEE et al. 2000). Multiple bilateral lesions are common (Fig. 12.10) (KNISELY et al. 1999). The lymphoma may show little or no change over a prolonged period, suggesting its indolent nature. Hilar and mediastinal lymphadenopathies and pleural fluid collection may be seen in more aggressive disease (Fig. 12.10).

12.5.1.6
Stomach

Although the stomach is the most frequently involved site of MALT lymphoma in patients who do not have Sjögren syndrome, the occurrence of MALT lymphoma in the stomach is less common in patients who have preexisting Sjögren syndrome (THIEBLEMONT et al. 1997). MALT in the stomach is acquired by the presence of *Helicobacter pylori* as a causative antigen (ISAACSON and WRIGHT 1984). On CT scans, various patterns may be observed including focal thickening of the gastric wall, lobulated inner gastric wall, and multinodular lesions (RODALLEC et al. 2002). Submucosal mass and ulcerative lesions are rare.

12.5.1.7
Lymph Nodes

Any nodal site can be involved in malignant lymphomas associated with Sjögren syndrome (ZUFFEREY

Fig. 12.5a–c. MALT lymphoma and pseudolymphoma of the lacrimal glands in a 50-year-old woman. The disease duration of Sjögren syndrome prior to the onset of malignant lymphoma was 3 years. **a** Axial unenhanced CT scan shows wedged-shaped enlargement of bilateral lacrimal glands (*arrows*). No obvious bone alterations are observed. **b** Axial spin-echo T1-weighted MR image shows both glands to be slightly hyperintense to extraocular muscles. Both glands show posterior extension and mold to globe. **c** Axial fast spin-echo T2-weighted MR image shows both glands to be slightly hyperintense to extraocular muscles. Histological examinations show MALT lymphoma on right and pseudolymphoma on left. (With permission from [TONAMI et al. 2002b])

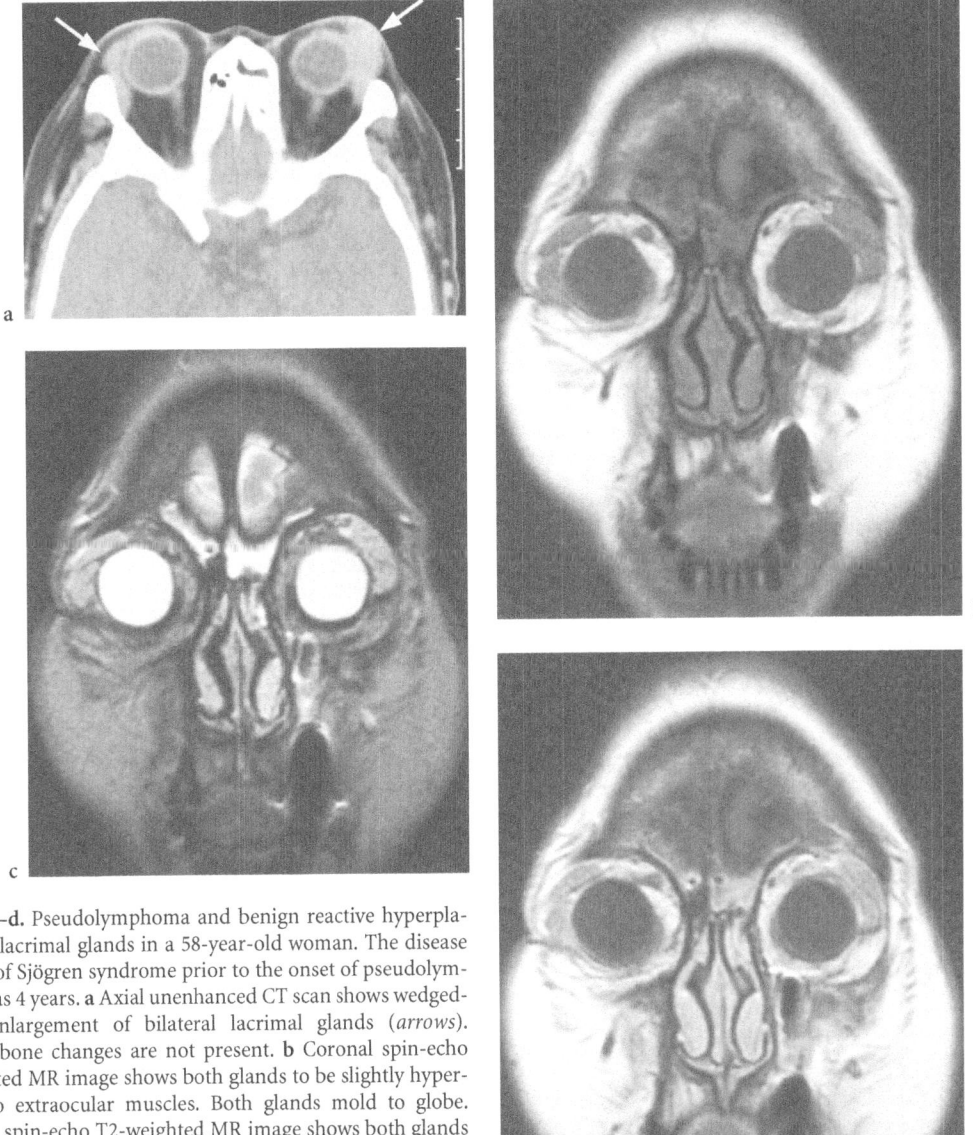

Fig. 12.6a–d. Pseudolymphoma and benign reactive hyperplasia of the lacrimal glands in a 58-year-old woman. The disease duration of Sjögren syndrome prior to the onset of pseudolymphoma was 4 years. **a** Axial unenhanced CT scan shows wedged-shaped enlargement of bilateral lacrimal glands (*arrows*). Adjacent bone changes are not present. **b** Coronal spin-echo T1-weighted MR image shows both glands to be slightly hyperintense to extraocular muscles. Both glands mold to globe. **c** Coronal spin-echo T2-weighted MR image shows both glands to be hyperintense to extraocular muscles. **d** Coronal contrast-enhanced spin-echo T1-weighted MR image shows speckled enhancement in both glands. Histological examinations show benign lymphoid hyperplasia on right and pseudolymphoma on left. (With permission from [Tonami et al. 2002b])

et al. 1995). However, nodal involvement is mostly peripheral, and cervical lymph nodes are highly involved (Fig. 12.11). Most of the nodal lymphomas observed in Sjögren syndrome are low-grade monocytoid B-cell lymphoma which is the nodal counterpart of the MALT lymphoma. The other nodal sites involved included supraclavicular and axillary regions (Voulgarelis et al. 1999). Exclusively abdominal or thoracic nodal involvement is rare (Fig. 12.12).

12.5.2
Follow-up Imaging Features

As previously described, more than half of the malignant lymphomas occurring in Sjögren syndrome are low-grade MALT lymphoma. MALT lymphoma has been known to have a tendency to remain localized within the affected MALT organ for prolonged times, to have a less aggressive course, and to respond well to

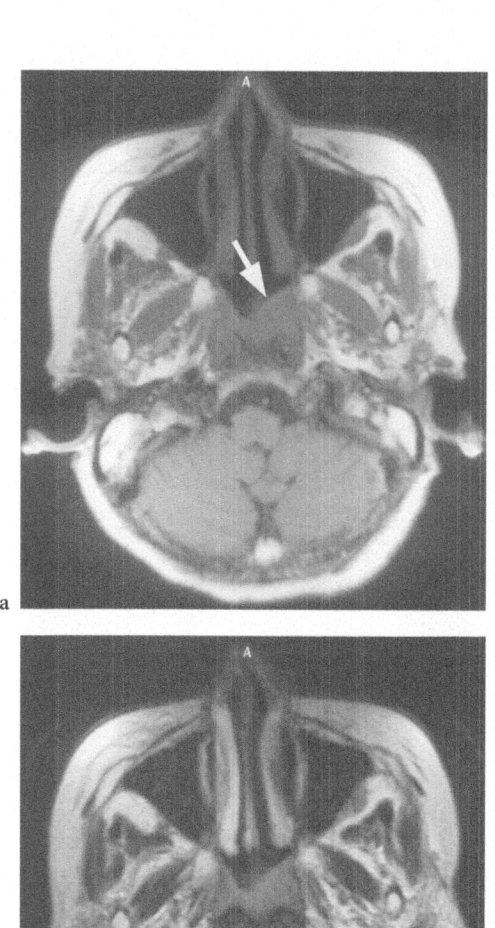

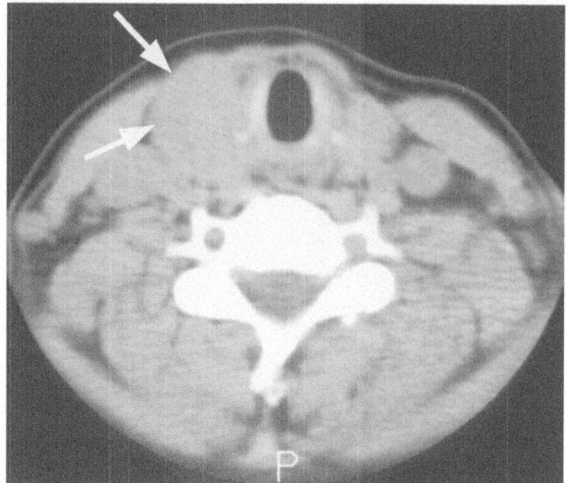

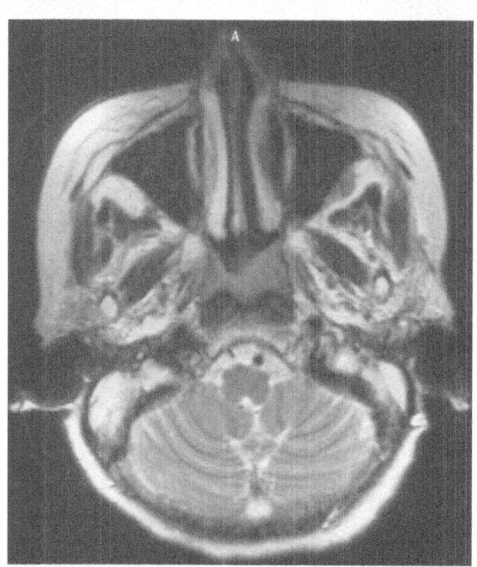

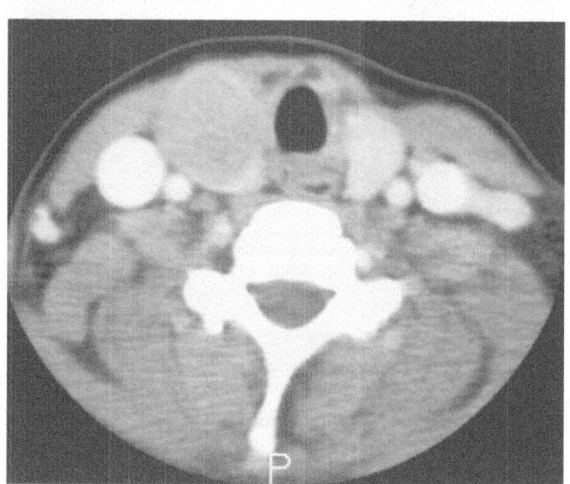

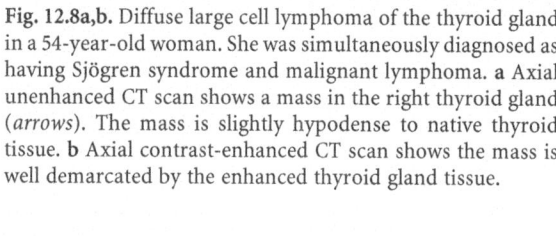

Fig. 12.8a,b. Diffuse large cell lymphoma of the thyroid gland in a 54-year-old woman. She was simultaneously diagnosed as having Sjögren syndrome and malignant lymphoma. **a** Axial unenhanced CT scan shows a mass in the right thyroid gland (*arrows*). The mass is slightly hypodense to native thyroid tissue. **b** Axial contrast-enhanced CT scan shows the mass is well demarcated by the enhanced thyroid gland tissue.

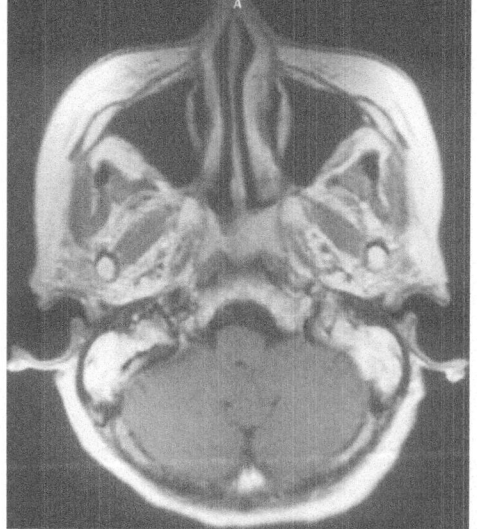

Fig. 12.7a–c. MALT lymphoma of the nasopharynx in a 75-year-old woman. The disease duration of Sjögren syndrome prior to the onset of malignant lymphoma was 10 years. **a** Axial spin-echo T1-weighted MR image shows an asymmetric thickening of nasopharyngeal mucosa mimicking the adenoidal hypertrophy (*arrow*). The mass is hyperintense to muscles. **b** Axial fast spin-echo T2-weighted MR image shows mass to be hyperintense to muscles. **c** Axial contrast-enhanced T1-weighted MR image shows diffuse enhancement of the mass. The distinction of between normal lymphoid tissue and lymphoma is difficult from these MR findings.

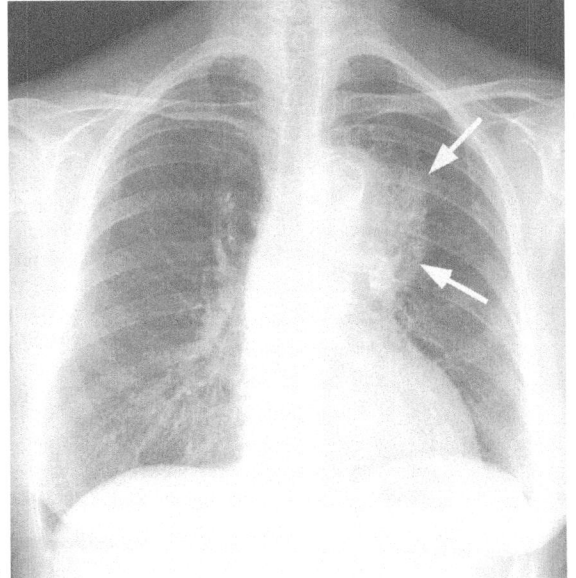

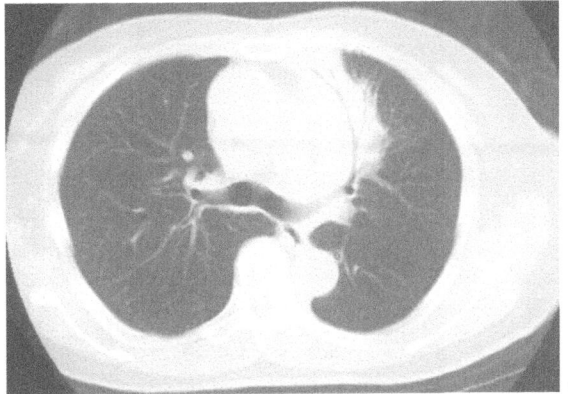

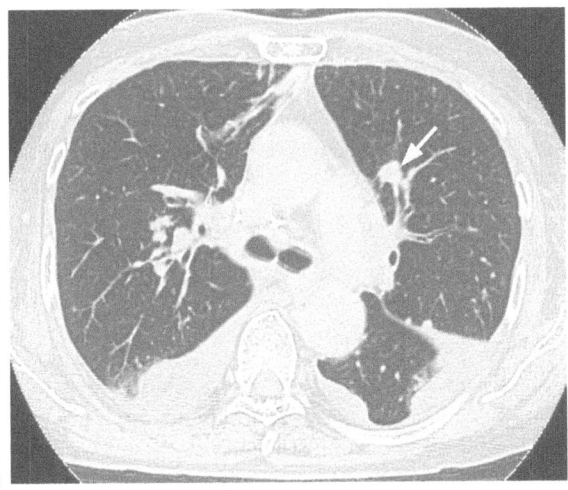

Fig. 12.9a–c. MALT lymphoma of the lung in a 79-year-old woman. She was simultaneously diagnosed as having Sjögren syndrome and malignant lymphoma. **a** Posteroanterior chest radiograph shows an extensive consolidation in the left upper lobe (*arrows*) with air bronchograms. Axial unenhanced CT scans with (**b**) mediastinal window and (**c**) lung window show an air-space consolidation in the left upper lobe (*arrows*) with prominent air bronchograms.

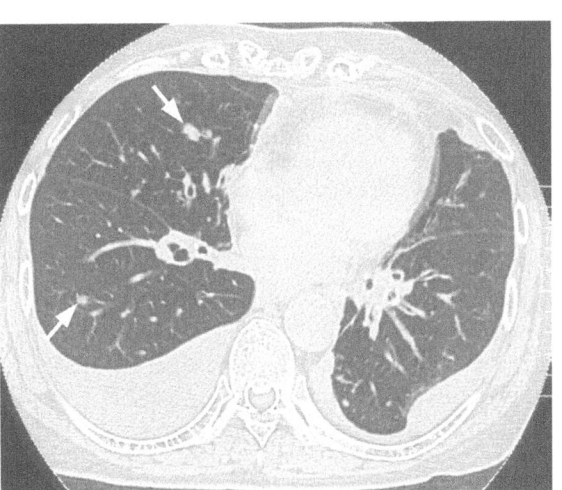

Fig. 12.10a,b. Diffuse medium cell lymphoma of the lung in a 72-year-old woman. The disease duration of Sjögren syndrome prior to the onset of malignant lymphoma was 26 years. **a, b** Axial thin section CT scans with lung window show multiple nodules with relatively smooth margin in the bilateral lung (*arrows*). Note bilateral pleural fluid collection suggestive aggressive condition.

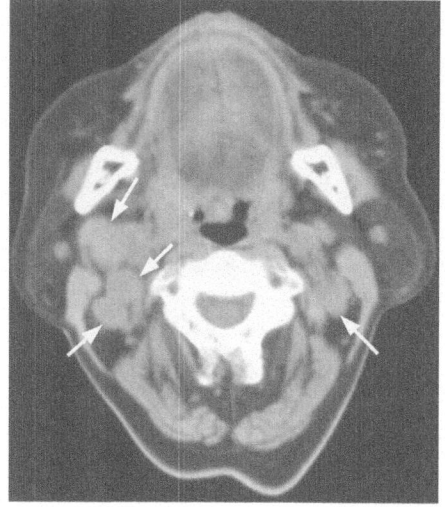 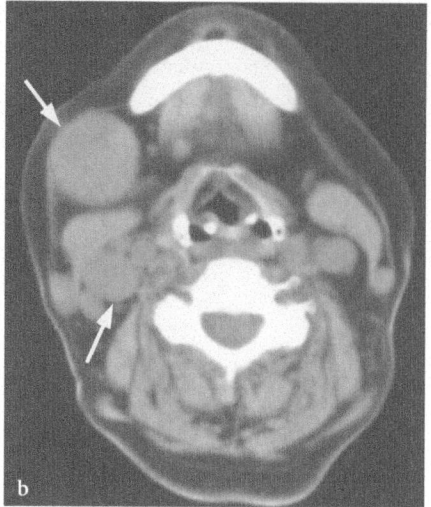

Fig. 12.11a,b. Monocytoid B-cell lymphoma of the cervical lymph nodes in a 62-year-old woman. The disease duration of Sjögren syndrome prior to the onset of malignant lymphoma was 2 years. **a, b** Axial unenhanced CT scans of the neck show multiple lymph nodes swelling bilaterally (*arrows*). The other nodal sites were not involved. She received chemotherapy and achieved complete remission. She is still alive in complete remission 10 years after the end of the treatment.

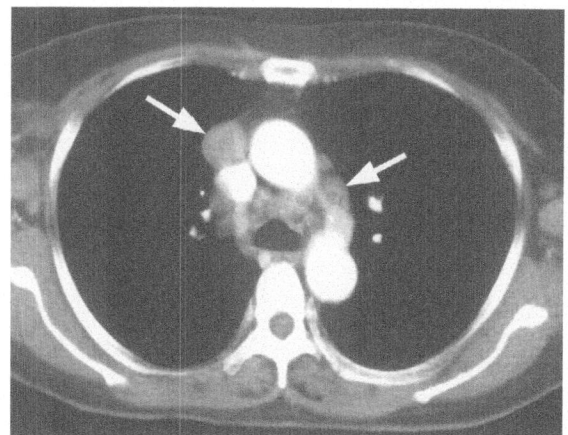 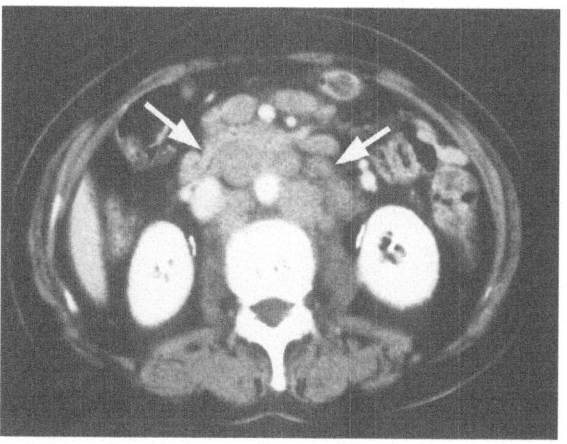

Fig. 12.12a,b. Generalized nodal involvement by mantle cell lymphoma in a 72-year-old woman. The disease duration of Sjögren syndrome prior to the onset of malignant lymphoma was 6 years. Axial contrast-enhanced CT scans of the (**a**) thorax and (**b**) abdomen show multiple lymph nodes swelling (*arrows*). She received systemic chemotherapy, only achieving partial remission and subsequently died of the disease 2 years after the initial diagnosis.

therapy (Fig. 12.13) (ARAKI et al. 1998). On the other hand, disease spread to other mucosal sites within the organ of origin (Fig. 12.14) or to the other mucosal sites of different MALT containing organ (Figs. 12.4, 12.15) is sometimes observed during the course of follow-up (GRAZIADEI et al. 1998). This "homing" phenomenon can be explained in part by the tendency of activated mucosal lymphocytes to preferentially recirculate to the mucosa by binding their surface receptor to the respective ligand on mucosal venule endothelium. From the clinical point of view, careful observation of the primary site as well as other mucosal sites is important even if complete remission has been obtained in the primary site (TONAMI et al. 2002a).

12.6
Treatment

The treatment and prognosis of malignant lymphoma in Sjögren syndrome depend on type and stage of the lymphoma. In patients with localized low-grade lymphomas especially marginal zone B-cell lymphoma, the principle of no initial therapy should be considered (PORTLOCK and ROSENBERG 1979). Survival rate at 5 years in these low-grade lymphomas in Sjögren syndrome generally is more than 50% (THIEBLEMONT et al. 1997). Surgical resection, if possible, is also curative in low-grade and lower stages lymphomas (HYJEK et al. 1988). If the tumor

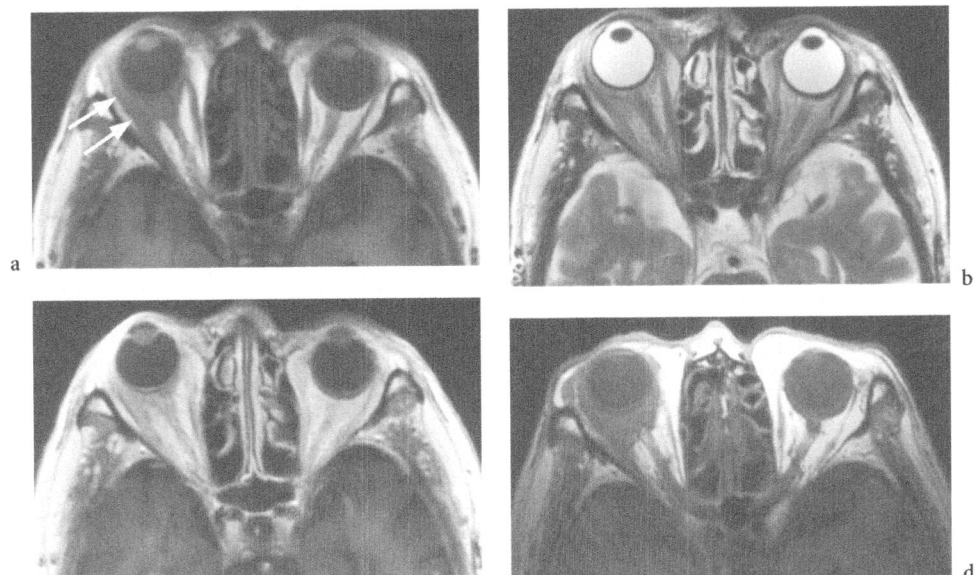

Fig. 12.13a–d. MALT lymphoma of the ocular adnexa in a 88-year-old man. He was simultaneously diagnosed as having Sjögren syndrome and malignant lymphoma. **a** Axial spin-echo T1-weighted MR image shows orbital mass (*arrows*) involving palpebral lobe of right lacrimal gland and extending to retrobulbar space. The mass is slightly hyperintense to extraocular muscles. **b** Axial fast spin-echo T2-weighted MR image shows mass to be slightly hyperintense to extraocular muscles. **c** Axial contrast-enhanced spin-echo T1-weighted MR image shows diffuse enhancement. He was put under close follow-up without treatment. **d** Axial unenhanced spin-echo T1-weighted MR image obtained 15 months later shows no progression of lesion. (With permission from [Tonami et al. 2002a])

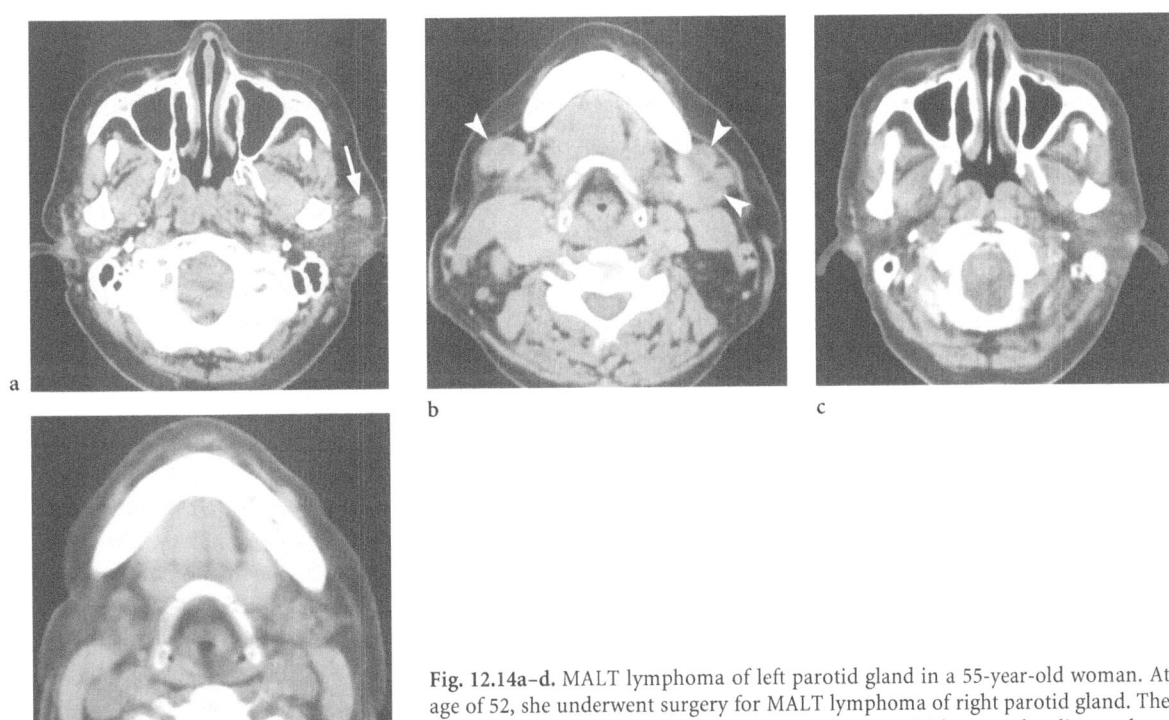

Fig. 12.14a–d. MALT lymphoma of left parotid gland in a 55-year-old woman. At age of 52, she underwent surgery for MALT lymphoma of right parotid gland. The disease duration of Sjögren syndrome prior to the initial onset of malignant lymphoma was 3 years. Axial contrast-enhanced CT scans show (**a**) a discrete mass in left parotid gland (*arrow*) with (**b**) multiple lymph nodes swelling (*arrowheads*). Superficial lobe of right parotid gland has been resected by previous surgery. She underwent radiation therapy followed by chemotherapy. Axial unenhanced CT scans obtained 2 years later show that (**c**) left parotid mass and (**d**) enlarged lymph nodes have disappeared. (With permission from [Tonami et al. 2002a])

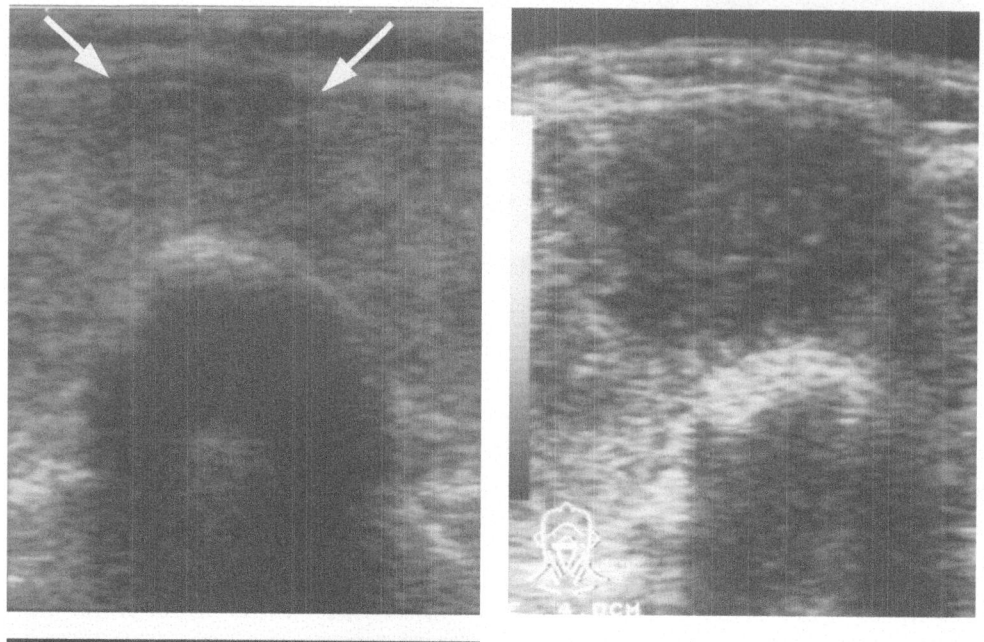

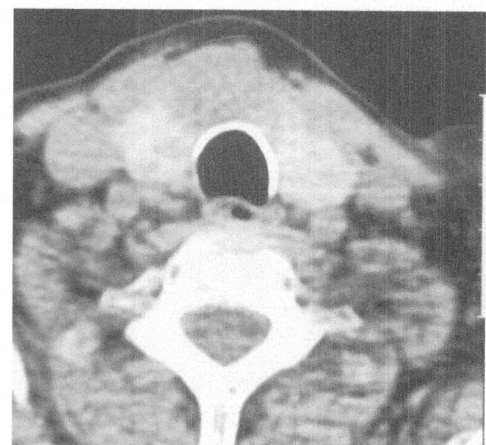

Fig. 12.15a–c. MALT lymphoma of the thyroid gland in a 79-year-old woman. At the age of 66, she underwent surgery for MALT lymphoma of the right parotid gland. The disease duration of Sjögren syndrome prior to the initial onset of malignant lymphoma was 10 years. **a** Transverse ultrasound image shows a hypoechoic mass in the thyroid gland (*arrows*). Close follow-up was performed without treatment. **b** Transverse ultrasound image and (**c**) axial unenhanced CT scan obtained 1 year later show the thyroid mass to be slightly enlarged. She then underwent chemotherapy, achieving complete remission.

cannot be totally resected, additional radiation therapy is justified. In patients with intermediate to high-grade lymphomas, a combination of radiation therapy and chemotherapy is recommended.

12.7
Conclusion

Patients with Sjögren syndrome are at increased risk of lymphoma development. Imaging features of malignant lymphomas in patients with Sjögren syndrome are not substantially different from those reported in the other lymphomas occurring in patients without an underlying Sjögren syndrome. Although both extranodal and nodal involvements are observed, extranodal manifestation is more common. The extranodal site is often the salivary gland, but other extranodal sites including the lacrimal gland, the thyroid gland, Waldeyer's ring, the lung, and the stomach are also involved. Nodal involvement is mostly peripheral, and cervical lymph nodes are highly involved. Histologically, more than half of the malignant lymphomas occurring in Sjögren syndrome are low-grade B-cell MALT lymphomas. Despite their indolent nature, MALT lymphomas tend to spread to other mucosal sites during the follow-up period. From the clinical point of view, therefore, careful observation of the primary site as well as other mucosal sites is important even if complete remission has been obtained in the primary site.

References

Anaya JM, McGuff HS, Banks PM, et al. (1996) Clinicopathological factors relating malignant lymphoma with Sjögren's syndrome. Semin Arthritis Rheum 25:337–346

Araki K, Kubota Y, Iijima Y, et al. (1998) Indolent behaviour of low-grade B-cell lymphoma of mucosa-associated lymphoid tissue involved in salivary glands, renal sinus and prostate. Scand J Urol Nephrol 32:234–236

Bhattacharyya N, Frankenthaler RA, Gomolin HI, et al. (1998) Clinical and pathologic characterization of mucosa-associated lymphoid tissue lymphoma of the head and neck. Ann Otol Rhinol Laryngol 107:801–806

Biasi D, Caramaschi P, Ambrosetti A, et al. (2001) Mucosa-associated lymphoid tissue lymphoma of the salivary glands occurring in patients affected by Sjögren's syndrome: report of 6 cases. Acta Haematol 105:83–88

Bloch KJ, Buchanan WW, Wohl MJ, et al. (1965) Sjögren's syndrome: a clinical, pathological, and serological study of sixty-two cases. Medicine 44:187–232

Bunim JJ, Talal N (1963) Development of malignant lymphoma in the course of Sjögren's syndrome. Trans Assoc Am Physicians 76:45–56

Chan JKC, Ng SC, Isaacson PG (1990) Relationship between high grade lymphoma and low grade B-cell mucosa-associated lymphoid tissue lymphoma (MALToma) of the stomach. Am J Pathol 136:1153–1164

Cummings NA, Schall GL, Asofsky R, et al. (1971) Sjögren's syndrome: newer aspects of research diagnosis and therapy. Ann Intern Med 75:937–950

Fishleder A, Tubbs R, Hesse B, et al. (1987) Uniform detection of immunoglobulin-gene rearrangement in benign lymphoepithelial lesions. N Engl J Med 316:1118–1121

Fox RI, Howell FV, Bone RC, et al. (1984) Primary Sjögren syndrome: clinical and immunopathologic features. Semin Arthritis Rheum 14:77–105

Graziadei G, Pruneri G, Carboni N, et al. (1998) Low-grade MALT lymphoma involving multiple mucosal sites and bone marrow. Ann Hematol 76:81–83

Grevers G, Ihrler S, Vogl TJ, et al. (1994) A comparison of clinical, pathological and radiological findings with magnetic resonance imaging studies of lymphomas in patients with Sjögren's syndrome. Eur Arch Otorhinolaryngol 251: 214–217

Harris NL, Jaffe ES, Stein H, et al. (1994) A revised European-American classification of lymphoid neoplasms: a proposal from the international lymphoma study group. Blood 84:1361–1392

Hornbaker JH, Foster EA, William GS, et al. (1966) Sjögren's syndrome and nodular reticulum-cell sarcoma. Arch Intern Med 118:449–452

Hyjek E, Smith WJ, Isaacson PG (1988) Primary B-cell lymphoma of salivary glands and its relationship to myoepithelial sialadenitis. Hum Pathol 19:766–776

Isaacson PG, Wright DH (1984) Extranodal malignant lymphoma arising from mucosa-associated lymphoid tissue. Cancer 53:2415–2524

Isaacson PG, Spencer J (1987) Malignant lymphoma of mucosa-associated lymphoid tissue. Histopathology 11: 445–462

Kassan SS, Thomas TL, Moutsopoulos HM, et al. (1978) Increased risk of lymphoma in sicca syndrome. Ann Intern Med 89:888–892

Kiratli H, Soylemezoglu F, Bilgic S, et al. (1999) Mucosa-associated lymphoid tissue lymphoma of the lacrimal gland. Ophthal Plast Reconstr Surg 15:272–276

Knisely BL, Mastey LA, Mergo PJ, et al. (1999) Pulmonary mucosa-associated lymphoid tissue lymphoma: CT and pathologic findings. AJR Am J Roentgenol 172:1321–1326.

Kruize AA, Hene RJ, van der Heide A, et al. (1996) Long-term followup of patients with Sjögren's syndrome. Arthritis Rheum 39:297–303

Lee DK, Im J-G, Lee KS, et al. (2000) B-cell lymphoma of bronchus-associated lymphoid tissue (BALT): CT features in 10 patients. J Comput Assist Tomogr 24:30–34

Liao Z, Ha CS, McLaughlin P, et al. (2000) Mucosa-associated lymphoid tissue lymphoma with initial supradiaphragmatic presentation: natural history and patterns of disease progression. Int J Radiation Oncology Biol Phys 48:399–403

Mariette X (1999) Lymphomas in patients with Sjögren's syndrome: review of the literature and physiopathologic hypothesis. Leuk Lymphoma 33:93–99

Nakano A, Fujisawa K, Mimura H, et al. (1999) Mucosa-associated lymphoid tissue (MALT) lymphoma of the thyroid: report of a case. Anticancer Res 19:811 814

Pariente D, Anaya JM, Combe B, et al. (1992) Non-Hodgkin's lymphoma associated with primary Sjögren's syndrome. Eur J Med 1:337–342

Pavlidis NA, Drosos AA, Papadimitriou C, et al. (1992) Lymphoma in Sjögren's syndrome. Med Pediatr Oncol 20: 279–283

Pisa EK, Pisa P, Kang H-I, et al. (1991) High frequency of t(14;18) translocation in salivary gland lymphomas from Sjögren's syndrome patients. J Exp Med 174:1245–1250

Polio E, Galieni P, Leccisotti A (1996) Clinical and radiological presentation of 95 orbital lymphoid tumors. Graefe's Arch Clin Exp Ophthalmol 234:504–509

Portlock CS, Rosenberg SA (1979) No initial therapy for stage III and IV non-Hodgkin's lymphomas of favorable histologic types. Ann Intern Med 90:10–13

Rodallec M, Guermazi A, Brice P, et al. (2002) Imaging of MALT lymphomas. Eur Radiol 12:348–356

Royer B, Cazals-Hatem D, Sibilia J, e al (1997) Lymphomas in patients with Sjögren's syndrome are marginal zone B-cell neoplasms, arise in diverse extranodal and nodal sites, and are not associated with viruses. Blood 90:766–775

Sato K, Kawana M, Sato Y, et al. (2002) Malignant lymphoma in the head and neck associated with benign lymphoepithelial lesion of the parotid gland. Auris Nasus Larynx 29:209–214

Scholefield JH, Quayle AR, Harris SC, et al. (1992) Primary lymphoma of the thyroid, the association with Hashimoto's thyroiditis. Eur J Surg Oncol 18:89–92

Shin SS, Sheibani K, Fishleder A, et al. (1991) Monocytoid B-cell lymphoma in patients with Sjögren's syndrome. Hum Pathol 22:422–430

Som PM, Brandwein MS, Silvers A (1995) Nodal inclusion cysts of the parotid gland and parapharyngeal space: a discussion of lymphoepithelial, AIDS-related parotid, and branchial cysts, cystic Warthin's tumors, and cysts in Sjögren's syndrome. Laryngoscope 1105:1122–1128

Som PM, Brandwein MS (2002) Salivary glands: anatomy and pathology. In: Som PM, Curtin HD (eds) Head and neck imaging. Mosby, St. Louis, pp 2109–2113

Stewart A. Bleukinsopp PT, Henry K (1994) Bilateral parotid MALT lymphoma and Sjögren's syndrome. Brit J Oral Maxillofac Surg 32:318–322

Sutcliffe N, Inanc M, Speight P, et al. (1998) Predictors of lymphoma development in primary Sjögren's syndrome. Semin Arthritis Rheum 28:80–87

Tagnon BB, Theate I, Weynand B, et al. (2002) Long-standing mucosa-associated lymphoid tissue lymphoma of the parotid gland: CT and MR imaging findings. AJR Am J Roentgenol 178:1563–1565

Talal N, Sokoloff L, Barth WF (1967) Extrasalivary lymphoid abnormalities in Sjögren's syndrome (reticulum-cell sarcoma, "pseudolymphoma" macroglobulinemia). Am J Med 43:50–65

Thieblemont C, Bastion Y, Berger F, et al. (1997) Mucosa-associated lymphoid tissue gastrointestinal and nongastrointestinal lymphomas behavior: analysis of 108 patients. J Clin Oncol 15:1624–1630

Tonami H, Matoba M, Yokota H, et al. (2002a) Mucosa-associated lymphoid tissue lymphoma in Sjögren's syndrome: initial and follow-up imaging features. AJR Am J Roentgenol 179:485–489

Tonami H, Matoba M, Yokota H, et al. (2002b) CT and MR findings of bilateral lacrimal gland enlargement in Sjögren syndrome. Clin Imaging 26:392–396

Vogl TJ, Dresel SHJ, Grevers G, et al. (1996) Sjögren's syndrome: MR imaging of the parotid gland. Eur Radiol 6: 46–51

Voulgarelis M, Dafni UG, Isenberg DA, et al. (1999) Malignant lymphoma in primary Sjögren's syndrome: a multicenter, retrospective, clinical study by the European concerted action on Sjögren's syndrome. Arthritis Rheum 42: 1765–1772

Wotherspoon AC, Ortiz-Hidalgo C, Falzon MR, et al. (1991) Hilicobacter Pylori-associated gastritis and primary B-cell gastric lymphoma. Lancet 338:1175–1176

Zucca E, Roggero E, Pileri S (1998) B-cell lymphoma of MALT type: a review with special emphasis on diagnostic and management problems of low-grade gastric tumors. Br J Haematol 100:3–14

Zufferey P, Meyer OC, Grossin M, et al. (1995) Primary Sjögren's syndrome (SS) and malignant lymphoma: a retrospective cohort study of 55 patients with SS. Scand J Rheumatol 24:342–345

Zulman J, Jaffe R, Talal N (1978) Evidence that the malignant lymphoma of Sjögren's syndrome is a monoclonal B-cell neoplasm. N Engl J Med 299:1215–122

13 Burkitt and Burkitt-like Lymphoma

KATHERINE B. M. COLQUHOUN, KEN TUNG

CONTENTS

13.1
Introduction

Burkitt and Burkitt-like lymphomas form part of the diverse spectrum of non-Hodgkin lymphoma (NHL). Both are classified as small non-cleaved cell lymphomas with B-cell monoclonal cell lines. Burkitt is further subdivided into endemic, African and non-endemic or American subtypes. These share pathological and some radiological features but are clinically distinct. Both conditions are rare, accounting for approximately 50% of all NHL in children, and only 1–3% in immunocompetent adults. However, with the advent of infection with the human immunodeficiency virus (HIV), first recognized in the mid 1980s, there has been an increase in incidence of all forms of NHL. The diagnosis has become a more important consideration, in particular because of the highly aggressive but potentially curable nature of these conditions.

KATHERINE B. M. COLQUHOUN, MD
Specialist Registrar Radiologist, Department of Clinical Radiology, C Level, Centre Block, Southampton University Hospitals Trust, Tremona Road, Southampton, S016 6YD, UK
KEN TUNG, MD
Consultant Radiologist, Department of Clinical Radiology, C Level, Centre Block, Southampton University Hospitals Trust, Tremona Road, Southampton, S016 6YD, UK

Burkitt-like lymphoma is less well-defined. It has been allocated a classification as a provisional entity in the Revised European American Lymphoma (REAL) classification. It is clinically similar to non-endemic Burkitt but is intermediate cytomorphologically between large cell (centroblastic/immunoblastic) and Burkitt lymphoma. Several studies have suggested an older age-group and the more frequent involvement of nodal sites than in Burkitt lymphoma (HARRIS et al. 1994). Certainly an increasing incidence has been observed among AIDS patients.

This chapter will consider the radiological features of Burkitt and Burkitt-like lymphomas, and in particular those imaging techniques which are helpful in their diagnosis and management.

13.2
Endemic Burkitt Lymphoma

The distinctive lymphoid malignancy of the jaw prevalent amongst east African children was first described by Burkitt in 1958. This disease entity has since been found to be endemic in parts of Africa, Papua New Guinea and South America (EPSTEIN and CRAWFORD 1996). Physical factors important in this geographic distribution are thought to be mean temperatures of greater than 17° C and annual rainfall of greater than 55 cm. There is also a well-recognized association with Epstein-Barr virus (EBV); raised titers of antibodies to EBV are found in > 90% of cases of endemic Burkitt lymphoma. In recent cytogenetic studies, EBV genomes have been identified in tumor cells from endemic cases. EBV sequences have also been found in 25–40% of cases in patients with AIDS-related Burkitt's, but less frequently in non-endemic, non-immunocompromised cases (HARRIS et al. 1994; EPSTEIN and CRAWFORD 1996).

An additional cofactor in the pathogenesis is thought to be malaria, which also favors warm, humid conditions that support populations of the anopheles mosquito. The precise relationship between the two factors has not been established. One theory proposes that malarial infection leads to an impaired immunity, which combined with EBV-driven proliferation of B-cells, results in a greater risk of mutations occurring, in particular the Burkitt lymphoma translocations (t8:14, t8:22, t2:8). These translocations activate the c-myc oncogene resulting in malignant changes in the cell line (EPSTEIN and CRAWFORD 1996).

The condition originally described by Burkitt was a highly aggressive lymphoid tumor of the jaw. It quickly became apparent that the condition was almost always multifocal at presentation. The disease predominantly involves extranodal sites. Tumors of the maxilla, mandible and salivary glands; both nodal and visceral sites in the abdomen; the gonads; axial and peripheral skeleton, and extradural spinal sites have been described (COCKSHOTT 1965; WHITTAKER 1973; DUNNICK et al. 1979; KRUDY et al. 1981; ZWANGER-MENDELSON et al. 1989). The commonest clinical presentation is of a rapidly expansile painless lesion of the jaw with minimal associated constitutional disturbance. The aggressive nature of the tumor results in a relentless clinical course and death within months in the absence of treatment. In a high proportion of cases the clinical presentation is highly suggestive and the diagnosis made, supported by histological evidence. In these circumstances radiology is more useful in staging the tumor than in primary diagnosis.

Fortunately, the tumors are usually exquisitely sensitive to chemotherapy. Prognosis depends less on the sites involved and more on the volume of disease at presentation. In cases where the tumor volume is small, a rapid and sustained response to chemotherapy may be anticipated. Larger tumor loads are more susceptible to the treatment induced metabolic disturbances associated with the acute tumor lysis syndrome (SENAPATI et al. 1994). This and the short doubling time underline the need for early imaging and histological diagnosis and expedient treatment.

13.2.1
Head and Neck Involvement

The commonest manifestations in the jaw are primary bone lesions involving the mandible and maxilla. Typical radiographic appearances are of localized bony destruction centered on the medullary cavity, without surrounding sclerosis. As the lesions enlarge they erode the cortex eventually leading to cortical destruction and pathological fracture. The lamina dura is also lost and soft tissue displaces the teeth causing the classical appearance of "floating teeth". There are commonly large soft tissue masses associated with the primary bone lesion; the commonest clinical presentation is with a rapidly enlarging, often painless, jaw mass (COCKSHOTT 1965; WHITTAKER 1973; SENAPATI et al. 1994). With tumors originating in the maxilla, exophthalmos may result from orbital spread of the expanding tumor. Head and neck tumors originating in the salivary glands and thyroid have also been described.

The soft tissue mass responds rapidly, often within days, to combination chemotherapy. The teeth return to their normal position and the architecture of the medullary bone is restored. Rarely, the appearances can mimic aggressive osteosarcomatous lesions, with radiating, spiculated periosteal reactions (COCKSHOTT 1965; WHITTAKER 1973).

Long bone deposits have also been described. These tend to have a diaphyseal or meta-diaphyseal locus and more often display amorphous or lamellated periosteal reactions than lesions located in the mandible (COCKSHOTT 1965; WHITTAKER 1973). Due to the multi-centric nature of the disease, once the primary lesion has been identified, there should be radiological review and staging, with imaging of any clinically suspicious sites.

13.2.2
Abdominal Involvement

Involvement of abdominal sites is a common finding at presentation. Liver, renal, small bowel, and gonadal involvement are common. Retroperitoneal adenopathy is also a feature, although interestingly the disease tends to spare the spleen and peripheral nodes. In addition, extradural spinal tumors presenting with rapid onset paraplegia have also been described.

In the past plain film radiograph was used to stage abdominal disease and to identify large soft tissue masses. This was combined with excretory urography to assess renal involvement. As with other abdominal malignancies, the mainstay of diagnostic and staging imaging has become computed tomography (CT) and/or magnetic resonance (MR) imaging.

The differential diagnosis depends very much on the location of the tumor. In children with facial bone tumors, rhabdomyosarcoma, extraocular extension of retinoblastoma, and neuroblastoma metastases should be considered. Nephroblastoma is an important differential diagnosis for renal tumors in this age group; but this is less commonly bilateral or multifocal at presentation. Ovarian malignancy should be considered in the differential diagnosis of abdominal and pelvic masses. In addition, in endemic areas tuberculosis and acute transverse myelitis are important considerations in patients presenting with precipitous paraplegia.

13.3
Non-Endemic Burkitt Lymphoma

Clinical and radiological features of Burkitt lymphoma in non-endemic parts of Africa and in other parts of the world differ from those in endemic areas. In published series of non-endemic Burkitt the mean age at presentation is 11 years, an older age group than the endemic form (EPSTEIN and CRAWFORD 1996; DUNNICK et al. 1979; HARRIS et al. 1994; EPSTEIN and CRAWFORD 1996; JOHNSON et al. 1998). Although head and neck tumors are documented, there is less predilection for the jaw and there is a higher incidence of abdominal and peripheral nodal disease (Figs. 13.1, 13.2). In addition thoracic disease,

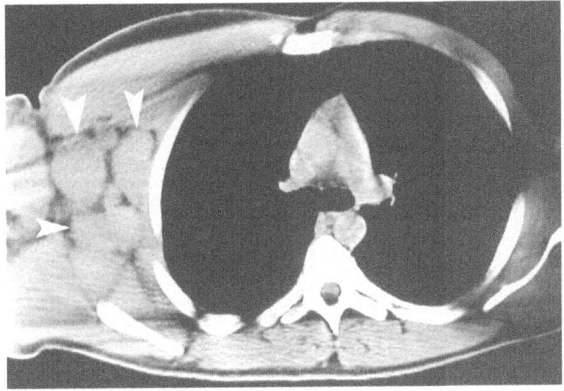

Fig. 13.2. Disseminated Burkitt lymphoma in a 41-year-old man. Axial unenhanced CT scan shows large volume right axillary lymphadenopathy (*arrowheads*).

usually in the form of malignant effusions, has been described (DUNNICK et al. 1979; KRUDY et al. 1981; JOHNSON et al. 1998).

13.3.1
Abdominal Involvement

In series published in North America, 45–92% of cases had abdominal or pelvic disease at presentation. The ileocecal region is the commonest site of primary bowel pathology (Figs. 13.3–13.6). Primary lesions are also described in the colon and stomach (Figs. 13.7, 13.8) (KRUDY et al. 1981; JOHNSON et al. 1998). In addition, the bowel may be involved secondary to lesions arising from the mesentery, and disseminated disease often involves the solid abdominal and pelvic organs as well as retroperitoneal and pelvic nodes (Figs. 13.9–13.12).

Tumor mass is frequently well shown on contrast-enhanced CT as well-defined areas of homogeneous soft tissue density (Fig. 13.13). Tumor may be difficult to distinguish from bowel, and the extent of disease has been underestimated in the past before the advent of safer and better tolerated oral and intravenous iodinated contrast, and rapid helical acquisition techniques.

Primary lesions arising from bowel may present with concentric thickening or polypoid endoluminal lesions (Fig. 13.5). Later these may cause an almost aneurysmal dilatation of the involved segment, which is likely to be related to loss of the integrity of the smooth muscle layers of the wall (Fig. 13.14). More diffuse infiltrative lesions and malignant ascites have also been described (Figs. 13.15, 13.16). Small bowel

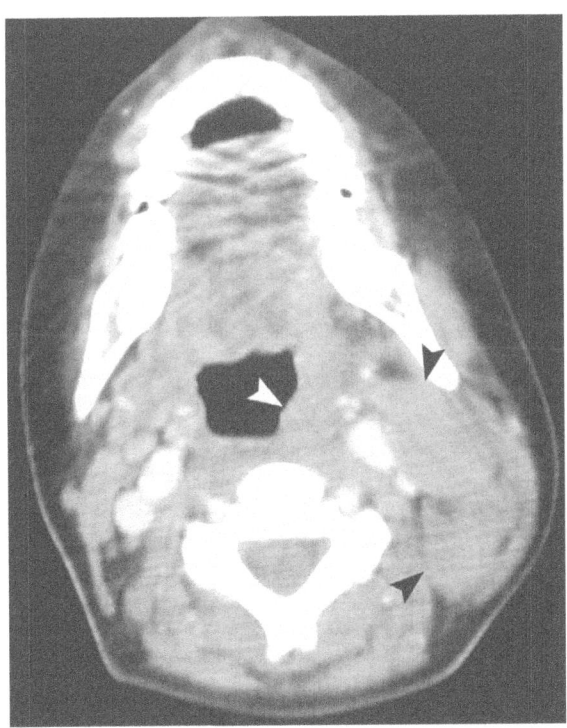

Fig. 13.1. Burkitt lymphoma in a 40-year-old man. Axial contrast-enhanced CT scan shows a left parapharyngeal soft tissue mass (*white arrowhead*) and high left cervical lymphadenopathy (*black arrowheads*).

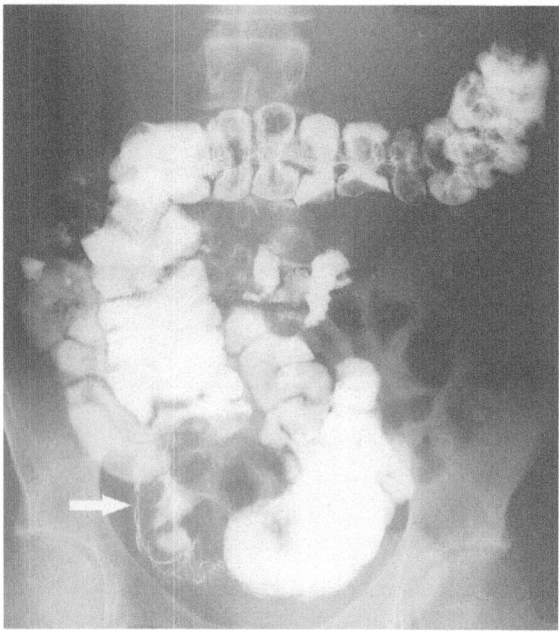

Fig. 13.3. Burkitt lymphoma in a 17-year-old boy. Barium follow-through examination demonstrates an ileal ulcerated mass (*arrow*).

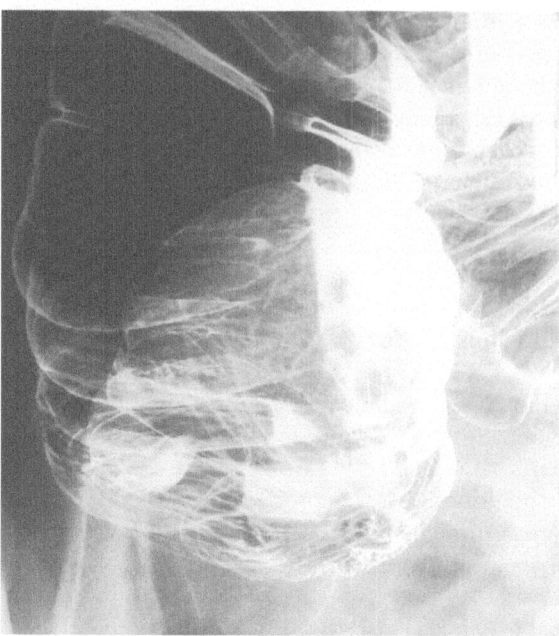

Fig. 13.4. Burkitt lymphoma in a 20-year-old man. Double contrast barium enema study showing an intussuscepting cecal mass.

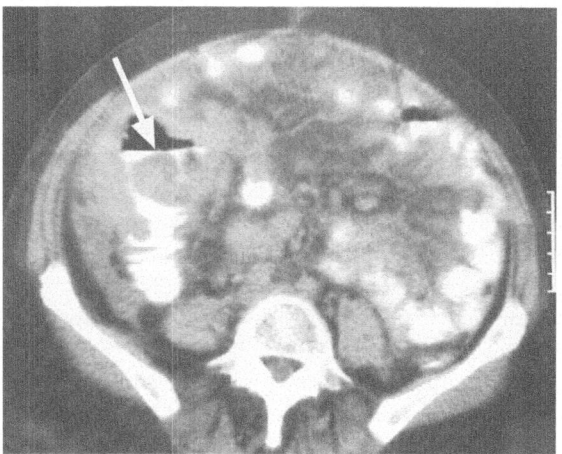

Fig. 13.5. Burkitt lymphoma in a 35-year-old man. Axial CT scan with oral opacification shows a polypoid ileocecal mass (*arrow*) with extensive peritoneal infiltration.

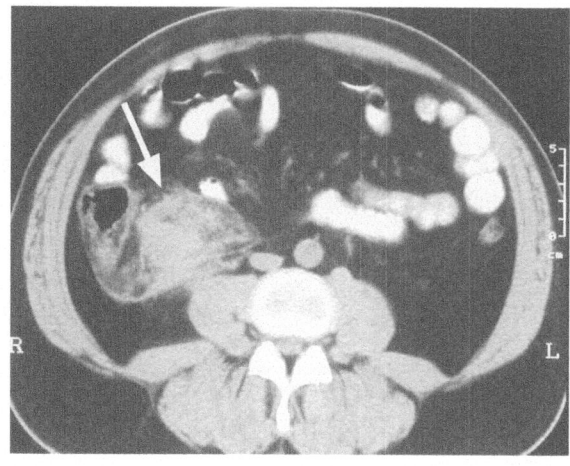

Fig. 13.6. Burkitt abdominal lymphoma in a 25-year-old man. Axial CT scan with oral opacification demonstrates an ileocecal mass infiltrating locally involving the appendix (*arrow*).

contrast studies show mucosal irregularity not demonstrated on CT (Fig. 13.3). This is particularly helpful in confirming gastric mucosal or wall thickening suspected on CT.

Abdominal and pelvic lesions often present with an acute abdomen, with perforation, intussusception, or obstruction, requiring emergency laparot-

omy prior to formal diagnosis or staging (Figs. 13.4, 13.17). In addition, following the initiation of treatment, there may be such a rapid destruction of the tumor bulk that perforation may occur. This is a particularly important consideration as it may be masked clinically by intercurrent immunosuppressive agents.

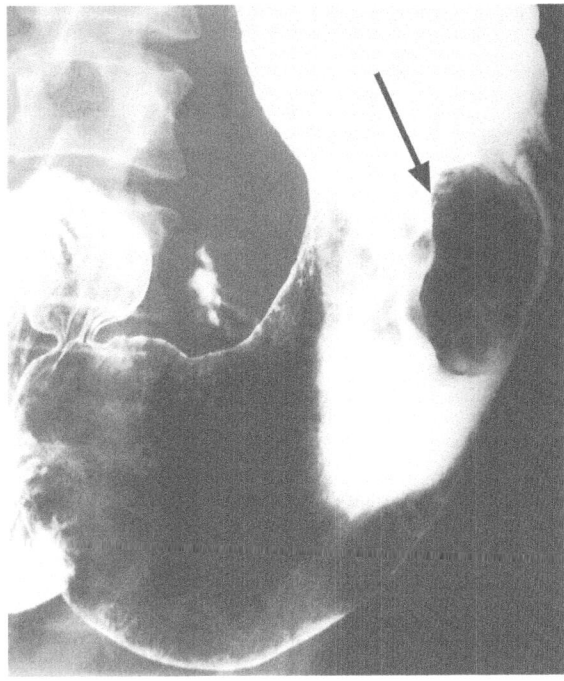

Fig. 13.7. Burkitt abdominal lymphoma in a 34-year-old woman. Double contrast barium meal demonstrates a polypoid ulcerating gastric mass (*arrow*).

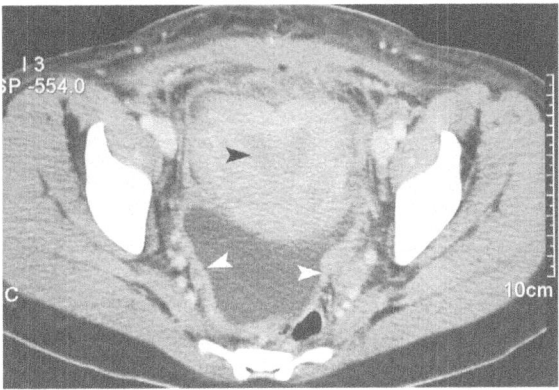

Fig. 13.9. Burkitt lymphoma in a 34-year-old woman. Axial contrast-enhanced CT scan of the pelvis shows a diffuse tumor involvement of the uterus with dilatation of the endometrial cavity (*black arrowhead*). There is also a thickening of the pelvic peritoneal reflection (*white arrowheads*) and free fluid in the pouch of Douglas.

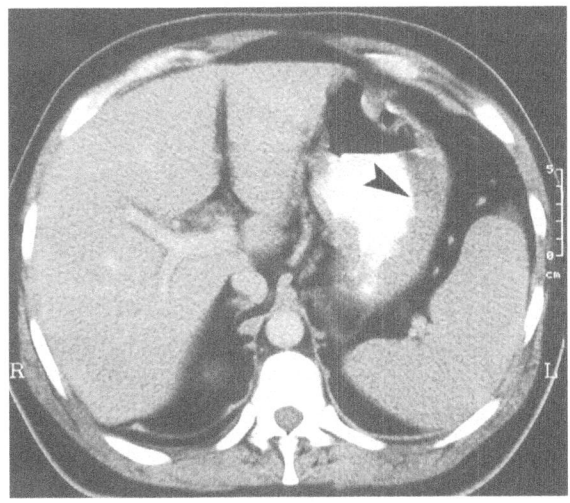

Fig. 13.8. Disseminated Burkitt lymphoma in a 32-year-old man. Axial contrast-enhanced CT scan with oral opacification shows eccentric mural thickening of the stomach (*arrowhead*).

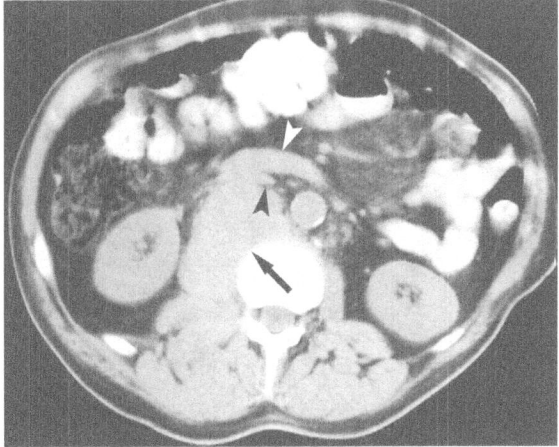

Fig. 13.10. Burkitt lymphoma in a 20-year-old man. Axial CT scan of the abdomen with oral opacification shows a right sided retroperitoneal nodal mass (*arrow*) encasing the inferior vena cava and displacing the right renal artery (*black arrowhead*) and unopacified duodenum anteriorly (*white arrowhead*).

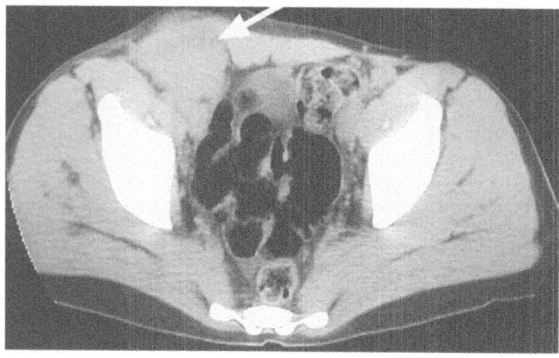

Fig. 13.11. Burkitt lymphoma in a 26-year-old man. Axial unenhanced CT scan of the pelvis shows a right inguinal node mass infiltrating the anterior abdominal wall (*arrow*).

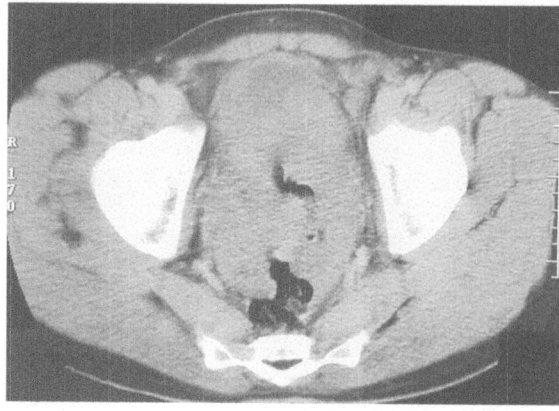

Fig 13.12. Extensive Burkitt lymphoma in a 17-year-old boy. Axial contrast-enhanced CT scan of the pelvis demonstrates pelvic tumor encasing the sigmoid colon.

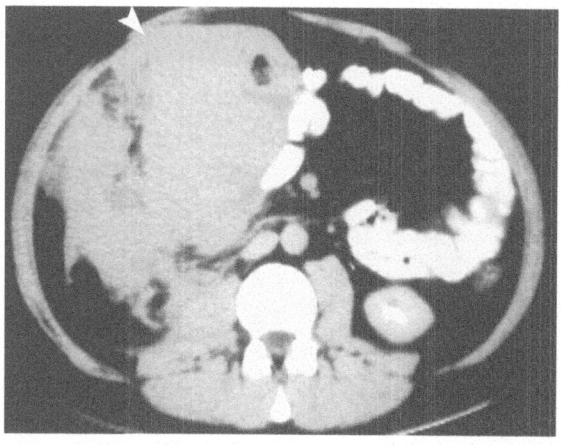

Fig. 13.13. Burkitt lymphoma in a 67-year-old woman. Axial contrast-enhanced CT scan of the abdomen with oral opacification shows a large right sided paracolic tumor mass that can be seen extending anteriorly to involve the anterior abdominal wall (*arrowhead*), and posteriorly to involve the right psoas. It is difficult to distinguish the encased loops of ascending colon, which are not opacified by oral contrast.

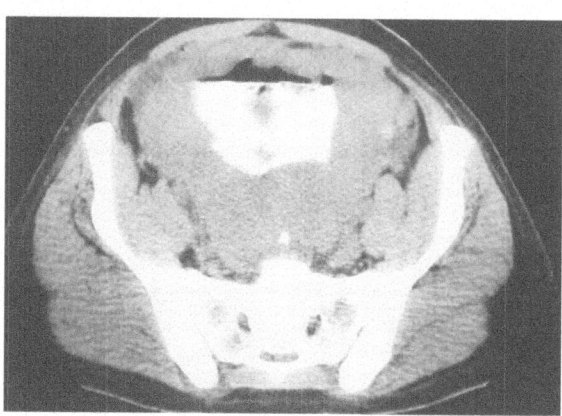

Fig. 13.14. Burkitt lymphoma in a 19-year-old woman. Axial unenhanced CT scan shows a large abdominal mass with central cavitation which is filled with oral contrast demonstrating due to pathologic connection with bowel.

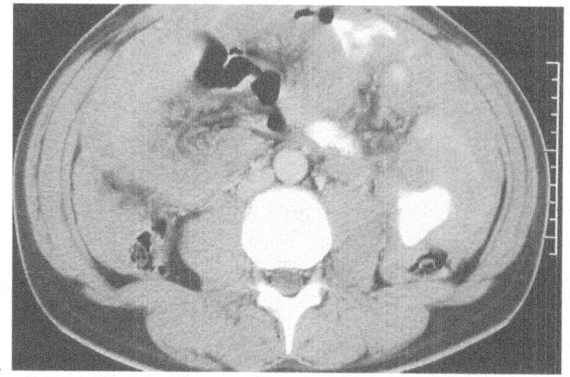

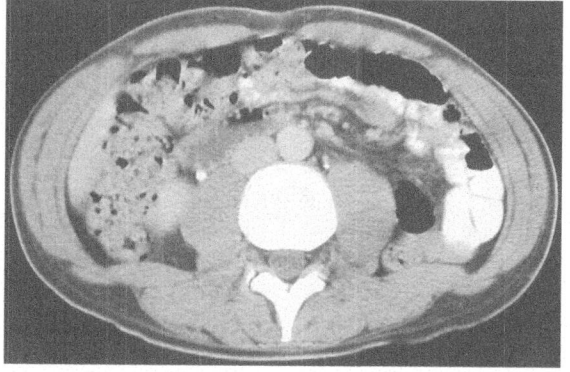

Fig. 13.15a,b. Burkitt lymphoma in a 17-year-old boy. Axial contrast-enhanced CT scans of the abdomen with oral opacification at the level of L2 show extensive mesenteric and peritoneal disease (**a**) prior to onset of chemotherapy, and resolution of these changes (**b**) following treatment.

Primary Burkitt lymphoma of the liver is exceptionally rare (CHIM et al. 2001), although the liver is commonly involved in disseminated disease (Figs. 13.18, 13.19). A case published in the literature described an insidious presentation with painless abdominal distension and weight loss, hepatomegaly, and deranged liver function biochemistry. CT examination revealed multiple discrete iso to hypodense lesions which were mildly or non-enhancing post iodinated intravenous contrast in the absence of lymphadenopathy. The diagnosis of Burkitt lymphoma was confirmed on Tru-Cut biopsy.

Renal involvement is an unusual imaging finding in most reported series, but is more prevalent in post mortem studies (KRUDY et al. 1981; STRAUSS et al. 1986). A retrospective review of 29 patients with biopsy proven Burkitt lymphoma assessed with renal ultrasound as part of their imaging work-up found 10 patients to have evidence of infiltration (STRAUSS et al. 1986). Findings included diffuse renomegaly, increased cortical reflectivity, and focal renal masses. Hydronephrosis is also described although this may be caused by distal ureteric involvement in pelvic and / or retroperitoneal disease. Focal renal lesions may be identified on contrast enhanced CT but ultrasound is a more sensitive modality for detecting more subtle changes in cortical reflectivity with diffuse infiltration (Fig. 13.20).

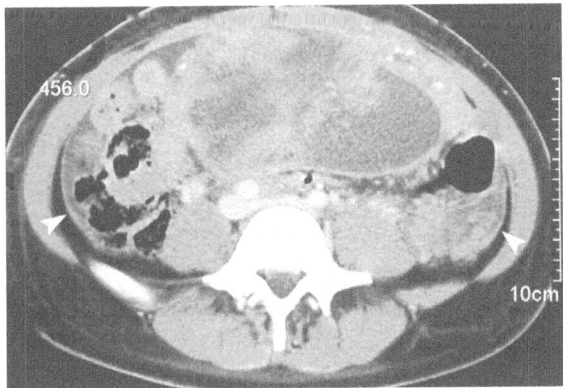
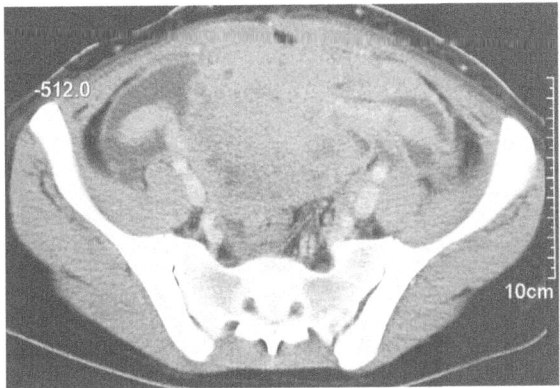

Fig. 13.16a,b. Burkitt lymphoma in a 27-year-old woman. Axial contrast-enhanced CT scans of the (a) abdomen and (b) pelvis show a large, heterogeneous part solid, part necrotic mesenteric mass. Ascites and diffuse peritoneal thickening can be seen in both paracolic gutters (*arrowheads*).

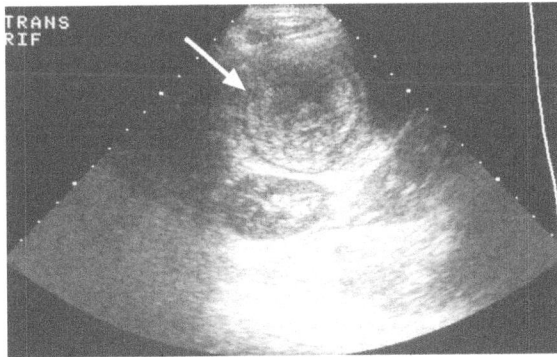

Fig. 13.17. Burkitt lymphoma in a 21-year-old man. Transverse ultrasound image of the right flank shows the alternating increased and reduced reflectivity layers of an ileocecal intussusception (*arrow*), secondary to an endoluminal lymphomatous mass.

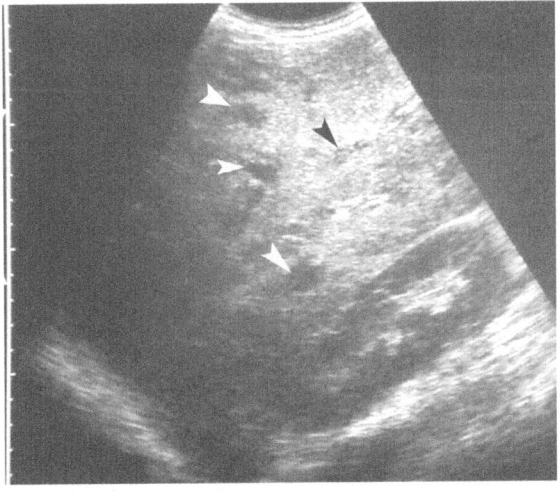

Fig. 13.18. Disseminated Burkitt lymphoma in a 35-year-old man. Longitudinal ultrasound image of the liver shows multiple hypoechoic hepatic nodules (*arrowheads*).

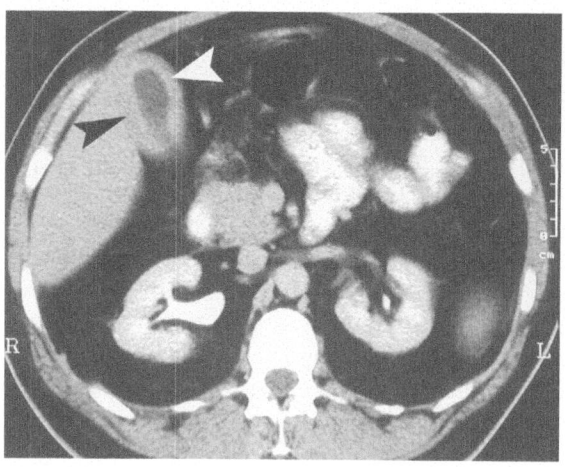

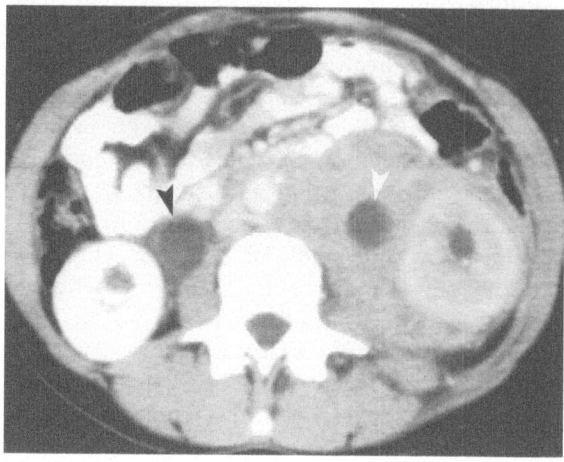

Fig. 13.19. Multifocal Burkitt lymphoma in a 32-year-old man. Axial contrast-enhanced CT scan of the upper abdomen with oral opacification shows concentric thickening of the gall bladder wall (*arrowheads*). This resolved completely after chemotherapy.

Fig. 13.20. Burkitt lymphoma in a 34-year-old woman. Axial contrast-enhanced CT scan with oral opacification shows recurrent retroperitoneal disease with extensive perirenal infiltration. There is bilateral hydronephrosis and dilatation of both proximal ureters (*arrowheads*). The left kidney is enlarged and poorly enhancing compared to the right suggesting diffuse renal involvement or renovascular compromise.

Gonadal involvement, either separately or via direct spread from pelvic disease is also well-described. Involvement of the testes has been reported in approximately 5% of a series of 557 male patients with endemic Burkitt lymphoma (ZWANGER-MENDELSON et al. 1989). Testicular, epididymal and spermatic cord involvement is even rarer in reported non-endemic cases and usually forms part of the presentation of atypical disseminated presentations in patients with underlying HIV infection. Ultrasound is the modality of choice for assessing local infiltration, with subtle changes in reflectivity and vascularity being well shown with high frequency phased-array transducers.

13.3.2
Extra-Abdominal Involvement

Thoracic involvement is uncommon in reported series of American Burkitt lymphoma. Pleural effusion is the most common intrathoracic abnormality but mediastinal and hilar abnormality are very rare findings (Fig. 13.21).

Head and neck pathology is a more common finding: 19% of patients reviewed in our center and 8–25% of patients in studies conducted elsewhere. In contrast to endemic or African Burkitt lymphoma, disease originating in the facial bones is uncommon

(0–33%) and nodal or soft tissue involvement is more usual (Figs. 13.22, 13.23) (DUNNICK et al. 1979; KRUDY et al. 1981; BAUER et al. 1993; VINAYAK et al. 1994; JOHNSON et al. 1998).

Central nervous system (CNS) involvement in disseminated Burkitt lymphoma is well described. Meningeal and cranial nerve infiltration are the commonest manifestations in non-endemic cases, while paraspinal masses are more frequent in the endemic group. MR imaging is the most useful modality for demonstrating the presence and extent of CNS disease. In particular, meningeal infiltration may only be detectable with contrast-enhanced T1-weighted MR imaging and easily overlooked on CT. In addition spinal MR imaging may also show extensive marrow involvement not obvious on plain film (Fig. 13.24) (DUNNICK et al. 1979; KRUDY et al. 1981; JOHNSON et al. 1998).

Disseminated disease is becoming a more common finding at presentation (JOHNSON et al. 1998). This may be related to the increasing incidence of non-endemic Burkitt lymphoma in immune compromised patients and patients with HIV infection. This emerging group of patients may have different clinical features to immune competent groups. In a series of 105 HIV positive patients presenting with lymphoma, 85% were found to have B-cell NHL, and of these, 40% had Burkitt or Burkitt-like small non-cleaved cell lymphoma. In this group only 8% presented with the typical abdomino-

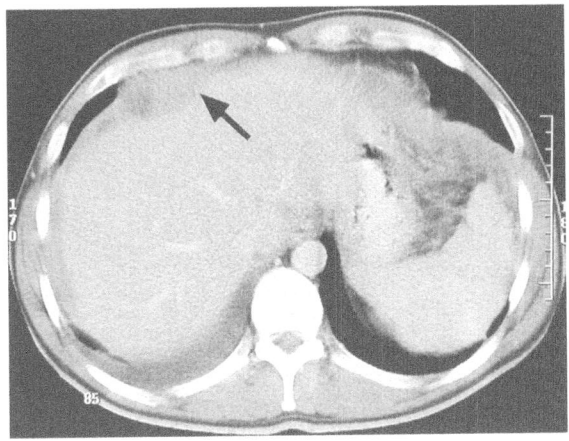

Fig. 13.21. Burkitt lymphoma in a 18-year-old man. Axial contrast-enhanced CT scan through the liver shows both right-sided pleural effusion and nodular hypodense peritoneal deposits over the anterior surface of the liver (*arrow*).

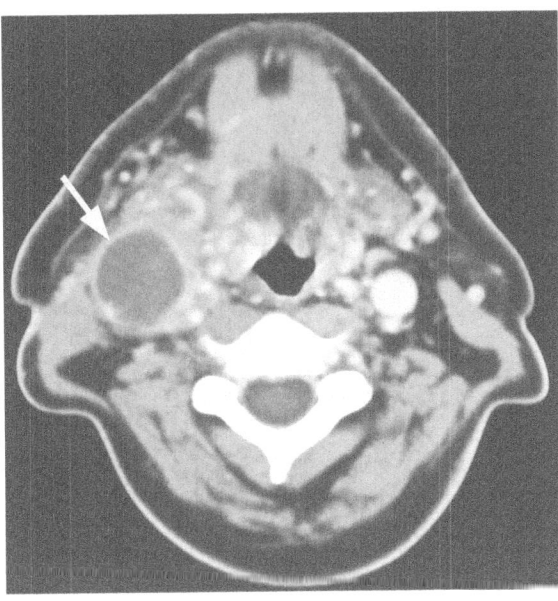

Fig. 13.22. Burkitt lymphoma in a 57-year-old man. Axial contrast-enhanced CT scan of the neck demonstrates a right-sided large necrotic jugulodigastric node (*arrow*) at presentation.

centric disease. Most cases presented with widespread lymphadenopathy, hepatic and splenic involvement and extranodal sites such as the testes. CNS and bone marrow involvement were common at presentation and at recurrence (BALTHAZAR et al. 1997; MUNN 2002). HIV-related disease is therefore more likely to have an atypical disseminated pattern at presentation and to have a more aggressive course.

13.4
Conclusion

Burkitt and Burkitt-like lymphoma, endemic and non-endemic forms, present with rapidly progressive disease. The presentation may involve a single organ system, however, disseminated disease is becoming more prevalent particularly among immune-incompetent patients. Although the diagnosis is often suggested clinically, imaging and in particular cross-sectional techniques has proved invaluable to characterize disease extent at presentation, guide the acquisition of biopsy material and monitor the response to treatment.

Acknowledgements:
The authors would like to thank Dr. K. A. Johnson for selected images; and the Medical Imaging and Photographic services at Southampton University Hospitals Trust for their kind assistance in the reproduction of the clinical images.

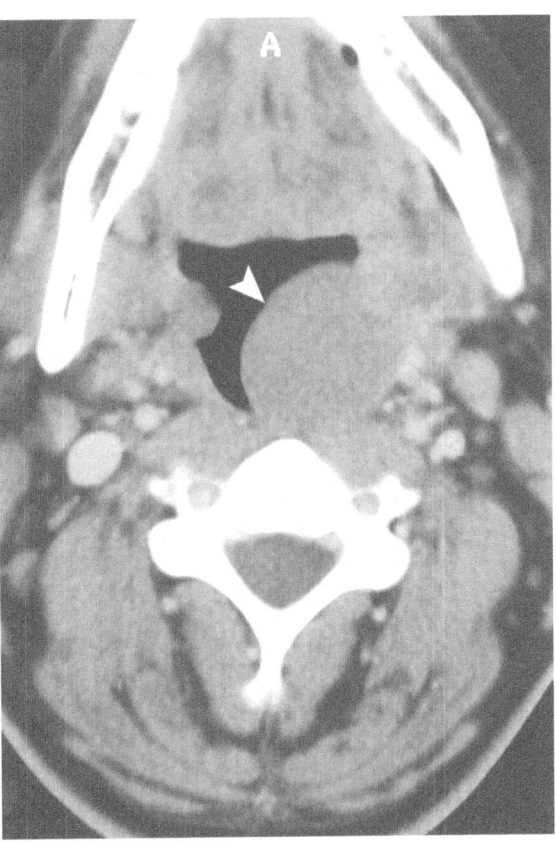

Fig. 13.23. Burkitt lymphoma in a 27-year-old man. Axial CT scan of the upper cervical region shows a left parapharyngeal mass expanding into the oropharynx (*arrowhead*).

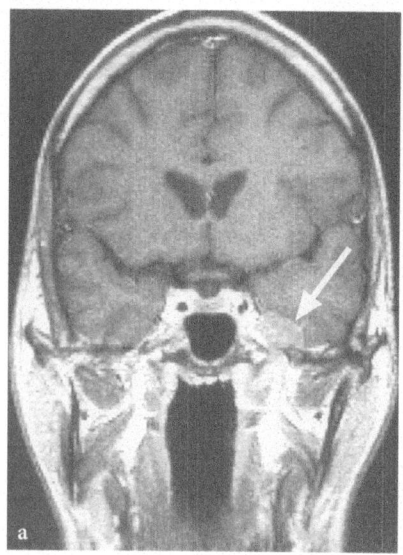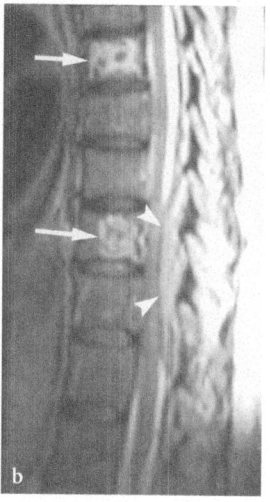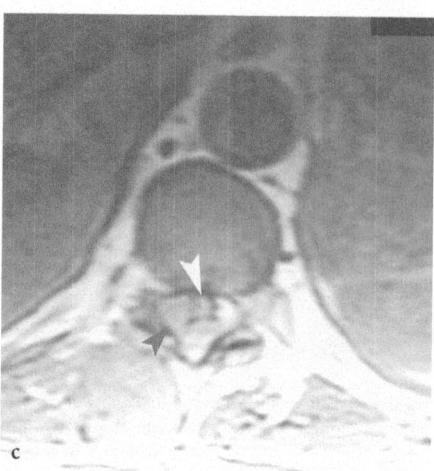

Fig. 13.24a–c. Burkitt lymphoma in a 33-year-old HIV positive man with hemophilia. **a** Coronal contrast-enhanced T1-weighted MR image of the head demonstrates enhancing meningeal lymphomatous mass of the floor of the left middle cranial fossa (*arrow*). **b** Sagittal T2-weighted MR image of the thoracic spine shows recurrent posterior extradural intraspinal disease (*arrowheads*) and widespread marrow involvement (*arrows*) with no history of previous radiation therapy. **c** Axial contrast-enhanced TI-weighted MR image shows mid-thoracic extradural tumor mass (*black arrowhead*) obliterating the right lateral recess and indenting the cord (*white arrowhead*).

References

Balthazar EJ, Noordhoorn M, Megibow AJ, Gordon RB (1997) CT of small-bowel lymphoma in immunocompetent patients and patients with AIDS: comparison of findings. AJR Am J Roentgenol 168:675–680

Bauer GP, Volk MS, Siddiqui SY, et al. (1993) Burkitt's lymphoma of the parapharygeal space. Arch Otolaryngol Head Neck Surg 119:117–120

Chim CS, Choy C, Ooi GC, Liang R (2001) Primary hepatic lymphoma. Leuk Lymphoma 40:667–670

Cockshott WP (1965) Radiological aspects of Burkitt's tumour. Br J Radiol 38:172–180

Dunnick NR, Reaman GH, Head GL, Shawker TH, Ziegler JL (1979) Radiological manifestations of Burkitt's lymphoma in American patients. AJR Am J Roentgenol 132:1–6

Epstein MA, Crawford DH (1996) The Epstein-Barr virus. In: Weatherall DJ, Ledingham JGG, Warrell DA (eds) The Oxford textbook of medicine. Oxford Medical Publications, Oxford, pp 352–357

Harris NL, Jaffe ES, Stein H, et al. (1994) A revised European-American classification of lymphoid neoplasms: A proposal from the international lymphoma study group. Blood 84:1361–1392

Johnson KA, Tung K, Mead G, Sweetenham J (1998) The imaging of Burkitt's and Burkitt's-like lymphoma. Clin Radiol 53:835–841

Krudy AG, Dunnick NR, Magrath IT, et al. (1981) CT of American Burkitt's lymphoma. AJR Am J Roentgenol 136: 747–754

Munn S (2002) Imaging HIV/AIDS. Burkitt's lymphoma. AIDS patient care STDS 16:395–399

Senapati SN, Samanta D, Mishra RC, et al. (1994) Burkitt's lymphoma. J Indian Med Assoc 92:126–127

Strauss S, Libson E, Schwartz E, et al. (1986) Renal sonography in American Burkitt lymphoma. AJR Am J Roentgenol 146: 549–552

Vinayak BC, Reddy KTV, Fulton J, Milford CA (1994) Pediatric nonendemic Burkitt's lymphoma of the head and neck. Ann Otol Rhinol Laryngol 103:238–240

Whittaker LR (1973) Burkitt's lymphoma. Clin Radiol 24: 339–346

Zwanger-Mendelsohn S, Shreck EH, Doshi V (1989) Burkitt lymphoma involving the epididymis and spermatic cord: sonographic and CT findings. AJR Am J Roentgenol 153: 85–86

14 Pediatric Lymphoma

R. Paul Guillerman and Bruce R. Parker

CONTENTS

14.1 Introduction

As the third most common malignant neoplasm in childhood and adolescence, lymphoma is of significant interest to physicians involved in the diagnosis and treatment of pediatric oncologic patients. Considered a frequently lethal disease until the late 1960's, lymphoma now represents one of the most curable of pediatric cancers with long-term survival expected in a large majority of children and adolescents treated according to contemporary regimens. Advances in imaging have played a seminal role in improving the assessment of lymphoma preceding, during, and following treatment, and have guided the design of clinical trials to evaluate novel treatments.

To serve as a foundation for subsequent coverage of imaging technique and clinical management, this chapter commences with a synopsis of pediatric lymphoma classification and epidemiology, and an overview of the tropism of lymphoma subtypes for certain patterns of anatomic distribution. The relative merits of the various imaging modalities for the evaluation of pediatric lymphoma are then addressed. A discussion of the role of imaging in the clinical management of pediatric lymphoma patients follows, with particular attention to the topics of emergency treatment, diagnosis, staging, risk stratification, response evaluation, and surveillance for relapse and late effects of therapy. The chapter concludes with an insight into future approaches to the imaging of pediatric lymphoma patients, including implementation of advances in

R. Paul Guillerman, MD
Assistant Professor of Radiology, Baylor College of Medicine, Department of Diagnostic Imaging, Texas Children's Hospital, 6621 Fannin Street, MC 2-2521, Houston, Texas 77030, USA
Bruce R. Parker, MD
Professor of Radiology, Baylor College of Medicine, Chief, Department of Diagnostic Imaging, Texas Children's Hospital, 6621 Fannin Street, MC 2-2521, Houston, Texas 77030, USA

functional and molecular imaging, and integration of clinical imaging research into cancer cooperative group study protocols.

14.2
Classification

Lymphoma is a neoplasm of the lymphocyte cell lineage that develops secondary to aberrations in the processes of cellular proliferation, differentiation, and apoptosis. The response of neoplastic cells to signals that influence these processes varies in different tissues and organs. This may lead to preferential growth of neoplasm in some parts of the body, accounting for distinctive patterns of tissue and organ distribution for each subtype of lymphoma (MAGRATH 2002). Such patterns can be useful in establishing a differential diagnosis on the basis of the clinical and imaging findings at the time of presentation.

The two major forms of lymphoma are HD and NHL. The myriad of different classification systems for lymphoma subtypes used over the past several decades created difficulty in communicating clinical and research findings. To address this problem, the International Lymphoma Study Group developed a practical classification scheme called the REAL. This classification scheme is based upon patterns of morphologic, immunophenotypic, genotypic, and clinical features (HARRIS et al. 1994), and has been adopted by the WHO (HARRIS et al. 1999; JAFFE et al. 2001). According to this scheme, there are three major categories of lymphoid malignancies: HD, B-cell neoplasms, and T or NK-cell neoplasms.

The characteristic feature of HD is the Reed-Sternberg cell, which is clonal in nature and thought to be derived from the B lymphocyte lineage. Reed-Sternberg cells account for only a small fraction of the tumor mass, with most of the mass composed of a reactive infiltrate of lymphocytes, plasma cells, histiocytes, eosinophils, and collagen deposition (GOLDSBY and CARROLL 1998). HD is traditionally classified histopathologically according to the Rye scheme, which includes four subtypes: lymphocyte predominant, mixed cellularity, lymphocyte depleted, and nodular sclerosis. The biological profile and clinical behavior of the lymphocyte predominant subtype is distinctive compared to the other subtypes. Acknowledging this distinction, the REAL classification proposes that HD be subdivided into lymphocyte predominant HD and classical HD, with

classical HD encompassing nodular sclerosis, mixed cellularity, lymphocyte depleted, and lymphocyte-rich classical HD subtypes (HARRIS et al. 1994).

NHL is divided into T and B-cell types, according to the predominant rearrangement of antigen receptor genes (T or B-cell receptors). The NK cell lineage lymphomas are exceptional because they do not have rearranged antigen receptor genes, and are encountered almost exclusively in pediatric anaplastic large cell lymphomas. NHL is also classified immunophenotypically as of immature or mature lymphoid origin (MAGRATH 2002).

The spectrum of NHL that occurs in children differs from that in adults. Adult NHL is most commonly of low or intermediate grade, while nearly all pediatric NHL in the United States and Europe occurs as one of four high grade categories with a tendency for early, widespread dissemination: lymphoblastic lymphoma, Burkitt and Burkitt-like lymphoma, anaplastic large cell lymphoma, and diffuse large B-cell lymphoma (HARRIS 1997). While there is some overlap, these categories are associated with distinctive molecular biological characteristics and clinical presentations. Burkitt lymphoma, Burkitt-like lymphoma, and large B-cell lymphoma have a mature B-cell immunophenotype. In the new WHO classification, the histologic entity of Burkitt-like lymphoma includes tumors that could be classified as large B-cell lymphoma on the basis of biologic features, particularly in older patients, but behave like Burkitt lymphoma with rapid proliferation and good response to Burkitt lymphoma therapy. In fact, Burkitt-like lymphoma may be composed of a mixture of Burkitt lymphoma and a rapidly proliferative variant of large B-cell lymphoma. Lymphoblastic lymphoma is predominantly of precursor T-cell origin. Anaplastic large cell lymphoma typically is of mature T-cell or null-cell phenotype, and is usually CD30 (Ki-1) positive (MAGRATH 2002). The anaplastic lymphoma kinase (ALK)-positive form of anaplastic large cell lymphoma is strongly related to younger age groups and portends a good prognosis (TEN BERGE et al. 2003). Rare childhood NHL forms include follicular lymphoma, which tends to be localized and has a proclivity for testicular involvement, marginal zone B-cell lymphoma, which is most common in HIV-infected children, and peripheral T-cell lymphoma, which is most common in Southeast Asia in the setting of EBV-associated hemophagocytic syndrome.

Lymphoma can present with diffuse bone marrow involvement. The arbitrary criterion of > 25% neoplastic cells in the bone marrow is considered requisite for the diagnosis of leukemia, but there is little biologic or prognostic significance to this distinction. Bone marrow involvement in lymphoma is more a sign of extensive disease than an indication of a different disease (MAGRATH 2002).

14.3
Epidemiology

According to recent data from the National Cancer Institute's Surveillance, Epidemiology, and End Results (SEER) program, approximately 15% of childhood malignancies in the United States are lymphomas, making lymphoma the third most frequent type of cancer in children, trailing only leukemia and malignant brain tumors. The incidence varies markedly with age, with lymphoma accounting for only 3% of cancer in children younger than 5 years of age, and 24% of cancer in 15–19 year olds. In the United States, approximately 1,700 children and adolescents are diagnosed with lymphoma each year, with 850–900 HD cases and 750–800 NHL cases (PERCY et al. 1999).

By far the most common subtype of HD in children and adolescents is nodular sclerosis (70%), followed by mixed cellularity (16%), lymphocyte predominant (7%), cases not otherwise specified (6%), and lymphocyte depleted (< 2%). The relative proportion of mixed cellularity is higher among children younger than 10 years of age and among males than females (PERCY et al. 1999). The lymphocyte depleted subtype is rare overall in children, although common in HIV patients. EBV-associated HD is correlated with mixed cellularity subtype, children from economically less developed regions, male sex, and young age at presentation (MAGRATH 2002).

The relative incidence of lymphoma subtypes is similar in the United States and Europe, but varies greatly in other regions of the world. In equatorial Africa, approximately 50% of pediatric cancers are lymphomas, due to the very high incidence of Burkitt lymphoma in this region (MAGRATH 1991). In the United States and Europe, approximately 35–50% of pediatric NHL is Burkitt lymphoma or Burkitt-like lymphoma, 30–40% is lymphoblastic lymphoma, and 15–25% is large cell lymphoma (50% large B-cell and 50% anaplastic large cell lymphoma) (MURPHY et al. 1989; MAGRATH 2002). In a small proportion of cases, childhood NHL is associated with various immunodeficiency states, including congenital immunodeficiency syndromes (e.g. ataxia-telangiectasia, severe combined immunodeficiency syndrome, Wiskott-Aldrich syndrome, X-linked lymphoproliferative syndrome), AIDS, and immunosuppressive therapy for solid organ and bone marrow transplantation.

There is a slight overall male predominance in HD. In NHL, 70% of cases occur in males, with a male predominance particularly notable in Burkitt lymphoma. NHL is more frequent than HD in younger children and the opposite is true in adolescents. HD is rare in children less than 5 years old. The incidence of NHL increases in the first three years of life, plateaus from 4–10 years of age, then increases again after age 10 years. Burkitt lymphoma predominates among 5–14 year olds, the incidence of diffuse large cell lymphoma increases steadily with age, and lymphoblastic lymphoma occurs at similar incidence across all pediatric age groups. The incidence of pediatric HD decreased slightly between 1975 and 1995, while the incidence of NHL among children less than 15 years of age remained fairly constant over this time period, and NHL incidence slightly increased for the 15–19 year old population (PERCY et al. 1999).

14.4
Anatomic Considerations

14.4.1
Hodgkin Disease

Hodgkin disease tends to spread in a contiguous manner. The most frequent site of involvement is the cervical and supraclavicular nodes (90%), followed by the mediastinum and thoracic nodes (85%), paraaortic nodes and spleen (35%). Hepatic, gastrointestinal tract and genitourinary tract involvement are uncommon (SIEGEL 1999). Statistical analysis of pathologically staged HD revealed that HD actually spreads predictably via functionally, not necessarily anatomically, contiguous nodes. In patients with right cervical node involvement, HD spreads via the upper mediastinum and hila to the upper abdominal nodes and spleen. In left cervical node involvement, HD spreads directly to the abdomen bypassing the mediastinum, then upward via the hila and mediastinum to the neck regions bilaterally and the axillary nodes, and finally to the inguinal nodes (ROTH et al. 1998).

The nodular sclerosis subtype has a striking propensity for lower cervical, supraclavicular, and anterior mediastinal lymph nodes (Fig. 14.1). The mixed

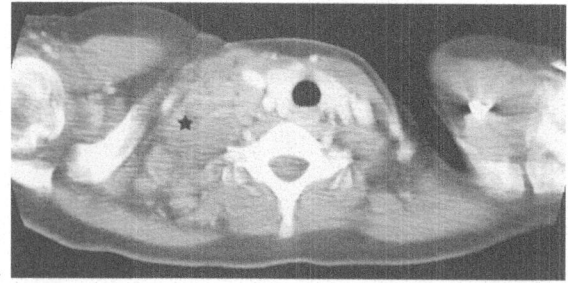

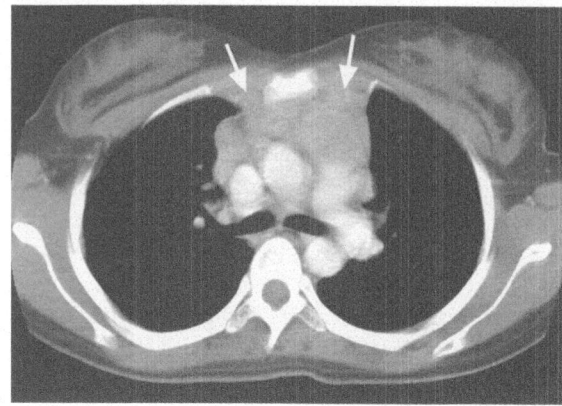

Fig. 14.1a,b. Nodular sclerosis Hodgkin disease in a 17-year-old girl with neck and mediastinal involvement. Axial contrast-enhanced CT scans of (**a**) the lower neck and (**b**) upper thorax show classic presentation with lower cervical, supraclavicular (*star*), and anterior mediastinal lymphadenopathy (*arrows*).

cellularity subtype frequently presents as advanced disease with extranodal involvement. The lymphocyte depleted subtype often presents as widespread disease with bone and bone marrow involvement. Lymphocyte predominant HD usually affects single cervical, axillary, or inguinal nodes rather than groups of nodes. In lymphocyte predominant HD, bone marrow involvement occurs only occasionally, and involvement of the thymus is unusual, unlike with other forms of HD (HUDSON and DONALDSON 2002).

14.4.2
Non-Hodgkin Lymphoma

Childhood NHL is much more often extranodal than adult NHL or childhood HD, and is frequently widespread at presentation, with a majority having abdominal disease, including involvement of mesenteric nodes in 50%, paraaortic nodes in 30%, bowel in 18%, spleen in 17%, liver in 17%, and kidney

in 5% (CASTELLINO et al. 1975). The most commonly involved sites are in the abdomen for B-cell lymphomas and in the thorax for T-cell lymphomas. Atypical sites of presentation, such as lung, skin, or muscle, are most common in anaplastic large cell lymphoma and HIV-associated NHL, and more common in T-cell lymphomas than B-cell lymphomas. Both B-cell and T-cell lymphomas frequently involve the nasopharynx, bone marrow, and CNS. Involvement of the thymus, the site of T-cell differentiation, is typical of immature T-cell lymphomas, such as lymphoblastic lymphoma (MAGRATH 2002).

14.4.2.1
Burkitt Lymphoma

Burkitt lymphoma is very fast growing, with a doubling time as short as 1–2 days (WOO et al. 1980). Consequently, Burkitt lymphoma typically presents with a large tumor burden and early dissemination. About half of patients have non-localized disease at presentation (HAMRICK-TURNER et al. 1994).

The abdomen is the most frequent site of involvement at time of presentation of sporadic Burkitt lymphoma. Involvement is most typical in the distal ileum, cecum, appendix, and mesenteric, iliac, and retroperitoneal lymph nodes (Fig. 14.2) (LAQUAGLIA et al. 1992). Common clinical presentations include abdominal pain, abdominal mass, intussusception, gastrointestinal bleeding, and bowel obstruction. It has been held that intussusception in a child greater than 4 years old is due to intestinal tract lymphoma until proven otherwise (Fig. 14.3) (PARKER 1997). The bone marrow, serous membranes, ovaries, kidneys, and pancreas are common sites of involvement, with liver and spleen involvement less frequent. There may be substantial ascites or effusions, potentially allowing diagnosis by paracentesis or thoracentesis (HAMRICK-TURNER et al. 1994). Bone marrow involvement occurs in 23% at presentation (CAIRO et al. 2003b), but there is evidence that occult bone marrow involvement occurs in another 20% (BENJAMIN et al. 1983), and involvement of the bone marrow is frequently present at relapse. Bone, pharyngeal, sinus, and cranial nerve involvement is occasionally seen, while thyroid, salivary gland, testicular, lung, CNS, epidural, and gastric involvement is uncommon, and skin, breast, and mediastinal involvement is rare at presentation (Fig. 14.4) (MAGRATH 2002, HAMRICK-TURNER et al. 1994). Epidural or CNS involvement is uncommon at the time of presentation, with CNS involvement in only 12% (CAIRO et al. 2003b), but dissemination to the

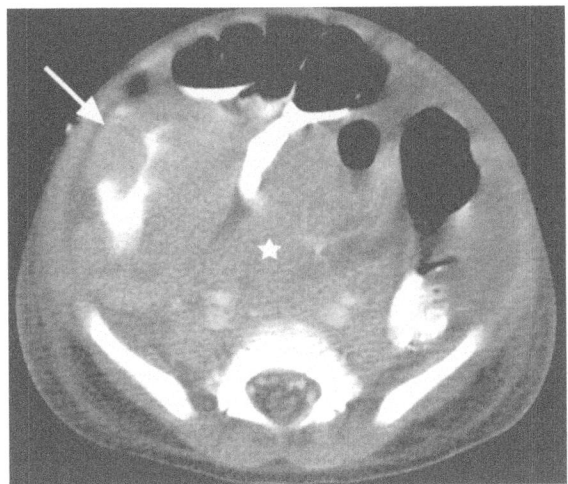

Fig. 14.2. Burkitt lymphoma in a 3-year-old boy with enteric and mesenteric involvement. Axial contrast-enhanced CT scan of the lower abdomen depicts the common presentation of marked bowel wall thickening in the right lower abdominal quadrant (*arrow*) and bulky mesenteric lymphadenopathy (*star*).

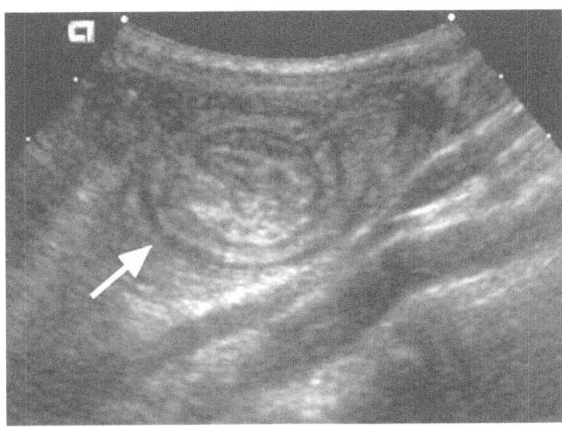

Fig. 14.3. Burkitt lymphoma in an 8-year-old boy presenting with abdominal pain due to intussusception. Longitudinal US image of the periumbilical region shows the characteristic sonographic appearance of an intussusception (*arrow*). The intussusception was not reduced by enema, and surgical exploration revealed an ileocolic intussusception with Burkitt lymphoma as the lead point mass.

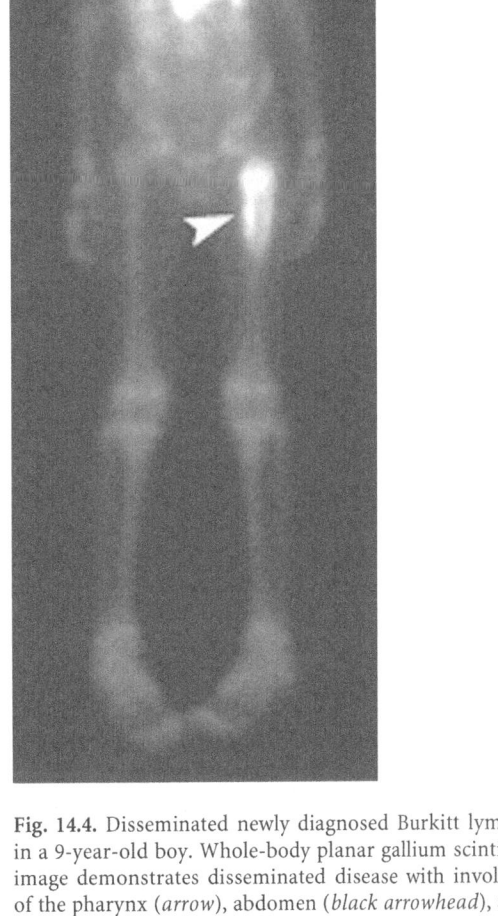

Fig. 14.4. Disseminated newly diagnosed Burkitt lymphoma in a 9-year-old boy. Whole-body planar gallium scintigraphy image demonstrates disseminated disease with involvement of the pharynx (*arrow*), abdomen (*black arrowhead*), and left femur (*white arrowhead*).

CNS occurs early. CNS involvement correlates with bone marrow involvement, with CNS involvement present in two-thirds of those with bone marrow involvement (MAGRATH 2002).

Perinatal infection with EBV increases the likelihood of endemic Burkitt lymphoma, and may contribute to the particularly high incidence of endemic Burkitt lymphoma in equatorial Africa. Endemic Burkitt lymphoma commonly presents in the facial skeleton, abdomen, paraspinal region, and CNS. Jaw involvement is the most frequent site of involvement, particularly in young children, with maxillary masses twice as frequent as mandibular masses (MAGRATH 2002). Abdominal involvement is present in slightly over half of patients, but involvement of the ileocecal region is uncommon (MAGRATH 1991). Thyroid and salivary gland involvement is occasionally present, liver and spleen involvement is infrequent, and isolated pharyngeal or mediastinal involvement is very rare. Ovarian involvement is frequent but testicular involvement is uncommon. Bone marrow involvement, with exception of the jaw, occurs in less than 10% at presentation (MAGRATH 1991). CNS disease occurs in one-third at presentation, and epidural involvement with paraplegia occurs in 15% at presentation (ZIEGLER et al. 1979). Compared to the sporadic form, endemic Burkitt lymphoma has much less frequent bone marrow and peripheral lymph node involvement, but much more frequent jaw and epidural involvement (MAGRATH 2002).

14.4.2.2
Large B-cell Lymphoma and Burkitt-Like Lymphoma

Large B-cell lymphoma and Burkitt-like lymphoma have a broader range of presentation than Burkitt lymphoma. Large B-cell lymphoma and Burkitt-like lymphoma frequently present with extranodal disease in locations typical of Burkitt lymphoma, particularly in the abdomen, but thoracic, abdominal, and peripheral lymph node involvement is much more frequent in large B-cell lymphoma and Burkitt-like lymphoma than in Burkitt lymphoma. The liver and spleen are involved more often in older individuals, and the older the patient, the more likely the presentation of Burkitt-like lymphoma will resemble large B-cell lymphoma rather than Burkitt lymphoma. Common sites of initial involvement are Waldeyer's ring, Peyer's patches, peripheral lymph nodes, skin, lung, and bone (SMITH et al. 1990). As with Burkitt lymphoma, there may be serous membrane involvement with substantial effusions and ascites with Burkitt-like lymphoma (Fig. 14.5). Large B-cell lymphoma uncommonly involves the bone marrow (8%) and CNS (2%) (CAIRO et al. 2003a), with the exception of isolated brain involvement by large B-cell lymphoma in immunocompromised patients. Mediastinal involvement occurs much more frequently than in Burkitt lymphoma. Primary mediastinal large B-cell lymphoma is a unique subtype that may be associated with superior vena cava syndrome and pleural and pericardial effusions, with spread beyond the mediastinum typically to the kidneys, adrenals, liver, and ovaries, and uncommonly to the bone marrow and extra-mediastinal lymph nodes (AISENBERG 1999).

14.4.2.3
Lymphoblastic Lymphoma

Lymphoblastic lymphoma is predominantly of precursor T-cell nature, and occasionally of precursor

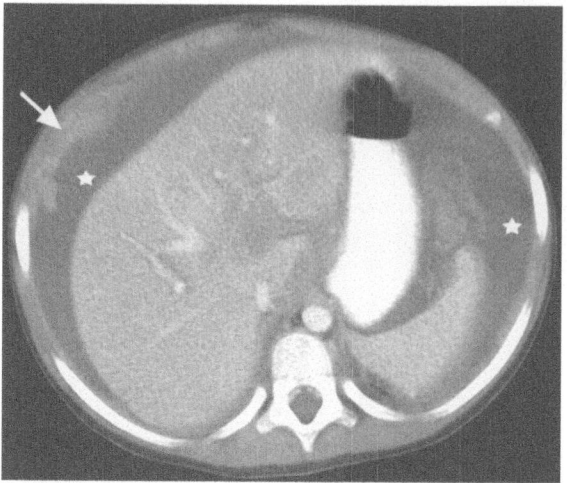

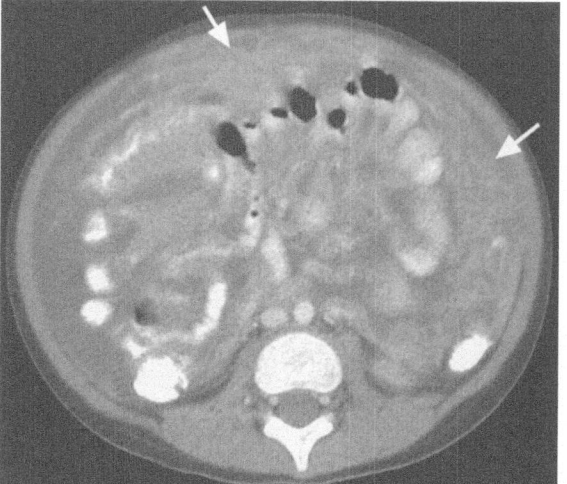

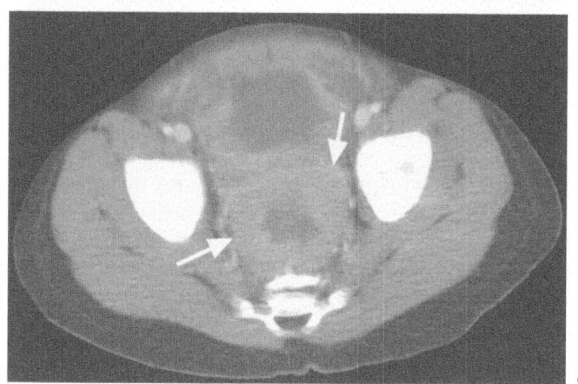

Fig. 14.5a–c. Burkitt-like lymphoma in a 5-year-old boy presenting with abdominal distention. Axial contrast-enhanced CT scans of (**a, b**) the abdomen and (**c**) pelvis reveal ascites (*stars*) and peritoneal implants along (**a**) the right hemidiaphragm (*arrow*), (**b**) omentum (*arrows*), and (**c**) pelvic rectovesicular cul-de-sac (*arrows*). This was found to represent intraperitoneal spread of Burkitt-like lymphoma.

B-cell nature. Reflecting the role of the thymus in T-cell development, a majority of precursor T-cell lymphoblastic lymphoma presents as a large anterior mediastinal mass with enlargement or replacement of the thymus, frequently with pleural effusions (Fig. 14.6) (MAGRATH 2002). Lymph node involvement occurs in 50–80% and is most common in the neck, supraclavicular regions, or axilla. Involvement of bone, testis, nasopharynx, skin, and bone marrow is occasionally seen at presentation, although usually without a large mediastinal mass. Abdominal involvement is uncommon and usually manifests as liver or spleen enlargement. Other uncommon sites include the orbits, sinuses, thyroid, and parotid glands. CNS involvement occurs in less than 10% at presentation. However, precursor T-cell lymphoblastic lymphoma has a strong tendency to rapidly spread to the CNS, bone marrow, and gonads (HAMRICK-TURNER et al. 1994). Apparently localized precursor T-cell lymphoblastic lymphoma is rare and may signify a failure to detect dissemination rather than representing a truly localized disease. On the other hand, precursor B-cell lymphoblastic lymphoma nearly always presents with limited disease, with frequent involvement of bone, lymph nodes, or skin (NETH

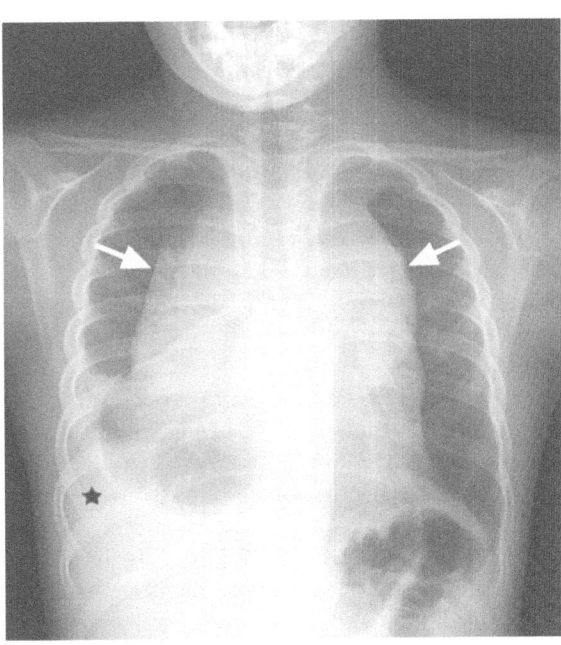

Fig. 14.6. T-cell lymphoblastic lymphoma in a 9-year-old boy with thoracic involvement. Anteroposterior chest radiograph shows a pleural effusion (*star*) and large anterior mediastinal mass (*arrows*). The frequent anterior mediastinal involvement in T-cell lymphoblastic lymphoma reflects the role of the thymus in T-cell development.

et al. 2000). The malignant cells of precursor T-cell lymphoblastic lymphoma are very similar to those in ALL. The frequency of bone marrow involvement varies with definition of T-cell ALL (typically defined as ALL if > 25% blasts in the bone marrow). Indeed, T-cell ALL acts much like leukemia with a mediastinal mass (MAGRATH 2002).

14.4.2.4
Anaplastic Large Cell Lymphoma

Anaplastic large cell lymphoma has a number of anatomic predilections that are distinctive compared to other childhood NHL. Anaplastic large cell lymphoma can present with a slowly progressive or even waxing and waning course, often with systemic symptoms such as fever and weight loss. The most frequent site of involvement of anaplastic large cell lymphoma is the lymph nodes, both peripheral and within the thorax and abdomen. Skin involvement is much more common than in other childhood NHL subtypes, particularly along the lateral thorax. Involvement of the skin and peripheral lymph nodes was the outstanding feature in the first series of children recognized with anaplastic large cell lymphoma (KADIN et al. 1986). Bone involvement is common, often multifocal, and sometimes is the primary site of involvement (Fig. 14.7). Mediastinal involvement and hepatosplenomegaly are frequently present (Fig. 14.8), and there may be involvement of unusual sites for lymphoma such as muscle, lung, and other soft tissues. The CNS and bone marrow are unusual sites of disease, and the gastrointestinal tract is rarely involved.

14.4.3
Lymph Nodes

Assessment of nodal involvement with lymphoma has traditionally been based on detection and measurement of nodal enlargement by physical exam and imaging. There is no consensus on whether lymph node long axis or short axis diameter should be used, although there is less variability with short axis measurements. The upper limit of normal nodal size has been cited as a diameter of 1 cm for short axis and 1.5 cm for long axis (LISTER et al. 1989), but the normal size range varies with location, ranging from an upper limit of 6 mm in the retrocrural region to 1.5 cm in the pelvis based on CT and autopsy series of adults (MAVROMATIS and CHESON 2002). Determination of nodal enlargement is limited by the paucity

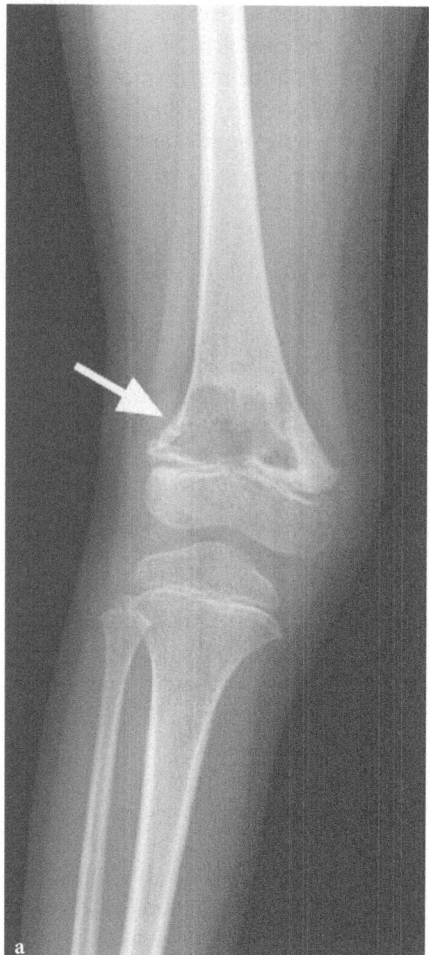

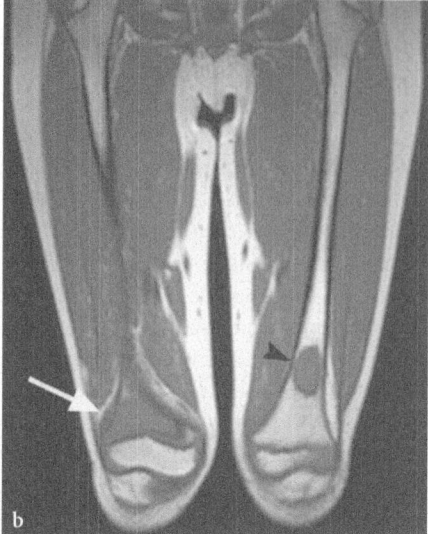

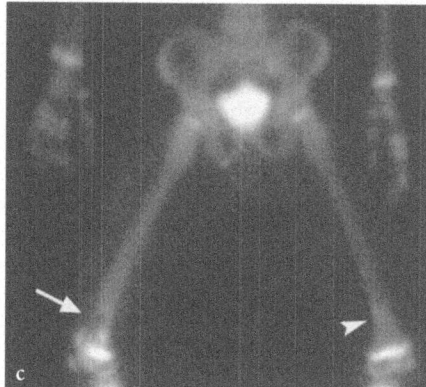

Fig. 14.7a–c. Anaplastic large cell lymphoma with multifocal skeletal involvement in a 6-year-old boy who presented with right lower extremity pain. **a** Anteroposterior radiograph of the right knee depicts a lytic destructive lesion of the distal right femoral metaphysis with permeation of the lateral cortex (*arrow*). **b** Coronal T1-weighted MR image further defines the right femoral lesion (*arrow*), and also identifies a distal left femoral metadiaphysis lesion (*arrowhead*) that was asymptomatic and occult to radiography. **c** On planar bone scintigraphy image, the distal right femoral lesion exhibits diminished uptake centrally and increased uptake peripherally (*arrow*), while the distal left femoral lesion exhibits subtle increased uptake (*arrowhead*). Biopsy of the right femur lesion revealed anaplastic large cell lymphoma.

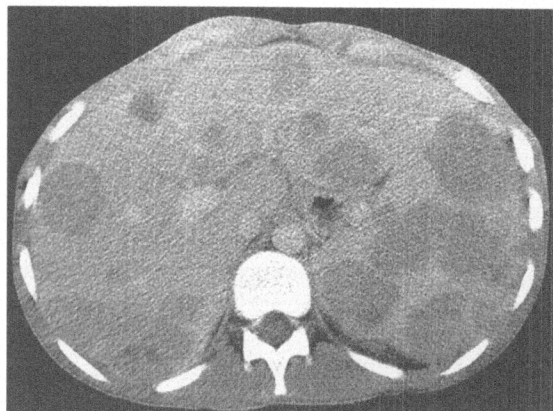

Fig. 14.8. Anaplastic large cell lymphoma in a 16-year-old boy who presented with abdominal pain and weight loss. Axial contrast-enhanced CT scan of the abdomen shows hepatosplenomegaly with numerous hypodense lesions in the liver and spleen. Hepatosplenic involvement is frequently present in anaplastic large cell lymphoma.

of studies on normal lymph node size in children. Hilar and retroperitoneal nodes rarely achieve a size of 1 cm in normal children, but axillary, inguinal, and mesenteric nodes may exceed this size in the absence of neoplasm.

In children, relatively large nodes may be encountered in the setting of benign reactive lymphoid hyperplasia, limiting the specificity of nodal enlargement as a criterion for nodal involvement with lymphoma. This is particularly problematic in children under 11 years of age, where the incidence of benign reactive nodal hyperplasia is almost 20%. In older children and adolescents, the incidence of benign reactive nodal hyperplasia drops to about 8% (PARKER 1997).

There is a trade-off of sensitivity and specificity with any node size threshold, since nodes may be enlarged due to reactive hyperplasia or neoplasm, and unenlarged nodes may contain tumor deposits.

Lymph node enlargement due to lymphoma must be differentiated from enlargement due to lymphoid hyperplasia, infection, and metastatic disease from other neoplasms. Correlation with the clinical evaluation and/or tissue sampling is often required for diagnosis (Fig. 14.9).

Lymphomatous nodes may appear as discrete nodes or conglomerate masses, and tend to show little enhancement on CT or MR imaging. Nodal calcification visible by imaging is rarely present in untreated lymphoma, occurring in less than 1% of cases, and is seen most often in the mediastinum, in NHL, and in aggressive disease (APTER et al. 2002). Calcification is more common in treated lymphoma, either after chemotherapy or radiation therapy (FISHMAN et al. 1991). Cystic changes related to necrosis may occur as a consequence of rapid tumor growth or treatment response (Fig. 14.10) (HOPPER

et al. 1990). On US, lymphomatous nodes are typically hypoechoic with moderate vascular flow on Doppler (LEWIS et al. 1989).

14.4.4
Central Nervous System

CNS involvement with lymphoma is uncommon at presentation. CNS involvement may manifest as a discrete cerebral mass, blasts in the cerebrospinal fluid, cranial nerve palsy, or meningeal infiltration (VAZQUEZ et al. 2002). CNS lymphoma is typically of B-cell lineage (EPSTEIN et al. 1988). Primary CNS lymphoma is the most common cause of focal brain mass lesions in children with AIDS, occurring with an incidence of 3–4% in pediatric HIV infection. The attenuation on unenhanced CT and signal intensity

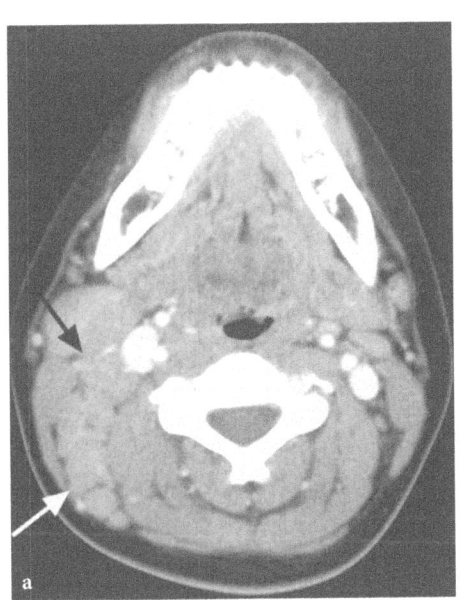
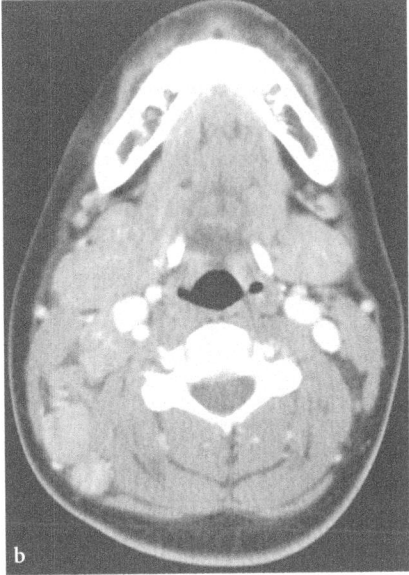

Fig. 14.9a,b. Nodular sclerosis Hodgkin disease in a 12-year-old boy with cervical lymphadenopathy mimicking lymphadenitis. a Axial contrast-enhanced CT scan of the neck shows enlarged jugular chain and posterior cervical lymph nodes (arrows) initially thought to represent infectious lymphadenitis. b Follow-up axial contrast-enhanced CT scan performed after a course of antibiotics demonstrates unresolving lymphadenopathy. Biopsy revealed nodular sclerosis Hodgkin disease.

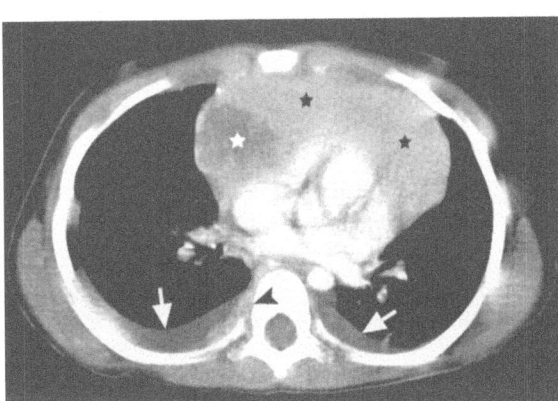

Fig. 14.10. T-cell lymphoblastic lymphoma in a 4-year-old girl. Axial contrast-enhanced CT scan of the thorax at the time of presentation shows a large anterior mediastinal mass in the region of the thymus (black stars), and pleural effusions (arrows). The finding of a pleural-based soft tissue mass (arrowhead) is relatively uncommon. The mediastinal mass contains a cystic-appearing hypodense component (white star) which may represent necrosis related to rapid tumor growth prior to treatment. Such cystic-appearing components may persist or even enlarge after therapy.

on MR imaging is typically heterogeneous, with marked enhancement with contrast and variable peritumoral edema. Primary CNS lymphoma tends to be multicentric, periventricular, and supratentorial. When solitary, the imaging features can overlap with those of gliomas (Fig. 14.11). Use of double-dose delayed contrast-enhanced CT scan technique or MR imaging increases the sensitivity of imaging for CNS lymphoma (Vazquez et al. 2002).

14.4.5
Extracranial Head and Neck

Lymphoma is the most common extracranial head and neck malignancy in childhood. Approximately 60–90% of children with HD and 30% of children with NHL have cervical node involvement at presentation. The internal jugular and spinal accessory nodal groups are the most frequently involved. Extranodal head and neck involvement at locations such as the paranasal sinuses, nasal cavity, Waldeyer's ring, and orbits is unusual in HD but common in NHL (Fig. 14.12) (Siegel 1999). Primary differential diagnostic considerations for an extracranial pediatric head and neck tumor include lymphoma and rhabdomyosarcoma.

14.4.6
Thorax

Lymphoma is the most common cause of a neoplastic mediastinal mass in a child, accounting for almost 70% of such masses (Bower and Kiesewetter 1977). HD is more common in the mediastinum than NHL. Approximately 70% of HD patients have mediastinal involvement at presentation. Over 95% of patients with intrathoracic HD have mediastinal lymphadenopathy, with superior mediastinal modes involved in nearly all, hilar nodes in a third, subcarinal nodes in 20%, cardiophrenic nodes in 8%, and posterior mediastinal nodes in 5% (Castellino et al. 1986). Intrathoracic disease exists in 40–45% of cases of NHL at presentation. Of these cases, the superior mediastinal nodes are involved in 75%, subcarinal nodes in 13%, posterior mediastinal nodes in 10%, hilar nodes in 9%, and cardiophrenic nodes in 7% (Castellino 1991b; Castellino et al. 1996).

In the anterior mediastinum, lymphoma can present as infiltration of the thymus or lymph nodes. Approximately 95% of patients with thymic infiltration by lymphoma have adenopathy elsewhere in the mediastinum (Siegel 1999). Anterior mediastinal adenopathy can be difficult to distinguish from normal thymus in younger children.

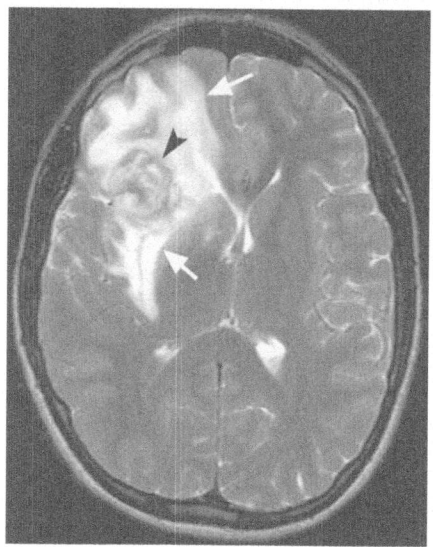 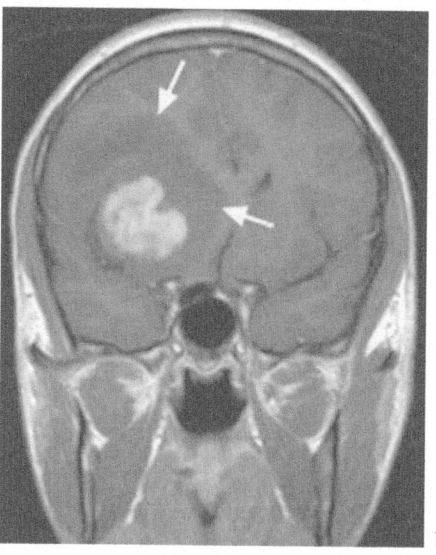

a · b

Fig. 14.11a,b. Primary central nervous system T-cell non-Hodgkin lymphoma mimicking a glioma in a 17-year-old boy who presented with headaches. **a** Axial T2-weighted MR image of the brain shows a heterogeneous mass lesion occupying the deep right frontal lobe (*arrowhead*). The mass shows marked enhancement on (**b**) coronal contrast-enhanced T1-weighted MR image. There is extensive peritumoral vasogenic edema (*arrows*), with mass effect effacing the frontal horn of the right lateral ventricle, and leftward shift of the midline structures. This aggressive-appearing tumor was thought to most likely represent a glioma by the imaging features, but biopsy revealed T-cell non-Hodgkin lymphoma.

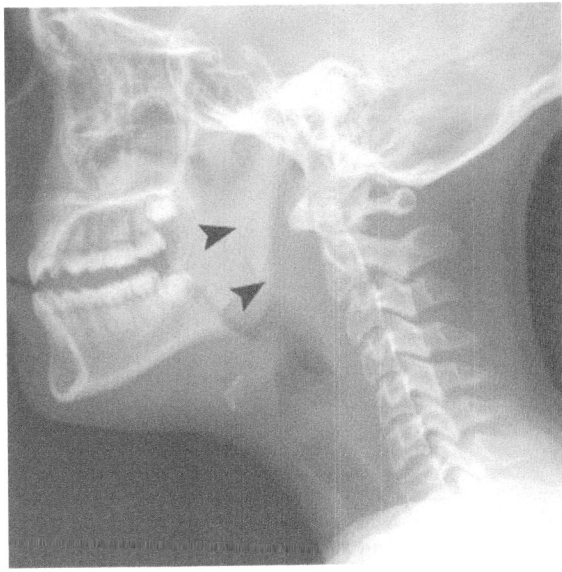
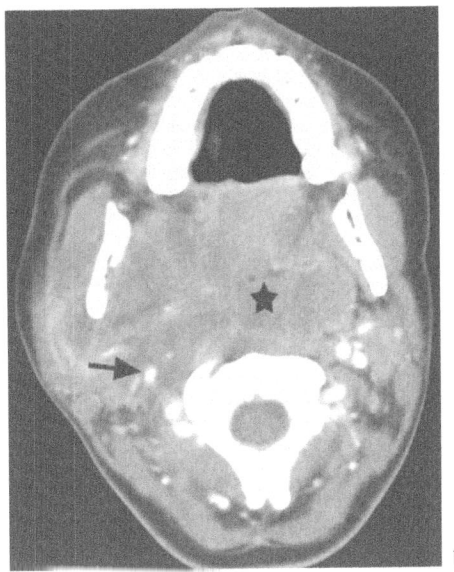

Fig. 14.12a,b. Waldeyer's ring large B-cell lymphoma in a 14-year-old girl who presented with neck swelling and trismus. a Lateral upper airway radiograph shows effacement of the upper pharyngeal airway by enlarged Waldeyer ring soft tissues (*arrowheads*). b Axial contrast-enhanced CT scan of the neck demonstrates lymphomatous infiltration of the pharyngeal mucosal space, soft palate, and retropharyngeal and parapharyngeal soft tissues with resulting pharyngeal airway effacement (*star*). There is also involvement of the right masticator and carotid spaces, with occlusion of the right internal jugular vein and narrowing of the right internal carotid artery (*arrow*).

The thymus is visible with cross-sectional imaging in virtually all normal children. In children less than 5 years of age, the thymus has a quadrilateral shape with convex lateral margins and undulating borders related to costal cartilage impressions. At ages above 5 years, the thymus progressively assumes a triangular shape with straight or concave margins. On CT, the density of the normal thymus approximates that of muscle. On MR imaging, the signal intensity of normal thymus is less than fat and slightly greater than muscle on T1-weighted images, and greater than muscle and slightly less than fat on T2-weighted images (Siegel et al. 1989). On US, the pediatric thymus has similar echotexture to liver parenchyma and lower echogenicity than the thyroid parenchyma (Adam and Ignotus 1993). Prior to puberty, the parenchyma of the thymus appears homogeneous. After puberty, heterogeneous fatty infiltration of the thymus can be present (St. Amour et al. 1987). The thymus is very variable in size in childhood. The thickness of the thymus decreases with advancing age and normal pediatric thymus size standards have been published using CT (St. Amour et al. 1987), MR imaging (Siegel et al. 1989), and US (Adam and Ignotus 1993). The normal thymus exerts little or no mass effect on adjacent structures. In most cases, a mediastinal mass or thymic infiltration can be dif-

ferentiated from normal thymus by imaging with attention to deviation from normal thymic shape and homogeneity. The normal thymus can extend superiorly into the thoracic inlet or posteriorly into the posterior mediastinum (Fig. 14.13). In these cases, normalcy can be established by the findings of homogeneous attenuation, absence of significant compression of adjacent tracheobronchial structures or mediastinal vessels, and continuity with thymus in the anterior mediastinum (Cory et al. 1987).

Thymic lymphoma occasionally has cystic-appearing components (Fig. 14.10). These components are usually identified at time of diagnosis rather than after treatment. These components can remain stable in size or even enlarge following treatment despite regression of disease elsewhere, and such behavior does not necessarily indicate residual or recurrent disease or an increased risk of relapse (Lindfors et al. 1985; Wernecke et al. 1991).

In studies of predominantly adult populations, the lung parenchyma is involved in 11–13% of cases of intrathoracic HD and NHL (Castellino et al. 1986; Castellino et al. 1996). Lung parenchymal involvement may appear as nodules or as an air space or interstitial infiltrate. A pleural effusion is present in 10% of cases of intrathoracic HD. Aspiration of a pleural effusion at the time of presentation

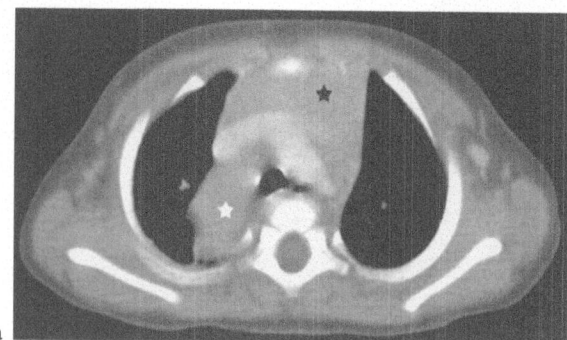
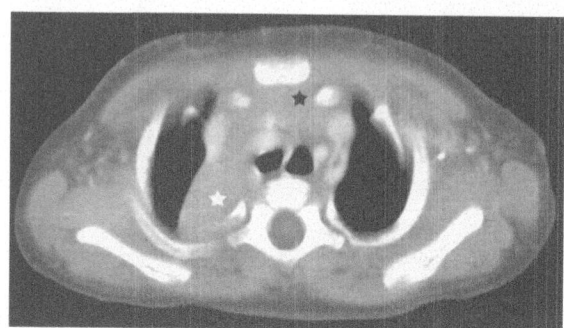

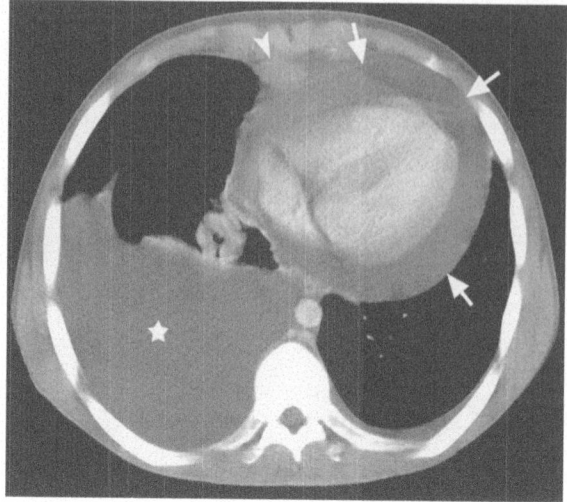

Fig. 14.14. Hodgkin disease in a 17-year-old boy with large pleural and pericardial effusions. Axial contrast-enhanced CT scan of the thorax demonstrates a large right pleural effusion (*star*), large pericardial effusion (*arrows*), and pericardial lymphadenopathy (*arrowhead*). Emergent drainage of such effusions may be required if there is associated compromise of respiratory or cardiac function.

Fig. 14.13a,b. Normal thymic variation in a 1-year-old girl with an upper mediastinal mass suspected on a chest radiograph. a, b Axial contrast-enhanced CT scans of the upper thorax show a soft tissue structure in the right paratracheal and posterior mediastinal region (*white star*). The structure has smooth borders and homogeneous density, with continuity between the superior vena cava and innominate artery with the thymus in the anterior mediastinum (*black star*), and no significant mass effect on the adjacent trachea or major mediastinal vessels. These findings are consistent with a normal variant in the positioning of the thymus.

of HD usually fails to reveal malignant cells, whereas the presence of a pericardial effusion in HD usually indicates malignant invasion of the pericardium (Fig. 14.14). Pleural effusions are common in some subtypes of NHL, most notably lymphoblastic lymphoma (Figs. 14.6, 14.10) and Burkitt lymphoma, even when the primary tumor is intra-abdominal. The effusions in pediatric NHL typically result from lymphatic obstruction, and, although the effusions may contain malignant cells, gross pleural soft tissue masses are unusual (Fig. 14.10) (WHITE 2001).

14.4.7
Abdomen and Pelvis

Lymphoma frequently involves the liver and spleen, either in the form of discrete lesions or diffuse infiltration. Hepatosplenic involvement is typically part of systemic disease. In the liver and spleen, high-grade NHL most frequently shows large nodular lesions (Fig. 14.8), while low grade NHL and HD have a tendency for small nodular or diffuse lesions (GORG et al. 1996).

Liver involvement is more common in NHL than HD. In HD, liver involvement is almost always associated with splenic involvement. Hepatic involvement most commonly appears as focal hypodense lesions on CT (Fig. 14.8), hypoechoic or anechoic lesions on US, and hypointense lesions on T1-weighted and hyperintense lesions on T2-weighted MR images. Hepatomegaly often indicates diffuse involvement (HALLIDAY and BAXTER 2003), although a liver of normal size can be diffusely infiltrated with lymphoma (WERNECKE et al. 1987).

Splenic involvement is found at staging laparotomy in one-third of children with HD and 15% of children with NHL. The involved spleen may or may not be enlarged. Mild to moderate splenomegaly may be present without involvement (MENDENHALL et al. 1993), although there is a high likelihood of involvement with marked splenomegaly (CASTELLINO 1986). Splenic involvement without associated para-aortic lymph node disease is unusual.

Pancreatic involvement by lymphoma is almost exclusively seen in NHL. Pancreatic involvement can appear as focal lesions, or diffuse infiltration mimicking pancreatitis. Even with large pancreatic masses, biliary or pancreatic duct obstruction is unusual (Fig. 14.15) (HALLIDAY and BAXTER 2003).

Lymphoma is the most common pediatric bowel malignancy, and bowel involvement occurs much more commonly with NHL than HD. Massive intraabdominal lymphoma in children is nearly always of B-cell origin, and most commonly is Burkitt lymphoma (Fig. 14.15) or Burkitt-like lymphoma. NHL of the bowel most frequently involves the small bowel, particularly the distal ileum, and multifocal involvement is not uncommon. Involvement may appear as nodular, polypoid, ulcerative, or infiltrative lesions (REZVANI et al. 1986; GOERG et al. 1990). Bowel wall thickening > 1 cm and aneurysmal bowel dilation are particularly suggestive of lymphoma (Fig. 14.2) (SIEGEL et al. 1988). Intussusception and fistula tracts may occur as complications (GUILLERMAN 2000). Mesenteric node involvement occurs in 50% of children with NHL and 5% of children with HD at the time of presentation (SIEGEL 1999). Conglomerate mesenteric nodal involvement with envelopment of mesenteric vessels and fat produces the "sandwich sign" on imaging (HARDY 2003).

Renal involvement with lymphoma detectable by imaging has an incidence of approximately 8%. Renal involvement is more common with NHL than HD, and is commonly bilateral with concomitant

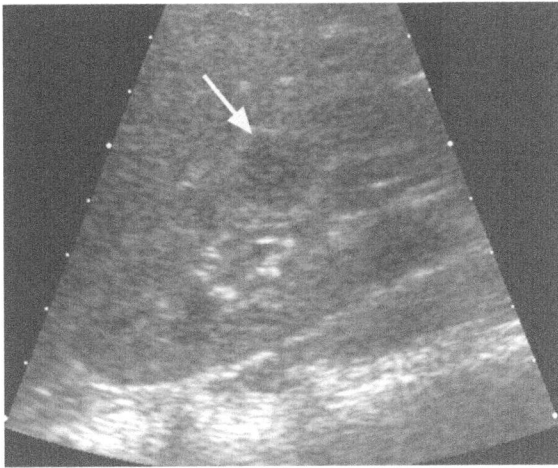

Fig. 14.16. Burkitt lymphoma in a 9-year-old boy with renal involvement. Longitudinal US image of the abdomen demonstrates a hypoechoic ovoid lesion (*arrow*) of the interpolar region of the right kidney, consistent with focal renal lymphoma. An additional lesion was discovered in the right renal upper pole (not depicted). The presence of multiple focal lesions is the most common imaging manifestation of renal lymphoma.

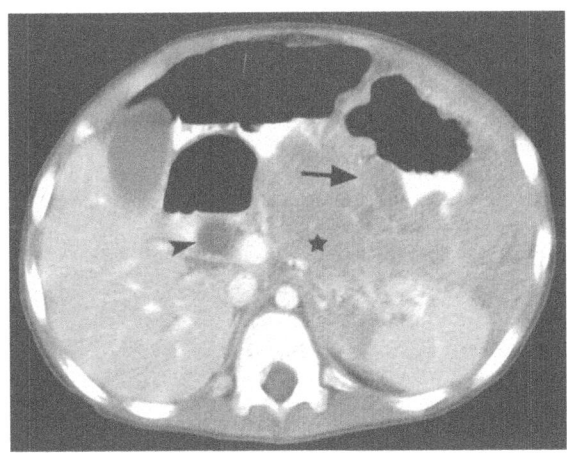

Fig. 14.15. Burkitt lymphoma in an 8-year-old boy with a history of renal transplantation and post-transplant lymphoproliferative disease. Axial contrast-enhanced CT scan of the abdomen shows massive abdominal involvement, with infiltration of the gastric wall (*arrow*), mesentery, and retroperitoneum, including the pancreas (*star*). There is associated bile duct obstruction with marked common bile duct dilation (*arrowhead*), an unusual manifestation with lymphoma. Biopsy of the abdominal mass revealed EBV-associated Burkitt lymphoma.

retroperitoneal lymphadenopathy (CHEPURI et al. 2003). CT is superior to US in depicting renal lymphoma (WEINBERGER et al. 1990). The most common imaging appearance of pediatric renal lymphoma is multiple soft tissue nodules that are hypoenhancing on CT and hypoechoic on US, occurring in 60–70% of cases (Fig. 14.16). Less common presentations include direct renal invasion from adjacent nodal masses (10–20%), a solitary renal mass (5–10%) or nephromegaly from diffuse infiltration (5–10%) (SIEGEL 1999; CHEPURI et al. 2003; NG et al. 1994). Diffuse renal enlargement in a lymphoma patient is more likely secondary to nephritis or tumor lysis than lymphoma infiltration (CHEPURI et al. 2003). Urinary tract symptomatology from renal lymphoma is rare, although hydroureteronephrosis may occur with ureteral compression by retroperitoneal or pelvic lymphadenopathy (Fig. 14.17).

14.4.8
Musculoskeletal System

Skeletal lymphoma most often occurs in the setting of disseminated disease. The incidence of bone involvement at presentation in children is 7% in NHL and 1–2% in HD (PARKER 1997). There is a predilection of lymphoma for sites with predominantly hemat-

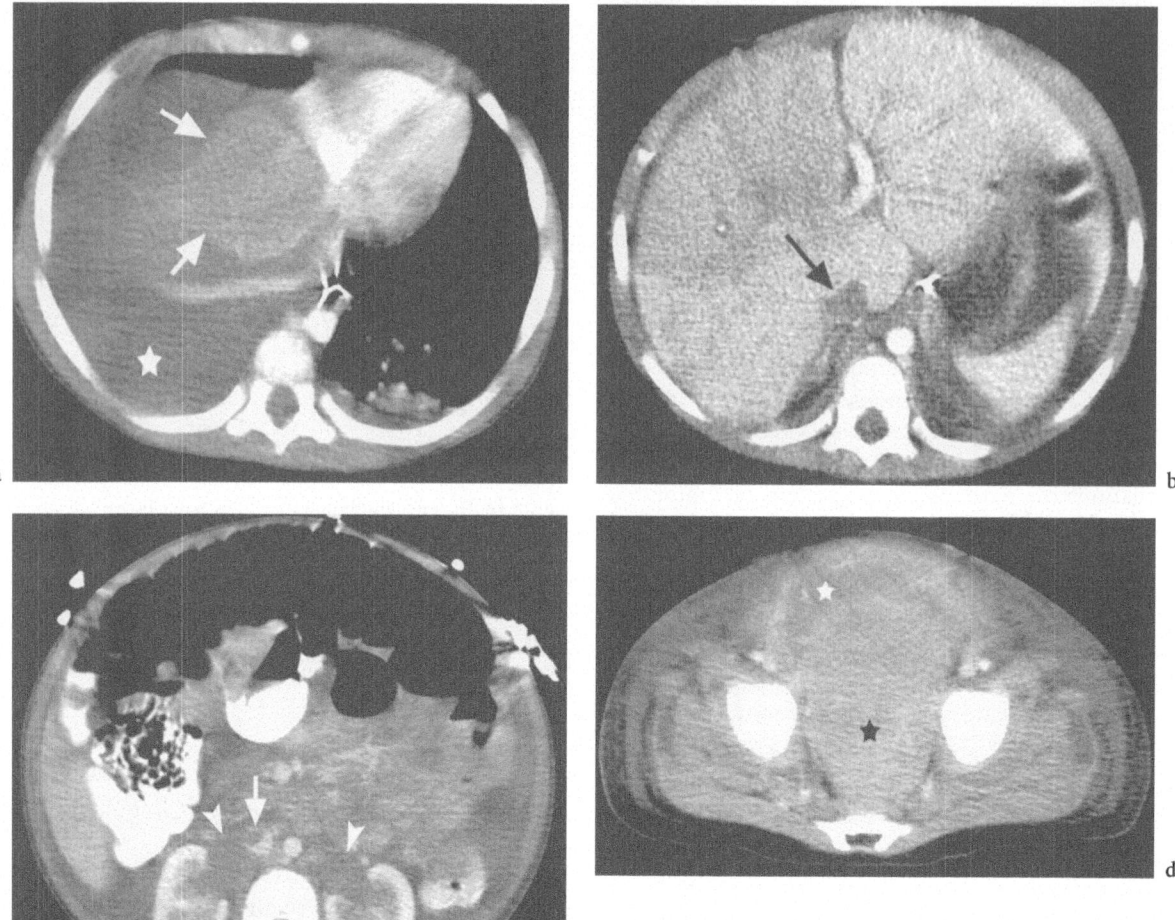

Fig. 14.17a–d. Burkitt lymphoma in a 3-year-old boy who presented with abdominal distention. **a** Axial contrast-enhanced CT scan of the chest shows a large mass that impresses on the right atrium (*arrows*), and a large right pleural effusion (*star*) associated with right lung atelectasis. **b** Axial contrast-enhanced CT scan of the upper abdomen demonstrates the intrahepatic inferior vena cava is occluded (*arrow*), with hepatomegaly, ascites, and inhomogeneous liver enhancement, consistent with Budd-Chiari syndrome. **c** Axial contrast-enhanced CT scan of the mid abdomen shows the intracaval thrombus extends inferiorly to the level of the kidneys (*arrow*). There is mild hydronephrosis (*arrowheads*), a consequence of a large pelvic mass (*black star*) seen on (**d**) axial contrast-enhanced CT scan of the pelvis. The mass impresses on the distal ureters and displaces the urinary bladder anteriorly (*white star*). Biopsy revealed Burkitt lymphoma.

opoietic marrow, such as the ribs, skull, pelvis, vertebra, and extremity long bones (Fig. 14.18) (WHITE 2001). Primary bone lymphoma is rare and usually affects a lower extremity (HALLIDAY and BAXTER 2003). Primary lymphoma of the bone has a propensity for the metaphysis but often crosses the growth plate into the epiphysis, and occasionally extends into the joint space (PARKER 1997).

Radiographically, skeletal NHL typically has a permeative pattern of destruction (Fig. 14.7), while HD typically has a sclerotic or mixed lytic and sclerotic pattern. MR imaging is the best imaging modality for revealing the extent of involvement of the bone marrow and extra-osseous soft tissues, when clinically indicated (Fig. 14.7). Whole-skeleton screening is traditionally done by bone scintigraphy (Fig. 14.18). The value of screening is limited, though, since the clinical outcome of pediatric NHL is not strongly correlated with the presence of bone involvement (ROSENTHAL et al. 2000). The utility of bone scintigraphy in evaluating response to treatment is confounded by the non-specificity of increased skeletal radiopharmaceutical uptake, since an osteoblastic response can relate to healing

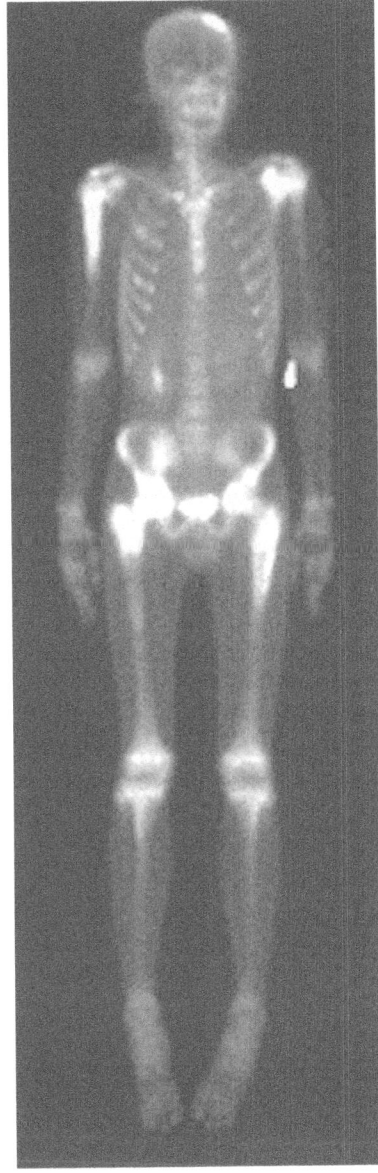

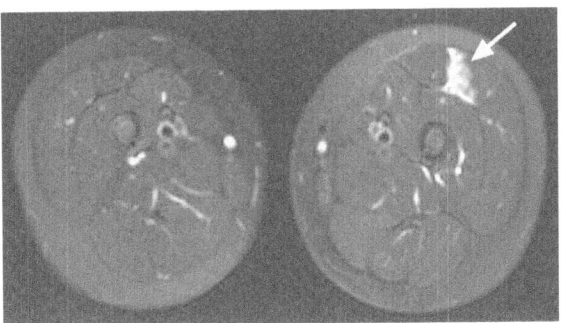

Fig. 14.19. Anaplastic large cell lymphoma in a 6-year-old boy with muscle involvement. Axial fat-suppressed T2-weighted MR image of the thighs demonstrates a focal hyperintense lesion of the anteromedial aspect of the left vastus lateralis muscle (*arrow*). Myositis or muscle strain could have a similar appearance.

Fig. 14.18. Anaplastic large cell lymphoma in a 16-year-old boy with multifocal skeletal involvement. Whole-body planar image from a ^{99m}technetium diphosphonate scintigraphy exam shows multiple bone lesions, including involvement of the left parietal skull, proximal right humerus, scapulae, posterior right ilium, and proximal femurs. This illustrates the propensity for lymphoma to involve the hematopoietic marrow bearing areas of the axial and appendicular skeleton.

14.4.9
Testicular

Testicular lymphoma can occur as primary disease or part of the spectrum of disseminated disease. Testicular lymphoma is most typically B-cell NHL (DALLE et al. 2001). The US appearance of testicular lymphoma is nonspecific, most commonly presenting as bilateral enlarged hypoechoic testes with or without focal masses, with increased Doppler flow (MAZZU et al. 1995). The testicles can serve as a sanctuary site since the blood-gonad barrier can prevent accumulation of high levels of intratesticular chemotherapeutic drugs (HADDY et al. 1988).

14.5
Imaging Modalities

Imaging plays a seminal role in the diagnosis, staging, restaging, and surveillance of pediatric lymphoma. While many imaging tests are requested according to the schedule of a clinical trial protocol or clinical practice guideline, clinical judgment must always be exercised by the oncologist and radiologist in selecting the imaging modality that is most appropriate for the specific clinical circumstance of the individual patient. Imaging tests for the evaluation of lymphoma include conventional radiography, fluoroscopy, lymphography, US, CT, MR imaging, and nuclear medicine (principally bone scintigraphy, gallium scintigraphy, and PET).

or disease progression. Interpretation of MR imaging of skeletal involvement after treatment can also be problematic, as bone marrow signal alterations have been reported to persist after successful therapy in up to 71% of cases (ROSENTHAL et al. 2000).

Primary muscle lymphoma is very rare and typically NHL. The involvement may occur as a discrete mass or diffuse infiltration. MR imaging of muscle lymphoma involvement shows hypointensity on T1-weighted images and hyperintensity on T2-weighted images (Fig. 14.19) (HALLIDAY and BAXTER 2003). This is a nonspecific pattern that must be differentiated from other processes such as myositis, muscle strain, muscle infarction, and rhabdomyolysis.

14.5.1
Conventional Radiography

Conventional chest radiography now has a limited role in the evaluation of lymphoma, due to the widespread practice of acquiring chest CT exams. Chest radiographs may still be useful for assessing for bulky mediastinal disease at presentation, providing a baseline for follow-up, detecting pulmonary infection in the febrile patient after treatment, estimating the degree of tracheal compression from a mediastinal mass prior to procedures requiring sedation or general anesthesia, and for identifying cardiopericardial silhouette enlargement suggesting a large pericardial effusion requiring emergency treatment to allay the risk of cardiac tamponade.

Apart from screening for ileus, bowel obstruction, pneumatosis, or free intraperitoneal air in a patient with acute abdominal symptoms at presentation or in the course of treatment, conventional abdominal radiography has little role in the evaluation of lymphoma. An occasional exception at a few institutions is the depiction of abdominal and pelvic nodes opacified by lymphography contrast for infradiaphragmatic radiation therapy portal planning, treatment response, and surveillance.

14.5.2
Fluoroscopy

Barium fluoroscopy studies are useful in the evaluation of gastrointestinal tract involvement. Barium fluoroscopy may be more sensitive for minimal bowel involvement than other imaging modalities. However, the overall practical utility of barium fluoroscopy is less than that of cross-sectional modalities such as CT, which can not only image the bowel but also the mesenteric and retroperitoneal lymph nodes and solid abdominal viscera.

14.5.3
Ultrasound

US has the advantages of low cost and virtually no risk. US is the modality of choice for evaluation of peripheral small parts (e.g., testicles, thyroid) and for imaging of the female pelvic structures. As a diagnostic test ordered for evaluation of an abdominal mass or abdominal pain, sonography may detect intestinal lymphoma presenting as an intussusception (Fig. 14.3) or as thick-walled bowel with the

appearance of a "pseudokidney" (Fig. 14.20) (DORAK et al. 1991) or "doughnut sign" (HASEGAWA et al. 1998). However, US is not well suiting as a staging or surveillance tool, due to technical limitations in depicting the mediastinum, lungs, deep abdominal nodal regions, and skeleton.

14.5.4
Computed Tomography

CT is the primary imaging modality used in the staging and follow-up of childhood lymphoma. CT provides a convenient method of globally surveying the neck, chest, abdomen, and pelvis for adenopathy and visceral organ involvement. Limitations of CT include insensitivity for involvement of normal-sized nodes, spleen, and bone marrow, as well as risks incurred with the use of intravenous contrast media and ionizing radiation exposure.

When clinically feasible, CT should be performed with intravenous and oral contrast to better discriminate bowel and vascular structures from lymph nodes, which otherwise can be a difficult task for even experienced observers due to the paucity of retroperitoneal and mesenteric fat in children. Section thickness and field of view is tailored to patient size. Follow-up studies should be performed and interpreted with parameters as close as possible to the baseline study to optimize validity of comparisons. For example, lesions should be measured at the same

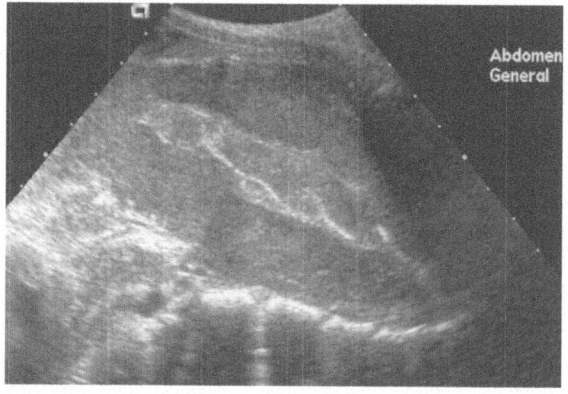

Fig. 14.20. "Pseudokidney" in Burkitt lymphoma in a 3-year-old boy who presented with abdominal distention. Longitudinal US image of the abdomen reveals a large mass of abnormal bowel resembling a hydronephrotic kidney, with a central fluid collection enveloped by a thick peripheral rind of soft tissue. This appearance is highly suggestive of lymphoma with intramural infiltration of the bowel, and in children is most commonly due to Burkitt lymphoma, as in this case.

window settings and reconstruction intervals. Attention should be paid to technical parameters such as mAs and pitch to keep radiation dose as low as reasonably achievable. This is particularly important given concerns over the risk of malignancy induction by ionizing radiation exposure from pediatric CT (BRENNER et al. 2001), and the relatively large number of CT scans received by pediatric lymphoma patients during the course of treatment and surveillance. A general principle is that the higher the anticipated lesion conspicuity, the higher the dose reduction permissible. A dose reduction of 90% with multidetector CT compared to standard technique has been reported to provide adequate image quality for evaluation of thoracic lymphoma, where a large lymphoma mass has high conspicuity when situated adjacent to aerated lung and contrast-enhanced mediastinal vessels (DINKEL et al. 2003). The same degree of dose reduction may not be achievable in other settings, for example, a CT obtained to evaluate for hepatic microabscesses in a neutropenic patient during treatment, due to the reduced conspicuity of tiny hepatic lesions at high image noise levels.

14.5.5
Magnetic Resonance Imaging

Due to its superior contrast resolution, MR imaging is the imaging modality of choice for evaluation of the CNS and musculoskeletal system, including the bone marrow (HAMRICK-TURNER et al. 1994). MR imaging is complementary to bone marrow biopsy, and up to one-third of patients evaluated with routine bone marrow biopsies may have otherwise occult marrow tumor visible on MR imaging (HOANE et al. 1991). Imaging cannot replace bone marrow biopsy, since imaging does not detail the status of normal bone marrow precursors or the histology of marrow involvement (MAVROMATIS and CHESON 2002). In those unable to receive intravenous contrast for CT due to conditions such as contrast allergy or renal insufficiency, MR imaging may be used as an alternative for body imaging. Compared to CT, MR imaging has the disadvantages of higher cost, lesser availability, and increased need for sedation.

14.5.6
Gallium Scintigraphy

The primary role of gallium scintigraphy is assessment of response and residual masses. [67]Gallium is a ferric ion analogue, with uptake that correlates with viable tumor. The efficacy of gallium scintigraphy for evaluation of infradiaphragmatic disease is limited by physiologic uptake in the liver and spleen, and by excretion into the gastrointestinal tract. Physiologic uptake in the thymus, nasopharynx, and bone marrow can complicate interpretation. Also, gallium has poor sensitivity for skeletal lymphoma compared to MR imaging and technetium-99[m] diphosphonate scintigraphy (ORZEL et al. 1988).

A dose range of 40–160 uCi/kg Gallium citrate is recommended in children. The growth plates are the critical tissue in dosing. Acquisition is initiated 48–72 hours after injection, and may be repeated after several days to allow clearance of bowel activity to improve evaluation of infradiaphragmatic disease. Gallium uptake may be affected by chemotherapy or radiation therapy, and gallium should be injected before initiating therapy to reduce potential false negative exams, but treatment should not be delayed in emergent cases (WHITE 2001; FRONT and ISRAEL 1995). The addition of single photon emission computed tomography (SPECT) increases the sensitivity of gallium for lymphoma over planar imaging, particularly for small lesions, and aids in the discrimination of pathologic uptake in the mediastinum from adjacent physiologic bone or soft tissue uptake (FRONT et al. 1990; TAN and GELFAND 1996).

14.5.7
Positron Emission Tomography

FDG-PET is a promising modality for evaluation of pediatric lymphoma. FDG is a glucose analogue and PET imaging with FDG detects malignant cells, including those of lymphoma, which avidly take up FDG due to increased glucose transporter activity and glycolysis. The patient should fast for at least 4 hours prior to injection of FDG, and the plasma glucose should be checked and appropriately treated with small doses of insulin to avoid false negative exams related to hyperglycemia. FDG is administered intravenously at a dose of 0.125–0.200 mCi/kg in children, with a minimum total dose of 2.0 mCi and maximum total dose of 10.0 mCi. The patient should drink water or receive intravenous fluids after injection to promote urinary FDG excretion. After injection, the patient is kept at rest for 45–60 minutes and imaging is then performed. The urinary bladder should be voided immediately prior to imaging. Although FDG-PET imaging can be achieved with a gamma camera adapted for co-incidence imaging,

imaging with a dedicated PET scanner is preferred. FDG activity should be corrected for attenuation. The level of tumor uptake is assessed subjectively by visual inspection and semi-quantitatively by determination of standardized uptake values (SUV).

Most studies to date of FDG-PET in lymphoma have been small series encompassing a heterogeneous group of histologies in predominantly adult patients, limiting conclusions on the efficacy of FDG-PET in the specific setting of pediatric lymphoma. Reviews and meta-analyses of the published studies imply superiority of FDG-PET over gallium and CT for staging, prediction of outcome, and assessment of response and residual masses in lymphoma (KOSTAKOGLU and GOLDSMITH 2000; SCHODER et al. 2001; TALBOT et al. 2001). Studies supporting the efficacy of FDG-PET in evaluating pediatric lymphoma are emerging (MONTRAVERS et al. 2002).

Pitfalls in FDG-PET interpretation include false positive exams due to inflammatory disease and physiological activity in the urinary tract, liver, bowel, thymus, brown fat, or tense muscle (Fig. 14.21) (BARRINGTON and O'DOHERTY 2003). FDG-PET is insensitive to extranodal MALT-type B-cell lymphoma. FDG-PET is inaccurate compared to MR imaging and bone marrow biopsy for evaluation of bone marrow disease, with false negatives on FDG-PET from minimal marrow involvement and false positives from hyperplastic marrow (KOSTAKOGLU and GOLDSMITH 2000)

Widespread application of FDG-PET is limited primarily by availability and cost, although these constraints are fading with the introduction of combined CT-PET units and increased reimbursement coverage by insurers. It is anticipated that FDG-PET will eventually supplant gallium in many instances. FDG-PET has a number of significant advantages compared to Gallium scintigraphy. Because of the short physical half-life of 1.8 hours for ^{18}F and its high photon energy of 511 keV, FDG-PET imaging may follow bone or Gallium scintigraphy on the same day, or FDG-PET imaging may be performed on the day preceding these studies. FDG-PET interpretation can be completed on the same day as the tracer injection, while Gallium scintigraphy interpretation is can not be completed for at least 48–72 hours after tracer injection. FDG-PET has superior spatial resolution, higher tumor to background uptake ratio, and several-fold lower radiation dose than Gallium scintigraphy. Gallium scintigraphy is more confounded by physiologic hepatosplenic uptake and bowel excretion than FDG-PET in the interpretation of infradiaphragmatic disease. FDG-

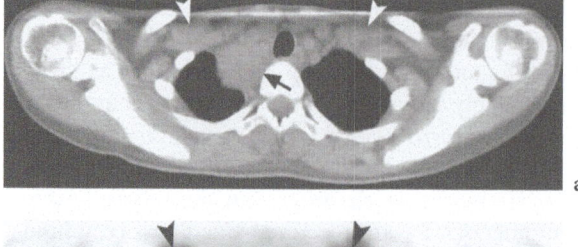

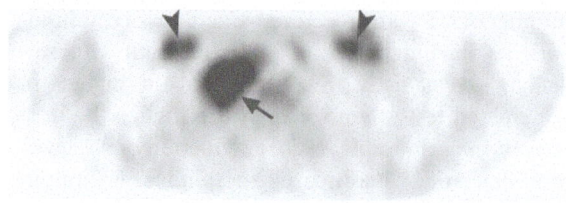

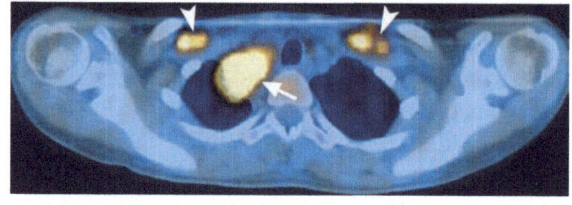

Fig. 14.21a–c. Staging evaluation for Hodgkin disease in an 18-year-old girl. a Axial unenhanced CT scan of the upper thorax shows a large right mediastinal mass (*arrow*). Axial (b) FDG-PET and (c) PET-CT fusion images of the upper thorax show intense FDG-PET uptake is present within the large right upper mediastinal lymphoma mass (*arrow*). Uptake is also present within muscle (*arrowheads*) anterior to the subclavian vessels bilaterally, postulated as due to muscle tension, and potentially mimicking uptake by lymphoma. *(Image courtesy of Dr. O. Israel)*

PET uptake is more readily quantified than Gallium uptake. (MONTRAVERS et al. 2002; KOSTAKOGLU and GOLDSMITH 2000).

14.5.8
Bone Scintigraphy

The performance of a bone scan with ^{99m}technetium diphosphonate scintigraphy may be indicated at staging or restaging when there is a reasonable likelihood of skeletal involvement. Such settings include the presence of skeletal symptoms, elevated alkaline phosphatase level, other sites of extranodal involvement, or lymphoma histology with a proclivity for skeletal involvement (e.g. large cell lymphoma). Due to the difficulty of discriminating between uptake related to healing from that of disease progression, bone scintigraphy has limited utility for assessing response to therapy.

14.5.9
Lymphography

Conventional lymphography with iodized oils once played a prominent role in the evaluation of Hodgkin lymphoma. Lymphography is capable of demonstrating internal nodal architecture, permitting identification of enlarged reactive nodes and normal sized involved nodes. Lymphography serves as a guide map for involved nodes for surgical sampling if laparotomy is planned or for treatment portals if subdiaphragmatic radiation therapy is planned. Follow-up radiographs allow assessment of relapse, with nodes remaining opacified for approximately 6–18 months in children, with the more rapid washout in younger children. Conventional lymphography has many disadvantages. These include the technically difficult nature of the exam, the inability to evaluate mesenteric, celiac axis, portal hepatic, and splenic hilar nodes not in the direct line of drainage, and the inability to evaluate organs such as the liver, spleen, and kidneys (PARKER 1997). Due to these disadvantages, conventional lymphography has been abandoned at many institutions.

14.6
Management

Imaging plays an important role in guiding the management of children with lymphoma. Management includes initial assessment to determine whether emergency procedures are necessary, definitive diagnosis, staging, risk stratification for determining prognosis and optimal therapy, initiation of therapy, assessment of response, completion of therapy, and surveillance for relapse and late effects. With contemporary management, pediatric lymphoma has become a curable disease in a high proportion of cases. According to recent SEER data, the overall 5-year survival rate for HD in American children less than 20 years of age is 91%, one of the highest survival rates of all childhood cancers. The histologic subtype of classic HD is not a major prognostic indicator. The overall 5-year survival rate for NHL in American children less than 20 years of age is 72%. Those with limited or localized NHL may achieve survival rates in excess of 90% (PERCY et al. 1999).

14.6.1
Emergency Management

Although prompt initiation of specific therapy is an important objective in treating lymphoma, especially in tumors with very rapid growth rates such as pediatric NHL, some patients have presentations which require emergency management before further diagnostic work-up and therapy. Imaging plays an important role in identifying these presentations. Among these are airway obstruction from pharyngeal, neck, or thoracic masses (Figs 14.12, 14.22, 14.23), cardiac tamponade from large pericardial effusions (Fig. 14.14), paraplegia or nerve palsies from epidural or perineural masses (Fig. 14.24), obstruction of the superior vena cava and other major chest vessels from mediastinal

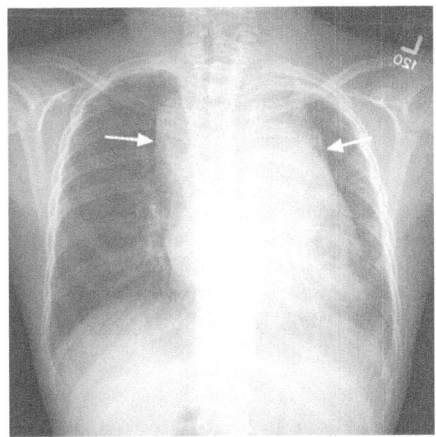
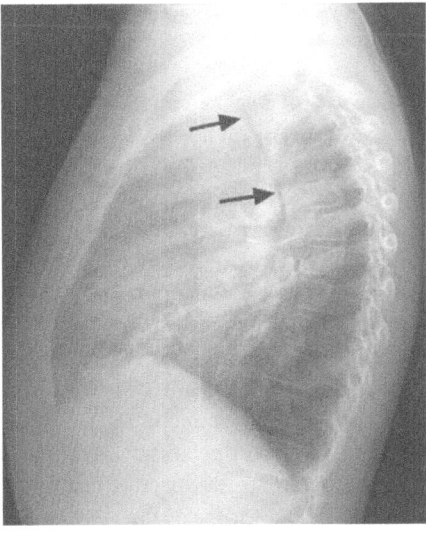

Fig. 14.22a,b. T-cell lymphoblastic lymphoma in a 9-year-old boy who presented with respiratory distress with large mediastinal mass and airway compression. **a** Anteroposterior chest radiograph demonstrates a large anterior mediastinal mass (*arrows*). **b** Lateral chest radiograph shows the mass has resulted in posterior displacement and marked narrowing of the compressed intrathoracic trachea (*arrows*).

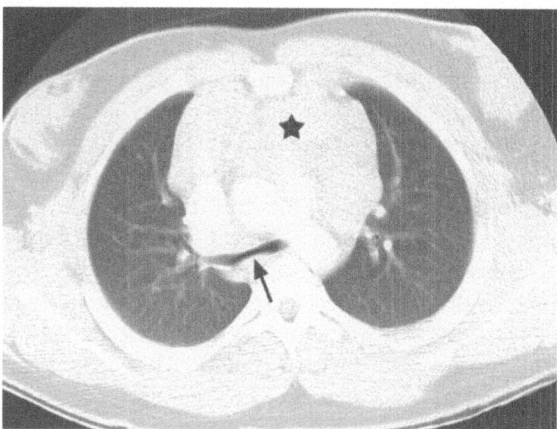

Fig. 14.23. Bulky mediastinal nodular sclerosis Hodgkin disease in a 16-year-old boy with airway compression. Axial CT scan of the thorax at lung windowing shows bulky anterior mediastinal mass (*star*). The mass effect displaces the tracheobronchial airway posteriorly and narrows the lumens of the carina and origins of the mainstem bronchi (*arrow*).

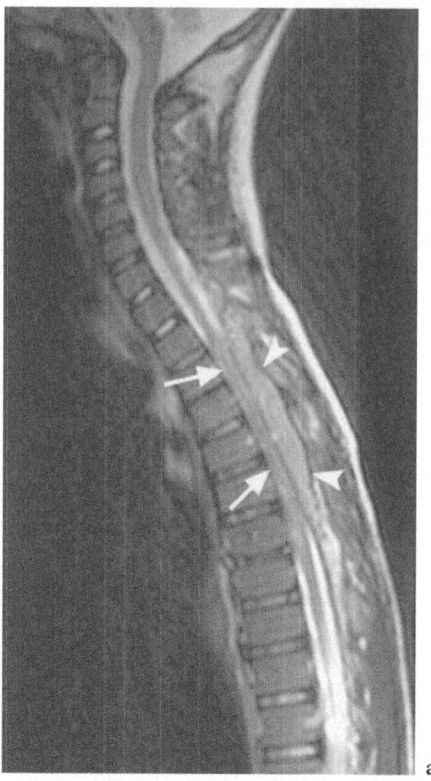

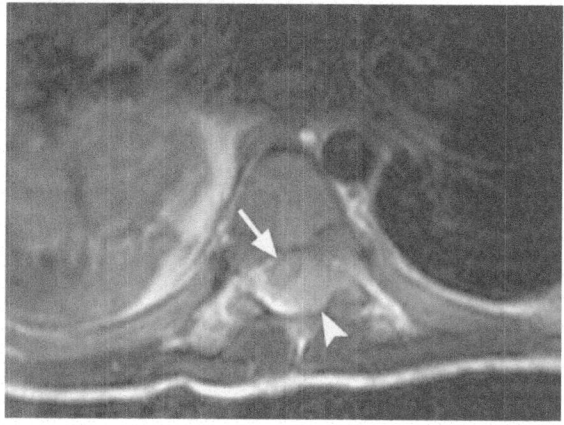

Fig. 14.24a,b. Epidural Burkitt lymphoma in an 8-year-old boy with a history of renal transplantation and post-transplant lymphoproliferative disease presenting with new onset paraparesis. **a** Sagittal and (**b**) axial T2-weighted MR images of the cervicothoracic spine show an epidural soft tissue mass (*arrowheads*) extending from the T2/3 to T7/8 levels, anterolaterally displacing and compressing the thoracic spinal cord (*arrows*). Biopsy revealed EBV-associated Burkitt lymphoma.

masses (Fig. 14.25), pulmonary compromise from large pleural effusions (Fig. 14.14), bowel obstruction, hemorrhage, or perforation from gastrointestinal tract masses, urinary tract obstruction from retroperitoneal or pelvic masses (Fig. 14.17), and obstruction of the inferior vena cava from extrinsic mass effect or intraluminal thrombus (Fig. 14.17). Because of differences in the typical patterns of presentation among the lymphoma subtypes, the frequency of emergent complications varies among the lymphoma subtypes. For example, compression of intra-thoracic structures is much more likely with lymphoblastic lymphoma or HD than Burkitt lymphoma, while intra-abdominal complications are much more likely with Burkitt lymphoma.

In lymphoma patients with a mediastinal mass, chest radiography including a lateral view can provide a gross estimate of the degree of airway compression (Fig. 14.22). The most accurate method of assessing the degree of airway compression is CT (Fig. 14.23). Life-threatening upper airway obstruction with induction of general anesthesia or heavy sedation is a potential complication of an anterior mediastinal mass, and patency of the airway should be determined before any procedure requiring general anesthesia or heavy sedation in a patient with an anterior mediastinal mass. It should be noted that substantial narrowing of the trachea or major bronchi can occur without significant compromise of breathing at rest. Abnormalities on pulmonary function tests correlate with the degree of tracheal narrowing, and it has been reported that general anesthesia can be safely used in children with a tracheal cross sectional area determined by CT and peak expiratory flow rate > 50% of predicted (SHAMBERGER et al. 1995).

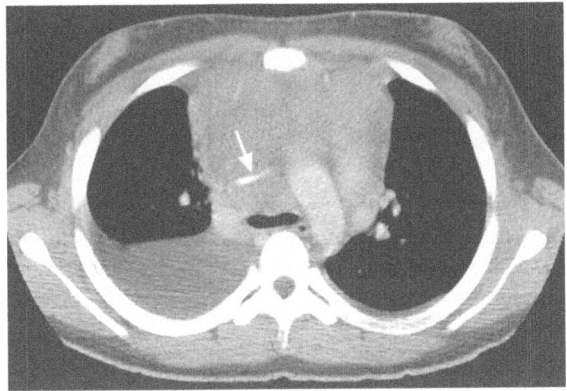

Fig. 14.25. Bulky mediastinal nodular sclerosis Hodgkin disease in a 13-year-old boy with superior vena cava compression. Axial contrast-enhanced CT scan of the thorax shows the compression of the anterior mediastinal venous structures by mass effect nearly completely effaces the lumen of the junction of the superior vena cava and left brachiocephalic vein (*arrow*).

For patients with significant respiratory compromise and high risk for general anesthesia or heavy sedation, there are several reasonable diagnostic approaches. These include thoracentesis under local anesthesia if a pleural effusion is present, biopsy under local anesthesia of accessible extrathoracic disease (especially peripheral nodes in the cervical, supraclavicular, axillary, or inguinal regions), bone marrow biopsy under local anesthesia, transthoracic anterior thoracotomy (Chamberlin procedure) under local anesthesia, and percutaneous imaging guided needle biopsy under local anesthesia. If these methods are not clinically feasible, options include corticosteroid or radiation therapy with shielding of the area to be used for future biopsy.

Large pericardial and pleural effusions are best managed by drainage and rapid institution of specific therapy. Prolonged tube drainage or pleurodesis is rarely needed, as specific therapy of the primary tumor usually suffices (WHITE 2001). Superior vena cava syndrome can be treated with radiation therapy, but in tumors such as lymphoblastic lymphoma that are highly responsive to chemotherapy, radiation therapy increases toxicity without therapeutic gain (MAGRATH 2002). While not necessarily requiring emergent treatment, occlusion or significant narrowing of the superior vena cava or of a brachiocephalic, subclavian, or internal jugular vein (Figs 14.12, 14.25) is important to note since this may influence planning of the approach to central vascular catheter placement.

Intestinal obstruction at presentation is most commonly due to intussusception (Fig. 14.3). This is often treated with pneumatic or hydrostatic reduction by a radiologist when the diagnosis of lymphoma is not certain, but this treatment is usually only a temporizing measure since surgery is eventually required to address the lead point mass. Surgical resection to prevent gastrointestinal bleed or perforation is not recommended in the setting of extensive bowel involvement since these complications may be even more likely after surgery (MAGRATH 2002).

Urinary tract obstruction is important to detect. Untreated urinary tract obstruction may impair the diuresis that is desired to reduce the effects of acute tumor lysis syndrome, especially with large tumor burdens. Detection of urinary tract obstruction by imaging prior to therapy allows remedial measures such as dialysis or urinary diversion to be instituted (Fig. 14.17) (MAGRATH 2002).

Occlusion of the inferior vena cava may arise from extrinsic mass effect or intraluminal thrombosis (Fig. 14.17). Differentiating these etiologies can influence the planning of corrective measures, but is not always possible by imaging. The risk of hemorrhagic complications with anticoagulation for suspected thrombosis is higher in the presence of gastrointestinal masses prone to ulceration, or thrombocytopenia and impaired hepatic warfarin metabolism induced by chemotherapy (MAGRATH 2002).

14.6.2
Diagnosis

Definitive diagnosis of lymphoma is traditionally established by histologic analysis. When unattainable on histologic grounds, distinction of lymphoma from other small round blue cell tumors and benign lymphoproliferative disorders is usually readily accomplished by immunophenotyping and cytogenetics demonstrating clonality and specific translocations of malignant lymphoma, with the occasional exception of anaplastic large cell lymphoma of null phenotype (MAGRATH 2002).

14.6.2.1
Percutaneous Biopsy

Open surgical excisional lymph node biopsy has been the standard approach to the diagnosis of lymphoma in children. Percutaneous fine needle aspiration and core needle biopsy are widely used in the diagnosis of lymphoma in adults, and can be accomplished with low-risk of complications with CT, US, or fluoroscopic guidance. If the results of bone marrow aspiration or bone marrow biopsy do not lead to a diagnosis in a case of suspected lymphoma in a child, percutaneous biopsy should be considered a safe, effective alternative to surgical biopsy. Percutaneous biopsy is often successful in establishing a diagnosis of NHL, but may be less helpful in confirming a diagnosis of HD due to the relative paucity of diagnostic Reed-Sternberg cells and sampling bias with percutaneous methods. Aspiration of a fluid collection under local anesthesia or light sedation in children with a large mediastinal mass can reduce the risk of airway compromise incurred by heavy sedation or anesthesia with more invasive diagnostic procedures (GARRETT et al. 2002). This may be most applicable in children with lymphoblastic lymphoma, who have a relatively high incidence of a mediastinal mass with an associated pleural effusion (CHAIGNAUD et al. 1998)

When percutaneous biopsy is pursued, the interventional radiologist, oncologist, and pathologist need to communicate in advance regarding the type and amount of specimen to be obtained and the transport medium desired if special studies, such as cytogenetics, flow cytometry, or immunophenotyping, are planned. Cooperative group protocols often require a relatively large quantity of tissue for biology studies. Material obtained by fine needle aspiration may not be in sufficient quantity for complete diagnostic characterization, while core needle biopsy specimens allow for cytogenetic, immunophenotypic, and histopathologic analyses (WHITE 2001).

14.6.3
Staging, Risk Stratification, and Therapeutic Planning

Staging and risk stratification are processes designed to categorize patients into different prognostic categories for risk adapted therapy. Stratification of patients by risk group is a fundamental feature of modern therapeutic protocols for pediatric lymphoma. By adjusting the intensity of therapy to the patient's risk category, treatment can be modulated to minimize toxicity in a low risk patient and maximize the probability of durable remission or cure in a high risk patient (MAGRATH 1997). The major determinants of prognosis are tumor biology, tumor volume and extent, and the treatment administered. Imaging plays a central role in determining tumor volume and extent for staging and risk stratification at the time of presentation and for assessment of treatment response during and after therapy. Also, insights into tumor biology are being provided by the emerging techniques of functional and molecular imaging.

14.6.3.1
Hodgkin Disease

Until the 1980's, high dose large field radiation therapy was the primary treatment for pediatric HD and surgical staging was required to accurately define disease extent. Appreciation of the adverse late effects of radiation therapy in children, especially musculoskeletal growth impairment and second malignancies, led to the development of combined modality protocols using lower dose, smaller field radiation therapy and systemic chemotherapy (HUDSON and DONALDSON 2002). Surgical staging was largely abandoned by the 1990's and replaced by clinical staging due to recognition of the risks of infection (CHILCOTE et al. 1976) and acute non-lymphocytic leukemia after splenectomy (TURA et al. 1993). Advances in diagnostic imaging now provide a non-invasive means to accurately evaluate abdominal involvement, and successful incorporation of systemic chemotherapy into protocols precludes the need for confirmation of microscopic abdominal disease. In the 1990's, therapy took on a risk-adapted approach, with treatment intensity modulated according to the prognostic factors at presentation, in an effort to optimize the chance of cure with reduced risk of late effects.

The current standard of care for a large majority of children and adolescents with HD is risk-adapted combined-modality therapy using low-dose involved-field radiation therapy and multi-agent chemotherapy. Possible exceptions include older adolescents with well-staged, favorable, non-bulky, localized disease in whom high-dose, extended-field radiation therapy alone can be curative, and lymphocyte predominant HD thought to be restricted to a single lymph node group and fully resected, where the need for further treatment is questionable (HUDSON and DONALDSON 2002). Pediatric HD patients may be "understaged" by clinical staging, but with the exception of the rare setting of a child receiving radiotherapy as a single modality, this is typically not a significant detriment in the vast majority of patients who are treated with combined modality therapy including systemic chemotherapy. Selection of risk-adapted therapy for pediatric HD is influenced by clinical stage and other prognostic variables, such as the presence or absence of bulk disease or B symptoms (HUDSON and DONALDSON 2002).

The Ann Arbor staging system for HD adopted in 1971 is based on the observation that HD has a tendency for contiguous spread along lymph nodes until late in the disease course (CARBONE et al. 1971). This staging system is still used with some modification (Table 14.1).

Table 14.1. Ann Arbor staging system for Hodgkin disease.

Stage I	Involvement of a single lymph node region (I) or of a single extralymphatic organ or site (I_E)
Stage II	Involvement of two or more lymph node regions on the same side of the diaphragm (II) or localized involvement of an extralymphatic organ or site and one or more lymph node regions on the same side of the diaphragm (II_E)
Stage III	Involvement of lymph node regions on both sides of the diaphragm (III), which may be accompanied by involvement of the spleen (III_S) or by localized involvement of an extralymphatic organ or site (III_E) or both (III_{SE})
Stage IV	Diffuse or disseminated involvement of one or more extralymphatic organs or tissues with or without associated lymph node involvement

Anatomic lymph node regions for the purpose of staging include Waldeyer's ring, cervical/supraclavicular / occipital / pre-auricular, infraclavicular, axillary / pectoral, mediastinal, hilar, splenic / splenic hilar, paraaortic / celiac / periportal, mesenteric, iliac, inguinal/femoral, and popliteal (KAPLAN and ROSENBERG 1966). HD substage classifications include the designation A for "asymptomatic disease", and B for the presence of unexplained fever exceeding 38°C orally for 3 consecutive days, drenching night sweats, or unexplained loss of at least 10% body weight over 6 months. The designation E is for minimal extralymphatic disease, originally devised to indicate extralymphatic disease limited enough to be subjected to definitive treatment by radiation therapy (HUDSON and DONALDSON 2002).

The concept of "bulk disease" is a tradition that has endured since the era before CT, with bulk mediastinal disease defined as existing when the ratio of the maximum transverse diameter of the tumor mass to the internal thoracic diameter at the level of T5/6 on an inspiratory upright chest radiograph equals or exceeds one-third (Fig. 14.26). Patients with bulk disease have been found to have worse outcomes than those without bulk disease (WHITE 2001). An excellent correlation exists between CT and chest radiograph for measurement of bulk disease. The presence of a mediastinal mass with a longest diameter of > 10 cm on CT correlates with an increased risk of progressive disease, carrying the same implication as the chest radiograph definition of bulk disease (BRA-

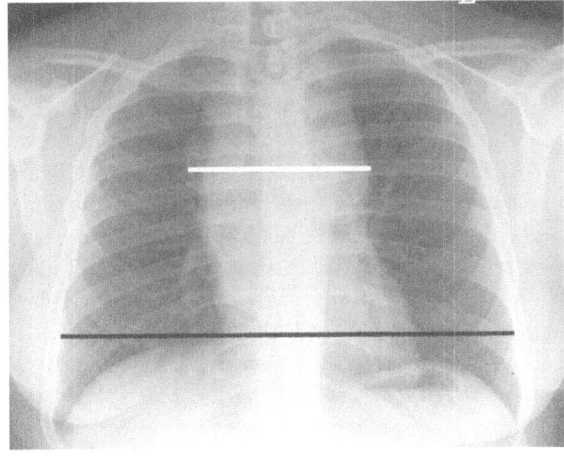

Fig. 14.26. "Bulk disease" in a 16-year-old boy with newly diagnosed mediastinal nodular sclerosis Hodgkin disease. Inspiratory anteroposterior upright chest radiograph shows the ratio of the maximum transverse width of the mediastinal tumor (*white line*) to the maximal transverse internal thoracic diameter at the level of T5/6 (*black line*) is approximately 0.38, slightly above the threshold of one-third required for the designation of mediastinal "bulk disease".

DLEY et al. 1999). The definition of bulk disease in the periphery has been less consistent in protocols, being variously defined as a mass > 6–10 cm diameter.

Imaging evaluation of pediatric HD for staging and risk stratification routinely includes chest radiograph, CT, and gallium scintigraphy. Bone scintigraphy and MR imaging are obtained in selected circumstances, while lymphography is very rarely performed. FDG-PET may become a frequent or even routine part of staging and risk stratification.

Supradiaphragmatic HD is typically evaluated by chest radiograph and CT. While cervical node involvement can be screened by physical exam, a neck CT is often obtained as a baseline to facilitate comparison of size and extent of cervical node involvement at follow-up. If enlarged high cervical nodes are detected at physical exam, attention should be paid on the neck CT exam to possible Waldeyer's ring involvement (HUDSON and DONALDSON 2002).

Chest radiography depicts a mediastinal mass in two-thirds of patients (PARKER 1997), and is primarily obtained to evaluate for bulk mediastinal disease. Chest CT is the best modality for assessing the most common sites of extranodal HD in the thorax, including the pulmonary parenchyma, chest wall, pleura, and pericardium (HUDSON and DONALDSON 2002). Approximately half of HD patients have disease depicted on chest CT that is occult on chest radiograph (ROSTOCK et al. 1983).

The impact of chest CT on therapy depends on disease distribution and the planned treatment protocol, with the impact greatest on the strategy for radiation therapy. The standard involved field is the minimum radiation field size used in combined modality protocols and includes both the lymph nodes with overt involvement and the nearby lymph nodes in the same nodal region. The mantle field is the most important treatment field and may include the submandibular, submental, cervical, supraclavicular, infraclavicular, axillary, mediastinal, and hilar nodes, with modifications to exclude uninvolved areas, particularly in females to reduce irradiation of the breasts (HUDSON and DONALDSON 2002). Demonstration of involvement of the chest wall, pericardium, or nodes in the subcarinal, cardiophrenic, or paravertebral regions not evident on chest radiograph has the greatest impact on planning of radiation therapy portals (CASTELLINO et al. 1986). Since the bronchopulmonary and subcarinal nodes directly drain the lungs, involvement of these nodes implies possible microscopic pulmonary involvement, and radiation therapy portals may need to be modified accordingly (PARKER 1997). In patients with renal insufficiency, iodinated contrast allergy, or other contraindications to contrast-enhanced CT, supradiaphragmatic disease can best be evaluated with unenhanced chest CT to assess the lungs and MR imaging to assess the neck, mediastinum, and chest wall structures.

Subdiaphragmatic HD is typically evaluated by abdominal and pelvic CT. Splenic involvement occurs in 30–40% and liver involvement in a smaller percentage, but the size of the spleen and liver as defined by CT does not correlate with the degree of involvement (HUDSON and DONALDSON 2002). Using staging laparotomy as a gold standard, the sensitivity of CT for splenic involvement and retroperitoneal lymph node involvement has been reported to be as low as 19% and 40%, respectively, in pediatric HD (BAKER et al. 1990). This limitation of CT is mitigated by the rarity of splenic involvement in children with the most common clinical presentation of cervical or supraclavicular lymphadenopathy, and by the standard use of systemic chemotherapy in pediatric treatment regimens (HUDSON and DONALDSON 2002)

MR imaging with use of a STIR sequence has been reported as more sensitive than CT for abnormal subdiaphragmatic nodes in pediatric HD, and more sensitive than lymphography for abnormal upper paraaortic nodes (HANNA et al. 1993). However, MR imaging is limited for evaluating mesenteric nodes due to lack of a consistently satisfactory oral contrast agent. The greater expense, lesser availability, and more frequent need for sedation relegate MR imaging to second line status behind CT for staging of infradiaphragmatic HD in children.

Conventional lymphography has a greater sensitivity for involved retroperitoneal nodes than CT in pediatric HD (BAKER et al. 1990). However, lymphography cannot evaluate nodal groups outside the line of drainage or extranodal disease, and is very operator dependent, with a limited number of institutions having the necessary expertise and resources to perform the procedure. In the institutions where lymphography is still available, lymphography can be useful for planning of subdiaphragmatic radiation therapy ports, and for monitoring response to therapy with abdominal radiographs.

Due to the infrequency of bone involvement, bone scintigraphy is not routinely indicated in pediatric HD patients. Bone scintigraphy and correlative radiographs should be reserved for children with bone pain, elevated alkaline phosphatase, or extranodal disease by other imaging studies (PARKER 1997; HUDSON and DONALDSON 2002). Bone marrow involvement at the time of presentation is uncommon and rarely occurs as an isolated site of extranodal disease. A bone marrow biopsy is not recommended with newly diagnosed clinical stage I to IIA disease, but is advocated with clinical stage III or IV disease, B symptoms, or disease recurrence (HUDSON and DONALDSON 2002). Although MR imaging is not part of routine evaluation of the bone marrow in pediatric HD patients, MR imaging has been advocated as a complementary test to bone marrow biopsy. In patients with negative bone marrow biopsies, MR imaging can detect bone marrow involvement distant from the iliac crest biopsy site, but cannot replace bone marrow biopsy since biopsy is needed to detect microscopic involvement (HOANE et al. 1991).

Gallium scintigraphy is frequently performed at the time of staging to serve as a baseline for later treatment response and residual disease assessment. Gallium scintigraphy has been reported to have 94% accuracy in evaluating mediastinal involvement and 86% accuracy in evaluating extramediastinal supradiaphragmatic involvement in newly diagnosed children and adolescents with HD (FLETCHER et al. 1995). However, gallium scintigraphy has limited efficacy for evaluation of subdiaphragmatic disease compared to CT.

Preliminary studies show FDG-PET to be more sensitive overall than CT or gallium for detection of lymphomatous involvement. FDG-PET is complementary to CT in staging lymphoma, with each modality capable of distinguishing involved and uninvolved sites not clarified by the other modality. In studies consisting of primarily adult subjects with HD and NHL, results of FDG-PET led to a change in staging in 17–44% of patients (TALBOT et al. 2001; SCHODER et al. 2001). In a small series of pediatric HD cases, FDG-PET resulted in upstaging of a majority of the cases (MONTRAVERS et al. 2002).

The cancer cooperative groups are actively engaged in refining treatment protocols for pediatric HD to better match risk-adapted therapy with precise risk groups. Definitions of favorable or low risk disease and unfavorable or high risk disease have varied according to the significance given to the various prognostic indicators in each protocol. Favorable or low risk disease has generally been applied to presentations with stage I–II disease involving less than 3 nodal groups, and no B symptoms or bulk disease, while unfavorable or high risk disease has generally been applied to presentations with stage III–IV disease and B symptoms, elevated erythrocyte sedimentation rate, extranodal disease or bulk disease. An intermediate risk category has also evolved, encompassing stage I–IIA/B bulky or extranodal disease and stage IIIA disease (HUDSON and DONALDSON 2002). Imaging plays an important role in defining risk groups by clarifying tumor burden and extent.

14.6.3.2
Non-Hodgkin Lymphoma

The principal treatment modality for NHL of childhood is chemotherapy, regardless of stage or disease site, based on the principle that NHL is a disseminated disease. Chemotherapy is adapted to the different subtypes of NHL, especially Burkitt lymphoma and lymphoblastic lymphoma. Therapy for Burkitt lymphoma is intensive, risk-adapted, short in duration, and includes CNS-directed therapy. Therapy for lymphoblastic lymphoma is derived from protocols designed for high risk acute lymphoblastic lymphoma (PATTE 1998). There is no routine role for radiation therapy in the primary treatment of childhood NHL, and the use of radiation therapy in any situation must be clearly justified (MAGRATH 2002). Apart from diagnosis and treatment of complications, surgery has a very limited role in the management of childhood NHL. Surgery may be beneficial in limited abdominal disease for complete resection of small tumors presenting acutely with intussusception or for isolated ovarian tumors (MAGRATH 2002).

Pediatric NHL is most commonly staged by the modified Murphy or St. Jude Children's Research Hospital system. The St. Jude staging system correlates disease stage with site(s) of disease and tumor burden, and separates patients with limited disease from those with extensive disease. Unlike the Ann Arbor staging system for HD, intrathoracic tumor upstages the disease to stage III in the St. Jude staging system for NHL (Table 14.2).

Table 14.2. St. Jude staging system for childhood non-Hodgkin lymphoma.

Stage I	A single tumor (extranodal) or single anatomic site (nodal), excluding mediastinum or abdomen
Stage II	A single tumor (extranodal) with regional node involvement
	Two or more nodal sites on the same side of the diaphragm
	Two single (extranodal) tumors with or without regional node involvement on the same side of the diaphragm
	A primary gastrointestinal tract tumor, usually ileocecal, with or without associated mesenteric nodes, grossly completely resected
Stage III	Two single tumors (extranodal) on opposite sides of the diaphragm
	Two or more nodal areas above and below the diaphragm
	All primary intrathoracic tumors (mediastinal, pleural, thymic)
	All extensive primary intra-abdominal disease, unresectable
	All paraspinal or epidural tumors regardless of other sites
Stage IV	Any of the above with initial central nervous system or bone marrow involvement (< 25%)

Staging laparotomy is not advocated for NHL patients, although some patients may have undergone a diagnostic laparotomy. Imaging has a major role in the staging of NHL, defining disease extent and bulk for prognostic information, and providing a baseline for response assessment. A chest radiograph, CT of the neck/chest/abdomen/pelvis, and often a gallium scan are performed as part of the staging work-up (WHITE 2001).

CT defines tumor size and anatomic extent of tumor for staging and provides a baseline for response assessment. CT of the neck/chest/abdomen/pelvis is typically performed at staging since disease spread in NHL can be unpredictable. Chest CT has greater sensitivity than chest radiograph for the detection of intrathoracic disease (COHEN et al. 1986), but has less impact on initial therapeutic planning for NHL than for HD since NHL tends to be more disseminated at the time of staging (CASTELLINO 1991b). Although

CT is insensitive for lymphomatous involvement of normal-sized nodes, nodal involvement in NHL usually presents as bulky masses (CASTELLINO 1991a).

Although gallium scintigraphy has not been considered as a compulsory imaging test in pediatric NHL by the cancer cooperative groups due to inconsistent uptake in adult NHL, gallium scintigraphy has greater value in pediatric NHL than in adult NHL because of the higher frequency of high grade NHL in children and the greater sensitivity of gallium scintigraphy in high grade NHL (SCOTT and LARSON 1993; WHITE 2001). The overall sensitivity of gallium scintigraphy for NHL may be less than CT, but gallium scintigraphy is complementary to CT, with gallium scintigraphy capable of identifying up to 10% of additional sites not detected with CT, such as involved normal-sized nodes (DELCAMBRE et al. 2000). Gallium scintigraphy is particularly valuable in Burkitt lymphoma, where the site sensitivity is 89% and the specificity is 91% (SANDROCK et al. 1993). Gallium scintigraphy obtained at the time of staging of NHL can serve as a baseline for response assessment and residual mass evaluation.

MR imaging is the preferred modality when CNS disease is suspected. Although MR imaging is a good modality for assessing the bone marrow, the presence of limited bone marrow disease may have no significant impact on outcome with current treatment protocols in patients who would otherwise be stage III (MAGRATH 2002). Ultrasound is not routinely indicated, but can be useful for evaluation of suspected gonadal masses. Bone scintigraphy is obtained in only in certain circumstances, as the yield is low, and it may be replaced by gallium scintigraphy (WHITE 2001).

Stage alone is an insufficient method of risk stratification of pediatric NHL patients for selection of therapy. Total tumor burden, which can by estimated with imaging studies and laboratory assays such as LDH levels, has been recognized for many years as the most important determinant of prognosis for Burkitt lymphoma (MAGRATH 1980). Although uncommon, patients with stage I disease occasionally have very large tumor burdens. Stage III disease encompasses a broad range of tumor burden, and the results of treatment of stage III and IV disease often do not differ significantly.

In recognition of the limitations of assigning risk on the basis of stage alone, pediatric NHL risk stratification schemes have been developed by the Children's Oncology Group (formerly Children's Cancer Group and Pediatric Oncology Group), FAB (French-American-British), and BFM (Berlin-Frank-furt-Munster) cooperative cancer groups, with two or three risk strata based on factors such as stage, LDH level, completeness of surgical resection of an abdominal mass, and presence or absence of involvement of the CNS. The status of certain other anatomic sites may also be relevant for risk stratification of anaplastic large cell lymphoma, where involvement of the skin, mediastinum, or lung is an indicator of poor prognosis (PATTE 1998). A means of identifying patients with limited disease who are likely to do poorly is very desirable, since treatment could then be intensified to improve the cure rate (MAGRATH 1997). Imaging assessment of the tumor volume at presentation or the rate of response to therapy may provide such a means.

14.6.4
Response Assessment

With any treatment regimen, there is an obvious desire to learn whether the treatment is effective. This process of tumor response assessment can have different endpoints, depending on the clinical setting, and it should be noted that objective tumor response and clinical improvement are distinct entities. In phase II clinical trials, tumor response assessment acts as a prospective end point to determine whether the treatment exhibits encouraging enough results to warrant further testing. In phase III clinical trials designed to estimate benefit, tumor response assessment may function as a surrogate end point of outcome. Outside the clinical trial setting, response assessment serves as a guide for the clinician to make decisions about continuation of current therapy (THERASSE 2002).

14.6.4.1
Response Criteria

To allow valid comparison of treatment efficacy in clinical trials, tumor response criteria must be uniform and reproducible. The revised WHO criteria held sway for many years as the basis for response assessment of solid tumors (MILLER et al. 1981). These criteria standardized tumor measurement techniques, with lesions measured bidimensionally and reported as the product of the longest diameter and greatest perpendicular diameter. These criteria also standardized treatment response into the categories of complete response (CR), partial response (PR), stable disease (SD), and progressive disease (PD), with CR requiring disappearance of all known disease, PR at least 50% decrease from baseline, and PD at least 25% increase in one or more lesions, or appearance of new lesions. Since the introduction of the revised WHO criteria there has been a proliferation of alternative response criteria for solid tumors adopted by the various cancer cooperative groups and other organizations conducting clinical trials.

The Cotswolds criteria (LISTER et al. 1989) were established in an attempt to standardize HD response criteria in recognition of advances in diagnostic imaging and treatment approach. By these criteria, CR is defined as no clinical, imaging, or other evidence of disease. Changes consistent with the effects of previous therapy (e.g. radiation therapy fibrosis) may be present. CRu, or CR(unconfirmed/uncertain) is defined as no clinical evidence of disease but some imaging abnormality not consistent with effects of therapy persists at a site of previous disease, attempts to resolve the dilemma should be made with other imaging studies, such as gallium scintigraphy, or pathologic exam. Partial remission is defined as a decrease by at least 50% in the sum of the products of the largest perpendicular diameters of all measurable lesions. Progressive disease is defined as 25% or more increase in the bi-dimensional size of at least one measurable lesion or the appearance of a new lesion. This system was not widely adopted, and HD protocols continued to vary with respect to response criteria.

Standardized response criteria for NHL were introduced in 1999 by a National Cancer Institute-sponsored international working group (CHESON et al. 1999). Response is based on radiological, clinical, and pathological (bone marrow) criteria. A lymph node size of > 1 cm in longest transverse diameter is proposed as compatible with involvement, with CT considered the standard for nodal size evaluation. CR is defined as complete disappearance of all detectable clinical and radiographic evidence of disease and disappearance of all disease-related symptoms, if present before therapy, and normalization of laboratory abnormalities definitely assignable to NHL. CRu (unconfirmed) is defined as a residual lymph node mass > 1.5 cm in maximal transverse diameter that has regressed more than 75% in the sum of the product of the perpendicular diameters (SPD). PR is defined as at least 50% decrease in SPD of the 6 largest nodal masses, no increase in size of other nodes or organs, regression of splenic and hepatic nodules by at least 50% in the SPD, and no new sites of disease. SD is defined as not PR or PD. PD (for PR and nonresponders) is defined as at least 50% increase from nadir in the SPD of any previously

identified node, or new lesions. Relapsed disease (for CR and CRu) is defined as new lesions or increase of at least 50% in size of previously identified sites, or at least 50% increase in maximal diameter of any node previously identified greater than 1 cm short axis diameter or in the SPD of more than one node. The cancer cooperative group CALGB (Cancer and Leukemia Group B) has adopted these criteria for NHL.

In an effort to more widely standardize tumor response criteria, the Response Evaluation Criteria in Solid Tumors (RECIST) Guidelines were developed by a joint effort of the European Organization for Research and Treatment of Cancer (EORTC), National Cancer Institute (NCI), and National Cancer Institute of Canada Clinical Trials Group (THERASSE et al. 2000). These guidelines are notable for stipulating that only a single dimension is to be used to express lesion size, with measurable disease defined as the presence of at least one measurable lesion, and measurable lesions defined as lesions that can be accurately measured in at least one dimension (greater than or equal to 1 cm with spiral CT). Nonmeasurable lesions include bone lesions, leptomeningeal spread, ascites, effusions, lymphangitic spread, cystic lesions, and lesions too small to measure accurately (< 1 cm). Target lesions are defined as all measurable lesions up to 5 per organ and 10 in total selected on the basis of size (longest diameters) and suitability for accurate repeated measurements. CR is defined as disappearance of all target lesions, PR as at least 30% decrease in sum of longest diameter of target lesions using the baseline sum as reference, PD as at least 20% increase in sum of longest diameters, with the smallest sum observed since treatment began as reference, or the appearance of new lesions, and stable disease as not CR, PR, or PD. For nontarget lesions, CR is disappearance of all nontarget lesions and normalization of tumor marker levels, incomplete response/SD is persistence of nontarget lesion(s) and/or the maintenance of tumor marker levels above normal, and PD is appearance of new lesions and/or progression of nontarget lesions. SD in nontarget lesions will reduce a CR in target lesions to an overall PR, while SD in nontarget lesions will not reduce a PR in target lesions. RECIST also provides specifications for imaging. For cross-sectional imaging, the minimum lesion size should be no less than double the slice thickness, the longest diameter of target lesions should be selected in the axial plane only for CT, and lesions should be measured at the same window setting. The cancer cooperative groups have been reluctant to adopt RECIST for lymphoma due to lack of consideration in RECIST for a complete response with a residual mass, and possible increase in response miscategorization from the method of measuring tumors in only one dimension. For tumors with a length:width ratio > 1.5, bi-dimensional measurements provide a significantly more accurate estimation of volume than uni-dimensional measurements (SAINI 2001; SPEARS 1984)

Existing response criteria have either neglected to address or varied in the threshold used for normal lymph node size, reflecting the arbitrary nature of such a threshold. The upper limit of normal for uninvolved nodal size may increase after treatment due to nodal fibrosis, but the trade-off of sensitivity and specificity will remain. The relatively high frequency of benign lymphoid hyperplasia further confounds response assessment in children. Decreasing the nodal size threshold will not decrease the overall response rate, but will decrease the complete response rate (GRILLO-LOPEZ et al. 2000).

The distinction of complete from partial response is important, since a true partial response indicates that the tumor is resistant to the therapy being used and continuation with the same therapy is unlikely to be successful. This is pertinent in B-cell NHL, for example, where partial response is a more frequent cause of treatment failure than recurrent disease after a period of complete remission (MAGRATH 2002).

It should be noted that both the WHO bi-dimensional and RECIST uni-dimensional methods of measuring tumor size are only crude surrogates for true tumor volume. The imprecision and inaccuracy of these methods is accentuated with tumors with irregular borders or ill-defined margins with adjacent structures, as is common with lobular or infiltrative lymphoma masses. Incorrect response category assignment can occur in up to 23% of cases as a result of using bi-dimensional rather than true volume measurements (HOPPER et al. 1996a; EGGLI et al. 1995). Inter-observer measurement variability with CT is approximately 15%, which compares with an intra-observer variability of 6%, suggesting that the same radiologist should perform the measurements on the baseline and follow-up exams, or that the radiologist should redo the measurements on the preceding exams if they were interpreted by a different radiologist (HOPPER et al. 1996b). Regardless of the measurement method utilized, it is difficult to quantitate response in a group of nodes that are conglomerate prior to therapy but break up into smaller discrete nodes after therapy (MAVROMATIS and CHESON 2002). Calculation of true volumes would seem to be the optimal method of size measurement,

but time constraints and lack of widespread access to image segmentation software have limited implementation of such calculation into routine clinical practice. The implementation of new multidetector CT scanners coupled with semi-automated volume calculation software promises to make obtaining true volume measurements more feasible.

Response criteria have traditionally focused on the degree of tumor size change occurring between the initiation and completion of therapy. Since a large proportion of treatment failures in pediatric lymphoma are caused by primary resistance to therapy or toxic death, it would be valuable to be able to identify early in the course of therapy patients destined to relapse or die from progressive disease when the current therapy is continued, so that treatment could be changed accordingly (MAGRATH 2002). As an example, the French Society of Pediatric Oncology has used poor response to pre-phase therapy (1st week of treatment) to identify high-risk NHL patients who are subsequently directed to intensification of therapy. Imaging may be able to serve in such a role, since the rapidity in reduction of tumor size or loss of avidity to gallium or FDG may be an independent predictor of ultimate response in pediatric lymphoma. In childhood T-cell lymphoblastic lymphoma, those with normalization of the chest radiograph within 60 days of starting treatment have a better 5-year event free survival those with prolongation of chest radiograph abnormality beyond 60 days (SHEPARD et al. 1995). A restaging gallium scan performed early during treatment is more accurate in predicting outcome than a gallium scan obtained at the end of treatment (Fig. 14.27) (SALLOUM et al. 1997). Normalization of the gallium scan early during therapy is a good predictor of outcome for NHL and HD (FRONT et al. 1999; JANICEK et al. 1997; ARMITAGE et al. 1986). By identifying rapid or slow early responders by imaging, those with a slow early response and presumed higher risk of relapse can have their treatment modified to improve the chance of a complete response. New Children's Oncology Group (COG) protocols for pediatric lymphoma are adopting this approach of stratifying treatment on the basis of early response, with imaging playing a central role in response assessment.

The limitations of size changes as a measure of tumor response must be recognized. Tumor volume provides only a rough estimate of the number of viable neoplastic cells, since tumor masses may be composed of variable proportions of viable neoplastic cells, infiltrating non-neoplastic cells, necrosis, fibrosis, and extracellular matrix. Also, the number

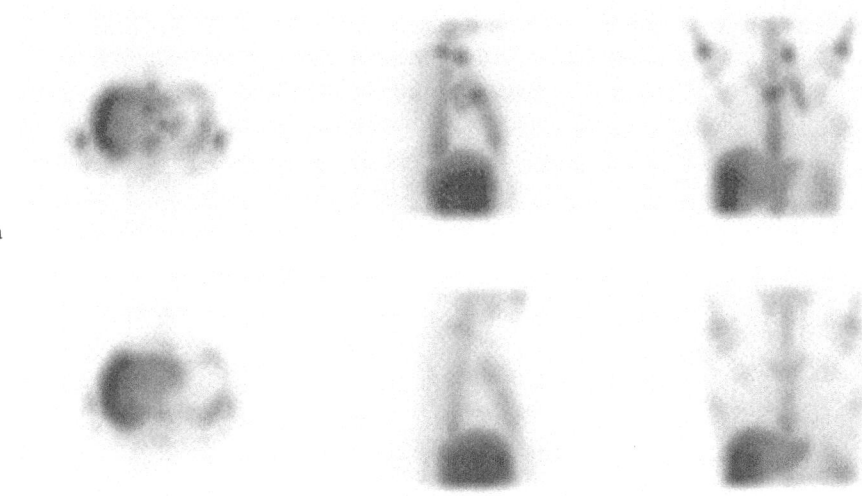

a

b

Fig. 14.27a,b. Early treatment response evaluation in a 16-year-old girl with Hodgkin disease. **a** Pre-treatment axial (*left*), sagittal (*middle*), and coronal (*right*) gallium SPECT images show several sites of abnormal gallium uptake with normalization (**b**) after one course of chemotherapy. A restaging gallium scan performed early during treatment of lymphoma may be more accurate in predicting outcome than a gallium scan obtained at the end of treatment. Those without early normalization and presumed higher risk of relapse can have their treatment modified to improve the chance of a complete response. *(Image courtesy of Dr. H. Nadel)*

of viable neoplastic cells may not be correlated with proclivity for malignant behavior such as invasion and metastasis. Some new therapeutic agents, such as those targeted against tumor angiogenesis, may be more cytostatic than cytotoxic, and better assessed by measures such as progression-free survival or time to progression than tumor size reduction. Response to therapy in terms of metabolic activity and expression of various molecular markers precedes changes in tumor size and is potentially assessable with functional and molecular imaging techniques. For these reasons, tumor response criteria must be adaptable to the specific biological mechanism and goal of therapy. While adoption of uniform response criteria facilitates comparison of trial results, a one method fits all approach is ultimately misguided.

14.6.4.2
Residual Mass

A common and vexing clinical dilemma is the detection of a residual mass by imaging after treatment for lymphoma, despite resolution of clinical symptoms and normalization of lab tests. This is particularly frequent in the mediastinum, where residual masses occur in 22–47% of children and adolescents treated for lymphoma (BRISSE et al. 1998; LUKER and SIEGEL 1993). The abdomen is also a frequent site,

with residual masses occurring in 21% of children with abdominal Burkitt lymphoma (KARMAZYN et al. 2001).

A residual mass after treatment may be composed of lymph node tissue, fibrosis, necrosis, and inflammation with or without residual neoplasm (LEWIS et al. 1982). Lymphomas that are associated with large amounts of fibrosis, such as nodular sclerosis HD, are more frequently associated with residual masses than more cellular lymphomas (Fig. 14.28). Residual masses on CT commonly appear as a soft tissue mass, occasionally with calcifications, with a slight increase in density of the adjacent fat. Even when benign, the mass may persist for years, eventually stabilizing in size or involuting (WHITE 2001).

In children treated for NHL in clinical remission, only 20% of residual abdominal masses contain viable neoplasm as determined by laparotomy (FUKS et al. 1982). Also, the majority of residual masses in HD are benign (WEIHRAUCH et al. 2001). The size of the tumor mass at diagnosis correlates with the size of the residual mass, with larger tumors involuting less than small tumors. Although the degree of tumor size reduction correlates with the risk of relapse, the size of the residual mass does not correlate with the risk of relapse. Also, relapse occurs as frequently outside the mass as within the mass (RODRIGUEZ 1998; RODRIGUEZ-CATARINO et al. 2000).

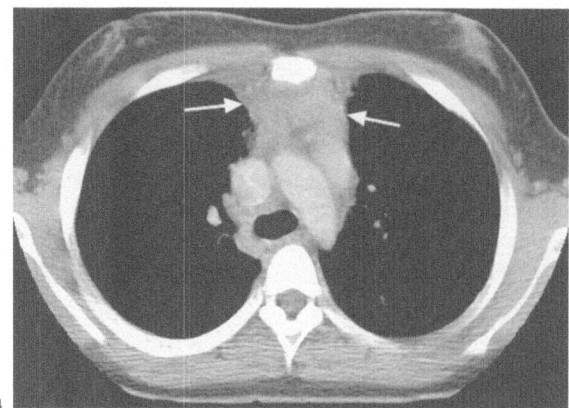

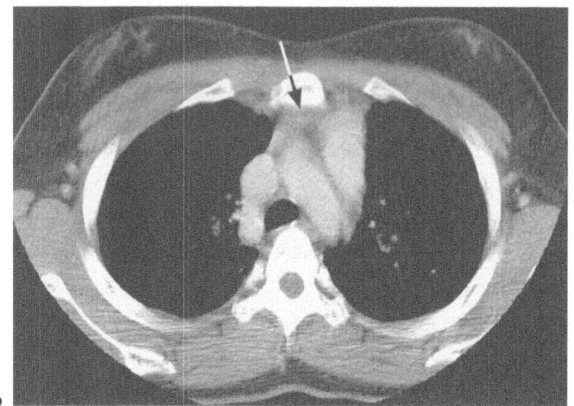

Fig. 14.28a,b. Residual mediastinal mass in a 13-year-old boy with treated nodular sclerosis Hodgkin disease. **a** Axial contrast-enhanced CT scan of the thorax following therapy shows a large residual anterior mediastinal mass (*arrows*). The residual mass demonstrated a loss of avidity for gallium and progressively involuted in size on (**b**) follow-up axial contrast-enhanced CT scan (*arrow*), implying a probable benign nature of the mass.

The criterion for assigning patients with residual masses into complete or partial response categories has varied widely in studies (MAVROMATIS and CHESON 2002). Characterizing a residual mass is important, as active residual neoplasm portends a poor prognosis with the therapy being used and alternative therapy needs to be pursued, while a benign residual mass confers a good prognosis without further treatment. If the residual mass is in the periphery, biopsy can readily be performed, but residual masses are typically in the mediastinum and abdomen where a noninvasive method of diagnosis is desirable. CT, MR imaging, gallium, and FDG-PET have been evaluated as noninvasive methods of determining whether residual masses contain active residual neoplasm.

On CT, the attenuation values of neoplastic and non-neoplastic elements such as fibrosis overlap.

This prevents reliable discrimination of benign and malignant residual masses by CT. The sensitivity of CT in detecting recurrence in a residual mass is also limited, since the neoplastic component must grow enough to visibly increase the volume of the mass. It is unknown at present whether dynamic contrast-enhanced CT techniques will be of value in evaluating residual masses.

On MR imaging, fibrosis shows hypointensity on both T1-weighted images and T2-weighted images, while residual neoplasm displays intermediate or high signal intensity on T2-weighted images and enhancement on contrast-enhanced T1-weighted images. However, these features are not specific. Intermediate or high signal intensity on T2-weighted images and enhancement on contrast-enhanced T1-weighted images can also be seen with infection, radiation mediastinitis, and fibrotic tissue in the first several months post-treatment (Fig. 14.29). Also, residual neoplasm can be present in hypointense areas on T1-weighted images (ELKOWITZ et al. 1993).

Gallium scintigraphy can help discriminate post-treatment fibrosis and residual neoplasm. Increased avidity for gallium is present in 60–80% of patients with previously untreated mediastinal HD, and

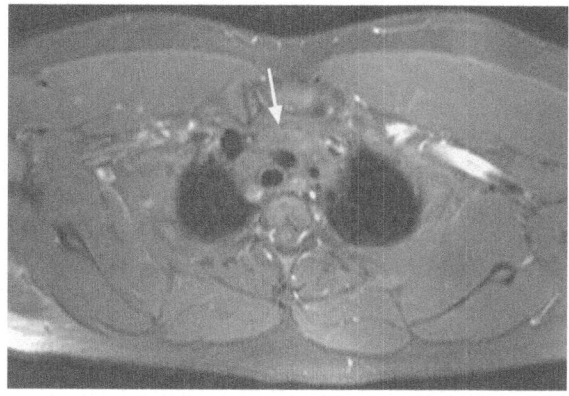

Fig. 14.29. Residual mediastinal mass in a 16-year-old boy with treated nodular sclerosis Hodgkin disease. MR imaging was obtained rather than CT due to a history of iodinated contrast allergy. Anterior bulk mediastinal disease was present prior to treatment. Axial fat-suppressed contrast-enhanced T1-weighted MR image of the thorax shows a slightly enhancing residual soft tissue (*arrow*) remains present in the anterior superior mediastinum following treatment. As with CT, MR imaging cannot consistently distinguish residual neoplasm from fibrosis or radiation mediastinitis in residual masses, and correlation with the patient's clinical status supplemented with gallium scintigraphy, FDG-PET, or follow-up imaging, and occasionally biopsy, is required to direct subsequent management.

persistent avidity in a residual mass after therapy suggests residual disease, while loss of gallium avidity suggests the absence of residual neoplasm (Fig. 14.30) (WEINER et al. 1991). Gallium scintigraphy has been reported to have a sensitivity of up to 92% and a specificity of up to 99% for the evaluation of active neoplasm in residual masses (FRONT et al. 1992; FRONT et al. 1990). A positive gallium scan after therapy has a high positive predictive value for

residual active neoplasm, and additional therapy can often be pursued without the need for further confirmation. A negative gallium scan after therapy has a lower negative predictive value in HD patients with stage III and IV disease than stage I or II disease. In one study, the negative predictive value of gallium was found to be only 64.5% for children and adults with stage III or IV disease (SALLOUM et al. 1997), indicating that the absence of residual active

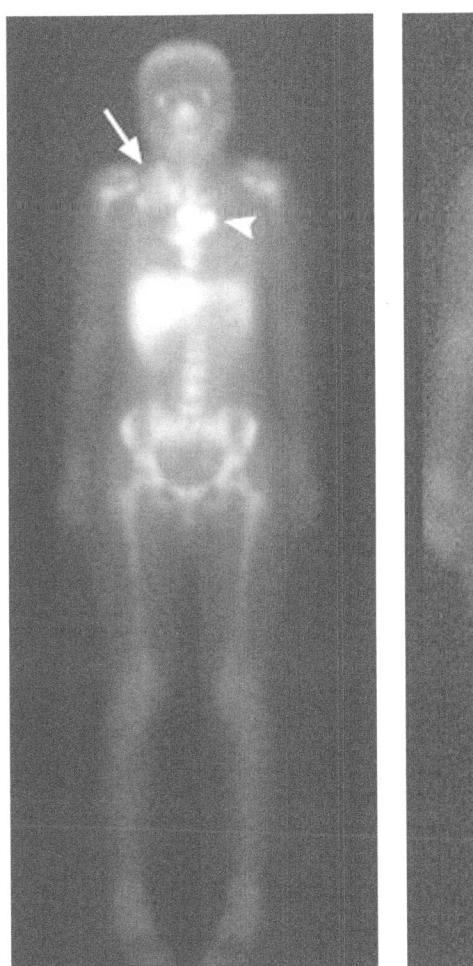
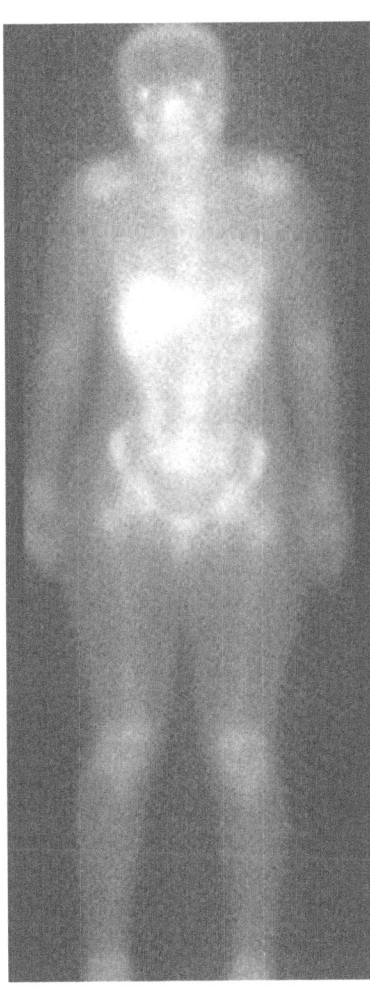

a

c

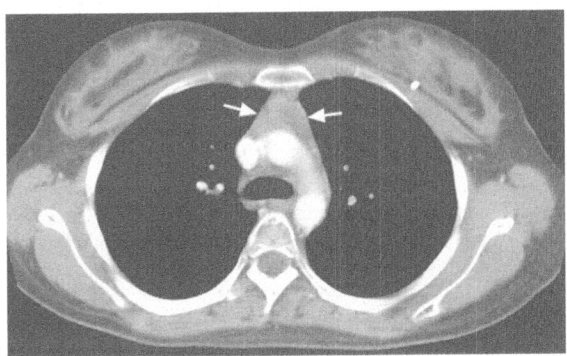

b

Fig. 14.30a-c. Treatment response evaluation in a 17-year-old girl with nodular sclerosis Hodgkin disease. **a** Whole-body planar gallium scintigraphy image prior to treatment demonstrates avid gallium uptake consistent with lymphoma in the mediastinum (*arrowhead*), right infraclavicular, right supraclavicular, and lower right cervical regions (*arrow*). **b** Axial contrast-enhanced CT scan of the thorax after treatment shows a small residual anterior mediastinal mass (*arrows*). **c** Whole-body planar gallium scintigraphy after treatment is normal, suggesting but not confirming the absence of viable residual neoplasm. Gallium scintigraphy after treatment of lymphoma has a higher positive predictive value than negative predictive value regarding the presence or absence of viable residual neoplasm.

neoplasm cannot be assumed with a negative gallium scan in this setting.

FDG-PET is under investigation as a promising method to evaluate residual masses. While most studies on FDG-PET to date have focused on predominantly adult populations, FDG-PET was found to have a 93% negative predictive value in a pediatric series evaluating the assessment of response to therapy and characterization of residual masses (MONTRAVERS et al. 2002). In a review of recently published studies, FDG-PET was touted as the most accurate noninvasive method for differentiating scar tissue from viable neoplasm in residual masses (RESKE 2003). FDG-PET at the completion of therapy may be able to separate patients into good and poor prognostic groups based on the presence or absence of uptake in residual masses.

No imaging test can predict with certainty which patients with residual masses will relapse. However, with the high frequency of residual masses without viable neoplasm, negative imaging of a residual mass with gallium scintigraphy or FDG-PET in a patient in clinical remission may allow for observation and imaging follow-up rather than biopsy (BRISSE et al. 1998; KARMAZYN et al. 2001). In some cases, such as clinical trial protocol requirements, biopsy may be required for verification of disease status. In this setting, a thoracoscopic approach is more sensitive than image-guided percutaneous biopsy for residual mediastinal neoplasm (GOSSOT et al. 2001).

14.6.4.3
Pitfalls in Response Assessment

In addition to the quandary posed by residual masses, there are multiple potential pitfalls in response assessment of pediatric lymphoma. These include rebound thymic hyperplasia, physiologic thymic gallium and FDG uptake, benign hilar gallium uptake, and physiologic muscle or brown fat FDG uptake. The practitioner should become familiar with these to avoid false positive readings and resultant unnecessary additional diagnostic and therapeutic measures.

Special attention must be paid to the anterior mediastinum in children with lymphoma since the thymus and anterior mediastinal lymph nodes are frequent sites of lymphoma involvement, and imaging features of the thymus, particularly with rebound thymic hyperplasia, can simulate residual or recurrent neoplasm on CT, gallium, and FDG-PET scans (DROSSMAN et al. 1990). Rebound thymic hyperplasia most characteristically presents in children

as an enlarging thymic mass within 6–8 months of completion of therapy with no other evidence of relapse (Fig. 14.31) (PARKER 1997). Rebound thymic hyperplasia can demonstrate avidity for gallium, with a frequency as high as 43% in high-grade pediatric NHL (Fig. 14.32) (PEYLAN-RAMU et al. 1989). The finding is usually transient, although in rare cases it may persist for several years (EVEN-SAPIR and ISRAEL 2003). The thymus may demonstrate uptake on FDG-PET physiologically or as a result of rebound thymic hyperplasia after treatment for lymphoma (Fig. 14.33) (WEINBLATT et al. 1997; BRINK et al. 2001; YOON et al. 2001). The pattern of physiologic thymic FDG uptake consists of weak diffuse uptake in an inverse V shape, whereas lymphomatous involvement of the thymus appears as intense discrete foci of uptake (PATEL et al. 1996; MONTRAVERS et al. 2002). If a child or adolescent treated for

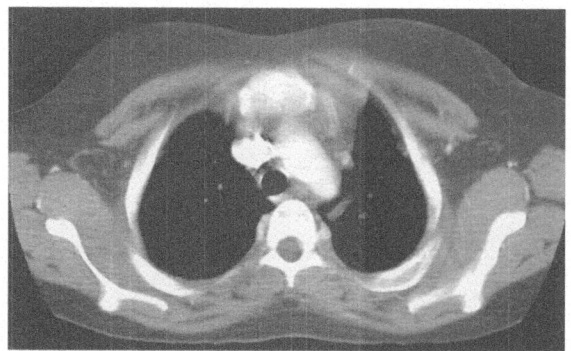

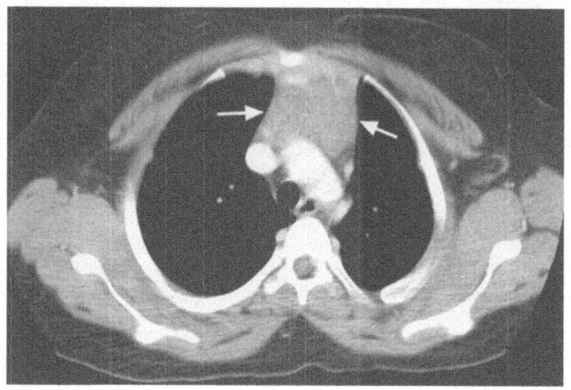

Fig. 14.31a,b. Rebound thymic hyperplasia in a 15-year-old boy with a history of large B-cell lymphoma. **a** Axial contrast-enhanced CT scan of the thorax after completion of therapy shows no residual mediastinal mass. **b** Axial contrast-enhanced CT scan of the thorax obtained 4 months after completion of therapy demonstrates development of a homogeneous soft tissue mass with smooth contours in the anterior mediastinum (*arrows*). In the clinical context of a normal clinical evaluation and absence of other soft tissue masses, this is most consistent with rebound thymic hyperplasia.

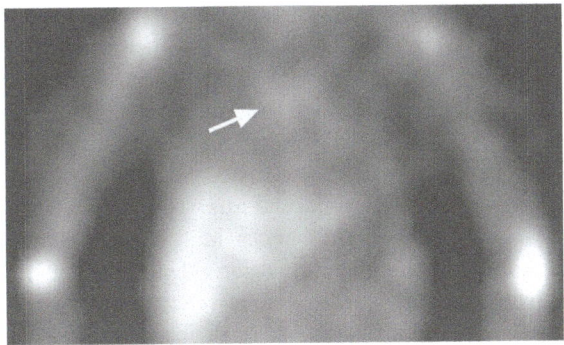

Fig. 14.32. Rebound thymic hyperplasia in an 11-year-old boy with a history of Hodgkin disease. Coronal Gallium SPECT image obtained several months after completion of treatment shows a "V" shaped pattern of increased mediastinal uptake (*arrow*), consistent with uptake related to rebound thymic hyperplasia in the appropriate clinical context.

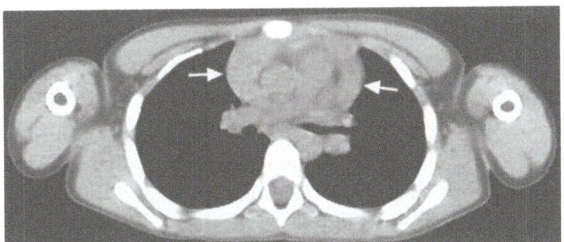

a

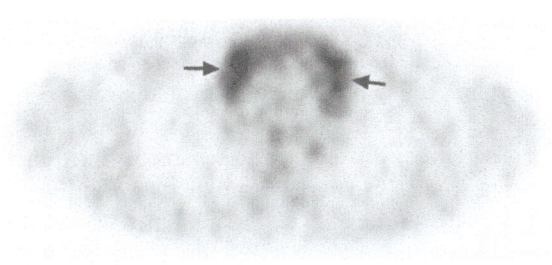

b

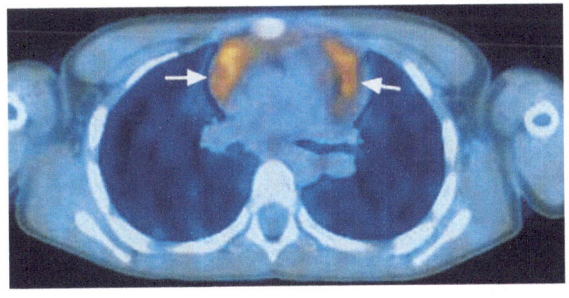

c

Fig. 14.33a–c. Rebound thymic hyperplasia in an 11-year-old boy in complete remission after treatment for non-Hodgkin lymphoma. **a** Axial unenhanced CT scan of the thorax shows a smooth-bordered anterior mediastinal soft tissue structure with homogeneous density (*arrows*). The mass demonstrates diffuse FDG uptake (*arrows*) on axial (**b**) FDG-PET and (**c**) PET-CT fusion images. These findings are consistent with rebound thymic hyperplasia in the appropriate clinical context. (*Image courtesy of Dr. O. Israel*)

lymphoma has imaging findings compatible with rebound thymic hyperplasia or physiologic thymic radiopharmaceutical uptake, especially if there is no other evidence of lymphoma recurrence or prior involvement of the region of the thymus, observation and imaging follow-up are advised rather than biopsy (PARKER 1997).

Hilar uptake is often seen at gallium scintigraphy in lymphoma patients. Symmetric hilar uptake with less intense uptake than the original lymphoma mass is most consistent with benign hilar uptake. Asymmetric uptake of similar intensity to the original lymphoma mass is suggestive of lymphoma involving the hilum (FROHLICH et al. 2000).

Increased FDG uptake in the neck and thoracic paraspinous region can be seen in the absence of neoplasm, particularly in low body mass patients, perhaps related to muscle tension or brown fat metabolism in response to cold. This can be intense and asymmetric, potentially causing false positive or false negative readings, by mimicking or masking involvement of cervical, mediastinal, and paravertebral lymph nodes (Fig. 14.21) (BARRINGTON and O'DOHERTY 2003).

14.7
Surveillance

14.7.1
Relapse

The primary objective of tumor surveillance is early detection of relapse, based on the assumption that salvage therapy is more effective if initiated early. Imaging surveillance after treatment has been largely based on ad hoc assumptions, with the frequency of recommended evaluations tapering as the perceived risk of relapse wanes. For HD, follow-up every 3 months for 2 years, every 4 months for the third year, every 6 months for the following 2 years, then annually has been proposed (LISTER et al. 1989). For NHL, reassessment after treatment completion every 3 months for 2 years, then every 6 months for 3 years, and then annually for at least 5 years has been suggested (CHESON et al. 1999). Such protocols can result in a high cumulative number of imaging exams over the course of surveillance, and the efficacy of these protocols in pediatric lymphoma has not been established by outcomes research or cost-effectiveness studies.

The efficacy of routinely scheduled imaging tests for surveillance in asymptomatic lymphoma patients after treatment has been questioned. In a study of adult large cell NHL, virtually all relapses were detected at unscheduled evaluations prompted by symptoms, despite routine post-treatment follow-up at 6 months intervals, with only 6% of relapses detected before the advent of symptoms. The median time interval since the previous CT scan for patients with a clinical relapse was 5.6 months, suggesting the rate of detection would have been higher if the interval between studies had been shorter (WEEKS et al. 1991). In a study of adult follicular NHL, only 14% of relapses were detected solely by abdominal and pelvic CT performed at 3–6 months intervals for the first 5 years and annually thereafter (OH et al. 1999). In studies of adult patients with intermediate or high-grade NHL (ELIS et al. 2002) and patients with early stage HD treated primarily with radiation therapy (TORREY et al. 1997), follow-up strategies consisting mainly of history and physical exam were deemed most cost-effective. Similar analyses have not yet been performed for pediatric lymphoma populations, although there is the perception that too many imaging studies are obtained in the follow-up of pediatric lymphoma patients (COHEN et al. 1986).

A more evidence-based approach to imaging surveillance than the traditional ad hoc approach is warranted in the interests of reducing the costs, patient and parental anxiety, false positive exams, and potential radiation risks associated with numerous surveillance imaging tests, without adversely impacting outcomes. The efficacy of surveillance is dependent upon the testing strategy. A rational surveillance strategy should be based upon knowledge of the frequency and timing of relapse, sites of relapse, risk factors for relapse, efficacy of diagnostic testing, and efficacy of salvage therapy.

Diagnostic tests, including imaging exams, obtained during surveillance should be concentrated when the risk of relapse is highest and taper in frequency as the risk of relapse wanes. In pediatric HD, most relapses occur within the first 3 years, with the exception of lymphocyte predominant disease which has an indolent course and relatively high proportion of late relapse. The need for surveillance in pediatric HD is being reduced by the progressively diminishing relapse rate related to improvements in staging and therapy (HUDSON and DONALDSON 2002). Relapses of Burkitt lymphoma nearly always occur during the first year of treatment. Relapsed B-cell NHL is now rare and usually presents within 6 to 8 months after the cessation of therapy. In the rare case of B-cell NHL relapse presenting beyond 1 year after

therapy, the relapse may actually represent a clonally distinct new neoplasm rather than recurrence of the initial neoplasm (MAGRATH 2002). Relapse occurs in approximately a third of lymphoblastic lymphoma cases, with a higher frequency of late relapse than other pediatric NHL types (SMITH et al. 1990), but those who have not relapsed after 30 months from the start of treatment have a high probability of remaining in complete remission (MAGRATH 2002).

The anatomic pattern of recurrence can influence the sensitivity of imaging exams chosen for surveillance and restaging. In HD, the mediastinum is the most common site of relapse, and the retroperitoneal lymph nodes are the most common site of subdiaphragmatic relapse (TORREY et al. 1997), although relapse of pediatric HD is less common at the sites of initial involvement if radiation therapy is part of the treatment regimen than if chemotherapy alone is used (HUDSON and DONALDSON 2002). Relapsed pediatric B-cell NHL is usually disseminated. Relapse in lymphoblastic lymphoma is not uncommon in the CNS or gonads (HAMRICK-TURNER et al. 1994). Although the focus of testing should be on anatomic sites with the highest incidence of recurrence, a majority of relapses are found to involve both new and original disease sites (ELIS et al. 2002; WEEKS et al. 1991), and global surveys with a full body CT and/or gallium scintigraphy are typically performed during surveillance and restaging.

Certain prognostic indicators should also be considered when planning surveillance strategies. Stage at presentation, histology, and results of functional imaging studies can serve as predictors of ultimate relapse. The results of FDG-PET obtained at the end of treatment for lymphoma are more predictive than gallium scintigraphy or CT. Patients with a negative FDG-PET exam and low-stage HD may require no further imaging unless relapse is clinically suspected, while those with a negative FDG-PET exam but NHL or high-stage HD may benefit from close imaging surveillance (SPAEPEN et al. 2003).

The efficacy of a surveillance strategy is dependent upon the lead time afforded by the diagnostic test. The lead time is a measure of the ability of a diagnostic test to detect clinically occult disease, and is defined as the interval between when a tumor is detectable with and without the diagnostic test. The time between when a scheduled diagnostic test is obtained and when the tumor would become clinically overt approaches the lead time as the frequency of testing increases. The lead time depends upon both the natural growth rate of the tumor and the inherent ability of the test to detect tumor. Lead time can be estimated by analyzing the relative proportion of relapses first detected by imaging alone, clinical evaluation alone, and imaging and clinical evaluation simultaneously as a function of testing interval. The lead time of chest radiography in the detection of recurrent intrathoracic pediatric HD has been estimated at 2.5 months (CHANG et al. 1989). The lead time of other imaging modalities for pediatric lymphoma remains to be defined.

Even if diagnostic imaging is efficacious in detecting relapse earlier than the clinical evaluation, the costs can be prohibitive if the risk of relapse is very small, and a beneficial impact on survival is unlikely unless there is an option of curative salvage therapy that is more effective if initiated early. For example, patients with B-cell NHL and lymphoblastic lymphoma who relapse shortly after completion of treatment are resistant to therapy and have poor prognosis (MAGRATH 2002). However, even if survival is unlikely to be affected, surveillance when there is no proven curative salvage therapy may serve to identify disease in unsuspected sites so that morbid complications may possibly be prevented with palliative therapy (WEEKS et al. 1991).

An optimal solution to the problem of cancer surveillance can be identified with operations research methodology by using hazard rate analysis to determine when relapse is most likely to occur; lead time estimation to assess how good the imaging test to be used is; and utility/risk analysis to define the importance of early detection of relapse (DWYER et al. 1983; DWYER 1989; CHANG et al. 1989). An optimal surveillance strategy for chest radiography in pediatric HD has been proposed as every 3 months for 17 months after remission, every 5–6 months for 17–54 months, and cessation of testing at 54 months (CHANG et al. 1989). This strategy is based on limited data from two institutions and may not be generally applicable to other practice settings, particularly with differences in relapse rates and efficacy of salvage therapy, as well as advances in imaging technology since the study. To achieve the goal of a more evidence-based strategy for tumor surveillance in pediatric lymphoma patients, the clinical trial protocols organized by the various cancer cooperative groups should provide a mechanism for collection and analysis of appropriate relapse data for the various tumor subtypes and risk categories, so that the optimal surveillance strategies can be derived.

It should be noted that the way in which patients are followed after treatment may differ considerably between a clinical trial and clinical practice. In a clinical trial setting, uniformity of surveillance intervals is mandated to allow comparison of outcome measures such as event-free survival, disease-free survival, and progression-free survival, since these outcome measures may appear to differ if the protocols differ in timing of surveillance testing, even if there is no true difference (MAVROMATIS and CHESON 2002). It should also be noted that the optimal surveillance schedule is independent of imaging indications other than relapse detection, such as detection of opportunistic infection or other complications related to treatment (CHANG et al. 1989).

14.7.2
Late effects

The relatively high cure rates for pediatric lymphoma have not come without cost. With the increased lifespan of children treated for lymphoma, there has been increased recognition of morbidity and mortality related to late effects of treatment regimen toxicity. Deaths from late effects begin to exceed those from HD itself in patients who survive for 15 years after diagnosis (HOPPE 1997). Late effects where imaging may play a role in surveillance include second malignant neoplasms and complications involving the cardiovascular and musculoskeletal systems.

The risk of second malignant neoplasm (SMN) largely relates to a history of radiation therapy or combined radiation therapy and chemotherapy for HD, with additional risk factors including younger age and female gender (NEGLIA et al. 2001). Unlike HD, SMN has not been a significant problem in patients with NHL (HADDY et al. 1998). Solid tumors comprise approximately 80% of SMN in treated HD, with an absolute risk of 6.5% at 15 years from diagnosis (METAYER et al. 2000) and nearly 30% at 30 years (BHATIA et al. 1996). Breast and thyroid cancer are the most common solid SMN, with breast cancer accounting for nearly 50% of cases in women. Solid SMN most often develop in relation to the radiation therapy field, although the present trend of risk-adapted therapy with reduced radiation therapy in low risk patients and heightened intensity of chemotherapy in high-risk patients may alter the pattern of second malignant neoplasms.

The risk of thyroid cancer is highest in girls who received larger doses of radiation therapy at younger ages. The Children's Oncology Group Late Effects Screening Guidelines recommend annual physical exam of the thyroid, with US of any palpable nodules. The risk of breast cancer in women previously treated for HD as children or adolescents is strikingly elevated, with a standardized incidence ratio of 75 compared to the general population, and a cumulative probability of 35% by 40 years of age (BHATIA et al. 1996). An increased risk is detectable approximately 10 years after HD treatment, with a median time from HD treatment to breast cancer diagnosis of 14–19.5 years (MUNKER et al. 1999; DILLER et al. 2002), and a median age of 31.5 years at time of breast cancer diagnosis (BHATIA et al. 1996). The risk of breast cancer increases with increased radiation therapy dose, and the highest risk is incurred when radiation therapy is administered at 10–16 years of age when breast growth is most active (BHATIA et al. 1996).

Recommendations for breast cancer surveillance in those treated for HD as children or adolescents vary among experts. A baseline mammogram is generally advocated at age 25–40 years or 5–8 years after radiation therapy to the thorax, with subsequent mammograms every 1–3 years until age 30–40 years, then annually (DILLER et al. 2002; DERSHAW et al. 1992; YAHALOM et al. 1992; CLEMONS et al. 2000; PETERS et al. 1995; KASTE et al. 1998). The recently published Children's Oncology Group Late Effects Screening Guidelines advise mammograms yearly beginning 8 years after radiation therapy or at age 25, whichever is later.

The limitations of screening young women for breast cancer with conventional film-screen mammography must be acknowledged. Sensitivity is decreased by the dense breast tissue of young women. There is also concern of potential breast cancer induction by the cumulative radiation dose to the relatively radiosensitive breasts of young women during the course of screening mammography. Potential alternatives to conventional film-screen mammography that are undergoing evaluation for screening include digital mammography and breast MR imaging. Digital mammography incurs less radiation dose than conventional film-screen mammography, and diagnostic efficacy may be enhanced by the use of post-processing algorithms, tomosynthesis, and computer-assisted diagnosis (PISANO et al. 2001). Breast MR imaging has the advantages of excellent contrast resolution in radiographically dense breasts, no ionizing radiation exposure, and greater sensitivity for invasive carcinoma than mammography (TILANUS-LINTHORST et al. 2000; WARNER et al. 2001), but is disadvantaged by a low sensitivity for ductal carcinoma in situ (KINKEL and VLASTOS 2001), only moderate specificity for carcinoma, and by lack of established biopsy and post-biopsy specimen exam procedure (WARREN

and CRAWLEY 2002). Both digital mammography and breast MR imaging are currently constrained by relatively high costs and limited availability.

Cardiac complications of therapy for childhood and adolescent lymphoma are increasingly recognized as more patients experience long term remission. Cardiotoxicity may affect as many as 25% of children treated with anthracyclines with the risk of congestive heart failure higher in younger patients and in those treated with both anthracyclines and radiation therapy for lymphoblastic lymphoma (MESSINGER and UCKUN 1999). For those treated with anthracyclines, a baseline evaluation of cardiac function with echocardiography or radionuclide ventriculography is recommended, with the frequency of recommended periodic follow-up dependent upon cumulative anthracycline dose, according to the Children's Oncology Group Late Effects Screening Guidelines.

Cardiovascular disease ranks behind only HD itself and second malignant neoplasms as the cause of mortality in those treated for HD, with ischemic heart disease accounting for over two-thirds of the cardiac mortality in these patients. Risk factors include younger age at exposure, increased time since radiation therapy, and higher radiation therapy dose, although increased risk has been demonstrated in HD survivors without a history of radiation therapy. The increased relative risk for cardiac-related death is 2–7, with the absolute risk increasing with age. The increase over baseline risk may occur as soon as 5 years after radiation therapy, with a rapid increase over baseline risk after about 10 years. The pathophysiology of the ischemic heart disease is postulated as coronary artery fibrosis and accelerated atherosclerosis, and there is a relatively high rate of silent ischemia, possibly secondary to autonomic nerve damage (ADAMS et al. 2003). Cardiac CT with coronary artery calcification scoring has emerged as a sensitive screening test for angiographically significant coronary artery stenosis due to atherosclerotic plaque (NALLAMOTHU et al. 2001), but the efficacy and cost-effectiveness for predicting cardiac events is currently unknown in the setting of coronary artery disease related to lymphoma treatment toxicity.

Musculoskeletal late effects of the treatment of pediatric lymphoma do not pose the mortality risk of second malignant neoplasms and cardiovascular complications, but can result in considerable morbidity. Radiation therapy, especially in those treated the longest before skeletal maturity, induces skeletal growth deformities. MR imaging has been advocated to screen for osteonecrosis, which can occur in children receiving intensive prednisone therapy for NHL and leads to premature degenerative joint disease (Fig. 14.34) (RIBEIRO et al. 2001). Bone mineral density and height are reduced in survivors of childhood lymphoma, consequent to effects of sex hormone and growth hormone deficiency, skeletal irradiation, and treatment with corticosteroids and methotrexate (AISENBERG et al. 1998; NYSOM et al. 2001). Monitoring of bone mineral density after completion of therapy using quantitative computed tomography (QCT) or dual-energy absorptiometry (DXA) may be warranted to identify those with bone mineral density deficits that would benefit from institution of corrective therapy.

Late effects account for substantial morbidity and mortality in those treated for HD as children, and screening programs for late effects should be investigated and instituted where cost-effective. However, it should be noted that recurrent HD accounts for one-half of deaths and second malignant neoplasms related to treatment account for one-fifth of deaths in those with a history of childhood HD (WOLDEN et al. 1998). Since the greatest risk to life in these patients is relapse of HD, the primary goal must remain curative treatment with initial therapy (HUDSON and DONALDSON 2002).

14.8
Conclusion

The contribution of radiology to the evaluation and management of children with lymphoma promises to expand with further innovations in imaging technol-

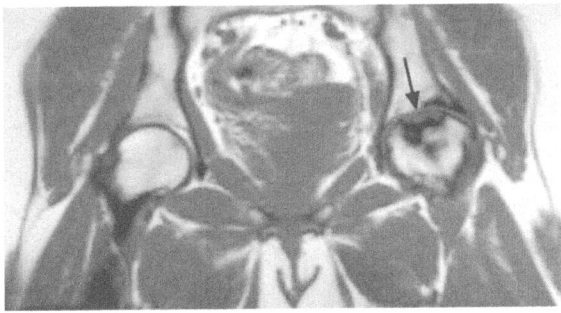

Fig. 14.34. Femoral head osteonecrosis in a 25-year-old girl after treatment for Hodgkin disease. Coronal T1-weighted MR image of the hips show osteonecrosis of the left femoral head (*arrow*) with subchondral cortical collapse and flattening of the weight-bearing surface, predisposing to morbidity from degenerative hip joint disease. (*Image courtesy of Dr. S. Kaste*)

ogy. Multidetector CT scanners are capable of acquiring a body CT exam within a few seconds, reducing motion artifact and the need for sedation in children. Isotropic voxel imaging with multidetector CT scanners allows multiplanar images to be reconstructed with minimal artifacts, permitting more precise and accurate tumor size measurements. Coupled with image segmentation software, true tumor volumes can be obtained in a semi-automated fashion, facilitating quantitation of tumor burden for risk stratification and response assessment. Combined CT-PET scanners and image fusion software improve the ability to anatomically localize sites of abnormal FDG uptake. Active disease in normal-sized lymph nodes and residual masses, and enlarged reactive nodes or residual masses without active disease may be more readily identified, increasing the accuracy of staging and restaging.

The burgeoning fields of functional and molecular imaging are especially promising, since they provide techniques to evaluate in vivo metabolic changes which precede morphologic changes. FDG-PET is being incorporated into the Children's Oncology Group lymphoma protocols, with anticipation that the benefit of FDG-PET demonstrated in the evaluation of adult lymphoma will also be shown in children. While FDG-PET is the most widely recognized application of functional imaging in lymphoma, other techniques are under active investigation. Apoptosis, a mechanism of tumor cell death in lymphoma, is amenable to imaging with ^{99m}Technitium annexin-V (BLANKENBERG and STRAUSS 2002). Antigen and cell surface receptors specific to lymphoma or lymphoma subtypes, such as CD20, can potentially be targeted with Gadolinium or radiopharmaceutical conjugated peptides, monoclonal antibodies, polymerized vesicles, or nanoparticles, and subsequently imaged (SHARMA et al. 2002). Superparamagnetic iron oxide nanoparticle contrast agents taken up by reticuloendothelial cells and imaged by MR imaging improve the evaluation of tumor infiltration of the bone marrow, lymph nodes, and spleen (DALDRUP-LINK et al. 2002; MACK et al. 2002; WEISSLEDER et al. 1989). Tumor perfusion and angiogenesis can be assessed by dynamic contrast-enhanced CT or MR imaging (PADHANI 2002). The tumor masses of lymphoma have increased microvascularity, which decreases with treatment leading to cell death. As measured by dynamic contrast-enhanced CT, tumor perfusion > 0.5 ml/min/ml implies active and intermediate/high-grade disease, while perfusion < 0.2 ml/min/ml implies inactive disease (DUGDALE et al. 1999). These techniques may prove useful for guiding treatment selection in risk-adapted, response-based protocols, although these techniques will need to show cost-effective, incremental value over existing conventional imaging techniques before they can be advocated for routine use.

As the success of treatment of pediatric lymphoma continues to improve and a decrease in late effects is emphasized, efforts should also be made to reduce the risks and costs of imaging (WHITE 2001). With the potential increased risk in children of induction of malignancy by ionizing radiation from imaging studies (BRENNER et al. 2001), radiation dose should be kept as low as possible without compromising diagnostic efficacy, according to the ALARA (As Low As Reasonably Achievable) principle. Studies are needed to better determine the degree to which radiation dose can be reduced for individual imaging studies in specific clinical settings while maintaining adequate image quality for diagnosis. Studies are also needed to determine the optimal schedule of imaging studies for adequate surveillance of relapse and late effects after therapy.

Cancer cooperative groups possess the resources to carry out multi-institutional clinical trials on pediatric lymphoma patients. Many of these trials are conducted on large numbers of patients in a prospective, randomized design with standardized protocols for management, maximizing the statistical power and scientific rigor. These protocols have a profound influence on the selection and timing of imaging studies for staging, tumor response assessment, and surveillance (WHITE 2001). The Children's Oncology Group (COG) is the largest cancer cooperative group devoted exclusively to children and adolescents and is supported by the United States National Cancer Institute (NCI) to organize clinical oncology trials at more than 200 member institutions, including cancer centers at the major universities and teaching hospitals in the United States and Canada, and at sites in Europe and Australia. Pediatric radiologists are actively involved with Children's Oncology Group protocol development and implementation, and central review of pertinent imaging studies.

By participating in the clinical trial activities of the cancer cooperative groups, radiologists can transcend the traditional focus of radiology on optimization of technical parameters and diagnostic efficacy of imaging, and address the impact of imaging on therapeutic planning, patient outcomes, and costs to better promote evidence-based care of children and adolescents with lymphoma. Even if not involved directly with clinical oncology trials, it is incumbent for radiologists participating in the care of children with cancer to have a working knowledge of the most current approaches to imaging and management of pediatric lymphoma patients. It is hoped that the resources in this chapter can serve as a valuable reference to guide the selection and interpretation of imaging studies and support the role of the radiologist as a vital member of the pediatric oncology team.

References

Adam EJ, Ignotus PI (1993) Sonography of the thymus in healthy children: frequency of visualization, size, and appearance. Am J Roentgenol AJR 161:153–155

Adams MJ, Hardenbergh PH, Constine LS et al. (2003) Radiation–associated cardiovascular disease. Crit Rev Oncol Hematol 45:55–75

Aisenberg AC (1999) Primary large cell lymphoma of the mediastinum. Semin Oncol 26:251–258

Aisenberg J, Hsieh K, Kalaitzoglou G et al. (1998) Bone mineral density in young adult survivors of childhood cancer. J Pediatr Hematol Oncol 20:241–245

Apter S, Avigdor A, Gayer G et al. (2002) Calcification in lymphoma occurring before therapy: CT features and clinical correlation. Am J Roentgenology 178:935–938

Armitage JO, Weisenberger DD, Hutchins M et al. (1986) Chemotherapy for diffuse large–cell lymphoma – rapidly responding patients have more durable remissions. J Clin Oncol 4:160–164

Baker LL, Parker BR, Donaldson SS et al. (1990) Staging of HodgkinHodgkin's disease in children: comparison of CT and lymphography with laparotomy. Am J Roentgenol AJR 154:1251–1255

Barrington SF, O'Doherty MJ (2003) Limitations of PET for imaging lymphoma. Eur J Nucl Med Mol Imaging 30 Suppl 1:117–127

Benjamin D, Magrath IT, Douglass EC et al. (1983) Derivation of lymphoma cell lines from microscopically normal bone marrow in patients with undifferentiated lymphomas: evidence of occult bone marrow involvement. Blood 61:1017–1019

Bhatia S, Robison LL, Oberlin O et al. (1996) Breast cancer and other second neoplasms after childhood Hodgkin's disease. N Engl J Med 334:745–751

Blankenberg FG, Strauss HW (2002) Nuclear medicine applications in molecular imaging. J Magn Reson Imaging 16:352–361

Bower RJ, Kiesewetter WB (1977) Mediastinal masses in infants and children. Arch Surg 112:1003–1009

Brenner DJ, Elliston CD, Hall EJ et al (2001) Estimated risk of radiation–induced fatal cancer from pediatric CT. Am J Roentgenol AJR 176:289–296

Bradley AJ, Carrington BM, Lawrance JA et alBradley AJ, Carrington BM, Lawrance JA et al. (1999) Assessment and significance of mediastinal bulk in Hodgkin's disease: comparison between computed tomography and chest radiography. J Clin Oncol 17:2493–2498

Brenner DJ, Elliston CD, Hall EJ et al. (2001) Estimated risk of radiation–induced fatal cancer from pediatric CT. Am J Roentgenol AJR 176:289–296

Brink I, Reinhardt MJ, Hoegerle S et al. (2001) Increased metabolic activity in the thymus gland studied with 18F–FDG

PET: age dependency and frequency after chemotherapy. J Nucl Med 42:591–595

Brisse H, Pacquement H, Burdairon E et al. (1998) Outcome of residual mediastinal masses of thoracic lymphomas in children: impact on management and radiological follow-up strategy. Pediatr Radiol 28:444–450

Cairo MS, Sposto R, Hoover-Regan M et al. (2003a) Childhood and adolescent large cell lymphoma (LCL): a review of the Children's Cancer Group experience. Am J Hematol 72:53–63

Cairo MS, Sposto R, Perkins SL et al. (2003b) Burkitt's and Burkitt-like lymphoma in children and adolescents: a review of the Children's Cancer Group experience. Br J Hematol 120:660–670

Carbone PP, Kaplan HS, Husshoff K et al. (1971) Report of the committee on Hodgkin's disease staging classification. Cancer Res 31:1860–1861

Castellino RA (1986) Hodgkin disease: practical concepts for the diagnostic radiologist. Radiology 159:305–310

Castellino RA (1991a) Diagnostic imaging evaluation of Hodgkin Hodgkin's disease and non-HodgkinHodgkin's lymphoma. Cancer 67 Suppl 67:1177–1180

Castellino RA (1991b) The non-Hodgkin's lymphomas: practical concepts for the diagnostic radiologist. Radiology 178:315–321

Castellino RA, Bellani FF, Gasparini M et al. (1975) Radiographic findings in previously untreated children with non-Hodgkin's lymphoma. Radiology 117:657–663

Castellino RA, Blank N, Hoppe RT et al. (1986) Hodgkin disease: contributions of chest CT in the initial staging evaluation. Radiology 160:603–605

Castellino RA, Hilton S, O'Brien JP et al. (1996) Non-Hodgkin Hodgkin's lymphoma: contribution of chest CT in the initial staging evaluation. Radiology 199:129–132

Chaignaud BE, Bonsack TA, Kozakewich HP et al. (1998) Pleural effusions in lymphoblastic lymphoma: a diagnostic alternative J Pediatr Surg 33:1355–1357

Chang PJ, Parker BR, Donaldson SS, Thompson EI (1989) Dynamic probabilistic model for determination of optimal timing of surveillance chest radiography in pediatric Hodgkin's disease. Radiology 173:71–75

Chepuri NB, Strouse PJ, Yanik GA (2003) CT of renal lymphoma in children. Am J Roentgenol AJR 180:429–431

Cheson BD, Horning SJ, Coiffier B et al. (1999) Report of an international workshop to standardize response criteria for non-Hodgkin's lymphomas. J Clin Oncol 17:1244–1253

Chilcote RR, Baehner RL, Hammond D (1976) Septicemia and meningitis in children splenectomized for Hodgkin's disease. N Engl J Med 295:798–800

Clemons M, Loijens L, Goss P (2000) Breast cancer risk following irradiation for Hodgkin'sHodgkin's disease. Cancer Treat Rev 26:291–302

Cohen MD, Siddiqui A, Weetman R et al. (1986) Hodgkin disease and non-Hodgkin lymphomas in children: utilization of radiological modalities. Radiology 158:499–505

Cory DA, Cohen MD, Smith JA (1987) Thymus in the superior mediastinum simulating adenopathy: appearance on CT. Radiology 162:457–459

Daldrup-Link HE, Rummeny EJ, Ihssen B et al. (2002) Iron-oxide-enhanced MR imaging of bone marrow in patients with non-Hodgkin's lymphoma: differentiation between tumor infiltration and hypercellular bone marrow. Eur Radiol 12:1557–1566

Dalle JH, Mechinaud F, Michon J et al. (2001) Testicular disease in childhood B-cell non-Hodgkin's lymphoma: the French Society of Pediatric Oncology experience. J Clin Oncol 19:2397–2403

Delcambre C, Reman O, Henry-Amar M et al. (2000) Clinical relevance of gallium-67 scintigraphy in lymphoma before and after therapy. Eur J Nucl Med 27:176–184

Dershaw DD, Yahalom J, Petrek JA (1992) Breast carcinoma in women previously treated for Hodgkin disease: mammographic evaluation. Radiology 184:421–423

Diller L, Medeiros Nancarrow C, Shaffer K et al. (2002) Breast cancer screening in women previously treated for Hodgkin's disease: a prospective cohort study. J Clin Oncol 20:2085–2091

Dinkel H-P, Sonnenschein M, Hoppe H et al. (2003) Low-dose multislice CT of the thorax in follow-up of malignant lymphoma and extrapulmonary primary tumors. Eur Radiol 13:1241–1249

Dorak AC, Alp E, Deviren MU (1991) Hydronephrotic pseudokidney sign: is it specific for intestinal lymphoma? J Clin Ultrasound 19:561–563

Drossman SR, Schiff RG, Kronfeld GD et al. (1990) Lymphoma of the mediastinum and neck: evaluation with Ga-67 imaging and CT correlation. Radiology 174:171–175

Dugdale PE, Miles KA, Bunce I et al. (1999) CT measurement of perfusion and permeability within lymphoma masses and its ability to assess grade, activity, and chemotherapeutic response. J Comput Assist Tomogr 23:540–547

Dwyer AJ (1989) Time and disease: the fourth dimension of radiology. Radiology 173:17–21

Dwyer AJ, Prewitt JM, Ecker JG et al. (1983) Use of the hazard rate to schedule follow-up exams efficiently. An optimization approach to patient management. Med Decis Making 3:229–244

Eggli KD, Close P, Dillon PW et al. (1995) Three-dimensional quantitation of pediatric tumor bulk. Pediatr Radiol 25:1–6

Elis A, Blickstein D, Klein O et al. (2002) Detection of relapse in non-Hodgkin's lymphoma: role of routine follow-up studies. Am J Hematol 69:41–44

Elkowitz SS, Leonidas JC, Lopez M et al. (1993) Comparison of CT and MRI in the evaluation of therapeutic response in thoracic Hodgkin disease. Pediatr Radiol 23:301–304

Epstein LG, DiCarlo FJ Jr, Joshi VV et al. (1988) Primary lymphoma of the central nervous system in children with acquired immunodeficiency syndrome. Pediatrics 82:355–63

Even-Sapir E, Israel O (2003) Gallium-67 scintigraphy: a cornerstone in functional imaging of lymphoma Eur J Nucl Med Mol Imaging 30 Suppl 1:65–81

Fishman EK, Kuhlman JE, Jones RJ (1991) CT of lymphoma: spectrum of disease. Radiographics 11:647–669

Fletcher BD, Kauffman WM, Kaste SC et al. (1995) Use of Tl-201 to detect untreated pediatric Hodgkin disease. Radiology 196:851–855

Frohlich DE, Chen JL, Neuberg D et al. (2000) When is hilar uptake of 67Ga-citrate indicative of residual disease after CHOP chemotherapy? J Nucl Med 41:269–274

Front D, Israel O (1995) The role of Ga-67 scintigraphy in evaluating the results of therapy of lymphoma patients. Semin Nucl Med 25:60–71

Front D, Bar-ShalomIsrael O, Epelbaum R, Mor M et al (1999) Hodgkin disease: prediction of outcome with 67Ga scintigraphy after one cycle of chemotherapy.. (1990) Ga–676 SPECT before and after treatment of lymphoma. Radiology 210:487–491175:515–519

Front D, Ben–Haim S, Israel O et al. (1992) Lymphoma: predictive value of Ga–67 scintigraphy after treatment. Radiology 182:359–363

Front D, Israel O, EpelbaumBar–Shalom R, Mor M et al (1990) Ga–676 SPECT before and after treatment of lymphoma.. (1999) Hodgkin disease: prediction of outcome with 67Ga scintigraphy after one cycle of chemotherapy. Radiology 175:515–519210:487–491

Fuks JZ, Aisner J, Wiernik PH (1982) Restaging laparotomy in the management of the non–Hodgkin lymphomas. Med Pediatr Oncol 10:429–438

Garrett KM, Hoffer FA, Behm FG et al. (2002) Interventional radiology techniques for the diagnosis of lymphoma or leukemia. Pediatr Radiol 32:653–662

Goerg C, Schwerk WB, Goerg K (1990) Gastrointestinal lymphoma: sonographic findings in 54 patients. Am J Roentgenol AJR 155:795–798

Goldsby RE, Carroll WL (1998) The molecular biology of pediatric lymphomas. J Pediatr Hematol Oncol 20:282–296

Gorg C, Weide R, Schwerk WB (1996) Sonographic patterns in extranodal abdominal lymphomas. Eur Radiol 6:855–864

Gossot D, Girard P, de Kerviler E et al. (2001) Thoracoscopy or CT–guided biopsy for residual intrathoracic masses after treatment of lymphoma. Chest 120:289–94

Grillo–Lopez AJ, Cheson B, Horning S et al. (2000) Response criteria for NHL: importance of 'normal' lymph node size and correlations with response rates. Ann Oncol 11:399–408

Guillerman RP (2000) Primary Intestinal Lymphoma.intestinal lymphoma. J Pediatr Hematol Oncol 22: 476–478

Haddy T, Adde M, McAlla J et al. (1998) Late effects in long–term survivors of high–grade non–Hodgkin's lymphoma. J Clin Oncol 16:2070–2079

Haddy TB, Sandlund JT, Magrath IT (1988) Testicular involvement in young patients with non–Hodgkin's lymphoma. Am J Pediatr Hematol Oncol 10:224–229

Halliday T, Baxter G (2003) Lymphoma: pictorial review. Eur Radiol 13:1224–1234

Hamrick–Turner JE, Saif MF, Powers CI et al. (1994) Imaging of childhood non–Hodgkin lymphoma: assessment of histologic subtype. Radiographics 14:11–28

Hanna SL, Fletcher BD, Boulden TF et al. (1993) MR imaging of infradiaphragmatic lymphadenopathy in children and adolescents with Hodgkin disease: comparison with lymphography and CT. J Magn Reson Imaging 3:461–470

Hardy SM (2003) The sandwich sign. Radiology 226:651–652

Harris NL (1997) Principles of the revised European–American Lymphoma Classification (from the International Lymphoma Study Group). Ann Oncol 8 Suppl 2:11–16

Harris NL, Jaffe ES, Diebold J et alHarris NL, Jaffe ES, Stein H et al. (1994) A revised European–American classification of lymphoid neoplasms: a proposal from the International Lymphoma Study Group. Blood 84:1361–1392

Harris NL, Jaffe ES, Diebold J et al. (1999) The World Health Organization classification of hematologic malignancies. Report of the Clinical Advisory Committee meeting, Airlie House, Virginia, November, 1997. J Clin Oncol 17:3835–3849

Harris NL, Jaffe ES, Stein H et al (1994) A revised European–American classification of lymphoid neoplasms: a proposal from the International Lymphoma Study Group. Blood 84:1361–1392

Hasegawa T, Sumimura J, Mizutani S et al. (1998) The doughnut sign: an ultrasound finding in pediatric intestinal Burkitt's lymphoma. Pediatr Surg Int 13:297–298

Hoane BR, Shields AF, Porter BA (1991) Detection of lymphomatous bone marrow involvement with magnetic resonance imaging. Blood 78:728–738

Hoppe RT (1997) Hodgkin's disease: complications of therapy and excess mortality. Ann Oncol 8 Suppl:115–118

Hopper KD, Diehl LF, Cole BA et al. (1990) The significance of necrotic mediastinal lymph nodes on CT in patients with newly diagnosed Hodgkin disease. Am J Roentgenol AJR 155:267–270

Hopper KD, Kasales CJ, Eggli KD et al. (1996a) The impact of 2D versus 3D quantitation of tumor bulk determination on current methods of assessing response to treatment. J Comput Assist Tomogr 20:930–937

Hopper KD, Kasales CJ, Van Slyke MA et al. (1996b) Analysis of interobserver and intraobserver variability in CT tumor measurements Am J Roentgenol AJR 187:851–854

Hudson MM, Donaldson SS (2002) Hodgkin' Hodgkin's disease. In: Pizzo PA, Poplack DG (eds) Principles and practice of pediatric oncology. Lippincott Williams & Wilkins, Philadelphia, pp 637–660

Janicek M, Kaplan W, Neuberg D et al (1997) Early restaging gallium scans predict outcome in poor–prognosis patients with aggressive non–Hodgkin's lymphoma with high–dose CHOP chemotherapy. J Clin Oncol 15:1631–1637

Jaffe ES, Harris NL, Stein H et alJaffe ES, Harris NL, Stein H et al. (2001) Pathology and genetics of tumours of haematopoietic and lymphoid tissues. In: Kleihues P, Sobin LH (eds) World Health Organization classification of tumours. IARC Press, Lyon, pp 75–117

Janicek M, Kaplan W, Neuberg D et al. (1997) Early restaging gallium scans predict outcome in poor–prognosis patients with aggressive non–Hodgkin's lymphoma with high–dose CHOP chemotherapy. J Clin Oncol 15:1631–1637

Kadin ME, Sako D, Berliner N et al. (1986) Childhood Ki–1 lymphoma presenting with skin lesions and peripheral lymphadenopathy. Blood 68:1042–1049

Kaplan HS, Rosenberg SA (1966) The treatment of Hodgkin's disease. Med Clin North Am 50:1591–1610

Karmazyn B, Ash S, Goshen Y et al. (2001) Significance of residual abdominal masses in children with abdominal Burkitt's lymphoma. Pediatr Radiol 31:801–805

Kaste SC, Hudson MM, Jones DJ et al. (1998) Breast masses in women treated for childhood cancer: incidence and screening guidelines. Cancer 82:784–792

Kinkel K, Vlastos G (2001) MR imaging: breast cancer staging and screening. Semin Surg Oncol 20:187–196

Kostakoglu L, Goldsmith SJ (2000) Fluorine–18 fluorodeoxyglucose positron emission tomography in the staging and follow–up of lymphoma: is it time to shift gears? Eur J Nucl Med 27:1564–1578

LaQuaglia MP, Stolar CHJ, Krailo M et al. (1992) The role of surgery in abdominal non–Hodgkin's lymphoma: experience from the Children's Cancer Study Group. J Pediatr Surg 27:230–235

Lewis E, Bernardino ME, Salvador PG et al. (1982) Post therapy CT detected mass in lymphoma patients: is it viable tissue? J Comput Assist Tomogr 6:792–795

Lewis GJS, Leithiser RE Jr., Glaxier CM et al. (1989) Ultrasonography of pediatric neck masses. Ultrasound Q 7: 315–355

Lindfors KK, Meyer JE, Dedrick CG et al. (1985) Thymic cysts in mediastinal Hodgkin disease. Radiology 156:37–41

Lister TA, Crowther D, Sutcliffe SB et al. (1989) Report of a committee convened to discuss the evaluation and staging of patients with Hodgkin's disease: Cotswolds Meeting. J Clin Oncol 7:1630–1636

Luker GD, Siegel MJ (1993) Mediastinal Hodgkin disease in children: response to therapy. Radiology 189:737–740

Mack MG, Balzer JO, Straub R et al. (2002) Superparamagnetic iron-oxide enhanced MR imaging of head and neck lymph nodes. Radiology 222:239–244

Magrath IT (1991) African Burkitt's lymphoma: history, biology, clinical features, and treatment. Am J Pediatr Hematol Oncol 13:222–246

Magrath IT (1997) Limiting therapy for limited childhood non-Hodgkin's lymphoma. N Engl J Med 337:1304–1306

Magrath IT (2002) Malignant non-Hodgkin's lymphomas in children. In: Pizzo PA, Poplack DG (eds) Principles and practice of pediatric oncology. Lippincott Williams & Wilkins, Philadelphia, pp 661–704

Magrath IT, Lee YJ, Anderson T et al. (1980) Prognostic factors in Burkitt's lymphoma: importance of total tumor burden. Cancer 45:1507–1515

Mavromatis BH, Cheson BD (2002) Pre- and post-treatment evaluation of non-Hodgkin's lymphoma. Best Pract Res Clin Haematol 15:429–447

Mazzu D, Jeffrey RB, Ralls PW (1995) Lymphoma and leukemia involving the testicles: findings on gray-scale and color Doppler sonography. Am J Roentgenol AJR 164:645–647

Mendenhall NP, Cantor AB, Williams JL et al. (1993) With modern imaging techniques, is staging laparotomy necessary in pediatric Hodgkin's disease? A pediatric oncology group study. J Clin Oncol 11:2218–2225

Messinger Y, Uckun FM (1999) A critical risk-benefit assessment argues against the use of anthracyclines in induction regimens for newly diagnosed childhood acute lymphoblastic lymphomas. Leuk Lymphoma 34:415–432

Metayer C, Lynch CF, Clarke EA et al. (2000) Second cancers among long-term survivors of Hodgkin's disease diagnosed in childhood and adolescence. J Clin Oncol 18:2435–2443

Miller AB, Hogestraeten B, Staquet M, Winkler A (1981) Reporting results of cancer treatment. Cancer 47:207–214

Montravers F, McNamara D, Landman-Parker J et al. (2002) [18F]FDG in childhood lymphoma; clinical utility and impact on management. Eur J Nuc Med 29:1155–1165

Munker R, Grutzner S, Hiller E et al. (1999) Second malignancies after Hodgkin's disease: the Munich experience. Ann Hematol 78:544–554

Murphy SB, Fairclough DL, Hutchison RE et al. (1989) Non-Hodgkin's lymphomas of childhood: an analysis of the histology, staging, and response to treatment of 338 cases at a single institution. J Clin Oncol 7:186–193

Nallamothu BK, Saint S, Bielak LF et al. (2001) Electron-beam computed tomography in the diagnosis of coronary artery disease: a meta-analysis. Arch Intern Med 161:833–838

Neglia JP, Friedman DL, Yasui Y et al. (2001) Second malignant neoplasms in five-year survivors of childhood cancer: childhood cancer survivor study. J Natl Cancer Inst 93:618–629

Neth O, Seidemann K, Jansen P et al. (2000) Precursor B-cell lymphoblastic lymphoma in childhood and adolescence: clinical features, treatment, and results in trials NHL–BFM 86 and 90. Med Pediatr Oncol 35:20–27

Ng YY, Healy JC, Vincent JM et al. (1994) The radiology of non-Hodgkin's lymphoma in childhood: a review of 80 cases. Clin Radiol 49:594–600

Nysom K, Holm K, Michaelsen KF et al. (2001) Bone mass after treatment of malignant lymphoma in childhood. Med Pediatr Oncol 37:518–524

Oh YK, Ha CS, Samuels BI et al. (1999) Stages I–III follicular lymphoma: role of CT of the abdomen and pelvis in follow-up studies. Radiology 210:483–486

Orzel JA, Sawaf NW, Richardson ML (1988) Lymphoma of the skeleton: scintigraphic evaluation. Am J Roentgenol AJR 150:1095–1099

Padhani AR (2002) Dynamic contrast-enhanced MRI in clinical oncology: current status and future directions. J Magn Reson Imaging 16:407–422

Parker BR (1997) Leukemia and lymphoma in childhood. Radiol Clin North Am 35:1495–1516

Patel PM, Alibazoglu H, Ali A et al. (1996) Normal thymic uptake of FDG on PET imaging. Clin Nucl Med 21:772–775

Patte C (1998) Non-Hodgkin's lymphoma. Eur J Canc Cancer 34:359–363

Percy CL, Smith, MA, Linet M et al. (1999) Lymphomas and reticuloendothelial neoplasms. Chapter II. In: Cancer incidence and survival among children and adolescents: United States SEER Program, 1975–1995; NCI monograph

Peters MH, Sonpal IM, Batra MK (1995) Breast cancer in women following mantle irradiation for Hodgkin's disease. Am Surg 61:763–766

Peylan-Ramu N, Haddy TB, Jones E et al. (1989) High frequency of benign mediastinal uptake of gallium–67 after completion of chemotherapy in children with high-grade non-Hodgkin's lymphoma. J Clin Oncol 7:1800–1806

Pisano ED, Kuzmiak C, Koomen M et al. (2001) What every surgical oncologist should know about digital mammography. Semin Surg Oncol 20:181–186

Reske SN (2003) PET and restaging of malignant lymphoma including residual masses and relapse. Eur J Nucl Med Mol Imaging. 30 Suppl 1:89–96

Rezvani L, Tully RJ, Levine C et al. (1986) Computed tomography in the diagnosis and follow-up of American Burkitt's lymphoma. Gastrointest Radiol 11:36–40

Ribeiro RC, Fletcher BD, Kennedy W et al. (2001) Magnetic resonance imaging detection of avascular necrosis of the bone in children receiving intensive prednisone therapy for acute lymphoblastic leukemia or non-Hodgkin lymphoma. Leukemia 15:891–897

Rodriguez M (1998) Computed tomography, magnetic resonance imaging and positron emission tomography in non-Hodgkin's lymphoma. Acta Radiol 417 Suppl:1–36

Rodriguez-Catarino M, Jerkeman M, Ahlstrom H et al. (2000) Residual mass in aggressive lymphoma– - does size, measured by computed tomography, influence clinical outcome? Acta Oncol 39:485–489

Rosenthal H, Kolb R, Gratz KF et al. (2000) Bone manifestations in non-Hodgkin's lymphoma in childhood and adolescence. Radiologe 40:737–744

Rostock RA, Siegelman SS, Lenhard RE et al. (1983) Thoracic CT scanning for mediastinal Hodgkin's disease: results and therapeutic implications. Int J Radiat Oncol Phys 9:1451–1457

Roth SL, Sack H, Havemann K et al. (1998) Contiguous pattern spreading in patients with Hodgkin's disease. Radiother Oncol 47:7–16

Saini S (2001) Radiologic measurement of tumor size in clinical trials: past, present, and future. Am J Roentgenol AJR 176:333–334

Salloum E, Brandt DS, Caride VJ et al. (1997) Gallium scans in the management of patients with Hodgkin's disease: a study of 101 patients. J Clin Oncol 15:518–527

Sandrock D, Lastoria, Magrath IT et al. (1993) The role of gallium-67 tumor scintigraphy in patients with small, non-cleaved cell lymphoma. Eur J Nucl Med 20:119–122

Schoder H, Meta J, Yap C et al. (2001) Effect of whole-boy (18)F-FDG PET imaging on clinical staging and management of patients with malignant lymphoma. J Nucl Med 42:1139–1143

Scott AM, Larson SM (1993) Tumor imaging and therapy. Radiol Clin North Am 31:859–880

Shamberger RC, Holzman RS, Griscom NT et al. (1995) Prospective evaluation by computed tomography and pulmonary function tests of children with mediastinal masses. Surgery 118:468–471

Sharma V, Luker GD, Piwnica-Worms D (2002) Molecular imaging of gene expression and protein function in vivo with PET and SPECT. J Magn Reson Imaging 16:336–351

Shepard SF, A'Hern RP, Pinkerton CR (1995) Childhood T-cell lymphoblastic lymphoma – does early resolution of mediastinal mass predict for final outcome? Br J Cancer 72:752–756

Siegel MJ (1999) Pediatric body CT, 1st edn. Lippincott Williams & Wilkins, Philadelphia

Siegel MJ, Evans SJ, Balfe DM (1988) Small bowel disease in children: diagnosis with CT. Radiology 169:127–130

Siegel MJ, Glazer HS, Wiener JI et al. (1989) Normal and abnormal thymus in childhood: MR imaging. Radiology 172:367–371

Smith SD, Rubin CM, Horvath A et al. (1990) Non-Hodgkin lymphoma in children. Semin Oncol 17:113–119

Spaepen K, Stroobants S, Verhoef G et al. (2003) Positron emission tomography with [(18)F]FDG for therapy response monitoring in lymphoma patients. Eur J Nucl Med Mol Imaging. 30 Suppl 1:97–105

Spears CP (1984) Volume doubling measurement of spherical and ellipsoidal tumors. Med Pediatr Oncol 12:212–217

St. Amour TE, Siegel MJ, Glazer HS et al. (1987) CT appearances of the normal and abnormal thymus in children. J Comput Assist Tomogr 11:645–650

Talbot JN, Haioun C, Rain JD et al. (2001) [18F]-FDG positron imaging in clinical management of lymphoma patients. Crit Rev Oncol Hematol 38:193–221

Tan TX, Gelfand MJ (1996) Ga-67 scintigraphy in pediatric patients. Comparison of extended SPECT of the chest and abdomen with planar imaging. Clin Nucl Med 21:717–719

ten Berge RL, Oudejans JJ, Ossenkoppele GJ et al. (2003) ALK-negative systemic anaplastic large cell lymphoma: differential diagnostic and prognostic aspects – a review. J Pathol 200:4–15

Therasse P (2002) Measuring the clinical response. What does it mean? Eur J Cancer. 38:1817–1823

Therasse P, Arbuck SG, Eisenhauer EA et al. (2000) New guidelines to evaluate the response to treatment in solid tumors. J Natl Cancer Inst 92:205–216

Tilanus-Linthorst MM, Obdeijn IM, Bartels KC et al. (2000) First experiences in screening women at high risk for breast cancer with MR imaging. Breast Cancer Res Treat 63:53–60

Torrey MJ, Poen JC, Hoppe RT (1997) Detection of relapse in early-stage Hodgkin's disease: role of routine follow-up studies. J Clin Oncol 15:1123–1130

Tura S, Fiacchini M, Zinzani PL et al. (1993) Splenectomy and the increasing risk of secondary acute leukemia in Hodgkin's disease. J Clin Oncol 11:925–930

Vazquez E, Lucaya J, Castellote A et al. (2002) Neuroimaging in pediatric leukemia and lymphoma: differential diagnosis. Radiographics 22:1411–1428

Warner E, Plewes DB, Shumak RS et al. (2001) Comparison of breast magnetic resonance imaging, mammography, and ultrasound for surveillance of women at high risk for hereditary breast cancer. J Clin Oncol 19:3524–3531

Warren RM, Crawley A (2002) Is breast MRI ever useful in a mammographic screening programme? Clin Radiol 57:1090–1097

Weeks JC, Yeap BY, Canellos GP et al. (1991) Value of follow-up procedures in patients with large-cell lymphoma who achieve a complete remission. J Clin Oncol 9:1196–1203

Weihrauch MR, Re D, Scheidhauer K et al. (2001) Thoracic positron emission tomography using 18F-fluorodeoxyglucose for the evaluation of residual mediastinal Hodgkin disease. Blood 98:2930–2934

Weinberger E, Rosenbaum DM, Pendergrass TW (1990) Renal involvement in children with lymphoma: comparison of CT with sonography. Am J Roentgenol AJR 155:347–349

Weinblatt ME, Zanzi I, Belakhlef A et al. (1997) False-positive FDG-PET imaging of the thymus of a child with Hodgkin's disease. J Nucl Med 38:888–890

Weiner MA, Leventhal BG, Cantor A et al. (1991) Gallium-67 scans as an adjunct to CT scans for the assessment of a residual mediastinal mass in pediatric patients with Hodgkin's disease: a Pediatric Oncology Group study. Cancer 68:2478–2480

Weissleder R, Elizondo G, Stark DD et al. (1989) The diagnosis of splenic lymphoma by MR imaging: value of superparamagnetic iron oxide. Am J Roentgenol AJR 152:175–180

Wernecke K, Peters PE, Kruger KG (1987) Ultrasonographic patterns of focal hepatic and splenic lesions in Hodgkin's and non-Hodgkin's lymphoma. Br J Radiol 60:655–660

Wernecke K, Vassalo P, Rutsch F et al. (1991) Thymic involvement in Hodgkin disease: CT and sonographic findings. Radiology 181:375–383

White KS (2001) Thoracic imaging of pediatric lymphomas. J Thorac Imaging 16:224–237

Wolden SL, Lamborn KR, Cleary SF et al. (1998) Second cancers following pediatric Hodgkin's disease. J Clin Oncol 16:536–544

Woo KB, Funkhouser WK, Sullivan C et al. (1980) Analysis of the proliferation kinetics of Burkitt's lymphoma cells. Cell Tissue Kinet 13:591–604

Yahalom J, Petrek JA, Biddinger PW et al. (1992) Breast cancer in patients irradiated for Hodgkin's disease: a clinical and pathologic analysis of 45 events in 37 patients. J Clin Oncol 10:1674–81

Yoon SN, Park CH, Kim MK et al. (2001) False-positive F-18 FDG gamma camera positron emission tomographic imaging resulting from inflammation of an anterior mediastinal mass in a patient with non-Hodgkin's lymphoma. Clin Nuc Med 26:461–462

Ziegler J, Magrath IT, Olweny CLM (1979) Cure of Burkitt's lymphoma: 10 -year follow-up of 157 Ugandan patients. Lancet 2:936–938

15 Waldenström Macroglobulinemia

Lia A. Moulopoulos and Ali Guermazi

CONTENTS

15.1
Introduction

Waldenström macroglobulinemia (WM) is a low-grade lymphoma characterized by malignant proliferation of mature plasmacytoid lymphocytes, which produce a monoclonal immunoglobulin M (IgM). According to the revised European-American classification of lymphoid neoplasms, most of the cases included under the diagnosis of Lymphoplasmacytoid Lymphoma/Immunocytoma are cases of WM (Harris et al. 1994).

Lia A. Moulopoulos, MD
Assistant Adjunct Professor, MD Anderson Cancer Center, Assistant Professor, Department of Radiology, Areteion Hospital, University of Athens, Medical School, 76 Vas. Sophias Avenue, G-11528, Athens, Greece
Ali Guermazi, MD
Visiting Associate Professor, Department of Radiology, University of California San Francisco, 350 Parnassus Avenue, Suite 150, San Francisco, CA 94117, USA

WM was first described in 1944 by Waldenström, who reported two patients with anemia, a tendency to bleed, enlarged lymph nodes, infiltration of the bone marrow by abnormal cells with lymphoid and plasma cell characteristics and marked elevation of a high molecular weight gamma globulin in the serum (Waldenström 1944).

The incidence rate of WM is 6.1 cases per million in white men and 2.5 cases per million in white women. WM is considerably less common than multiple myeloma or chronic lymphocytic leukemia. Incidence rates increase with age (median age of 63). Men are affected slightly more often than women, and whites significantly more often than blacks (Herrington and Weiss 1993; Groves et al. 1998).

The cause of WM is not known, but a genetic influence has been reported in some families (Renier et al. 1989). No specific chromosome abnormality has been associated with WM but the presence of multiple cytogenetic abnormalities heralds a poor prognosis. Occupational exposure to leather, rubber dyes, and paints has been implicated in some studies (Tepper and Moss 1994).

The clinical features of WM are related to direct infiltration of various tissues by malignant cells, circulating IgM, and tissue-deposition of IgM. Patients may present with fatigue, anemia, hyperviscosity, B symptoms, bleeding, neurological manifestations, splenomegaly, and enlarged lymph nodes (Kyrtsonis et al. 2001; Garcia-Sanz et al. 2001). Symptomatic cryoglobulinemia, cold agglutinin anemia and amyloidosis may be seen in occasional patients. The hallmark of the disease is the presence of monoclonal IgM. The light chain is kappa in two-thirds of patients and light chain proteinuria, usually of small amounts, is present in approximately one-half of patients (Dimopoulos et al. 2000). About a third of patients with WM, are asymptomatic at diagnosis and half of them may not require treatment for many years (Garcia-Sanz et al. 2001).

15.2
Bones and Bone Marrow

15.2.1
Bones

Lytic lesions are rare in patients with WM and, when present, they are radiologically indistinguishable from either multiple myeloma or lytic bone metastases. They have been reported in less than 5% of patients with this disease (Kyle and Garton 1987). For the unusual patient who presents with lytic bone lesions and monoclonal IgM, the diagnosis of either WM with bone lesions or IgM multiple myeloma should rely on specific morphologic and immunophenotypic changes of the bone marrow. It may be worth mentioning here that flow cytometric studies in a single patient with WM and lytic bone lesions showed a hybrid phenotype with strong expression of CD38, CD20 and FMC7 but absence of CD45 and DR (Haghighi et al. 1998).

15.2.2
Bone Marrow

The bone marrow is always involved in WM. It shows a diffuse proliferation of small lymphocytes, plasmacytoid lymphocytes (i.e. cells with abundant basophilic cytoplasm but lymphocyte-like nuclei) and plasma cells. Mast cells and Dutcher bodies (i.e. PAS positive intranuclear and intracytoplasmic inclusions of IgM) may be seen. Histological patterns of bone marrow infiltration in 22 patients with WM were diffuse (45%), nodular-interstitial (22%), mixed paratrabecular-nodular (20%) and paratrabecular (13%) (Andriko et al. 1997).

Magnetic resonance (MR) imaging has been applied to the study of the bone marrow in patients with WM. Duhem et al. (1994) reported bone marrow abnormalities in all 7 patients with WM who were studied with MR imaging. We found MR imaging evidence of marrow involvement in 91% of 23 patients with WM (Moulopoulos et al. 1993). MR imaging patterns of marrow involvement were diffuse or variegated (Figs. 15.1, 15.2). In diffuse patterns there was complete absence of normal bone marrow signal intensity. On T1-weighted images the signal intensity of the abnormal marrow was equal to or lower than that of muscle (in the spine the signal intensity of the abnormal marrow was equal to or even lower than that of the intervertebral disc which is usually hypointense to normal bone marrow). On T2-weighted MR images the signal intensity of the abnormal bone marrow increased and on T1-weighted images obtained after the intravenous administration of contrast, abnormal marrow enhanced. Variegated patterns consisted of innumerable small foci of abnormal signal intensity

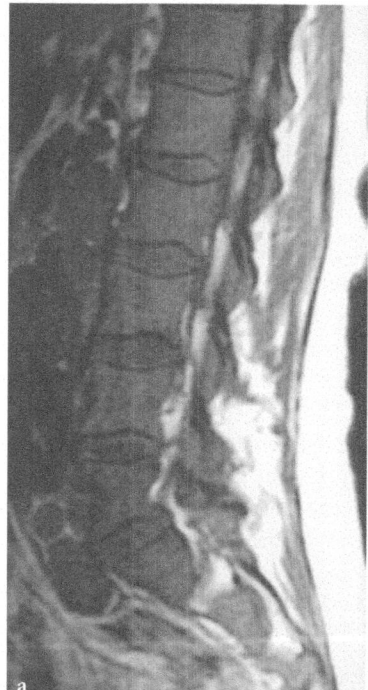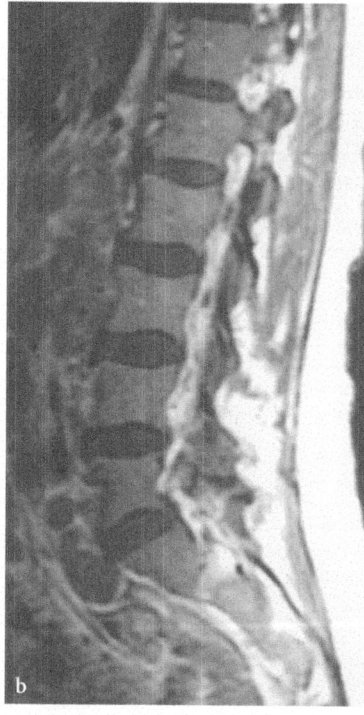

Fig. 15.1a,b. Waldenström macroglobulinemia and diffuse bone marrow involvement in a 52-year-old man. Sagittal fast spin-echo T1-weighted MR images of the lumbosacral spine (a) before and (b) after contrast administration show (a) hypointensity of bone marrow (note similar signal intensity of vertebral bodies to intervertebral discs) which take up contrast homogeneously on the (b) enhanced image. There are also multiple enlarged retroperitoneal nodes.

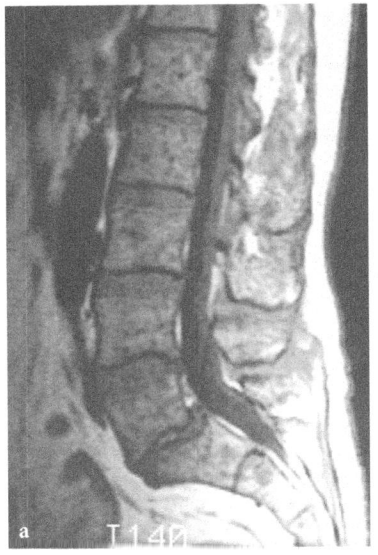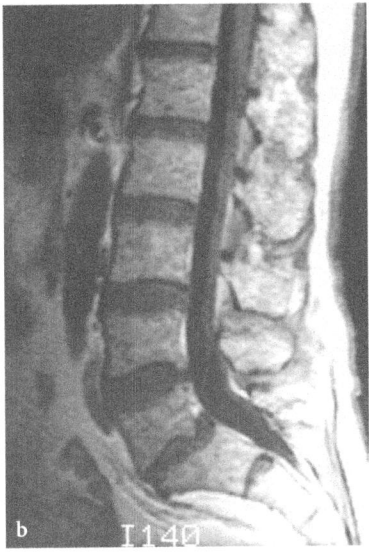

Fig. 15.2a,b. Waldenström macroglobulinemia and variegated bone marrow involvement in a 57-year-old man. Sagittal fast spin-echo T1-weighted MR images of the lumbosacral spine (**a**) before and (**b**) after contrast administration show (**a**) innumerable small hypointense foci which take up contrast on the (**b**) enhanced image.

on a background of intact bone marrow. These small foci were hypointense to uninvolved bone marrow on T1-weighted images, hyperintense on T2-weighted images and they enhanced on post contrast images. The absence of focal patterns of bone marrow involvement is in keeping with the rarity of lytic bone lesions in WM and with the more dispersed pattern of malignant infiltration of the bone marrow observed in this disease. In multiple myeloma, focal patterns are more common and they are more frequently associated with focal areas of bone destruction. The appearance of bone marrow involvement in WM may not be differentiated from that of other causes of diffuse or variegated bone marrow infiltration.

A close correlation of the MR imaging appearance of the bone marrow with laboratory parameters of tumor burden has been shown (MOULOPOULOS et al. 1993). Diffuse MR imaging patterns of bone marrow involvement in WM are observed in patients with more advanced disease. An association exists between MR imaging patterns and values of hemoglobin and marrow-lymphoplasmacytoid indices but not between MR imaging patterns and values of β2-microglobulin or monoclonal protein. Increased grades of contrast uptake on enhanced MR images are associated with lower hemoglobin values and higher lymphoplasmacytoid indices, i.e. more advanced disease. MR imaging assessment or response to therapy was consistent with clinical and laboratory staging in 7 patients who were studied before and after treatment, indicating a potential role for this modality as a noninvasive means of staging WM (MOULOPOULOS et al. 1993).

15.3
Reticuloendothelial System

The reticuloendothelial system is involved in one third of patients with WM. Enlarged nodes are not painful or tender and occur at several superficial sites. Retroperitoneal lymph nodes are involved more often than mediastinal nodes (Figs. 15.3–15.5). We identified enlarged lymph nodes on computed tomography (CT) scans of the abdomen and pelvis in 43% of 23 patients with WM (MOULOPOULOS et al. 1993). In most patients multiple nodal groups were involved along the retrocrural, retroperitoneal, iliac and inguinal nodal chains. Nodal involvement was indicative of increased tumor burden.

Splenomegaly is observed in up to 30% of patients with WM and is usually of mild or moderate degree (Fig. 15.6). Occasional patients present or develop massive and symptomatic splenomegaly, which causes pancytopenia. Limited case reports suggest that splenectomy may be helpful for managing symptomatic splenomegaly. Furthermore, in patients with massive splenomegaly who underwent splenectomy, a significant decrease or even disappearance of the monoclonal IgM has been reported (DIMOPOULOS et al. 2000).

Mild or moderate hepatomegaly is present in one-fifth of patients with WM. It is not usually associated with focal lesions on imaging studies or impairment of liver function tests (DIMOPOULOS et al. 2000).

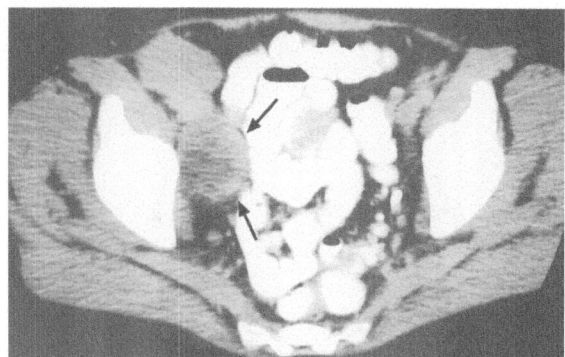

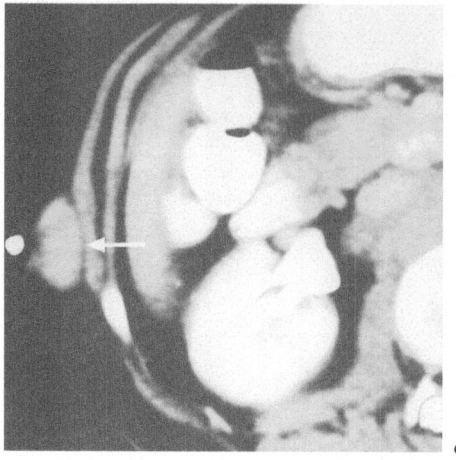

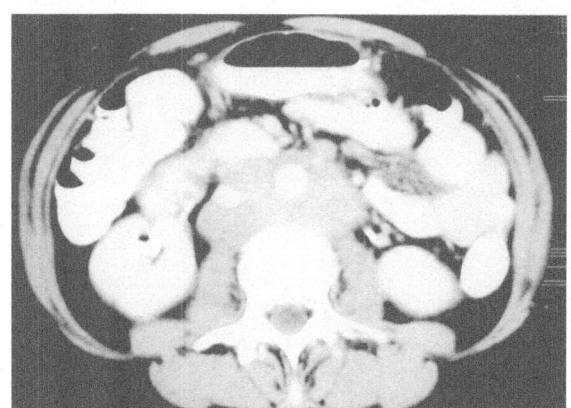

Fig. 15.3a–c. Waldenström macroglobulinemia with enlarged lymph nodes and subcutaneous lesions in a 65-year-old man. a Axial unenhanced CT scan of the pelvis shows enlarged right obdurator lymph nodes (*arrows*). b Axial contrast-enhanced CT scan of the abdomen shows enlarged retroperitoneal lymph nodes surrounding the aorta and the inferior vena cava. c Axial contrast-enhanced CT scan of the abdomen in the same patient shows 2 cm subcutaneous nodule (*arrow*).

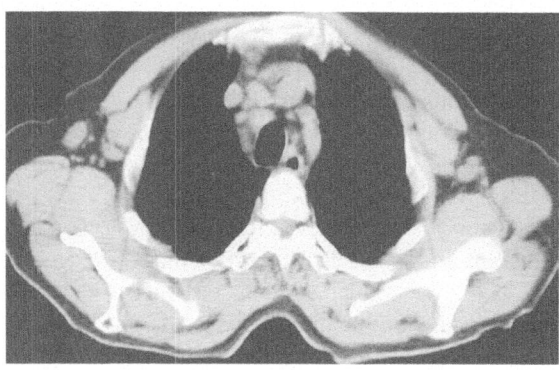

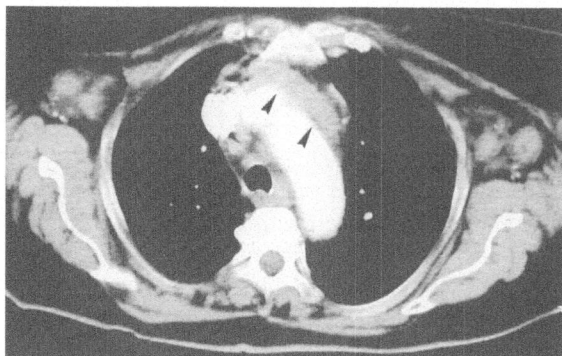

Fig. 15.4. Waldenström macroglobulinemia with enlarged lymph nodes in an 82-year-old man. Axial CT scan of the chest shows enlarged anterior mediastinal and axillary lymph nodes.

Fig. 15.5. Waldenström macroglobulinemia and lymph node involvement in a 78-year-old woman. Axial contrast-enhanced CT scan of the chest shows small right paratracheal nodes, an enlarged thymus (*arrowheads*) and large axillary lymph nodes.

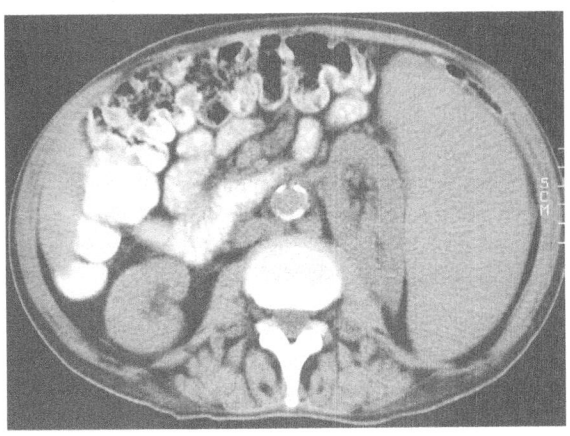

Fig. 15.6. Waldenström macroglobulinemia and marked splenomegaly in an 80-year-old man. Axial unenhanced CT scan of the abdomen shows markedly enlarged spleen displacing left kidney medially.

15.4
Central Nervous System

About 10% of patients with WM suffer from a chronic, sensorimotor peripheral neuropathy, which is, in most cases, a demyelinating process. Peripheral neuropathy may develop as a result of the monoclonal IgM protein acting as an antibody against myelin or various gangliosides or it may be caused by cryoglobulinemia, amyloidosis or direct infiltration of the nerves by malignant cells.

Central manifestations such as stroke, subarachnoid hemorrhage, and multifocal leukoencephalopathy are rare in patients with WM (KYLE and GARTON 1987). Infiltration of the meninges simulating meningioma or leptomeningeal disease has been reported (RICHARDS 1995; ABAD et al. 1999).

15.5
Genitourinary System

Renal disease is less common in WM and it is usually due to subendothelial deposition of circulating IgM. Patients may present with mild proteinuria, which is usually reversible. Nephrotic syndrome may be caused by amyloid deposition complicating the disease (DIMOPOULOS and ALEXANIAN 1994). Renal or perirenal infiltration by malignant cells are unusual presentations of WM observed in only 4 (6%) of 64 patients with WM (MOORE et al. 1995). Renal involvement consisted of renal nodules in one

patient and renal masses in another (Fig. 15.7). Perirenal involvement manifested as a mass enveloping an otherwise normal kidney in one patient and as small tumorous nodules in another. All 4 patients had enlarged retroperitoneal lymph nodes.

15.6
Gastrointestinal Tract

Gastrointestinal manifestations are infrequent and nonspecific; patients may present with diarrhea and symptoms of malabsorption. Radiological examination of the small bowel may show thickening of the valvulae conniventes and a granular appearance due to punctate filling defects representing the distended villi (KYLE 1998). Histological examination may show infiltration of the lamina propria by cells that appear cytologically benign but are polyclonal on immunohistochemical stains (VELOSO et al. 1988). Gastric involvement is exceedingly rare, with less than 10 cases reported in the literature (Fig. 15.8). A case of localized gastric lymphoplasmacytoid involvement was reported in a patient with high serum monoclonal IgM lambda paraprotein (ROSENTHAL et al. 1998). CT scan showed diffuse thickening of the gastric wall. The disease responded well to treatment with chemotherapy and local radiotherapy.

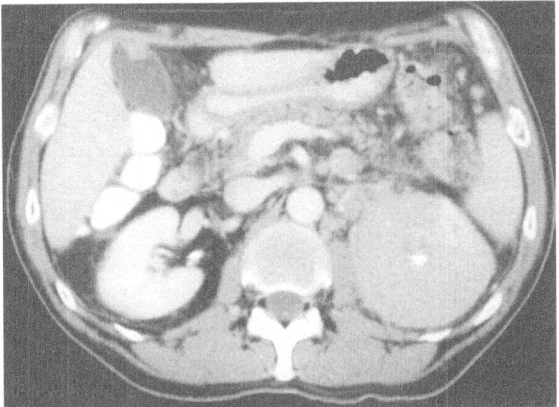

Fig. 15.7. Waldenström macroglobulinemia and renal involvement in a 70-year-old man. Axial contrast-enhanced CT scan of the abdomen shows hypodense left renal mass, which conforms to the contour of the kidney.

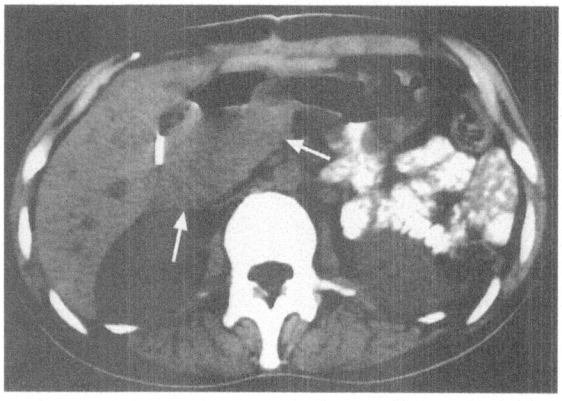

Fig. 15.8. Waldenström macroglobulinemia and gastric involvement in a 37-year-old woman. Axial unenhanced CT scan of the abdomen shows large mass of pyloric antrum (*arrows*).

15.7
Thorax

Although uncommon, a variety of pulmonary manifestations have been described in patients with WM. Symptoms of pulmonary involvement include dyspnea, nonproductive cough and chest pain. Manifestations from the lungs include pulmonary infiltrates, isolated masses and pleural effusions (Fig. 15.9) (RAUSCH and HERION 1980). These abnormalities may regress with the application of effective treatment and they do not affect disease prognosis.

15.8
Skin

IgM skin deposits may cause flesh-colored papules (LOWE et al. 1996; WHITTAKER et al. 1996). Urticarial lesions may be caused by lymphoplasmacytoid infiltration of the dermis or by IgM expression of antiepidermal basement membrane antibodies (SCHNITZLER et al. 1974).

15.9
Other Organ Involvement

Ocular manifestations of WM are usually limited to the retina and are produced by the increased plasma viscosity. A retroorbital aggregate of lymphoplasmacytoid cells may cause proptosis and reduced eye motility (ETTL et al. 1992; SHEN et al. 2000). Lacrimal gland involvement and infiltration of the conjunctiva and vitreous have been reported (KRISHNAN and ADAMS 1995).

Involvement of the breast in the form of a nodule was reported in a patient with WM and was best shown on CT scans and color Doppler ultrasound. The patient had extensive nodal disease in the chest, abdomen and pelvis (LAMB et al. 1999).

15.10
Treatment

Patients who are diagnosed with WM by chance and who do not have anemia, organomegaly, hyperviscosity or other IgM-related complications, should not be treated at presentation but should be followed with serial clinical and laboratory assessments. Plasmapheresis, which reduces the amount of circulating IgM, and chemotherapy, which inhibits tumor growth, are the standard treatment for WM. Primary chemotherapy for symptomatic patients consists of oral chlorambucil. Combinations of alkylating agents do not offer any further benefit. Chlorambucil, combined with plasmapheresis when symptomatic hyperviscosity is present, is usually adequate treatment for elderly patients without other life-threatening complications. Nucleoside analogues such as cladribine or fludarabine are highly active agents, which can induce responses more rapidly than chlorambucil (DIMOPOULOS et al. 2000). Although it is not known whether primary therapy with nucleoside analogues may prolong patients' survival, these agents may be

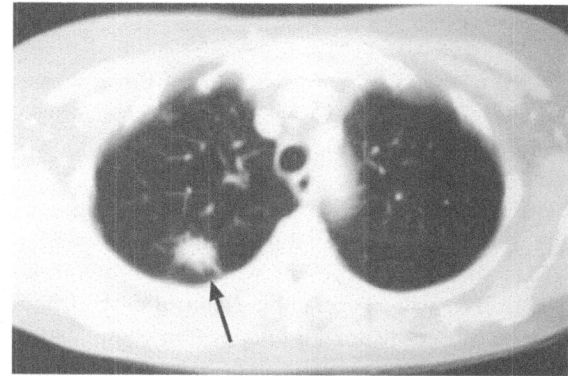

Fig. 15.9. Waldenström macroglobulinemia and lung involvement in a 65-year-old woman. Axial CT scan of the chest shows spiculated right upper lobe lung nodule (*arrow*). Multiple other lung nodules were present (*not shown*).

the primary treatment of choice when rapid control of the disease is necessary. For disease resistant to alkylating agents either fludarabine or cladribine can induce responses in about one-third of patients. Recent evidence suggests that the anti-CD20 monoclonal antibody rituximab, is active in approximately 40% of patients with WM (DIMOPOULOS et al. 2002). This treatment option is of particular interest because it is not associated with myelosuppression. Finally, high dose therapy with autologous stem cell support may induce disease control even in patients resistant to chemotherapy (ANAGNOSTOPOULOS and GIRALT 2002). The use of plasmapheresis is indicated for the treatment of symptomatic hyperviscosity and limited data support its use for the treatment of certain complications associated with IgM monoclonal proteins, such as neuropathy or cryoglobulinemia. In such cases, plasmapheresis should be regarded as interim therapy until definitive treatment can be initiated (DIMOPOULOS et al. 2000).

15.11
Prognosis

WM is a relatively indolent disease with a median survival of 5 to 10 years in different series. Most studies have indicated that advanced age, anemia, hypoalbuminemia and elevated levels of serum β-microglobulin are associated with inferior outcome (KYRTSONIS et al. 2001; GARCIA-SANZ et al. 2001; MOREL et al. 2000). Most patients with WM die of progressive disease, which has become refractory to treatment. In advanced stages of the disease, many patients suffer from the complications of pancytopenia (i.e. infections, bleeding), which is usually due to the heavily infiltrated bone marrow. However, some patients develop myelodysplastic syndrome or secondary acute myelogenous leukemia, and in others the disease may transform into a diffuse large cell lymphoma (DIMOPOULOS et al. 2000).

15.12
Conclusion

Waldenström macroglobulinemia is due to a malignant lymphoplasmacytic infiltrate of the bone marrow, which produces monoclonal IgM. Patients more often present with anemia, splenomegaly and enlarged lymph nodes. Unique features of this

disease rarely seen in other lymphoproliferative disorders include hyperviscosity, cryoglobulinemia, cold-agglutinin disease and peripheral neuropathy. MR imaging will show bone marrow involvement in most patients and it may provide information on tumor burden and assessment of response to therapy. Unlike multiple myeloma, focal bone lesions are rarely seen on conventional radiographs or on MR imaging studies. CT of the abdomen and pelvis will show enlarged lymph nodes in over one third of patients. Occasionally, patients with WM have been reported with lung, renal, gastrointestinal, and other organ involvement. Standard primary treatment for symptomatic patients consists of chemotherapy such as oral chlorambucil or a nucleoside analogue (fludarabine, cladribine). Plasmapheresis may be required when a hyperviscosity syndrome is prominent.

References

Abad S, Zagdanski AM, Brechgnac S, et al. (1999) Neurolymphomatosis in Waldenström's macroglobulinaemia. Br J Haematol 106:100–103

Anagnostopoulos A, Giralt S (2002) Stem cell transplantation for Waldenström's macroglobulinemia. Bone Marrow Transplant 29:943–947

Andriko JA, Aguilera NS, Chu WS, et al. (1997) Waldenström's macroglobulinemia: a clinicopathologic study of 22 cases. Cancer 15:1926–1935

Dimopoulos MA, Alexanian A (1994) Waldenström's macroglobulinemia. Blood 83:1452–1459

Dimopoulos MA, Panayotidis P, Moulopoulos LA, et al. (2000) Waldenström's macroglobulinemia: clinical features, complications and management. J Clin Oncol 18:214–226

Dimopoulos MA, Zervas C, Zomas A, et al. (2002) Treatment of Waldenström's macroglobulinemia with rituximab. J Clin Oncol 20:2327–2333

Duhem C, Ries F, Dicato M (1994) Accuracy of magnetic resonance imaging (MRI) of bone marrow in Waldenström's macroglobulinemia (abstract 2598). Blood 84:653

Ettl AR, Birbamer GG, Philipp W (1992) Orbital involvement in Waldenström's macroglobulinemia: ultrasound, computed tomography and magnetic resonance findings. Ophthalmologica 205:40–45

Garcia-Sanz R, Montoto S, Torrequebrada A, et al. (2001) Waldenström macroglobulinaemia: presenting features and outcome in a series with 217 cases. Br J Haematol 115:575–582

Groves FD, Travis LB, Devesa SS, et al. (1998) Waldenström's macroglobulinemia: incidence patterns in the United States, 1988–1994. Cancer 82:1078–1081

Haghighi B, Yanagihara R, Cornbleet PJ (1998) IgM myeloma: case report with immunophenotypic profile. Am J Hematol 59:302–308

Harris NL, Jaffe ES, Stein H, et al. (1994) A revised European-American classification of lymphoid neoplasms: a proposal from the International Lymphoma Study Group. Blood 84:1361–1392

Herrington LJ, Weiss NS (1993) Incidence of Waldenström's macroglobulinemia. Blood 82:3148–3150

Krishnan K, Adams PT (1995) Bilateral orbital tumors and lacrimal gland involvement in Waldenström's macroglobulinemia. Eur J Hematol 55:205–206

Kyle RA (1998) Waldenström's macroglobulinemia. In: Malpas JS, Bergsagel DE, Kyle R, Anderson K (eds) Myeloma: biology and treatment. Oxford University Press, New York, pp 639–662

Kyle RA, Garton JP (1987) The spectrum of IgM monoclonal gammopathy in 430 cases. Mayo Clin Proc 62:719–731

Kyrtsonis MC, Vassilakopoulos TP, Angelopoulou MK, et al. (2001) Waldenström's macroglobulinemia: clinical course and prognostic factors in 60 patients. Experience from a single hematology unit. Ann Hematol 80:722–727

Lamb PM, Perry NM, Mulele CK (1999) Waldenström's macroglobulinemia of the breast detected by colour Doppler ultrasound. Br J Radiol 72:82–84

Lowe L, Fitzpatrick JE, Huff JC, et al. (1996) Cutaneous macroglobulinosis. Arch Dermatol 135:283–286

Moore DF, Moulopoulos LA, Dimopoulos MA (1995) Waldenström's macroglobulinemia presenting as a renal or perirenal mass: clinical and radiographic features. Leuk Lymphoma 17:331–334

Morel P, Monconduit M, Jacomy D, et al. (2000) Prognostic factors in Waldenström's macroglobulinemia: a report in 232 patients with the description of a new scoring system and its validation on 253 other patients. Blood 96: 852–858

Moulopoulos LA, Dimopoulos MA, Varma DGK, et al. (1993) Waldenström's macroglobulinemia: MR imaging of the spine and CT of the abdomen and pelvis. Radiology 188: 669–673

Rausch PG, Herion JC (1980) Pulmonary manifestations of Waldenström's macroglobulinemia. Am J Hematol 9: 201–209

Renier G, Ifrah N, Chevalier A, et al. (1989) Four brothers with Waldenström's macroglobulinemia. Cancer 64:1554–1559

Richards AI (1995) Response of meningeal Waldenström's macroglobulinemia to 2-chlorodeoxyadenosine. J Clin Oncol 13:2476

Rosenthal JA, Curran WJ Jr, Schuster SJ (1998) Waldenström's macroglobulinemia resulting from localized gastric lymphoplasmacytoid lymphoma. Am J Hematol 58:244–245

Schnitzler L, Schubert B, Boasson M, et al. (1974) Urticaire chronique, lesions osseuses, macroglobulinemie IgM: maladie de Waldenström? Bull Soc Fr Dermatol Syphiligr 81:363

Shen DF, Fardeau C, Roberge FG, et al. (2000) Rearrangement of immunoglobulin gene in metastatic Waldenström macroglobulinemia to the vitreous. Am J Ophthalmol 129: 395–396

Tepper A, Moss CE (1994) Waldenstrom's macroglobulinemia: search for occupational exposure. J Occup Med 36: 133–136

Veloso FT, Fraga J, Saleiro JV (1988) Macroglobulinemia and small intestine disease. A case report with review of the literature. J Clin Gastroenterol 10:546–550

Waldenström J (1944) Incipient myelomatosis or "essential" hyperglobulinemia with fibrinogenopenia–A new syndrome? Acta Med Scand 117:216–222

Whittaker SJ, Bhogla BS, Black MM (1996) Acquired immunobullous disease: a cutaneous manifestation of IgM macroglobulinemia. Br J Dermatol 135:283–286

16 Multiple Myeloma

Bruno C. Vande Berg, Frédéric E. Lecouvet, Baudouin E. Maldague, Jacques Malghem

CONTENTS

Bruno C. Vande Berg, MD, PhD
Associate Professor, Department of Radiology and Medical Imaging, Saint Luc University Hospital, Université Catholique de Louvain, 10 Avenue Hippocrate, B-1200 Brussels, Belgium
Frédéric E. Lecouvet, MD, PhD
Assistant Professor, Department of Radiology and Medical Imaging, Saint Luc University Hospital, Université Catholique de Louvain, 10 Avenue Hippocrate, B-1200 Brussels, Belgium
Baudouin E. Maldague, MD
Professor, Department of Radiology and Medical Imaging, Saint Luc University Hospital, Université Catholique de Louvain, 10 Avenue Hippocrate, B-1200 Brussels, Belgium
Jacques Malghem, MD
Professor, Department of Radiology and Medical Imaging, Saint Luc University Hospital, Université Catholique de Louvain, 10 Avenue Hippocrate, B-1200 Brussels, Belgium

16.1 Introduction

Multiple myeloma (or Kahler disease, plasma cell myeloma) is the most severe form of several diseases known as plasma cell dyscrasias or monoclonal gammopathies. These diseases share two features: uncontrolled proliferation and accumulation of plasma cells in the bone marrow and the presence in serum and/or in urine of a monoclonal immunoglobulin (known as "paraprotein" or "M component" – M for monoclonal or myeloma) or immunoglobulin fragments (the light chain or Bence-Jones protein). Multiple myeloma is a disease of the late middle-aged and elderly, with a median age at diagnosis of 65 years, and a slight male preponderance. It has an average incidence of about 3 per 100,000 but an approximately double incidence in blacks compared to the white population. It accounts for approximately 10% of hematological malignancies and 1% of all cancers (Kapadia 1980; Salmon and Cassady 1995; Malpas and Caroll 1995).

16.2 Clinical Features

16.2.1 Pathophysiology and Diagnosis

Typically, multiple myeloma includes marrow infiltration by abnormal plasma cells and plasmablasts, overproduction of monoclonal immunoglobulin, and presence of light chains (Bence-Jones protein) in the urine and bone destruction. The presence of at least 10% plasma cells in bone marrow aspirates or biopsies obtained at blind bone marrow biopsy is the minimum criterion for diagnosis of multiple myeloma (Terpstra et al. 1992; Greipp 1992; Boccadoro and Pileri 1997). Several authors distinguish smoldering, indolent and overt myeloma with respective threshold levels of marrow plasmacytosis of 10, 20 and 30% (MALPAS and CAROLL 1995). Serum monoclonal components determine a sharp peak (or spike, "M" band) in the γ globulin region on electrophoresis. Urinary monoclonal components are usually detected in concentrates of 24-hour urine collection and migrate similarly on electrophoresis. The most commonly produced monoclonal protein is IgG (about 60% of cases), followed by IgA (about 20%), light chains only (15–20%) and IgD (about 1%). IgE and IgM myeloma are rare. In 1–2%, no monoclonal component can be detected in either serum or urine ("non secretory myeloma") (SALMON and CASSADY 1995).

Excessive bone resorption is a characteristic feature of the disease: focal osteolytic lesions and diffuse osteoporosis are present alone or in association in up to 85% of patients, on radiographic skeletal surveys and at autopsy (KAPADIA 1980; BATAILLE et al. 1992). Bone destruction may result from increased osteoclastic resorption and inhibition of new bone formation. Bone biopsies and histomorphometric studies from myeloma patients demonstrate increased numbers of osteoclasts and increased proportion of bone surface undergoing resorption in close vicinity to the abnormal plasma cells (BATAILLE et al. 1986). These cells or their microenvironment synthesize and release "osteoclast activating factors" that stimulate the resorption process (MUNDY et al. 1974). Several cytokines have been identified, among which interleukin (IL)-1β, IL-6 and tumor necrosis factor seem to play a key role in promoting osteoclast formation and bone resorption (CROUCHER and APPERLEY 1998; KLEIN et al. 1995). Osteoclastic bone resorption is generally an early phenomenon in the disease course; inhibition of bone formation occurs later and leads to further aggravation of osteoporosis (BATAILLE et al. 1992). In addition, glucocorticoids that are often included in therapy regimen may also contribute to bone loss. The lack of lytic bone lesions in some patients or the rare cases presenting sclerotic lesions could reflect the combination of increased bone resorption with a normal or even increased bone formation (BATAILLE et al. 1992).

16.2.2
Clinical Presentation

Prominent symptoms observed in myeloma patients result from monoclonal protein secretion and from abnormal plasma cell accumulation in the marrow spaces. Bone pain is one of the commonest present-ing symptoms, being present in 37–87% of patients and frequently involves the back and ribs (KAPADIA 1980; MALPAS and CAROLL 1995; RICCARDI et al. 1991). Pain most likely results from fractures or increased medullary pressure. Isolated lesions, for example in the skull, do not appear painful. Vertebral compression fractures are present in 55–80% of myeloma during disease course. Spinal cord or nerve root compression occurs in 10–15% of cases (RICCARDI et al. 1991; SPIESS et al. 1988). They are the initial clinical symptom in 34–64% of cases. Repeated vertebral fractures may lead to a loss of height or exaggerated kyphosis. Non-vertebral fractures are seen in more than 30% of patients.

Weakness and fatigue are frequent and correlate closely with the level of anemia (RICCARDI et al. 1991; KYLE 1975). Other consequences of bone marrow suppression include chronic bleeding or purpura on the skin due to thrombocytopenia, and infection and fever due to leukopenia and depletion of normal immunoglobulins (MALPAS and CAROLL 1995). Hypercalcemia due to bone resorption is observed in one third of patients and may be the presenting feature (WEINSTEIN 1992). Acute or chronic renal failure may be observed as a consequence of Bence-Jones proteinuria, hypercalcemia, hyperuricemia, amyloidosis or renal infection.

16.2.3
Staging and Prognostic Factors

Survival in untreated patients with MM is extremely variable and ranges from a few months to many years (KYLE 1983). Indeed, the diagnosis of myeloma does not represent an absolute mandate for immediate treatment. The variability in the pace of disease progression and in individual symptoms, and the need to optimize the therapeutic strategy to the aggressiveness of the disease has raised the need for staging systems. The clinical staging system proposed by DURIE and SALMON (1975) is still commonly used because of its easy application. This staging system is based on blood levels of calcium, hemoglobin, immunoglobulin and of radiographic evidence of lytic bone lesions. It distinguishes different patient subsets in terms of tumor mass and disease aggressiveness (Table 16.1). Smoldering and indolent or Durie and Salmon stage I myeloma are considered to be associated with low tumor burden, evolve slowly, and are generally not treated until careful clinical follow up is performed to detect significant evolution and trigger treatment (KYLE and

Table 16.1. The Durie and Salmon myeloma staging system (Durie and Salmon 1975)

Stage*	Criteria
I	All of the following: 　Hemoglobin value: > 10 g/dl (100 g/L) 　Normal serum calcium value 　　(≤ 12 mg/dl [3 mmol/L]) 　At radiography, normal bone structure or solitary 　　bone plasmacytoma 　Only low monoclonal component production rates 　IgG value: < 5 g/dL (50 g/L) 　IgA value: < 3 g/dL (30 g/L) 　Urine light chain M component at electrophoresis: 　　< 4 g/24h
II	Fitting neither stage I nor stage III
III	One or more of the following: 　Hemoglobin value: < 8,5 g/dL (85 g/L) 　Serum calcium value: > 12 mg/dL (3 mmol/L) 　Advanced lytic bone lesion 　High monoclonal component production rates 　　IgG value: > 7 g/dL (70 g/L) 　　IgA value: > 5 g/dL (50 g/L) 　　Urine light chain M component at 　　electrophoresis: > 12 g/24h

*Subclassifications: A: relatively normal renal function (serum creatinine < 2.0 mg/dl [175 µmol/l]). B: abnormal renal function (serum creatinine ≥ 2.0 mg/dl [175 µmol/l])

Greipp 1980; Alexanian and Dimopoulos 1995). Durie and Salmon stages II and III and symptomatic overt MM are associated with high tumor mass and systemic therapy is mandatory.

However, within these different groups, prognosis is variable and many efforts have been made to define additional factors that help predict survival and response to therapy in individual patients. The serum levels of β2-microglobulin and C-reactive protein (CRP), the plasma cell labeling index, the number of circulating plasma cells, and more recently molecular biology and cytogenetic markers seem the most relevant predictors of clinical outcome (Davies et al. 1997; Boccadoro and Pileri 1995; Tricot et al. 1997). The potential for MR imaging of the bone marrow in this field also appears promising (Moulopoulos et al. 1995; Vande Berg et al. 1996; Weber et al. 1997).

16.2.4
Role of Imaging

In patients without known disease and bone symptoms, conventional radiography, CT or MR imaging can be the first line tools for their workup. In patients with newly diagnosed plasma cell

neoplasms, the radiographic skeletal survey plays a crucial role in staging. The radiographic skeletal survey includes radiographs of the skull and ribs, spine, humeri and femora. Examination of the distal aspects of the lower and upper limbs is not necessary because these areas generally contain yellow marrow and do not contain myeloma lesions. Demonstration of plasma cells containing lytic lesions in a patient with a monoclonal gammopathy is an indirect sign of high tumor mass and suggests poor spontaneous outcome. Patients with monoclonal gammopathy of undetermined significance (MGUS) and those with solitary bone plasmacytoma or early stage myeloma have no or only one lytic lesion respectively. Patients with at least two lytic foci are classified in advanced disease subgroups and aggressive systemic treatment is indicated (Durie and Salmon 1975; de Gramont et al 1985). The radiographic skeletal survey may be decisive for the therapeutic decision and clinical management in up to one third of patients with advanced myeloma who show only moderate alteration of blood parameters (Lecouvet et al. 1999).

16.3
Imaging Features of Osseous Involvement

16.3.1
Imaging Features in Untreated Multiple Myeloma

16.3.1.1
Radiographic Findings

Typical radiographic findings include focal lytic lesions, diffuse osteoporosis, and fractures alone or in association. However, normal radiographic skeletal surveys are seen in up to 20% of patients (Kapadia 2003; Kyle 1975; Carson and Ackerman 1955; Heiser and Schartzmann 1952).

16.3.1.1.1
Focal Lytic Lesions

The most common appearance of myeloma-associated focal lytic lesions is that of "punched-out", well circumscribed, round or oval translucencies (Fig. 16.1). Generally the bone trabeculae within the lesions are completely destroyed. These lesions are typically of small (up to 20 mm) and relatively homogeneous size when multiple. Their margins are sharply demarcated and surrounding sclerotic rim or periosteal reaction are exceptional. Rounded lytic

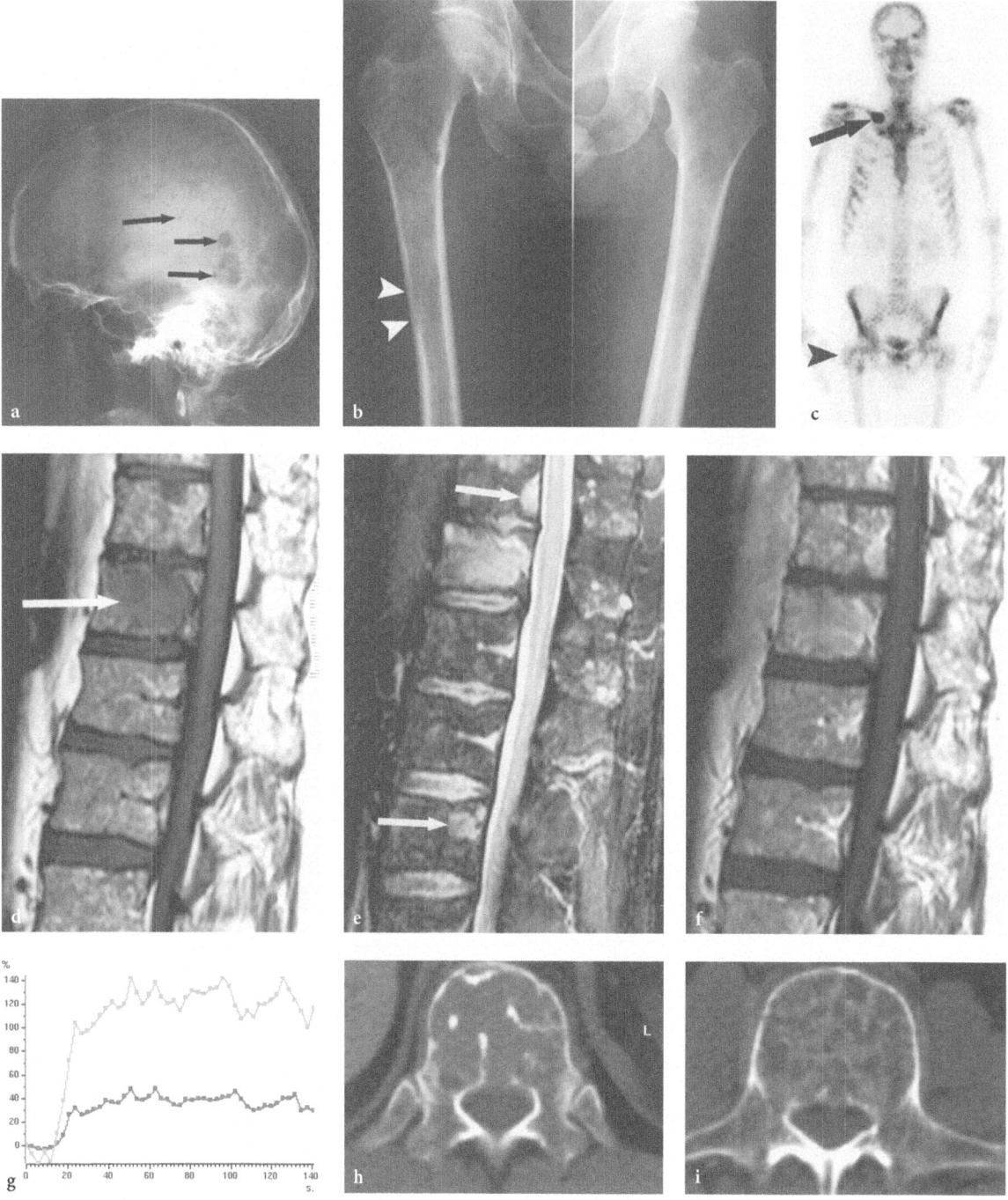

Fig. 16.1a–i. Multiple myeloma in a 44-year-old man. **a** Lateral radiograph of the skull shows multiple punched-out lytic lesions (*arrows*). **b** Comparative anteroposterior radiographs of both femurs show thinning of the cortex of the right femur with endosteal scalloping (*arrowheads*). Note the lack of periosteal reaction. The distal aspect of the right femur is spared. **c** Bone scintigraphy obtained before the diagnosis of multiple myeloma shows one definite area of increased uptake in the right clavicle (a recent fracture) (*arrow*) and a questionable area of increased uptake in the proximal right femur (*arrowhead*). The skull lesions seen on radiographs are not detected on the bone scintigraphy. **d** Sagittal T1-weighted MR image of the lumbar spine shows a hypointense lesion in the T12 vertebral body (*arrow*). Adjacent marrow shows minor signal heterogeneities. **e** On the corresponding sagittal fat-suppressed fast spin-echo T2-weighted MR image, the large T12 lesion shows hyperintensity. Multiple other hyperintense lesions are present in all vertebral bodies including the T11 and L3 vertebral bodies (*arrows*). These lesions show normal signal intensity on the sagittal T1-weighted spin-echo MR image (**d**), which is not rare in multiple myeloma. **f** The corresponding sagittal contrast-enhanced spin-echo T1-weighted MR image shows diffuse and focal enhancement of the marrow with disappearance of the lesions. **g** Enhancement curves derived from dynamic enhanced MR imaging demonstrate rapid and intense enhancement in the T12 lesion (*upper curve*) and rapid and less intense enhancement in the L3 marrow (*lower curve*). **h** Axial CT scan of the T12 lesion shows destruction of the central trabeculae and thickening of residual cortical and trabecular bone. **i** Axial CT scan of L3 vertebral body shows another pattern of bone osteolysis with poorly-delimited areas of cancellous bone destruction.

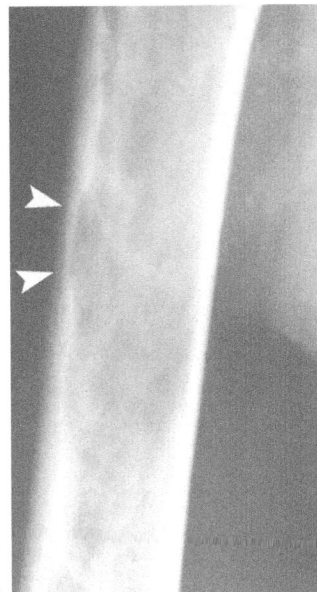
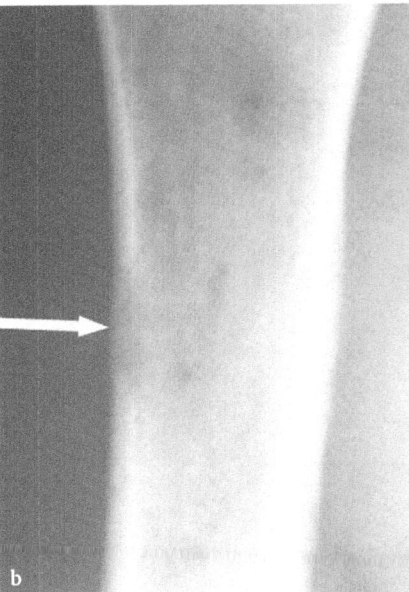

Fig. 16.2a,b. Patterns of focal lytic lesions of the humeral diaphyses in a 56-year-old and a 48-year-old woman with multiple myeloma. **a** Endosteal scalloping of the cortex (*arrowheads*) without intracortical lucencies or periosteal reaction. The intraosseous margins of the lesions are not seen. **b** Permeative osteolysis of the humeral diaphyses (*arrow*) without periosteal reaction. This pattern is relatively uncommon in multiple myeloma.

foci are found most often in the calvarium, ribs and proximal femora and humeri on conventional radiographs. In the long bones, myeloma-associated lysis involves the endosteal aspect of the cortex (Figs. 16.1, 16.2) and scalloping of the endosteal aspect of the long bones can be a unique finding, without periosteal reaction or intracortical lucencies.

Occasionally, osteolytic foci in MM patients are ill-defined leading to a "moth-eaten" or permeative appearance of the bone destruction (Fig. 16.2) (HEISER and SCHARTZMANN 1952). This pattern generally indicates a rapidly progressive lesion and is frequently associated with cortical disruptions and soft tissue mass, especially in the ribs and vertebra.

Focal osteolysis in patients with multiple myeloma can lead to the formation of a benign-looking expansive lesion with preservation of a "cortical shell", especially in the spine, ribs and pelvis (Fig. 16.3). These lesions generally grow slowly.

Radiographs frequently show predominant involvement of the skull and ribs with evident osteolysis in up to 70% of patients (Fig. 16.4) (DE GRAMONT et al. 1985; LECOUVET et al. 1999; CARSON and ACKERMAN 1955; HEISER and SCHARTZMANN 1952). This high frequency of involvement of the skull and ribs is most likely due to the thinness of these bones and to their high cortex/trabeculae bone ratio. Focal areas of trabecular bone destruction as large as 1 cm in diameter or more may not be detectable on radiographs (HEALY and ARMSTRONG 1994; ARDRAN 1951). Spine radiographs show lytic lesions in less than 50% of patients, probably because an important propor-

tion of the mineral content of a vertebra (40 to 50%) must be lost before significant bone destruction is detected on plain films.

16.3.1.1.2
Osteoporosis

Diffuse osteopenia is a frequent finding on radiographs of patients with multiple myeloma (Fig. 16.5). Autopsy findings show diffuse marrow infiltration by myeloma cells, with lesser degrees of bone destruction compared to focal osteolytic lesions. This generalized osteopenia may be homogeneous without focal translucencies and with or without accentuation of the residual vertical trabeculae. Superimposition of poorly circumscribed small areas of osteolysis may be responsible for a heterogeneous appearance, or spotty osteoporosis, often missed in the spine, but more easily detected in the ribs, skull and long bones (Fig. 16.2).

16.3.1.1.3
Sclerotic Bone Lesions

Spontaneous sclerosis is observed in 1–3% of myeloma patients (HALL and GORE 1988). Nodular or punctate sclerotic foci or diffuse osteosclerosis of the axial skeleton may be observed as isolated abnormalities, or very rarely in association with more classic "punched-out" or ill-defined osteolytic lesions (Fig. 16.6). Osteosclerotic myeloma has several distinctive clinical features compared to common myeloma: patients are generally younger at onset, the

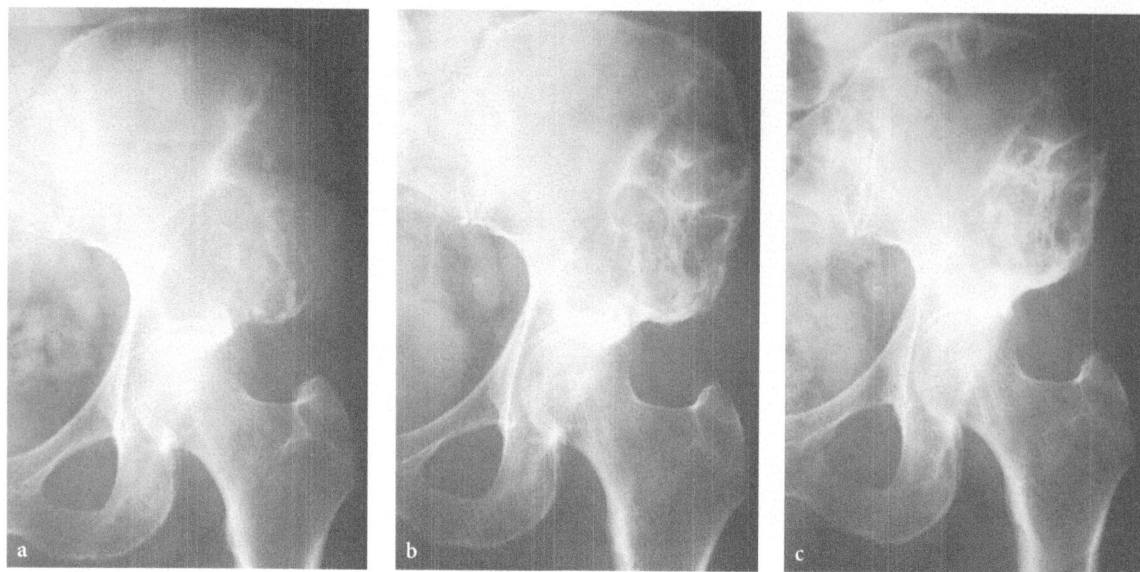

Fig. 16.3a–c. Expansile lytic lesion in a 52-year-old woman at diagnosis of multiple myeloma and during treatment. **a** Initial radiograph of the left iliac bone shows a large expansile lytic lesion. **b** Two and (**c**) six-year follow-up radiographs obtained during treatment show reappearance of the cortex and progressive decrease in size of the expansile extraosseous component. The intraosseous margins remain unchanged. Six years later, new lesions are visible in the proximal femur, that indicate active disease.

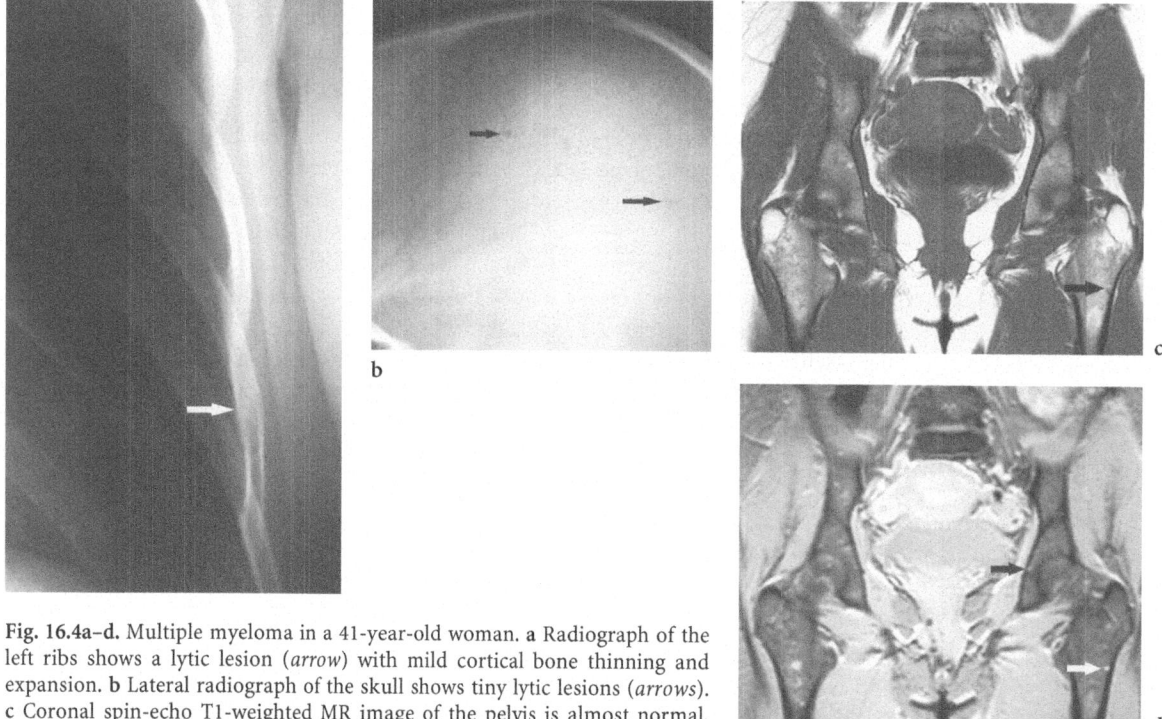

Fig. 16.4a–d. Multiple myeloma in a 41-year-old woman. **a** Radiograph of the left ribs shows a lytic lesion (*arrow*) with mild cortical bone thinning and expansion. **b** Lateral radiograph of the skull shows tiny lytic lesions (*arrows*). **c** Coronal spin-echo T1-weighted MR image of the pelvis is almost normal, except for a possible lesion adjacent to the cortex in the left femur (*arrow*). **d** Corresponding coronal gradient-echo T2*-weighted MR image shows multiple hyperintense areas that probably correspond to myeloma lesions (*arrows*). Gradient-echo T2*-weighted MR images occasionally better show the marrow lesions that the T1-weighted MR images because of focal osteolysis and subsequent disappearance of the trabecular bone-dependent decrease in signal intensity of the normal medullary cavity.

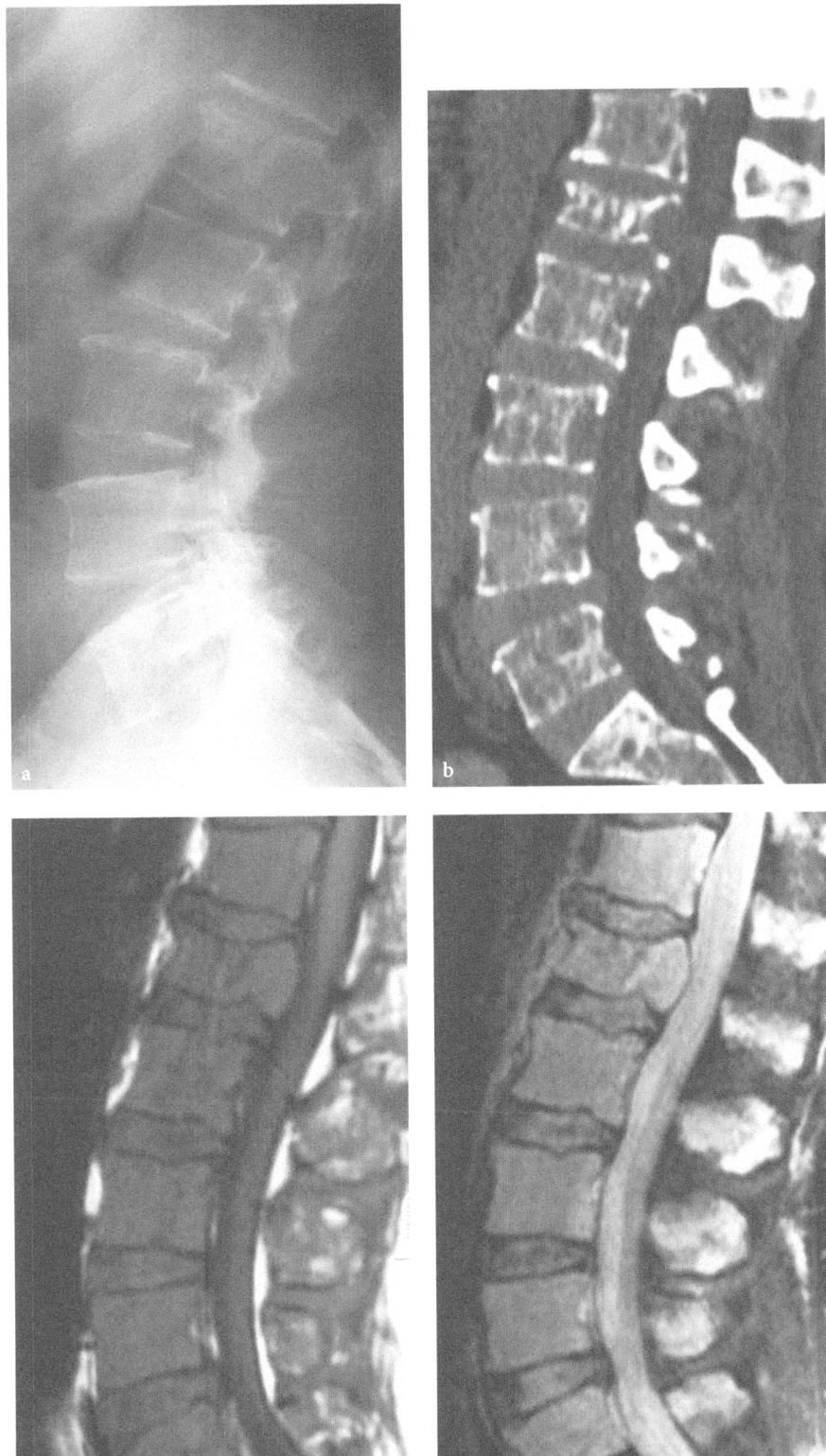

Fig. 16.5a–d. Bone and marrow lesions in a 54-year-old man with multiple myeloma. **a** Lateral radiograph of the lumbar spine shows heterogeneous osteoporosis with deformity of the T12 vertebral body. No definite bone lesions can be seen. **b** Sagittal reconstruction from spiral CT scan of the corresponding lumbar spine demonstrates multiple lytic lesions and fracture of T12. Sagittal (**c**) spin-echo T1 and (**d**) fat-suppressed fast spin-echo T2-weighted MR images show diffuse marrow infiltration, with marrow signal intensity lower than that of the intervertebral disks on T1-weighted images. Bulging of the posterior wall of T12 is well seen. On T2-weighted images, the signal of the abnormal marrow is diffusely increased, but there is no internal standard of reference with which to compare the signal intensity of the marrow.

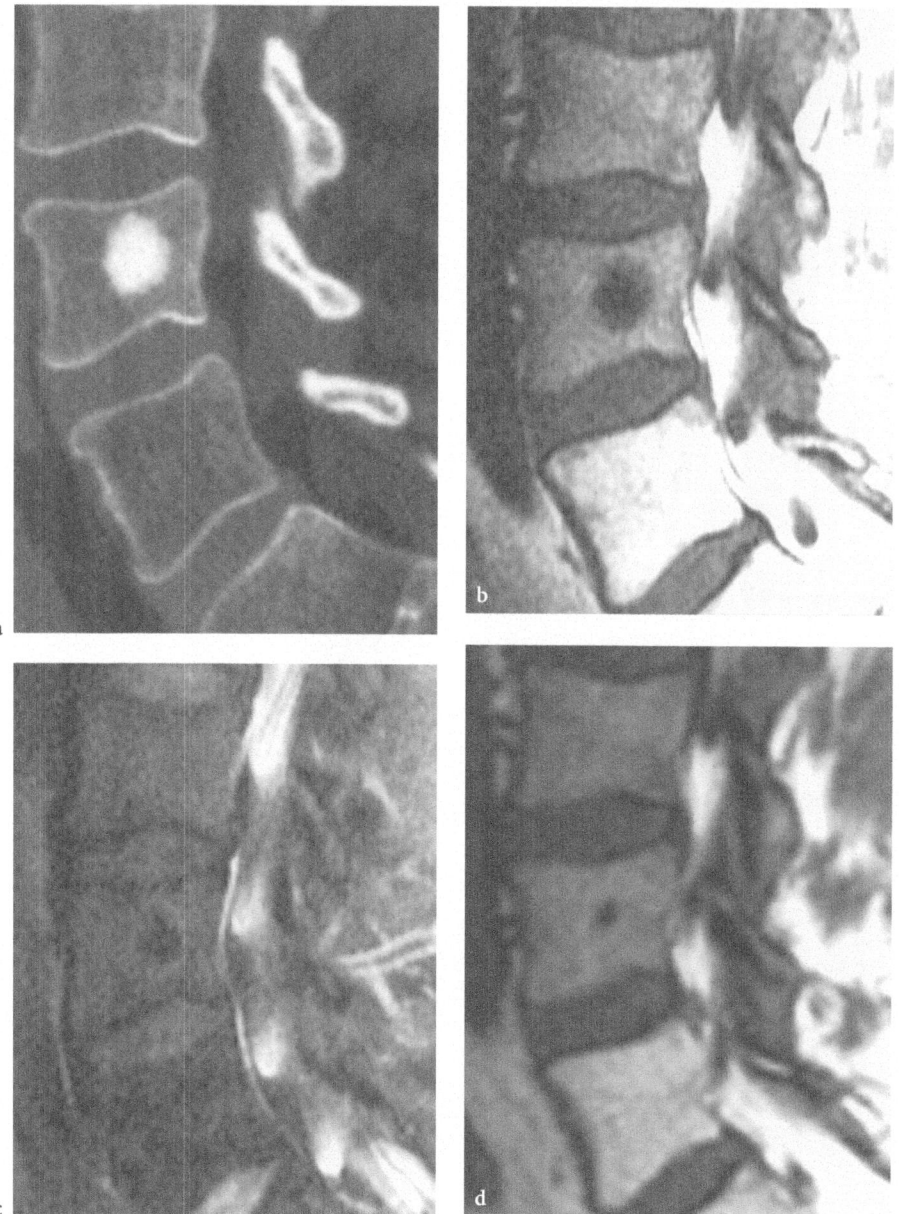

Fig. 16.6a–d. Sclerotic multiple myeloma in a 57-year-old man. He presented with polyneuropathy and monoclonal gammopathy. a Sagittal reformatted CT image of the lumbar spine shows a sclerotic bone lesion within the L4 vertebral body. The lesion is similar to a bone island, but the central location is unusual for a simple bone island that is generally near the vertebral walls. Other sclerotic lesions were seen and in association with the polyneuropathy, a diagnosis of POEMS syndrome was suggested. Sagittal (b) T1 and (c) fat-suppressed fast spin-echo T2-weighted MR images of the lumbar spine show hypointense lesion in the L4 vertebral body, surrounded by discrete edema. d Sagittal spin-echo T1-weighted MR image of the lumbar spine obtained 4 years ago demonstrates that the L4 lesion was much smaller.

male/female ratio is higher, serum levels of monoclonal immunoglobulins and marrow plasmacytosis are lower, and survival is usually longer. Polyneuropathy may be observed in up to 50% of patients whereas its frequency in lytic myeloma is about 3% (IWASHITA et al. 1977). Although polyneuropathy is the most frequent presenting feature associated with the sclerotic myeloma, a spectrum of other manifestations may be observed. These abnormalities have been summarized by the acronym POEMS, which stands for polyneuropathy (P), organomegaly (O) (hepatosplenomegaly, adenopathy), endocrinopathy, (E), monoclonal (M) protein, and skin (S) changes. Beside

nodular or more diffuse osteosclerosis, the presence of a sclerotic rim surrounding a radiolucent center is common in this entity (HALL and GORE 1988).

16.3.1.2
CT Findings

On CT images, an extremely wide spectrum of osteolysis patterns can be seen, even in the same patient (LECOUVET et al. 2001; LAROCHE et al. 1996). Complete destruction of trabecular and cortical bone with expansion of bone contours without periosteal reaction or sclerotic margins can be seen

(Figs 16.1, 16.7). Permeative osteolysis may result from the dissemination of poorly-delimited areas of trabecular bone destruction (Figs 16.1, 16.7). In vertebral bodies, scalloping of the endosteal aspect of the vertebral wall may help differentiate normal variants from merely focal lesions in the cervical spine. It may also help in the differential diagnosis between benign senile or post-menopausal osteoporosis and myeloma in patients with bone loss and a monoclonal component in the blood (KYLE et al. 1985). Dissemination of submillimeter foci of osteolysis can also be seen, even in patients with normal radiographs and MR images (Fig. 16.8). Finally, lytic lesions with preserved cortical shell and thickening of some residual trabeculae suggestive of a slowly progressive lesion can be seen (Figs. 16.1, 16.9).

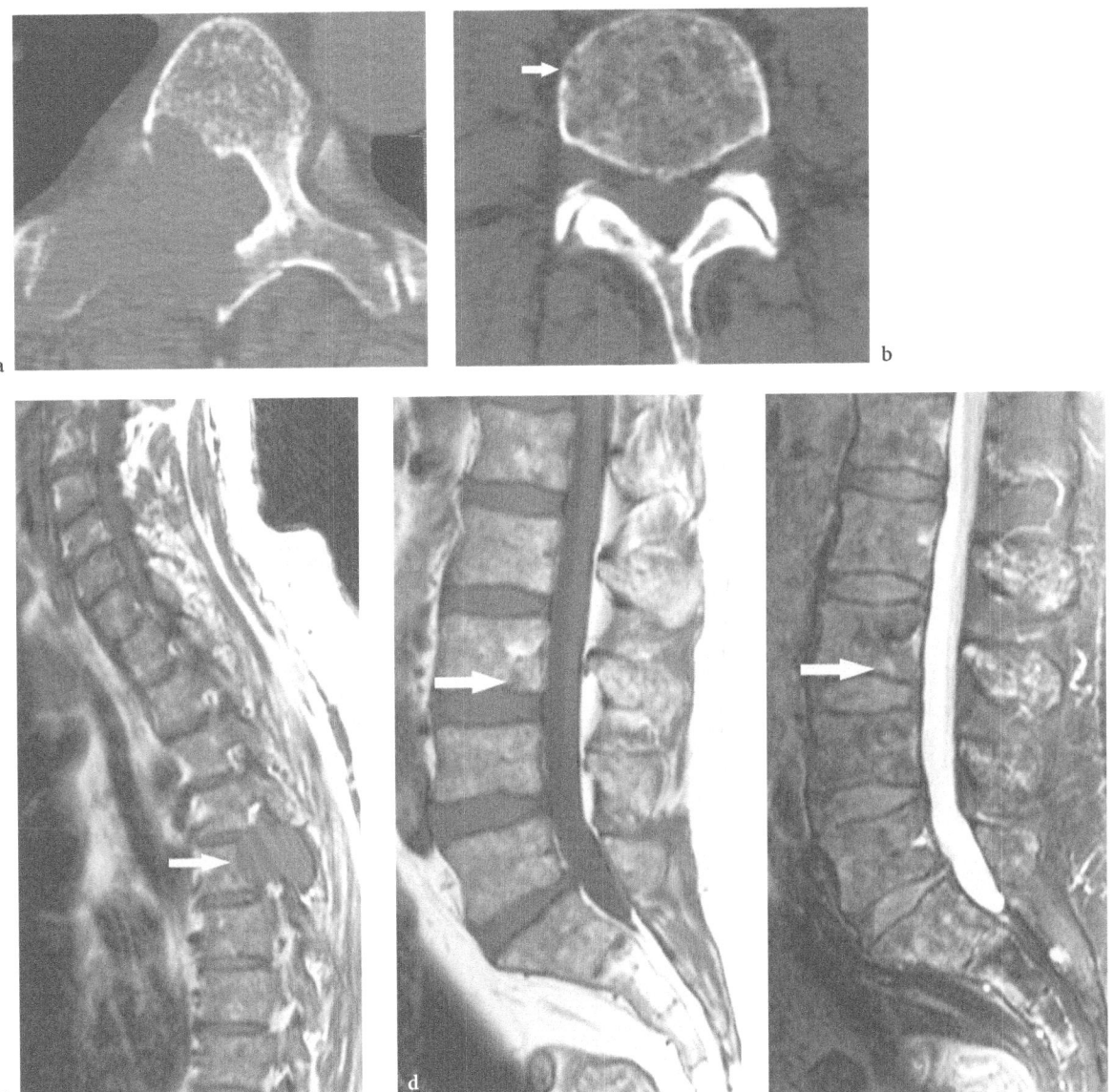

Fig. 16.7a–e. Multiple myeloma in a 43-year-old woman. **a** Axial CT scan of a thoracic vertebral body shows a large expansile lytic lesion of the right posterior arch without surrounding cortex or trabecular bone sclerosis. **b** Axial CT scan of the L3 vertebral body shows unquestionable trabecular bone osteolysis with endosteal scalloping (*arrow*) of the cortical bone. **c** Sagittal spin-echo T1-weighted MR image of the thoracic spine shows a large lesion involving the posterior arch of a vertebral body (*arrow*). Sagittal (**d**) T1 and (**e**) fat-suppressed fast spin-echo T2-weighted MR images show a roughly normal marrow appearance with a possible small lesion adjacent to the inferior vertebral end-plate of L3 (*arrow*). Occasionally, diffuse plasma cell infiltration of the marrow does not cause obvious marrow changes on T1 and T2-weighted MR images but is nonetheless responsible for trabecular bone osteolysis, visible on the CT scans.

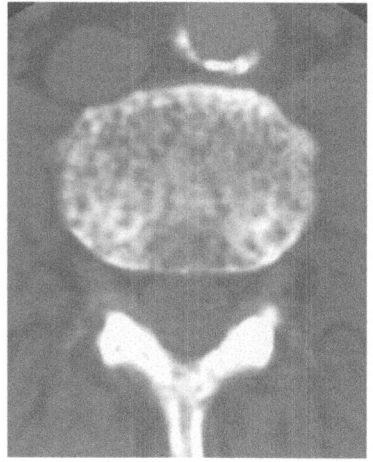

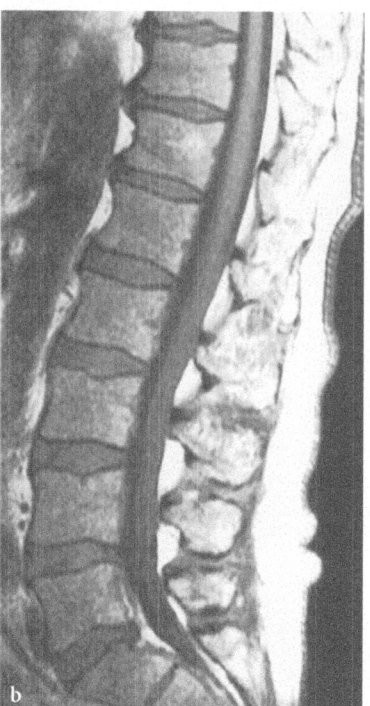

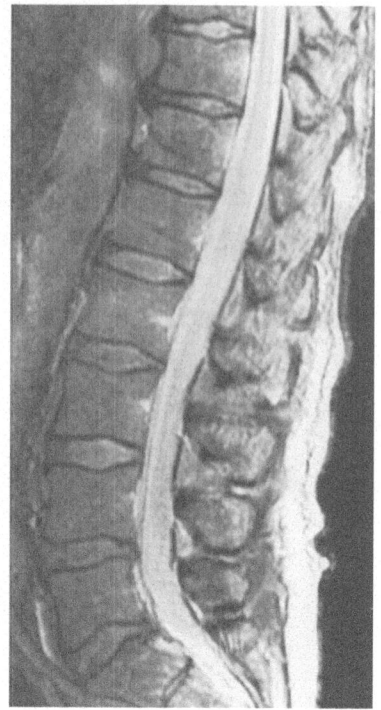

Fig. 16.8a–c. Multiple myeloma in a 54-year-old woman. **a** Axial CT scan shows diffuse alteration of the trabecular bone network with multiple tiny areas of osteolysis. **b** Sagittal spin-echo T1-weighted and (**c**) gradient-echo T2*-weighted images of the spine show a normal marrow pattern.

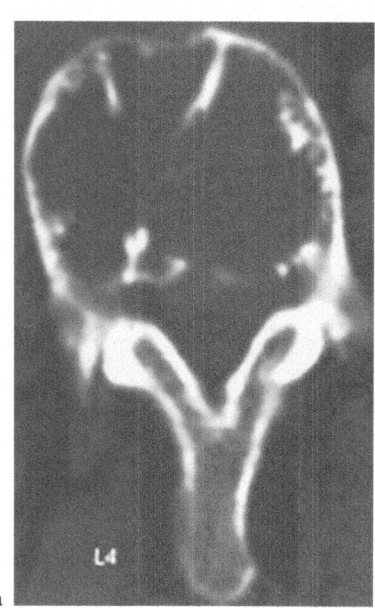

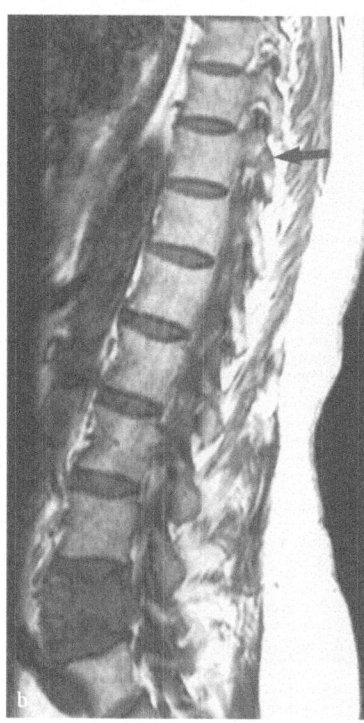

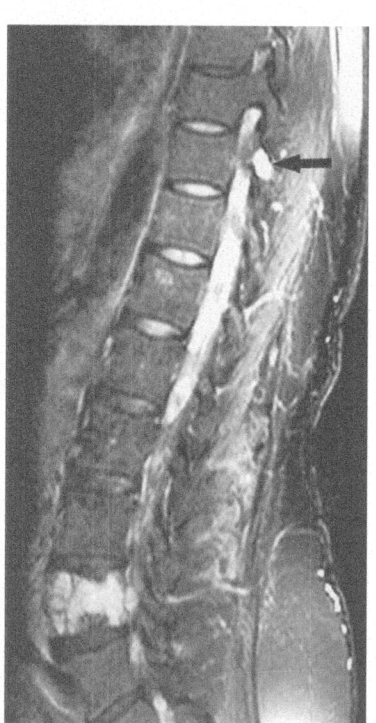

Fig. 16.9a–c. Multiple myeloma in a 42-year-old man. **a** Axial CT scan of L4 shows a chronic lytic lesion with thickening of some trabeculae. Sagittal (**b**) T1 and (**c**) fat-suppressed spin-echo T2-weighted MR images show a focal lesion in the L4 vertebral body, with posterior wall deformity. They also show a marrow lesion (*arrow*) in the posterior arch of the T10 vertebral body. Lesions of the posterior arch are frequently more easily detected on fat-suppressed fast spin-echo T2-weighted than on the T1-weighted MR images. Presence of the T10 lesion modified the treatment of that patient and chemotherapy rather than local radiation therapy of the L4 lesions was prescribed.

Due to necessary limitations in the anatomic areas involved, CT does not play the role of a screening imaging tool in myeloma. However, it enables more precise analysis of bone destruction and soft tissue involvement than radiographs. It is important to be familiar with the CT appearance because CT may be the initial imaging study in patients with back symptoms and not yet recognized plasma cell dyscrasia.

16.3.1.3
Differential Diagnosis of Radiographic and CT Findings

Differential diagnosis of multiple lytic foci encompasses bone metastases and lymphoma. Homogeneity in lesion size and the presence of sharp margins are suggestive of myeloma. Focal lytic lesions with cortical expansion may be observed in myeloma but also in other slowly growing lesions including metastases from kidney or thyroid cancer, aneurismal bone cysts and osteoblastoma. The poorly circumscribed "moth-eaten" osteolytic lesions may be observed in more rapidly progressive lesions including lung and breast cancer metastases and lymphoma.

Diffuse osteoporosis, especially if isolated and homogeneous, may be indistinguishable from postmenopausal and senile osteoporosis. Radiographs of the distal aspects of the limbs may help in this particularly difficult differential diagnosis because the bone architecture should be normal in multiple myeloma (neoplastic disease involving the red marrow containing skeleton) and should demonstrate osteopenia in the case of osteoporosis (metabolic disease involving the entire skeleton, whatever its marrow content) (LECOUVET at al. 2001).

The differential diagnosis of nodular sclerotic foci includes osteoblastic metastases, solitary bone islands, osteopoikilosis, sarcoidosis and tuberous sclerosis. Diffuse osteosclerosis may be observed in widespread carcinomatosis, myelofibrosis, mastocytosis, renal osteodystrophy, fluorosis and osteopetrosis.

Moreover, no characteristic radiographic picture permits an unquestioned diagnosis of multiple myeloma. Biological and histological data remain mandatory for a definite diagnosis. In addition, blind biopsy of the bone marrow (iliac crest-sternum) should always precede the eventual guided-biopsy of a focal bone lesion because multiple myeloma is generally a diffuse disease, even if it appears focal on radiographs, CT and MR images. If the blind bone marrow biopsy indicates multiple myeloma, then biopsy of the focal bone lesion may become unnecessary.

16.3.1.4
MR Imaging Findings

MR imaging appearance of the normal bone marrow merely results from the respective contribution of fat cells and more hydrated cellular components whereas bone trabeculae play little role (VOGLER and MURPHY 1988). The difference in fat proportion between yellow and red (or hematopoietic) marrow enables mapping of their respective distribution in the skeleton. Throughout adult life, hematopoietic marrow is typically located in the axial skeleton and proximal humeri and femora. Since myeloma affects the hematopoietic compartment, MR studies should focus on those areas and aim at detecting signal alterations due to localized or more diffuse changes in the fat/non fat balance.

16.3.1.4.1
Anatomic Areas and Imaging Protocols

The spine is the most frequently investigated anatomic area in myeloma patients. Sagittal studies enable screening of a high proportion of hematopoietic marrow in a limited time and detection of potential spinal cord compression (JOFFE et al. 1988; LUDWIG et al. 1987). Imaging of pelvic and proximal femur marrow by using coronal images provides additional information. The pelvic girdle contains about one more third of the red marrow capital (CRISTY 1981) and isolated lesions can be found there. In patients with a normal or equivocal spinal bone marrow MR appearance, imaging of the pelvis may demonstrate unquestionable diffuse changes and therefore increase the confidence with which diffuse abnormalities are identified (VANDE BERG et al. 1996; VANDE BERG et al. 1998). Imaging of the pelvic girdle may also enable detection of lesions in the femoral heads, necks and proximal shafts that may be at risk for fracture.

The T1-weighted spin-echo pulse sequence currently remains the cornerstone of bone marrow MR imaging. This sequence can be obtained easily, rapidly, and reproducibly on all MR imaging units. T1-weighted MR images will often be sufficient to detect marrow alterations, showing focal or diffuse decrease of the normal marrow signal. In richly cellular red marrow (spontaneous or treatment induced), contrast between lesions and adjacent marrow is less favorable and lesion conspicuity decreases (DAFFNER et al. 1986). In this situation, additional sequences and contrast material injection may be helpful, although in most cases, contrast injection does not appear mandatory for focal lesion detection (RAHMOUNI et al. 1993a). T2-weighted fast spin-echo MR images with selective fat signal saturation, short inversion time recovery (STIR) and fast-STIR images are preferred on high-field MR imaging units, and T2*-weighted gradient-echo sequences has been used successfully on low and mid-field-strength MR imagers. All these sequences may show focal or diffuse marrow abnormalities as areas of relatively higher signal intensity than that of red and yellow marrow (MOULOPOULOS et al. 1995; VANDE BERG et al. 1996; LUDWIG et al. 1987; MOULOPOULOS et al. 1992; AVRAHAMI et al. 1993).

Normal adult marrow shows no or barely perceptible enhancement on T1-weighted MR images obtained after intravenous administration of gadolinium derivatives. Contrast-enhanced T1-weighted MR images and fast dynamic imaging after contrast injection may be helpful to differentiate normal richly cellular marrow from discrete diffuse myeloma infiltration (STABLER et al. 1996). However the clinical impact of MR imaging in the detection of diffuse marrow infiltration is less than that in the detection of focal marrow lesion because diffuse marrow infiltration is always detected by blind bone marrow biopsy. MR plays a crucial role in the detection of focal marrow lesions when the findings of blind bone marrow biopsy are normal or equivocal.

16.3.1.4.2
MR Imaging Patterns of Marrow Involvement

Qualitative analysis of the spinal and pelvic bone marrow MR imaging appearance has lead to the recognition of three different patterns of marrow abnormalities. These patterns may be associated in the same patients. One must keep in mind that bone marrow may maintain a normal MR imaging appearance despite biopsy proven plasma cell infiltration of marrow spaces on microscopic examination (MOULOPOULOS et al. 1995; VANDE BERG et al. 1996; LIBSHITZ et al. 1992; LECOUVET et al. 1998b).

The focal pattern consists of a localized area of hypointensity on T1-weighted MR images and intermediate signal intensity to hyperintensity on T2-weighted MR images (Figs. 16.1, 16.7, 16.9). Lesion margins are generally sharply demarcated, on a background of an otherwise normal appearing bone marrow. Enhancement of untreated lesions is the rule and appears homogeneous on T1-weighted MR images obtained after contrast injection (Fig. 16.1). At biopsy or autopsy, focal lesions generally correspond to osteolytic areas with numerous packed abnormal plasma cells, although rounded foci may be seen on

MR images without evident osteolysis. Occasionally, focal myeloma lesions show relative hyperintensity and may be overlooked on T1-weighted MR images (Fig. 16.1). T2 or T2*-weighted MR images are necessary to detect these lesions.

The diffuse pattern of marrow involvement is characterized on T1-weighted MR images by a diffuse and homogeneous decrease in marrow signal intensity which becomes identical to or lower than that of adjacent intervertebral discs (Figs. 16.5, 16.10). On T2-weighted MR images, diffuse or patchy hyperintensity can be seen (STABLER et al. 1996; LECOUVET et al. 1998b). Contrast enhancement is usually evident on post contrast T1-weighted images. If diffuse changes are subtle, signal enhancement will be appreciated on the basis of an increased signal contrast between the enhanced marrow signal and the unenhanced intervertebral disks due to the combination of subtle increase in the signal of the vertebral marrow and a "paradoxical" decrease in the intervertebral disk signal due to a technical rescaling effect (Fig. 16.11).

The variegated or "salt and pepper" pattern is characterized by the presence of multiple tiny foci of hypointensity on T1-weighted MR images, intermediate signal intensity to hyperintensity on T2-weighted MR images, with enhancement on contrast-enhanced T1-weighted MR images (Fig. 16.12). This pattern is frequently seen in early stages of the disease (MOULOPOULOS et al. 1995; VANDE BERG et al. 1996).

A normal marrow MR imaging appearance of the spine on T1 and T2-weighted images is present at diagnosis in 50 to 75% of patients with early untreated (stage I) myeloma and in about 20% of patients with advanced and treated (stage III) disease (Fig. 16.11). Most likely, MR images fail to demonstrate alterations in marrow signal intensity, as long as the variation in the ratio of hematopoietic (and neoplastic) to fat cells in the bone marrow does not exceed the ratio observed in healthy individuals (MOULOPOULOS et al. 1992; STABLER et al. 1996; BAUR et al. 1997). The other patterns of marrow involvement seen at MR imaging also seem to correlate with some laboratory parameters. Patients with the normal or variegated patterns tend to have lower tumor burden than those with the focal or diffuse marrow involvement patterns. Higher cellularity and plasmacytosis in marrow specimens and more severe signs of bone marrow failure have been repeatedly found in patients with the diffuse MR imaging pattern (MOULOPOULOS et al. 1992; STABLER et al. 1996; LECOUVET et al. 1998b; CARLSON et al. 1995; LECOUVET et al. 1997b).

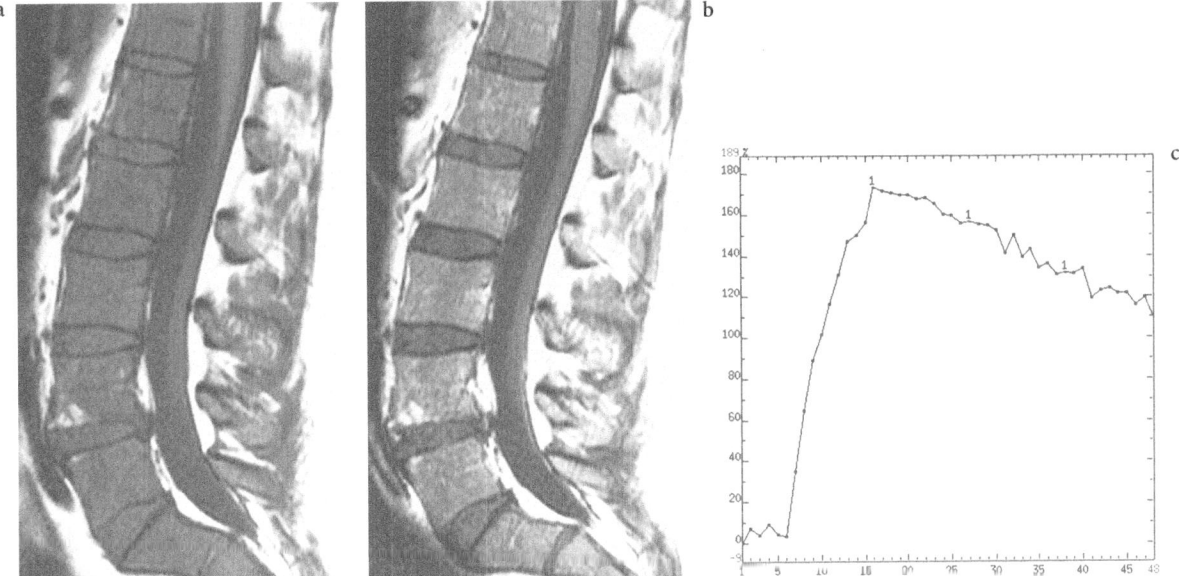

Fig. 16.10a–c. Multiple myeloma in a 53-year-old man. Sagittal spin-echo T1-weighted MR images of the spine obtained (a) before and (b) after contrast injection show a marked hypointense marrow on T1-weighted image and marked increase in signal intensity after contrast injection. c Diagrammatic representation of signal intensity enhancement after contrast injection demonstrates rapid and intense enhancement of the marrow.

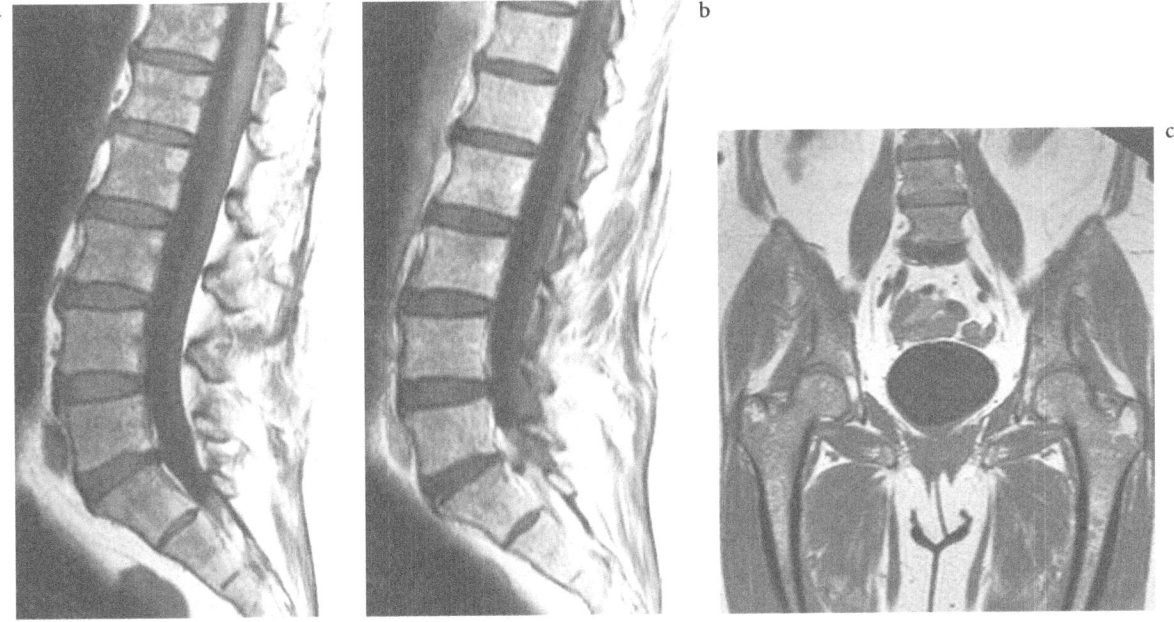

Fig. 16.11a–c. Multiple myeloma in a 65-year-old man. **a** Sagittal spin-echo T1-weighted MR image of the lumbar spine shows moderate heterogeneity of the marrow. **b** The corresponding sagittal contrast-enhanced spin-echo T1-weighted MR image shows signal intensity enhancement. Visual analysis of enhancement is subjective and depends on several parameters. **c** Coronal T1-weighted MR image of the pelvis shows unquestionable abnormal marrow distribution with presence of red marrow in the epiphyses and greater trochanter. Heterogeneity of the marrow is more obvious in the pelvis than in the spine.

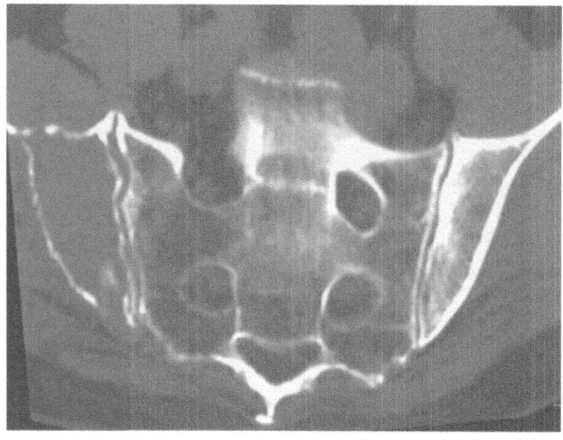
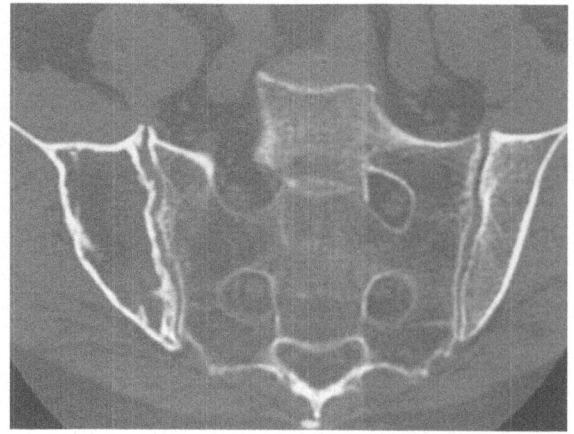

a
b

Fig. 16.12a,b. Multiple myeloma in a 56-year-old woman. Axial CT scans of a focal myeloma lesion obtained (**a**) before and (**b**) after chemotherapy. Before treatment, there is a lytic lesion in the right iliac wing with trabecular bone destruction and cortical interruption. After treatment, the cortex is thickened and continuous but the trabecular bone is still absent.

16.3.1.4.3
Differential Diagnosis of MR Imaging Patterns

The lack of specificity of MR imaging findings must be emphasized. The focal and diffuse MR patterns may be observed in metastatic disease from primary solid tumors and in other hematologic malignancies, including leukemias and lymphomas. Differentiation between red marrow hyperplasia – in relation to anemia, infection or treatment – and neoplastic marrow infiltration can be extremely difficult or even impossible. Normal marrow heterogeneities may mimic the variegated pattern, although in most cases hyperintensity on T2-weighted images and contrast enhancement help distinguish myeloma-associated marrow abnormalities from normal hematopoietic foci which generally show intermediate signal intensity on T2-weighted images and no contrast enhancement on T1-weighted images.

16.3.1.4.4
Prognostic Value of MR Imaging

In early asymptomatic stages of the disease with no or only one lytic lesion on bone radiographs, patients with relevant abnormalities on MR imaging have a significantly shorter time lag before the onset of more aggressive disease (and necessary initiation of systemic treatment) than those with normal appearing marrow at MR imaging (MOULOPOULOS et al. 1995; VANDE BERG et al. 1996; WEBER et al. 1997). Among patients with advanced disease stages treated with conventional chemotherapy, patients with normal MR imaging findings on T1 and T2-

weighted images at diagnosis have a better response to treatment and survive longer than those with focal or diffuse marrow abnormalities on MR imaging (LECOUVET et al. 1998a). This prognostic value has still to be assessed in patients treated with marrow transplantation.

MR imaging of the spine and pelvis consistently demonstrates more numerous marrow lesions and more patients with marrow involvement than the corresponding conventional radiographs (LECOUVET et al. 1999; LUDWIG et al. 1987; FRUEHWALD et al. 1988; TERTTI et al. 1995). However, despite this superiority over radiographs for spinal and pelvic lesion detection, an MR imaging survey limited to these areas may be less sensitive than the conventional radiographic skeletal survey for the detection of patients with bone lesions, especially in the skull and ribs (LECOUVET et al. 1999). Bone radiographs seem to retain an important place in myeloma staging (LECOUVET et al. 1999; TERTTI et al. 1995).

16.3.1.5
Bone Scintigraphy

Technetium disphosphonate radionuclide imaging is of little interest in myeloma, although it may be helpful in patients with pain or suspected fractures. Its sensitivity is inferior to that of radiographs, CT and MR imaging (Fig. 16.1) (LUDWIG et al. 1982; WOOLFENDEN et al. 1980) probably because isotopes are markers of osteoblastic activity that is considerably inhibited in myeloma (BATAILLE et al. 1982). Large lytic lesions may even show local "cold spots" due to the lack of local isotope uptake. Isotope uptake mostly occurs in reactive bone changes at fracture sites, in relation to local repair, or less frequently due to calcification in treated lesions or in soft tissue amyloid deposits.

16.3.2
Imaging Findings in Complicated Multiple Myeloma

Both osteolytic lesions and diffuse osteoporosis predispose to bone fractures that most commonly involve the spine and ribs, followed by the pelvis, clavicle and long bones. Vertebral compression fractures occur in the majority of patients during the course of the disease. Compression of neurological structures may occur secondary to bone displacement or soft tissue masses.

16.3.2.1
Neurological Complications

MR imaging is the diagnostic procedure of choice for the work-up of myeloma patients with neurological symptoms (JOFFE et al. 1988; MOULOPOULOS and DIMOPOULOS 1997). This technique enables prompt and accurate diagnosis of focal complicated spinal lesions, delineation of soft-tissue or epidural extension, and assessment of the level and extent of spinal cord or nerve root compression.

16.3.2.2
Spinal Fractures

Although pathologic in origin, the majority of myeloma related fractures differ from those observed in metastases and lymphoma. Their distribution is closely similar to that of osteoporotic fractures, with a peak at the thoraco-lumbar junction and uncommon involvement of the upper three thoracic vertebrae (LECOUVET et al. 1997b). MR imaging criteria have been developed for the differentiation of benign and malignant vertebral fractures, which can be difficult and sometimes impossible with conventional radiographs and even CT (CUENOD et al. 1996; MOULOPOULOS et al. 1996). Application of these criteria to vertebral fractures seen in myeloma has shown that up to two thirds appear benign on MR imaging, despite their association with a malignancy (Fig. 16.10) (MOULOPOULOS et al. 1992; LIBSHITZ et al. 1992; FRUEHWALD et al. 1988; LECOUVET et al. 1997b). The frequent similarity in MR imaging appearance and distribution between vertebral fractures seen in

myeloma and those seen in benign osteoporosis, most likely results from the key role of diffuse osteopenia in fracture pathogenesis, which leads to diffuse alteration of vertebral resistance to biomechanical stresses, whereas this alteration is more focal in metastatic disease and lymphoma (LECOUVET et al. 1997a). At least one third of myeloma-associated fractures are malignant-looking, with possible soft tissue extension and spinal cord or nerve root compression (Figs. 16.5, 16.9).

Correlation of the MR imaging appearance of the bone marrow at diagnosis to the subsequent occurrence of vertebral fractures in patients with advanced disease has shown that patients with numerous focal spinal lesions or diffuse marrow abnormalities had six-times higher fracture risk than those with less than ten focal lesions or a normal marrow MR imaging appearance (LECOUVET et al. 1997a). Although MR imaging could identify patients at high risk for spinal fractures, it does not help predict the level of fracture (LECOUVET et al. 1998a).

16.3.3
Imaging Findings in Treated Multiple Myeloma

Treatment monitoring generally relies on serial assessment of biological markers of disease (monoclonal protein levels and bone marrow plasmacytosis). Difficulties may arise in the rare cases of non-secretory multiple myeloma and in relapse after treatment in which recurrence may be non-secretory (MOULOPOULOS and DIMOPOULOS 1997). On radiographs, focal lesions generally show no sclerosis on serial radiographs. Expansion of the lesion may regress with the reappearance of an intact cortex (Fig. 16.3). Diffuse osteopenia may remain unchanged or may show moderate sclerosis on follow-up radiographs. Serial bone densitometry has shown significant changes during treatment (MARIETTE et al. 1992; MARIETTE et al. 1995). Appearance of new lesions during treatment or follow-up is an unequivocal sign of disease progression. CT images of treated focal lytic lesions may highlight subtle changes that are not seen with conventional radiographs including disappearance of soft tissue masses, reappearance of a continuous cortical contour and appearance of a peripheral fatty rim (Fig. 16.13).

Interpretation of post-treatment MR images is difficult given the wide spectrum of possible treatment-induced changes in MR imaging findings for each pattern of marrow involvement, and given the lack of correlation of these changes to long-term

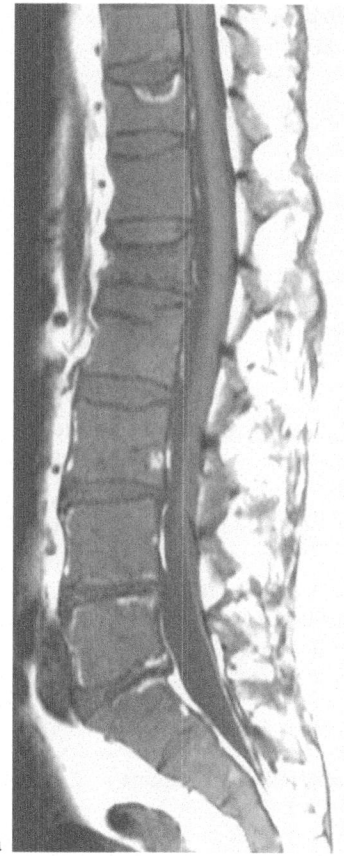
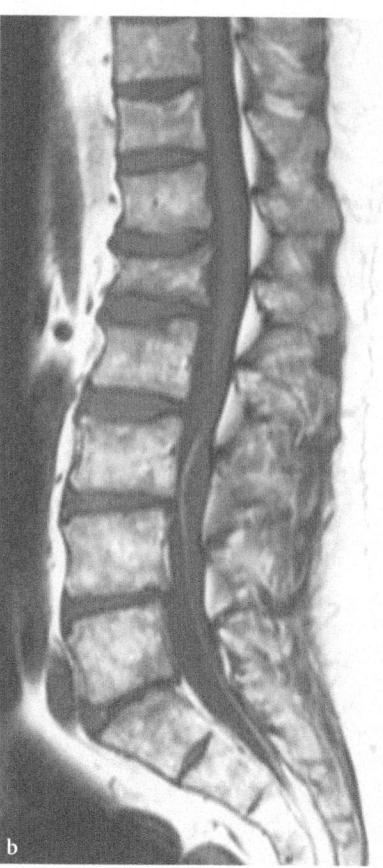

a

b

Fig. 16.13a,b. Multiple myeloma in a 63-year-old man. Sagittal T1-weighted MR images of the lumbar spine obtained (a) before and (b) after 8 months of chemotherapy show diffuse marrow infiltration before treatment and reappearance of normal marrow signal intensity after treatment.

follow-up of patients. After treatment, focal marrow lesions may remain identical or decrease in size, with possible appearance of a peripheral "fatty halo". Changes in contrast enhancement between the pre and post-treatment MR imaging examinations include appearance of no or peripheral enhancement (RAHMOUNI et al. 1993b; MOULOPOULOS et al. 1994). Local radiation therapy of focal complicated lesions induces rapid and important decrease in the soft tissue extension and appearance of presumably necrotic, avascular central areas within the lesion on contrast-enhanced T1-weighted MR images, with a later decrease in lesion size. In patients with diffuse marrow changes, a diffuse increase in the marrow signal is usually observed on T1-weighted MR images obtained after treatment. The transformation of a diffuse pattern of marrow involvement before treatment to a focal pattern of marrow involvement after treatment should not be considered to indicate disease progression. Actually, the focal abnormalities seen on post-treatment MR images were present initially on pre-treatment T2-weighted images, and were not seen on T1-weighted images because of the associated diffuse changes.

After bone marrow transplantation, bone marrow generally is hyperintense on T1-weighted MR images in relation to the aggressive cytotoxic therapy, but focal residual lesions are frequent (AGREN et al. 1998). Post-treatment marrow appearance may also be influenced by the use of marrow stimulating factors, which increase marrow cellularity, and by multiple transfusions, which may lead to marrow hemosiderosis and to a decrease in the marrow signal on gradient-echo MR images due to susceptibility artifacts associated with iron deposition.

16.4
Imaging Features of Extraosseous Involvement

As a rule, multiple myeloma involves the medullary cavity of bones. Extraosseous involvement that is not secondary to soft tissue invasion from an osseous lesion is a relatively rare event (MOULOPOULOS et al. 1993). In the vast majority of cases, dissemination to other tissues than bone marrow is a pre-terminal event (KAPADIA 1980). Rarely, when extraosseous manifestations occur early in the disease course, they are associated with an aggressive form of multiple myeloma (Fig. 16.14) (BARLOGIE et al. 1989).

Extraosseous involvement generally involves the spleen, liver and lymph nodes, although almost any organ can be involved. Lymph node involvement in multiple myeloma is similar to that of lymphoma, with involvement of multiple nodal groups (MOULOPOULOS et al. 1993). Spleen and liver involvement usually causes spleen or liver enlargement without focal lesions. In the lung, myeloma deposits usually appear as masses or nodules similar to metastases, with occasional enlarged lymph nodes (SHIN et al. 1992). Involvement of the central nervous system is also rare, and includes diffuse leptomeningeal dissemination or less frequently meningeal nodules (LEIFER et al. 1992).

16.5
Conclusion

Conventional radiographs, CT and MR images demonstrate extremely variable patterns of bone destruction and marrow involvement among patients with multiple myeloma and even within the same patient. Most likely this variable behavior stems from the variable pace of evolution of these lesions. This wide spectrum of imaging findings mirrors that of the clinical course observed in patients with monoclonal gammopathy.

References

Agren B, Rudberg U, Isberg B, Svensson L, Aspelin P (1998) MR imaging of multiple myeloma patients with bone-marrow transplants. Acta Radiol 39:36–42

Alexanian R, Dimopoulos MA (1995) Management of multiple myeloma. Semin Hematol 32:20–30

Ardran G (1951) Bone destruction not demonstrable by radiography. Brit J Radiol 24:107–115

Avrahami E, Tadmor R, Kaplinsky N (1993) The role of T2-weighted gradient echo in MRI demonstration of spinal multiple myeloma. Spine 18:1812–1815

Barlogie B, Smallwood L, Smith T, Alexenian R (1989) High levels of lactic dehydrogenase identify a high grade lymphoma-like myeloma. Ann Intern Med 110:521–525

Bataille R, Chevalier J, Rossi M, Sany J (1982) Bone scintigraphy in plasma-cell myeloma. A prospective study of 70 patients. Radiology 145:801–804

Bataille R, Chappard D, Alexandre C, Dessauw P, Sany J (1986) Importance of quantitative histology of bone changes in monoclonal gammopathy. Br J Cancer 53:805–810

Bataille R, Chappard D, Klein B (1992) Mechanisms of bone lesions in multiple myeloma. Hematol Oncol Clin North Am 6:285–295

Baur A, Stabler A, Bartl R, Lamerz R, Scheidler J, Reiser M (1997) MRI gadolinium enhancement of bone marrow: age-related changes in normals and in diffuse neoplastic infiltration. Skeletal Radiol 26:414–418

Boccadoro M, Pileri A (1995) Prognostic factors in multiple myeloma. In: Malpas JS, Bergasagel DE, Kyle RA (eds) Myeloma: biology and management. Oxford University Press, New York, pp 251–270

Boccadoro M, Pileri A (1997) Diagnosis, prognosis, and standard treatment of multiple myeloma. Hematol Oncol Clin North Am 11:111–131

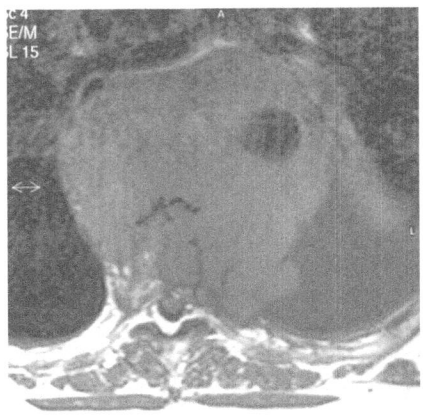
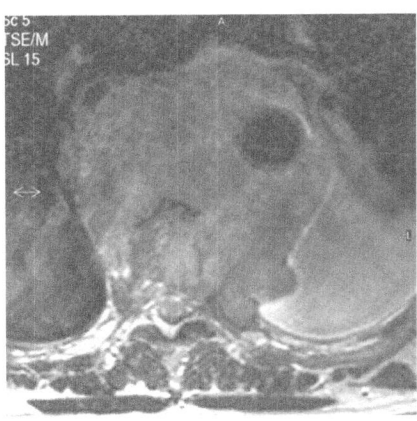
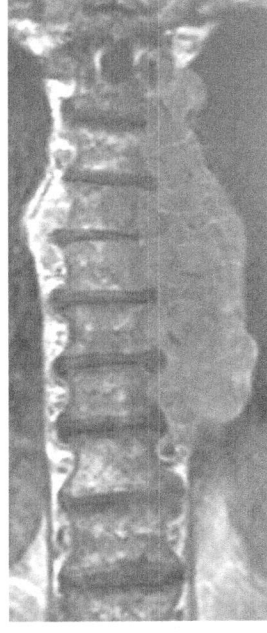

a

b

c

Fig. 16.14a-c. Multiple myeloma in a 71-year-old woman. She presented with enlarged mediastinum on chest radiograph. Axial (a) T1 and (b) T2-weighted MR images of the thoracic spine show a large mass involving the posterior mediastinal space with secondary bone involvement. Transtracheal biopsy demonstrated multiple myeloma. Blind iliac crest was normal. c Coronal contrast-enhanced T1-weighted MR image of the thoracic spine shows the predominant involvement of the mediastinum and secondary osseous involvement.

Carlson K, Astrom G, Nyman R, et al. (1995) MR imaging of multiple myeloma in tumour mass measurement at diagnosis and during treatment. Acta Radiol 36:9

Carson CP, Ackerman R (1955) Plasma cell myeloma. A clinical, pathologic and roentgenologic review of 90 cases. Am J Clin Pathol 25:849

Cristy M (1981) Active bone marrow distribution as a function of age in humans. Phys Med Biol 26:389–400

Croucher PI, Apperley JF (1998) Bone disease in multiple myeloma. Br J Haematol 103:902

Cuenod CA, Laredo JD, Chevret S, et al. (1996) Acute vertebral collapse due to osteoporosis or malignancy: appearance on unenhanced and gadolinium-enhanced MR images. Radiology 199:541–549

Daffner RH, Lupetin AR, Dash N, Deeb ZL, Sefczek RJ, Schapiro RL (1986) MRI in the detection of malignant infiltration of bone marrow. AJR Am J Roentgenol 146:353–358

Davies FE, Jack AS, Morgan G (1997) The use of biological variables to predict outcome in multiple myeloma. Br J Haematol 99:719

de Gramont A, Benitez O, Brissaud P, et al. (1985) Quantification of bone lytic lesions and prognosis in myelomatosis. Scand J Haematol 34:78–82

Durie BG, Salmon SE (1975) A clinical staging system for multiple myeloma. Correlation of measured myeloma cell mass with presenting clinical features, response to treatment, and survival. Cancer 36:842–854

Fruehwald FX, Tscholakoff D, Schwaighofer B, et al. (1988) Magnetic resonance imaging of the lower vertebral column in patients with multiple myeloma. Invest Radiol 23:193–199

Greipp PR (1992) Advances in the diagnosis and management of myeloma. Semin Hematol 29:24–45

Hall FM, Gore SM (1988) Osteosclerotic myeloma variants. Skeletal Radiol 17:101–105

Healy JC, Armstrong P (1994) Radiology of myeloma. In: Malpas JS, Bergasagel DE, Kyle RA (eds) Myeloma:biology and management. Oxford University Press, New York, pp 222–250

Heiser S, Schartzmann JJ (1952) Variation in the Roentgen appearance in the skeletal system in myeloma. Radiology 58:178

Iwashita H, Ohnishi A, Asada M, Kanazawa Y, Kuroiwa Y (1977) Polyneuropathy, skin hyperpigmentation, edema, and hypertrichosis in localized osteosclerotic myeloma. Neurology 27:675–681

Joffe J, Williams MP, Cherryman GR, Gore M, McElwain TJ, Selby P (1988) Magnetic resonance imaging in myeloma. Lancet 1:1162–1163

Kapadia SB (1980) Multiple myeloma: a clinicopathologic study of 62 consecutively autopsied cases. Medicine Baltimore 59:380

Klein B, Zhang 19G, Lu ZY, Bataille R (1995) Interleukin-6 in human multiple myeloma. Blood 85:863–872

Kyle RA (1975) Multiple myeloma: review of 869 cases. Mayo Clin Proc 50:29–40

Kyle RA (1983) Long-term survival in multiple myeloma. N Engl J Med 308:314–316

Kyle RA, Greipp PR (1980) Smoldering multiple myeloma. N Engl J Med 302:1347–1349

Kyle RA, Schreiman JS, McLeod RA, Beabout JW (1985) Computed tomography in diagnosis and management of multiple myeloma and its variants. Arch Intern Med 145:1451–1452

Laroche M, Assoun J, Sixou L, Attal M (1996) Comparison of MRI and computed tomography in the various stages of plasma cell disorders: correlations with biological and histological findings. Clin Exp Rheumatol 14:171–176

Lecouvet FE, Malghem J, Michaux L, et al. (1997a) Vertebral compression fractures in multiple myeloma. Part II. Assessment of fracture risk with MR imaging of spinal bone marrow. Radiology 204:201–205

Lecouvet FE, Vande Berg BC, Maldague BE, et al. (1997b) Vertebral compression fractures in multiple myeloma. Part I. Distribution and appearance at MR imaging. Radiology 204:195–199

Lecouvet FE, Vande Berg BC, Michaux L, Jamart J, Maldague BE, Malghem J (1998a) Development of vertebral fractures in patients with multiple myeloma: does MRI enable recognition of vertebrae that will collapse? J Comput Assist Tomogr 22:430–436

Lecouvet FE, Vande Berg BC, Michaux L, Jamart J, Maldague BE, Malghem J (1998b) Stage III multiple myeloma: clinical and prognostic value of spinal bone marrow MR imaging. Radiology 209:653–660

Lecouvet FE, Malghem J, Michaux L, et al. (1999) Skeletal survey in advanced multiple myeloma: radiographic versus MR imaging survey. Br J Haematol 106:35–39

Lecouvet FE, Vande Berg BC, Maldague BE, Malghem J (2001) Magnetic resonance and computed tomography imaging in multiple myeloma. Semin Musculoskelet Radiol 5:43–55

Leifer D, Grabowski T, Simonian N, Demirjian ZN (1992) Leptomeningeal myelomatosis presenting with mental status changes and other neurologic findings. Cancer 70:1899–1904

Libshitz HI, Malthouse SR, Cunningham D, MacVicar AD, Husband JE (1992) Multiple myeloma: appearance at MR imaging. Radiology 182:833–837

Ludwig H, Kumpan W, Sinzinger H (1982) Radiography and bone scintigraphy in multiple myeloma: a comparative analysis. Br J Radiol 55:173–181

Ludwig H, Fruhwald F, Tscholakoff D, Rasoul S, Neuhold A, Fritz E (1987) Magnetic resonance imaging of the spine in multiple myeloma. Lancet 2:364–366

Malpas JS, Caroll JJ (1995) Myeloma: clinical presentation and diagnosis. In: Malpas JS, Bergasagel DE, Kyle EA (eds) Myeloma: biology and management. Oxford University Press, New York, pp 169–190

Mariette X, Khalifa P, Ravaud P, et al. (1992) Bone densitometry in patients with multiple myeloma. Am J Med 93:595–598

Mariette X, Bergot C, Ravaud P, et al. (1995) Evolution of bone densitometry in patients with myeloma treated with conventional or intensive therapy. Cancer 76:1559–1563

Moulopoulos LA, Varma DG, Dimopoulos MA, et al. (1992) Multiple myeloma: spinal MR imaging in patients with untreated newly diagnosed disease. Radiology 185:833–840

Moulopoulos LA, Granfield CAJ, Dimopoulos MA, Kim EE Alexenian R, Libshitz HI (1993) Extraosseous multiple myeloma: imaging features. AJR Am J Roentgenol 161:1083–1087

Moulopoulos LA, Dimopoulos MA, Alexanian R, Leeds NE, Libshitz HI (1994) Multiple myeloma: MR patterns of response to treatment. Radiology 193:441–446

Moulopoulos LA, Dimopoulos MA, Smith TL, et al. (1995) Prognostic significance of magnetic resonance imaging in patients with asymptomatic multiple myeloma. J Clin Oncol 13:251–256

Moulopoulos LA, Yoshimitsu K, Johnston DA, Leeds NE, Libshitz HI (1996) MR prediction of benign and malignant vertebral compression fractures. J Magn Reson Imaging 6:667–674

Moulopoulos LA, Dimopoulos MA (1997) Magnetic resonance imaging of the bone marrow in hematologic malignancies. Blood 90:2127–2147

Mundy GR, Raisz LG, Cooper RA, Schechter GP, Salmon SE (1974) Evidence for the secretion of an osteoclast stimulating factor in myeloma. N Engl J Med 291:1041–1046

Rahmouni A, Divine M, Mathieu D, et al. (1993a) Detection of multiple myeloma involving the spine: efficacy of fat-suppression and contrast-enhanced MR imaging. AJR Am J Roentgenol 160:1049–1052

Rahmouni A, Divine M, Mathieu D, et al. (1993b) MR appearance of multiple myeloma of the spine before and after treatment. AJR Am J Roentgenol 160:1053–1057

Riccardi A, Gobbi PG, Ucci G, et al. (1991) Changing clinical presentation of multiple myeloma. Eur J Cancer 27:1401–1405

Salmon SE, Cassady JR (1995) Plasma cell neoplasms. In: De Vita VT (ed) Cancer: principles and practice of oncology. Philadelphia, pp 1984–2024

Shin MS, Carcelen MF, Kang-Yeh H (1992) Diverse roentgenographic manifestations of the rare pulmonary involvement in myeloma. Chest 102:946–948

Spiess JL, Adelstein DJ, Hines JD (1988) Multiple myeloma presenting with spinal cord compression. Oncology 45:88–92

Stabler A, Baur A, Bartl R, Munker R, Lamerz R, Reiser MF (1996) Contrast enhancement and quantitative signal analysis in MR imaging of multiple myeloma: assessment of focal and diffuse growth patterns in marrow correlated with biopsies and survival rates. AJR Am J Roentgenol 167:1029–1036

Terpstra WE, Lokhorst HM, Blomjous F, Meuwissen OJ, Dekker AW (1992) Comparison of plasma cell infiltration in bone marrow biopsies and aspirates in patients with multiple myeloma. Br J Haematol 82:46–49

Tertti R, Alanen A, Remes K (1995) The value of magnetic resonance imaging in screening myeloma lesions of the lumbar spine. Br J Haematol 91:658–660

Tricot G, Sawyer JR, Jagannath S, et al. (1997) Unique role of cytogenetics in the prognosis of patients with myeloma receiving high-dose therapy and autotransplants. J Clin Oncol 15:2659–2666

Vande Berg BC, Lecouvet FE, Michaux L, et al. (1996) Stage I multiple myeloma: value of MR imaging of the bone marrow in the determination of prognosis. Radiology 201:243–246

Vande Berg BC, Lecouvet FE, Michaux L, Ferrant A, Maldague B, Malghem J (1998) Magnetic resonance imaging of the bone marrow in hematological malignancies. Eur Radiol 8:1335–1344

Vogler JB, III, Murphy WA (1988) Bone marrow imaging. Radiology 168:679–693

Weber DM, Dimopoulos MA, Moulopoulos LA, Delasalle KB, Smith T, Alexanian R (1997) Prognostic features of asymptomatic multiple myeloma. Br J Haematol 97:810–814

Weinstein RS (1992) Bone involvement in multiple myeloma. Am J Med 93:591–594

Woolfenden JM, Pitt MJ, Durie BG, Moon TE (1980) Comparison of bone scintigraphy and radiography in multiple myeloma. Radiology 134:723–728

17 Solitary Plasmacytoma

Lia A. Moulopoulos and Meletios A. Dimopoulos

CONTENTS

17.1
Introduction

Plasmacytomas are localized proliferations of malignant monoclonal plasma cells. They are found in bones or in soft tissues. These tumors may be single or multiple; they are more frequently found in patients with multiple myeloma but they may occur in patients with no bone marrow abnormality. The term solitary plasmacytoma is reserved for those plasma cell tumors that arise in bone (solitary plasmacytoma of bone, SBP) or in extraosseous soft tissues (extramedullary plasmacytoma, EMP) with no evidence of disease elsewhere.

17.2
Solitary Plasmacytoma of Bone

Solitary plasmacytoma of bone is a very rare tumor. It occurs in 3 to 7% of patients with plasma cell dys-

Lia A. Moulopoulos, MD
Assistant Adjunct Professor, MD Anderson Cancer Center, Assistant Professor, Department of Radiology, Areteion Hospital, University of Athens, Medical School, 76 Vas. Sophias Avenue, 11528, Athens, Greece
Meletios A. Dimopoulos, MD
Professor, Department of Medical Oncology, Alexandra Hospital, University of Athens, Medical School, 80 Vas. Sophias Avenue and Lourou Street, 11528, Athens, Greece

crasias and more often affects men (Conklin and Alexanian 1975; Knowling et al. 1983). The diagnosis of SBP requires histologic evidence of a monoclonal plasma cell infiltrate in a single bone lesion, no other bone lesions on conventional radiographs and absence of bone marrow plasmacytosis. Moreover, there should be no evidence of anemia, hypercalcemia or renal dysfunction that could be attributed to the plasma cell proliferative disorder (Table 17.1).

Table 17.1. Diagnostic criteria for solitary bone plasmacytoma

1. Single area of bone marrow infiltration by monoclonal plasma cells
2. Normal bone marrow aspiration and biopsy
3. Normal skeletal survey and MR imaging of the spine and pelvis
4. No anemia, hypercalcemia, or abnormal renal function related to a plasma cell dyscrasia

SBP affects younger patients than multiple myeloma (median age of 56, about a decade younger) and it may even occur in children (Frassica et al. 1989; Dimopoulos et al. 1992). It more often affects the axial skeleton and, in particular, the thoracic spine, because active bone marrow is found there. Involvement of the appendicular skeleton distal to the proximal femur or humerus is rare. In the Mayo Clinic series, 54% of SBPs were located in the spine; the thoracic spine was more often involved, followed by the lumbar spine and ribs (Figs. 17.1, 17.2) (Frassica et al. 1989). Electrophoresis of serum and urine shows monoclonal protein in 24% to 72% of patients with SBP. The levels of monoclonal protein are much lower than in patients with multiple myeloma and the levels of uninvolved immunoglobulins are almost always normal in SBP (Frassica et al. 1989).

The most frequent presentation of SBP is that of a painful bone lesion. If the tumor is localized in the spine, the patient may complain of back pain or may develop neurological symptoms related to compression of the spinal cord or nerve roots. Patients with SBP may also present with fractures or

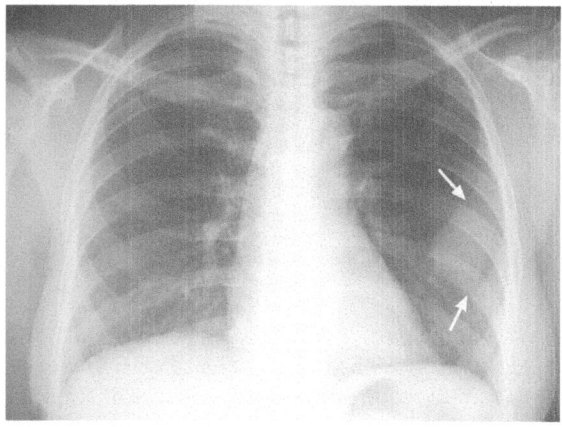
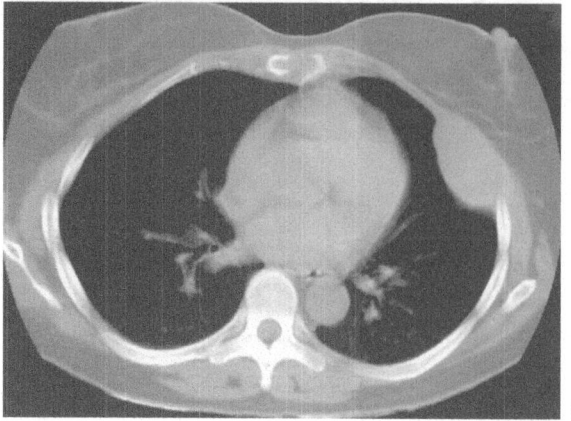

Fig. 17.1a,b. Solitary plasmacytoma of bone of the rib in a 49-year-old woman. **a** Posteroanterior radiograph of the chest reveals an expanding and destructive lesion of the left fourth rib (*arrows*). **b** Axial CT scan of the chest shows the well-defined and lytic mass of the rib.

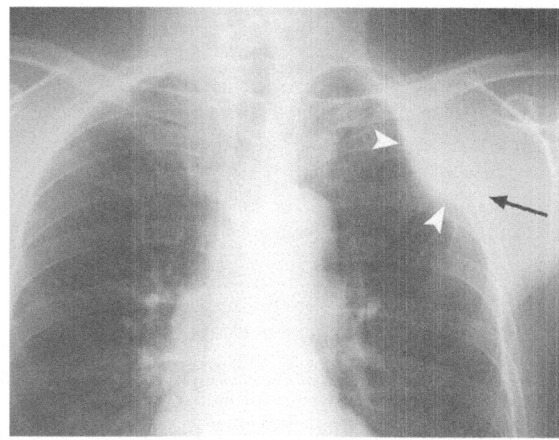
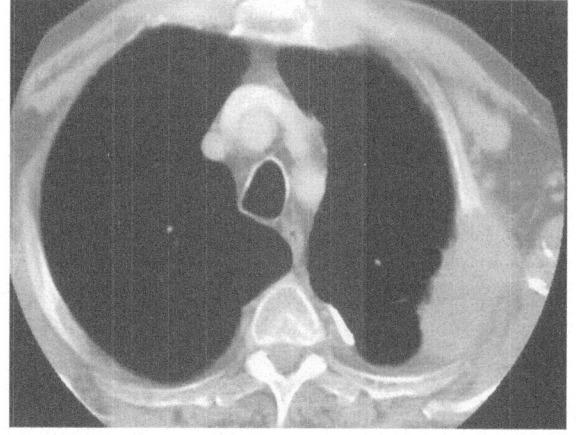

Fig. 17.2a,b. Solitary plasmacytoma of bone of the rib in a 69-year-old man. **a** Posteroanterior radiograph of the chest demonstrates an elongated and destructive mass of the second rib (*arrowheads*). There is also a fracture of the third rib (*arrow*). **b** Axial CT scan of the chest demonstrates the destructive soft-tissue mass of the rib extending into the surrounding tissues.

a palpable mass if the tumor is superficially located. Occasional patients with SBP present with symptoms and signs of peripheral polyneuropathy (FRASSICA et al. 1989).

On conventional radiographs, SBP appears as a multicystic, expansile lytic lesion with thickened trabeculae. More rarely, it may appear as an area of pure bone destruction resembling a lytic bone metastasis (Fig. 17.3). Occasionally it may present as a sclerotic lesion. Extraosseous extension of the bone lesion occurs in about 40% of lesions (FRASSICA et al. 1989). Although in most cases SBP is clearly demonstrated with conventional radiographs, cross

sectional imaging with computed tomography (CT) or magnetic resonance (MR) imaging is necessary to assess the extent of any associated extraosseous mass and to define the portals for local radiation therapy which is the treatment of choice for SBP.

On MR imaging, SBP does not have a characteristic appearance. On T1-weighted images the tumor is hypointense to fat and nearly isointense to muscle and it enhances after the administration of intravenous paramagnetic contrast (Figs. 17.3–17.5). On T2-weighted fast spin echo images with fat saturation or on STIR images the tumor is hyperintense to both muscle and fat. MR imaging does delineate

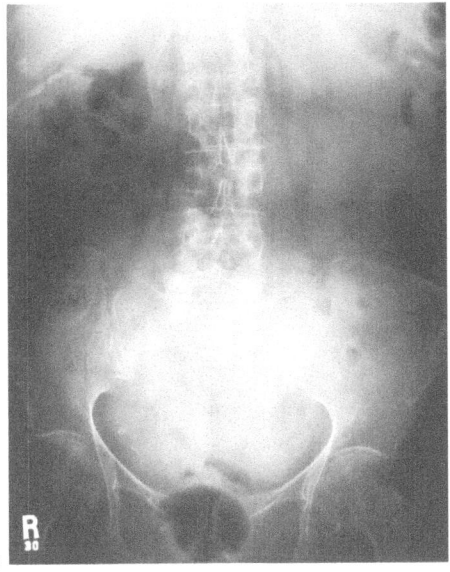
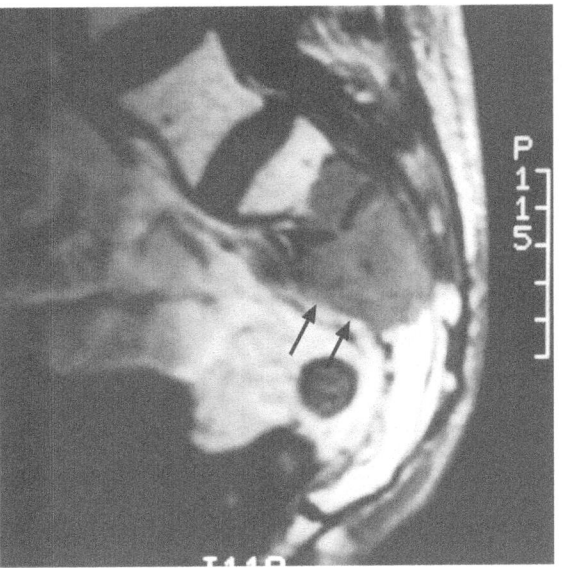

Fig. 17.3a,b. Solitary plasmacytoma of bone of the sacrum in a 64-year-old woman. a Anteroposterior radiograph of the pelvis shows lytic destruction of the sacrum. b Sagittal spin echo T1-weighted MR image of the sacrum shows mass in upper sacrum and anterior paraspinal space (*arrows*).

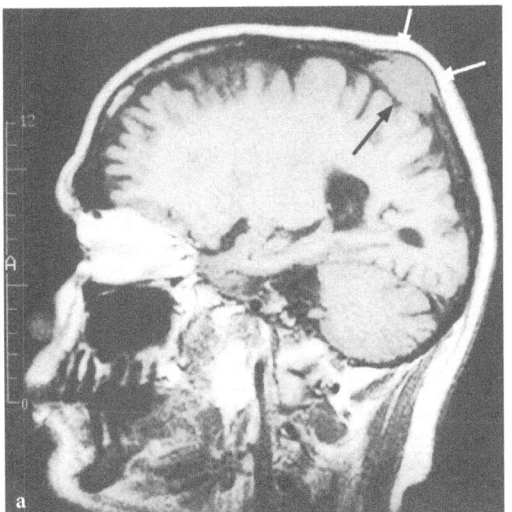
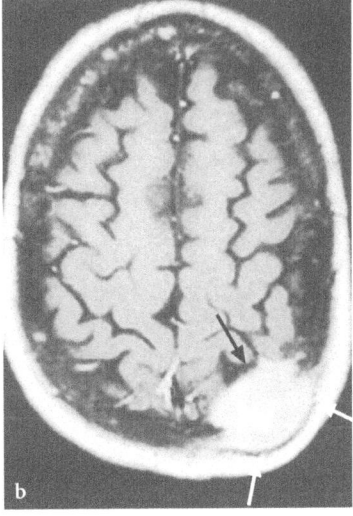

Fig. 17.4a,b. Solitary plasmacytoma of bone of the skull in a 67-year-old man. a Sagittal unenhanced and (b) axial contrast-enhanced spin echo T1-weighted MR images of the brain show marrow-replacing abnormality at the left parietal bone with soft-tissue mass in the epidural space and subcutaneous fat (*arrows*).

the soft-tissue extent better than CT because of increased contrast resolution, although with state of the art enhanced CT it is unlikely that any vital information concerning the extent of the bone tumor will be missed. The value of MR imaging in patients with SBP is the search for occult sites of bone marrow involvement (Figs. 17.6, 17.7) (MOULOPOULOS et al. 1993; MATHIEU et al. 1993).

Definitive treatment for SBP consists of local radiotherapy with approximately 45 Gy. Treatment fields should be designed to encompass all disease shown by CT or preferably by MR imaging, and should include a margin of normal tissue. For spinal lesions, the margin should include at least one uninvolved vertebra. After radiation therapy symptomatic relief occurs in virtually all patients. Signs of response to radiation therapy on conventional radiographs, consist of sclerosis and bone remineralization and are observed in up to 50% of patients (LIEBROSS et al. 1998). On MR images, abnormalities of the bone

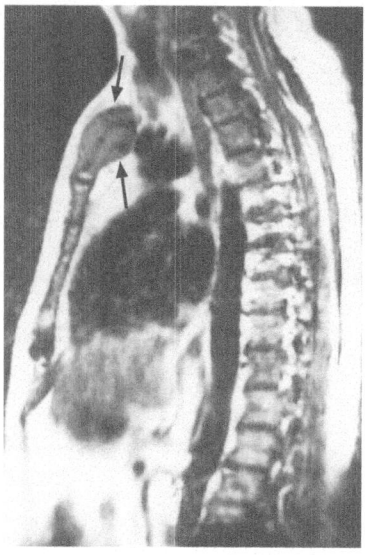

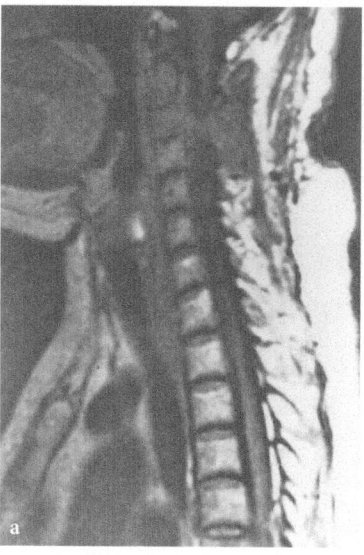

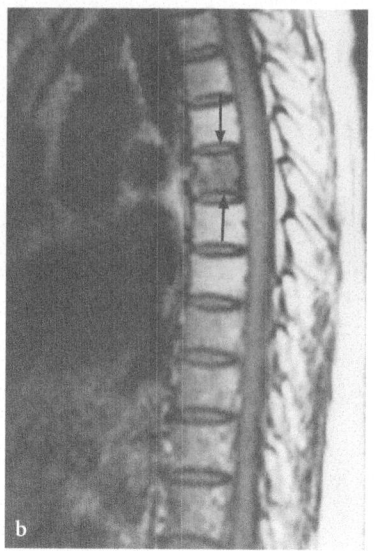

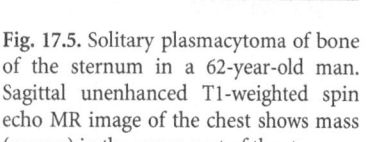

Fig. 17.5. Solitary plasmacytoma of bone of the sternum in a 62-year-old man. Sagittal unenhanced T1-weighted spin echo MR image of the chest shows mass (*arrows*) in the upper part of the sternum.

Fig. 17.6a,b. Solitary plasmacytoma of bone of the second cervical vertebra in a 40-year-old woman, treated with surgery and unsuspected focus of disease. Sagittal unenhanced spin-echo T1-weighted MR images of the (**a**) cervical and (**b**) thoracic spine show postoperative changes at site of primary tumor and a second focus of disease at T6 (*arrows*) for which the patient was treated with local radiation therapy.

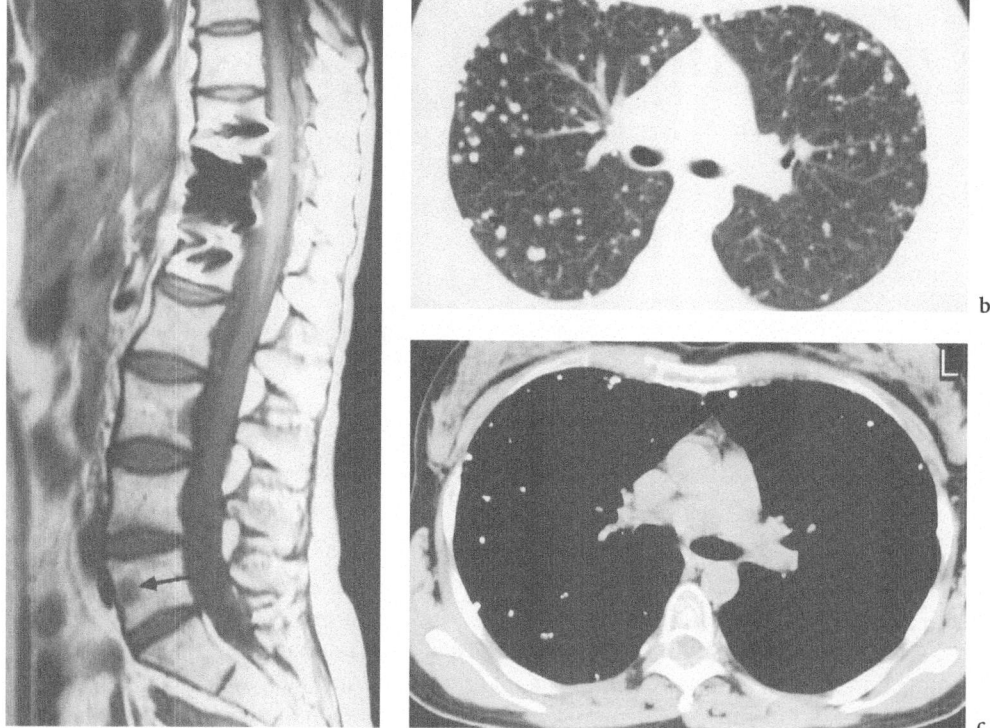

Fig. 17.7a–c. Solitary plasmacytoma of bone of T12 in a 38-year-old woman, treated with surgery and local radiation therapy and unsuspected focus of disease. **a** Sagittal unenhanced fast spin-echo T1-weighted MR image of the lumbosacral and lower thoracic spine shows postoperative changes of the lower thoracic spine and an unexpected focus of disease at L5 (*arrow*). Shortly after the MR study, the patient developed overt multiple myeloma with multiple bone lesions. Patient also developed amyloidosis of the lungs with multiple partially calcified lung nodules on (**b, c**) axial CT scans of the chest.

marrow and an associated soft tissue mass may persist even after successful treatment (Fig. 17.8) (LIEBROSS et al. 1998). With modern radiotherapy techniques and with adequate doses, local control, defined as long-term clinical and radiographic stability is expected in at least 90% of patients (FRASSICA et al. 1989). In most patients with evaluable monoclonal protein, this marker is reduced substantially after radiotherapy. The rate of reduction may be slow and a continuous decrease of the monoclonal protein may be noted for several years (DIMOPOULOS et al.

1992). Complete disappearance of the protein occurs in less than half of evaluable patients. Persistence of an M-protein following tumoricidal radiation is associated with increased risk of disease progression even though some of these patients may remain stable for a long time (DIMOPOULOS et al. 1992). Tumors that are greater than 5 cm also have an increased risk for disease progression. Overall, the majority of patients with SBP progress to systemic disease and the 10-year disease-free survival ranges from 20–45% (DIMOPOULOS et al. 1992).

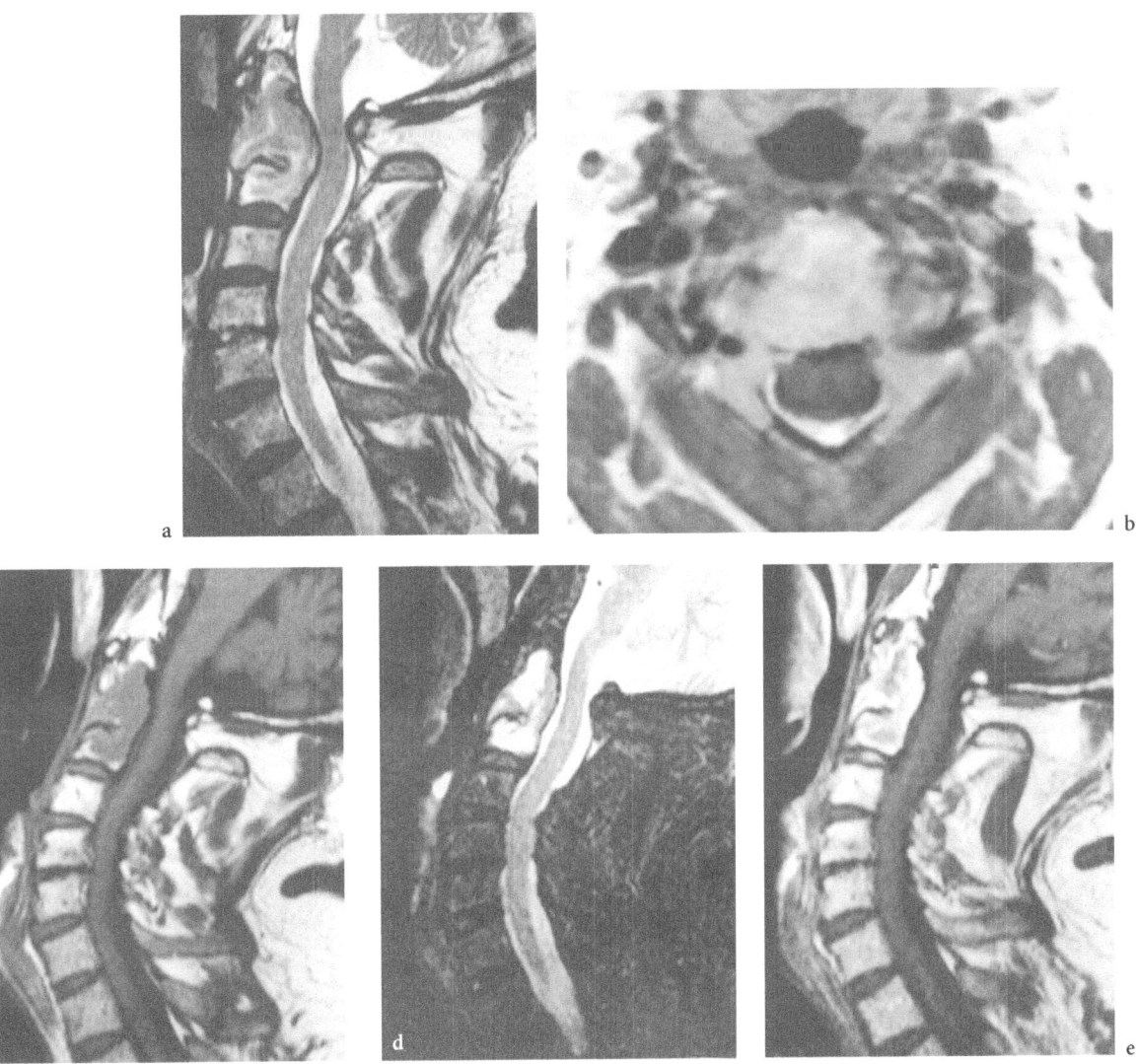

Fig. 17.8a–e. Posttreatment MR imaging changes in a 50-year-old man with solitary plasmacytoma of bone of the upper cervical spine. **a** Sagittal spin-echo T2-weighted and (**b**) axial contrast-enhanced T1-weighted MR images of the cervical spine show tumor involving the first two cervical vertebrae causing mild narrowing of the spinal canal. Sagittal (**c**) unenhanced fast spin-echo T1-weighted, (**d**) short tau inversion recovery (STIR) and (**e**) contrast-enhanced fast spin-echo MR images were obtained a year after treatment with local radiation therapy. Note central necrosis with hyperintensity at (**d**) and peripheral enhancement at (**e**). Two years after treatment, patient is well with no evidence of monoclonal protein in serum.

Progression to multiple myeloma in patients with SBP has been attributed to growth of previously undetected disease. MR imaging detected unsuspected foci of bone marrow involvement in 4 of 12 patients who, otherwise, fulfilled all the criteria for the diagnosis of SBP (MOULOPOULOS et al. 1993). All 4 patients with additional foci of disease on MR imaging, developed multiple myeloma within 18 months from the initial diagnosis of SBP. In another similar study, 4 of 6 patients with SBP and MR imaging lesions not shown on bone survey, developed systemic disease (MATHIEU et al. 1993). In 23 patients with SBP of the thoracolumbar spine, multiple myeloma developed in 7 of 8 patients who were staged with conventional radiographs but in only 1 of 7 patients who were staged with both conventional radiographs and MR imaging (MOULOPOULOS et al. 1993). A recent update of the M.D. Anderson data indicated that 26% of patients initially diagnosed with SBP based on standard criteria, which included normal skeletal surveys, had been misdiagnosed because MR imaging of the spine showed abnormal lesions (WILDER et al. 2002).

MR imaging is the imaging modality of choice for the assessment of response of SBP to local radiotherapy. It should be noted here that persistence of an associated soft-tissue mass does not have any prognostic significance; it may well represent fibrosis (WILDER et al. 2002). Comparison of dynamic pre- and post treatment MR imaging studies may help look for viable tumor by studying changes in the pharmacokinetic profile of the intravenously administered paramagnetic contrast (MOULOPOULOS et al. 2003).

17.3
Extramedullary Plasmacytoma

Extramedullary plasmacytoma (EMP) is even more rare than SBP. It is a plasma cell tumor, which can arise from any site outside the bone marrow in patients with no evidence of myeloma elsewhere (Table 17.2). In a small number of patients (< 25%), monoclonal protein may be present in the serum or urine. Immunohistochemistry and flow cytometry may be required to distinguish EMP from reactive plasmacytosis, plasma cell granuloma, poorly differentiated neoplasms, immunoblastic lymphoma, lymphoplasmacytic lymphoma and MALT lymphoma. Some investigators believe EMP to be a form of dedifferentiated, marginal extranodal lymphoma which tends to affect the mucosa and spread to other soft tissues (HUSSONG 1999; WILTSHAW 1976).

Patients with EMP are younger than patients with multiple myeloma with a mean age of 55 years. Men are affected more often than women. There have been reports of EMPs arising from various sites in the body but over two thirds of such tumors arise in the head and neck region (Fig. 17.9); they are submucosal tumors which frequently affect the upper respiratory tract. Patients with EMP of the head and neck, may present with epistaxis, nasal discharge or nasal obstruction, sore throat, hoarseness or hemoptysis (BATSAKIS et al. 2002; DIMOPOULOS et al. 1999; SUSNERWALA et al. 1997). The second most common site of EMP is the gastrointestinal system (HOLLAND 1997). Other sites of EMP include the parotid gland (Fig. 17.10), the thyroid, lungs, breast (Figs. 17.11, 17.12), testis,

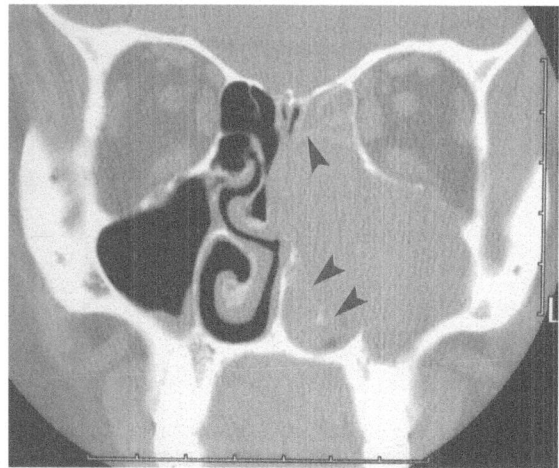
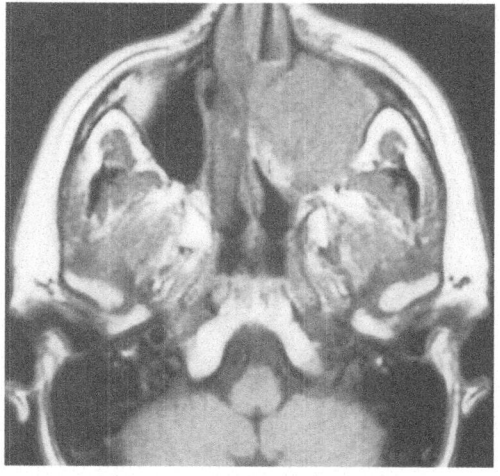

Fig. 17.9. Extramedullary plasmacytoma of the maxillary sinus in a 37-year-old man. **a** Coronal CT scan and (**b**) axial unenhanced fast spin-echo T1-weighted MR image of the paranasal sinuses show mass filling the left maxillary sinus and extending into the ipsilateral ethmoid air cells and nasal turbinates (*arrowheads*).

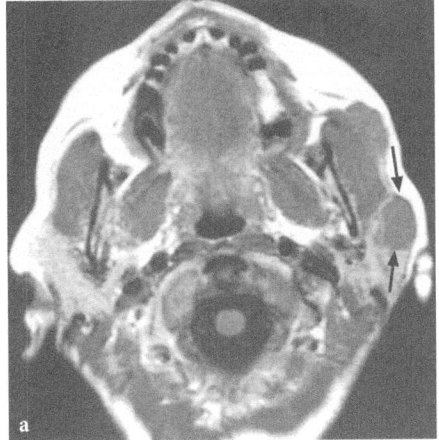
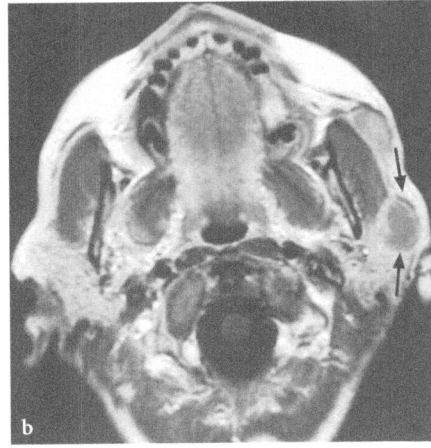

Fig. 17.10a,b. Extramedullary plasmacytoma of the parotid in a 40-year-old woman. Axial (**a**) unenhanced and (**b**) contrast-enhanced fast spin-echo T1-weighted MR images of the neck show a 1.5 cm hypointense lesion (*arrows*) which enhances peripherally, at the superficial portion of the left parotid gland.

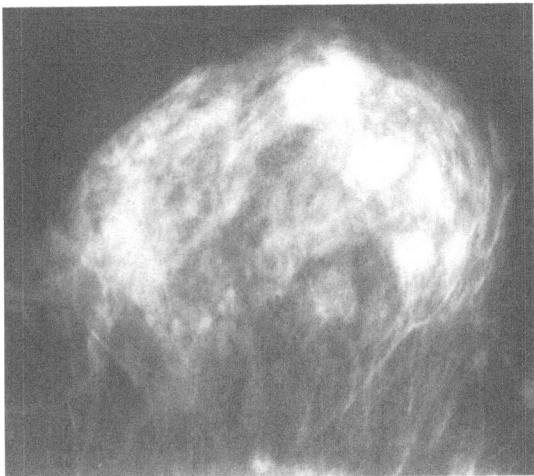
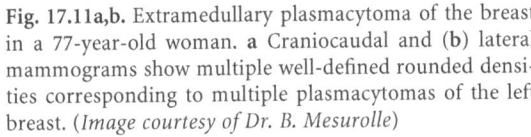
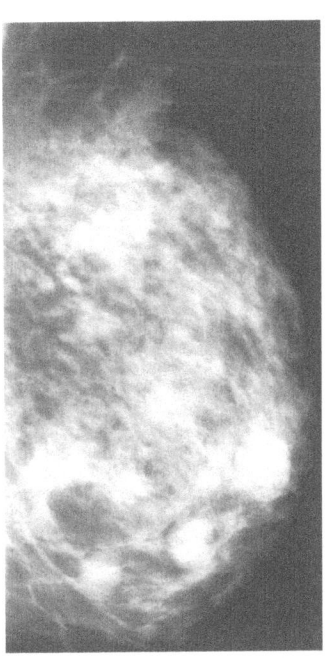

Fig. 17.11a,b. Extramedullary plasmacytoma of the breast in a 77-year-old woman. **a** Craniocaudal and (**b**) lateral mammograms show multiple well-defined rounded densities corresponding to multiple plasmacytomas of the left breast. (*Image courtesy of Dr. B. Mesurolle*)

Table 17.2. Diagnostic criteria for extramedullary plasmacytoma

1. Extramedullary mass with evidence of monoclonal plasma cells
2. Exclusion of reactive plasmacytosis, poorly differentiated epithelial tumors, lymphoplasmacytoid disorders
3. Normal bone marrow aspiration and biopsy
4. Normal skeletal survey and (?) MR imaging of the spine and pelvis
5. No anemia, hypercalcemia or abnormal renal function related to a plasma cell dyscrasia

meninges (Fig. 17.13), kidney (Fig. 17.14) and skin (DE CHIARA et al. 2001; GONZALEZ-GARCIA et al. 1998; KOSS et al. 1998; RAMADAN et al. 2000; RUBIN et al. 1990; TUTLING and BORK 1996).

CT or MR imaging is employed for the depiction of these tumors and for delineation of their extent. Fine needle aspiration of the tumor can be performed under CT guidance. EMPs do not have specific tomographic characteristics and differential diagnosis from other soft tissue tumors is usually difficult. Involvement of adjacent lymph nodes or bony structures may be noted and does not exclude the diagnosis of EMP.

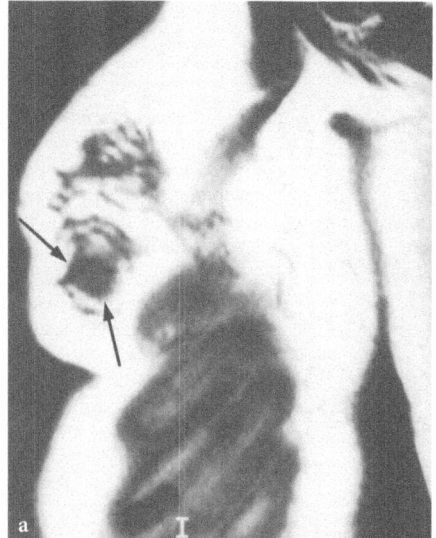
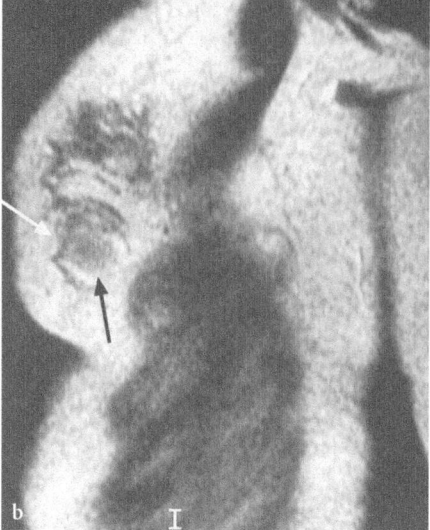

Fig. 17.12a,b. Extramedullary plasmacytoma of the breast in a 41-year-old woman. Sagittal (**a**) unenhanced T1-weighted and (**b**) T2-weighted spin-echo MR images of the breast show lesion (*arrows*) which is hypointense in (**a**) and becomes hyperintense to fat in (**b**). EMP cannot be differentiated from other solid breast lesions.

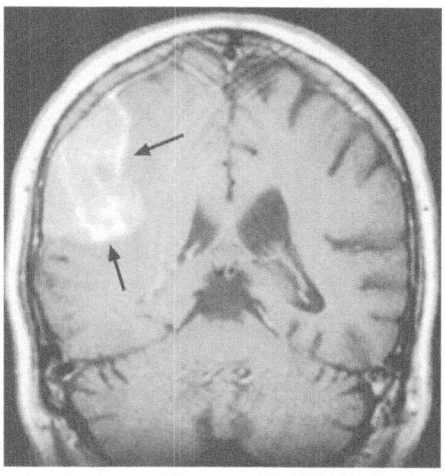

Fig. 17.13. Extramedullary plasmacytoma of the meninges in a 64-year-old man. Coronal contrast-enhanced spin echo T1-weighted MR image of the brain shows enhancing extraaxial mass at right parietal region (*arrows*). The mass was initially diagnosed as meningioma; surgical removal of the tumor revealed a plasmacytoma arising from the meninges without involvement of the adjacent bone.

Fig. 17.14. Extramedullary plasmacytoma of the perirenal space in a 55-year-old man. Axial unenhanced CT scan of the abdomen at the level of the renal hilum shows mass in the left posterior perirenal space (*arrows*).

EMPs are treated with local radiotherapy (at least 4000 cGy). Tumors outside the head and neck region may be surgically removed if possible. About 5% of tumors will recur locally. A small number of patients may develop multiple extramedullary tumors without evidence of plasmacytosis of the bone marrow. Distant recurrence is seen in less than 30% of patients with EMP (GALIENI et al. 2000). Ten-year disease-free survival for patients with EMP is 70%.

17.4 Conclusion

SBPs are rare plasma cell tumors, characterized by involvement of a single bone and no evidence of multiple myeloma. Definitive treatment of these tumors consists of local radiotherapy; both CT and MR imaging can be used to define the radiation portals. MR imaging of the bone marrow may detect unsuspected additional bone marrow lesions in about a third of patients with SBP. It should therefore be part of the initial staging of patients with SBP since it can identify those patients who have occult multiple myeloma and who may benefit from the institution of systemic treatment.

EMPs are even more rare plasma cell tumors, which occur outside the bone marrow, most often in the head and neck region. They do not have characteristic imaging features and either CT or MR imaging may be used to assess the extent of the tumor. Treatment for EMPs consists of local radiotherapy or surgical excision when this is possible.

References

Batsakis JG, Medeiros JL, Luna MA, et al. (2002) Plasma cell dyscrasias and the head and neck. Ann Diagn Pathol 6: 129–140

Conklin R, Alexanian R (1975) Clinical classification of plasma cell myeloma. Arch Intern Med 135:139–143

De Chiara A, Lositi S, Terracciano L, et al. (2001) Primary plasmacytoma of the breast. Arch Pathol Lab Med 125: 1078–1080

Dimopoulos MA, Doldstein J, Fuller L, et al. (1992) Curability of solitary bone plasmacytoma. J Clin Oncol 10:587–590

Dimopoulos MA, Kiamouris C, Moulopoulos LA (1999) Solitary plasmacytoma of bone and extramedullary plasmacytoma. Hematol Oncol Clin North Am 13: 1219–1257

Frassica DA, Frassica FJ, Schray MF, et al. (1989) Solitary plasmacytoma of bone: Mayo Clinic experience. Int J Radiat Oncol Biol Phys 16:43–48

Galieni P, Cavo M, Pulsoni A, et al. (2000) Clinical outcome of extramedullary plasmacytoma. Haematologica 85:47–51

Gonzalez-Garcia J, Ghufoor K, Sandhu G, et al. (1998) Primary extramedullary plasmacytoma of the parotid gland: a case report and review of the literature. J Laryngol Otol 112: 179–181

Holland AJ, Kubacz GJ, Warren JR (1997) Plasmacytoma of the sigmoid colon associated with a diverticular stricture:

case report and review of the literature. J R Coll Surg Edinb 42:47–51

Hussong JW, Perkins SL, Shnitzer B, et al. (1999) Extramedullary plasmacytoma. A form of marginal zone lymphoma. Am J Clin Pathol 111:111–116

Knowling MA, Harwood AR, Bergsagel DE (1983) Comparison of extramedullary plasmacytomas with solitary and multiple plasma cell tumors of bone. J Clin Oncol 1:255–262

Koss MH, Hochholzer L, Moran CA, et al. (1998) Pulmonary plasmacytomas: a clinico-pathologic and immunohistochemical study of five cases. Ann Diagn Pathol 2:1–11

Liebross RH, Ha CS, Cox JD, et al. (1998) Solitary bone plasmacytoma: outcome and prognostic factors following radiotherapy. Int J Radiat Oncol Biol Phys 41:1063–1067

Mathieu D, Rahmouni A, Divine M, et al. (1993) MR imaging of the spine in presumed solitary plasmacytoma (abstract). Radiology 189:S119

Moulopoulos LA, Dimopoulos MA, Weber D, et al. (1993) Magnetic resonance imaging in the staging of solitary plasmacytoma of bone. J Clin Oncol 11:1311–1315

Moulopoulos LA, Maria TG, Papanikolaou N, et al. (2003) Detection of malignant bone marrow involvement with dynamic contrast-enhanced magnetic resonance imaging. Ann Oncol 14:152–158

Ramadan A, Naab T, Frederick W, et al. (2000) Testicular plasmacytoma in a patient with acquired immunodeficiency syndrome. Tumori 86:480–482

Rubin J, Johnson S, Kileen R (1990) Extramedullary plasmacytoma of the thyroid associated with a serum monoclonal gammopathy. Arch Otolaryngol Head Neck Surg 116:855–858

Susnerwala SS, Shanks JH, Banerjee SS, et al. (1997) Extramedullary plasmacytoma of the head and neck region: clinicopathological correlation in 25 cases. Br J Cancer 75:921–927

Tuting T, Bork K. Primary plasmacytoma of the skin (1996) J Am Acad Dermatol 34:386–390

Wilder RB, Ha CS, Cox JD, et al. (2002) Persistence of myeloma protein for more that one year after radiotherapy is an adverse prognostic factor in solitary plasmacytoma of bone. Cancer 94:1532–1537

Wiltsaw E (1976) The natural history of extramedullary plasmacytoma and its relation to solitary plasmacytoma of bone and myelomatosis. Medicine 55:217–238

18 Amyloidosis

Shuichi Monzawa and Tsutomu Araki

CONTENTS

Shuichi Monzawa, MD
Staff Radiologist, Department of Radiology, Hyogo Medical Center for Adults, Kitaohji 13–70, Akashi City, Hyogo 673-8558, Japan
Tsutomu Araki, MD
Professor and Chairman, Department of Radiology, University of Yamanashi School of Medicine, Shimokatou 1110, Tamaho, Nakakoma, Yamanashi 409-3898, Japan

18.1
Introduction

Amyloidosis is characterized by the extracellular deposition of abnormal proteins, called amyloid, in various organs and tissues. Progressive accumulation of amyloid compresses and replaces normal tissues, and it leads to organ dysfunction (SIPE and COHEN 2001). Amyloid deposits are largely composed of protein fibrils and are insoluble and fairly resistant to normal proteolytic digestion. Glycosaminoglycans are always tightly associated with the fibrils; the term amyloid (from the Latin "amylum" and Greek "amylon" meaning starch) is attributed to the propensity of the glycosaminoglycans component in the proteins to turn blue with iodine, which is characteristic of starch. In addition, a non-fibrillary glycoprotein, amyloid P component, is present as a minor constituent in all forms of amyloid (HAWKINS 1995). Protein precursors consisting of amyloid of major types are derived from normally occurring serum proteins, such as immunoglobulin light chains and acute phase reactant proteins. Although an exact mechanism has not been fully elucidated, these protein precursors are produced excessively by a certain type of blood disorder and circulate through blood flow, and then accumulate in tissues where they are converted into amyloid. Patients susceptible to amyloidosis seem to have a reduced capacity for degrading and mobilizing amyloids, once amyloid has formed.

Amyloid deposits may occur in a systemic (generalized) form involving virtually every organ system of the body, or may occur in a localized form involving a single organ (organ-limited amyloidosis) or producing a mass lesion (amyloidoma). Systemic amyloidosis and some localized forms are progressive diseases that are frequently fatal. Amyloidoses are classified according to the biochemical nature of the amyloid proteins. AL amyloidosis represents the most common type of systemic amyloidosis, and occurs in a primary (idiopathic) form or in association with multiple myeloma. AA amyloidosis is another major type of systemic amyloidosis, and occurs in association with chronic diseases that may be infectious, inflammatory, inherited, or neoplastic. Aβ_2M amyloidosis occurs in patients undergoing long-term hemodialysis and involves osteoarticular tissues.

Serious complications such as infarction, bleeding, perforation, and rupture may occur in various organs. Common causes of death in systemic amyloidosis are cardiac and renal failure.

Diagnosis is usually initiated by clinical suspicion on the basis of symptoms, signs and imaging findings and confirmed by histologic demonstration of amyloid deposits in tissues. Imaging studies can depict a wide spectrum of amyloid deposits in various organ systems. Imaging findings, however, are often variable and nonspecific, and simulate those of inflammatory and neoplastic diseases. The presence of calcification on CT scans and decreased signal intensity on T2-weighted MR images can aid differential diagnosis.

18.2
Classification of Amyloidosis

Amyloidosis has been classified based on anatomic sites of involvement (i.e., localized to one specific site, or generalized throughout the body – systemic) and whether it is a primary (in the sense of idiopathic) process without known antecedent or secondary to some other condition or familial. Amyloidosis is now classified according to its biochemical nature. Types of amyloid deposits are designated by two letters: a capital A for amyloid followed by an abbreviation for the fibril protein. There are two major, biochemically distinct types of amyloid protein fibrils designated AL and AA, as well as minor types unrelated to AL and AA (Table 18.1) (Hawkins 1995; Sipe and Cohen 2001).

18.2.1
AL Amyloidosis

AL is derived from immunoglobulin light chains (abbreviated L) produced by abnormal clones of

immunoglobulin-secreting plasma cells (B-cells). AL amyloidosis (light chain amyloidosis) is the most common form of systemic amyloidosis seen in current clinical practice. Less than 20% of patients with AL amyloidosis have preexisting or coexisting multiple myeloma. The majority of patients who develop AL amyloidosis apparently do so in the absence of clinically overt myeloma or other predisposing disease, and such cases are commonly referred to as primary or idiopathic amyloidosis. However, there is evidence now that many cases thought to have been primary amyloidoses are actually caused by an immunocyte dyscrasia, whether clinically recognized or not. About 15–20% of patients with multiple myeloma have amyloidosis (Sipe and Cohen 2001). Primary amyloidosis and amyloidosis associated with multiple myeloma have similar clinical behaviors. Amyloid is deposited principally in mesenchymal tissues, though it may affect any other tissue except the brain. The heart, spleen, kidney, liver, bone marrow, nerves, skin, vascular walls, and gastrointestinal tract are frequently involved. Clinical manifestations of AL amyloidosis are varied and depend on the area of the body involved. Proteinuria is often the first symptom associated with AL amyloidosis (Sipe and Cohen 2001).

18.2.2
AA Amyloidosis

AA is considered to be a product of enzymatic cleavage of an acute phase reactant protein (non-immunoglobulin) synthesized by hepatic cells. AA amyloidosis (amyloid A amyloidosis) has been termed secondary or reactive amyloidosis in the past because the deposits occur in association with chronic diseases. Associated diseases can be infectious, inflammatory, inherited, or neoplastic. The deposits occur most frequently in association with rheumatoid arthritis (about 5–10% of rheumatoid patients) and also occur with tuberculosis, inflammatory bowel disease, renal cell carcinoma, and Hodgkin disease (Sipe and Cohen 2001). Amyloid is commonly deposited in the kidney, and patients show proteinuria and nephrotic syndrome, and may have renal failure in advanced stages, which is one of the major causes of death. The spleen is infiltrated heavily in every case and may be functionally impaired. The adrenal gland and liver are frequently involved, although the function of these organs is usually well preserved (Hawkins 1995). However, no organ system is spared and vascular involvement may be widespread, though clinically significant involvement of the heart is rare.

18.2.3
Aβ₂M Amyloidosis

Aβ₂M is derived from β₂-microglobulin, a 100 amino acid protein that exists on the surface of most nucleated cells as the light chain of the class I major histocompatibility antigens, and is found in the serum of normal individuals. Aβ₂M amyloidosis (β₂-microglobulin amyloidosis), called dialysis-related amyloidosis (DRA), occurs almost exclusively in patients undergoing long-term hemodialysis but can also occur in patients receiving continuous ambulatory peritoneal dialysis. β₂-microglobulin is normally filtered by the glomerulus, and is reabsorbed and catabolized by the proximal tubules in the kidney. In patients with renal failure, the protein accumulates in the serum. Conventional dialysis membranes do not remove β₂-microglobulin from the bloodstream. As a result, serum levels become elevated, and deposits form in a variety of tissues (HAWKINS 1995). Aβ₂M amyloidosis is relatively common in patients who have been on dialysis for more than 5 years, especially among the elderly. Clinical manifestations almost never appear before 5 years of dialysis therapy, but after 10 years, up to 80% of patients may be affected. In contrast to other types of amyloidosis, Aβ₂M deposits are confined largely to osteoarticular sites. Patients often present with a characteristic triad of carpal tunnel syndrome, shoulder pain, and scapulohumeral arthropathy (JANSSEN et al. 2000). Visceral deposits are rare, occurring after 10 or more years of dialysis, and do not cause symptoms in most patients, although patients with perforation of the colon and heart failure have been reported (KAWANO et al. 1998; SHINDO et al. 2001). Many other protein precursors have been identified (Table 18.1).

18.2.4
Localized Amyloidosis

Localized amyloidosis comprises both organ-limited amyloidosis and amyloidoma (focal amyloidosis), both without associated systemic manifestations. In organ-limited amyloidosis, amyloid deposits are limited to a single organ such as the brain, lung, heart and pancreas without evidence of systemic involvement (SIPE and COHEN 2001). Aβ (β-amyloid protein) deposits are likewise confined to the brain and cerebral blood vessels, and may develop into Alzheimer disease or cerebral amyloid angiopathy. Many tumors of amine precursor uptake deamination (APUD) cells that produce peptide hormones have amyloid deposits in their stroma. These are probably composed of hormone peptides and include procalcitonin in medullary carcinoma of the thyroid and islet amyloid polypeptide (IAPP) in insulinomas. AIAPP (IAPP-amyloid) deposits may also occur in the pancreatic islets of Langerhans as a complication of type II diabetes mellitus (Table 18.1). Amyloidoma is a localized focus of amyloid deposits and is usually composed of AL (HAWKINS 1995). The etiology of amyloidoma remains unclear. Some investigators have suggested that amyloidoma arises from isolated clones of plasma cells in localized lymphoid tissues, serving as the local producers of immunoglobulin light chains which, through enzymatic degradation, are converted into amyloid fibrils in a connective tissue stroma (KYLE and GREIPP 1983). Others believe that amyloidoma may arise from burnt-out extramedullary plasmacytoma (GLENNER 1980a; 1980b). Amyloidoma may occur in a variety of locations, including the upper airways, skin, lymph nodes, skull, gastrointestinal tracts, kidney, urinary tract, lung, orbit, breast, soft-tissues, brain, gasserian ganglia, pituitary gland and nasopharynx (HAWKINS 1995).

Table 18.1. Classification of common types of amyloid and amyloidosis

Amyloid protein	Precursor	Systemic or Localized	Syndrome or Involved tissue
AL	Immunoglobulin light chain	Systemic, Localized	Primary, Myeloma-associated
AA	Serum amyloid A	Systemic	Secondary (reactive)
Aβ₂M	β₂-microglobulin	Systemic	Chronic hemodialysis
ATTR	Transthyretin	Systemic	Senile systemic, Familial amyloid polyneuropathy
Aβ	β-amyloid protein	Localized	Alzheimer disease, Cerebral amyloid angiopathy
APrP	Prion protein	Localized	Spongiform encephalitis of kuru, Jakob-Creutzfeldt disease, Gerstmann Sträussler syndrome.
ACal	Procalcitonin	Localized	Medullary thyroid carcinoma
AIAPP	Islet amyloid polypeptide	Localized	Islets of Langerhans in type II diabetes mellitus, Insulinoma

18.3
Diagnosis

Accurate diagnosis is often delayed up to a year or more. Diagnosis is usually initiated by clinical suspicion on the basis of symptoms, signs and imaging findings; however, it must be confirmed by histologic examination of tissue. Subcutaneous abdominal fat pad aspiration and biopsy of rectal mucosa are the best screening tests for systemic amyloidosis. Other useful biopsy sites are gingiva, skin, nerve, kidney, and liver. For $A\beta_2M$, biopsy specimens obtained from bone and synovial lesions or centrifuged synovial fluid sediments are usually tested; the most common site for biopsy is the sternoclavicular joint. Unlike other types of amyloidosis, rectal biopsy and subcutaneous fat aspiration are less valuable.

Microscopically, amyloid shows an amorphous eosinophilic appearance after staining with hematoxylin and eosin, orange by light microscopy and green birefringence by polarizing light microscopy in tissue sections stained with Congo-red dye. Because different types of amyloidosis require different approaches to treatment, determining only that a patient has amyloidosis is no longer adequate. Confirmation of the type of amyloid deposits by specific immunostaining using monoclonal antibody is necessary.

A unique protein called amyloid P component is universally associated with all types of amyloid and forms the basis of a diagnostic test. I-123 serum amyloid P component scintigraphy is a sensitive noninvasive means of diagnosing amyloid in most organs and has been used for quantitative evaluation of amyloid deposition and monitoring the response to therapy in many settings (HAWKINS 2002).

18.4
Treatment and Prognosis

KYLE et al. (1999) reported survival of 810 patients with primary systemic (AL) amyloidosis was 51% at 1 year, 16% at 5 years, and 4.7% at 10 years. In AL amyloidosis, standard treatment aims to suppress the precursor production by chemotherapy or, occasionally, by radiation therapy. Alkylating agents have been used for patients with AL amyloidosis; however, these agents are toxic and not very effective. The most effective form of treatment currently is stem cell transplantation and immunosuppressive drugs (melphalan). Several long-term remissions have been reported, but serious complications, even death, can occur. Cardiac transplanta-

tion has been successful in carefully selected cases. The major causes of death are heart disease (arrhythmias or intractable heart failure) and renal failure. An average survival period after diagnosis is 1 year. Amyloidosis associated with multiple myeloma has a very poor prognosis, and life expectancy is usually less than 6 months (SIPE and COHEN 2001).

In AA amyloidosis, treatment is directed first to the underlying disease. Remission may be achieved by eradication of the disease. Renal replacement therapy is performed in patients with end-stage renal disease and may improve the prognosis. Renal transplantation is a viable option in patients with AA amyloidosis when the underlying disease has been successfully treated (O'MEARA et al. 2001).

The treatment for $A\beta_2M$ amyloidosis is largely supportive, directed toward controlling symptoms. Renal transplantation is the treatment of choice for $A\beta_2M$ amyloidosis as it lowers the blood concentration of β_2-microglobulin, halting the progression of the disease and may result in the complete alleviation of osteoarticular symptoms, such as joint pain and swelling. Unfortunately, no cure for $A\beta_2M$ amyloidosis has been found; osteolytic lesions usually remain unchanged, and regression of amyloid deposits probably does not occur (JANSSEN et al. 2000).

Localized amyloid tumors may be removed without recurrence. Colchicine has been used effectively in preventing acute attacks and amyloidosis in patients with familial Mediterranean fever. It has been shown that in hereditary amyloidosis due to transthyretin mutations, liver transplantation, which removes the site of synthesis of the mutant protein, is very effective (SIPE and COHEN 2001).

18.5
Central Nervous System

The central nervous system (CNS) is not affected in systemic amyloidosis presumably because of the blood-brain barrier (HAWKINS 1995).

18.5.1
Aβ Amyloidosis and Prion Diseases

β-amyloid protein (Aβ) varies in length from 39 to 43 amino acids and is derived from a large transmembrane glycoprotein called amyloid β-precursor protein. Deposits of Aβ commonly occur in blood vessel walls and cause a pathological condition known as cerebral amyloid angiopathy (CAA) that is one of the major causes of brain hemorrhage. CAA is present in approximately 4–10% of patients with cerebral hemorrhages, whereas cerebral hemorrhage has been reported in 40% of autopsy-proven cases of CAA. In contrast to hypertensive hemorrhage, hemorrhages in CAA are characteristically multiple, spare basal ganglia and brainstem, and are located at the corticomedullary junction (CAULO et al. 2001).

Alzheimer's disease, the most common cause of dementia, is also thought to be closely related to Aβ deposits. Common manifestations are a slow progressive decline in memory and orientation. The findings of CT and MR imaging are not specific and may be normal early in the course of the disease. However, these imaging studies help to exclude other disorders, such as primary and secondary neoplasms, multiinfarct dementia, diffuse white matter disease, and normal-pressure hydrocephalus. As Alzheimer's disease progresses, diffuse cortical atrophy including the hippocampus becomes apparent (BIRD 2001).

Prions are a unique class of infectious proteins and cause a group of neurodegenerative diseases related to prion protein amyloid (APrP) deposits, such as the spongiform encephalitis of kuru, Jakob-Creutzfeldt disease, Gerstmann-Sträussler syndrome. APrP is derived from a prion protein, which is a plasma membrane glycoprotein similar to Aβ (SIPE and COHEN 2001).

18.5.2
Amyloidoma in Central Nervous System

Within CNS, amyloidoma has been reported in the brain, gasserian ganglion, pituitary gland, and spinal cord. Previously reported amyloidomas of the brain parenchyma were usually seen in the cerebral white matter and were solitary or multiple, and ranged in size from several millimeters to 8 cm. They showed typically hyperdensity on unenhanced CT scans and enhancement on contrast-enhanced CT scans. On MR imaging, they showed hypo or hyperintensity on T1-weighted images, and mixed or hyperintensity on T2-weighted images, and intense but inhomogeneous enhancement after contrast administration (LEE et al. 1995; CAERTS et al. 1997).

Amyloidoma may occur in the gasserian ganglion and usually cause trigeminal neuropathies. Calcification may be seen on CT scans. MR imaging shows a mass in Meckel's cave, which is isointense on T1-weighted images and iso- to hypointense on T2-weighted images (Fig. 18.1) (ISHIKURA 1998; VORSTER 1998). Although the exact mechanism has not been

disclosed, the short T2-relaxation time may be due to rapid phase dispersion and/or spin-spin interaction derived from the beta-pleated sheet structure of amyloid fibrils (GEAN-MARTON et al. 1991). Also it is thought to result from the hydrophobicity, hypocellularity, and tightly packed configuration of amyloid deposits (JANSSEN et al. 2000). Unlike amyloidoma in other sites, the mass usually enhances homogeneously on both CT scans and MR images after contrast administration (ISHIKURA 1998; VORSTER 1998).

18.6
Head and Neck

18.6.1
Tongue

The tongue is the most common site of amyloidosis in the head and neck. Unlike amyloidosis of other head and neck organs, tongue amyloidosis often represents systemic disease and appears in 15–20% of patients with AL amyloidosis (KYLE and GREIPP 1983). The tongue may be enlarged with smooth or nodular appearance and extrude through gaps between the teeth; macroglossia is a classic feature of AL amyloidosis. Since, in addition to its large size, the tongue becomes adynamic, firm and friable, problems with deglutition, speech, and breathing, and sialorrhea may be seen (FRIEDMAN and JANOWITZ 1998). There have been a few reports describing radiological findings. CT scans may show an enlarged tongue base (wider than 50 mm) and enlarged genioglossus muscles (wider than 11 mm) in patients with tongue involvement and macroglossia (LARSSON et al. 1986). In a reported case with localized amyloidosis of the tongue, the lesion showed marked enhancement on contrast-enhanced CT scans, and hypointensity on T1-weighted MR images, hyperintensity on T2-weighted MR images and marked enhancement on early phase images followed by gradually decreased enhancement on late phase images of dynamic MR imaging (Fig. 18.2) (ASAUMI et al. 2001). Surgical reduction of the tongue is not recommended because of high risk of hemorrhage, airway compromise, and poor healing (FRIEDMAN and JANOWITZ 1998).

18.6.2
Larynx

The larynx is the next most common site in the head and neck. In most instances laryngeal amyloidosis

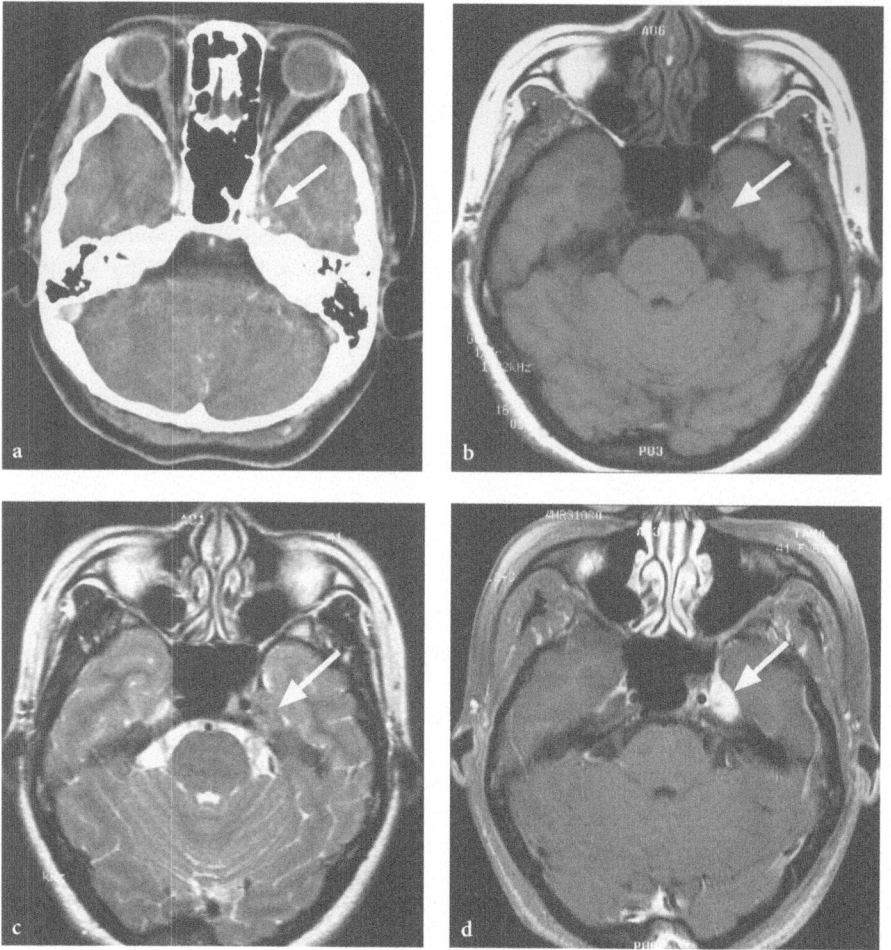

Fig. 18.1a–d. Amyloidoma of the gasserian ganglion in a 41-year-old woman. a Axial contrast-enhanced CT scan shows a hypodense mass (*arrow*) with a small focus of calcification in the Meckel's cave on the left. The mass (*arrow*) is isointense compared to the gray matter on (b) T1 and (c) T2-weighted MR images and marked enhancement (d) after contrast administration. The calcification seen on CT scan (a) is depicted as a hypointense area on MR images (b–d). Surgical removal was performed and histological study of the mass showed deposits of AL. (With permission from [ISHIKURA et al. 1998])

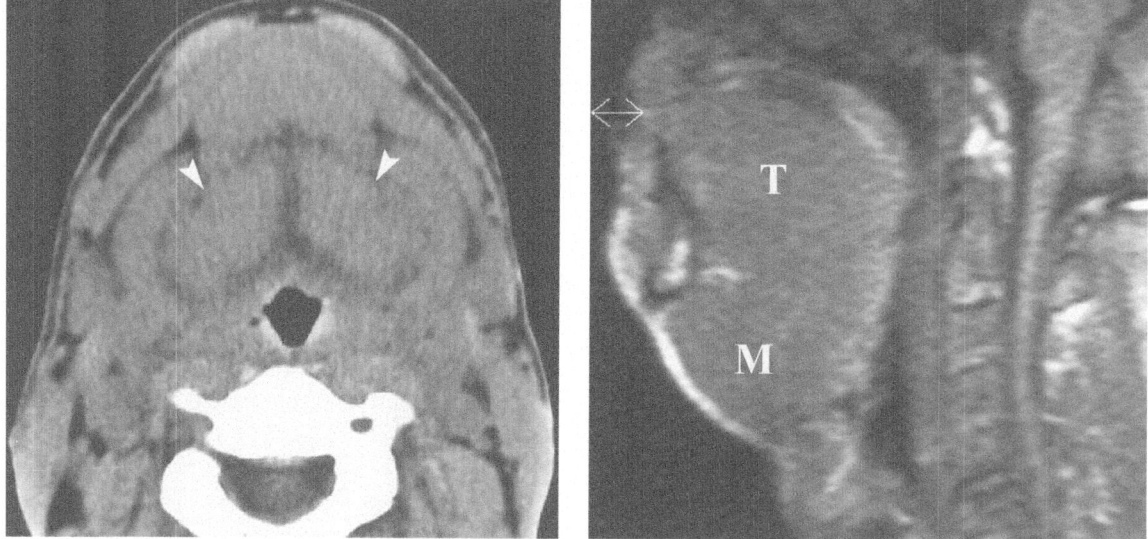

Fig. 18.2a,b. Macroglossia associated with systemic amyloidosis in a 65-year-old man. a Axial unenhanced CT scan shows marked and symmetric enlargement of genioglossus muscles (*arrowheads*). b Sagittal T1-weighted MR image shows diffuse enlargement of the tongue (*T*) and extrinsic tongue muscles (*M*). Biopsy of the tongue showed deposits of AL. (*Image courtesy of Dr. M. Karikomi*)

results from localized AL deposits and is not associated with or followed by systemic disease. Amyloidosis represents 0.5–1% of benign laryngeal diseases with a peak occurrence between the ages of 40 and 60 years and a male predominance (RODRIGUEZ-ROMERO et al. 1996). Diffuse infiltrative and nodular (amyloidoma) forms of laryngeal amyloidosis have been described. Amyloid deposits occur most commonly in the supraglottic larynx, especially the false cords, and usually present with hoarseness or breathing difficulty. The diffuse form with an intact mucosa is more common, sometimes with tracheobronchial extension (GILLMORE and HAWKINS 1999). The nodular form is depicted as a relatively well-defined, submucosal mass commonly with calcification on CT scans. Contrast enhancement is absent or minimal (RODRIGUEZ-ROMERO et al. 1996). The disorder is usually relatively benign but can be progressive or recur after treatment. Fatal hemorrhage has been reported (GILLMORE and HAWKINS 1999).

18.6.3
Thyroid Gland

The most common amyloid deposits are localized amyloidosis associated with medullary carcinoma of the thyroid. Amyloid (ACal) deposits occur in the tumor stroma. Amyloid goiter is thyroid enlargement due to massive amyloid deposits and an extremely rare manifestation of systemic amyloidosis (LIVOLSI et al. 1999). Patients show a progressively growing neck mass associated with dyspnea, dysphagia, or hoarseness. The thyroid is most commonly affected in a bilateral and diffuse manner and no thyroid hormone function abnormalities are usually identified. Histologically, diffuse amyloid deposition is found in perifollicular and interfollicular spaces (HAMED et al. 1995) and foreign body giant cell response and fat tissue infiltration may be observed (LIVOLSI et al. 1999). Patients with amyloid goiter often show multiple solid lesions or cystic changes in a diffusely enlarged thyroid gland on ultrasonography, CT and MR imaging. The solid lesions show low or high attenuation on CT scans and marked enhancement after contrast administration. The cystic changes may be associated with hemorrhage and show variable appearance on CT scans and MR images (HATABU et al. 1990; FONTAN et al. 1995). Calcification may be seen on CT scans (HATABU et al. 1990). Sometimes striking fatty infiltration is seen in the lesion, and it is depicted as areas of hyperechogenicity on ultrasound and of hypodensity on CT scans (MIYAKE et al. 1988).

The prognosis of patients with amyloid goiter depends on the severity of systemic disease rather than of the thyroid lesion. Surgical treatment may be performed if it is necessary to relieve symptoms or if the diagnosis is not clear (HAMED et al. 1995).

18.6.4
Other Head and Neck Organs

In the orbit, amyloid deposits may cause oculomotor palsies resulting from involvement of the extraocular muscles. CT scans may show enlarged extraocular muscles with or without calcifications. On MR imaging, T2-weighted images may show hypointensity in the muscles. Marked enhancement may be seen in the muscles after contrast administration (OKAMOTO et al. 1998). When the lacrimal gland is involved, the disease resembles a lacrimal gland tumor. CT scans may occasionally show calcification in amyloid deposits. On MR imaging, the lesion shows signal intensities similar to those of skeletal muscles on all imaging sequences (MAFEE 2003). Amyloidoma may rarely occur in the nasopharynx. CT scans may show calcification and relatively homogeneous enhancement in the lesion after contrast material administration (GEAN-MARTON et al. 1991). On MR imaging, amyloidoma show signal intensity equal to that of surrounding muscle on T1-weighted images and are isointense to slightly hyperintense on T2-weighted images (HEGARTY and RAO 1993). LEACH et al. (1999) reported a patient with bilateral massive adenopathy of cervical lymph nodes caused by primary systemic amyloidosis (AL type). Other sites of involvement include the nose, paranasal sinuses, Waldeyer's ring, major salivary glands, and temporal bone.

18.7
Trachea and Bronchus

Tracheobronchial amyloidosis occurs almost exclusively in the absence of systemic amyloidosis. Patients are often asymptomatic but can demonstrate hemoptysis, cough, dyspnea, or recurrent pneumonia (GILLMORE and HAWKINS 1999). Amyloid deposits occur in the submucosal and muscular layers of the trachea and bronchi and may lead to luminal narrowing and ulceration. Two forms of tracheobronchial amyloid deposits have been described: focal and diffuse. The focal form manifests as a submucosal focal mass, protruding from the wall of the trachea or bronchi, and partially or completely occluding the airway. There is often infiltration of adjacent peritracheal or bronchial tissue, frequently with calcified foci. This form may mimic both benign and malignant tracheal tumors (SASSON et al. 2003). The diffuse form is more common and shows elevated mucosa forming ridges and nodules. CT scans show circumferential thickening of the tracheobronchial wall with calcification or ossification and severe involvement can result in obstruction (URBAN et al. 1993; GILLMORE and HAWKINS 1999; SASSON et al. 2003). One of the conditions requiring differential diagnosis is tracheopathia osteoplastica, which also shows diffuse calcification in the tracheobronchial wall but spares the posterior membrane (PRINCE et al. 2002). Increased accumulation of ^{99m}Tc hydroxymethylene diphosphonate (HMDP) may be seen in tracheobronchial involvement (Fig. 18.3) (YOSHIDA et al. 1993). Although tracheobronchial amyloidosis is not associated with primary systemic amyloidosis, its course may not be benign. Fatal respiratory failure or recurrent pneumonia secondary to bronchial obstruction may occur. Five-year survival rates range from 30% to 50%, although bronchoscopic surgical and laser resection of airway amyloid deposits may improve prognosis (URBAN et al. 1993; GILLMORE and HAWKINS 1999).

18.8
Lungs

Two forms of involvement have been described: nodular and diffuse parenchymal.

18.8.1
Nodular Form

The nodular form is usually a localized AL type and is not associated with systemic amyloidosis. It is frequently seen in older patients, with an average age in the sixth decade. Patients are usually asymptomatic, rarely presenting with cough or shortness of breath. Nodules may be single or multiple, and show smooth or lobulated contours. The largest reported nodule was 15 cm; the size of most nodules ranges from 4 mm to 5 cm; and the average nodule is 3 cm (UTZ et al. 1996; PICKFORD et al. 1997). The nodules usually vary in size when multiple. They may occur more frequently in the lower lobes, and reveal asymmetric distribution when bilateral involvement is present. They may grow slowly, often over years, and there is no regression. Calcification is seen in about half of the cases often centrally or in an irregular pattern within the nodule. Cavitation may also occur (GROSS et al. 1986). CT is especially helpful in the demonstration of subtle calcification, which is often the only finding that can help suggest the diagnosis (Figs. 18.4, 18.5). The differential diagnosis includes primary or metastatic neoplasm and granulomatous disease.

18.8.2
Diffuse Parenchymal Form

Diffuse parenchymal amyloidosis (also called diffuse alveolar septal amyloidosis) is much less common and usually a manifestation of systemic amyloidosis. Patients commonly demonstrate symptoms of

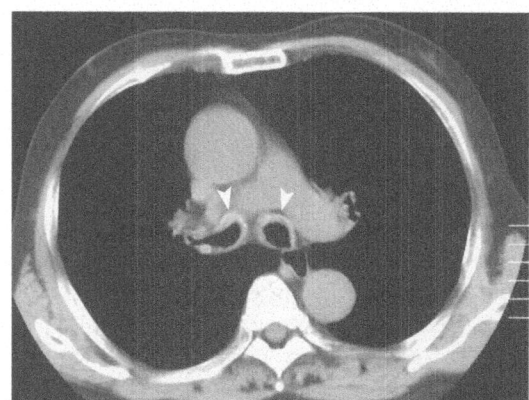
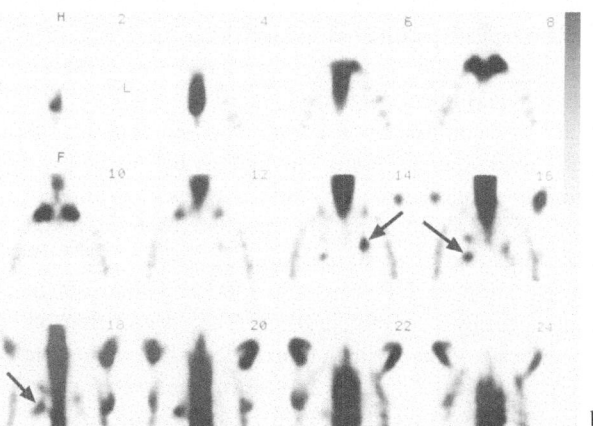

Fig. 18.3a,b. Tracheobronchial amyloidosis in a 70-year-old man with recurrent hemoptysis and pneumonia. a Axial unenhanced CT scan shows circumferential thickening and calcification of the main bronchi (*arrowheads*). b ^{99m}Tc-HMDP bone SPECT images show increased accumulation in the bilateral hilar bronchi (*arrows*). Transbronchial biopsy showed amyloid deposits. (With permission from [YOSHIDA et al. 1993])

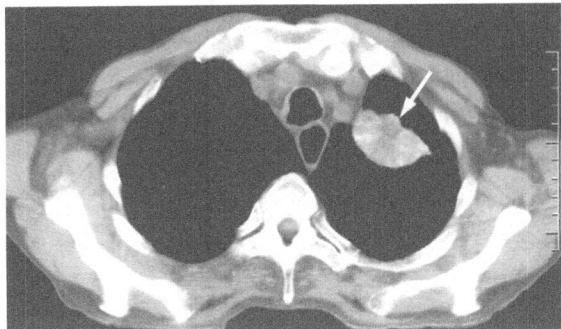

Fig. 18.4. Nodular form of pulmonary amyloidosis in a 60-year-old man. Axial unenhanced CT scan shows a solitary large mass (*arrow*) with multiple small foci of calcification in the upper lobe of the left lung. The diagnosis was confirmed by transbronchial biopsy. (*Image courtesy of Dr. T. Kudo*)

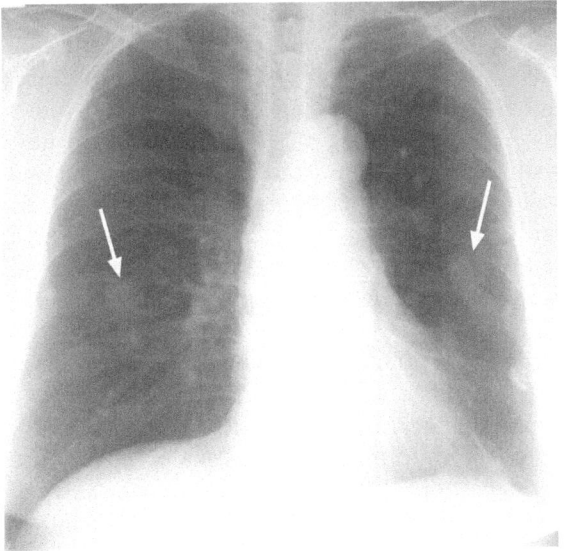

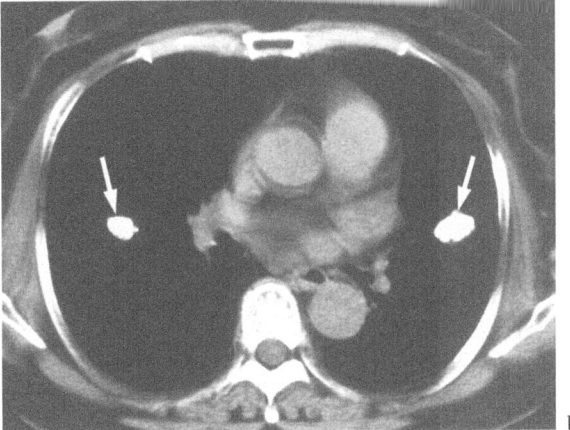

Fig. 18.5a,b. Nodular form of pulmonary amyloidosis in a 70-year-old woman. a Chest radiograph shows multiple bilateral pulmonary nodules (*arrows*). b Axial unenhanced CT scan shows marked calcification within the nodules (*arrows*). The diagnosis was confirmed by biopsy. (*Image courtesy of Dr. S. Noma*)

coughing and shortness of breath and may die of respiratory failure (URBAN et al. 1993). Patients with systemic amyloidosis and pulmonary involvement have a poor long-term prognosis with a median survival of 16 months (PICKFORD et al. 1997).

Histologically, amyloid deposits in the interstitial alveolar septa. Pulmonary arteries are also infiltrated and rarely, pulmonary hypertension may result (PATCHEFSKY 1999). CT findings of diffuse parenchymal amyloidosis include interlobular septal thickening, diffuse irregular lines, ground-glass opacity and honeycombing. These findings are seen predominantly in the peripheral and basilar regions. Calcification may be seen in the lesions. Hilar or mediastinal lymph adenopathies are common. The differential diagnosis includes pneumonia and many interstitial lung diseases (e.g., interstitial fibrosis, rheumatoid lung, or scleroderma). The presence of adenopathy with calcification or multiple small pulmonary nodules may lead to the correct diagnosis (PICKFORD et al. 1997).

18.9 Heart

The heart is commonly compromised by AL amyloidosis and approximately one-third of patients with amyloidosis develop congestive heart failure from mainly left ventricular involvement, the leading cause of death (KYLE and GREIPP 1983). Cardiac amyloidosis of AA type is uncommon, and usually does not result in significant myocardial dysfunction. Amyloid infiltrates between the myocardial fibers, often with extensive deposition within the papillary muscles. The walls of both ventricles become typically firm, rubbery, noncompliant and thickened (WYNNE and BRAUNWALD 2001). Calcification has not been seen in the heart (URBAN et al. 1993). Cardiac amyloidosis typically causes restrictive cardiomyopathy, characterized by abnormalities of diastolic ventricular function with normal to subnormal systolic function. Much less frequently, cardiac amyloidosis leads to dilated cardiomyopathy. In some cases, amyloid deposits result in interruption or in disturbances of the conduction system of the heart with resultant heart block or arrhythmias (WYNNE and BRAUNWALD 2001).

Reported findings of CT and MR imaging include cardiac wall thickening, enlargement of the overall heart size, and pleural and pericardial effusions. Although the wall thickening of cardiac amyloidosis may be suggestive of hypertrophic cardiomyopathy, systolic function, as measured by ejection fraction and wall motion, is normal or increased, in hypertrophic cardiomyopathy but decreased in amyloidosis (Fig. 18.6) (FRANK and GLOBITS 1999). Despite apparent ventricular hypertrophy, electrocardiography shows diffusely decreased voltages in amyloidosis (WYNNE and BRAUNWALD 2001). MR imaging may help in differentiation between cardiac amyloidosis and hypertrophic cardiomyopathy (FATTORI et al. 1998). Scintigraphy with technetium-99m pyrophosphate is often strongly positive with prominent amyloid involvement, although in some patients it is falsely negative (WYNNE and BRAUNWALD 2001).

18.10
Gastrointestinal System

18.10.1
Esophagus

In the esophagus, amyloid deposits occur in muscular layers and nerve tissues, and usually cause motility disorder. Patients with esophageal involvement often present with dysphagia and symptoms of esophageal reflux (FRIEDMAN and JANOWITZ 1998).

Bleeding and rupture may occur (KHAN et al. 1997). Upper gastrointestinal series may show a coarse mucosal pattern with fine granular elevations, polypoid protrusions, reflux, decreased peristalsis and dilated esophagus with tapering of the distal end, mimicking achalasia (ESTRADA et al. 1990; TADA et al. 1994; FRIEDMAN and JANOWITZ 1998).

18.10.2
Stomach

Gastric involvement is common in AL and AA amyloidosis and often results in impaired motility, with delayed gastric emptying and decreased pliability. Patients may have bleeding, epigastric pain, symptoms resulting from pyloric obstruction, and perforation (FRIEDMAN and JANOWITZ 1998). Amyloid deposits occur in the walls of submucosal arteries, and within the muscularis mucosae and muscularis propria, and are prominent in the antrum and body of stomach. Marked deposits in the lamina propria may cause enlarged gastric folds (OWEN 1999). Focal deposition of amyloid (amyloidoma) can occur. The findings of upper gastrointestinal series include coarse mucosal pattern with fine granular elevations, thickening of the folds, polypoid protrusions, rigidity of the gastric wall, marked gastric retention of barium, and, occasionally, obstruction associated with narrowing in the prepyloric and pyloric areas (Fig. 18.7) (FRIEDMAN and JANOWITZ 1998). CT findings includes focal or diffuse gastric wall thickening,

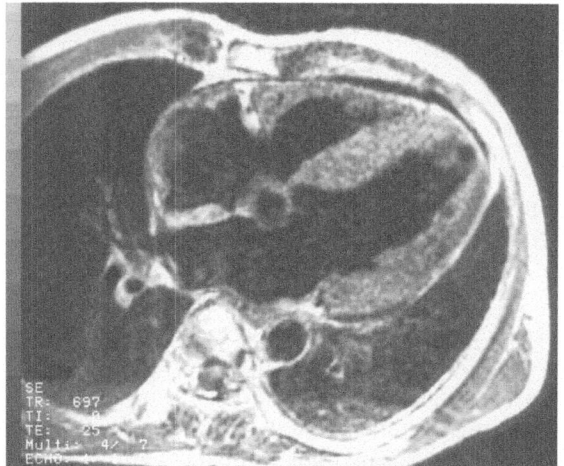 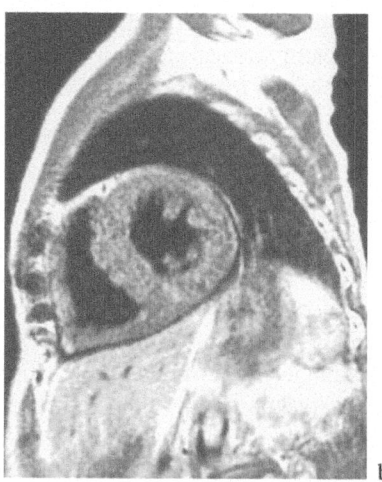

a   b

Fig. 18.6a,b. Cardiac amyloidosis associated with primary systemic amyloidosis in a 53-year-old man. **a** Axial and (**b**) sagittal T1-weighted MR images obtained at end diastole show cardiomegaly and thickened myocardium of the right and left ventricle. At autopsy, the heart was enlarged and abnormally stiff, and both atria were dilated and both ventricles hypertrophied. Diffuse deposits of AL were seen in the myocardium. (*Image courtesy of Drs. H. Tanaka, T. Kawaguchi and A. Hasegawa*)

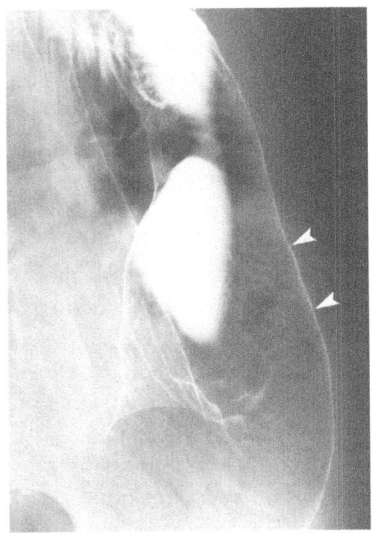

Fig. 18.7. Amyloidosis of the stomach in a 70-year-old man with primary systemic amyloidosis. Double-contrast study of the stomach taken in prone position shows multiple fine granular pattern (*arrowheads*) in the anterior wall of the gastric antrum. The diagnosis was confirmed by endoscopic biopsy. (*Image courtesy of Dr. K. Miyakawa*)

with or without ulcerations, gastric wall calcifications, and a focal mass (URBAN et al. 1993). Drainage operations such as gastrojejunostomies may be performed for decreased motility or obstruction.

18.10.3
Small Intestine

AL and AA amyloidosis commonly infiltrate the small intestine. Amyloid deposits occur in the wall of submucosal blood vessels, and within the lamina propria mucosae and muscularis propria. GILAT et al. (1969) reported amyloid deposits were found more frequently in the small intestine than in the stomach and colon. Patients show diarrhea, bleeding, malabsorption or a motility disturbance mimicking obstruction. On small bowel follow-through examination, approximately 40% of patients with primary amyloidosis exhibit radiographic abnormalities, including diminished motility, delay in barium passage, nodular folds, focal ulceration, transient intussusception, and acute perforations (FRIEDMAN and JANOWITZ 1998). A double-contrast study of the small intestine may show a granular mucosal pattern, polypoid protrusions, erosions and thickened mucosal folds. A granular mucosal pattern may reflect expansion of the lamina propria mucosae due to amyloid deposits,

and may be more common in AA amyloidosis. Polypoid protrusions and fold thickening may be due to massive deposits in the submucosa and muscularis mucosae, and they are seen in AL amyloidosis. Ischemic changes caused by vascular impairment may result in erosions and fold thickening due to edema (Fig. 18.8) (TADA et al. 1991; TADA et al. 1994). CT scans may show diffuse symmetrical wall thickening of the small intestine. Bowel wall calcifications may be seen and help point to correct diagnosis (HORTON et al. 1999). Most patients, however, show normal findings on CT scans (ARAOZ et al. 2000).

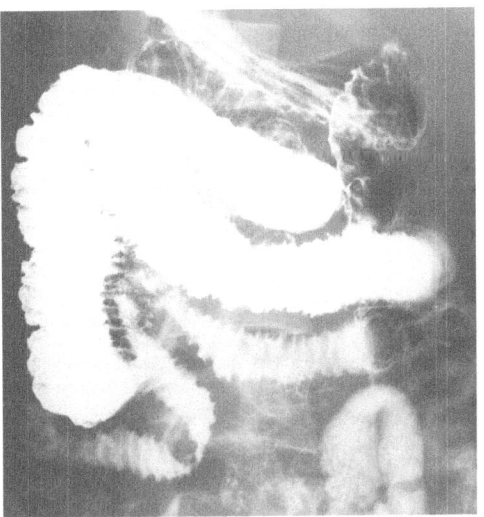

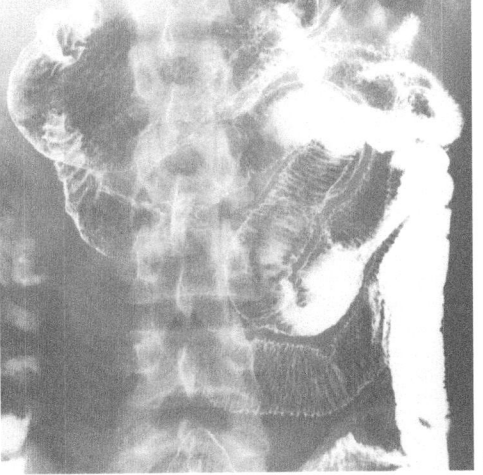

Fig. 18.8a,b. Amyloidosis of the small intestine complicated by ischemia in a 22-year-old man. **a** In acute phase, follow-through examination of the small intestine taken in prone position shows marked fold thickening probably due to ischemia. **b** On follow-up, double-contrast study taken one and half months later, the fold thickening is improved and becomes mild. Amyloid deposits were found by endoscopic biopsy. (*Image courtesy of Dr. K. Murakami*)

18.10.4
Colorectum

The colorectum is also commonly involved by AL and AA amyloidosis. Amyloid deposits occur in blood vessels and muscular layers. Colorectum amyloidosis may present with abdominal pain, diarrhea, constipation, bleeding, and intestinal pseudoobstruction. Amyloid deposits in the colorectum are rarely radiographically evident. The radiographic manifestations of colonic amyloidosis are varied and unspecific, and appear to result not only directly from amyloid deposition, but also in part from ischemia derived from vascular impairment by amyloid. Common findings of barium enema examinations are a granular mucosal pattern, thickened mucosal folds, luminal narrowing, loss of colonic haustrations, delay in barium passage and diverticulum formation (Fig. 18.9). Ischemic changes caused by vascular impairment may occur and result in ulceration, infarction and perforation. Radiologic appearances may resemble those of ischemic colitis or ulcerative colitis. The descending colon and rectosigmoid colon are the commonest areas demonstrating radiographic abnormalities (TRINH et al. 1991). On CT scans, thickening of the colonic wall and luminal narrowing may be seen (DIAZ CANDAMIO et al. 1999).

18.10.5
Liver

AL and AA amyloidosis often involves the liver. Amyloid is deposited in the parenchyma, along the sinusoids within the space of Disse, or in blood vessel walls. Chopra, et al. reported that hepatic-parenchymal amyloid deposition was seen in 100% of patients with AL amyloidosis and 77% with AA amyloidosis, and vascular amyloid deposition in 68% with AL amyloidosis and 100% with AA amyloidosis (CHOPRA et al. 1984). Hepatocytes are severely compressed by extensive accumulation of amyloid and they may atrophy or nearly disappear. In advanced cases with massive infiltration, the liver is enlarged with rubbery elastic consistency, and may show a 'lardaceous liver' appearance on cut surfaces. The clinical manifestations of hepatic involvement are usually mild. Hepatomegaly and minimally abnormal liver function test are the most frequent findings in patients with hepatic amyloidosis. However, serious symptoms such as hepatic failure, portal hypertension, spontaneous rupture and massive hemorrhage may occur (GASTINEAU et al. 1991; GERTZ et al. 1997).

Ultrasound shows heterogeneous echogenicity in the liver in patients with AL amyloidosis (MONZAWA et al. 2002). Conventional precontrast and contrast-enhanced CT shows enlarged liver with heterogeneous decreased attenuation. The hepatic parenchyma highly infiltrated by amyloid may appear as focal hypoattenuating areas on contrast-enhanced CT scans (SUZUKI et al. 1986; URBAN et al. 1993). Calcifications may be seen rarely in the hepatic parenchyma (Fig. 18.10) (JACOBS et al. 1997; KOBAYASHI et al. 2002). On dynamic CT, portal phase images show heterogeneous enhancement in the hepatic parenchyma in patients with AL amyloidosis. Delayed phase images taken 5 minutes after administration of contrast material show delayed enhancement with the presence of some focal hypoattenuating areas in the liver; these focal hypoattenuating areas may

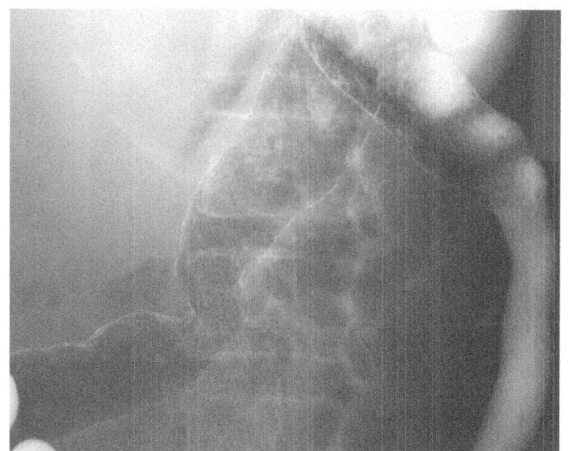
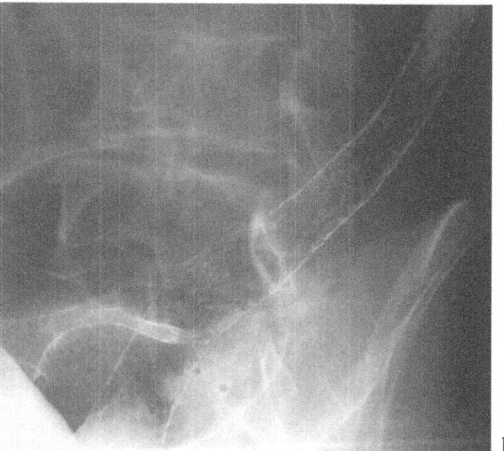

a   b

Fig. 18.9a,b. Amyloidosis of the colon in a 65-year-old man. a, b Double-contrast barium enema studies show a granular mucosal pattern and loss of haustration. The diagnosis was confirmed by endoscopic biopsy. (*Image courtesy of Dr. K. Murakami*)

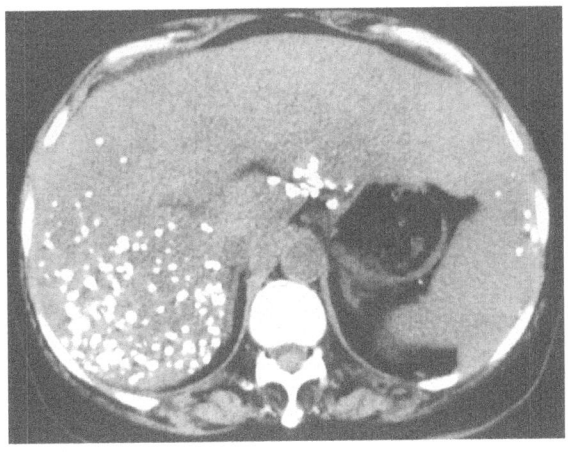

Fig. 18.10. Hepatic amyloidosis with calcifications in a 65-year-old woman with primary systemic AL amyloidosis. Axial unenhanced CT shows an enlarged liver with multiple small foci of calcification. The diagnosis was confirmed by biopsy from the liver, kidney and rectum. (With permission from [Kobayashi et al. 2002])

may occur and potentially increase the risk of serious infection (Powsner et al. 1998). Spontaneous splenic rupture is a known consequence of splenic amyloidosis (Tanno et al. 2001).

Reported findings of conventional CT in splenic amyloidosis include splenomegaly, calcification, and poor parenchymal enhancement after administration of contrast material (Suzuki et al. 1986; Urban et al. 1993). On dynamic CT, arterial phase images show lack of enhancement in the spleen, which may be a result of vascular involvement and diffuse parenchymal infiltration of amyloid. Delayed phase images taken 5 minutes after administration of contrast material show mild delayed enhancement in the spleen (Monzawa et al. 2002). T2-weighted MR images show low signal intensity in the spleen; this T2 shortening may be due to decreased blood content secondary to increased amyloid deposition (Benson et al. 1987). On T1-weighted MR images, no signal abnormalities may be seen in the spleen (Fig. 18.11) (Monzawa et al. 2002).

represent highly infiltrated hepatic parenchyma. MR imaging findings have not been well described. Monzawa et al. (2002) showed that significant signal abnormalities were not observed in the liver on T1-weighted or on T2-weighted MR images. Increased accumulation of ^{99m}Tc methylene diphosphonate (MDP) may be seen in involvement of the liver (Fig. 18.11) (Rosello et al. 1988).

18.10.6
Spleen

The spleen is frequently involved by AL and AA amyloidosis. Iwata and Ishihara showed that splenic deposits were identified in 83% of patients with AL amyloidosis and 87% of those with AA amyloidosis at autopsy (Iwata and Ishihara 1985). Amyloidosis of the spleen is seen in two forms. Most commonly, amyloid deposits are largely limited to the splenic follicles, producing tapioca-like granules on gross inspection. This form is designated "sago" spleen and is more commonly seen in AA amyloidosis than in AL amyloidosis. In the other form, amyloid deposits may spare the follicles and mainly infiltrate the red pulp sinuses, producing large, maplike areas of amyloid deposits. This form is designated "lardaceous" spleen and is characteristic of AL amyloidosis. In both of these forms, blood vessels are commonly involved (Iwata and Ishihara 1985). Splenic involvement is usually asymptomatic. Hyposplenism

18.10.7
Pancreas

Pancreatic amyloid may be massively deposited in the pancreas and cause marked acinar destruction. Pancreatic acinar atrophy may lead to pancreatic insufficiency and steatorrhea. This may contribute to the malabsorption caused by amyloidosis of the small bowel (Friedman and Janowitz 1998). Also diabetes mellitus may occur. Segovia Garcia et al. (2002) described radiologic findings seen in a case with pancreatic involvement by systemic AL amyloidosis. Ultrasonograms showed a hypoechoic and enlarged pancreas. On contrast-enhanced CT scans, the pancreas showed enlargement and very low attenuation. On MR imaging, the pancreas showed hypointensity on fat-suppressed T1-weighted images, hyperintensity on T2-weighted images, and a patchy pattern of enhancement after contrast administration. Later, this patient showed calcification in the pancreas.

18.11
Urogenital System

18.11.1
Kidney

The kidneys may be affected in any of the systemic forms of amyloidosis. Involvement of the kidney

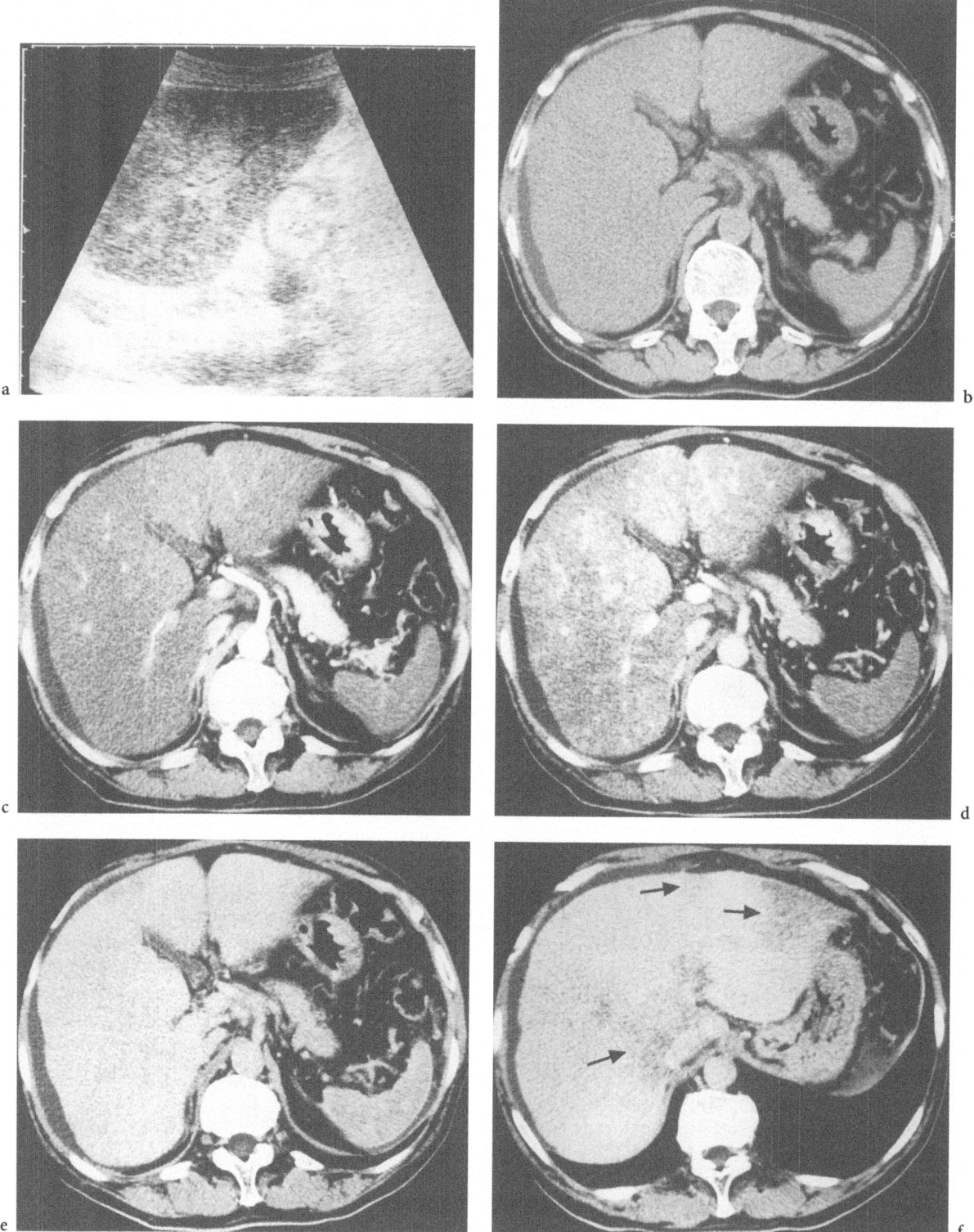

Fig. 18.11a–f...

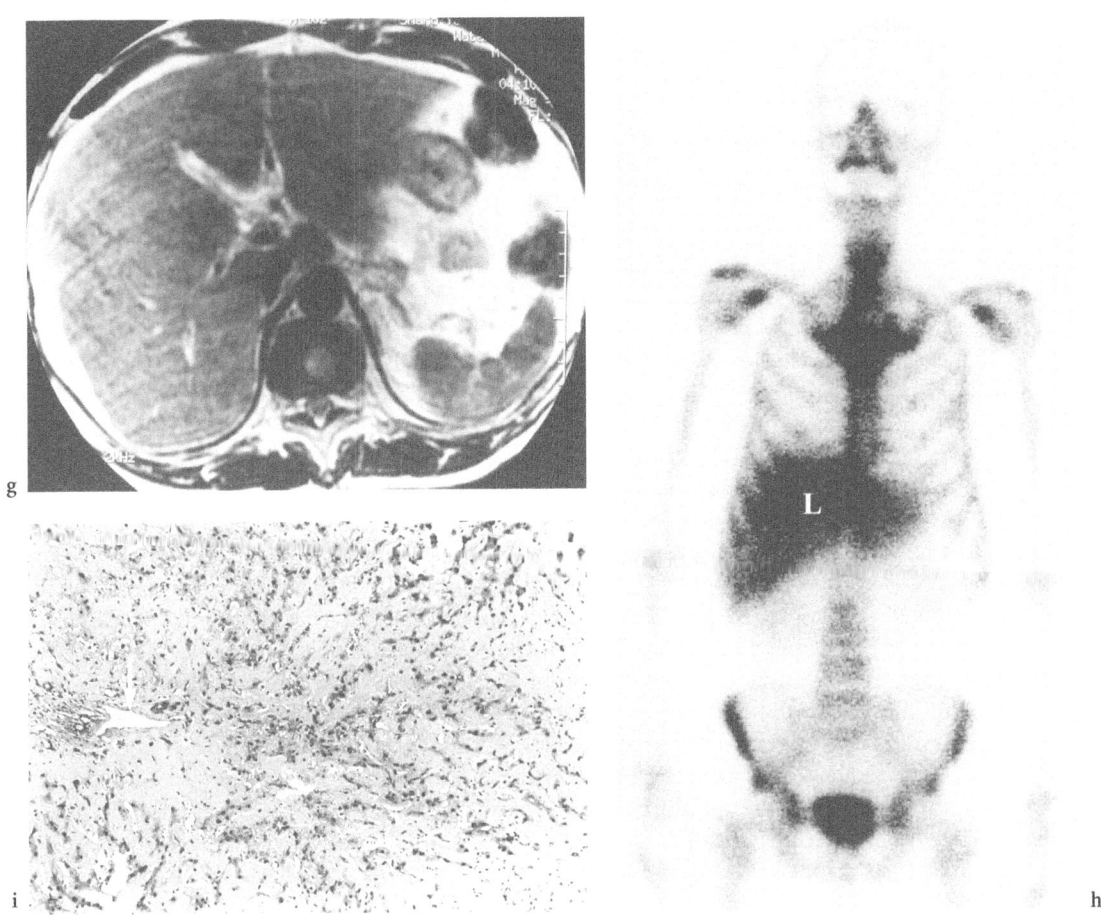

Fig. 18.11a–i. Amyloidosis of the liver and spleen in a 73-year-old man with primary systemic AL amyloidosis. The patient presented general fatigue and abdominal fullness. **a** Ultrasound image shows heterogeneous echogenicity in the liver. **b** Precontrast phase scan of dynamic CT shows an enlarged liver of decreased attenuation (attenuation value of the hepatic parenchyma is 43 HU and that of the splenic parenchyma is 44 HU). Collection of ascitic fluid is seen in the subphrenic space. **c** Arterial phase CT scan shows the lack of parenchymal enhancement in the spleen (49 HU). **d** Portal phase CT scan shows heterogeneous enhancement in the liver. **e, f** Delayed phase CT scans show homogeneous delayed enhancement of the hepatic parenchyma (89 HU) with focal hypodense areas (*arrows*; 58 HU). The spleen is enhanced mildly and heterogeneously (71 HU). **g** Axial T2-weighted spin-echo MR image shows hypointensity in the spleen. Signal loss is present in the deep portion of the abdomen because of decreased sensitivities of a surface coil. **h** Bone scintigram using ^{99m}Tc HMDP shows abnormal accumulation in the entire liver (*L*). **i** Photomicrograph of biopsy specimen from the liver shows extensive deposits of amyloid in the perisinusoidal space (the space of Disse). Hepatocytes are compressed severely by amyloid and have become atrophic. The portal venous tract (*arrow*) is also involved and distorted by massive amyloid deposition (hematoxylin and eosin staining; original magnification ×25). (With permission from [MONZAWA et al. 2002])

occurs in 76–92% of patients with AA amyloidosis and in about 35% of patients with AL amyloidosis, and sometimes in ATTR amyloidosis. Involvement in $A\beta_2M$ amyloidosis is rare (PORTER 1992). Amyloid deposits occur in the glomerular mesangia and glomerular basement membranes, and make glomerular filter leaky to plasma proteins e.g. albumin. Amyloid is also deposited in the interstitium and vascular walls (KYLE and GREIPP 1983). The kidney is usually normal in size or slightly enlarged. In advanced stages, the kidney may be small and shrunken due to vascular

compromise. Initially renal amyloidosis usually manifests as proteinuria, often resulting in nephrotic syndrome. A minority of patients present with renal failure due to vascular involvement, etc (O'MEARA et al. 2001). Treatment by hemodialysis or kidney transplantation improves the prognosis considerably. There have been a few reports describing the imaging findings of renal amyloidosis. The kidney is enlarged in the acute stage of renal involvement, and becomes small in advanced renal failure. Ultrasonography may show increased cortical echogenicity with preservation of corticomedullary contrast (Moon et al. 1995). In advanced cases, calcification may be seen on CT scans (Levine 1994; Apter et al. 2001).

18.11.2
Ureter

Amyloidosis of the ureter may occur as a localized lesion or as part of systemic amyloidosis. Both forms are extremely rare. Patients generally present with chronic obstructive uropathy, sometimes with flank pain and hematuria. Amyloid deposits occur more frequently in the lower third and only rarely in the middle third of the ureter. Instances of bilateral involvement have been reported. Calcification or ossification may occur. Intravenous urography may show a stricture in the distal ureter and CT may show a mass lesion at the site of stricture (Fig. 18.12). Radiologically it is difficult to distinguish from ureteric cancer and most reported cases have resulted in inappropriate nephroureterectomy (Hayashi et al. 1998). Calcification may aid in the diagnosis, if present. When involved in systemic amyloidosis, the ureter is usually diffusely narrowed and irregular from extensive amyloid deposits. In children, especially those with familial Mediterranean fever, there may be narrowing, rigidity, and an apparent shortening of the ureter.

18.11.3
Bladder

Amyloidosis of the urinary bladder is rare, and most cases are of the localized AL type, with fewer cases of the secondary AA type. Amyloidosis of the urinary bladder most commonly occurs in the fifth to seventh decades. There is no predilection of sex. Patients typically present with gross painless hematuria and urinary frequency. Amyloid deposits are most abundant in the mucosa and submucosa of the bladder, but commonly are also present within the muscularis propria. Cystoscopy shows irregular exophytic lesions, which bleed readily and may be ulcerated. Intravenous urography shows nonspecific filling defects projecting into the bladder lumen, and distorting the bladder outline (Petersen 1986). CT shows diffuse thickening of the urinary bladder wall. Occasionally, calcification may be present. Amyloid deposits show low signal intensity on T2-weighted images and are not enhanced after intravenous administration of gadolinium: MR imaging may be useful in differentiating the disease from bladder tumor or inflammation (Amano and Kumazaki 1996). Treatment usually consists of transurethral resection and fulguration, although segmental resection is sometimes required (Petersen 1986). Intravesical instillation of dimethyl sulfoxide (DMSO) has been reported to be successful in some cases (Tirzaman 2000).

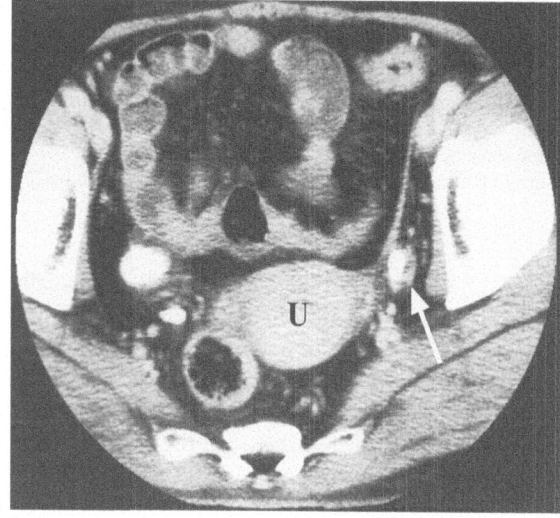
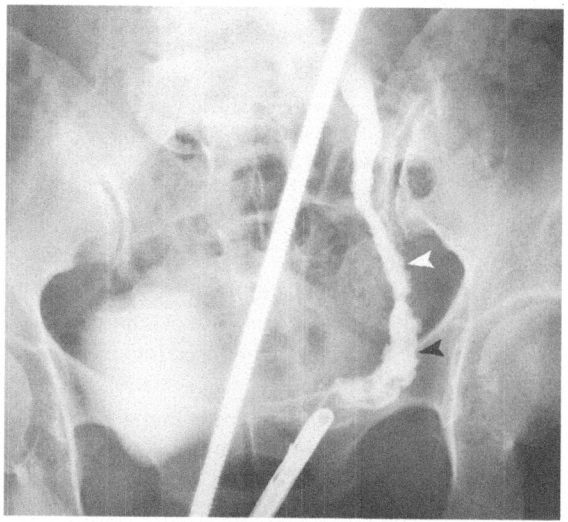

Fig. 18.12a,b. Amyloidosis of the ureter in a 51-year-old woman. **a** Axial contrast-enhanced CT scan shows diffuse wall thickening (*arrow*) in the lower ureter on the left. (*U = Uterus*) **b** Retrograde urograph shows multiple filling defects with irregularity in the left distal ureter (*arrowheads*). The diagnosis was confirmed by surgery. (*Image courtesy of Dr. K. Murakami*)

18.11.4
Seminal Vesicles

Amyloidosis of the seminal vesicles is a senile localized disorder and seldom causes clinical problems although it is rarely associated with systemic AA amyloidosis. The incidence of amyloid deposits in the seminal vesicles increases with increasing age, and they are found in 21% of men over 75 years. Amyloid deposits are located in the lamina propria of the seminal vesicle and are occasionally prominent leading to narrowing of the lumen. Both seminal vesicles are usually symmetrically involved. Compromised seminal vesicles show low signal intensity on T2-weighted MR images due to narrowing of the lumen and thickening of the wall of seminal vesicles due to amyloid deposits. Gadolinium may be helpful in making the diagnosis because amyloid does not enhance, whereas tumor invasion shows enhancement (Fig. 18.13) (KAJI et al. 1992; RAMCHANDANI et al. 1993).

18.11.5
Retroperitoneum

Diffuse involvement of the retroperitoneum by systemic AL amyloidosis has been reported. Amyloid deposits may show paraaortic or perirenal soft-tissue infiltration, thickening of renal fascia, calcification, and heterogeneous enhancement after contrast material administration on CT scans (SUEOKA et al. 1989; GLYNN et al. 1989). On MR imaging, the lesions may be isointense to slightly hyperintense on T1-

weighted images and hypointense on T2-weighted images compared to the renal cortex. Extrinsic ureteral narrowing may be evident on retrograde urography (SUEOKA et al. 1989).

18.12
Musculoskeletal System

18.12.1
Aβ₂M Amyloidosis

Aβ₂M amyloidosis usually invades osteoarticular, tendinous and periarticular sites, and causes osteoarthropathies that resemble inflammatory destructive processes. Large joints, such as the shoulders, wrists, hips and knees, are frequently affected (JANSSEN et al. 2000). Although the mechanism of involvement remains unclear, it is postulated that in the peripheral joints amyloid deposits progress from synovial fluid into the synovial membrane and finally to the bone, eventually causing lytic lesions and destruction. Patients with Aβ₂M amyloidosis commonly present severe joint pain, especially in the shoulder joint, carpal tunnel syndrome, and less frequently, trigger finger, flexor tendon contracture, spontaneous tendon rupture and pathological fracture (KURER et al. 1991).

Typical radiographic features include bilaterally symmetric arthropathies with soft-tissue masses, osteopenia, and focal osteolytic lesions, and occasionally extensive joint destruction (MURPHEY et al. 1993). Osteolytic lesions involve the medullary and

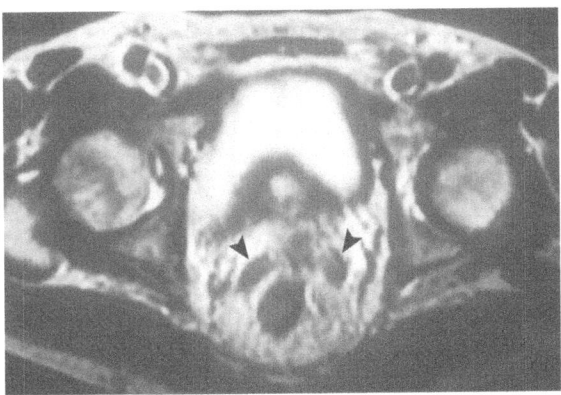 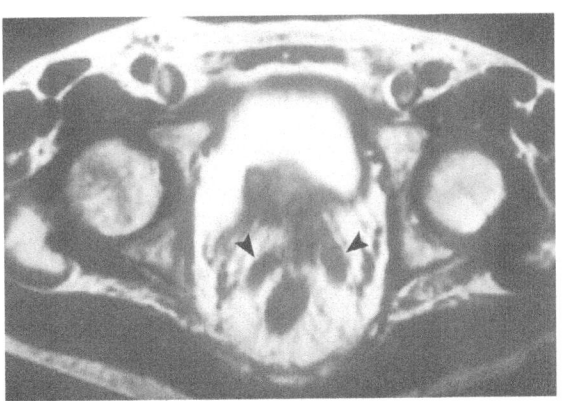

a   b

Fig. 18.13a,b. Localized amyloidosis of the seminal vesicles in a 78-year-old man with urinary bladder cancer. **a** Axial T2-weighted MR image shows the seminal vesicles to be hypointense (*arrowheads*). **b** Axial contrast-enhanced T1-weighted MR image shows no contrast enhancement of the seminal vesicles which remain hypointense (*arrowheads*). A radical cystectomy with seminal vesicle resection was performed for the urinary bladder cancer. Marked amyloid deposits were found in the lamina propria of the seminal vesicles histologically. (With permission from [KAJI et al. 1992])

cortical bone with variable size, and produce scalloping along the endosteal margin of the cortex. The lesions are frequently multiple and may be bilateral, and can increase in size and number. They are well-defined subarticular radiolucent lesions, usually with thin sclerotic margins. CT allows detailed depiction of these features and may be better for evaluating bone involvement. These lesions may accumulate bone-seeking radiopharmaceutical agents. MR imaging is useful for demonstrating the extent of soft-tissue and intraosseous lesions. T2-weighted MR sequences can distinguish amyloid deposits from inflammatory processes. Amyloid deposits usually show low signal intensity whereas inflammatory or infectious diseases show hyperintensity on T2-weighted MR images. Some amyloid lesions, however, can show foci of increased signal intensity within the intraosseous and soft-tissue lesions. Mixed results are also reported regarding the enhancement patterns of amyloid deposits. Thus the diagnosis of amyloid osteoarthropathy is suggested by clinical history and corroborated with imaging. The ultimate diagnosis may require biopsy (KURER et al. 1991; JANSSEN et al. 2000).

18.12.2
Carpal Tunnel Syndrome

Patients with $A\beta_2M$ amyloidosis commonly develop carpal tunnel syndrome, which is a neuropathy caused predominantly by compression of the median nerve due to amyloid deposits at the wrists. Patients with this disorder may experience pain, dysesthesias, weakness, and sensory changes in the hands. It is often bilateral and progressive. Radiographs show well-defined subarticular osteolytic lesions, usually with thin sclerotic margins in the carpal bones. T1 and T2-weighted MR images show soft tissues of low to intermediate signal intensity within the carpal canal, surrounding and displacing the flexor tendons. Widening of the scapholunate and distal radioulnar articulations, disruption of the triangular fibrocartilage complex, and numerous erosions may be seen (COBBY et al. 1991). Carpal tunnel release surgery for decompression of the median nerve may be effective in alleviating pain and restoring function (KURER et al. 1991).

18.12.3
Shoulder and Hip Joints

Involvement of the shoulder joints is common. Amyloid deposits occur in and around the rota-

tor cuff, and may cause rubbery, hard soft-tissue masses in the shoulder, resembling the shoulder pads worn by football players (referred to as the shoulder pad sign). Patients often show shoulder pain and decreased mobility. On MR images, the supraspinatus tendon shows thickening, irregularity and heterogeneous signal intensity. Periarticular osseous lesions are common in the humerus, which range in size from 1–2 mm to a few cm and show low to intermediate signal intensity on T1-weighted MR images and variable signal intensity on T2-weighted MR images. Joint and bursal effusions are commonly seen (Fig. 18.14). Ultrasound may be useful in the detection of thickening of the rotator cuff.

$A\beta_2M$ may involve the hip joint. Osteolytic lesions are seen in the femoral heads and acetabulum. Subsequent pathologic fractures may occur in the femoral neck (KURER et al. 1991). On MR images, thickening and irregularity are commonly found in the ilio-femoral portion of the joint capsules. Joint effusion and peritendinous or bursal effusions are also seen (Fig. 18.15) (ESCOBEDO et al. 1996). Thickening of joint capsules may be observed on ultrasound.

18.12.4
Destructive Spondyloarthropathy

$A\beta_2M$ may cause destructive spondyloarthropathy. The most common site is the lower segment of the cervical spine, although the atlantoaxial region may be affected. Amyloid deposits are found in the disks, paravertebral ligaments, and synovial tissues. Patients commonly present with neck and back pain (RESNICK 2002a; THEODOROU et al. 2002). Characteristic findings on radiographs include endplate and vertebral body destruction and progressive narrowing of the disk space, and absence of osteophytes. These changes may progress rapidly over a period of months. Findings may mimic those of infectious spondylodiscitis or inflammatory arthritis. On MR imaging, involved spinal segments have been reported to show various signal intensities on T2-weighted images: Generally the absence of hyperintensity on T2-weighted MR images may be helpful in eliminating the diagnosis of infectious diseases (Fig. 18.16) (JANSSEN et al. 2000; THEODOROU et al. 2002). With progression of the disease, collapse of the vertebral body, spinal instability and severe neurologic compromise related to compression of the spinal cord may occur. In patients with these complications, surgical treatment including decompression and spinal stabilization may be considered (THEODOROU et al. 2002).

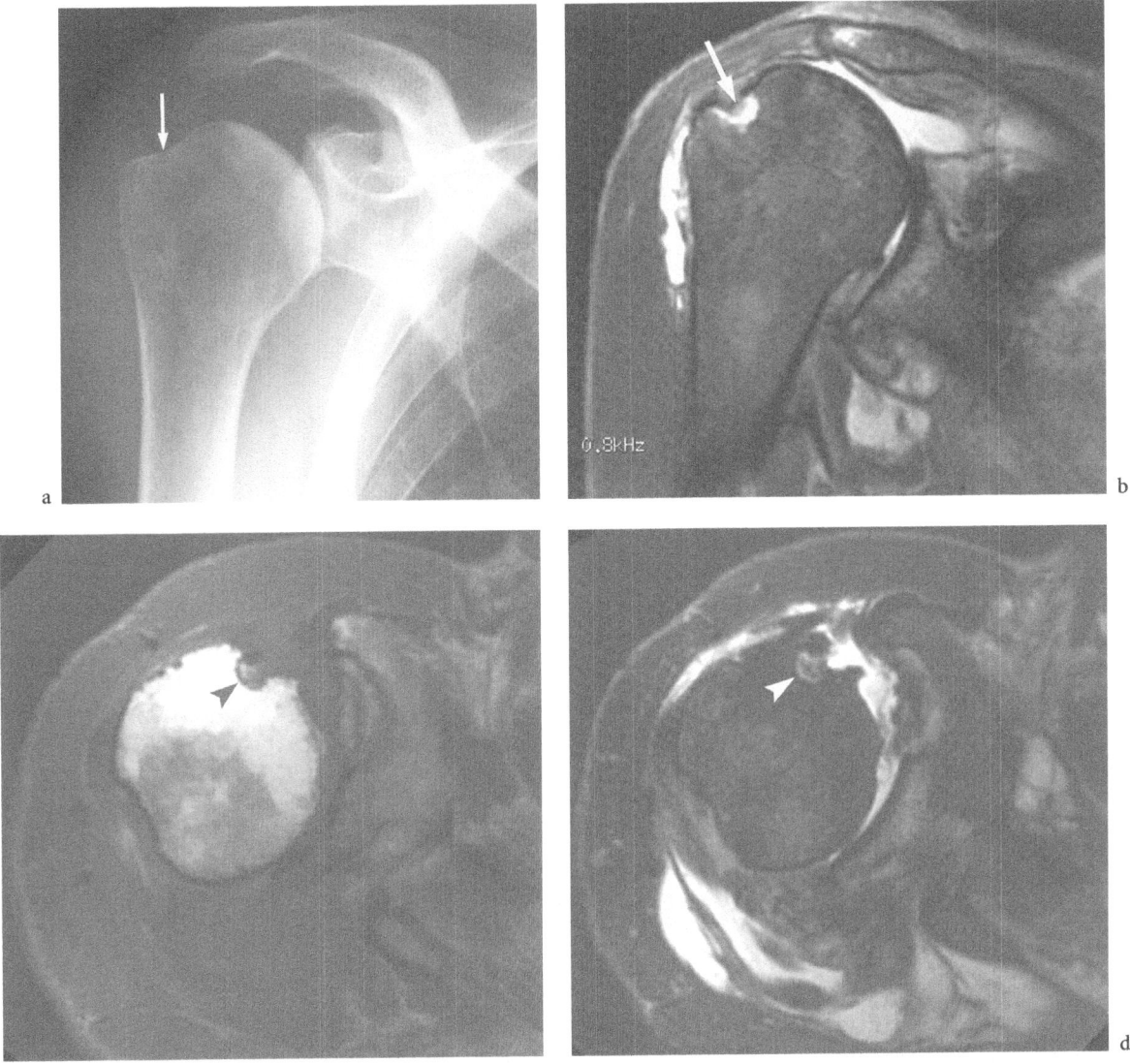

Fig. 18.14a–d. Aβ₂M amyloidosis of the shoulder joint in a 67-year-old man with end-stage renal failure receiving hemodialysis. **a** Radiograph shows a radiolucent lesion (*arrow*) with reactive sclerosis and osteoporosis in the humeral head. **b** Coronal fat-suppressed T2-weighted MR image shows a small periarticular osseous lesion in the head of the humerus (*arrow*). Axial (**c**) T1 and (**d**) fat-suppressed T2-weighted MR images show another small periarticular osseous lesion in the humeral head (*arrowhead*). Prominent bursal and joint effusions are seen. The diagnosis was confirmed by endoscopy and biopsy. (*Image courtesy of Dr. H. Oba*)

18.12.5
AL Amyloidosis

AL amyloidosis may involve the musculoskeletal system and show a number of characteristic appearances that are similar to Aβ₂M amyloidosis. AL deposits are found in bone, synovium, and soft tissue. Osteolytic lesions of variable size are detected particularly in the proximal portion of the humerus and proximal portion of the femur. Amyloid deposits in soft tissue are particularly prominent in the olecranon region and about the joints of the hand and wrist. Carpal tunnel syndrome is seen in 10 to 30% of patients with AL amyloidosis (RESNICK 2002b). Amyloid deposits in joints show hypointensity on T1-weighted MR images and low or mixed signal intensity on T2-weighted MR images (SHIM et al. 1997). These lesions may accumulate bone-seeking radiopharmaceutical agents (RESNICK 2002b). Amyloid myopathy is a rare manifestation of AL

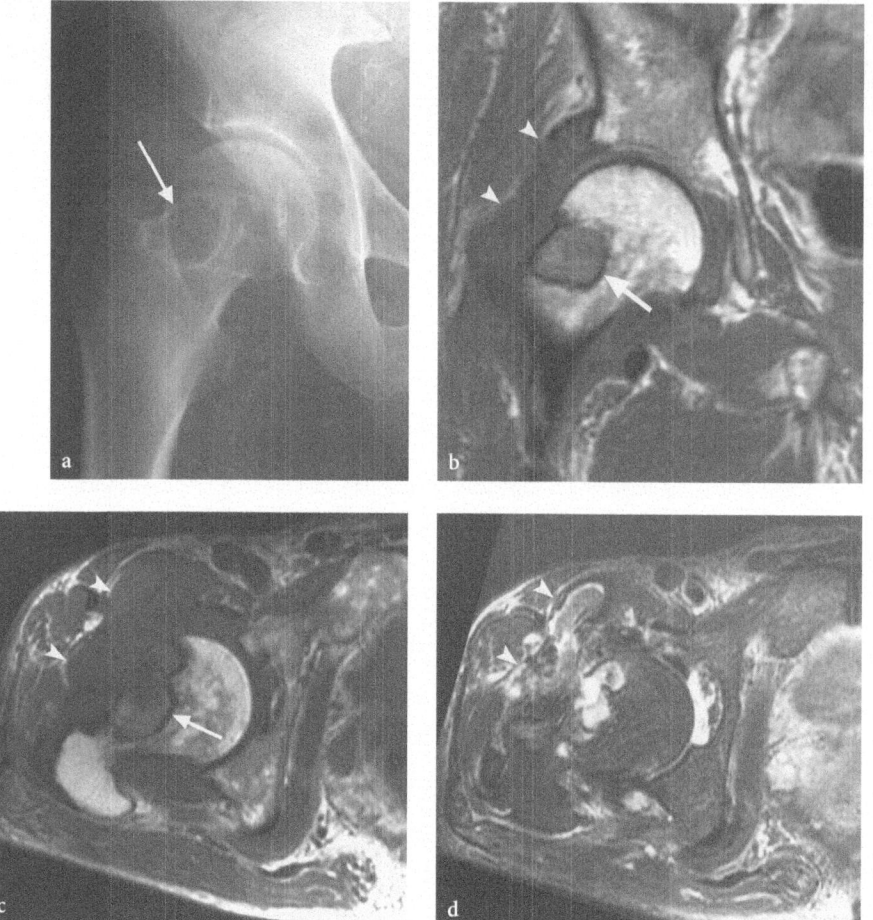

Fig. 18.15a–d. Aβ₂M amyloidosis of the hip joint in a 67-year-old man (same patient as in Fig. 18.14). **a** Radiograph shows a large radiolucent lesion with reactive sclerosis in the femoral neck (*arrow*). **b** Coronal and (**c**) axial T1-weighted MR images show a large periarticular osseous lesion in the humeral head (*arrow*), which is depicted as an intermediate signal intensity area with a rim of hypointensity. Marked capsular thickening (*arrowheads*) of hypointensity is also seen. **d** Axial fat-suppressed T2-weighted MR image shows the osseous lesion to be heterogeneously hyperintense, and the capsule to be heterogeneously hypointense (*arrowheads*). (*Image courtesy of Dr. H. Oba*)

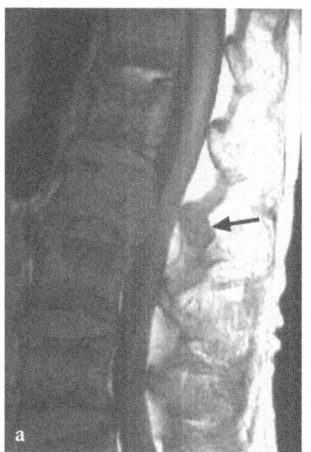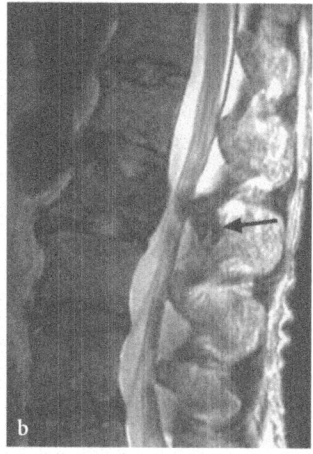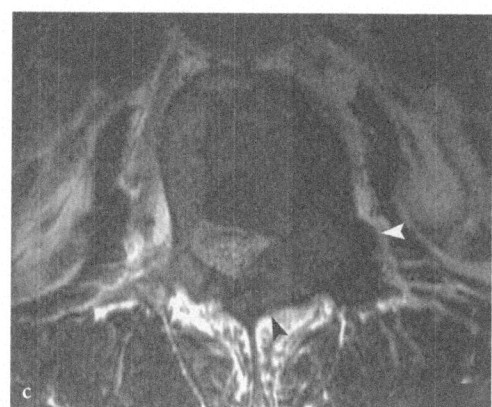

Fig. 18.16a–c. Destructive spondyloarthropathy in a 53-year-old woman with end-stage renal failure receiving hemodialysis. Sagittal (**a**) T1 and (**b**) T2-weighted MR images show mild collapse of the body and enlargement of the lamina (*arrow*) with hypointensity in the second lumbar vertebra. **c** Axial T2-weighted MR image shows a hypointense area infiltrating in the body and enlarged left arch (*arrowheads*) in the second lumbar vertebra. Histological studies of specimens obtained by surgical intervention revealed Aβ₂M deposits in the lesions. (*Image courtesy of Dr. K. Kimura*)

amyloidosis and is caused by deposits in interstitial connective tissues, blood vessels, and nerves. Patients show muscle weakness, stiffness, generalized muscle enlargement, and a woody consistency of the limbs. On MR images, affected muscles show minimal signal changes in contrast to a wide variety of other myopathy in which fat or edema usually show remarkable MR appearances (METZLER, et al. 1992).

18.13
Conclusion

Amyloidosis can demonstrate a wide spectrum of disease in nearly every organ and tissue type. Imaging modalities can depict these changes. Most imaging findings, however, are variable and nonspecific, and simulate those of other diseases. Knowledge of patient's clinical data and familiarization with clinicopathological and radiological findings of amyloidosis may be crucial for timely and correct diagnosis.

Acknowledgments
We thank The Fund of Cancer Research from Hyogo Prefecture Health Promotion Association, Kobe, Japan, for their financial support of our work.

We also thank Doctors Kazuro Sugimura, Shuji Adachi, Yoshiki Takada, Reiichi Ishikura, Masato Karikomi, Hideo Tanaka, Takeo Kawaguchi, Akio Hasegawa, Takehumi Kudo, Satoshi Noma, Koji Murakami, Kunihisa Miyakawa, Akihiko Kobayashi, Hiroshi Oba, and Kazuhiko Kimura.

References

Amano Y, Kumazaki T (1996) MR appearances of urinary bladder in amyloidosis associated with multiple myeloma. Abdom Imaging 21:468–469
Apter S, Zemer D, Terhakopian A, et al. (2001) Abdominal CT findings in nephropathic amyloidosis of familial Mediterranean fever. Amyloid 8:58–64
Araoz PA, Batts KP, MacCarty RL (2000) Amyloidosis of the alimentary canal: radiologic-pathologic correlation of CT findings. Abdom Imaging 25:38–44
Asaumi J, Yanagi Y, Hisatomi M, et al. (2001) CT and MR imaging of localized amyloidosis. Eur J Radiol 39:83–87
Benson L, Hemmingsson A, Ericsson A, et al. (1987) Magnetic resonance imaging in primary amyloidosis. Acta Radiol 28:13–15
Bird TD (2001) Alzheimer's disease and other primary dementias In: Braunwald E, Fauci AS, Hauser SL, Longo DL,

Jameson JL (eds) Harrison's principles of internal medicine. McGraw-Hill Companies, New York, pp 2391–2395
Caerts B, Mol V, Sainte T, et al. (1997) CT and MRI of amyloidoma of the CNS. Eur Radiol 7:474–476
Caulo M, Tampieri D, Brassard R, et al. (2001) Cerebral amyloid angiopathy presenting as nonhemorrhagic diffuse encephalopathy: neuropathologic and neuroradiologic manifestations in one case. AJNR Am J Neuroradiol 22:1072–1076
Chopra S, Rubinow A, Koff RS, et al. (1984) Hepatic amyloidosis. A histopathologic analysis of primary (AL) and secondary (AA) forms. Am J Pathol 115:186–193
Cobby MJ, Adler RS, Swartz R, et al. (1991) Dialysis-related amyloid arthropathy: MR findings in four patients. AJR Am J Roentgenol 157:1023–1027
Diaz Candamio MJ, Pombo F, Yebra MT (1999) Amyloidosis presenting as a perforated giant colonic diverticulum. Eur Radiol 9:715–718
Escobedo EM, Hunter JC, Zink-Brody GC, et al. (1996) Magnetic resonance imaging of dialysis-related amyloidosis of the shoulder and hip. Skeletal Radiol 25:41–48
Estrada CA, Lewandowski C, Schubert TT, et al. (1990) Esophageal involvement in secondary amyloidosis mimicking achalasia. J Clin Gastroenterol 12:447–450
Fattori R, Rocchi G, Celletti F, et al. (1998) Contribution of magnetic resonance imaging in the differential diagnosis of cardiac amyloidosis and symmetric hypertrophic cardiomyopathy. Am Heart J 136:824–830
Fontan FJ, Cordido F, Mosquera J, et al. (1995) Amyloid goitre: CT and MR findings. Clin Radiol 50:409–411
Frank H, Globits S (1999) Magnetic resonance imaging evaluation of myocardial and pericardial disease. J Magn Reson Imaging 10:617–626
Friedman S, Janowitz HD (1998) Systemic amyloidosis and the gastrointestinal tract. Gastroenterol Clin North Am 27:595–614
Gastineau DA, Gertz MA, Rosen CB, et al. (1991) Computed tomography for diagnosis of hepatic rupture in primary systemic amyloidosis. Am J Hematol 37:194–196
Gean-Marton AD, Kirsch CF, Vezina LG, et al. (1991) Focal amyloidosis of the head and neck: evaluation with CT and MR imaging. Radiology 1181:521–525
Gertz MA, Kyle RA (1997) Hepatic amyloidosis: clinical appraisal in 77 patients. Hepatology 25:118–121
Gilat T, Revach M, Sohar E (1969) Deposition of amyloid in the gastrointestinal tract. Gut 10:98–104.
Gillmore JD, Hawkins PN (1999) Amyloidosis and the respiratory tract. Thorax 54:444–451
Glenner GG (1980a) Amyloid deposits and amyloidosis: the beta-fibrilloses (first of two parts). N Engl J Med 302:1283–92
Glenner GG (1980b) Amyloid deposits and amyloidosis: the beta-fibrilloses (second of two parts). N Engl J Med 302:1333–1343
Glynn TP Jr, Kreipke DL, Irons JM (1989) Amyloidosis: diffuse involvement of the retroperitoneum. Radiology 170:726
Gross BH, Felson B, Birnberg FA (1986) The respiratory tract in amyloidosis and the plasma cell dyscrasias. Semin Roentgenol 21:113–127
Hamed G, Heffess CS, Shmookler BM, et al. (1995) Amyloid goiter. A clinicopathologic study of 14 cases and review of the literature. Am J Clin Pathol 104:306–312
Hatabu H, Iida Y, Kasagi K, et al. (1990) Amyloid goiter: radiologic findings. AJR Am J Roentgenol 155:193–194

Hawkins PN (1995) Amyloidosis. Blood Rev 9:135–142

Hawkins PN (2002) Serum amyloid P component scintigraphy for diagnosis and monitoring amyloidosis. Curr Opin Nephrol Hypertens 11:649–655

Hayashi T, Kojima S, Sekine H, et al. (1998) Primary localized amyloidosis of the ureter. Int J Urol 5:383–385

Hegarty JL, Rao VM (1993) Amyloidoma of the nasopharynx: CT and MR findings. AJNR Am J Neuroradiol 14:215–218

Horton KM, Corl FM, Fishman EK (1999) CT of nonneoplastic diseases of the small bowel: spectrum of disease. J Comput Assist Tomogr 23:417–428

Ishikura R, Ando K, Morikawa T (1998) Amyloidoma of the gasserian ganglion. Nippon Igaku Hoshasen Gakkai Zasshi 58:S4–S8

Iwata T, Ishihara T (1985) Pathology of AA and AL amyloidosis. Rinsho Byori 3:141–151

Jacobs JE, Birnbaum BA, Furth EE (1997) Abdominal visceral calcification in primary amyloidosis: CT findings. Abdom Imaging 22:519–521

Janssen H, Weissman BN, Aliabadi P, et al. (2000) MR imaging of arthritides of the cervical spine. Magn Reson Imaging Clin N Am 8:491–512

Kaji Y, Sugimura K, Nagaoka S, et al. (1992) Amyloid deposition in seminal vesicles mimicking tumor invasion from bladder cancer: MR findings. J Comput Assist Tomogr 16:989–991

Kawano M, Muramoto H, Yamada M, et al. (1998) Fatal cardiac beta2-microglobulin amyloidosis in patients on long-term hemodialysis. Am J Kidney Dis 31:E4

Khan GA, Lewis FI, Dasgupta M (1997) Beta 2-microglobulin amyloidosis presenting as esophageal perforation in a hemodialysis patient. Am J Nephrol 17:524–527

Kobayashi A, Saitoh Y, Tada A, et al. (2002) Hepatic amyloidosis with calcification: a case report. Jpn J Diagn Imag 22:776–780

Kurer MH, Baillod RA, Madgwick JC (1991) Musculoskeletal manifestations of amyloidosis. A review of 83 patients on haemodialysis for at least 10 years. J Bone Joint Surg Br 73:271–276

Kyle RA, Greipp PR (1983) Amyloidosis (AL) Clinical and laboratory features in 229 cases. Mayo Clin Proc 58:665–683

Kyle RA, Gertz MA, Greipp PR, et al. (1999) Long-term survival (10 years or more) in 30 patients with primary amyloidosis. Blood 93:1062–1066

Larsson SG, Benson L, Westermark P (1986) Computed tomography of the tongue in primary amyloidosis. J Comput Assist Tomogr 10:836–840

Leach DB, Hester TO, Farrell HA, et al. (1999) Primary amyloidosis presenting as massive cervical lymphadenopathy with severe dyspnea: a case report and review of the literature. Otolaryngol Head Neck Surg 120:560–564

Lee J, Krol G, Rosenblum M (1995) Primary amyloidoma of the brain: CT and MR presentation. AJNR Am J Neuroradiol 16:712–714

Levine E (1994) Abdominal visceral calcification in secondary amyloidosis: CT findings. Abdom Imaging 19:554–555

LiVolsi VA, Montone K, Sack M (1999) Pathology of thyroid disease. In: Sternberg SS (ed) Diagnostic surgical pathology. Lippincott Williams and Wilkins, Philadelphia, pp 529–575

Mafee MF (2003) Orbit: embryology, anatomy, and pathology. In: Som PM, Hugh HD (eds) Head and neck imaging. Mosby, St Louis, pp 529–654

Metzler JP, Fleckenstein JL, White CL 3rd, et al. (1992) MRI evaluation of amyloid myopathy. Skeletal Radiol 21:463–465

Miyake H, Maeda H, Isomoto I, et al. (1988) Computed tomography in amyloid goiter. J Comput Assist Tomogr 12:621–622

Monzawa S, Tsukamoto T, Omata K, et al. (2002) A case with primary amyloidosis of the liver and spleen: radiologic findings. Eur J Radiol 41:237–241

Moon WK, Kim SH, Im JG, et al. (1995) Castleman disease with renal amyloidosis: imaging findings and clinical significance. Abdom Imaging 20:376–378

Murphey MD, Sartoris DJ, Quale JL, et al. (1993) Musculoskeletal manifestations of chronic renal insufficiency. Radiographics 13:357–379

Okamoto K, Ito J, Emura I, et al. (1998) Focal orbital amyloidosis presenting as rectus muscle enlargement: CT and MR findings. AJNR Am J Neuroradiol 19:1799–1801

O'Meara YM, Brady HR, Brenner BM (2001) Glomerulopathies associated with multisystem diseases. In: Braunwald E, Fauci AS, Hauser SL, et al. (eds) Harrison's principles of internal medicine. McGraw-Hill Companies, New York, pp 1594–1595

Owen DA (1999) The stomach In: Sternberg SS (ed) Diagnostic surgical pathology. Lippincott Williams and Wilkins, Philadelphia, pp 1311–1347

Patchefsky AS (1999) Nonneoplastic pulmonary disease. In: Sternberg SS (ed) Diagnostic surgical pathology. Lippincott Williams and Wilkins, Philadelphia, pp 1011–1066

Petersen RO (1986) Amyloidosis in urinary bladder. In: Petersen RO (ed) Urologic pathology. JB Lippincott, Philadelphia, pp 320–321

Pickford HA, Swensen SJ, Utz JP (1997) Thoracic cross-sectional imaging of amyloidosis. AJR Am J Roentgenol 168:351–355

Porter KA (1992) The kidneys. In: Symmers WSC (ed) Systemic pathology. Churchill Livingstone, Edinburgh, pp 344–369

Powsner RA, Simms RW, Chudnovsky A, et al. (1998) Scintigraphic functional hyposplenism in amyloidosis. J Nucl Med 39:221–223

Prince JS, Duhamel DR, Levin DL, et al. (2002) Nonneoplastic lesions of the tracheobronchial wall: radiologic findings with bronchoscopic correlation. Radiographics 22:S215–S230

Ramchandani P, Schnall MD, LiVolsi VA, et al. (1993) Senile amyloidosis of the seminal vesicles mimicking metastatic spread of prostatic carcinoma on MR images. AJR Am J Roentgenol 161:99–100

Resnick D (2002a) Parathyroid disorders and renal osteodystrophy. In: Resnick D (ed) Diagnosis of bone and joint disorders. WB Saunders, Philadelphia, pp 2043–2111

Resnick D (2002b) Plasma cell dyscrasia and dysgammaglobulinemias. In: Resnick D (ed) Diagnosis of bone and joint disorders. WB Saunders, Philadelphia, pp 2188–2231

Rodriguez-Romero R, Vargas-Serrano B, Cortina-Moreno B, et al. (1996) Calcified amyloidoma of the larynx. AJNR Am J Neuroradiol 17:1491–1493

Rosello R, Lomena F, Pons F, et al. (1988) Bone scan in systemic amyloidosis. Nucl Med Commun 9:879–890

Sasson JP, Abderlrahman NG, Aquino S, et al. (2003) Trachea: anatomy, and pathology. In: Som PM, Hugh HD (eds) Head and neck imaging. Mosby, St Louis, pp 1700–1726

Segovia Garcia C, Quilez Barrenechea JI, Vidales Arechaga L, et al. (2002) Pancreatic involvement in primary amyloidosis: radiologic findings. Eur Radiol 12:774–778

Shim JC, Lee YW, Lee GJ, et al. (1997) MR finding of primary amyloid arthropathy associated with multiple myeloma. J Comput Assist Tomogr 21:800–802

Shindo H, Ishikawa H, Mine Y, et al. (2001) Gastrointestinal amyloidosis causing perforation of the colon–report of two cases. Nihon Rinsho Geka Igakkai Zasshi 62:2957–2961

Sipe JD, Cohen AS (2001) Amyloidosis. In: Braunwald E, Fauci AS, Hauser SL, Longo DL, Jameson JL (eds) Harrison's principles of internal medicine. McGraw-Hill Companies, New York, pp 1974–1979

Sueoka BL, Kasales CJ, Harris RD, et al. (1989) MR and CT imaging of perirenal amyloidosis. Urol Radiol 11:97–99

Suzuki S, Takizawa K, Nakajima Y, et al. (1986) CT findings in hepatic and splenic amyloidosis. J Comput Assist Tomogr 10:332–334

Tada S, Iida M, Matsui T, et al. (1991) Amyloidosis of the small intestine: findings on double-contrast radiographs. AJR Am J Roentgenol 156:741–744

Tada S, Iida M, Yao T, et al. (1994) Gastrointestinal amyloidosis: radiologic features by chemical types. Radiology 190:37–42

Tanno S, Ohsaki Y, Osanai S, et al. (2001) Spontaneous rupture of the amyloid spleen in a case of usual interstitial pneumonia. Intern Med 40:428–431

Theodorou DJ, Theodorou SJ, Resnick D (2002) Imaging in dialysis spondyloarthropathy. Semin Dial 15:290–296

Tirzaman O, Wahner-Roedler DL, Malek R, et al. (2000) Primary localized amyloidosis of the urinary bladder: a case series of 31 patients. Mayo Clin Proc 75:1264–1268

Trinh TD, Jones B, Fishman EK (1991) Amyloidosis of the colon presenting as ischemic colitis: a case report and review of the literature. Gastrointest Radiol 16:133–136

Urban BA, Fishman EK, Goldman SM, et al. (1993) CT evaluation of amyloidosis: spectrum of disease. Radiographics 13:1295–1230

Utz JP, Swensen SJ, Gertz MA (1996) Pulmonary amyloidosis. The Mayo Clinic experience from 1980 to 1993. Ann Intern Med 124:407–413

Vorster SJ, Lee JH, Ruggieri P (1998) Amyloidoma of the gasserian ganglion. AJNR Am J Neuroradiol 19:1853–1855

Wynne J, Braunwald E (2001) The cardiomyopathies and myocarditis. In: Zipes DP, Libby P, Braunwald E (eds) Heart disease: a textbook of cardiovascular medicine. WB Saunders Company, Philadelphia, pp 1775–1777

Yoshida S, Suematsu T, Koizumi T, et al. (1993) Demonstration of primary tracheobronchial amyloidosis by 99mTc-HMDP bone SPECT. Ann Nucl Med 7:269–272

19 Leukemia

NOBUYUKI TANAKA, TSUNEO MATSUMOTO, MATAKAZU FURUKAWA, OSAMU TOKUDA

CONTENTS

NOBUYUKI TANAKA, MD
Assistant professor, Chest Radiologist, Department of Radiology, Yamaguchi University School of Medicine, 1-1-1 Minamikogushi, Ube, Yamaguchi 755-8505, Japan
TSUNEO MATSUMOTO, MD
Associate Professor, Chest Radiologist, Department of Radiology, Yamaguchi University School of Medicine, 1-1-1 Minamikogushi, Ube, Yamaguchi 755-8505, Japan
MATAKAZU FURUKAWA, MD
Clinical Attending, Neuroradiologist, Department of Radiology, Yamaguchi University School of Medicine, 1-1-1 Minamikogushi, Ube, Yamaguchi 755-8505, Japan
OSAMU TOKUDA, MD
Clinical Attending, Musculoskeletal Radiologist, Department of Radiology, Yamaguchi University School of Medicine, 1-1-1 Minamikogushi, Ube, Yamaguchi 755-8505, Japan

19.1
Introduction

Leukemia is a malignant proliferation of hematopoietic cells, characterized by replacement of bone marrow by neoplastic cells. The leukemic cells usually are present in peripheral blood, and may infiltrate reticuloendothelial system, such as liver, spleen, lymph nodes, and other organs such as kidney, testes, bowel, lung, and central nervous system. In general, even in the state of remission, leukemic infiltration to several organs should be taken into consideration. In an autopsy study of NIES et al. (1965), leukemic infiltration was found in 10 of 15 patients in bone marrow remission who died from other causes. This chapter gives an overview of the common imaging appearances, and suggests imaging modalities to be utilized in leukemic patients.

19.2
Lymph Nodes

In pediatric patients with leukemia, mediastinal or hilar lymphadenopathy is relatively common. In adult patients, mediastinal lymphadenopathy is less common. However, in patients with acute lymphocytic leukemia (ALL), mediastinal lymphadenopathy is not infrequent. Among patients with chronic lymphocytic leukemia (CLL), mediastinal lymphadenopathy is relatively frequent. In patients with adult T-cell leukemia (ATL), which is common in Japan, mediastinal lymphadenopathy, as well as intraabdominal lymphadenopathy, is relatively common.

Computed tomography (CT) is superior to chest radiography in delineation of the exact location of enlarged lymph nodes. The pattern of lymphadenopathy is almost the same as in lymphoma. The anterior mediastinal and paratracheal lymph node are most frequently involved. In most cases, the lymphadenopathy is bilateral but asymmetrical. Hilar lymphadenopathy is rare unless mediastinal lymphadenopathy is present. CT is also valuable in assessing treatment responses.

However, follow-up CT examination may demonstrate some persistent, enlarged lymph nodes with no viable leukemic cells within. In such cases, magnetic resonance (MR) imaging may be able to differentiate non-viable lymph nodes from viable ones. The former shows hypointensity on both T1 and T2-weighted images. Concerning the criterion of lymph node enlargement for leukemic lymph node involvement, most reports suggest that a lymph node size of 2 cm is diagnostic and 1–2 cm is suspicious. However, it should be noted that use of even a 1-cm-diameter criterion will generate the possibility of false-negative results for pathologically enlarged lymph nodes (HARELL 1983). Furthermore, it might be inappropriate to apply the criteria of size for lymph node involvement of leukemia. Depiction of multiple small lymph nodes should sometimes be considered a positive finding for leukemic lymph node infiltration. Gallium (Ga-67) scintigraphy may be a useful modality for delineating multiple lymphade-nopathies in patients with leukemia (Fig. 19.1). Several studies have reported the utility of Ga-67 scintigraphy in patients with leukemia (FLORES et al. 1998).

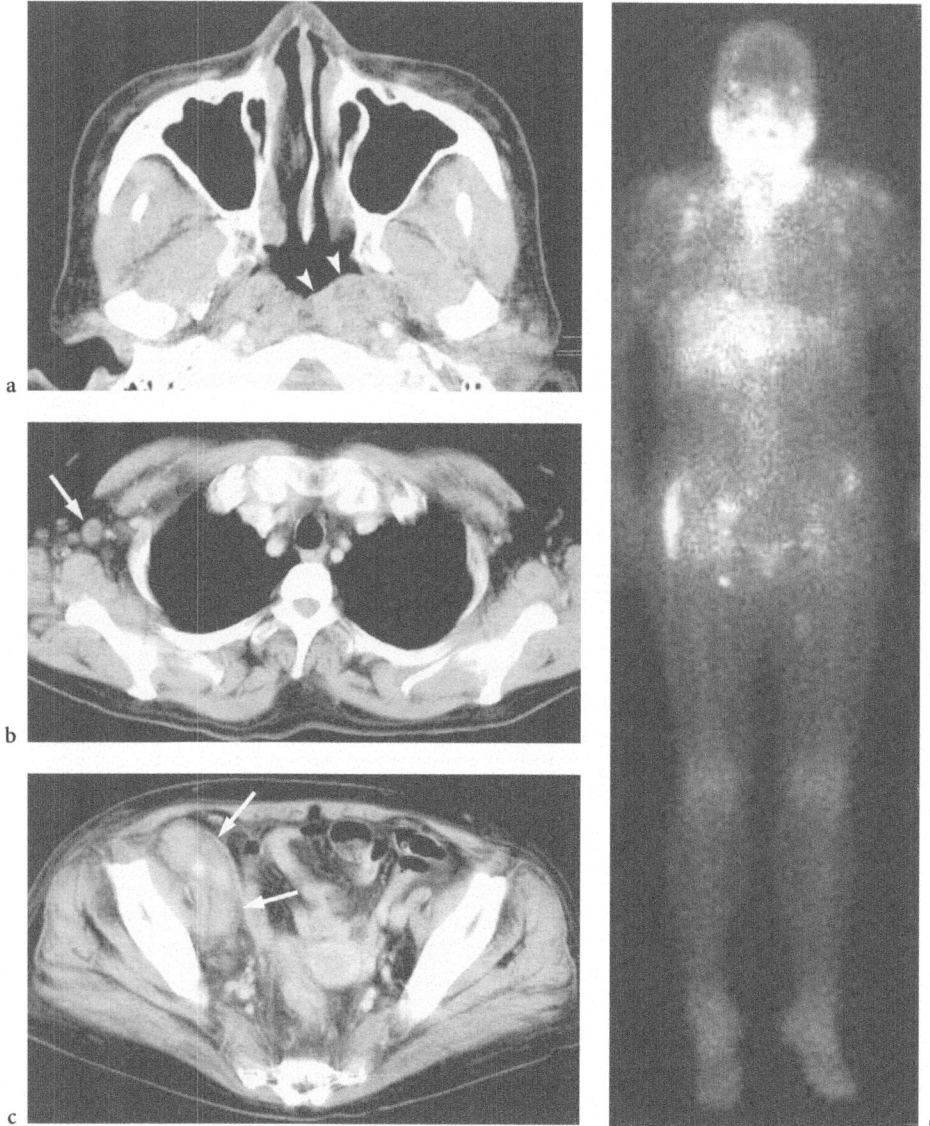

Fig. 19.1a–d. Multiple lymphadenopathies in a 60-year-old woman patient with adult T-cell leukemia. **a** Axial contrast-enhanced CT scan at the nasopharyngeal level shows asymmetrical thickening of the nasopharyngeal wall (*arrowheads*). This image shows leukemic infiltration into the nasopharyngeal tonsil. **b** Axial contrast-enhanced CT image of the chest shows right axillary lymphadenopathy (*arrow*). **c** Axial contrast-enhanced CT image of the pelvis shows multiple lymphadenopathies along the right external iliac artery (*arrows*). **d** Ga-67 scintigraphy shows multiple increased accumulations corresponding to above mentioned lymphadenopathy.

19.3
Chest

19.3.1
Pleura

Pleural thickening and effusions due to pleural leukemic infiltration are found in a significant percentage of patients at autopsy. Green and Nichols reviewed autopsy findings in 109 adult patients with leukemia (GREEN and NICHOLS 1959). Twenty-seven percent had pleural or pulmonary infiltration with leukemia, but symptomatic or radiographically evident pleural leukemic infiltration occurred in only 7%. VIADANA et al. (1978) identified leukemic pleural infiltration most frequently in ALL. Thirty-nine of 145 patients with ALL had pleural infiltration, and two of 66 patients with CLL had pleural infiltration. On CT, pleural infiltration was recognized as a plaque-like pleural thickening (KIM and FENNESSY 1994). Thickening of interlobular septa also extended from the thickened pleural surface. Microscopic examination showed that the infiltration of pleura and subpleural interlobular septa or peribronchial interstitium by leukemic cells was evident on autopsy. Pleural effusion may sometimes be seen. Although pleural effusion can be induced by hemorrhagic or infectious causes, some cases have been reported to show positive for leukemic cells in the pleural effusion, shown by HEIBERG et al. (1984).

19.3.2
Heart

Although clinically evident or grossly cardiac leukemic infiltration is rare, autopsy studies have demonstrated that 34 to 53% of patients with leukemia had pathologic evidence of cardiac involvement. A case of massive cardiac leukemic infiltration has been reported by MCADAMS et al. (1989). Bolus contrast-enhanced CT or MR imaging may be superior to ultrasound (US) and chest radiograph because these modalities can show the extent of disease.

19.3.3
Lung

Among the wide variety of pulmonary complications in patients with leukemia, leukemic pulmonary infiltration is one of the major complications. Microscopic pulmonary infiltration is frequent.

Autopsy series have demonstrated frequencies of up to 64%. However, clinically and radiographically significant leukemic pulmonary infiltration has been supposed to be rare. Clinically significant leukemic pulmonary infiltration may occur in less than 7% of leukemic patients (KLATTE et al. 1963) and fewer than 5% of patients may show leukemic infiltration on chest radiography (MAILE et al. 1983). In our experience, there are, in fact, cases of leukemic infiltration that showed respiratory distress or respiratory failure. The chest radiographic findings of leukemic pulmonary infiltration have been described as a diffuse reticular pattern, nodules and focal homogeneous opacities. Although leukemic pulmonary infiltration usually occurs mostly in the terminal stage of the illness, it can also occur during the initial stage prior to treatment. The occurrence of leukemic infiltration seems to depend on the number of leukemic cells in the peripheral blood. It usually occurs when the number of leukemic cells is high, in our experience. Because clinical symptoms of leukemic pulmonary infiltration are non-specific, such as cough, pyrexia and dyspnea, it is often difficult to correctly diagnose this entity. Although lung biopsy or bronchoalveolar lavage (BAL) is usually needed for an accurate diagnosis, these procedures are often contraindicated in such patients because of hypoxia or thrombocytopenia. CT is very useful in the correct diagnosis of chest complications in patients with leukemia. This modality is apparently superior to chest radiography because it can depict tiny lesions which cannot be depicted on chest radiography (HEUSSEL et al. 1999).

Furthermore, high resolution CT (HRCT) can show the correlation of lesions with secondary pulmonary lobules. Leukemic cells tend to infiltrate along the lymphatic routes surrounding the peribronchial and perivascular regions in the lung parenchyma (HARRIS. 1996). HRCT can reflect these pathological abnormalities more precisely than chest radiography. In the report of 10 patients with leukemic pulmonary infiltration by HEYNEMAN et al. (2000), all patients (100%) showed thickening of interlobular septa (ILS) and nine (90%) showed thickening of bronchovascular bundles (BVB). In the report of 11 patients by TANAKA et al. (2002), the thickening of BVB and ILS were frequently observed in nine (81.8%) and six cases (54.5%), respectively (Figs. 19.2–19.4). TANAKA et al. (2002) also showed CT-pathologic correlation in seven cases. Among these seven cases, thickening of BVB was seen in six patients and all showed, pathologically, leukemic cell infiltration around the small and large pulmonary arteries, bronchi or bronchioles (Fig. 19.2). The thickening of ILS was seen in five among seven cases and three showed leukemic cell infiltration within ILS. Other frequent findings were nodules/masses (Fig. 19.5) and ground-glass opacity (GGO)/airspace consolidation (Fig. 19.6). Nodules/masses were seen in all cases (100%) in Heyneman's study and in six cases (54.5%) in Tanaka's study. In Heyneman's study, centrilobular or peribronchovascular nodules were seen in seven cases, and the authors speculated that they probably showed the focal accumulation of leukemic cells in a perilymphatic distribution. Interestingly, in Tanaka's study, large nodules corresponded pathologically to the hemorrhagic infarction in one case (Fig. 19.7). GGO/airspace consolidation was seen in seven cases (70%) in Heyneman's study and in all cases (100%) in Tanaka's study. GGO/airspace consolida-

tion was frequently seen along the thickened BVB in both studies. CT-pathologic correlation by TANAKA et al. (2002), found that GGO/airspace consolidation was due to edema, hemorrhage or hemorrhagic infarction (Fig. 19.2) as well as leukemic cell infiltration within the alveolar spaces adjacent to the pulmonary arteries or bronchi. GGO/airspace consolidation in such cases may be due to the obstructive nature of massive infiltration of leukemic cells within the pulmonary small vasculature. The aggregates of leukemic cells within the vasculature may create pulmonary infarcts, hemorrhagic edema, or diffuse alveolar damage (DAD). This mechanism may be associated with the unusual pulmonary complications of leukemia reported previously: leukostasis and leukemic cell lysis pneumopathy.

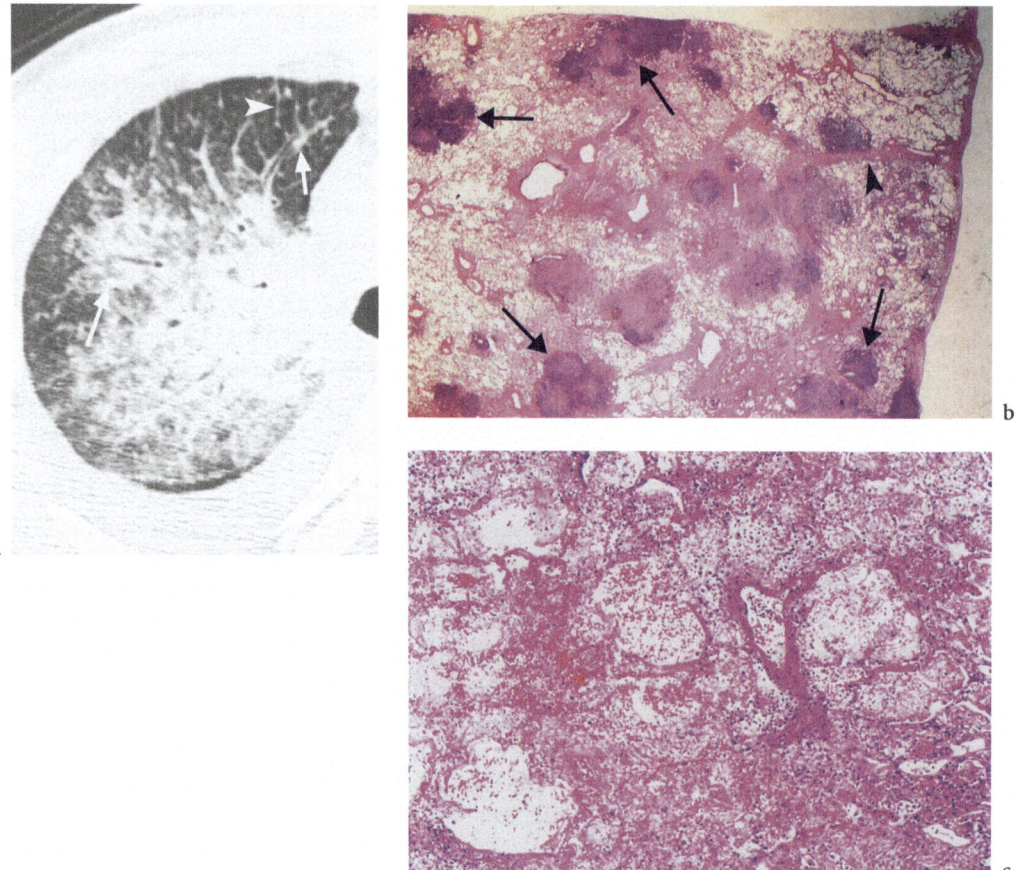

Fig. 19.2a–c. Leukemic pulmonary infiltration in a 39-year-old man patient with adult T-cell leukemia. **a** Axial HRCT shows marked and widespread thickening of bronchovascular bundles (*arrows*). Ground-glass opacities and airspace consolidation are distributed along the bronchovascular bundles. Thickening of the interlobular septa (*arrowhead*) are also noted at the subpleural region. **b** Autopsied specimen shows leukemic cell infiltration along the pulmonary arteries, bronchi, and bronchioles (*arrows*), which corresponds to the thickening of bronchovascular bundles on HRCT images. Thickening of interlobular septa due to leukemic cell infiltration and fibrosis is also shown (*arrowhead*). **c** Autopsied specimen of another region shows a marked exudative lesion of pulmonary edema and hemorrhage within alveolar spaces, which may correspond to ground-glass opacity/airspace consolidation around the thickened bronchovascular bundles. (With permission from [TANAKA et al. 2002])

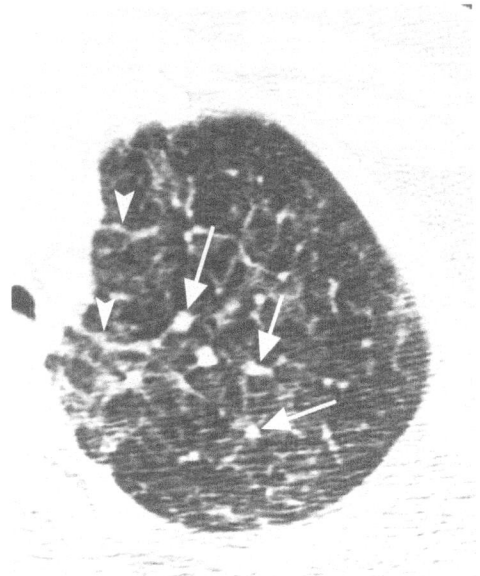

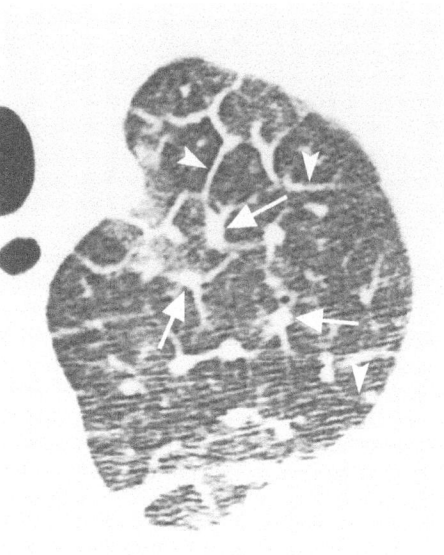

Fig. 19.3. Leukemic pulmonary infiltration in a 57-year-old woman patient with acute myeloid leukemia. Axial HRCT shows thickening of interlobular septa (*arrowheads*) and bronchovascular bundles (*arrows*). Patchy ground-glass opacity distributed along the thickened bronchovascular bundles.

Fig. 19.4. Leukemic pulmonary infiltration in a 43-year-old man patient with acute myeloid leukemia. Axial HRCT shows widespread thickening of interlobular septa (*arrowheads*) and bronchovascular bundles (*arrows*). Patchy ground-glass opacity is also noted.

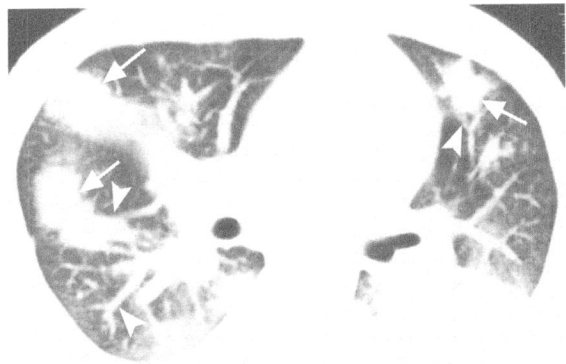

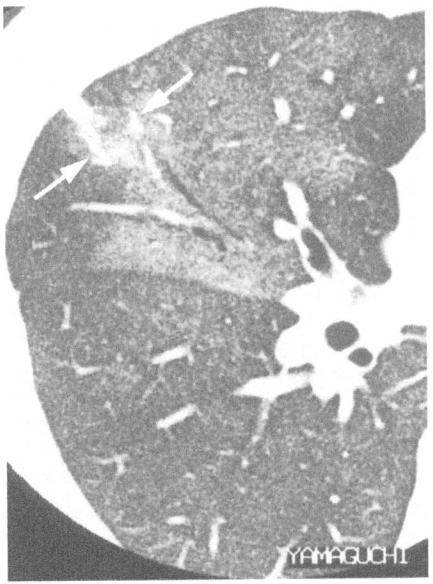

Fig. 19.5. Leukemic pulmonary infiltration in a 20-year-old man patient with acute myeloid leukemia. Axial CT scan shows multiple masses (*arrows*) distributed along the thickened bronchovascular bundles (*arrowheads*). Segmental airspace consolidation in the left lower lobe is also noted.

Fig. 19.6. Leukemic pulmonary infiltration in a 38-year-old woman patient with adult T-cell leukemia. Axial HRCT shows segmental ground-glass opacity, within which thickening of bronchovascular bundles (*arrows*) is noted.

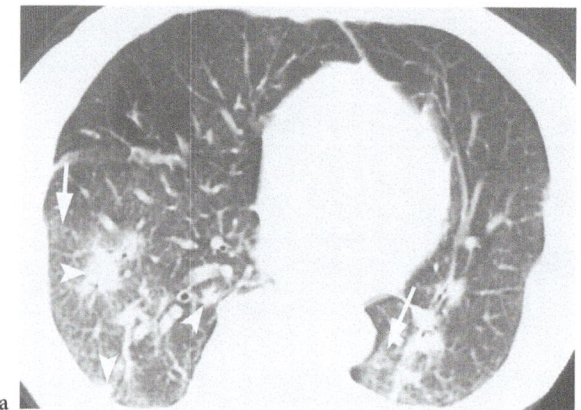 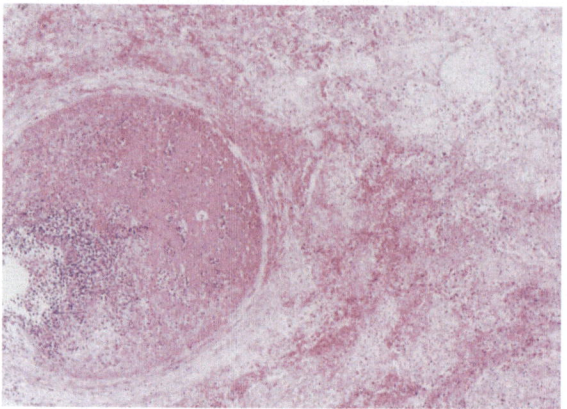

Fig. 19.7a,b. Leukemic cell lysis pneumopathy in a 73-year-old woman patient with acute myeloid leukemia. **a** Axial CT scan shows widespread ground-glass opacity (*arrows*), thickening of bronchovascular bundles and multiple nodules (*arrowheads*). This patient showed leukocytosis (white blood count 93300/mm³ and blast count 88600/mm³) at the initial examination and became severely hypoxic (PO2: 54.9mmHg) after chemotherapy. **b** This patient died 14 days after CT examination. Autopsied specimen corresponding to the peripheral nodules shows hemorrhagic infarction, within which a thrombosed pulmonary vessel is seen. (With permission from [TANAKA et al. 2002])

Leukemic patients with a high leukocyte count frequently encounter acute respiratory failure. In an autopsy study of 206 patients with leukemia, McKee et al. (1974) mentioned pulmonary vascular "leukostasis" or small vessel infiltration and occlusion by leukemic cell aggregates in all patients with a leukocyte count greater than 200,000/mm³. Pulmonary leukostasis is generally found in about 40% of autopsy series. Chest radiographic abnormalities include diffuse parenchymal opacities corresponding to pulmonary edema. In a study of 10 leukemic patients with leukostasis confirmed by autopsy by von Buchem et al. (1987), four patients showed pulmonary edema, recognized as diffuse bilateral alveolar consolidation on chest radiography. They speculated on the cause of pulmonary edema as follows: pulmonary edema was induced as the result of diffuse endothelial damage in the lungs from either simple embolic ischemia aggravated by continuing oxygen consumption of the sloughed leukemic cells or the release of proteolytic enzymes from those cells. Interestingly, six of 10 patients with leukostasis showed normal chest radiography in their study. Although their study was not based on CT findings, leukostasis has to be considered when no or minimal abnormalities are visible on the chest radiography or CT of patients with dyspnea (Fig. 19.8). In such patients with normal chest radiography or CT, lung perfusion scans may be useful. SZYPER-KRAVITZ et al. (2001) reported a patient with leukostasis and normal chest radiographic findings who showed a homogeneous diffuse pattern of low perfusion

in both lungs without segmental or subsegmental defects on lung perfusion scans. They mentioned that this pattern could be compatible with a diffuse vascular occlusive process like pulmonary leukostasis. It should also be noted that leukostasis could be present in patients with a leukocyte count less than 50,000/mm³, as reported by SOARES et al. (1992).

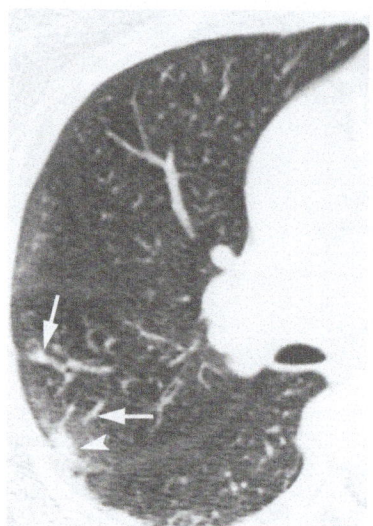

Fig. 19.8. Leukostasis in a 68-year-old woman patient with acute myeloid leukemia. Axial HRCT scan shows minimal abnormal findings including thickening of bronchovascular bundles (*arrows*) and focal airspace consolidation (*arrowhead*). This patient showed severe hypoxia (PO2: 50.5mmHg) and leukocytosis (white blood count 90200/mm³ and blast count 36500/mm³). After chemotherapy, the hypoxia disappeared.

Leukemia

357

Leukemic cell lysis pneumopathy was described by MYERS et al. (1983). They found four patients with acute nonlymphocytic leukemia and a leukocyte count of more than 200,000/mm³ who developed respiratory failure within 10–48 hours after initiation of chemotherapy. Chest radiography showed diffuse pulmonary infiltrates, vascular enlargement, cardiomegaly, and pleural effusion. Pathologic examination of three patients showed thrombi composed of leukemic cells which obstructed and distended the lumens of pulmonary arteries, capillaries and venules, with associated small infarctions, perivascular hemorrhage, and interstitial edema. Electron microscopy showed pulmonary endothelium and basement membrane damage and interstitial edema. Five similar cases have been reported by TRYKA et al. (1982). Each patient had an open lung biopsy, which revealed diffuse alveolar damage, and all recovered without specific therapy. The mechanism of this entity has been speculated to be that the leukostasis causes local tissue damage and hypoxemia as a result of vascular obstruction and oxygen consumption by blast cells, with the injury being accentuated by toxic and thromboplastic substances immediately released by these leukemic cells as a result of chemotherapy. There has been no report concerning the CT of this entity. In our experience, widespread GGO, thickening of BVB and multiple nodules were present (Fig. 19.7).

19.4
Abdomen

In general, 90% of patients with ALL and 60% of patients with acute myeloid leukemia (AML) are supposed to have visceral enlargement at the first examination of patients. Enlargement of the liver, spleen or kidney are frequent. CT will depict irregular low enhanced areas and MR imaging will depict hypointense areas on T1-weighted images and hyperintense areas on T2-weighted images. Paraaortic lymphadenopathy is also a frequent finding (Fig. 19.9).

19.4.1
Liver

Leukemic infiltration in the liver can take a form of infiltration along Glisson's sheath pathologically. Therefore, the finding of focal areas as space-occupying lesions is unlikely on US, CT or MR images.

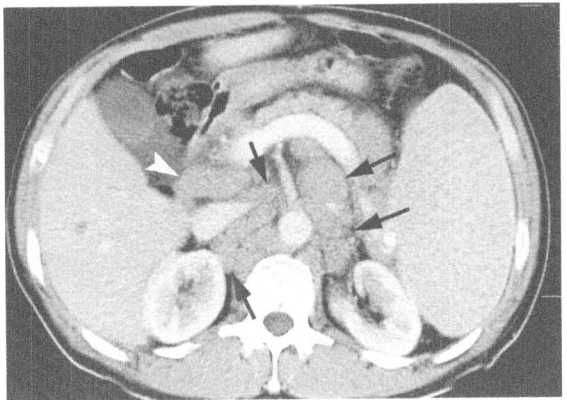

Fig. 19.9. Paraaortic lymphadenopathy in a 66-year-old man patient with chronic lymphocytic leukemia. Axial contrast-enhanced CT scan shows multiple lymphadenopathy at the paraaortic (*arrows*) and hepatic hilar (*arrowhead*) regions. Note that splenomegaly is also seen.

Hepatomegaly, not as frequent as splenomegaly, may sometimes be seen. Periportal low attenuation on CT images, characterized by areas of low attenuation around the portal vein and its branches, has been reported. Periportal infiltration with leukemic cells was noted at autopsy and biopsy in patients with CML. Periportal lymphadenopathy may be present as well as periportal low attenuation (SIEGEL and HERMAN 1992). Rarely, leukemic infiltration to the liver can lead to infarction or rupture. Ascites and esophageal varices have been reported. These complications may result from diffuse infiltration of leukemic cell into the liver or from direct, focal compression of extrahepatic portal vessels by leukemic cells (HUNTER and BJELLAND 1984).

19.4.2
Spleen

Splenomegaly is the most frequent complication as a form of leukemic infiltration to the spleen. In the report of HEIBERG et al. (1984), splenomegaly was detected in 27 patients among 43 patients with leukemia. In CML, splenomegaly may be marked, sometimes extending to the pelvic cavity (Fig. 19.10). In Heiberg's study, the spleen was massively enlarged with the tip below the iliac crest in seven of 27 patients with splenomegaly. The finding of focal areas in the spleen is quite rare except for splenic infarction. In the study of 22 patients showing focal lesions within the spleen by HESS et al. (1988), only one patient was a leukemic patient. In this patient, a focal

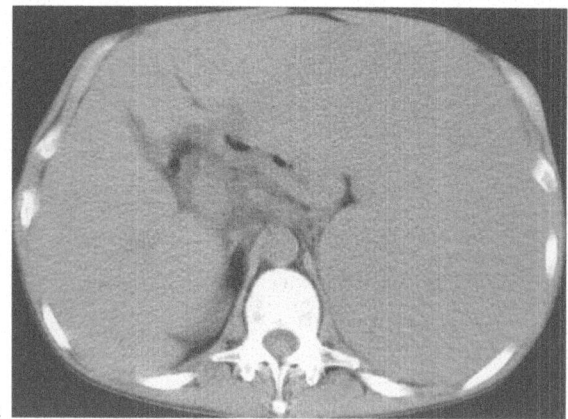
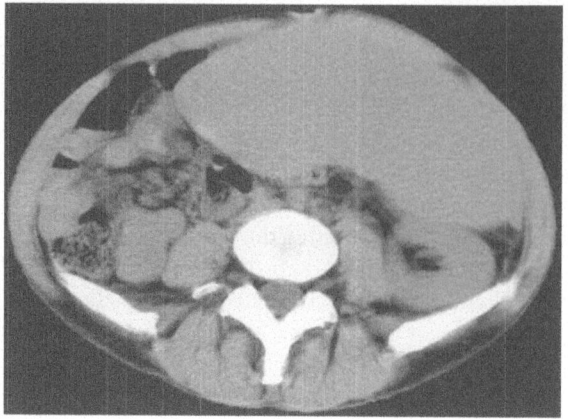

Fig. 19.10a,b. Splenomegaly due to leukemic infiltration in a 54-year-old man patient with chronic lymphocytic leukemia. Axial unenhanced CT scan shows marked splenomegaly (**a**), extending into the pelvic cavity (**b**).

hypointense area was detected on MR images and hypoechoic lesions were detected on US; however, CT was negative. Splenic infarcts may sometimes be seen. On CT images, infarct areas will appear as a wedge-shaped low enhanced area (Fig. 19.11). These areas may be seen as more linear low enhanced areas (HEIBERG et al. 1984).

19.4.3
Kidney

The kidney is one of the most frequent sites of leukemic infiltration, and leukemia is the most common malignant cause of bilateral global renal enlargement. It is reported that microscopic renal infiltration could be seen in approximately 60% of patients with leukemia at autopsy. Renal involvement in leukemia is also more common at relapse than at onset. Just as with the CNS and testes, the kidneys are considered "sanctuary sites" where relapse may occur even in the face of bone marrow remission. The leukemic cells infiltrate the interstitial tissue and crowd out normal structures. All portions of the renal parenchyma may be involved. The kidneys are usually symmetrically enlarged and the contour is smooth (Fig. 19.12) (HEIBERG et al. 1984; PARKER 1997). Focal lesions are relatively uncommon, however, one or more focal renal masses have been reported in B-cell and T-cell leukemia (Fig. 19.13). It should be noted that hemorrhagic complicating leukemic renal disease can appear as a focal mass or masses.

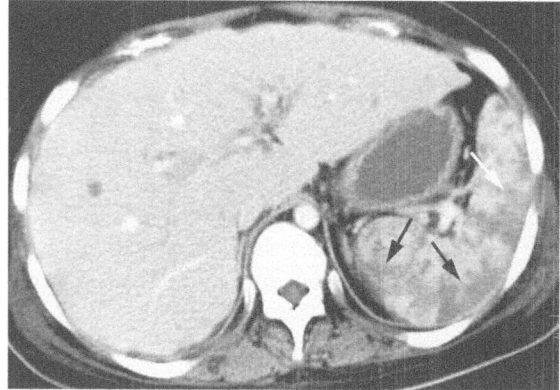
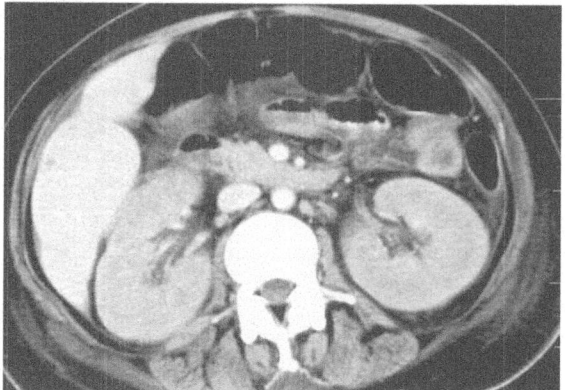

Fig. 19.11. Splenic infarction in an 18-year-old woman patient with acute myelocytic leukemia. Axial contrast-enhanced CT scan shows enlargement of spleen and multiple wedge-shaped or irregular low enhanced areas (*arrows*) within it.

Fig. 19.12. Leukemic renal infiltration in an 18-year-old woman patient with acute myelocytic leukemia. Axial contrast-enhanced CT image of the abdomen shows enlargement of the bilateral kidney. No focal abnormalities are seen. This finding disappeared after chemotherapy.

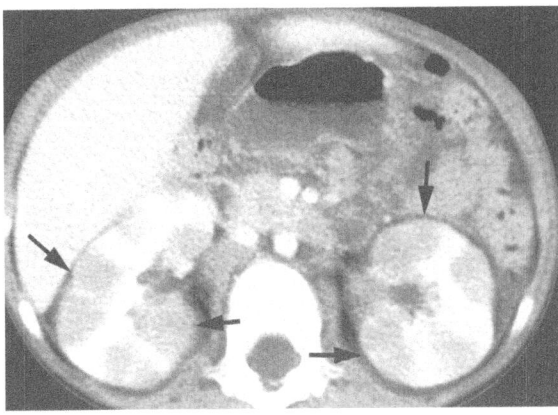

Fig. 19.13. Leukemic renal infiltration in a 3-year-old boy patient with acute lymphocytic leukemia. Axial contrast-enhanced CT scan shows enlargement of the bilateral kidney and multiple low enhanced areas (*arrows*) within them. The result of renal biopsy showed leukemic renal infiltration. These findings also disappeared immediately after chemotherapy.

19.4.4
Testis

Testicular involvement is more common at relapse than at onset. At US, the involved testis typically appears enlarged and hypoechoic (MAZZU 1995). Usually enlargement is more unilateral than bilateral.

19.4.5
Gastrointestinal Tract

Lymphoid tissue is distributed widely in the bowel and mesentery, especially in the ileum, appendix, and colon. Therefore, leukemic infiltration to these gastrointestinal tracts is common in later or progressive stages of the disease. The frequency of leukemic infiltration to these organs ranges from 9 to 62%. The involvement of stomach, ileum or colon is common. In a study by HUNTER and BJELLAND (1984), apparent gastrointestinal involvement was seen in 9% of patients. In an autopsy study of 148 patients with acute and chronic leukemia by PROLLA and KIRSNER (1964), gross leukemic gastrointestinal infiltration was seen in 25% of patients. In a study of WINTON et al. (1975), almost 50% of children with acute leukemia who die due to relapse show at least microscopic evidence of gastrointestinal leukemic involvement at postmortem examination. Leukemic gastrointestinal infiltration may show plaque-like thickening of the bowel wall, raised nodular lesions, diffuse mucosal or submucosal infiltration, polyp formation, and ulceration. On CT images, leukemic infiltration may be depicted as thickening of the gastrointestinal wall (Fig. 19.14) (HEIBERG et al. 1984; KHALIL and SINGER 1997). The differential diagnosis for diffuse bowel wall thickening includes neutropenic enterocolitis (typhlitis), characterized as a localized inflammation of the terminal ileum, appendix, or cecum. It is a rare but fatal complication. It is almost always seen in patients undergoing intensive chemotherapy. In most cases, the pathogenesis appears to be cecal ulceration from opportunistic bacterial overgrowth secondary to chemotherapy. The radiographic appearance of typhlitis is variable. Barium enema findings may include edematous change of cecum and ileum, showing the "thumb-print" sign. On CT images, thickening of the bowel wall is observed (HUNTER and BJELLAND 1984; HEIBERG et al. 1984). It may be difficult to distinguish this entity from leukemic infiltration into the bowel wall. However, in the clinical context, typhlitis is seen in the period of neutropenia after intensive chemotherapy. Fever and right lower quadrant pain is typically observed.

In a patient with leukemic bowel infiltration, an air contrast barium examination will show a constricting annular lesion. In addition, perforation, peritonitis or gross hemorrhage can occur as complications of leukemic infiltration. Gastrointestinal hemorrhage could be accentuated by thrombocytopenia secondary to the leukemia itself or its therapy, microscopic vascular insufficiency, neutropenia, and miscellaneous coagulation abnormalities. Severe hemorrhage often is the major contributing cause of death. Massive leukemic infiltration may cause not only bowel, but also biliary or pancreatic duct obstruction or cause intussusceptions (HUNTER and BJELLAND 1984).

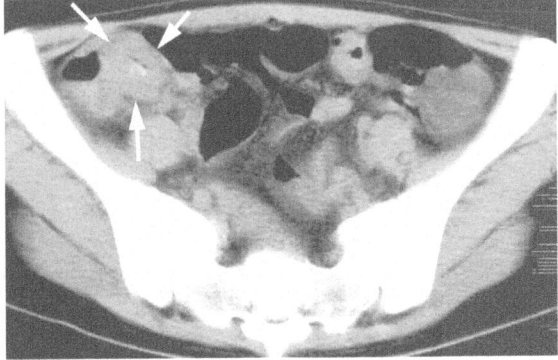

Fig. 19.14. Leukemic bowel infiltration in a 30-year-old woman patient with acute lymphocytic leukemia. Axial unenhanced CT scan of the pelvis shows thickening of the ileal wall (*arrows*). This finding diminished after intensive chemotherapy.

19.4.6
Miscellaneous

A 35-year-old man with leukemic infiltration of the gallbladder wall that mimicked acute cholecystitis has been reported. US showed a diffusely thickened gallbladder wall containing hypoechoic zones. CT showed an abnormal, septate area of fluid density around the gallbladder lumen. Pathologic examination revealed a distended gallbladder with evidence of hemorrhage within the wall, consistent with acute hemorrhagic cholecystitis. Microscopic sections revealed leukemic infiltration involving the entire thickness of the gallbladder wall (FINLAY et al. 1993).

19.5
Central Nervous System

In earlier years, central nervous system (CNS) complications of leukemia were rare because of the rapid fatality of the disease. More recently, with advances in treatment methods and consequent prolonged survival, the frequency of neurological complications has increased (CHEN et al. 1996; EVANS et al. 1970; NIEMEYER et al. 1985). CNS complications are caused either by the primary disease or by the therapy. The primary effects of the disease may include leukemic involvement of the leptomeninges, brain parenchyma, and cerebrovasculature (WALKER 1991).

CNS involvement during the course of acute leukemia is not infrequent, and it is well recognized that the CNS may be infiltrated by myeloid or lymphoid leukemia cells, either as meningeal leukemia or as nodular masses (PAGANO et al. 1999; BLEYER 1988). CNS leukemia is believed to develop as a result of leukemic metastases resulting either from hematogenous spread or from direct extension from involved cranial bone marrow (AZZARELLI and ROESSMAN 1977). Infiltration of the meninges by leukemic cells can affect the dura, the leptomeninges, or both.

MR imaging is useful for the diagnosis of meningeal infiltration, which appears as linear or small nodular enhanced lesions after contrast administration. But it is often difficult to differentiate meningeal infiltration by leukemic cells from infectious meningitis because of the resembling imaging findings in both conditions.

On CT scans, intra-axial leukemic masses are usually isodense or slightly hyperdense on precontrast scans and enhance brightly (Fig. 19.15). Multiple lesions are also seen. MR imaging of the CNS leukemic masses are well-delineated, strongly enhancing tumors with or without surrounding edema (Fig. 19.16). Imaging findings of intraaxial CNS leukemic mass resemble other primary CNS tumors, especially CNS lymphoma.

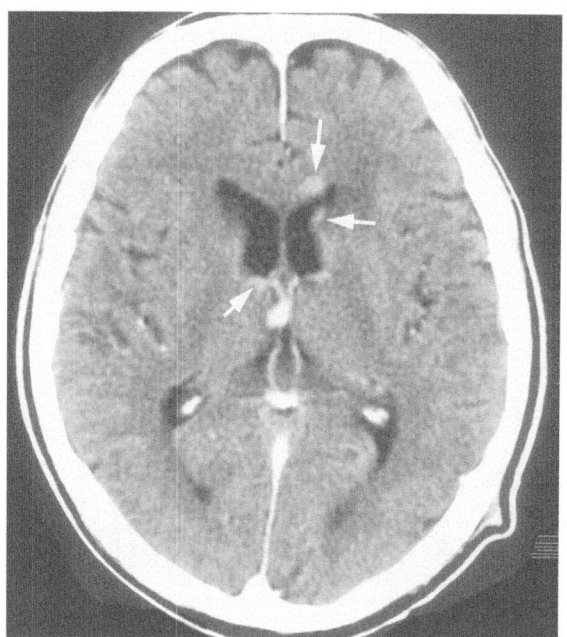
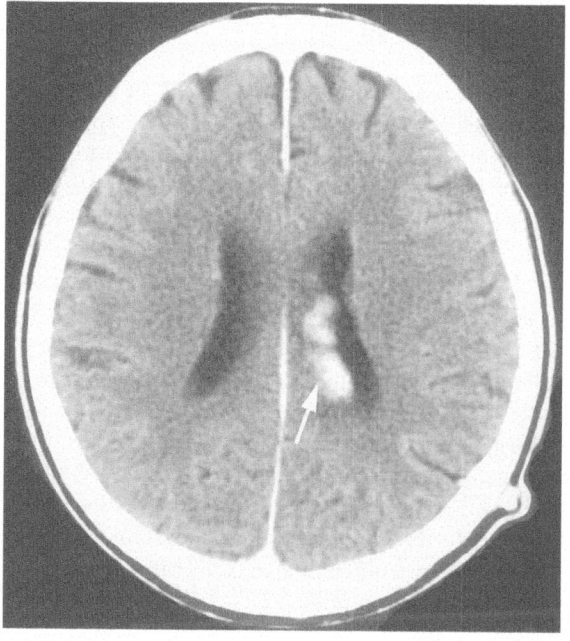

a   b

Fig. 19.15a,b. Leukemic central nervous system involvement in a 66-year-old man with adult T-cell leukemia. **a, b** Axial contrast-enhanced CT scans show multiple enhanced lesions around the lateral ventricles (*arrows*).

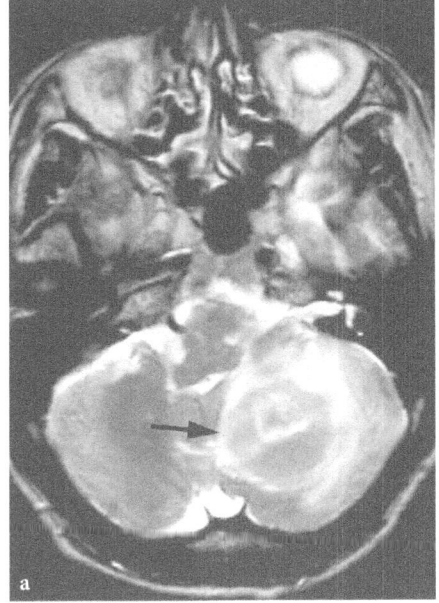 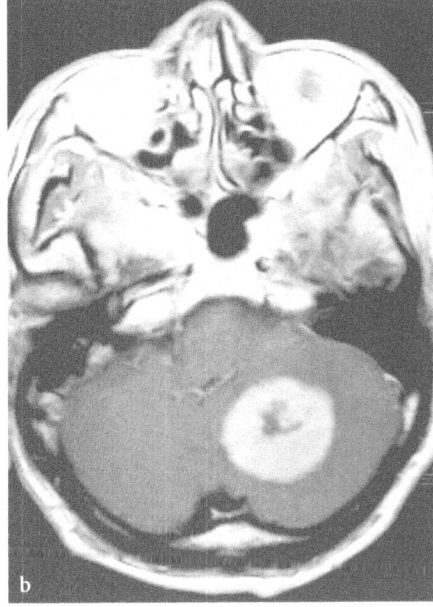

Fig. 19.16a,b. Leukemic cerebellar involvement in an 80-year-old man with acute myeloblastic leukemia. **a** Axial T2-weighted MR image reveals isointense mass in left cerebellum (*arrow*). **b** This mass enhances strongly on contrast-enhanced T1-weighted MR image. Tumor resection was performed, and the histological diagnosis was central nervous system leukemia.

19.6
Bone and Musculoskeletal

19.6.1
Acute Childhood Leukemia

Bone and joint pain, tenderness, and swelling are common findings. Arthralgias and arthritis are common, having been reported in 12–65% of patients. The disappearance of joint complaints is suggested as an early sign of improvement after treatment (Spilberg and Meyer 1972).

Diffuse Osteopenia
A diffuse decrease in the radiodensity of the skeleton may result from an alteration in mineral metabolism or from leukemic infiltration of the bone marrow (Simmons et al. 1968; Cohn et al. 1987). Medullary widening in tubular bones may be seen (Cohn et al. 1987).

Radiolucent and Radiodense Metaphyseal Bands
Symmetric metaphyseal band-like radiolucent areas, which probably reflect a nutritional deficit, are observed in leukemia and other chronic childhood illnesses. Histologically, the radiolucent lesions of the metaphysis are not always associated with leukemic cell infiltration. These areas in the metaphysis can lead to fracture and epiphyseal separation and displacement (Simmons et al. 1968). These findings are common at the capital femoral and proximal

humeral epiphysis (Manson et al. 1989). In some cases, the entire metaphysis is radiodense. Abnormally large and coarse trabeculae with areas of unresorbed calcified cartilaginous matrix are evident on histological examination. They may be observed in 50% of children with leukemia.

Osteolytic Lesions
The medial cortex of the proximal portion of the humerus is a characteristic site of involvement (Melhem and Saber 1980). Larger areas of bone destruction may represent a combination of leukemic infiltration in the bone marrow, hemorrhage, and osteonecrosis (Simmons et al. 1968).

Periostitis
Proliferating leukemic cells in the marrow invade the cortex via haversian canals and extend to subperiosteal locations (Fig. 19.17) (Simmons et al. 1968). Subperiosteal hemorrhage may be associated with this finding. Symmetric periostitis in some leukemic children simulates the appearance of secondary hypertrophic osteoarthropathy, syphilis, and other conditions.

Other Skeletal Abnormalities
Sutural diastasis is common in infants and children with leukemia (Nixon and Gwinn 1973). It is produced by an increase in intracranial pressure due to leukemic cell infiltration of the meninges or cerebrum.

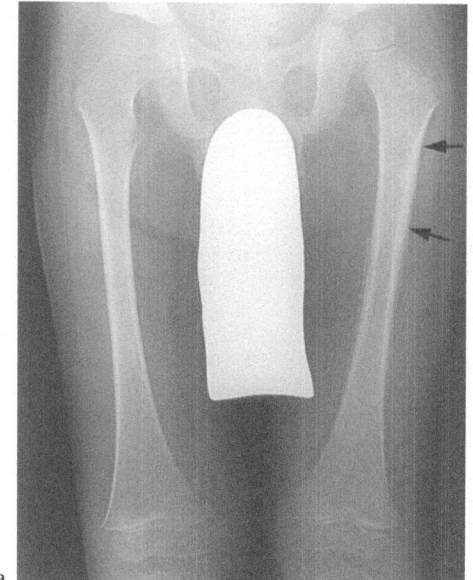
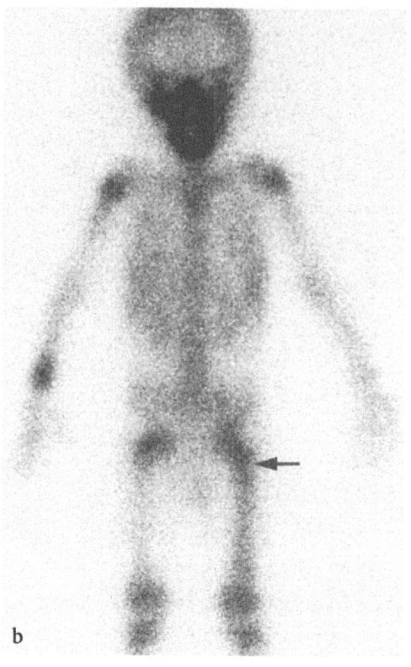

Fig. 19.17a,b. Periostitis in a 6-year-old boy with acute lymphoid leukemia. a Periostitis is apparent in the metaphysis of the left femur (*arrows*). b ^{99m}Tc MDP bone scan showing abnormal accumulation in the proximal femur (*arrow*).

Course of the Skeletal Lesions

The disappearance of lucent metaphyseal bands during remission has been noted and may be associated with transient metaphyseal sclerosis (ROSENFIELD and MCINTOSH 1977). However, there is poor correlation between the extent of bone lesions and the progress of leukemia.

Articular Abnormalities

Soft tissue swelling, effusion, and juxta-articular osteoporosis are seen occasionally (SPILBERG and MEYER 1972). The identification of leukemic involvement in a joint requires synovial biopsy, which reveals leukemic infiltration in the synovial membrane (HARDEN 1984). On rare occasions, calcium pyrophosphate dehydrate crystals have been identified in the symptomatic joints of patients with acute leukemia (WEINBERGER et al. 1981). Osteonecrosis occurring in association with leukemia typically affects the femoral epiphyses and condyles and the proximal portion of the humerus.

19.6.2
Acute Adult Leukemia

Clinical and radiologic evidence of skeletal involvement in leukemia is less common in adults than in children. Skeletal pain and tenderness are most frequent in the vertebral column and ribs. The radiologic findings are diffuse osteopenia, discrete osteolytic lesions, and metaphyseal radiolucency. Diffuse osteopenia resembles osteoporosis and other metabolic disorders. Osteolytic lesions may be evident in the skull, pelvis, and proximal long bones (VAN SLYCK 1972). Metaphyseal radiolucent bands are not so frequently observed in adult as those in children with acute leukemia.

19.6.3
Chronic Leukemia

The skeletal lesions in chronic leukemia are less common and less severe than those in acute leukemia. Occasionally, large and aggressive lesions may be encountered (SPENGLER et al. 1976). Rarely, widespread bone sclerosis is evident, perhaps related to diffuse marrow fibrosis (DEBECK et al. 1984). The radiographic manifestations of skeletal involvement in chronic leukemia can be more prominent during a blast crisis, in which a large number of leukemic cells appear in the bone marrow and peripheral blood (BRAUNSTEIN et al. 1980). SPILBERG and MEYER (1972) noted arthritis related to the primary disease in 12% of patients with chronic leukemia. Polyarticular involvement is more frequent than monoarticular involvement. Leukemic cell infiltration of the synovium may be seen. Secondary gout is a well known complication of chronic leukemia.

19.6.4
Magnetic Resonance Imaging

MR imaging has proved to be very sensitive for depicting changes in the bone marrow in patients with acute leukemia. Because the evaluation of response to treatment requires serial bone marrow biopsies during the course of therapy in patients with acute leukemia, investigators have focused on the prospect of MR imaging as a noninvasive method for assessing the post-treatment status of the bone marrow. TANAKA et al. (1996) concluded that MR imaging of the femoral marrow could be useful in the assessment of tumor volume in adult acute leukemia cases; however, there were limitations to predicting prognosis on the basis of the MR imaging manifestations.

Initial reports showed that serial measurements of bulk T1 relaxation times and serial measurements of fat and water proportion were helpful in differentiating patients responding to the therapy from those not responding (HENKELMAN et al. 1988; JENSEN et al. 1990). In general, leukemic marrow demonstrates a prolongation of the T1 relaxation value, leading to diminution of marrow signal intensity on spin-echo T1-weighted MR images (Figs. 19.18, 19.19) (OLSON et al. 1986). T2 changes are more variable and less dramatic and, in some studies, measured values of T2 relaxation times in leukemic marrow have not been significantly different from those of control groups (MOORE et al. 1986).

Quantitative chemical shift imaging (CSI) can help distinguish the individual contributions of fat and water to the total signal intensity, thus rendering a more quantitative assessment of the bone marrow (MOORE et al. 1986; ROSEN et al. 1988; GERARD et al. 1992). With successful therapy, the fat fraction and

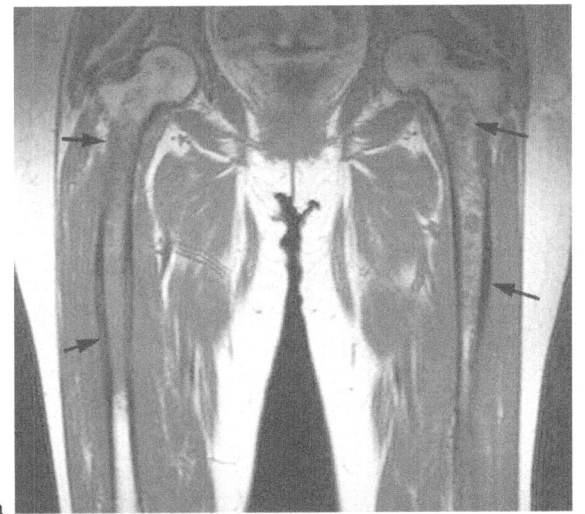

a

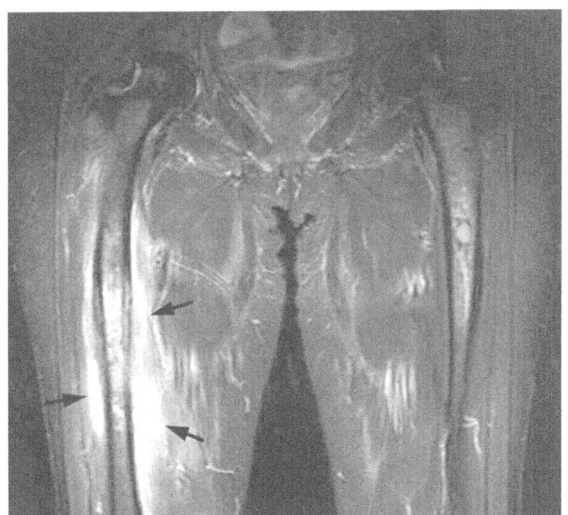

b

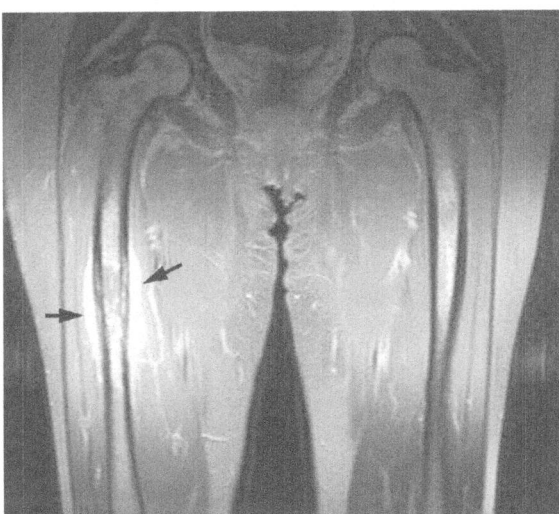

c

Fig. 19.18a–c. Leukemic bone marrow involvement in a 67-year-old man with acute myeloid leukemia. a Coronal spin-echo T1-weighted MR image of the thighs reveals diffuse hypointensity in the femoral metaphysis and diaphysis (*arrows*). b Coronal short tau inversion recovery (STIR) MR image reveals hyperintensity in the marrow of the diaphysis and metaphysis of the femur. Inhomogeneous hyperintense mass surrounding the right femur is also seen (*arrows*). c Coronal contrast-enhanced spin-echo T1-weighted MR image with fat suppression technique shows inhomogeneous signal intensity in the marrow of the diaphysis and metaphysis of the femur. The mass surrounding the right femur shows strong enhancement (*arrows*).

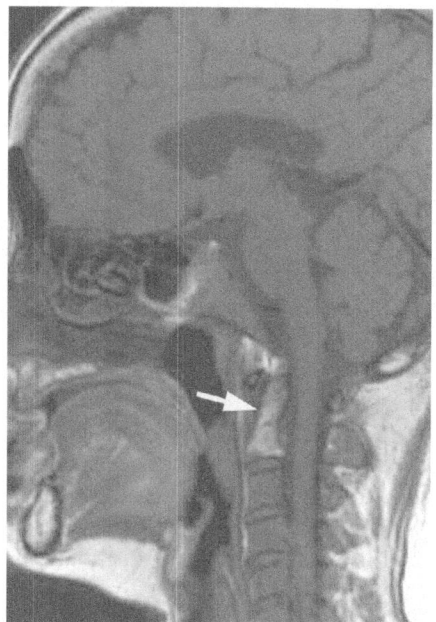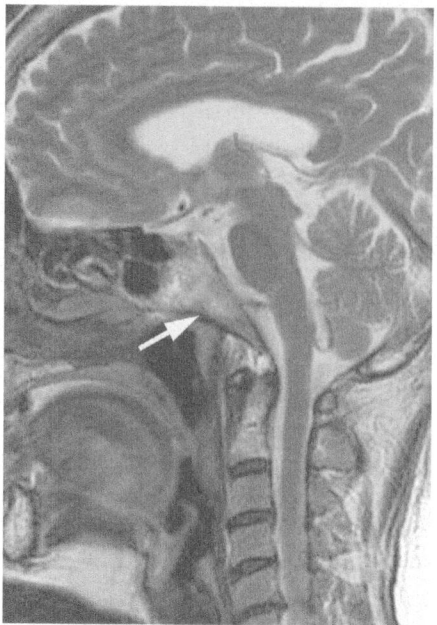

a   b

Fig. 19.19a,b. Leukemic bone marrow involvement in a 66-year-old woman with chronic lymphoid leukemia. **a** Sagittal spin-echo T1-weighted MR image of cervical spine shows hypointensity of the bone marrow of the clivus and cervical vertebral bodies except C2 (*arrow*) consistent with replacement of the fat tissue by leukemic cells. **b** Sagittal fast spin-echo T2-weighted MR image shows inhomogeneous hyperintensity in the clivus (*arrow*).

the number of hematopoietic cells increases, leading to significant changes in the fat and water composition of the marrow. Consequently, the quantitative assessment of fat fraction by CSI could be used to monitor the response to therapy in patients with leukemia.

MR spectroscopy may have a potential role, allowing analysis of water and lipid content in the bone marrow. BONGERS et al. (1992) reported that the fat signal increase was paralleled by a decrease of cellularity or leukemic cells in the marrow biopsies. Because leukemic patients with normocellular marrow can present normal MR spectroscopy and CSI findings, CSI and MR spectroscopy cannot replace a histologic diagnosis. However, there might be an important application of these methods in following up patients.

19.6.5
Acute Lymphoid Leukemia versus Acute Myeloid Leukemia

VANDE BERG et al. (1996) reported that a statistically significant difference in the initial bulk T1 values and in the changes of bulk T1 during treatment was observed between patients with ALL and those with AML. Sequential quantitative MR imaging during chemotherapy appears valuable for prediction of response in patients with ALL but not in those with AML.

19.7
Conclusion

Due to the improvement of therapy for leukemia, patients with leukemia can live longer. The importance of the diagnosis of leukemic infiltration into organs as well as complications due to the therapy should be stressed. Leukemic infiltration into organs is reported to occur even at the stage of bone marrow remission. In the diagnosis of leukemic infiltration, CT or MR imaging is superior to plain chest and abdominal radiography. Several CT and MR imaging findings are considered to be characteristic which may facilitate the correct diagnosis of leukemic infiltration into several organs. Nevertheless, few imaging patterns are absolutely specific for a particular pathology, and the final diagnosis is almost based on histological studies.

References

Azzarelli B, Roessman U (1977) Pathogenesis of central nervous system infiltration in acute leukemia. Arch Pathol Lab Med 191:203–205
Bleyer WA (1988) Central nervous system leukemia. Ped Clin North Am 35:789–814

Bongers H, Schick F, Skalej M, et al. (1992) Localized in vivo 1H spectroscopy and chemical shift imaging of the bone marrow in leukemic patients. Eur Radiol 2:350–356

Braunstein EM, Hammond B, Schniter B (1980) Bone destruction in myelogeneous marrow crisis. J Can Assoc Radiol 31:69–70

Chen CY, Zimmerman RA, Faro S, et al. (1996) Childhood leukemia: central nervous system abnormalities during and after treatment. AJNR Am J Neuroradiol 17:295–310

Cohn SL, Morgan ER, Mallote LE (1987) The spectrum of metabolic bone disease in lymphoblastic leukemia. Cancer 59:346–350

Debeck M, Peters O, Van Camp B, et al. (1984) Monocytic leukemia associated with myeloid metaplasia resembling metastatic bone disease. Skeletal Radiol 11:9–12

Evans AE, Gilbert ES, Zandstra R (1970) The increasing incidence of central nervous leukemia in children. Cancer 26:404–409

Finlay DE, Mitchell SL, Letourneau JG, et al. (1993) Leukemic infiltration of the gallbladder wall mimicking acute cholecystitis. AJR Am J Roentgenol 160:63–64

Flores LG 2nd, Nagamachi S, Nishii R, et al. (1998) Gallium-67 scintigraphy in the treatment and prognosis of acute adult T-cell lymphoma. Ann Nucl Med 12:105–108

Gerard EL, Ferry JA, Amrein PC, et al. (1992) Compositional changes in vertebral bone marrow during treatment for acute leukemia: assessment with quantitative chemical shift imaging. Radiology 183:39–46

Green RA, Nichols NJ (1959) Pulmonary involvement in leukemia. Am Rev Respir Dis 80:833–844

Harden EA, Moore JO, Haynes BF (1984) Leukemia-associated arthritis: identification of leukemic cells in synovial fluid using monoclonal and polyclonal antibodies. Arthritis Rheum 27:1306–1308

Harell GS (1983) The retroperitoneum. In: Haaga JR, Alfidi RJ (eds) Computed tomography of the whole body. Mosby, St. Louis, pp 753–773

Harris M (1996) Pulmonary lymphoproliferative disorders and related conditions. In: Hasleton PS (ed) Spencer's pathology of the lung. McGraw-Hill, New York, pp 1111–1129

Heiberg E, Wolverson MK, Sundarem M, et al. (1984) CT findings in leukemia. AJR Am J Roentgenol 143:1317–1323

Henkelman RM, Messner H, Poon PY, et al. (1988) Magnetic resonance imaging for monitoring relapse of acute myeloid leukemia. Leuk Res 12:811–816

Hess CF, Griebel J, Schmiedl U, et al. (1988) Focal lesions of the spleen: preliminary results with fast MR imaging at 1.5T. J Comput Assist Tomogr 12:569–574

Heussel CP, Kauczor HU, Heussel GE, et al. (1999) Pneumonia in febrile neutropenic patients and in bone marrow and blood stem-cell transplant recipients: use of high-resolution computed tomography. J Clin Oncol 17:796–805

Heyneman LE, Johkoh T, Ward S, et al. (2000) Pulmonary leukemic infiltrates: high-resolution CT findings in 10 patients. AJR Am J Roentgenol 174:517–521

Hunter TB, Bjelland JC (1984) Gastrointestinal complications of leukemia and its treatment. AJR Am J Roentgenol 142:513–518

Jensen KE, Sorensen PG, Christoffersen P, et al. (1990) Magnetic resonance imaging of the bone marrow in patients with acute leukemia during and after chemotherapy; changes in T1 relaxation. Acta Radiol 31:361–369

Khalil RM, Singer AA (1997) CT appearance of direct leukemic invasion of bowel. Abdom Imaging 22:464–465

Kim FM, Fennessy JJ (1994) Pleural thickening caused by leukemic infiltration: CT findings. AJR Am J Roentgenol 162:293–294

Klatte EC, Yardley J, Smith EB, et al. (1963) The pulmonary manifestations and complications of leukemia. AJR Am J Roentgenol 89:598–609

Maile CW, Moore AV, Ulreich S, et al. (1983) Chest radiographic-pathologic correlation in adult leukemia patients. Invest Radiol 18:494–499

Manson D, Martin RF, Cockshott WP (1989) Metaphyseal impaction fractures in acute lymphoblastic leukemia. Skeletal Radiol 17:561–564

Mazzu D, Jeffrey RB, Ralls PW (1995) Lymphoma and leukemia involving the testicles: findings on gray-scale and color Doppler sonography. AJR Am J Roentgenol 164:645–647

McAdams HP, Schaefer PS, Ghaed VN (1989) Leukemic infiltrates of the heart: CT findings. J Comput Assist Tomogr 13:525–527

McKee LC Jr, Collins RD (1974) Intravascular leukocyte thrombi and aggregates as a cause of morbidity and mortality in leukemia. Medicine (Baltimore) 53:463–478

Melhem RE, SaberTJ (1980) Erosion of the medial cortex of the proximal humerus: a sign of leukemia on the chest radiograph. Radiology 137:77–79

Moore SG, Gooding CA, Brash R, et al. (1986) Bone marrow in children with acute lymphocytic leukemia. Radiology 160:237–240

Myers TJ, Cole SR, Klatsky AU, et al. (1983) Respiratory failure due to pulmonary leukostasis following chemotherapy of acute nonlymphocytic leukemia. Cancer 51:1808–1813

Niemeyer CM, Kitchcock-Bryan S, Sallen SE (1985) Comparative analysis of treatment programs for childhood acute lymphoblastic leukemia. Semin Oncol 12:122–130

Nies BA, Bodey GP, Thomas LB, et al. (1965) The persistence of extramedullary leukemic infiltrates during bone marrow remission of acute leukemia. Blood 26:133–141

Nixon GW, Gwinn JL (1973) The roentgen manifestations of leukemia in infancy. Radiology 107:603–609

Olson PO, Schields AF, Scheurich CJ, et al. (1986) Magnetic resonance imaging of the bone marrow in patients with leukemia, aplastic anemia, and lymphoma. Invest Radiol 21:540–546

Pagano L, Larocca LM, Vaccario ML, et al. (1999) Acute hemorrhagic leukoencephalitis in patients with acute myeloid leukemia in hematologic complete remission. Hematologica 84:270–274

Parker BR (1997) Leukemia and lymphoma in childhood. Radiol Clin North Am 35:1495–1516

Prolla JC, Kirsner JB (1964) The gastrointestinal lesions and complications of the leukemias. Ann Intern Med 61:1084–1103

Rosen BR, Fleming DM, Kushner DC, et al. (1988) Hematologic bone marrow disorders: quantitative chemical shift MR imaging. Radiology 169:799–804

Rosenfield NS, McIntosh S (1977) Prospective analysis of bone changes in treated childhood leukemia. Radiology 123:413–415

Siegel MJ, Herman TE (1992) Periportal low attenuation at CT in childhood. Radiology 183:685–688

Simmons CR, Harle TS, Singleton EB (1968) The osseous

manifestations of leukemia in children. Radiol Clin North Am 6:115–130

Soares FA, Landell GAM, Cardoso MCM et al. (1992) Pulmonary leukostasis without hyperleukocytosis: a clinicopathologic study of 16 cases. Am J Hematol 40:28–32

Spengler DM, Leiberg OU, Bailey RW (1976) Rapid diaphyseal destruction. An unusual osseous manifestation of chronic granulocytic leukemia. Clin Orthop 115:231–235

Spilberg I, Meyer GJ (1972) The arthritis of leukemia. Arthritis Rheum 15:630–635

Szyper-Kravitz M, Strahilevitz J, Oren V, et al. (2001) Pulmonary leukostasis: role of perfusion lung scan in diagnosis and follow up. Am J Hematol 67:136–138

Tanaka N, Matsumoto T, Miura G, et al. (2002) CT findings of leukemic pulmonary infiltration with pathologic correlation. Eur Radiol 12:166–174

Tanaka O, Takagi S, Kobayashi Y et al. (1996) MR imaging of the femoral marrow in adult acute leukemia: correlation of MRI patterns with FAB subtype and prognosis. Nippon Acta Radiol 56:967–973

Tryka AF, Godleski JJ, Fanta CH (1982) Leukemic cell lysis pneumopathy. A complication of treated myeloblastic leukemia. Cancer 50:2763–2770

Vande Berg BC, Michaux L, Scheiff JM, et al. (1996) Sequential quantitative MR analysis of bone marrow: differences during treatment of lymphoid versus myeloid leukemia. Radiology 201:519–523

Van Slyck EJ (1972) The bony changes in malignant hematologic disease. Orthop Clin North Am 3:733–734

Viadana E, Bross DJ, Pickren JW (1978) An autopsy study of the metastatic patterns of human leukemias. Oncology 35: 87–96

von Buchem MA, Wondergem JH, Kool LJS, et al. (1987) Pulmonary leukostasis: radiologic-pathologic study. Radiology 165:739–741

Walker RW (1991) Neurologic complications of leukemia. Neurol Clin 9:989–999

Weinberger A, Schumacher HR, Schimmer BM, et al. (1981) Arthritis in acute leukemia: clinical and histopathological observation. Arch Inter Med 141:1183–1187

Winton RR, Gwynn AM, Roberts JC, et al. (1975) Leukemia and the bowel. Med J Aust 4:89–90

20 Granulocytic Sarcoma

Clara G. C. Ooi and Ali Guermazi

CONTENTS

20.1
Introduction

Granulocytic sarcoma (GS) is a rare solid malignant tumor, which consists of extramedullary primitive precursors of white blood cells including myeloblasts, promyelocytes and myelocytes (Pui et al. 1994). It is most commonly associated with acute myeloid leukemia (AML), in which 2.5–8% of patients will develop GS before, during or after the onset of systemic leukemia (Pui et al. 1994; Liu et al. 1973; Muss and Maloney 1973). It can predate leukemia by up to 49 months (mean of 10 months) (Frohna and Quint 1993), but most often, it is concurrent with systemic disease. GS may herald leukemia transformation in chronic myeloid leukemia and myelodysplastic disorders, such as polycythemia rubra vera, myeloid metaplasia and hypereosinophilia (Liu et al. 1973; Frohna and Quint 1993; Neiman et al. 1981; Au et al. 1999b; Rottenberg and Thomas 1994; Novick et al. 1998; Turner et al. 1991; Au et al. 1998). Primary GS presenting without existing hematological diseases is extremely rare (Wright et al. 1992; Fruauff et al. 1988). It carries a poor prognostic significance if GS is found in patients with chronic myeloid leukemia or myeloproliferative disorders as it indicates blastic transformation (Neiman et al. 1981; Guermazi et al. 2002). A similar negative sentiment is also attached to presentation of GS in patients with AML who are in remission (Neiman et al. 1981; Orlandi et al. 1989) or have been treated with bone marrow transplantation (BMT) (Békássy et al. 1996; Au et al. 1999a).

Originally described in 1811 by Burns (1821), the term "chloroma" was first used in 1853 to refer to the green color of the tumor caused by high content of myeloperoxidase (King 1853). As a significant proportion (30%) of GS were white, gray or brown and not green, depending on the state of oxidation or cellular concentrations of the pigmented enzyme, Rappaport in 1966 coined the term "granulocytic sarcoma" to describe these tumors (Muss and Maloney 1973; King 1853).

Clara G. C. Ooi, MD
Associate Professor, Department of Radiology, Room 405, Block K, Queen Mary Hospital, University of Hong Kong, Pokfulam Road, Hong Kong SAR, China
Ali Guermazi, MD
Visiting Associate Professor, Department of Radiology, University of California at San Francisco, 350 Parnassus Avenue, Suite 150, San Francisco, CA 94117, USA

20.2
Clinical Features

GS is most commonly found in childhood and adolescence without sex predilection (Liu et al. 1973), with up to 60% of all GS occurring in children under 15-years old. Radiologic and clinical presentations are protean but in general occur as a consequence of local tissue destruction, compression and obstruction (Liu et al. 1973; Ooi et al. 2001). Pain, reported in 78% of cases, is usually an early feature followed by motor disturbances, which may include urinary incontinence in cases of intracranial or intraspinal involvement (Liu et al. 1973). Cord compression, and painful radicular-spinal cord or syringomyelic syndromes may be presenting symptoms in patients with intraspinal involvement (Graham et al. 2001). Visible or palpable tumor nodules and exophthalmos are also common presenting features (Brock et al. 2001; Davis et al. 1985). Orbital involvement will also result in chemosis, diplopia and epiphora in addition to proptosis and pain. Occasionally, symptoms relating to biliary or renal obstruction are encountered when intraabdominal GS masses are present (Books et al. 1974). Occult asymptomatic GS tumors however can be found in up to 50% of cases at autopsy (Guermazi et al. 2002).

Although GS has been reported to arise from virtually any organ, bone and perineural tissues including the brain appear to be the commonest sites (Liu et al. 1973; Frohna and Quint 1973; Neiman et al. 1981) followed by subcutaneous tissues, breast, paranasal sinuses, bowel and lymph nodes (Pui et al. 1994; Liu et al. 1973; Guermazi et al. 2002; Ooi et al. 2001; Guermazi et al. 2000). In a series of 338 autopsied cases of myeloid leukemia with granulocytic sarcoma between 1949 and 1969 in Hiroshima and Nagasaki, granulocytic sarcoma of the bone accounted for 91.3% of cases, while lymph node, kidney and dural disease was found in 56.1%, 47.8% and 39.1% of cases respectively (Liu et al. 1973). These GS tumors are frequently multiple and may be metachronous and sequential (Novick et al. 1998; Ooi et al. 2001).

20.3
Pathogenesis

GS is postulated to arise from the bone marrow migrating via Haversian canals to reach the periosteum and henceforth to invade other structures such as the orbit, adjacent soft tissues, lymph nodes and epidural space (Azzarelli and Roesasman 1977). Central nervous system (CNS) involvement has been similarly theorized to occur via perivascular or perineural routes, direct extension from the dura or through capillary migration (Pui et al.

1994; Pochedly 1977). GS has also been postulated to arise de novo from rests of hematopoietic cells at extramedullary sites other than perineural tissue such as the gastrointestinal or genitourinary system (Pochedly 1977). In the bowel, lymph nodes sited within the bowel and mesentery are thought to represent the focus from which infiltration of bowel wall occurs (Prolla and Kirsner 1964).

20.4
Imaging Techniques

Cross-sectional imaging is most useful for characterizing GS masses. Plain films are of limited benefit apart from perhaps evaluating bone or lung involvement, and bowel wall thickening and obstruction. Ultrasound (US) evaluation of superficial structures, such as skin, testes and breast, may yield additional features. However, MR imaging and CT are most often required, particularly when intracranial, intraspinal or intraabdominal GS lesions are suspected in patients with leukemia. Enhancement characteristics and anatomic relationship with adjacent structures are best depicted with these modalities, and may allow distinction from abscesses, hematoma and secondary tumor (Pui et al. 1994). Most GS tumors show variable intensities of enhancement on both MR imaging and CT (Pui et al. 1994; Ooi et al. 2001) in addition to being multiple, multi-sited and metachronous. Although radionuclide studies such as Gallium (^{65}Ga) and positron emission tomography (PET) scans may be used to show activity and multiplicity of these tumors, the imaging features are generally nonspecific (Pui et al. 1994; Turner et al. 1991; Luddy et al. 1980).

20.5
Central Nervous System

20.5.1
Intracranial Lesions

Intracranial intraaxial GS lesions are rare (Parker et al. 1996) with most intracranial tumors sited near or at the epidural tissue presenting as extraaxial intracranial masses (Fig. 20.1). The most likely mode of leukemic transmission to account for this extraaxial position is spread from calvarial bone marrow to the dura and subarachnoid space via perivascular leu-

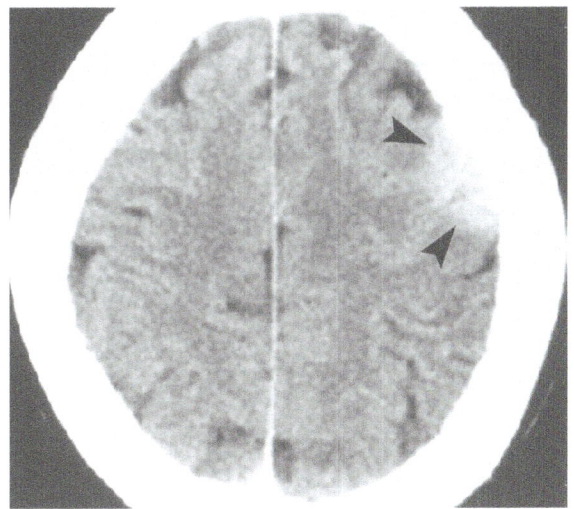

Fig. 20.1. Intracranial granulocytic sarcoma in a 55-year-old woman with essential thrombocytopenia who presented with headache. Axial unenhanced CT scan of the brain shows a hyperdense epidural lesion (*arrowheads*) abutting the left high frontoparietal lobe. At surgical resection a dural mass, later confirmed to be granulocytic sarcoma, was found without infiltration of the brain parenchyma. (With permission from [OOI and KHONG 2001])

kemic infiltration of arachnoidal venules. Breach of the pia-glial membrane would allow further leukemic penetration into brain parenchyma to become intra-axial GS (POCHEDLY 1977; FREEDY and MILLER 1991). The CT and MR imaging appearances of intracranial GS tumors are consistent, appearing hyperdense relative to normal brain tissue on CT (Figs. 20.1, 20.2), and hypo to isointense to gray matter on both T1 and T2-weighted MR sequences (Figs. 20.2, 20.3) (PUI et al. 1994; FROHNA and QUINT 1993; WRIGHT et al. 1992; FRUAUFF et al. 1988; OOI et al. 2001; OOI and KHONG 2001; PARKER et al. 1996; KAO et al. 1987; WENDLING et al. 1979; SOWERS et al. 1979; FITOZ et al. 2002; ROMANIUK 1992). GS tumors also typically show marked and homogeneous enhancement after contrast injection on CT and MR imaging (Fig. 20.4), with edema and mass effect (PUI et al. 1994; FRUAUFF et al. 1988; OOI et al. 2001). Although the imaging features of intracranial GS are fairly characteristic, it may still be indistinguishable from an acoustic neuroma if sited at the cerebello-pontine angles, and from meningioma or lymphoma (PUI et al. 1994; MUSS and MALONEY 1973; WRIGHT et al. 1992; FRUAUFF et al. 1988; PARKER et al. 1996; ROMANIUK 1992). However a careful search for presence of hyperostosis and calcification in a dural-based intracranial tumor in patients with myeloid leukemia may

help to differentiate GS lesion from a meningioma. A lack of both characteristics would point away from a diagnosis of meningioma. It may also be prudent to be aware that intracranial GS lesions, on the rare occasion, will have a central hypodense area with/without peripheral rim enhancement, akin to an abscess (OOI et al. 2001; WANG et al. 1987; BARNETT and ZUSSMAN 1986; VINTERS and GILBERT 1982; NIKOLIC et al. 2003). The central hypodense area has been attributed to tumor necrosis (BARNETT and ZUSSMAN 1986; VINTERS and GILBERT 1982; NIKOLIC et al. 2003), and a temporal change from hyperdensity to hypodensity on CT scan has been observed with treatment in intracranial GS lesions (NIKOLIC et al. 2003).

20.5.2
Intraspinal Lesions

Similar to intracranial GS, intraspinal lesions are also usually epidural (PUI et al. 1994; FROHNA and QUINT 1993; AU et al. 1999a; GRAHAM et al. 2001; PROULX and MCCARTHY 1998; RIPP et al. 1989) in origin, whilst intramedullary (OOI et al. 2001; KOOK et al. 1993) or intradural extramedullary (GRAHAM et al. 2001; ANG and VIRAPONGESE 1990; SCOTTI et al. 1985; KIM et al. 1990) lesions are rare (Figs. 20.5, 20.6). In general, the imaging characteristics on MR are similar to intracranial lesions, being primarily isointense on T1, and either iso or mildly hyperintense to muscle or spinal cord on T2-weighted images, with enhancement (PUI et al. 1994; FROHNA and QUINT 1993; OOI and KHONG 2001; GRAHAM et al. 2001; KOOK et al. 1993; ANG and VIRAPONGESE 1990; EELKEMA et al. 1989). The presence of homogeneous enhancement helps distinguish intraspinal GS from hematomas and abscesses, which are more frequent associations in myeloid leukemias. Hematomas do not enhance and abscesses tend to enhance peripherally. However, as with intracranial GS, intraspinal lesions may be indistinguishable from meningioma, neurofibroma or schwannoma.

20.6
Head and Neck

In the head and neck region, the orbits and paranasal sinuses are the most common sites of GS involvement (DAVIS et al. 1985; FREEDY and MILLER 1991; ANG and VIRAPONGESE 1990; DUNNICK and HEASTON

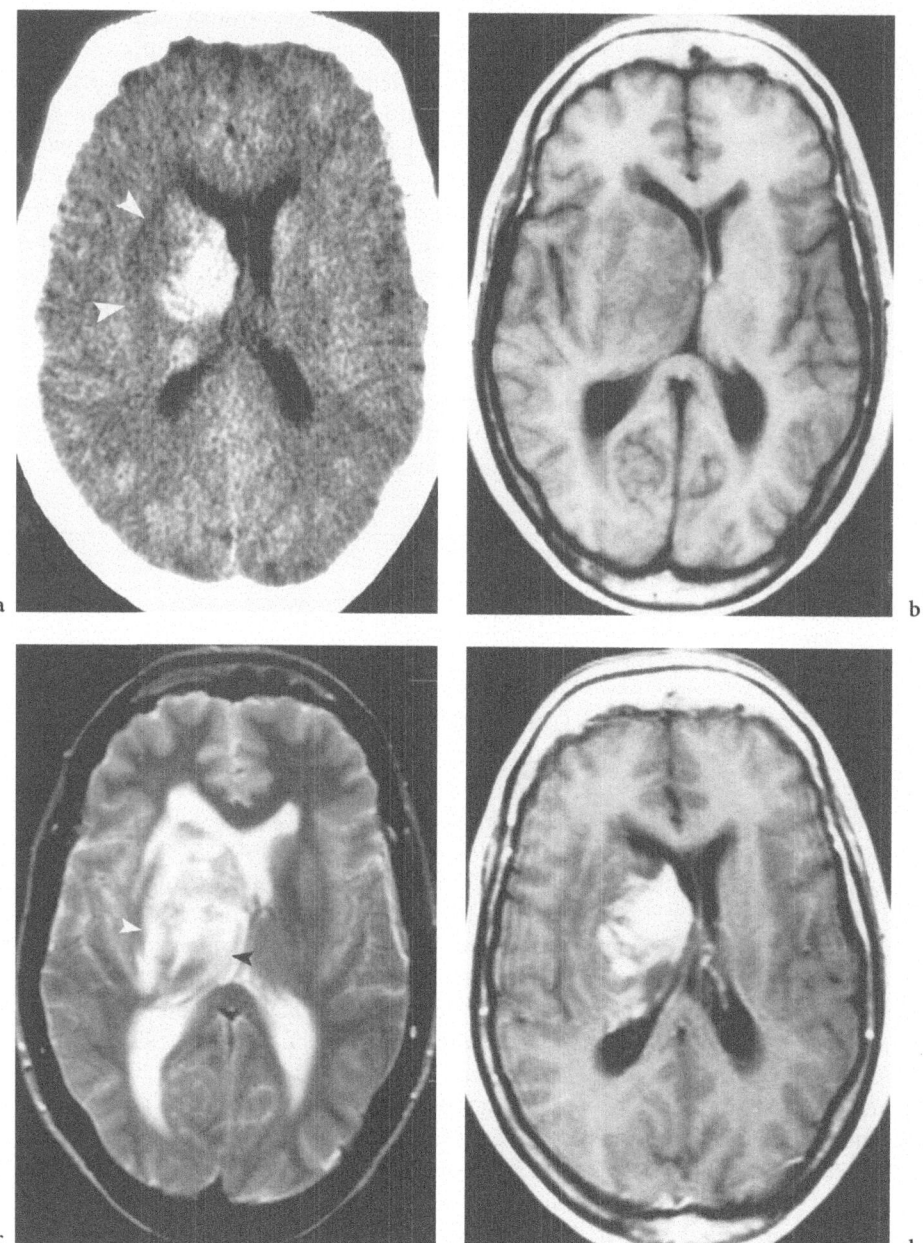

Fig. 20.2a–d. Intracranial granulocytic sarcoma in a 58-year-old woman who presented with a 2-month history of headache. **a** Axial unenhanced CT scan of brain shows right periventricular hyperdense mass surrounded by edema (*arrowheads*). **b** Axial unenhanced T1-weighted MR image shows poorly defined right periventricular lesion that is isointense with gray matter, with periventricular mass effect. **c** Axial T2-weighted MR image shows surrounding edema much better than (**b**) and shows relatively hypointense rim of lesion (*arrowheads*). **d** Axial contrast-enhanced T1-weighted MR image reveals marked homogeneous enhancement of the lesion. Examination of cerebrospinal fluid revealed blasts, and histologic examination revealed brain granulocytic sarcoma. No evidence of medullary or systemic disease was found. Seven months later, patient was diagnosed with systemic acute myeloblastic leukemia with eosinophils. (With permission from [GUERMAZI et al. 2002])

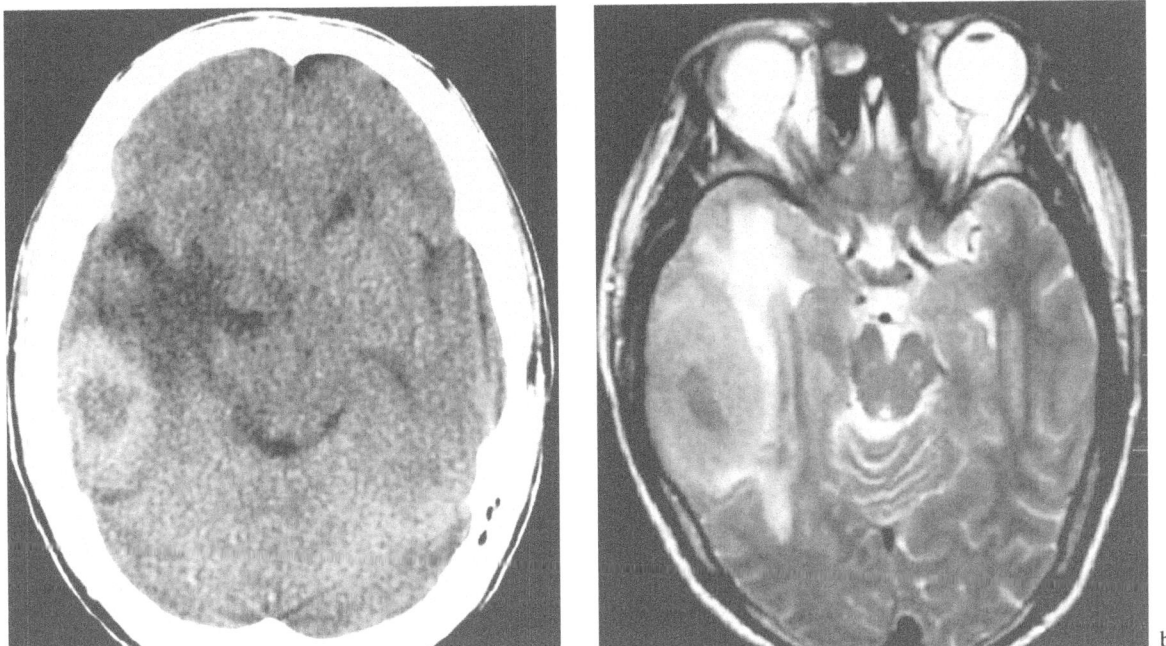

Fig. 20.3a,b. Intracranial granulocytic sarcoma in a 33-year-old man who had acute myeloid leukemia in bone marrow remission. **a** Axial unenhanced CT scan shows a mass in the right temporal lobe with adjacent vasogenic edema and central hypodensity consistent with necrosis. **b** The mass has a thick hyperintense rim that is isointense to normal gray matter on axial fast spin-echo T2-weighted MR image. (With permission from [Ooi and Khong 2001])

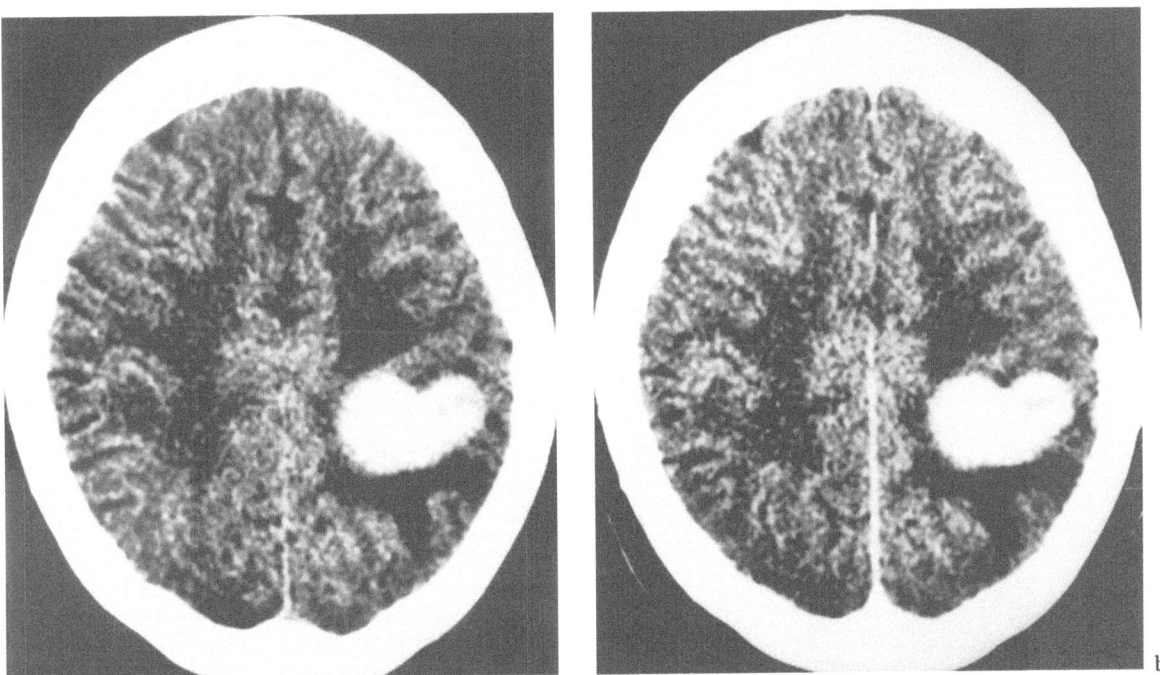

Fig. 20.4a,b. Intracranial granulocytic sarcoma in a 28-year-old woman with acute myeloblastic leukemia. She was readmitted to hospital 8 months after first remission with a 1-week history of headache, vomiting and dysphasia. **a** Axial unenhanced CT scan of brain shows irregular hyperdense mass with hypodense peritumoral edema in left parietal lobe. **b** Axial contrast-enhanced CT scan shows homogeneous enhancement of the mass after contrast administration. Biopsy subsequently revealed brain granulocytic sarcoma. (With permission from [Guermazi et al. 2002])

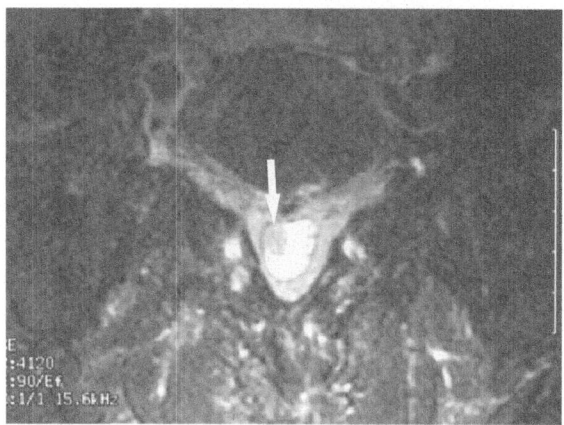
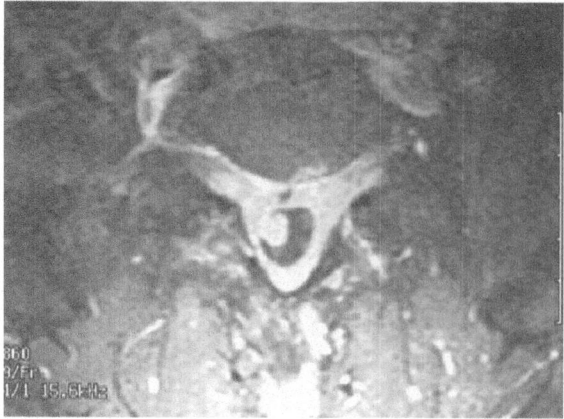

Fig. 20.5a,b. Intraspinal granulocytic sarcoma in a 78-year-old man with acute myeloid leukemia in his seventies who presented with bilateral lower leg weakness and pain. **a** Axial fast spin-echo T2-weighted MR image of the lumbar spine demonstrates abnormally thickened and mildly hyperintense nerve roots (*arrow*) and spinal epidural tissue. **b** Axial contrast-enhanced T1-weighted MR image shows marked enhancement in the abnormal nerve roots and epidural tissue. (With permission from [OOI and KHONG 2001])

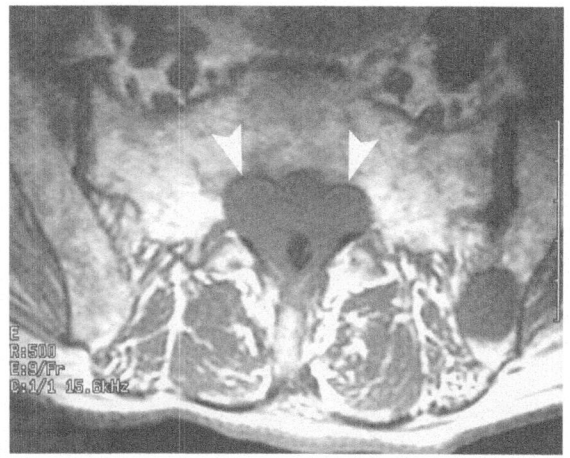
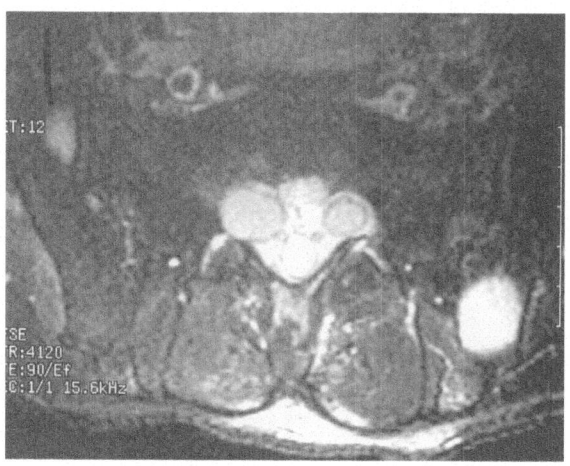

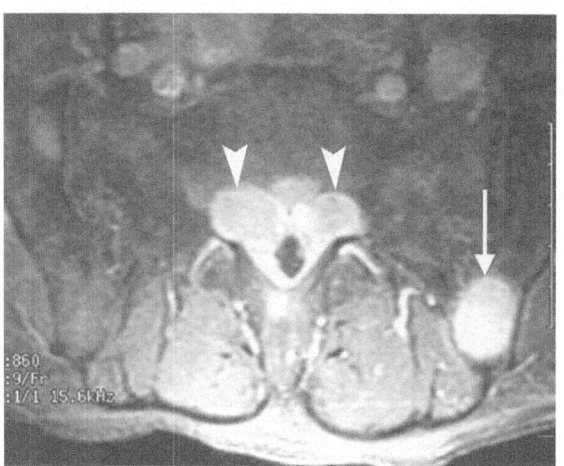

Fig. 20.6a–c. Intraspinal granulocytic sarcoma in a 68-year-old man with acute myeloid leukemia who had bone marrow relapse and complained of symptoms ascribed to the cauda equina during chemotherapy. **a** Axial spin-echo T1-weighted MR image shows intraspinal masses (*arrowheads*), isointense to muscle, with thickened epidura. **b** Axial fast spin-echo T2-weighted MR image shows these masses to be enlarged and hyperintense nerve roots with thickened spinal epidural tissue. **c** Axial contrast-enhanced fat-suppressed spin-echo T1-weighted MR image shows enhancement of both thickened nerve roots and epidural tissue (*arrowheads*). Note abnormal bone lesion in left sacrum (*arrow*), which shares similar signal changes with nerve roots and epidura. (With permission from [OOI and KHONG 2001; OOI et al. 2001])

1982; Prades et al. 2001). Orbital GS tends to affect patients in the first decade of life with a male preponderance (Zimmerman and Bilaniuk 1980; Banna et al. 1991), and can present as bilateral or unilateral disease. It usually arises from subperiosteal tissues (Pui et al. 1994; Cohen et al. 1988; Pomeranz et al. 1985; Uyesugi et al. 2000) and less commonly from the lacrimal gland and intraorbital muscles (Pui et al. 1994; Zimmerman and Bilaniuk 1980; Bulas et al. 1995). Other orbital manifestations of GS include optic nerve and intraocular infiltration (Guermazi et al. 2002; Ooi et al. 2001; Brock et al. 2001). GS orbital involvement is said to have a predilection for the lateral aspects of the orbits with sparing of the globe and optic nerve (Banna et al. 1991; Uyesugi et al. 2000). Lesions may arise primarily within the orbit (Fig. 20.7), or may extend from disease within the sinuses (Fig. 20.8) and infratemporal fossa, in which case destruction of the orbital walls may be associated (Guermazi et al. 2002; Cohen et al. 1988; Uyesugi et al. 2000). On CT scan, orbital GS lesions are of soft tissue density with homogenous enhancement (Pui et al. 1994; Brock et al. 2001; Uyesugi et al. 2000; Bulas et al. 1995), and if associated with adjacent bone, a "hair-on-end" periosteal reaction and cortical destruction may be found (Zimmerman and Bilaniuk 1980; Cohen et al. 1988). On MR imaging, the lesions are iso and mildly hyperintense to normal muscle on T1 and T2-weighted MR sequences respectively (Fig. 20.7) (Ooi et al. 2001). Differential diagnoses of a retrobulbar orbital mass in a child include rhabdomyosarcoma, metastatic neuroblastoma, inflammatory pseudotumor and lymphoma.

Paranasal sinus involvement by GS may be focal and well defined but with extensive and infiltrative disease, adjacent bone destruction may be associated (Figs 20.8, 20.9) (Freedy and Miller 1991; Prades et al. 2001). Other less usual head and neck sites of GS involvement include the nasopharynx (Fig. 20.10), maxillary gingiva, cavernous sinus, palate and cheek (Lee et al. 2001; Ficarra et al. 1987; Rodriguez et al. 1990; Carmona et al. 2000; Tong and Lam 2000). Leukemic infiltration can also involve the inner and middle ears, including the temporal bone and mastoid, which will invariably affect the adjacent facial and cochlear-vestibular nerves (Ooi et al. 2001; Ooi and Khong 2001; Au et al. 2000; Wuillemain et al 1993; Thompson et al. 1982; Almadori et al. 1996; Zappia 1990; Lee et al. 2002). Presenting complaints will often include post-auricular pain, hearing impairment, otalgia and facial nerve weakness. The CT and MR imaging characteristics of head and neck GS are broadly similar to those of orbital lesions, being masses that are primarily isodense on CT scan, and iso to hypointense on T1 and T2-weighted MR images (Ooi et al. 2001; Freedy and Miller 1991; Lee et al. 2001; Cankaya et al. 2001).

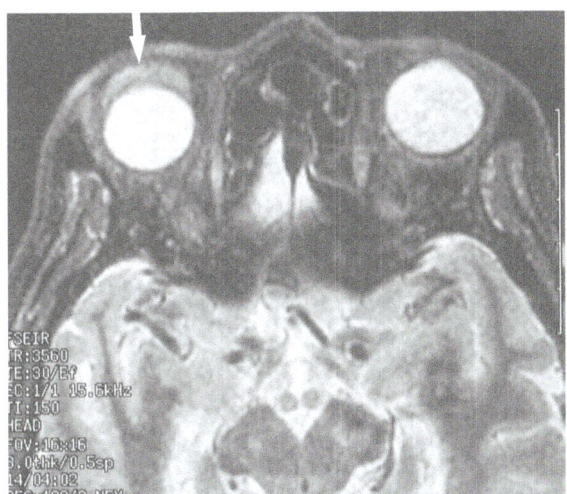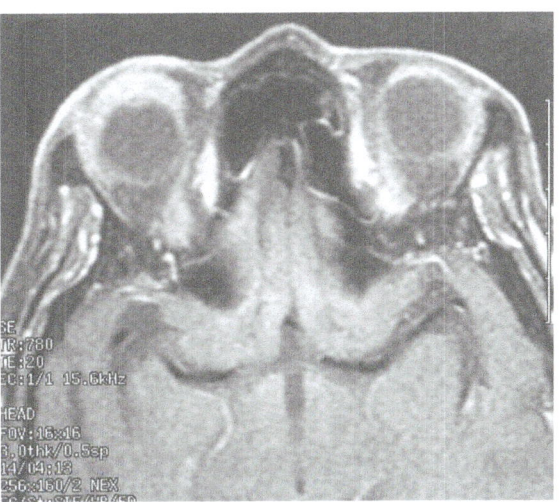

Fig. 20.7a,b. Orbital granulocytic sarcoma in a 68 year-old man with 2-year history of acute myeloid leukemia with active disease, who presented with a painful, swollen and red eye. **a** Axial fat-suppressed fast spin-echo T2-weighted MR image of the orbits shows thickened and mildly hyperintense (to muscle) conjunctiva (*arrow*) of right globe. **b** The conjunctiva is noted to be enhancing on the axial contrast-enhanced fat-suppressed spin-echo T1-weighted MR image of the orbits. This lesion was histologically confirmed to be granulocytic sarcoma. (With permission from [Ooi and Khong 2001; Ooi et al. 2001])

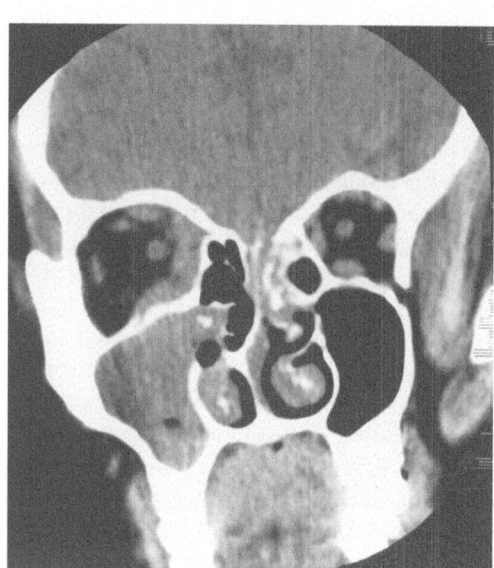
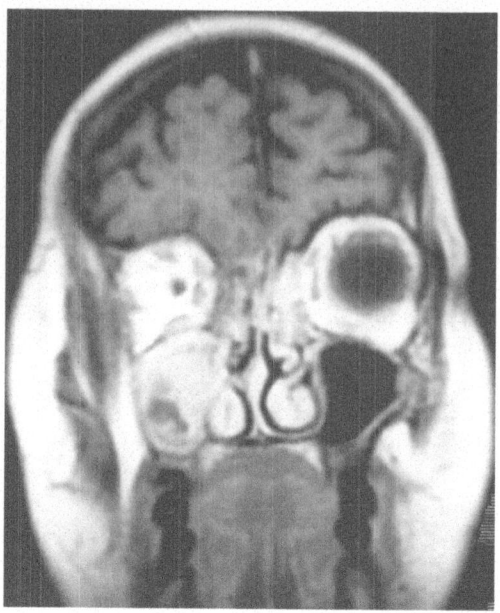

Fig. 20.8a,b. Paranasal sinus granuloytic sarcoma with orbital involvement in a 65-year-old woman with acute myeloblastic transformation of 1-year history of aplastic anemia. She presented with a 2 week history of ptosis of right eye. **a** Coronal contrast-enhanced CT scan through mid orbit reveals soft-tissue mass involving right medial rectus muscle and right maxillary sinus. Ethmoid mass with bony destruction of left ethmoid cells also can be seen. **b** Coronal contrast-enhanced T1-weighted MR image shows dense and heterogeneous enhancement of lesions. Biopsy subsequently showed right orbital and paranasal sinus granulocytic sarcoma. Despite therapy, patient died 6 months later. (With permission from [GUERMAZI et al. 2002])

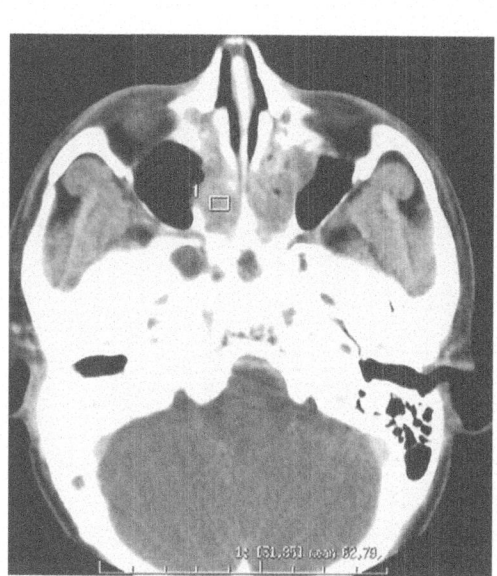
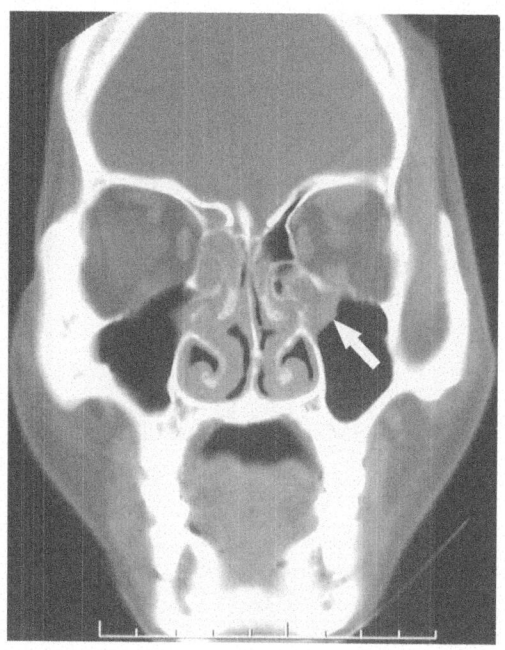

Fig. 20.9a,b. Granulocytic sarcoma of the nose in a 31-year-old man with acute myeloid leukemia that was in remission after chemotherapy. He complained of nasal obstruction. Bone marrow trephine biopsy was normal. **a** Axial contrast-enhanced CT scan performed through the skull base shows mildly enhancing soft tissue mass in the superior aspects of the nasal passages. **b** Coronal CT scan in bone algorithm illustrates more clearly the mass in both superior nasal passages extending into the left maxillary sinus via a widened osteomeatal complex (*arrow*). Endoscopic examination showed the mass in the nasal passage, which was confirmed to be a granulocytic sarcoma. (With permission from [OOI and KHONG 2001])

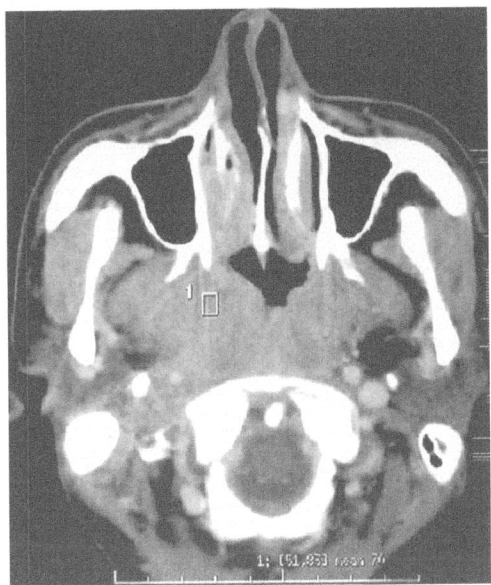

Fig. 20.10. Granulocytic sarcoma of the nasopharynx in a 32-year-old man with relapse of acute myeloid leukemia. Axial contrast-enhanced CT of nasopharynx shows soft tissue mass, which is obliterating right fossa of Rosenmuller. This granulocytic lesion was treated with local radiation therapy and chemotherapy. (With permission from [Ooi et al. 2001])

20.7
Musculoskeletal System

20.7.1
Bone

Bone is one of the most frequent sites of GS, occurring in 91.3% of GS lesions in one review of patients with myelogenous leukemia autopsied in Hiroshima and Nagasaki during 1949–1969 (Liu et al. 1973). Usually subperiosteal, bone GS commonly arises in the cranium, sacrum, sternum, ribs (Fig. 20.11) and spine (Liu et al. 1973; Frohna and Quint 1993; Neiman et al. 1981; Novick et al. 1998; Dunnick and Heaston 1982). On plain radiographs, it is usually lytic with ill-defined margins, but may have a mixed sclerotic and lytic pattern (Bulas et al. 1995; Laufer et al. 1996; Hermann et al. 1991; Cho et al. 1990; Libson et al. 1986). However a purely sclerotic lesion is rare (Laufer et al. 1996; Libson et al. 1986). Radiographic differential diagnosis includes metastatic neuroblastoma, Ewing sarcoma, eosinophilic granuloma and primitive neuroectodermal tumor in children, and metastasis, plasmacytoma, malignant fibrous histiocytoma, lymphoma and osteomyelitis in adults (Guermazi et al. 2002). On CT scan, a

soft tissue component is often seen in association with the bony lesion (Fig. 20.12) (Novick et al. 1998; Turner et al. 1991; Ooi et al. 2001; Laufer et al. 1996; Hermann et al. 1991; Levy et al. 1989). MR imaging features are non-specific: isointense on T1 and iso or mildly hyperintense on T2-weighted images with homogeneous enhancement (Figs. 20.6c, 20.12) (Turner et al. 1991; Ooi et al. 2001; Freedy and Miller 1991; Lee et al. 2002; Cho et al. 1990; Gómez et al. 1997). These signal characteristics may be similar to other bone tumors such as lymphoma, or osteomyelitis particularly if T2 time is prolonged. However when the GS lesion is isointense on both T1 and T2-weighted MR images, pathologies such as other bone tumors, synovitis and arthritis can be excluded with reasonable confidence. Conditions that are frequently found in myeloid leukemias such as abscess and hematoma can also be discounted based on their very different signal intensities.

20.7.2
Muscle

GS predominantly affecting the muscles have also been reported (Ooi et al. 2001; Dunnick and Heaston 1982; Bassichis et al. 2000). These appear as infiltrative enlargement of the affected muscle,

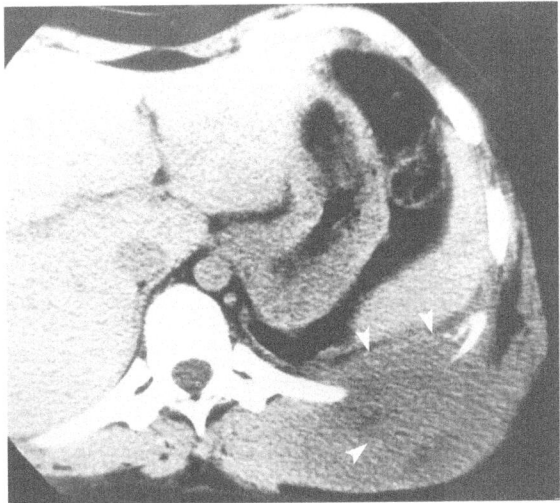

Fig. 20.11. Intrathoracic granulocytic sarcoma in a 40-year-old woman with relapse of acute myeloblastic leukemia who presented with left thoracic pain. Axial contrast-enhanced CT scan of chest shows soft-tissue mass of chest wall with rib lysis (arrowheads), which corresponded to granulocytic sarcoma at biopsy. Complete remission was obtained after chemotherapy and radiation therapy. (With permission from [Guermazi et al. 2002])

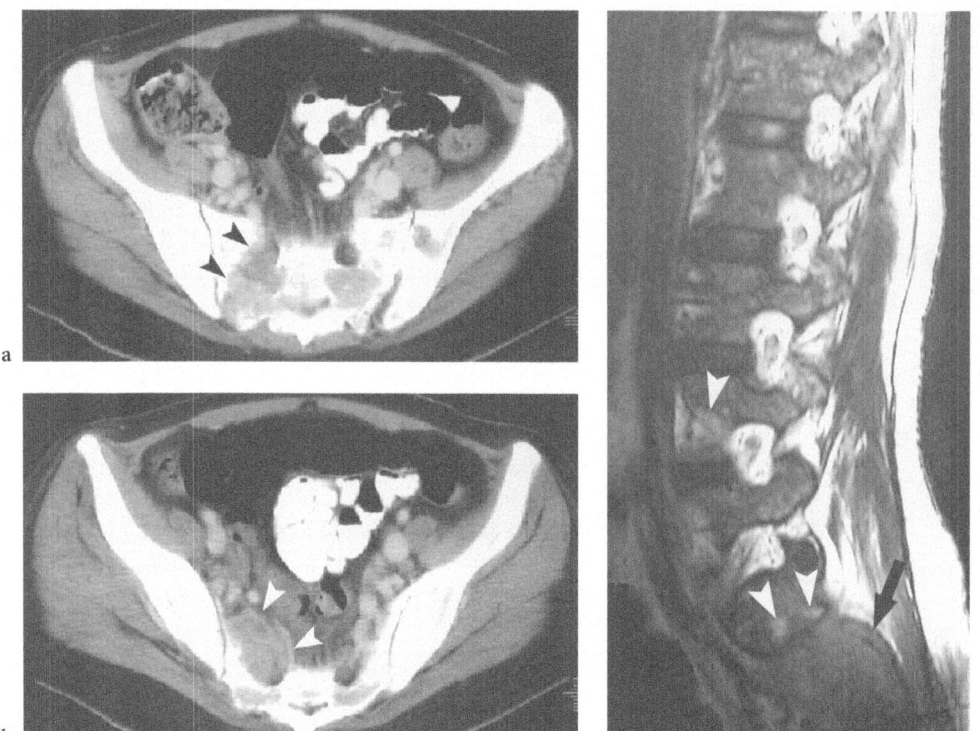

Fig. 20.12a–c. Granulocytic sarcoma of the bone in a 33 year-old woman with acute myeloid leukemia. Axial contrast-enhanced CT scans through the sacrum show (a) a lytic lesion in the right ala (*arrowheads*) with (b) a presacral soft tissue component (*arrowheads*). c Parasagittal fast spin-echo T2-weighted MR image of the lumbar spine shows abnormal hyperintense foci at L3 and L5 vertebral bodies (*arrowheads*), and mildly hyperintense pre-sacral soft tissue (*arrow*). (With permission from [Ooi and Khong 2001])

isodense to normal muscle and are heterogeneously enhancing on CT scan (Fig. 20.13) (Ooi et al. 2001; Dunnick and Heaston 1982; Bassichis et al. 2000). They may cause cortical erosion of adjacent bone. On MR imaging, muscle GS may share similar signal characteristics as infiltrated bone marrow (Turner et al. 1991). Appearances resembling abscess may be found on CT scan with hypodense center and peripheral enhancement in bone and muscle GS (Fig. 20.14) (Ooi et al. 2001; Laufer et al. 1996). In such lesions aspiration biopsies may be unavoidable.

20.8
Subcutaneous Tissues

20.8.1
Skin

Extramedullary leukemia can also manifest in subcutaneous tissues including the breast (Liu et al. 1973; Békássy et al. 1996). Although breast involvement

is rare, the skin is quite frequently involved with a reported incidence ranging from 20–50% (Neiman et al. 1981; Jakobiec 1991; Meis et al. 1986). Skin nodules usually appear as firm papulonodular lesions, which are often solitary (Harris et al. 1992;

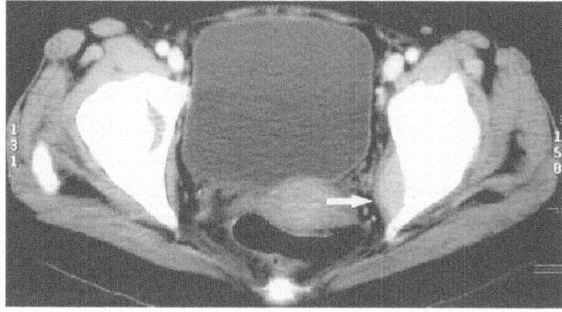

Fig. 20.13. Granulocytic sarcoma of the muscle in a 19-year-old woman with acute myeloid leukemia who had hematologic and extramedullary leukemic relapse at multiple sites after bone marrow transplantation. Axial contrast-enhanced CT scan of the pelvis shows an enlarged and enhancing left internal obturator muscle (*arrow*) with minimal cortical erosion of the adjacent ischium. (With permission from [Ooi and Khong 2001])

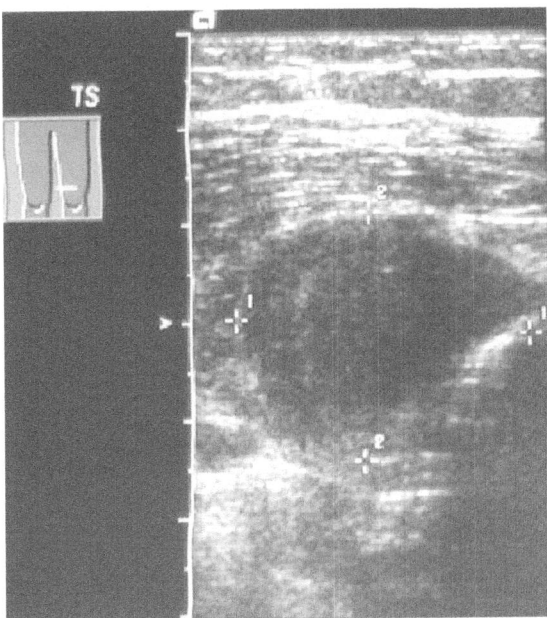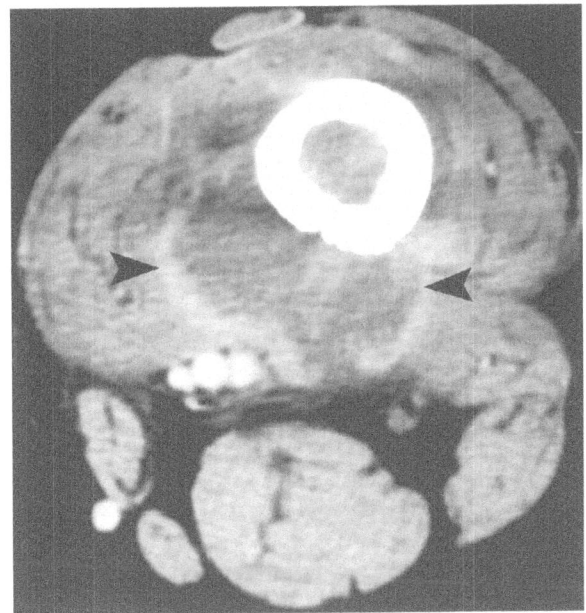

a

b

Fig. 20.14a,b. Granulocytic sarcoma of the muscle in a 33-year-old woman with chronic myeloid leukemia who complained of painful swollen left thigh. **a** Transverse US image of thigh shows heterogeneous hypoechoic mass. **b** Axial contrast-enhanced CT image shows the mass (*arrowheads*) to be hypodense with peripheral rim enhancement. Mass is noted to arise deep within vastus lateralis and intermedius muscles, abutting femoral shaft with adjacent cortical erosion. This lesion was thought to be an abscess based on imaging findings. Aspiration biopsy was performed, which confirmed the lesion to be granulocytic sarcoma and not an abscess. (With permission from [Ooi et al. 2001])

Fridus et al. 1993) but can be disseminated (Lin et al. 1990). They are rarely imaged, as they are easily palpable and biopsied. On CT scan, they can appear well defined or slightly spiculated with enhancement (Fig. 20.15) (Ooi et al. 2001; Ooi and Khong 2001).

20.8.2
Breast

Breast GS occurs more frequently in women than men and children with AML (Au et al. 1999b; Ahrar et al. 1998), although lymphoma remains the most common hematologic breast malignancy (Paulus and Libshitz 1972; Lin et al. 1997). On mammography, US and MR imaging, the imaging features of breast GS universally suggest a malignant pathology (Fig. 20.16). On mammography, breast GSs can appear either solitary or multiple, and are usually uncalcified, irregular, spiculated and poorly defined (Guermazi et al. 2000; Barloon et al. 1993; Son and Oh 1998). The US appearances have been described to be lobulated or irregular with an essentially hypoechoic texture, which can be either homogeneous or heterogeneous, and showing acoustic shadowing (Guermazi et al.

2000; Fitoz et al. 2002; Ahrar et al. 1998; Barloon et al. 1993; Son and Oh 1998; Hiorns and Murfitt 1997). The signal intensity of breast GS on MR imaging indicates a malignant lesion with prominent T2-hyperintensity, and a marked and heterogeneous enhancement after contrast administration (Guermazi et al. 2000; Fitoz et al. 2002). Tumor vascularity has also been demonstrated on Doppler US (Fitoz et al. 2002; Ahrar et al. 1998). Differentiation from other malignant breast disease such as carcinoma, lymphoma and metastasis cannot rest on imaging alone and biopsy is often required for definitive diagnosis.

20.9
Thorax

Thoracic GS is rare but can arise in the mediastinum, hila, paraspinal area, pleura or the lungs (Liu et al. 1973; Takasugi et al. 1996; Lee et al. 1991). In a review of 41 patients, thoracic GS preceded or was concurrent with myeloid leukemia in 80% cases while the remaining 20% followed the diagnosis of leukemia (Takasugi et al. 1996). In that review,

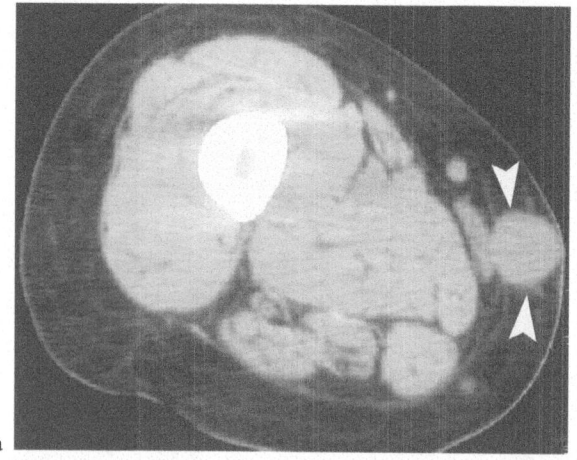
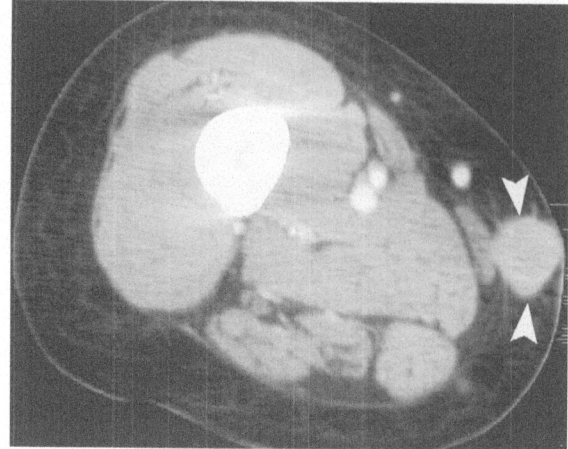
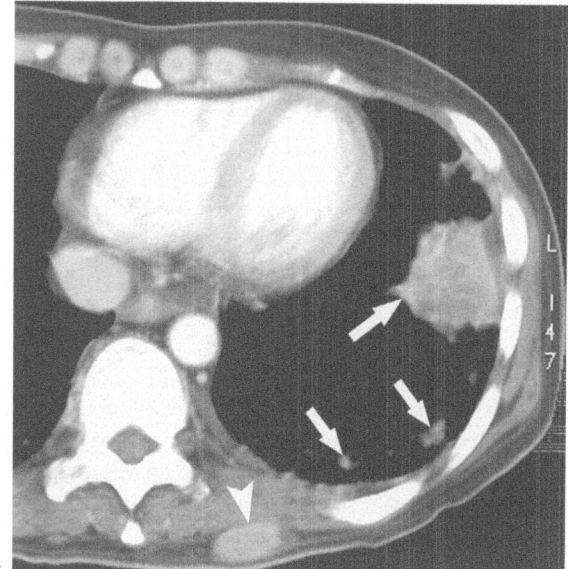

Fig. 20.15a–c. Multi-sited granulocytic sarcoma lesions affecting the muscle, lung and subcutaneous tissues in a 49-year-old woman with bone marrow and extramedullary leukemic relapse. Axial (a) unenhanced and (b) contrast-enhanced CT scans of the thigh show a mildly enhancing granulocytic sarcoma nodule (*arrowheads*) with slightly spiculated borders in the subcutaneous tissues of the thigh. c Axial contrast-enhanced CT scan of the thorax shows multiple left pulmonary granulocytic sarcoma nodules (*arrows*). Note another subcutaneous granulocytic sarcoma nodule on the posterior chest (*arrowhead*). (With permission from [OOI and KHONG 2001])

mediastinal involvement was the commonest manifestation of intrathoracic GS accounting for 50% of cases, followed by pleural (22%) and pericardial effusion (20%) (TAKASUGI et al. 1996).

20.9.1
Mediastinum

Mediastinal involvement on chest radiographs is similar to that of lymphoma, seen either as focal or diffuse mediastinal widening, as a result of which misdiagnosis on initial evaluation is not unusual (Fig. 20.17) (TAKASUGI et al. 1996). On CT scan, however, diffuse infiltration rather than focal masses are noted, a feature that may help distinguish GS from other causes of mediastinal masses such as fungal

and mycobacterial infection (TAKASUGI et al. 1996). GS may on the rare occasions, compress mediastinal structures resulting in superior vena cava and bronchial obstruction (RAVANDI-KASHANI et al. 2000; LIU et al. 1988). Paraspinal disease may extend anteriorly to involve the mediastinum, erode adjacent vertebrae or extend posteriorly into intraspinal epidural space (Figs. 20.17b, 20.18) (OOI and KHONG 2001; TAKASUGI et al. 1996). In such cases, MR imaging may be helpful in further evaluation of the posterior mediastinum.

20.9.2
Lung

Lung parenchymal lesion per se is rare, and can present as airspace shadowing (Fig. 20.19) (GUERMAZI et

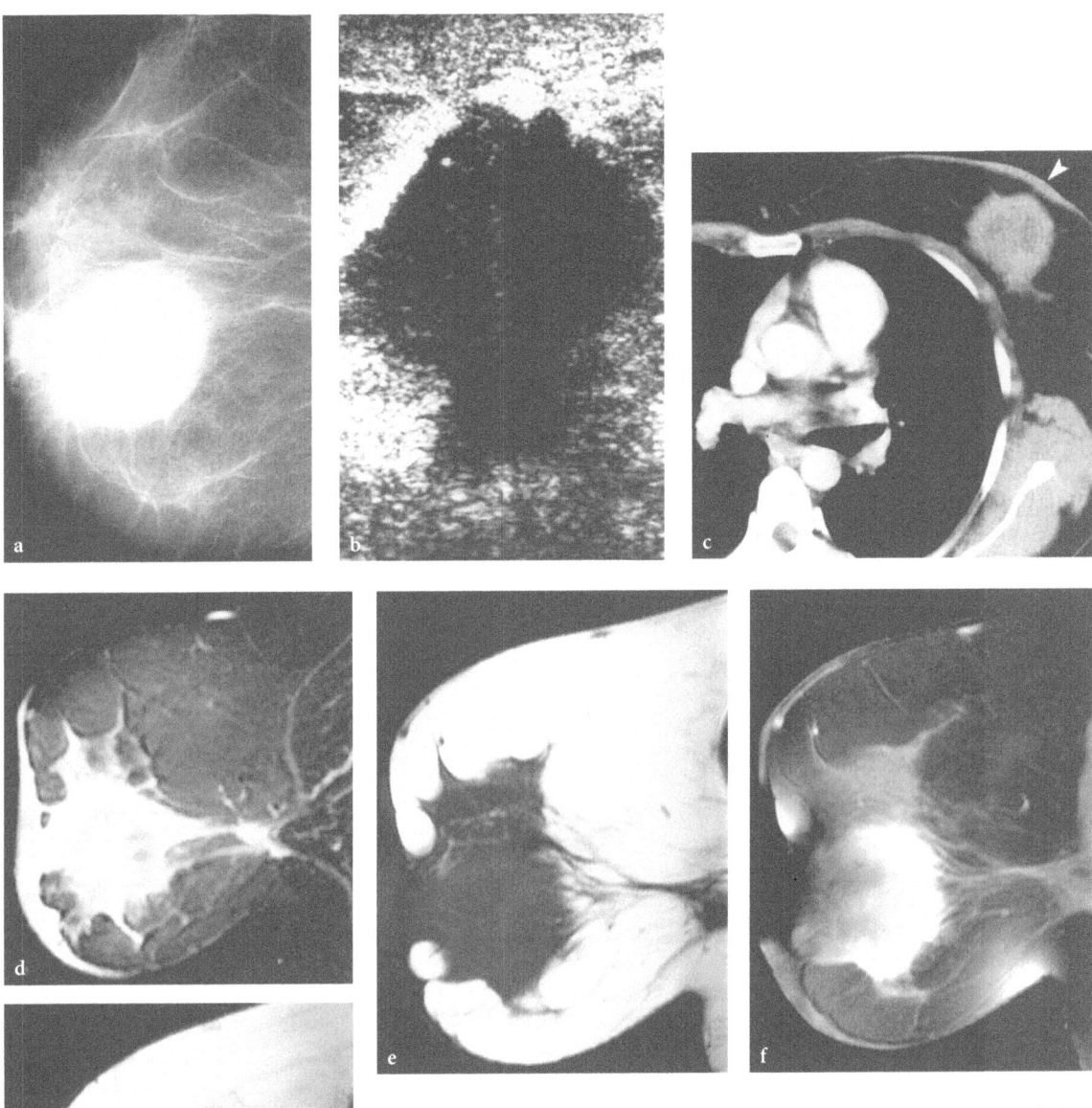

Fig. 20.16a–g. Breast granulocytic sarcoma in a 41-year-old woman with history of acute myeloblastic leukemia associated with abnormal eosinophils who presented with palpable mass in left breast. **a** Left lateral mammogram discloses dense, rounded, and spiculated mass of 3-cm diameter with irregular margins and skin retraction. **b** Axial US image shows irregularly shaped nonhomogeneous hypoechoic mass with ill-defined margins and posterior acoustic shadow. **c** Axial contrast-enhanced CT scan of thorax obtained 3 days after (**b**) shows spiculated mass that contains small foci of necrosis. Skin wall is thickened (*arrowhead*). On sagittal MR imaging the mass is inhomogeneous and hyperintense on (**d**) STIR image, hypointense on (**e**) T1-weighted image, and enhances markedly but inhomogeneously (**f**) after contrast administration and fat suppression. Note spiculation of mass and adjacent skin thickening. Fine-needle breast biopsy revealed granulocytic sarcoma. Patient received two courses of chemotherapy. Five weeks later, mass was no longer palpable. **g** Sagittal unenhanced T1-weighted MR image shows marked reduction of tumor size. (With permission from [GUERMAZI et al. 2002])

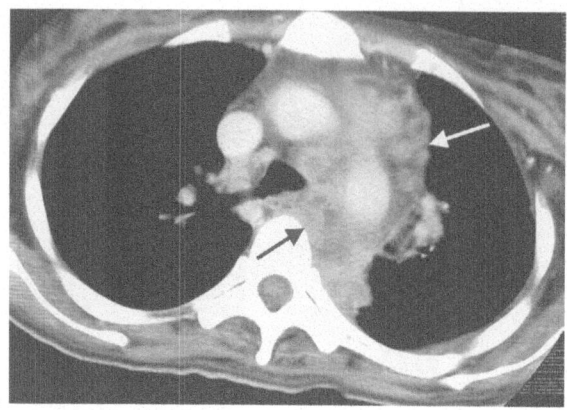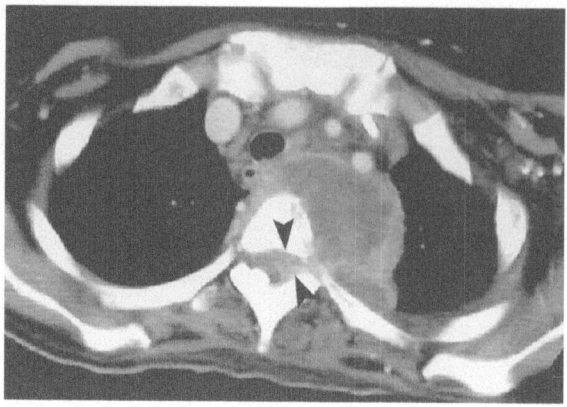

Fig. 20.17a,b. Intrathoracic granulocytic sarcoma in a 33-year-old woman with chronic myeloid leukemia. Axial contrast-enhanced CT scans of the chest show (**a**) the granulocytic sarcoma lesions manifested as diffusely enlarged mediastinal lymph nodes (*arrows*) and (**b**) a left paraspinal mass. Note intraspinal extension of the mass (*arrowheads*) via the neural foramen. She had concurrent bone marrow relapse and was treated with combination of chemotherapy and radiotherapy to no avail. (With permission from [OOI and KHONG 2001])

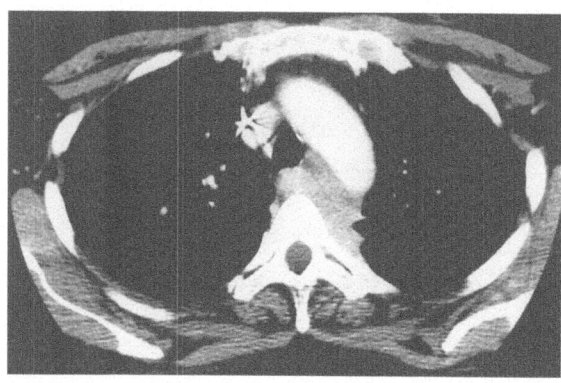

Fig. 20.18. Intrathoracic granulocytic sarcoma in a 44-year-old woman with history of acute myeloblastic leukemia. She had medullary and systemic relapse 6 months after autologous bone marrow transplantation. Axial contrast-enhanced CT scan of chest shows left paraspinal soft-tissue mass without bone destruction or epidural extension, which corresponded to granulocytic sarcoma at biopsy. Complete resolution was obtained within 2 months of chemotherapy. (With permission from [GUERMAZI et al. 2002])

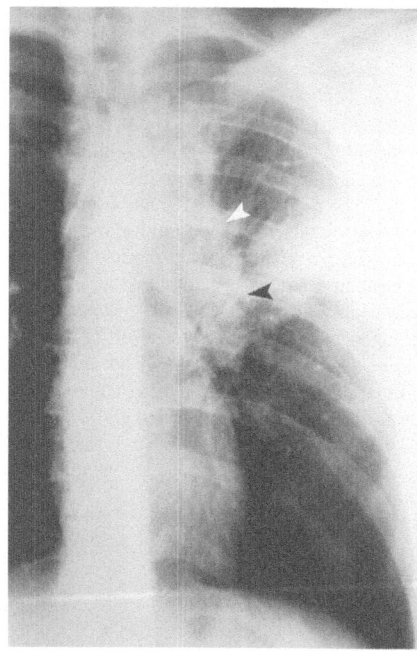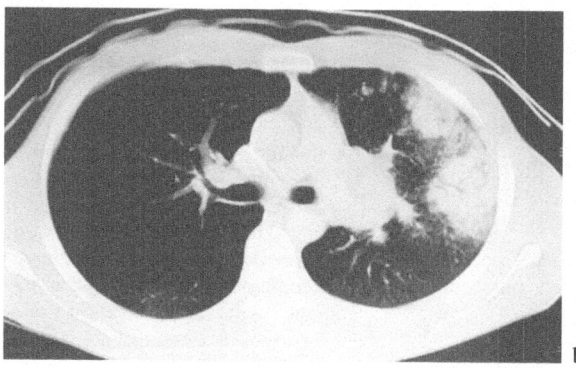

Fig. 20.19. Intrathoracic granulocytic sarcoma in a 24-year-old man with acute myeloblastic leukemia who presented with thoracic pain and hemoptysis. **a** Posteroanterior radiograph of chest shows left hilar lymph node enlargement (*arrowheads*) associated with left upper air-space consolidation. **b** Axial unenhanced CT scan of chest reveals large irregular nodular opacities. Subsequent biopsy showed granulocytic sarcoma infiltrating hilar lymph nodes and involving lung parenchyma. Complete resolution was obtained after chemotherapy and radiation therapy. (With permission from [GUERMAZI et al. 2002])

al. 2002; TAKASUGI et al. 1996; BHATI and COPPAGE 1995; DAVEY et al. 1986; TARYLE and SAHN 1979; WONG et al. 1993; DE PAZ et al. 2003), nodules (Fig. 20.15c) (GUERMAZI et al. 2002; OOI et al. 2001; WANG et al. 1987; KUMAR 1980; CALLAHAN et al. 1987) or more rarely interstitial lines (Fig. 20.20) (TAKASUGI et al. 1996; CALLAHAN et al. 1987). Pleural involvement shares similar features with mesothelioma and metastatic pleural disease and manifests itself primarily as pleural effusions or pleural thickening on chest radiographs (LEE et al. 1991; SIEGEL et al. 1981; HICKLIN and DREVYANKO 1988). On CT scan, focal or diffuse pleural thickening may be seen in association with the pleural effusion (LEE et al. 1991; KIM and FENNESSY 1994; HEIBERG et al. 1984).

20.10
Abdomen

20.10.1
Bowel

GS can affect any intraabdominal organ including the retroperitoneal lymph nodes (Fig. 20.21) (LIU et al. 1973; NEIMAN et al. 1981; AU et al. 1999b; POMERANZ et al. 1985; ROTTER et al. 1992; RAVANDI-KASHANI et al. 1999). Bowel involvement is the most common (17.4% to 50%) gastrointestinal manifestation in autopsy studies of leukemic patients, due to the close proximity of lymphoid tissue in the bowel and bowel mesentery (LIU et al. 1973; PROLLA and KIRSNER 1964; HUNTER and BJELLAND 1984; DEWAR et al. 1981). Both the large and small bowel can be involved (ROTTENBERG and THOMAS 1994; OOI et al. 2001; CORPECHOT et al. 1998; DABBAGH et al. 1999). Weight loss, abdominal pain and obstructive symptoms and even perforation may herald the presence of bowel GS (ROTTENBERG and THOMAS 1994; HUNTER and BJELLAND 1984), which manifests macroscopically as polypoid (GILDENHORN et al. 1962), nodular (ROTTENBERG and THOMAS 1994), diffuse (Fig. 20.22) (GUERMAZI et al. 2002; HUNTER and BJELLAND 1984), plaque-like (Fig. 20.23) (OOI et al. 2001) or ulcerated mucosal thickening (PROLLA and KIRSNER 1964; LIMBERAKIS et al. 1978). Despite being a relatively common autopsy finding, imaging examples of these lesions are not widely reported in the

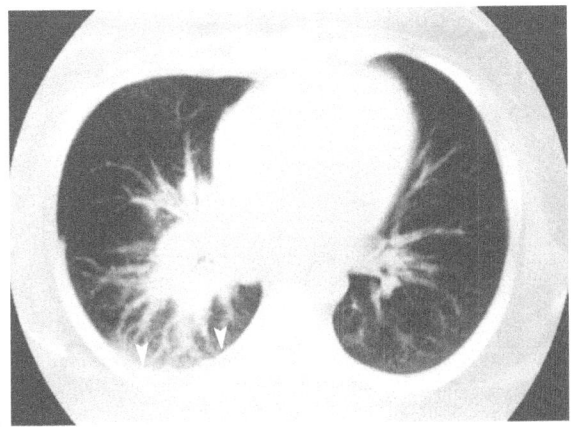

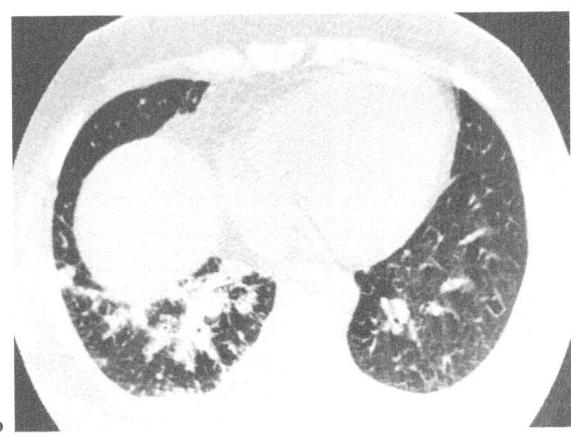

Fig. 20.20a,b. Intrathoracic granulocytic sarcoma in a 36-year-old woman with acute myeloblastic leukemia associated with myelofibrosis, who presented with dyspnea. a Axial unenhanced CT scan of chest shows large right hilar mass associated with small pleural effusion (*arrowheads*). b Axial CT slice 20-mm caudal to (a) shows right nodular peribronchial consolidations and some interstitial septal lines. Biopsy subsequently showed granulocytic sarcoma involving peribronchial spaces. Patient died 8 days later. (With permission from [GUERMAZI et al. 2002])

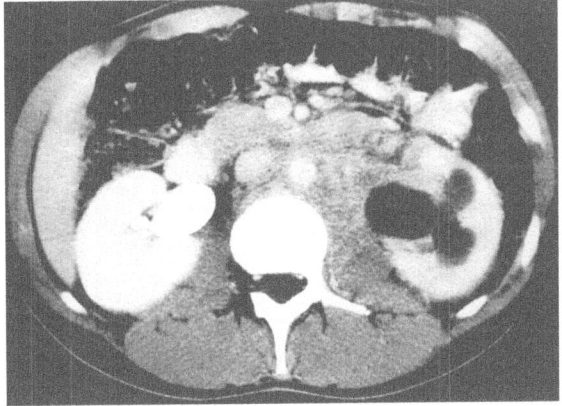

Fig. 20.21. Retroperitoneal granulocytic sarcoma in a 16-year-old boy with relapse of acute myeloblastic leukemia. The patient was admitted for intermittent left flank pain. Axial contrast-enhanced CT scan of abdomen shows left retroperitoneal mass invading psoas and kidney hilum associated with hydronephrosis. Subsequent biopsy confirmed retroperitoneal granulocytic sarcoma. Remission was obtained after chemotherapy. (With permission from [GUERMAZI et al. 2002])

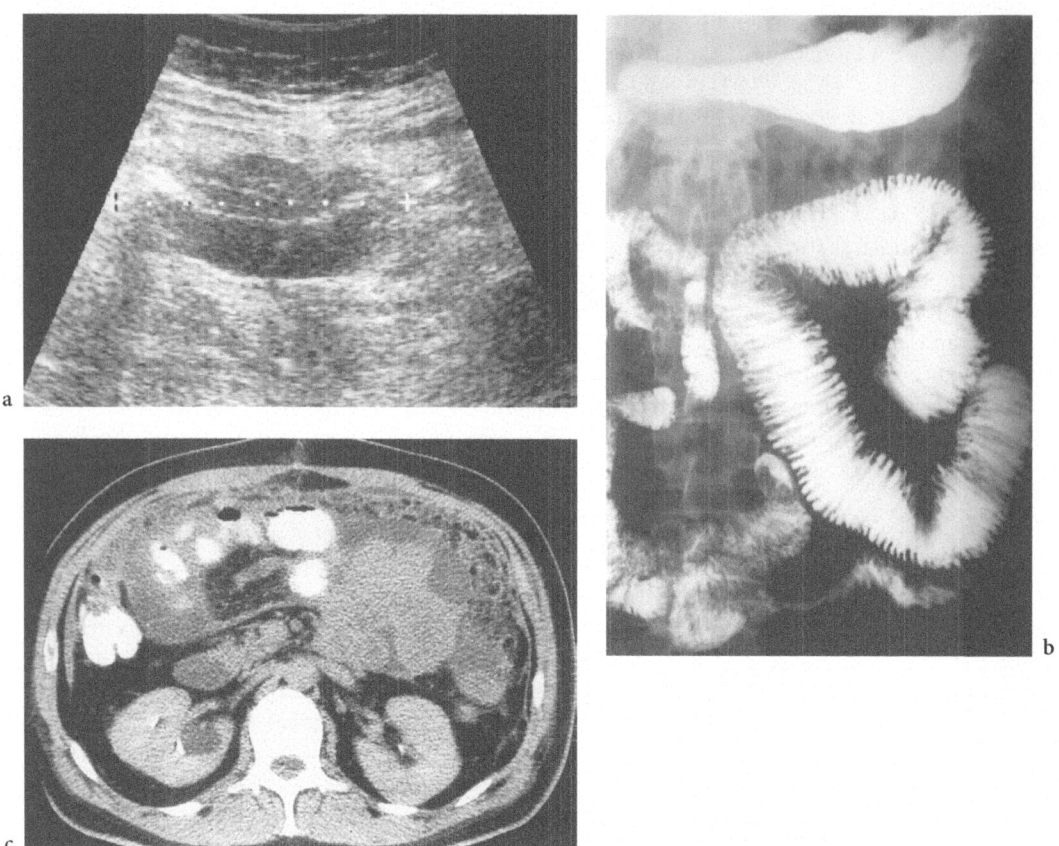

Fig. 20.22a–c. Granulocytic sarcoma of small bowel in a 40-year-old man with unremarkable medical history, who was admitted with small bowel obstruction. **a** Transverse US image shows marked mucosal thickening of the jejunum approximately 5-cm in length. **b** Barium examination of small bowel shows stricture of mid jejunum with up-stream dilatation. **c** Axial contrast-enhanced CT scan of abdomen shows intestinal involvement with stenosis and parietal thickening associated with ascites and peritoneal carcinosis. Diagnosis at biopsy was granulocytic sarcoma of small intestine without evidence of blood or bone marrow involvement. Twenty-one months later, patient was diagnosed with acute myeloblastic leukemia with central nervous system and bone marrow involvement. (With permission from [GUERMAZI et al. 2002])

literature. The various forms of bowel wall thickening described above can be appreciated on plain radiographs (HUNTER and BJELLAND 1984; LIMBERAKIS et al. 1978), US (GUERMAZI et al. 2002), barium studies (ROTTENBERG and THOMAS 1994; HUNTER and BJELLAND 1984; LIMBERAKIS et al. 1978), or CT scans (GUERMAZI et al. 2002; OOI et al. 2001).

20.10.2
Hepatobiliary System

Pancreatic and peribiliary lesions may cause upper abdominal pain and obstructive jaundice (OOI et al. 2001; ROTTER et al. 1992; RAVANDI-KASHANI et al. 1999; MATSUEDA et al. 1998). On US, peribiliary lesions have been described to be hypoechoic although

they can be iso or hypodense to soft tissue on CT scan (POMERANZ et al. 1985; RAVANDI-KASHANI et al. 1999; MATSUEDA et al. 1998). Similarly pancreatic GS are of soft tissue density (Figs. 20.23, 20.24), and on MR imaging are reported to be hypointense on T1 and hyperintense on T2-weighted images with minimal enhancement after contrast administration (OOI et al. 2001; RAVANDI-KASHANI et al. 1999; MARCOS et al. 1997).

20.11
Genitourinary System

Although rare, any organ in the genitourinary system can be affected by GS (LIU et al. 1973). The ovary may

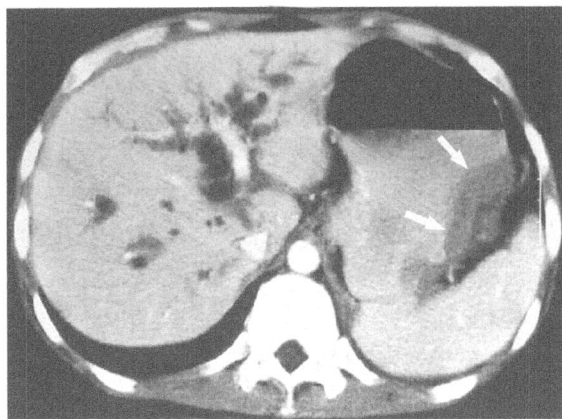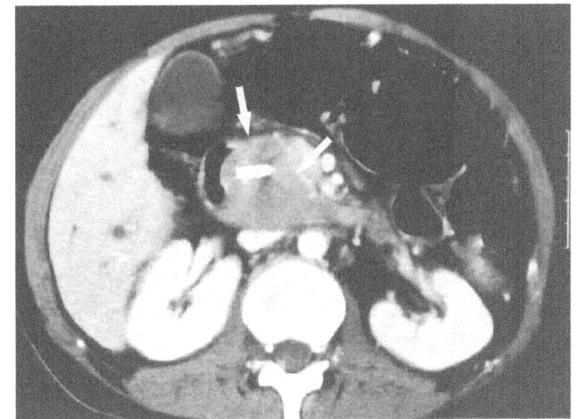

a   b

Fig. 20.23a,b. Intraabdominal granulocytic sarcoma affecting the stomach and pancreas in a 20-year-old man with acute myeloid leukemia who had medullary relapse concurrent to extramedullary disease. Axial contrast-enhanced CT scans of the abdomen show (**a**) plaque-like mucosal thickening found in the greater curve of the stomach (*arrows*) which was confirmed to be granulocytic sarcoma. **b** Dilated intrahepatic ducts are due to another granulocytic mass in the head of pancreas (*arrows*). Internal biliary drainage has been performed. (With permission from [Ooi and Khong 2001])

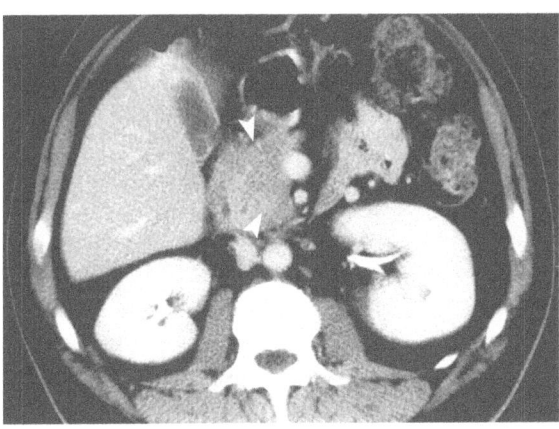

Fig. 20.24. Granulocytic sarcoma of the pancreas in a 53-year-old man with acute myeloblastic leukemia who presented with acute abdominal pain. Axial contrast-enhanced CT scan of abdomen obtained concurrently with diagnosis shows hypodense mass of head of pancreas (*arrowheads*). Biopsy subsequently confirmed diagnosis of pancreatic granulocytic sarcoma. Six weeks later, after chemotherapy and radiation therapy, repeated CT showed resolution of pancreatic mass. (With permission from [Guermazi et al. 2002])

be the first site of manifestation of GS (Ooi et al. 2001; Sreejith et al. 2000; Oliva et al. 1997; Jung et al. 1999). Other sites of involvement include the kidneys (Breatnach et al. 1985; Bagg et al. 1994), bladder (Ooi et al. 2001; Kerr et al. 2002), vagina (Oliva et al. 1997), uterus (Oliva et al. 1997) and testes (Pui et al. 1994; Liu et al. 1973; Guermazi et al. 2002;

Békássy et al. 1996; Ooi et al. 2001). Uterine involvement occurs less frequently than ovarian, while the cervix is more commonly affected than the uterine corpus. Primary and secondary involvement of the vagina or vulva is rare. Clinical symptoms depend on the site of genitourinary GS involvement. Ovarian GS may be asymptomatic or present as hydronephrosis, abdominal pain or mass, while abnormal vaginal bleeding is common with vaginal or uterine GS (Oliva et al. 1997). Hematuria, hydronephrosis, abdominal mass and pain are symptoms associated with renal and bladder GS lesions. Renal involvement is usually reported in autopsy rather than clinical series (Liu et al. 1973).

20.11.1
Genitals

Ovarian lesions on imaging can appear lobulated, solid, multiseptate, or mixed with solid and cystic components (Sreejith et al. 2000; Oliva et al. 1997; Jung et al. 1999), with variable enhancement on CT and MR imaging (Fig. 20.25) (Jung et al. 1999; Ooi and Khong 2001). Differential diagnosis include germ cell tumors in children, epithelial tumors such as cystadenoma and cystadenocarcinoma, granulose cell carcinoma, lymphoma and metastatic carcinoma The appearances can be similar to primary carcinoma.

Testicular GS is rarely reported and may present as testicular swelling, which may be painful (Ooi

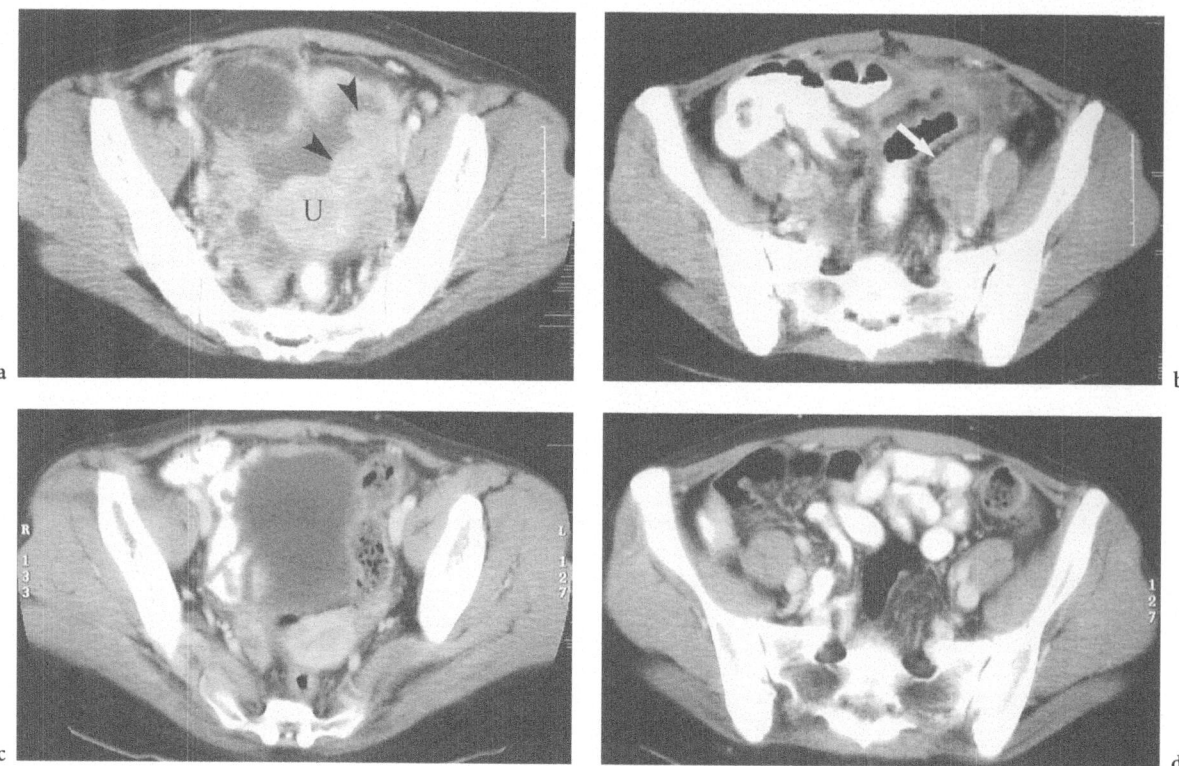

Fig. 20.25a–d. Primary granulocytic sarcoma arising in the ovary of a 33-year-old woman. She underwent chemotherapy and resection of the left ovary. There was no medullary involvement. **a** Axial contrast-enhanced CT scans of the pelvis show a lobulated heterogeneously enhancing left ovary (*arrowheads*) with parametrial and peritoneal disease. The uterus (*U*) is diffusely enlarged. A small amount of loculated ascites and (**b**) enlarged left pelvic nodes (*arrow*) are also noted. Axial contrast-enhanced CT scans after chemotherapy shows (**c**) normalization of the uterus and (**d**) resolution of enlarged lymph nodes. (With permission from [OOI and KHONG 2001])

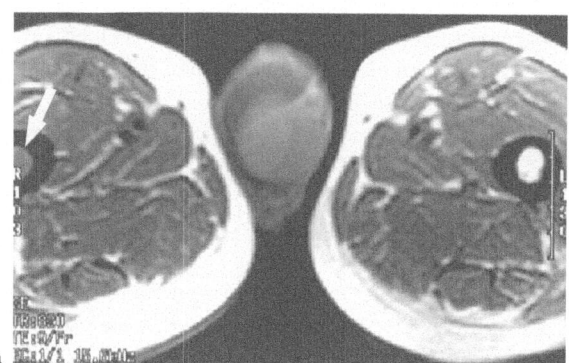

Fig. 20.26a,b. Granulocytic sarcoma lesion in a testis of a 69-year-old man with acute myeloid leukemia who presented with painful swelling of his testis. He had concurrent medullary relapse. **a** Axial spin-echo T1-weighted MR image shows mildly hyperintense testis relative to muscle with a hydrocele. Note abnormal bone marrow signal in the right femoral shaft (*arrow*). **b** Sagittal contrast-enhanced spin-echo T1-weighted MR image demonstrates marked enhancement of thickened tunica albuginea (*arrowheads*) with moderate testicular enhancement. He achieved partial response with chemotherapy with further medullary relapse a year later. (With permission from [OOI and KHONG 2001])

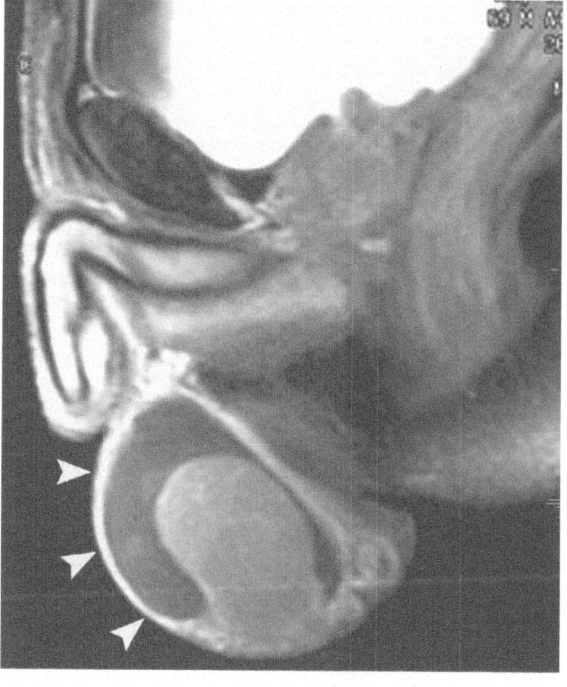

et al. 2001). On imaging diffuse enlargement of the organ is noted appearing as a heterogeneous mass on US (Fig. 20.26), and on MR imaging is mildly hyperintense to muscle on T1-weighted images, with loss of normal testicular hyperintensity on T2-weighted images (Fig. 20.27) (GUERMAZI et al. 2002; OOI et al. 2001). Epididymal involvement and hydroceles may be associated.

20.11.2
Urinary system

Imaging descriptions of renal GS are equally rare. Bragg et al described CT and MR imaging appearances of a renal GS that caused diffuse renal enlargement with infiltration of the renal pelvis and ureter (BAGG et al. 1994). The tumor was isointense on T1-weighted MR image with heterogeneous enhancement after contrast administration. Renal lymphoma was the main differential diagnosis. GS simulating an atypical transitional cell carcinoma has also been reported in which the tumor appeared to arise from the renal pelvis causing extrinsic compression on uroradiographic study with infiltration of the upper ureter (BREATNACH et al. 1985). CT confirmed a soft tissue mass within the renal sinus enveloping the ureter. Infiltration of pararenal fat from retroperitoneal GS can involve the kidneys and cause hydronephrosis (Fig. 20.21).

Bladder GS has been shown to manifest as diffuse or focal soft tissue infiltration of the bladder, with contrast enhancement (Fig. 20.28) (OOI et al. 2001; OOI and KHONG 2001; KERR et al. 2002).

20.12
Conclusion

The radiological manifestations of GS are variable, as with clinical presentation. There is often an overlap of imaging features with other complications of leukemia such as hematoma, abscesses and other pri-

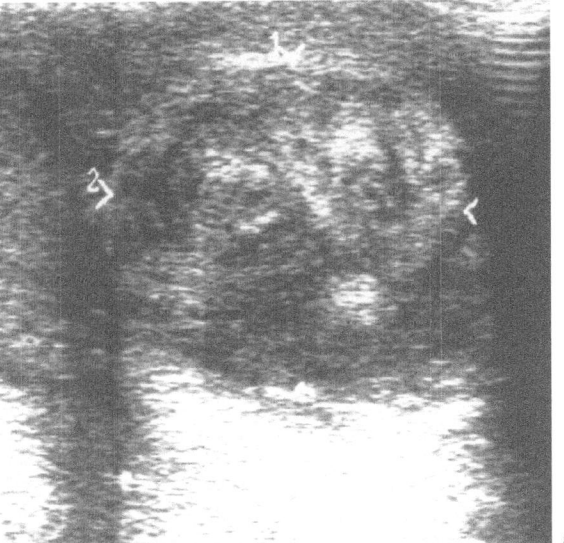

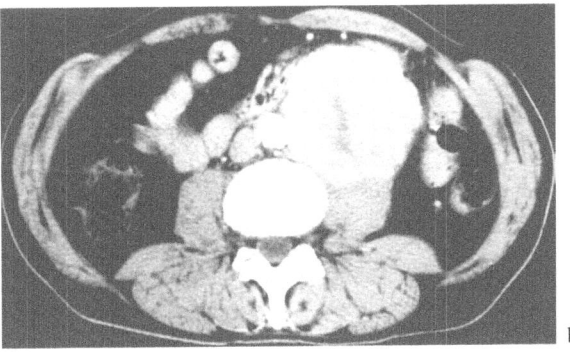

Fig. 20.27a,b. Testicular granulocytic sarcoma in a 58-year-old man with unremarkable medical history who presented with swelling of left testicle. a Transverse US image shows heterogeneous mass of testis and epididymis. Orchidectomy specimens revealed granulocytic sarcoma, without blood or bone marrow involvement. b Axial contrast-enhanced CT scan at 3 months revealed abdominal relapse with large partially necrotic lateroaortic mass. At same time, acute myeloblastic leukemia was diagnosed. CT-guided biopsy (not shown) revealed retroperitoneal granulocytic sarcoma. Patient died 1 month later of liver failure resulting from chemotherapy. (With permission from [GUERMAZI et al. 2002])

Fig. 20.28. Bladder granulocytic sarcoma in a 35-year-old woman with acute myeloid leukemia. Axial contrast-enhanced CT scan shows diffuse thickening of the bladder wall with variable enhancement. This lesion was histologically proven to be granulocytic sarcoma. Complete response was achieved with combination of bone marrow transplantation and chemotherapy. (With permission from [OOI and KHONG 2001])

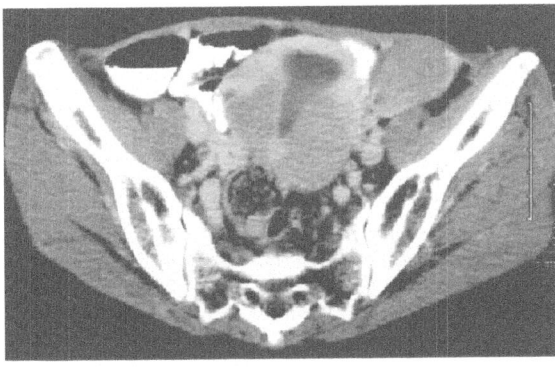

mary tumors such as lymphoma. Aspiration biopsies are therefore required in most cases. However the presence of soft tissue masses with variable contrast enhancement, which often occur sequentially at different sites in a patient with known leukemia or myelodysplastic disorders, should alert the radiologist to the possibility of GS. CT and MR imaging are useful for lesion detection and delineation, guiding needle biopsy and monitoring therapeutic response.

References

Ahrar K, McLeary MS, Young LW, Masotto M, Rouse GA (1998) Granulocytic sarcoma (chloroma) of the breast in an adolescent patient: ultrasonographic findings. J Ultrasound Med 17:383–384

Almadori G, Del Ninno M, Cadoni G, Di Mario A, Ottaviani F (1996) Facial nerve paralysis in acute otomastoiditis as presenting symptom of FAB M2, T8;21 leukemic relapse: case report and review of literature. Int J Pediatr Otorhinolaryngol 36:45–52

Ang P, Virapongese C (1990) Magnetic resonance imaging of spinal intradural granulocytic sarcoma. Magn Reson Imag 8:95–100

Au WY, Chan ACL, Lie AKW, So JCC, Liang R, Kwong YL (1998) Isolated extramedullary relapse after allogeneic bone marrow transplantation for chronic myeloid leukemia. Bone Marrow Transplant 22:99–102

Au WY, Kwong YL, Lie AKW, Ma SK, Liang R (1999a) Extramedullary relapse of leukemia following allogeneic bone marrow transplantation. Haemat Oncol 17:45–52

Au WY, Ma SK, Kwong YL, Lie AKW, Shek WH, Chow WC, Liang R (1999b) Acute myeloid leukemia relapsing as gynecomastia. Leuk Lymphoma 36:191–194

Au WY, Ma SK, Ooi GC, Liang R, Kwong YL (2000) Unusual manifestations of acute leukemia. J Clin Oncol 18: 3435–3437

Azzarelli V, Roesasman U (1977) Pathogenesis of central nervous system infiltration in acute leukemia. Arch Pathol Lab Med 101:203–205

Bagg MD, Wettlaufer JN, Willadsen DS, Ho V, Lane D, Thrasher JB (1994) Granulocytic sarcoma presenting as diffuse renal mass before hematological manifestations of acute myelogenous leukemia.. J Urol 152:2092–2093

Banna M, Aur R, Akkad S (1991) Orbital granulocytic sarcoma. Am J Neuroradiol 12:255–258

Barloon TJ, Young DC, Bass SH (1993) Mulitcentric granulocytic sarcoma (chloroma) of the breast: mammographic findings. Am J Roentgenol 161:963–964

Barnett MJ, Zussman WV (1986) Granulocytic sarcoma of the brain: a case report and review of the literature. Radiology 160:223–225

Bassichis B, McClay J, Wiatrak B (2000) Chloroma of the masseteric muscle. Int J Pediatr Otorhinolaryngol 53: 57–61

Békássy AN, Hermans J, Gorin NC, Gratwohl A (1996) Granulocytic sarcoma after allogeneic bone marrow transplan-

tation: a retrospective European multicenter survey. Bone Marrow Transplant 17:801–808

Bhati M, Coppage L (1995) Roentgenogram of the month: Dyspnoa nonproductive cough and blasts on peripheral blood smear. Chest 107:269–270

Books HW, Evans AE, Glass RM, Pang EM (1974) Chlromas of the head and neck in childhood. The initial manifestations of myeloid leukemia in three patients. Arch Otolaryngol. 100:306–308

Breatnach E, Stanley RJ, Carpenter JT Jr (1985) Intrarenal chloroma causing obstructive nephropathy: CT characteristics. J Comput Assist Tomogr 9:822–824

Brock WD, Brown HH, Westfall CT, Rock L (2001) Extramedullary myeloid cell tumor in an elderly man. Arch Opthalmol 119:1861–1864

Bulas RB, Laine FJ, Das Narla L (1995) Bilateral orbital granulocytic sarcoma (chloroma) preceding the blast phase of acute myelogenous leukemia: CT findings. Pediatr Radiol 25:488–489

Burns A (1821) Observations on the surgical anatomy of the head and neck, 2nd edn. Scorltan Wardlaw and Cumminghame, Glasgow, pp 386–397

Callahan M, Wall S, Askin F, Delaney D, Koller C, Orringer EP (1987) Granulocytic sarcoma presenting as pulmonary nodules and lymphadenopathy. Cancer 60:1902–1904

Cankaya H, Ugras S, Dilek I (2001) Head and neck granlocytic sarcoma with acute myeloid leukemia: three rare cases. Ear Nose Throat J 80:224–229

Carmona TI, Teijeiro CJ, Dioz DP, Feijoo FJ, Posse LJ (2000) Intra-alveolar granluocytic sarcoma developing after tooth xtraction. Oral Oncol 36:491–494

Cho JS, Kim EE, Ro JH, Pinkel DP, Goepfert H (1990) Mandibular chloroma demonstrated by magnetic resonance imaging. Head Neck 12:507–511

Cohen R, Segall HD, Nelson MD Jr, Zee CS, Ahmadi J (1988) Bilateral retro-orbital chloromas in a 16-month-old-child: CT features. J Comput Assist Tomogr 12:895–896

Corpechot C, Lémann M, Brocheriou I, Mariette X, Bonnet J, Daniel MT, Bertheau P, Lavergne A, Modigliani R (1998) Granulocytic sarcoma of the jejunum: a rare cause of small bowel obstruction. Am J Gastroenterol 93:2586–2588

Dabbagh V, Browne G, Parapia LA, Price JJ, Batman PA (1999) Granulocytic sarcoma of the rectum: a rare complication of myelodysplasia. J Clin Pathol 52:865–866

Davey DD, Foucar K, Burns CP, Goeken JA (1986) Acute myelocytic leukemia manifested by prominent generalized lymphadenopathy: report of two cases with immunological, ultrastructural and cytochemical studies. Am J Hematol 21:89–98

Davis JL, Parke DW, Font RL (1985) Granulocytsic sarcoma of the orbit: a clinico-pathooigc study. Opthalmology 92: 1758–1762

De Paz R, Canales MA, Hernandez-Navarro F (2003) Granulocytic sarcoma (chloroma) of the lung. Br J Haematol 120: 176–177

Dewar GJ, Lim NHC. Michalyshyn B, Akabutu J (1981) Gastrointestinal complications in patients with acute and chronic leukemia. Can J Surg 24:61–71

Dunnick NR, Heaston DK (1982) Computed tomography of extracranial chloroma. J Comput Assist Tomogr 6:83–85

Eelkema E, Johnson DW, Latchaw RE (1989) Multiple spinal granulocytic sarcomas simulating neurofibromatosis. Am J Neuroradiol 10:S42–44

Ficarra G, Silverman S Jr, Quivey JM, Hansen LS, Giannotti K (1987) Granulocytic sarcomc (chloroma) of the oral cavity: a case with aleukemic presentation. Oral Surg Oral Med Oral Pathol 62:709–714

Fitoz S, Atasoy C, Yavuz K, Gozdasoglu S, Erden I, Akyar S (2002) Granulocytic sarcoma: Cranial and breast involvement. J Clin Imag 26:166–169

Freedy RM, Miller KD (1991) Granulocytic sarcoma (chloroma): sphenoidal sinus and paraspinal involvement as evaluated by CT and MR. Am J Neuroradiol 12:259–262

Fridus SR, Rodman OG, Cyran SJ, Cardelli MB (1993) Multiple papules and plaques in a patient with ovarian carcinoma. Arch Dermatol 129:771–778

Frohna BJ, Quint DJ (1993) Granulocytic sarcoma (chloroma) causing spinal cord compression. Neuroradiology 35:509–511

Fruauff AA, Barasch ES, Rosenthal A (1988) Solitary myeloblast-oma presenting as acute hydrocephalus: review of literature, implications for therapy. Pediatr Radiol 18: 369–372

Gildenhorn HL, Springer EB, Amromin GD (1962) Necrotising enteropathy: roentgenography features. Am J Roentgenol 88:942–952

Gómez N, Elena O, Friera A, Penarrubia MJ, Acevedo A (1997) Magnetic resonance imaging features of chloroma of the shoulder. Skeletal Radiol 26:70–72

Graham A, Hodgson T, Jacubowski J, Norfolk D, Smith C (2001) MRI of perineural extramedullary granulocytic sarcoma. Neuroradiology 43:492–495

Guermazi A, Feger C, Rousselot P, Merad M, Benchaib N, Bourrier P, Mariette X, Frija J, de Kerviler E (2002) Granulocytic sarcoma (Chloroma): imaging findings in adults and children. Am J Roentgenol 178:319–325

Guermazi A, N'guyen-Quoc S, Socie G, Briere J, de Kerviler E, Solal-Celigny P, Frija J, Rousselot P (2000) Myeloblastoma (chloroma) in leukemia. J Clin Oncol 23:3993–3997

Harris DWS, Ostlere LS, Rustin MHA (1992) Cutaneous granulocytic sarcoma (chloroma) presenting as the first sign of relapse following autologous bone marrow transplantation for acute myeloid leukaemia. Br J Dermatol 127:182–184

Heiberg E, Wolverson MK, Sundaram M, Shields JB (1984) CT findings in leukemia. Am J Roentgenol 143:1317–1323

Hermann G, Feldman F, Abdelwahab IF, Klein MJ (1991) Skeletal manifestations of granulocytic sarcoma (chloroma). Skeletal Radiol 20:509–512

Hicklin GA, Drevyanko TF (1988) Primary granulocytic sarcoma presenting with pleural and pulmonary involvement. Chest 94:655–656

Hiorns MP, Murfitt J (1997) Granulocytic sarcoma (chloroma) of the breast: sonographic findings. Am J Roentgenol 169: 1639–1640

Hunter TB, Bjelland JC (1984) Gastrointestinal complications of leukaemia and its treatment. Am J Roentgenol 142:513–518

Jakobiec FA (1991) Granulocytic sarcoma. Am J Neuroradiol 12:263–264

Jung SE, Chun KA, Park SH, Lee EJ (1999) MR findings in ovarian granulocytic sarcoma. Br J Radiol 72:301–303

Kao SCS, Yuh WTC, Sato Y, Barloon TJ (1987) Intracranial granulocytic sarcoma (chloroma): MR findings. J Comput Assist Tomogr 11:938–941

Kerr P, Evely R, Pawade J (2002) Bladder chloroma complicating refractory anaemia with excess of blasts. Br J Haematol 118:688

Kim FM, Fennessy JJ (1994) Pleural thickening caused by leukemic infiltration: CT findings. Am J Roentgenol 162: 293–294

Kim FSC, Rutka JT, Bernstein M, Resch L, Warner E, Pantalony D (1990) Intradural granulocytic sarcoma presenting as lumbar radiculopathy. J Neurosurg 72:663–667

King A (1853) A case of chloroma. Monthly J Med 17:97

Kook H, Hwang TJ, Kang HK, Kim SH, Kim JH (1993) Spinal intramedullary granulocytic sarcoma: magnetic resonance imaging. Magn Reson Imag 11:135–137

Kumar R. (1980) Multiple pulmonary nodules in leukemia J Can Assoc Radiol 31:71–72

Laufer L, Benharroch D, Giryes H, Hertzanu Y (1996) Pelvic granulocytic sarcoma. Skeletal Radiol 25:693–695

Lee B, Fatterpekar GM, Kim W, Som PM (2002) Granulocytic sarcoma of the temporal bone. Am J Neuroradiol 23: 1497–1499

Lee MJ, Grogan L, Meehan S, Breatnach E (1991) Case report: pleural granulocytic sarcoma: CT characteristics. Clin Radiol 43:57–59

Lee SS, Kim HK, Choi SC, Lee JI (2001) Granulocytic sarcoma occurring in the maxillary gingiva demonstrated by magnetic resonance imaging. Oral Surg Oral Med Oral Pathol 92:689–693

Levy R, Shvero J, Sandbank J (1989) Granulocytic sarcoma (chloroma) of the temporal bone. Int J Pediatr Otorhinolaryngol 18:163

Libson E, Bloom RA, Galun E, Polliack A (1986) Granulocytic sarcoma (chloroma) of bone: the CT appearance. Comput Radiol 10:175–178

Limberakis AJ, Mossler JA, Roberts L Jr, Jackson DC, Thompson WM (1978) Leukemic infiltration of the colon. Am J Roentgenol 131:725–728

Lin CK, Liang R, Ma L, Tse PWT, Chan GTC, Liu HW (1990) Myelodysplastic syndrome presenting with generalized cutaneous granulocytic sarcomas. Acta Haematol 83: 89–93

Lin Y, Govindan R, Hess JL (1997) Malignant hematopoietic breast tumors. Hematopathology 107:177–186

Liu HW, Wong KL, Chan TYK, Lau CC, Liang R (1988) Superior vena cava syndrome: a rare presenting feature of acute myeloid leukaemia. Acta Haemat 79:213–216

Liu PI, Ishimaru T, McGregor DH, Okada H, Steer A (1973) Autopsy study of granulocytic sarcoma (chloroma) in patients with myelogenous leukemia, Hiroshima-Nagasaki 1949–1969. Cancer 31:948–955

Luddy RE, Levy BE, Schwartz AD (1980) 67Ga scintigraphy in granulocytic sarcoma. Cancer 46:1357–1359

Marcos HB, Semelka RC, Woosley JT (1997) Abdominal granulocytic sarcomas: demonstration by MRI. Magn Reson Imag 15:873–876

Matsueda K, Yamamoto H, Doi I (1998) An autopsy case of granulocytic sarcoma of the porta hepatis causing obstructive jaundice. J Gastroenterol 33:428–433

Meis JM, Butler JJ, Osborne BM, Manning JT (1986) Granulocytic sarcoma in nonleukemic patients. Cancer 58: 2697–2709

Muss HB, Maloney WC (1973) Chloroma and other myeloblastic tumors. Blood 42:721–728

Neiman RS, Barcos M, Berard C, Bonner H, Mann R, Rydell RE, Bennett JM (1981) Granulocytic sarcoma: a clinicopathologic study of 61 biopsied cases. Cancer 48: 1426–1437

Nikolic B, Feigenbaum F, Abbara S, Martuza RL, Schellinger D (2003) CT changes of an intracranial granulocytic sarcoma on short-term follow-up. Am J Roentgenol 180:78–80

Novick SL, Nicol TL, Fishman EK (1998) Granulocytic sarcoma (chloroma) of the sacrum: initial manifestation of leukemia. Skeletal Radiol 27:112–114

Oliva E, Ferry JA, Young RH, Prat J, Srigley JR, Scully RE (1997) Granulocytic sarcoma of the female genital tract: a clinicopathologic study of 11 cases. Am J Surg Pathol 21:1156–1165

Ooi GC, Khong PL (2001) Pictorial essay: imaging of granulocytic sarcomas. J HK Coll Radiol 4:89–96

Ooi GC, Chim CS, Khong PL, Lie AKW, AuWY, Tsang KWT, Kwong YL (2001) Radiologic manifestations of granulocytic sarcoma in adult leukemia. Am J Roentgenol 176:1427–1431

Orlandi E, Morra E, Lazzarino M, Castagnola C, Pauli M, Rosso R, Bernasconi C (1989) Multiple granulocytic sarcoma during complete remission of acute nonlymphovytic leukemia. Acta Haematol 81:41–43

Parker K, Hardjasudarma M, McClellan RL, Fowler MR, Milner JW (1996) MR features of an intracerebellar chloroma. Am J Neuroradiol 17:1592–1594

Paulus DD, Libshitz HI (1972) Metastsis to the breast. Radiol Clin North Am 20:561–568

Pochedly C (1977) Leukemia and lymphoma in the nervous system, vol 1. Charles C. Thomas, Springfield, pp 55–70

Pomeranz SJ, Hawkins HH, Towbin R, Lisberg WN, Clark RA (1985) Granulocytic sarcoma (chloroma): CT manifestations. Radiology 155:167–170

Prades JM, Alaani A, Mosnier JF, Dumollard JM, Martin C (2001) Granulocytic sarcoma of the nasal cavity. Rhinology 40:159–161

Prolla JC, Kirsner BJ (1964) The gastrointestinal lesions and complications of the leukemias. Ann Intern Med 61:1084–1103

Proulx GM, McCarthy P (1998) Case two: epidural chloroma of the lower spinal canal. J Clin Oncol 3201–3202

Pui MH, Fletcher BD, Langston JW (1994) Granulocytic sarcoma in childhood leukemia: imaging features. Radiology 190:698–702

Ravandi-Kashani F, Estey E, Cortes J, Medeiros LJ, Giles FJ (1999) Granulocytic sarcoma of the pancreas: a report of two cases and literature review. Clin Lab Haematol 21:219–224

Ravandi-Kashani F, Cortes J, Giles FJ (2000) Myelodysplasia presenting as granulocytic sarcoma of mediastinum causing superior vena cava syndrome. Leuk Lymphoma 36:631–637

Ripp DJ, Davis JW, Rengachary SS, Lotuaco LG, Watanabe IS (1989) Granulocytic sarcoma presenting as an epidural mass with cord compression. Neurosurgery 24:125–128

Rodriguez JC, Aeeanz JS, Forceledo MF (1990) Isolated granulocytic sarcoma: report of a case in the oral cavity. J Oral Maxillofac Surg 48:748–752

Romaniuk CS (1992) Case report: granulocytic sarcoma (chloroma) presenting as a cerebellopontine angle mass. Clin Radiol 45:284–285

Rottenberg GT, Thomas BM (1994) Case report: granulocytic sarcoma of the small bowel-a rare presentation of leukaemia. Clin Radiol 49:501–502

Rotter AJ, O'Donnell MR, Radin DR, Marx HF (1992) Peribiliary chloroma: a rare cause of jaundice after bone marrow transplantation. Am J Roentgenol 158:1255–1256

Scotti G, Scialfa G, Colombo N, Landoni L (1985) MR imaging of intradural extramdullary tumour of the cervical spine. J Comput Assist Tomogr 9:1037–1041

Siegel MJ, Shackelford GD, McAlister WH (1981) Pleural thickening: an unusual feature of childhood leukemia. Radiology 138:367–369

Son HJ, Oh KK (1998) Multicentric granulocytic sarcoma of the breast: mammographic and sonographic findings. Am J Roentgenol 171:274–275

Sowers JJ, Moody DM, Naidich TP, Ball MR, Laster DW, Leeds NE (1979) Radiographic features of granulocytic sarcoma (Chloroma). J Comput Assist Tomogr 3:226–233

Sreejith G, Gangadharan VP, Elizabath KA, Preetha S, Chithrathara K (2000) Primary granulocytic sarcoma of the ovary. Am J Clin Oncol 23:239–240

Takasugi JE, Godwin JD, Marglin SI, Petersdorf SH (1996) Intrathoracic granulocytic sarcomas. J Thorac Imag 11:223–230

Taryle DA, Sahn SA (1979) Rapidly progressive pulmonary infiltrates in chronic myelogenous leukemia. JAMA 242:15–16

Thompson DH, Ross DG, Reid JW (1982) Granulocytic sarcoma (chloroma) initially seen as acute mastoiditis. Arch Otolaryngol 108:388–391

Tong AC, Lam KY (2000) Granulocytic sarcomas presenting as an ulcerative mucogingival lesion: report of a case and review of the literature. J Oral Maxillofac Surg 58:1055–1088

Turner RM, Peck WW, Prietto C (1991) MR of soft tissue chloroma in a patient presenting with left pubic and hip pain. J Comput Assist Tomogr 15:700–702

Uyesugi WY, Watabe J, Petermann G (2000) Orbital and facial granulocytic sarcoma (chloroma): a case report. Pediatr Radiol 30:276–278

Vinters HV, Gilbert JJ (1982) Multifocal chloromas of the brain. Surg Neurol 17:47–51

Wang AM, Lin JCT, Power TC, Haykal HA, Zamani AA (1987) Chloroma of cerebellum, tentorium and occipital bone in acute myelogenous leukemia. Neuroradiology 29:590

Wendling LR, Cromwell LD, Latchaw RE (1979) Computed tomography of intracerebral leukemia masses. Am J Roentgenol 132:217–220

Wong KF, Chan JK, Chan JC, Lam SY (1993) Acute myeloid leukemia presenting as granulocytic sarcoma of the lung. Am J Haematol 43:77–78

Wright DH, Hise JH, Bauserman SC, Naul LG (1992) Intracranial granulocytic sarcoma: CT, MR and angiography. J Comput Assist Tomogr 16:487–489

Wuillemain WA, Vischer MW, Tobler A, Fey MF (1993) Relapse of acute myeloblastic leukemia presenting as temporal bone chloroma with facial nerve paralysis. Ann Onocol 4:339–340

Zappia JJ, Bunge FA, Koopmann CF, McClatchey KD (1990) Facial nerve paresis as the presenting sympton of leukemia. Int J Pediatr Otorhinolaryngol 19:259–264

Zimmerman RA, Bilaniuk LT (1980) CT of primary ad secondary craniocerebral neuroblastoma. Am J Roentgenol 135:1239–1242

21 Myelofibrosis

Ali Guermazi

CONTENTS

21.1
Introduction

Myelofibrosis, also called myeloid metaplasia, is a myeloproliferative disorder characterized by progressive bone marrow fibrosis, splenomegaly, extramedullary hematopoiesis, leukoerythroblastosis, anisopoikilocytosis, and teardrop poikilocytes. Most patients have moderate to severe anemia. Bone marrow in patients with myelofibrosis is usually hypocellular, with increased amounts of reticulin and collagen. Myelofibrosis may be primary (or idiopathic) or secondary, and usually affects adults, with only a few reports in children (GUERMAZI et al. 1999). Myelofibrosis is of unknown etiology, but association with an autoimmune diseases such as polyarteritis nodosa (CAMOS et al. 2003), ulcerative colitis (ARELLANO-RODRIGO et al. 2002), or primary biliary cirrhosis (HERNANDEZ-BOLUDA et al. 2002)

ALI GUERMAZI, MD
Visiting Associate Professor, Department of Radiology, University of California, San Francisco, 350 Parnassus Avenue, Suite 150, San Francisco, CA 94117, USA

gives support to the hypothesis of an immune basis of some idiopathic myelofibrosis cases. The average life expectancy of patients after diagnosis is 2 to 3 years. Only 8% of patients with the disease survive from 6 to 8 years. The common imaging findings in patients with myelofibrosis are osteosclerosis, hepatosplenomegaly, and lymphadenopathies. In addition, extramedullary hematopoiesis may develop in multiple sites such as chest, abdomen, pelvis, and central nervous system, simulating malignant disease (GUERMAZI et al. 1999). The purpose of this chapter is to illustrate the wide range of radiological abnormalities in patients affected by this serious, progressive and fatal disease.

21.2
Pathogenesis and Cytopathology

It is possible that autoimmune mechanisms are somehow involved in the pathogenesis of bone marrow fibrosis in a subgroup of patients. Circulating immune complexes have been described, but the pathogenetic significance of these findings is uncertain, since the occurrence of circulating immune complexes may solely reflect impaired clearance in the reticuloendothelial system owing to extramedullary hematopoiesis. Other observations favor the idea that circulating immune complexes, in some patients, may actually reflect autoimmune bone marrow damage. Thus, in the early phase of idiopathic myelofibrosis, the myeloproliferation may be accompanied by immune activity in bone marrow with a marked increase of lymphoid nodules. Another possibility is that megakaryocytes may play a pathogenetic part. This is supported by several observations: (a) early in the course of the disease, there is hyperplasia of morphologically abnormal megakaryocytes; (b) fibroblast proliferation is most pronounced around areas of megakaryocyte necrosis; and (c) functional and morphologic abnormalities of megakaryocytes and platelets are more pronounced in myelofibrosis than in the other myeloproliferative disorders.

Secondary myelofibrosis may be caused by chronic myeloproliferative disorders, systemic lupus erythematosus, nephrotic syndrome, lymphoma and other hematological diseases such as leukemia and myeloma (HASSELBALCH 1990; GUERMAZI et al. 1999).

Histological analysis of bone marrow biopsies is essential for the diagnosis and evaluation of the degree of medullary fibrosis. The evolution of myelofibrosis seems to be limited to an inappropriate release of growth factors from neoplastic megakaryocytes, especially platelet-derived growth factor (PDGF). The histological aspect progresses from a hypercellular stage with minimal fibrosis to an advanced stage with severe collagenization of bone marrow and osteomyelosclerosis:

- Stage I: early in the course of disease, the marrow is hypercellular with trilineage proliferation; the erythroid and granulocytic precursors appear normal, but megakaryocytes are large and dysplastic and tend to occur in a nest. Fibrosis is minimal during this cellular phase (Fig. 21.1a);
- Stage II: with the progression of the disease, the marrow becomes hypocellular and diffusely fibrotic. Clusters of atypical megakaryocytes are still found in fibrosis (Fig. 21.1b);

- Stage III: the presence of extensive collagen fibrosis and osteomyelosclerosis is accompanied by a decrease in bone marrow cellularity (Fig. 21.1c) (GUERMAZI et al. 1999).

21.3
Clinical and Laboratory Findings at the Time of Diagnosis

Myelofibrosis is an uncommon illness occurring with equal frequency in both sexes. It is a disease of adults, with few cases reported in children. The age range is 20 to 80 years (median age 60 years). The most common presenting symptoms are weakness, fatigue and weight loss. Other common presenting symptoms are, in order of frequency, dyspnea, pallor, edema, bleeding, infection, and bone pain. The duration of characteristic symptoms before diagnosis varies from 1 to 48 months. At physical examination, the most common finding is splenomegaly, present in 94% of the patients at the time of diagnosis. Hepatomegaly is also a prominent physical finding, seen in 72% of patients, whereas lymphadenopathy is seen in only 12%. Other initial physical findings

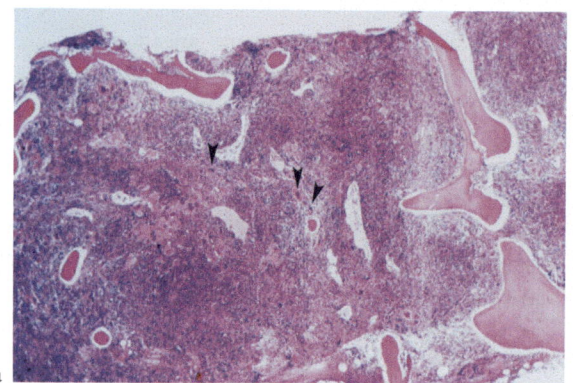
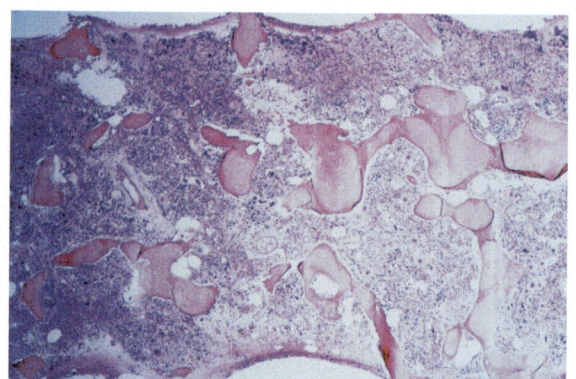
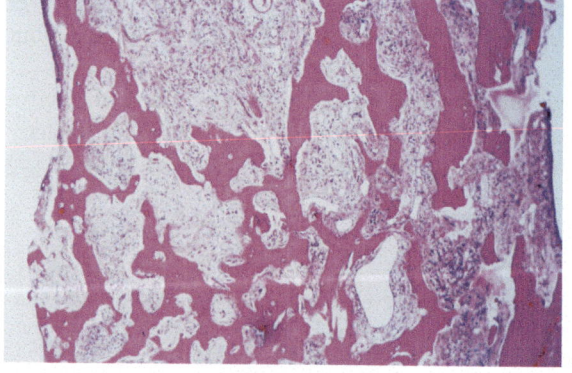

Fig. 21.1a–c. Histological studies with Hematoxylin and Eosin stain (original magnification, x40). **a** Myelofibrosis stage I: bone marrow biopsy shows a hypercellular bone marrow with megakaryocytic hyperplasia with atypical form (*arrowheads*). **b** Myelofibrosis stage II: Bone marrow cellularity is still increased and contains numerous clusters of dysplastic megakaryocytes. **c** Myelofibrosis stage III: Bone marrow biopsy shows prominent fibrosis with areas of collagenization and sparsely isolated residual hematopoietic elements. (With permission from [GUERMAZI et al. 1999])

are petechiae and purpura, cardiomegaly, jaundice, ascites and bone tenderness.

The peripheral blood findings demonstrate moderate anemia of the normocytic, normochromic type. The morphologic appearance of the erythrocytes is of some importance in the diagnosis of the disease. The red cells are characterized by poikilocytosis with numerous cells elongated into comma or teardrop shapes. Anisocytosis is also present, and reticulocyte counts are frequently elevated, even in cases where no frank hemolysis can be demonstrated. The majority of patients have leukocytosis, and in all of them, immature myeloid cells are found in peripheral blood differential counts. The platelet counts are variable: thrombocytopenia and thrombocytosis are most commonly seen. Giant platelets fragments of megakaryocytes are common in the peripheral blood (BOURONCLE and DUAN 1962, MALLOUH and SA'DI 1992; OZSOYLU 1994; GUERMAZI et al. 1999).

evident in the bones of the axial skeleton, including the ribs (Fig. 21.2), sternum, clavicles, scapulae, vertebrae (Fig. 21.3), pelvis (Fig. 21.4a), and metaphy-

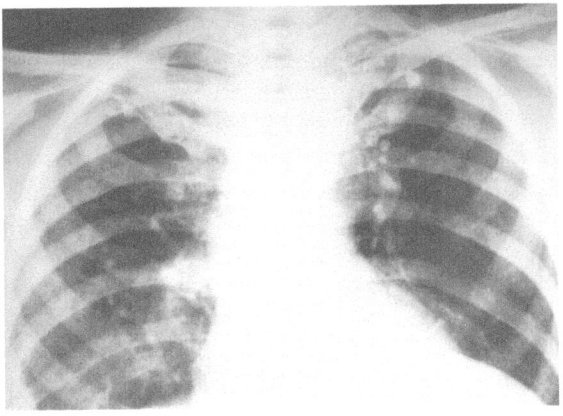

Fig. 21.2. Osteomyelosclerosis of the ribs in a 65-year-old-man with primary myelofibrosis. Anteroposterior radiograph of the thorax shows diffuse osteosclerosis of the ribs and clavicles.

21.4
Primary Myelofibrosis

Primary myelofibrosis (idiopathic myelofibrosis, splenic myelosis, megakaryocytic splenomegaly, chronic nonleukemic myelosis, or agnogenic myeloid metaplasia) is a chronic myeloproliferative disorder of unknown origin. It is characterized by anemia, hepatosplenomegaly, and extramedullary hematopoiesis. Before making a diagnosis of primary myelofibrosis, a thorough search is needed to exclude the secondary causes of bone marrow fibrosis. Myelofibrosis produces a stromal reaction of fibrosis of the marrow with replacement of the normal medullary fat and marrow elements. Splenomegaly is consistently present and may be massive. The most common medical complications are infection, cardiovascular disease, and thrombohemorrhagic complications. Therapy for asymptomatic individuals is generally supportive. Bone marrow transplantation, splenectomy, androgens, and chemotherapy have been used to treat some patients with limited success.

21.4.1
Musculoskeletal Abnormalities

Osteosclerosis
The predominant radiographic feature of myelofibrosis is osteosclerosis, a finding that occurs in approximately 30% to 70% of patients and is most

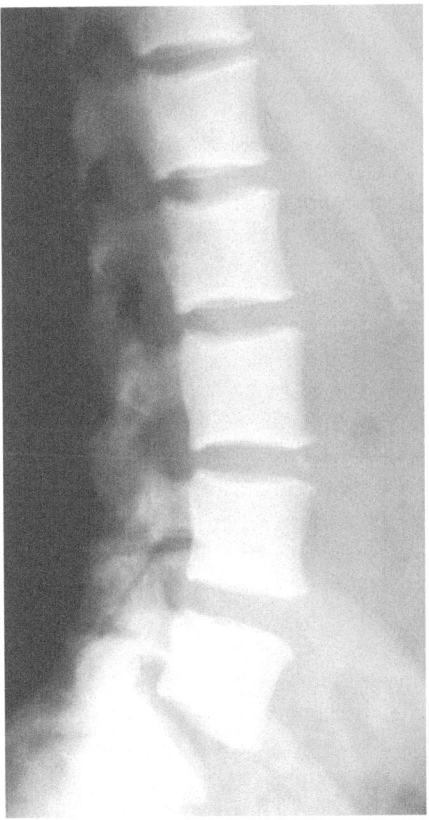

Fig. 21.3. Osteomyelosclerosis of the spine in a 54-year-old-woman with primary myelofibrosis. Lateral view of lumbar spine shows diffuse homogeneous osteosclerosis. (With permission from [GUERMAZI et al. 1999])

seal ends of the femur, humerus, and tibia (YU et al. 1994; GUERMAZI et al. 1999). Routine radiography usually does not detect the bone marrow changes in myelofibrosis until there is osteosclerosis. The osseous structures may be uniformly dense or demonstrate small areas of relative radiolucency. In the long bones, cortical thickening can be observed, due predominantly to endosteal sclerosis (Fig. 21.4b). This results in obliteration between cortical and medullary bone. In the spine, increased radiodensity or condensation of bone at the superior and inferior margins of the vertebral body (sandwich vertebrae) can be encountered (Fig. 21.5). Focal or diffuse sclerosis in the skull may obscure the interface between the tables and diploe (Fig. 21.6) (YU et al. 1994; GUERMAZI et al. 1999). Osteolytic lesions are extremely rare (KOSMIDIS et al. 1980; GUERMAZI et al. 1999).

Periosteal Reaction

Periosteal reaction is rarely associated with myelofibrosis but, when present, typically affects the medial aspect of the distal femur and proximal tibia (Fig. 21.7) and the bone around the ankle. On MR imaging, periosteal reaction is seen as diffuse periosteal thickening forming a sleeve around the shaft of the long bones (Fig. 21.8) (DIAMOND et al. 2002). Although it has been suggested that periosteal reaction may be indicative of more aggressive disease, recent studies do not support this position. The cause for the periosteal reaction is not known, but it may be related to subperiosteal extension of hypercellular marrow resulting in an increase in vascularity (YU et al. 1994).

MR Imaging Bone Marrow Assessment

MR imaging is useful for evaluating stage and progression of myelofibrosis as it is very sensitive to alterations in signal intensity of normal bone marrow (JONES 1992; KAPLAN et al. 1992; YU et al. 1994). Moreover, MR can assess the entire marrow compartment, overcoming sampling errors associated with aspiration and biopsy (JONES 1992; ROZMAN et al. 1999). On MR images, normal medullary marrow in adults is hyperintense on T1-weighted images and iso or slightly hyperintense on T2-weighted images, due to fatty bone marrow. In patients with myelofibrosis, MR imaging demonstrates a very low, mainly homogeneous signal intensity on both T1 and T2-weighted images (UEDA et al. 1994). Some areas of inhomogeneity may be due to areas of preserved marrow fat (Fig. 21.9). The decrease in signal intensity is a consequence of replacement of the hyperintense

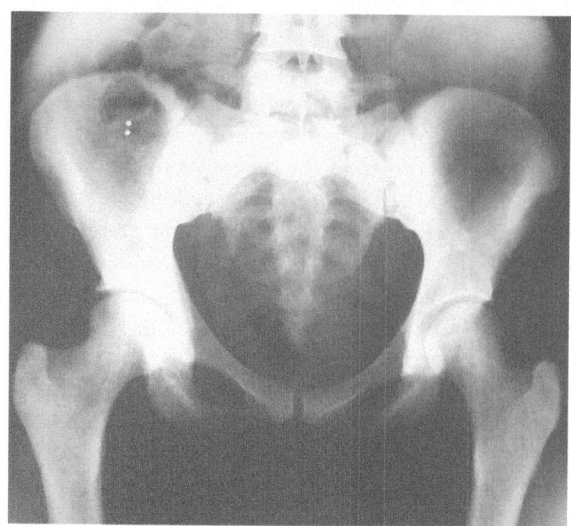

a

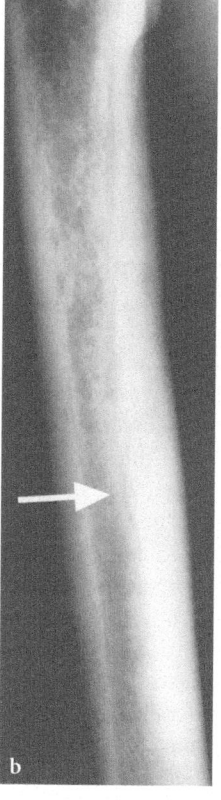

b

Fig. 21.4a,b. Osteomyelosclerosis in a 50-year-old-woman with primary myelofibrosis. a Anteroposterior radiograph of the pelvis shows patchy osteosclerosis of the entire pelvis associated with small radiolucent areas. b Anteroposterior radiograph of the right femur shows increased radiodensity of the bone caused predominantly by endosteal sclerosis (*arrow*). (With permission from [GUERMAZI et al. 1999])

marrow fat by collagen, reticulin fibers, and cellular material. This replacement affects both T1 and T2 values of marrow, and is compatible with late phase myelofibrosis and low hematopoietic activity (ALPDOGAN et al. 1998; GUERMAZI et al. 1999). However, in early stage myelofibrosis, the appearance is non specific, showing hypointensity on T1-weighted images and hyperintensity on T2-weighted and STIR

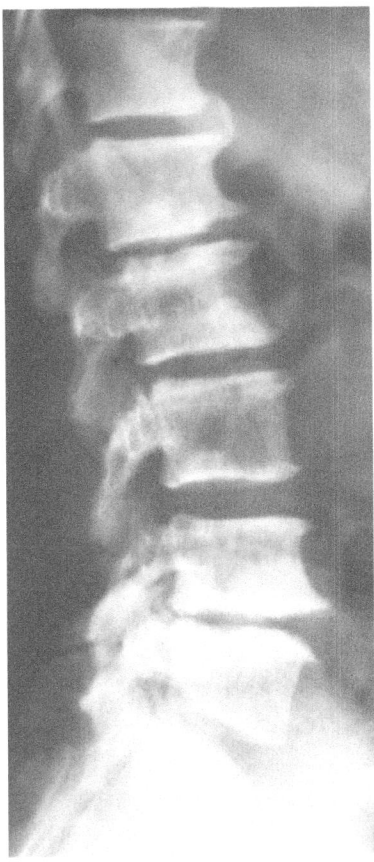

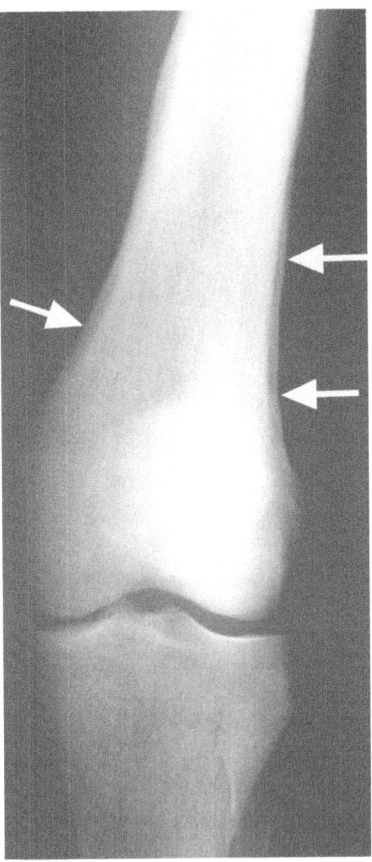

Fig. 21.5. Osteomyelosclerosis of the spine in a 49-year-old-man with primary myelofibrosis. Lateral view of lumbar spine shows condensation of bone at the superior and inferior margins of the vertebral bodies, known as "Sandwich vertebrae". (With permission from [GUERMAZI et al. 1999])

Fig. 21.7. Periosteal reaction in a 38-year-old-woman with primary myelofibrosis. Anteroposterior right knee radiograph discloses distal femur metadiaphysis mature periosteal reaction due to extramedullary hematopoiesis (*arrows*). (With permission from [GUERMAZI et al. 1999])

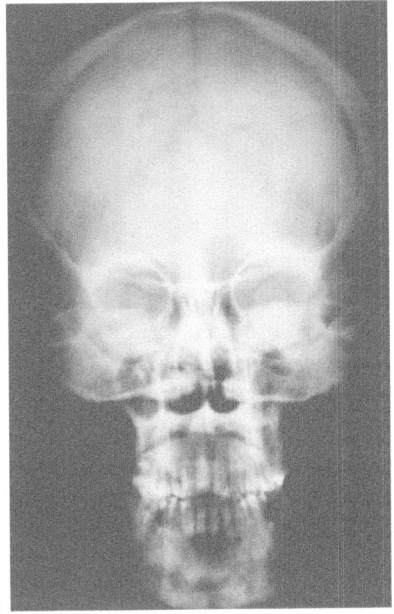

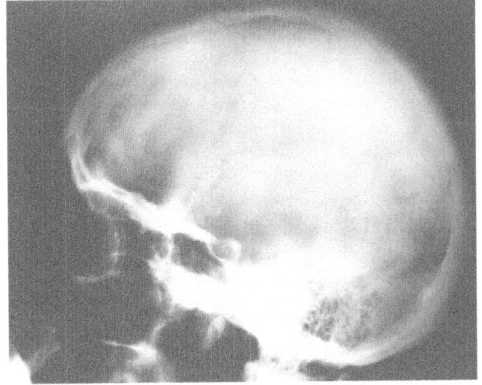

Fig. 21.6a,b. Osteomyelosclerosis of the skull in a 58-year-old-man with primary myelofibrosis. **a** Anteroposterior and (**b**) lateral radiographs of the skull show diffuse sclerosis in the skull that obscures the interface between the tables and diploe.

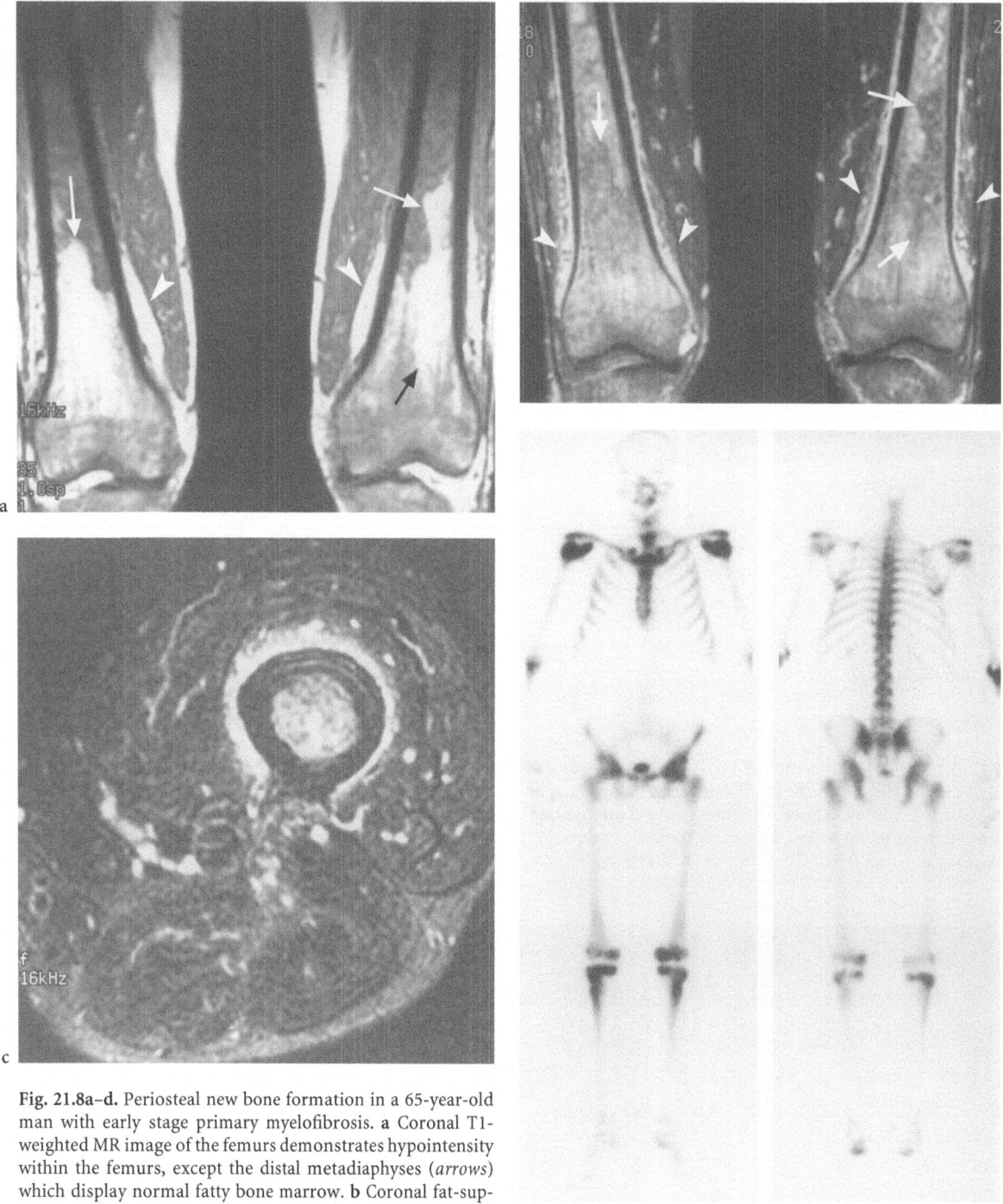

Fig. 21.8a–d. Periosteal new bone formation in a 65-year-old man with early stage primary myelofibrosis. a Coronal T1-weighted MR image of the femurs demonstrates hypointensity within the femurs, except the distal metadiaphyses (*arrows*) which display normal fatty bone marrow. b Coronal fat-suppressed T2-weighted MR image shows the abnormal bone marrow to be hyperintense and the normal bone marrow (*arrows*) to be hypointense due to fat suppression. These findings are related to the early hypercellular stage of myelofibrosis. There is also hyperintensity around the outer periosteum (*arrowheads*) on (a) and (b) suggestive of new bone formation. c Axial fat-suppressed T2-weighted MR image through the midshaft of the left femur better shows the periosteal new bone formation as hyperintensity measuring 3–10 mm in thickness, visible around the outer periosteum and forming a sleeve around the shaft of the long bone. d Anterior (*left*) and posterior (*right*) technetium labeled whole-body scans demonstrate increased tracer uptake within the thoracolumbar spine, sternum, pelvis and distal ends of the long bones such as femurs and tibias. The kidneys are not visualized. This is termed a "superscan", indicative of high bone turnover. The prominence of increased bone marrow activity in the distal ends of the long bones is suggestive of increased new bone formation. (With permission from [DIAMOND et al. 2002])

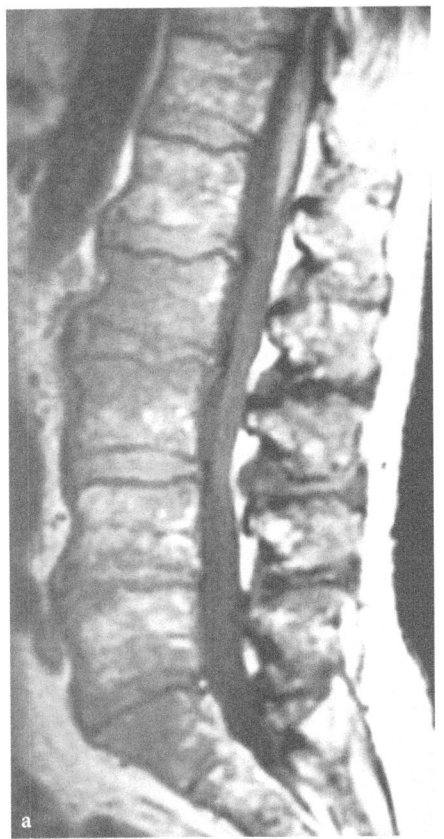 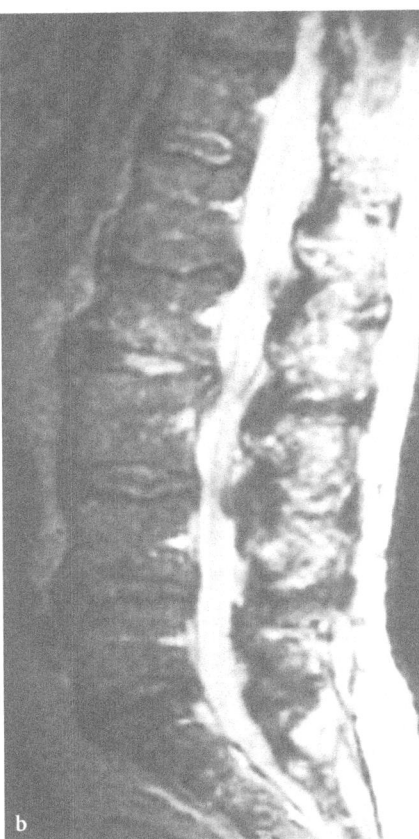

Fig. 21.9a,b. Spinal bone marrow involvement in a 56-year-old man with primary myelofibrosis. Sagittal (**a**) T1 and (**b**) T2-weighted MR images of the spine show diffuse marked heterogenous decreased signal of bone marrow due to myelosclerosis. (With permission from [GUERMAZI et al. 1999])

images. These findings are compatible with hypercellular bone marrow (Fig. 21.8) (ALPDOGAN et al. 1998; ROZMAN et al. 1999). It should be noted, however, that a homogeneous decrease in signal intensity of marrow on both T1 and T2-weighted images is not specific for myelofibrosis and has been demonstrated in children with leukemia and Gaucher disease. Prolongation of T1 and diminution of marrow signal intensity on T1 dependent pulse sequences is also shared by other pathologic processes such as tumors, osteomyelitis, and metastases of various origins. Therefore, shorter T1 times are less specific for bone pathologies. The T2-weighted images may be more specific since tumors and acute inflammation present longer T2 times, with increasing signal intensity, whereas fibrosis diminishes signal intensity. However, hypointense signal of the spine on T2-weighted images sometimes occurs in AIDS patients and with other causes of iron overload (LANIR et al. 1986). Recently, it has been reported that STIR and gadolinium-enhanced T1-weighted MR images, as well as MR spectroscopy, are useful in assessing the blood flow and extracellular space in bone marrow of myelofibrosis, and are also consistent with histopathological features (AMANO et al. 1997).

The spectrum of regional marrow abnormalities in the lower extremities ranges from replacement of the marrow in the femoral and tibial diaphyses with sparing of the marrow in the epiphyses around the knees, to replacement of all marrow. A correlation seems to exist between the signal patterns in the marrow of the proximal regions of the femur and the clinical severity of myelofibrosis (YU et al. 1994). Indeed, expansion of cellular marrow into the normal fatty marrow of both the femoral capital epiphyses and the greater trochanter is associated with more severe disease, as determined by serum lactate dehydrogenase and cholesterol values (KAPLAN et al. 1992).

21.4.2
Articular Abnormalities

Hemarthrosis
Hemarthrosis has been described in association with myeloproliferative disease and can be the presenting manifestation of the disease. Impaired platelet function presumably contributes to bleeding episodes (HARRIS and ROSS 1974).

Hyperuricemia

Hyperuricemia is relatively common in myelofibrosis. Secondary gout, which may antedate the diagnosis of this disorder, occurs in 5 to 20% of patients and may be associated with tophi and renal uric acid stones (Yu 1965).

Polyarthralgias and polyarthritis

Polyarthralgias and polyarthritis in myelofibrosis have also been related to an immune pathogenesis and to infiltration of the synovial membrane by bone marrow elements (Connelly et al. 1982; Heinicke et al. 1983).

21.4.3
Extramedullary Hematopoiesis

Extramedullary hematopoiesis is a compensatory mechanism by which the body attempts to maintain a level of erythrogenesis sufficient for its demands (Lund and Aldridge 1984). Extramedullary hematopoiesis can be primary, as in hematologic disorders like agnogenic myeloid metaplasia, or secondary, as in cases of marrow replacement by tumor or destruction by toxins. The most common sites of extramedullary hematopoiesis in myelofibrosis are the spleen, liver, and lymph nodes. Diverse areas of involvement, due to the presence of multipotential stem cells in mesenchymal tissues, have also been reported. Although foci of extramedullary hematopoiesis are often asymptomatic, occasionally they may be large enough to produce significant complications (Goodman et al. 1991), and extramedullary hematopoiesis may mimic neoplasms on imaging (Shaver and Clore 1981; Goodman et al. 1991).

21.4.3.1
Dura Mater Hematopoiesis

Dura mater hematopoiesis may occur in both cranial or spinal locations.

Brain

Cranial involvement can be revealed with headache, seizures, hemiplegia, and altered consciousness. On pathologic examination, the masses are vascular, usually multiple, and often cause a thickened falx cerebri (Urman et al. 1991). On CT, intracranial extramedullary hematopoiesis usually appears as multiple iso or hyperdense extra-axial masses, which exhibit T2 shortening on MR images. Marked homogenous enhancement is demonstrated after contrast administration on both CT and MR imaging. Differential diagnosis must include meningioma and chloroma (Ligumski et al. 1978; Lund and Aldridge 1984; Koch et al. 1994; Ohtsubo et al. 1994).

Spinal dural

Spinal dural proliferation is rare, and can result in spinal cord compression. The lesions are commonly localized to the mid-lower thoracic region, possibly because of the narrow diameter of the spinal cord in this region. Once the mass is formed in the thorax, invasion of the spinal canal can occur through the intervertebral canal (De Klippel et al. 1993; Guermazi et al. 1997). Both CT and MR imaging are useful diagnostic tools (Fig. 21.10); nevertheless, the superiority of MR imaging over CT has been demonstrated. MR imaging can facilitate the diagnosis and assessment of the extent of extramedullary hematopoiesis, and may allow differentiation of extramedullary hematopoiesis from epidural hemorrhage. On the spinal canal, signal intensity of extramedullary hematopoiesis is usually isointense to the spinal cord on T1-weighted images and may exhibit both T2 lengthening and shortening. These areas demonstrate marked enhancement after contrast administration. Radiotherapy is almost always sufficient to obtain good neurological recovery (Papavasiliou et al. 1990; Cook and Sharp 1994; Guermazi et al. 1997).

21.4.3.2
Abdominal Abnormalities

Spleen

Splenomegaly is the most common finding at physical examination, observed in about 94% of patients. The histopathology of the spleen reveals, in all cases, variable amounts of extramedullary hematopoiesis in the red pulp. The spleen is almost always massive (Fig. 21.11), and infarction is common (Shaver and Clore 1981; Siniluoto et al. 1992). Focal abnormalities in the spleen are commonly found at follow-up. Such lesions may be solitary or multiple, and are mostly hyperechoic on US (Fig. 21.12) (Guermazi et al. 1999; Yokoyama et al. 2000). Differential diagnosis of nontraumatic highly echogenic lesions includes metastases, malignant lymphomas, hemangiomas, and chronic infarcts. On CT, the focal lesions have well-defined margins with an internal mosaic pattern of low and high density. These lesions enhance very slightly after contrast administration (Fig. 21.13). These lesions are heterogeneously hypointense on T1 and T2-weighted MR images (Yokoyama et al.

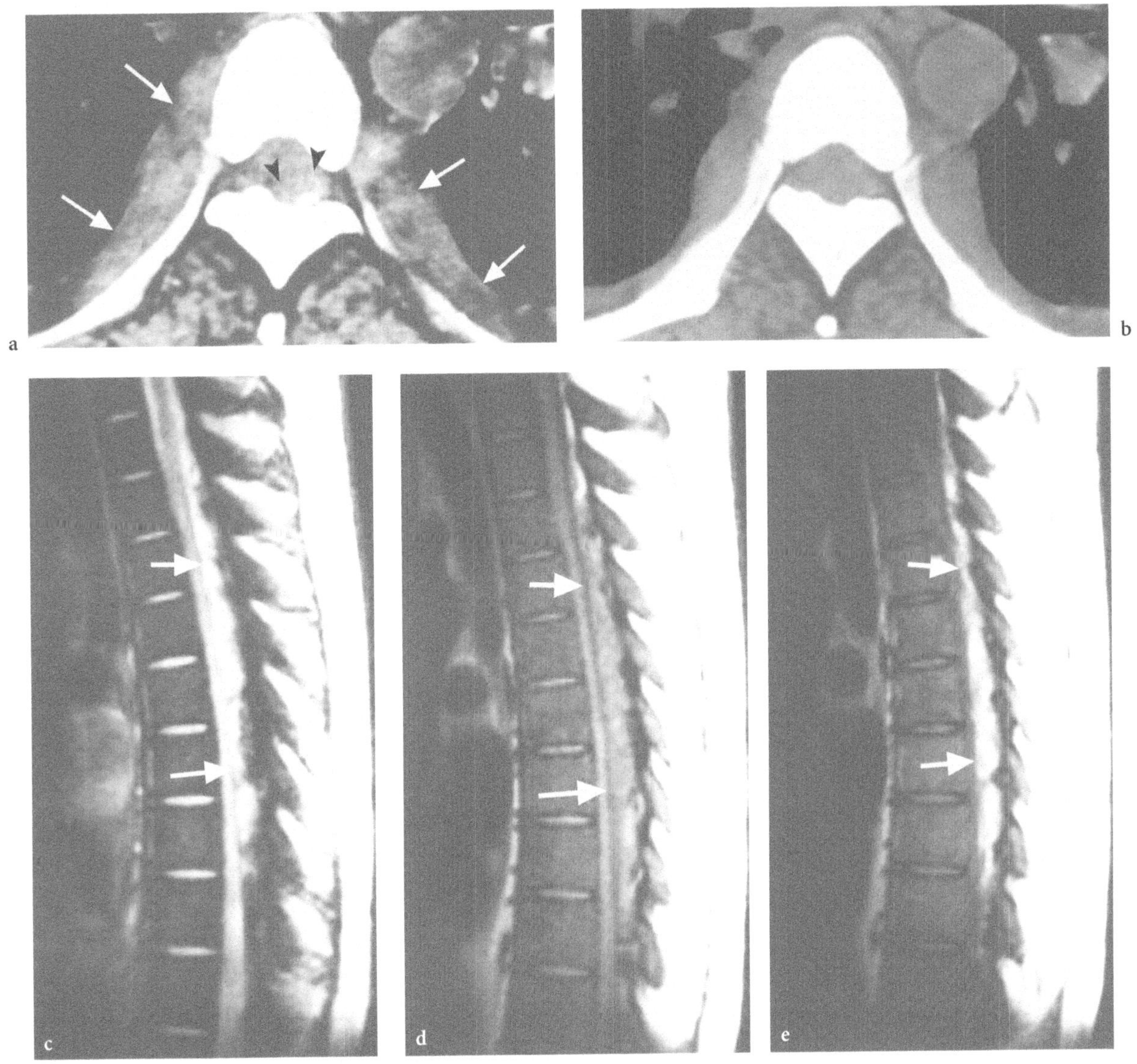

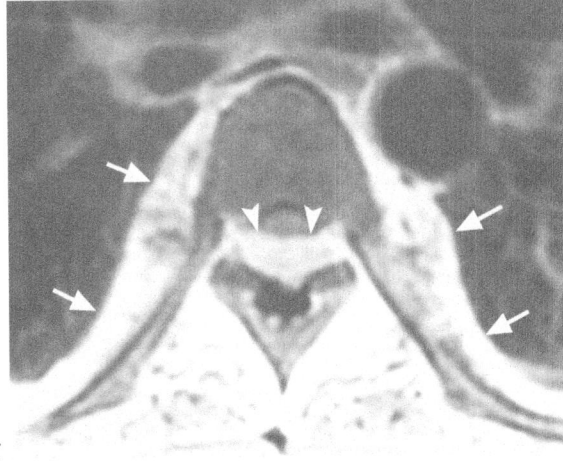

Fig. 21.10a–f. Spinal cord compression due to extramedullary hematopoiesis in a 36-year-old patient treated for primary myelofibrosis. **a** Axial contrast-enhanced CT scan at T6-level shows a soft-tissue mass filling the spinal canal (*arrowheads*). There is also a paravertebral mass (*arrows*). **b** Bone window setting shows a homogeneous increase in bone density due to myelosclerosis. There is no erosion or fracture. **c** Sagittal gradient-echo T2*-weighted MR image shows an intraspinal heterogeneous and predominantly hyperintense mass extending from T2 to T11 (*arrows*) and displacing the spinal cord anteriorly. The spinal cord is compressed mostly at the T5-8 level. The extradural mass is isointense (*arrows*) on sagittal (**d**) unenhanced spin-echo T1-weighted MR image and enhances strongly (**e**) after contrast administration (*arrows*). Note hypointense bone marrow on both T1 and T2*-weighted images secondary to myelofibrosis. **f** Axial contrast-enhanced spin-echo T1-weighted MR image at T6-level shows a hyperintense intraspinal mass infiltrating the spinal canal posteriorly (*arrowheads*) and compressing the spinal cord, with a symmetrical hyperintense paravertebral intrathoracic mass (*arrows*). The mass corresponds histologically to extramedullary hematopoiesis. (With permission from [Guermazi et al. 1997])

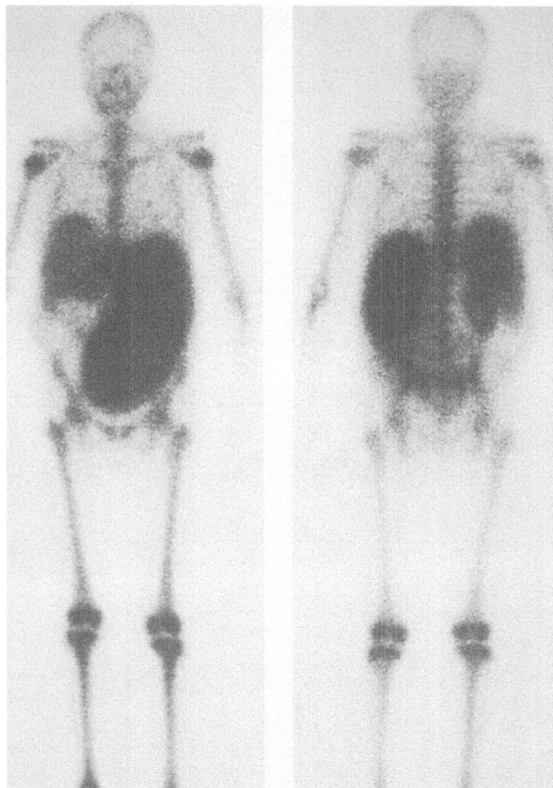

Fig. 21.11. Massive splenomegaly in a 46-year-old woman with primary myelofibrosis. Anterior (*left*) and posterior (*right*) technetium labeled whole body scan demonstrates increased tracer uptake within the increased size spleen, but also within the thoracolumbar spine, sternum, pelvis, and distal ends of long bones such as the femur and tibia. The prominence of increased bone marrow activity in the metaphyses of the long bones is suggestive of increased new bone formation.

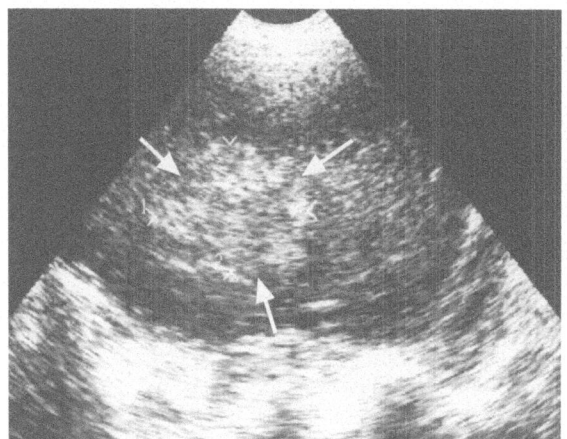

Fig. 21.12a–c. Focal intrasplenic extramedullary hematopoiesis in a 56-year-old woman with primary myelofibrosis. **a** Transverse US image shows heterogeneous hyperechoic well-defined large mass within the spleen (*arrows*). **b** Axial unenhanced CT scan of the upper abdomen shows 2 isodense masses within the spleen deforming the splenic surface. The largest contains small hyperdense areas probably due to hemorrhage (*arrowhead*). **c** Axial contrast-enhanced CT scan shows the masses enhance slightly following contrast administration (*arrows*). (With permission from [GUERMAZI et al. 1999])

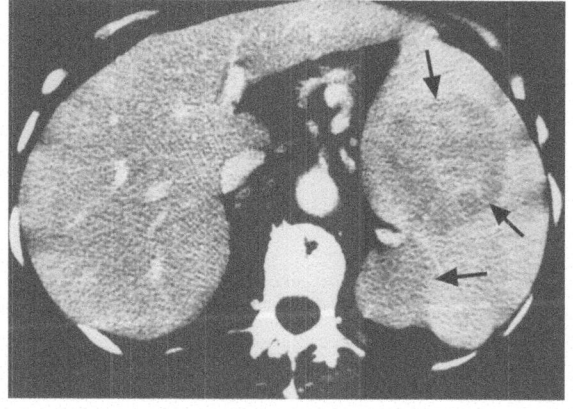

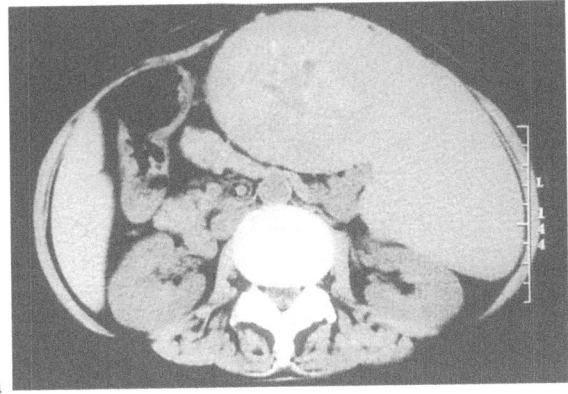
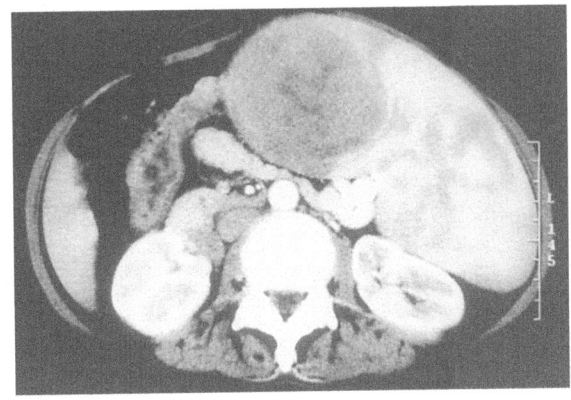

a

b

Fig. 21.13a,b. Splenic extramedullary hematopoiesis in a 61-year-old woman with secondary myelofibrosis developed from polycytemia vera. **a** Axial unenhanced CT scan shows a well defined margin on 7 cm diameter tumor-like lesion in the spleen with an internal mosaic pattern of low and high density. **b** This focal lesion enhances very slightly on axial contrast-enhanced CT scan. A partial splenectomy was performed and the histology of the splenic tumor yielded extensive extramedullary hematopoiesis. (With permission from [YOKOYAMA et al. 2000])

2000). Therefore, fine-needle biopsy, or histology after partial or total splenectomy is almost required for the diagnosis.

Liver

Hepatomegaly is a prominent physical finding, seen in 70% of cases. The hepatic involvement is almost always uniform. Nevertheless, focal intrahepatic masses and intrahepatic periportal anomalies have been reported. The focal hepatic disease can manifest as solitary or multiple lesions. The US features confirm the appearance of the focal hepatic lesions as a well-defined lesion or well-defined mass encircling the portal vein and its main branches (Fig. 21.14). These lesions can be hypoechoic or hyperechoic, frequently inhomogeneous, of variable size (2,5–15 cm), and their borders can be well defined or poorly defined (ABBITT and TEATES 1989; SINILUOTO et al. 1992; AYTAÇ et al. 1999; NAVARRO et al. 2000). Variation in ultrasonographic patterns can cause diagnostic difficulties. In the differential diagnosis, both infiltrative lesions such as leukemia and lymphoma, and non-infiltrative processes such as primary and metastatic tumors, hemangioma, focal nodular hypoplasia, and abscesses should be taken into consideration (AYTAÇ et al. 1999). Color Doppler US shows the lesion encircling a vascular structure, without vessel distortion or thrombosis (Fig. 21.15). This appearance favors mostly infiltrative lesions and benign processes (SINILUOTO et al. 1992; AYTAÇ et al. 1999). On CT, lesions of focal intrahepatic extramedullary hematopoiesis are hypodense, frequently heterogeneous,

and can show patchy or no enhancement after contrast administration (NAVARRO et al. 2000). On MR imaging, these focal masses show mild heterogeneous hyperintense lesions relative to the remaining liver parenchyma on T2-weighted sequences (Fig. 21.16) and present heterogeneous enhancement during contrast administration. No persistent enhancement has been observed on subsequent T1-weighted images (WARSHAUER and SCHIEBLER 1991; GIL-FERNANDEZ et al. 2001). Since the imaging findings are variable, percutaneous guided-biopsy is necessary for the diagnosis. No explanation is yet available for the variation in imaging patterns in myeloid metaplasia on the basis of hepatic and splenic cytology. The presence of variable amounts of fat and fibrosis is thought to be decisive for the imaging appearance (SHAVER and CLORE 1981; WIENER et al. 1987; KOBAYASHI et al. 1989; NAVARRO et al. 2000).

Lymph Nodes

Lymphadenopathy is found in 12% of patients. In general, it is of moderate degree, and hematopoiesis is present in its histologic studies. It may be abdominal or pelvic. If massive, adenopathy can mimic lymphoma (BOURONCLE and DOAN 1962; SHAVER and CLORE 1981; SINILUOTO et al. 1992). Unusual presentations may include a lack of nodular parenchymal masses in the liver and other organs that are frequent sites for extramedullary hematopoiesis, and the absence of typical fatty components in the extramedullary hematopoiesis lymph node masses (LA FIANZA et al. 2001).

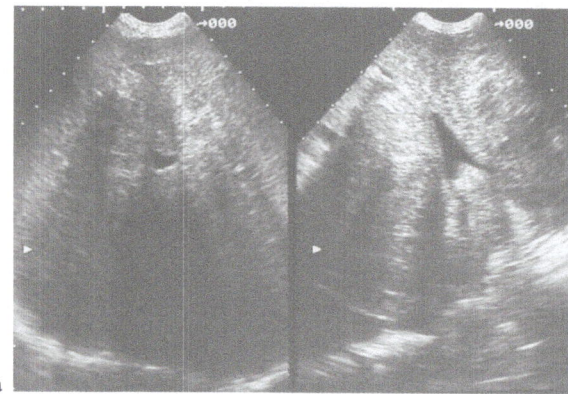
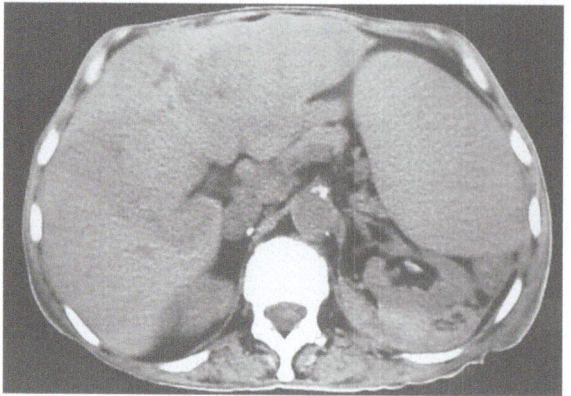

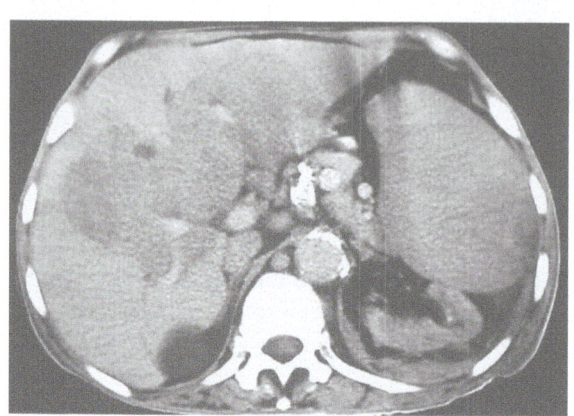

Fig. 21.14a–c. Periportal extramedullary hematopoiesis in a 82-year-old woman with primary myelofibrosis. **a** Transverse (*left*) and longitudinal (*right*) US images of the liver show a poorly defined hyperechoic mass in both lobes, which attenuated the sound in some areas. **b** Axial unenhanced CT scan of the upper abdomen shows a massive, well-defined, lobulated, hypodense intrahepatic mass with periportal location. The lesion displaced and encircled the main branches of the portal vein without signs of vascular invasion. **c** Axial contrast-enhanced CT image of the upper abdomen shows no enhancement of the mass. Note left posterior pararenal hematoma is seen and is attributed to the previous bone marrow biopsy. (With permission from [NAVARRO et al. 2000])

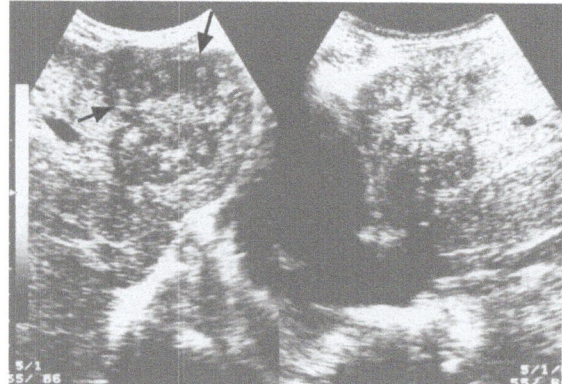

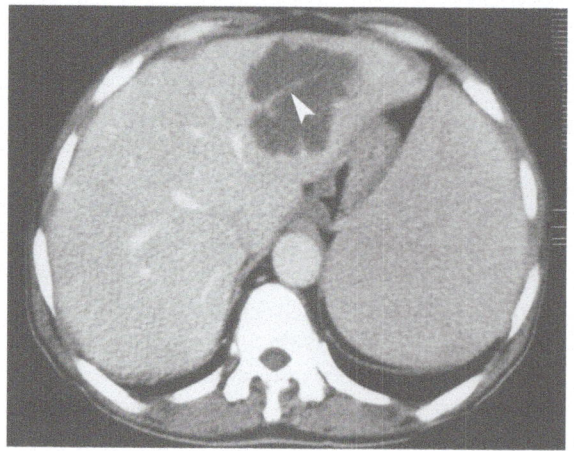

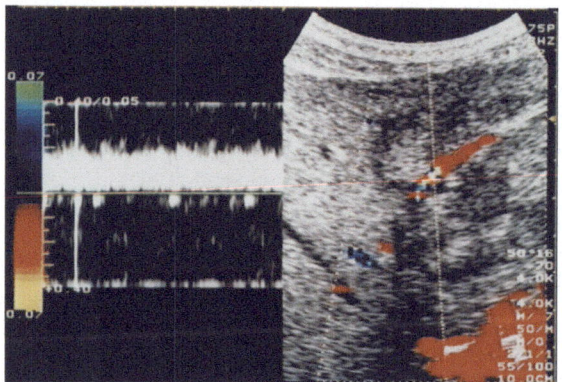

Fig. 21.15a–c. Focal intrahepatic extramedullary hematopoiesis in a 60-year-old man with primary myelofibrosis. **a** Oblique sagittal US image through the left lobe of the liver shows a hypoechoic heterogeneous solid mass (*arrows*). **b** Oblique sagittal color Doppler US image displays the left hepatic vein crossing the central part of the mass. **c** Axial contrast-enhanced CT scan of the upper abdomen show the well marginated hypodense lesion traversed by the left hepatic vein (*arrowhead*). (With permission from [AYTAÇ et al. 1999])

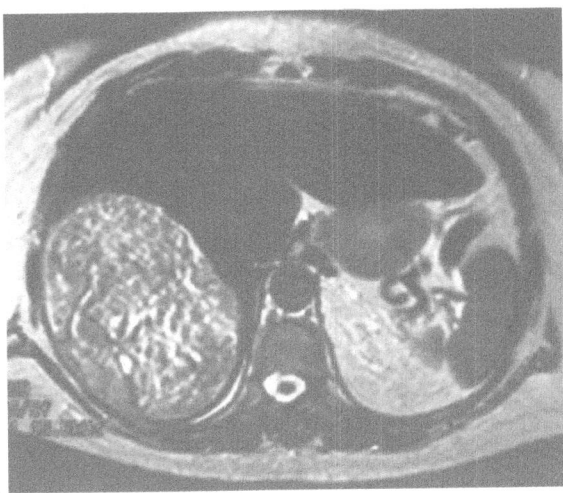
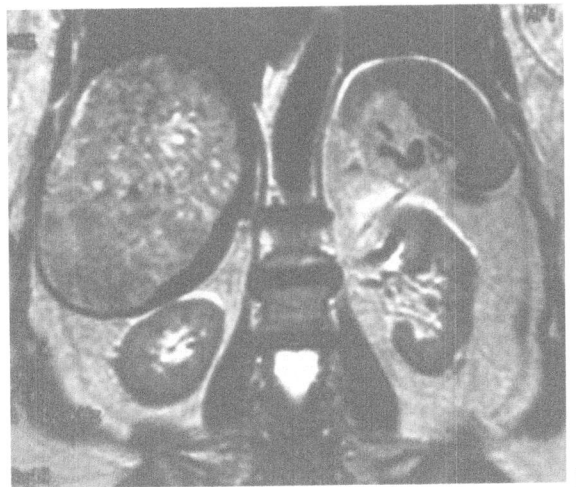

a   b

Fig. 21,16a,b. Giant hepatic mass of extramedullary hematopoiesis in a 74-year-old woman without myelofibrosis. a Axial and (b) coronal T2-weighted MR images of the liver show a giant well-defined, heteregeneous and hyperintense solid mass in the posterior segment of the right hepatic lobe. Biopsy of the mass disclosed foci of extramedullary hematopoiesis. (With permission from [GIL-FERNANDEZ et al. 2001])

Portal Hypertension

Portal hypertension develops in 10% of cases of myelofibrosis, and is almost always associated with ascites and varices (SHAVER and CLORE 1981). It can develop as a result of several mechanisms. Increased blood flow related to splenomegaly may contribute to the increased portal pressure, so-called "forward" portal hypertension (HUNG et al. 1999). Extensive infiltration of portal zones by primitive hematopoietic tissue is another possibility that may cause intrahepatic presinusoidal obstruction leading to portal hypertension (SHALDON and SHERLOCK 1962).

Ascites

Ascites can develop either secondary to portal hypertension or to the peritoneal proliferation of hematopoietic cells leading to a protein-rich exudate (SHAVER and CLORE 1981; JACOBS et al. 1991; HUNG et al. 1999). Ascites formation in myelofibrosis often occurs in the context of well-established disease. When caused by peritoneal implants of myeloid tissues, it may rarely be the initial manifestation of myelofibrosis (HUNG et al. 1999).

Intestines

Infiltration of the small or large intestines by hematopoietic tissue is rare, and may cause gastrointestinal complaints. Barium contrast studies and CT may be of value in establishing the presence, site, and extent of such changes (SHAVER and CLORE 1981; MACKINNON et al. 1986; SHARMA et al. 1986; SOLOMON et al. 1994).

Adrenal Glands

Adrenal glands may be bilaterally involved. CT demonstrates mildly inhomogeneous density mass within the adrenal gland. Biopsy is very useful for the differential diagnosis because the adrenals are often sites for metastatic and primary tumors. Furthermore, biopsy can distinguish extramedullary hematopoiesis from myelolipoma. The latter tumor is benign and contains considerable fat, whereas extramedullary hematopoiesis displays only small foci of fat tissue (KING et al. 1987; PAPAVASILIOU et al. 1990).

Intraabdominal and Pelvic Masses

Intraabdominal and pelvic masses of extramedullary hematopoiesis may be very large and exhibit invasive characteristics leading to serious complications (Fig. 21.17). These masses contain all the elements of hematopoiesis, and frequently one cell line dominates, usually the myeloid series (GLEW et al. 1973; CHAO et al. 1986; GUERMAZI et al. 1999).

21.4.3.3
Thoracic Manifestations

Breast

Extramedullary hematopoiesis in the breast is very rare, probably because the tissue masses do not show distinct malignant features and autopsies seldom include microscopic examination of the breasts. In the rare cases reported, mammography shows an asymmetric pattern of confluent densities and US reveals several smooth, homogeneous and hypoechoic masses of variable sizes in both breasts (Fig. 21.18). These masses are not distinguishable on the mammogram, and their imaging appearance is very similar to that of lymphoma. Nevertheless, the skin remains intact with out any signs of inflammation both clinically and radiologically (ZONDERLAND et al. 1991; CUFER and BRACKO 2001). Fine-needle aspiration biopsy is often required to exclude malignancy (SHAVER and CLORE, 1981; CUFER and BRACKO 2001).

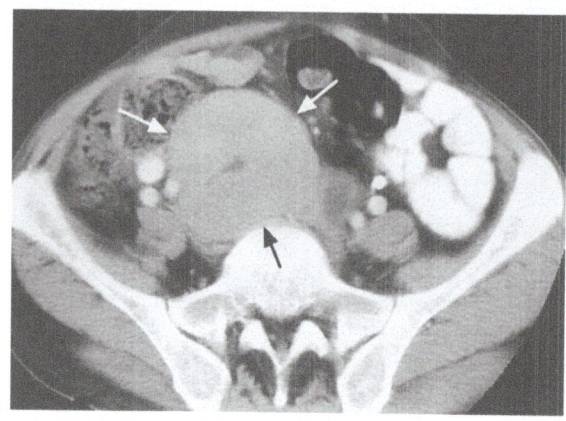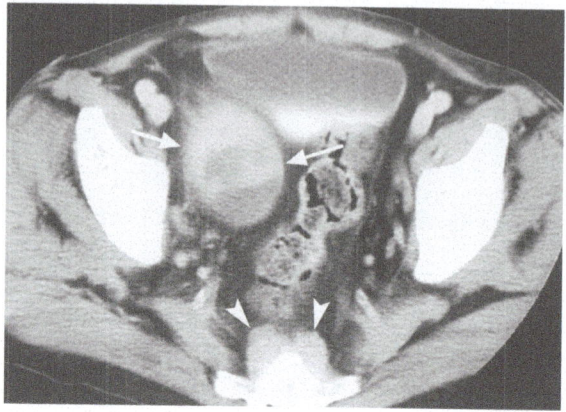

Fig. 21.17a,b. Pelvic extramedullary hematopoiesis in a 48-year-old man with primary myelofibrosis. Axial contrast-enhanced pelvic CT scans demonstrate (**a**) presacral (*arrows*), (**b**) pelvic (*arrows*) and coccygeal (*arrowheads*) heterogenous masses. CT guided-biopsy diagnosed extramedullary hematopoiesis. (With permission from [GUERMAZI et al. 1999])

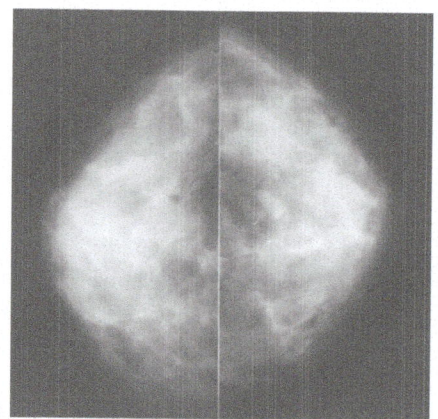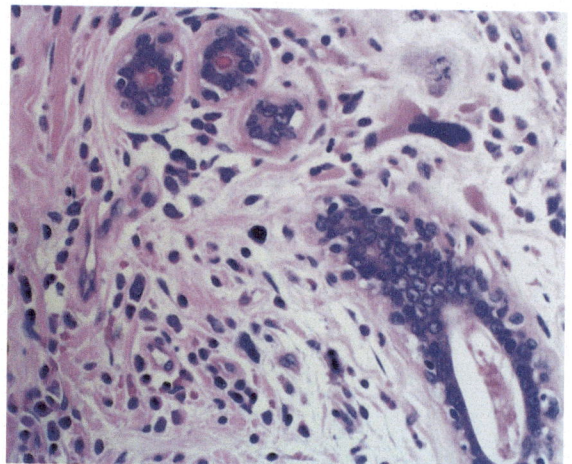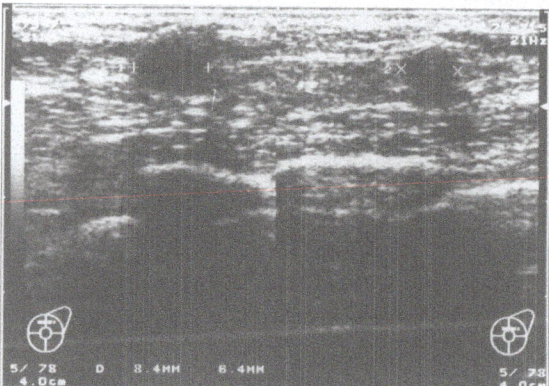

Fig. 21.18a–c. Extramedullary hematopoiesis of the breast in a 50-year-old woman with primary myelofibrosis. **a** Bilateral craniocaudal mammography shows an asymmetric pattern of confluent densities, which are prominent in the left breast. No circumscribed masses or microcalcifications are detected. **b** Transverse US image of the left breast shows two smooth, homogeneous and hypoechoic masses in the outer upper quadrant, measuring 8 and 6 mm in diameter, respectively. **c** Microscopic study (Hematoxylin-eosin stain; original magnification, ×400) shows the mammary stroma is infiltrated by immature and mature myeloid cells, erythroid cells and megakaryocytes. (With permission from [CUFER and BRACKO 2001])

Pleural Effusion

Pleural effusion contains immature cells of both the erythroid and myeloid lines and is transudate. It is usually microscopic and asymptomatic. When massive, pleural involvement produces a massive hemothorax which may require surgical evacuation (GLEW et al. 1973; LUND and ALDRIDGE 1984; KUPFERSCHMID et al. 1993).

Pulmonary Emboli

Pulmonary emboli probably originate from outside the lung in the spleen or other tissues. It is possible, however, that arterial occlusion follows invasion by interstitial hematopoietic precursors (GLEW et al. 1973; SHAVER and CLORE 1981; WYATT and FISHMAN 1994).

Interstitial Hematopoiesis

Interstitial hematopoiesis, mostly associated with small vessel involvement, is often found at autopsy and is sometimes noted on chest films with the clinical manifestation of dyspnea, pulmonary hypertension, and/or right heart failure. Chest radiographs may show prominence of the pulmonary vasculature. CT demonstrates ground glass opacities. Technetium-99m sulfur colloid bone marrow scintigraphy demonstrates diffuse lung uptake. Differential diagnosis must include pulmonary edema or hemorrhage, infection, drug reaction, and leukemic infiltration (SHAVER and CLORE 1981; COATES et al. 1994; WYATT and FISHMAN 1994).

Pericardium

Extramedullary hematopoiesis has rarely been associated with pericardial effusion resulting in cardiac tamponade and also with coronary arterial occlusion by hematopoietic emboli (SHAVER and CLORE 1981).

Mediastinal Mass

Mediastinal mass effect of extramedullary hematopoiesis is located posteriorly along the spine. No case of anterior or hilar adenopathy due to hematopoiesis has been reported. They are usually discovered during a screening examination for another problem. The masses are very well defined, do not erode bone, and are located along the paravertebral area at any thoracic level. Chest radiography shows posterior, most often bilateral, smooth rounded masses. The classic CT appearance of extramedullary hematopoiesis has been described as a homogeneous hyperdense or solid, round lobulated paravertebral soft tissue mass (Fig. 21.19). Widening of the vertebral ends of the ribs by medullary expansion and periosteal elevation can

often be detected on CT but not commonly on plain chest radiography. The masses have a high signal intensity rim on both T1 and T2-weighted images, which represents fatty tissue that may occur as a part of extramedullary hematopoiesis (SHAVER and CLORE 1981; SAVADER et al. 1988; PAPAVASILIOU et al. 1990; KUPFERSCHMID et al. 1993).

21.4.3.4
Genitourinary Manifestations

Kidneys

Renal hematopoietic involvement is rarely reported. The kidney may be homogeneously enlarged, unilaterally or bilaterally, and the involved areas may be nonenhancing or enhance homogeneously after contrast administration. Renal involvement is usually intraparenchymal (REDLIN et al. 1976; SHAVER and CLORE 1981) and characterized by interstitial focal infiltrates or tumor-like nodules extending into the pelvicalyceal system (GRYSPEERDT et al. 1995). In the latter presentation, distortion of the calyceal pattern with stretching and narrowing may be seen on excretory urography. These findings in some circumstances should be considered for differential diagnosis with hemorrhagic pelvic cysts, hypernephroma, and other kidney neoplasms. Perirenal localization is a very rare presentation, and imaging features may be indistinguishable from those of the rare perirenal lymphoma, metastases, hamartomas, amyloid or infection (Fig. 21. 20) (WRIGHT 1991; RAPEZZI et al. 1997). Organomegaly of both kidneys and expansion of the connective tissue around the capsule of the kidneys and the adventitial tissue around the renal tissue is another very rare imaging presentation (Fig. 21. 21) (SCHNUELLE et al. 1999). Biopsy or fine-needle aspiration is often necessary to confirm the diagnosis. Extramedullary hematopoiesis involving the kidneys may lead to renal failure. In such circumstances, radiotherapy is often effective (COHN et al. 1991; FERNBACH and FEINSTEIN 1992; HOLT et al. 1995; SCHNUELLE et al. 1999).

Ureters and Bladder

Extramedullary hematopoiesis of ureters and bladder has been reported. Intrinsic involvement of the upper and lower urinary tract results in obstruction of both kidneys and marked bladder dysfunction (OESTERLING et al. 1992).

Prostate

Prostate involvement is very rare. It induces bladder outlet obstruction and urinary retention (HUMPHREY and VOLLMER 1991).

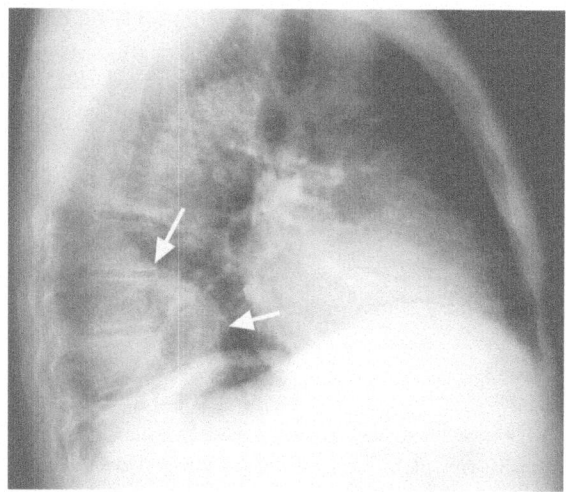

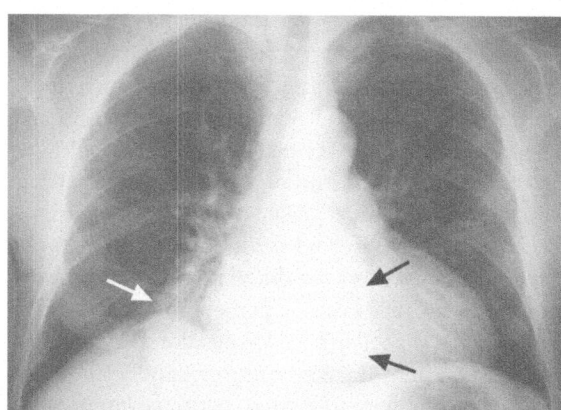

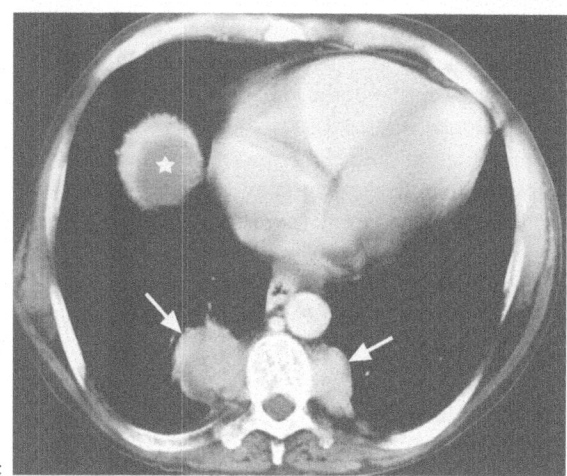

Fig. 21.19a–c. Thoracic extramedullary hematopoiesis in a 63-year-old man with primary myelofibrosis. **a** Lateral and (**b**) anteroposterior radiographs of the thorax show posterior bilateral opacities within the mediastinum (*arrows*). **c** Axial contrast-enhanced CT scan of the thorax demonstrates lobulated heterogeneous paravertebral masses (*arrows*) further identified as extramedullary hematopoiesis. Note a biliary cyst in the dome of the liver (*star*). (With permission from [GUERMAZI et al. 1999])

21.5
Secondary Myelofibrosis

Difficulties arise in the classification "secondary" as cases of marrow fibrosis have appeared in some patients initially diagnosed with primary disease. Whatever the associated disease, the musculoskeletal and articular abnormalities that are almost always associated with extramedullary hematopoiesis demonstrate the same characteristics as primary myelofibrosis (BOURONCLE and DOAN 1962; LANIR et al. 1986; HASSELBALCH 1990; COHN et al. 1991; MALLOUH and SA'DI 1992; OZSOYLU 1994; AMANO et al. 1997; YOKOYAMA et al. 2000), and no radiologic feature, even on MR imaging, is of value in differentiating between primary and secondary myelofibrosis (AMANO et al. 1997).

Malignant Diseases
– Acute leukemias
– Chronic myeloid leukemias
– Chronic lymphocytic leukemias
– Malignant lymphomas
– Other hemopathies: Vaquez disease, polycytemia vera, myeloma
– Systemic mastocytosis
– Metastatic carcinomas

Non Malignant Diseases
– Osseous diseases (rickets (Fig. 21.22), Paget disease)
– Auto-immune syndromes (renal failure, systemic lupus erythematosus)
– Infections (tuberculosis, viral infections)
– Congenital diseases (Gaucher disease)
– Toxins and chemical poisonings (Benzene, Thorium, busulphan)

21.6
Differential Diagnosis

The radiographic picture of myelofibrosis associates axial skeleton osteosclerosis and splenomegaly and almost always affects middle-aged or elderly patients.

Leukemia and lymphoma can lead to splenomegaly, but the extent of osteosclerosis in such diseases is not striking.

Systemic mastocytosis may be difficult to differentiate from myelofibrosis. It can produce hepatosplenomegaly and focal or diffuse osteosclerosis.

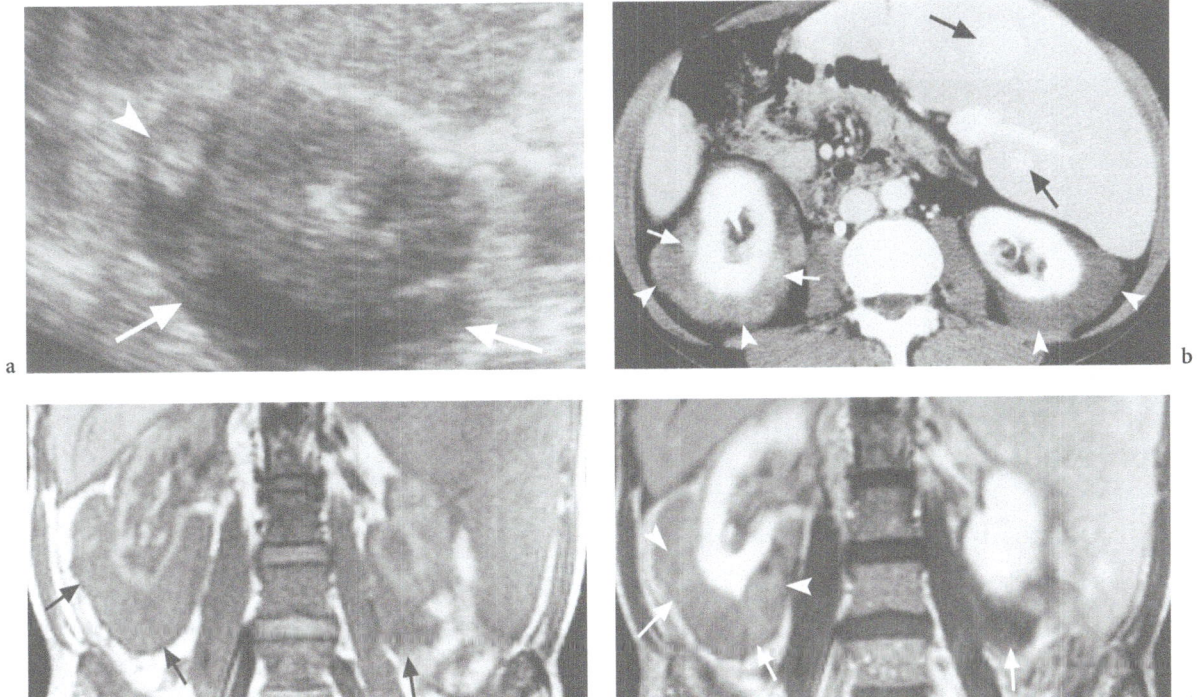

Fig. 21.20a–d. Perirenal extramedullary hematopoiesis in a 52-year-old man with primary myelofibrosis. **a** Transverse US image of the right kidney shows bilateral perirenal tissue (*arrows*) with several hyperechoic nodules (*arrowhead*) of extramedullary hematopoiesis. **b** Axial contrast-enhanced CT scan through the kidneys shows severe splenomagaly with multiple enhancing hemangioma-like nodules of extramedullary hematopoiesis (*black arrows*). The CT also shows bilateral perirenal rinds of tissue (*arrowheads*) with enhanced nodules of extramedullary hematopoiesis (*white arrows*). Coronal MR images of the renal area show the nodules (*arrowheads*), inside the bilateral perirenal tissue (*arrows*), are hypointense on (**c**) T1-weighted image and mild hyperintense on (**d**) T2-weighted image. A US-guided needle biopsy confirmed the presence of hematopietic tissue. (With permission from [RAPEZZI et al. 1997])

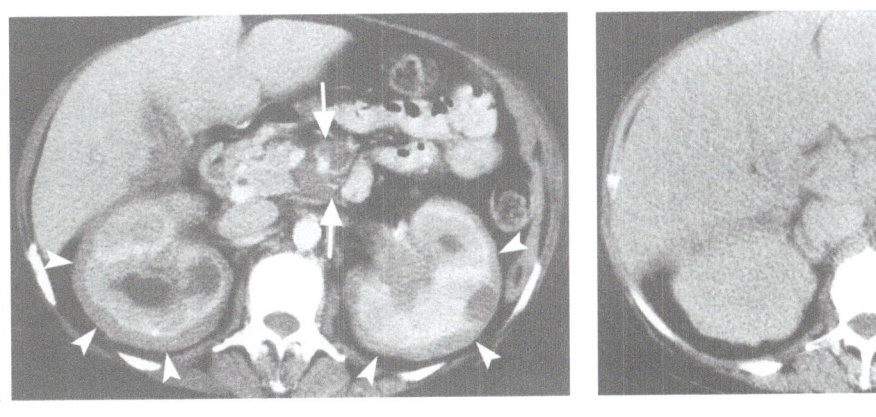

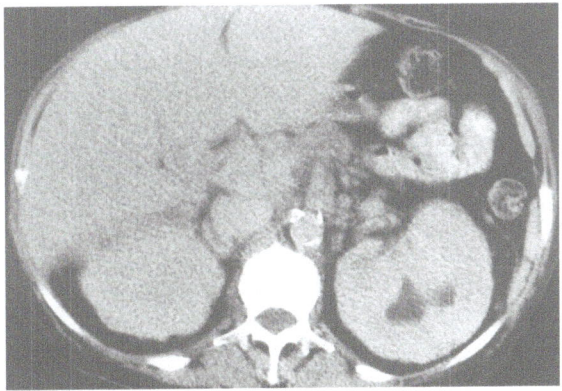

Fig. 21.21a–c. Extramedullary hematopoiesis in the kidneys in a 75-year-old woman with primary myelofibrosis. **a** Axial contrast-enhanced CT scan through the kidneys at early arterial phase shows enlargement of both kidneys with hypodense margin of additional soft tissue close to the capsule (*arrowheads*). The expansion of the connective tissue is also seen around the renal hilus and the superior mesenteric artery (*arrows*). **b** At late phase, contrast enhancement is poor causing isodense appearance of the additional soft tissue. Note a distension of renal pelvis and calyces. **c** Macroscopic postmortem specimen of the left kidney demonstrates distinct enlargement due to encasement and infiltration by myeloid metaplasia with fibrosis. (With permission from [SCHNUELLE et al. 1999])

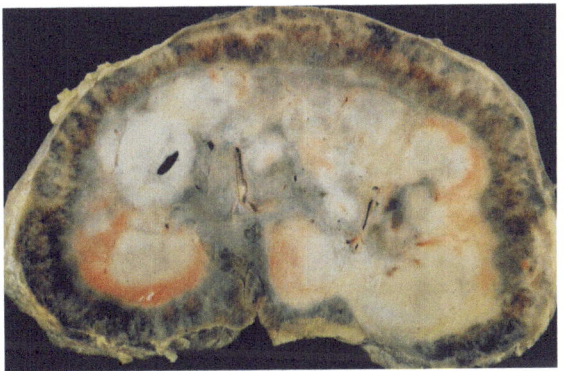

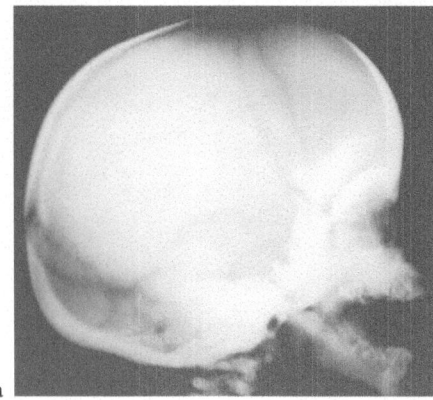

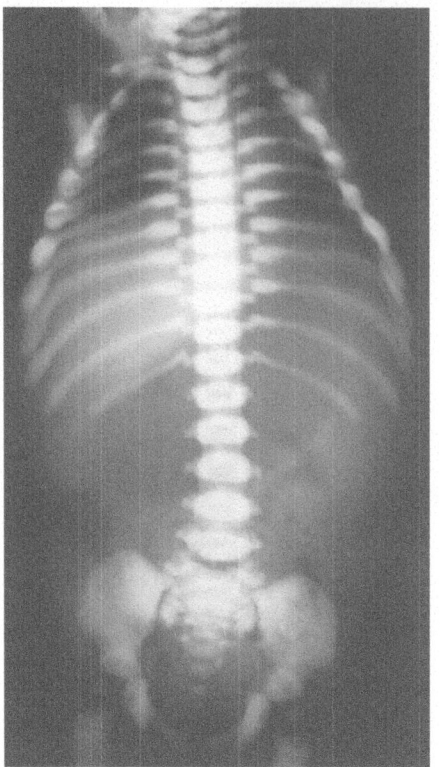

Fig. 21.22a,b. Diffuse osteomyelosclerosis in a 4-year-old boy with secondary myelofibrosis from chronic rickets. **a** Lateral skull and (**b**) anteroposterior thoracoabdominal radiographs show diffuse increased bone density due to myelofibrosis. (With permission from [GUERMAZI et al. 1999])

Metastasis, Paget disease, fluorosis, axial osteomalacia, and renal osteodystrophy can demonstrate osteosclerosis without splenomegaly. Association with other characteristic changes may help to diagnose each disease (GUERMAZI et al. 1999).

21.7
Conclusion

Myelofibrosis is an uncommon disease included in the myeloproliferative disorders. The main radiographic features are osteosclerosis, hepatosplenomegaly, and extramedullary hematopoiesis. At autopsy, extramedullary hematopoiesis is often found scattered through nearly all body tissues as an incidental finding. Extramedullary hematopoiesis can become clinically important both symptomatically and from the standpoint of differential diagnosis. The diagnosis is almost always established by guided-biopsy or fine-needle aspiration. In these situations, therapeutic intervention is necessary. The mainstay of treatment is radiation therapy, since myeloid tissue is extremely radiosensitive.

Acknowledgements
I would like to thank Drs C. Crespo, T. Cufer, T. Diamond, S. Fitoz, J.J. Gil-Fernandez, M. Navarro, D. Rapezzi, P. Schnuelle, and Y. Yano for their helpfulness and for providing me with their excellent images.

References

Abbitt PL, Teates CD (1989) The sonographic appearance of extramedullary hematopoiesis in the liver. J Clin Ultrasound 17:280–282

Alpdogan O, Budak-Alpdogan T, Bayik M, Akoglu T, Kodalli N, Gurmen N (1998) Magnetic resonance imaging in myelofibrosis. Blood 92:2995–2997

Amano Y, Onda M, Amano M, Kumazaki T (1997) Magnetic resonance imaging of myelofibrosis. STIR and gadolinium-enhanced MR images. Clin Imaging 21:264–268

Arellano-Rodrigo E, Esteve J, Gine E, Panes J, Cervantes F (2002) Idiopathic myelofibrosis associated with ulcerative colitis. Leuk Lymphoma 43:1481–1483

Aytaç S, Fitoz S, Akyar S, Atasoy C, Erekul S (1999) Focal intrahepatic extramedullary hematopoiesis: color Doppler US and CT findings. Abdom Imaging 24:366–368

Bouroncle BA, Doan CA (1962) Myelofibrosis: clinical, hematologic and pathologic study of 110 patients. Am J Med Sci 243:697–715

Camos M, Arellano-Rodrigo E, Abello D, Muntanola A, Ferrer A, Grau JM, Cervantes F (2003) Idiopathic myelofibrosis associated with classic polyarteritis nodosa. Leuk Lymphoma 44:539–541

Chao PW, Farman J, Kapelner S (1986) CT features of presacral mass: an unusual focus of extramedullary hematopoiesis. J Comput Assist Tomogr 10:684–685

Coates GG, Eisenberg B, Dail DH (1994) Tc-99m sulfur colloid demonstration of diffuse pulmonary interstitial extramedullary hematopoiesis in a patient with myelofibrosis. A case report and review of the literature. Clin Nucl Med 19:1079–1084

Cohn SL, Cohn RA, Chou P, Donaldson JS, Langman CB (1991) Infantile myelofibrosis with nephromegaly secondary to myeloid metaplasia. Clin Pediatr (Phila) 30:59–61

Connelly TJ, Abruzzo JL, Schwab RH (1982) Agnogenic myeloid metaplasia with polyarteritis. J Rheumatol 9:954–956

Cook G, Sharp RA (1994) Spinal cord compression due to extramedullary haemopoiesis in myelofibrosis. J Clin Pathol 47:464–465

Cufer T, Bracko M (2001) Myeloid metaplasia of the breast. Ann Oncol 12:267–270

De Klippel N, Dehou MF, Bourgain C, Schots R, De Keyser J, Ebinger G (1993) Progressive paraparesis due to thoracic extramedullary hematopoiesis in myelofibrosis. Case report. J Neurosurg 79:125–127

Diamond T, Smith A, Schnier R, Manoharan A (2002) Syndrome of myelofibrosis and osteosclerosis: a series of case reports and review of the literature. Bone 30:498–501

Fernbach SK, Feinstein KA (1992) Extramedullary hematopoiesis in the kidneys in infant siblings with myelofibrosis. Pediatr Radiol 22:211–212

Gil-Fernandez JJ, Martinez-Chamorro C, Tomas JF (2001) The irreplaceable image: A giant hepatic mass of myeloid metaplasia in a patient without myelofibrosis. Haematologica 86:445

Glew RH, Haese WH, McIntyre PA (1973) Myeloid metaplasia with myelofibrosis. The clinical spectrum of extramedullary hematopoiesis and tumor formation. Johns Hopkins Med J 132:253–270

Goodman P, Kumar R, Alperin JB (1991) Diffuse intraabdominal lymphoma complicating idiopathic myelofibrosis: CT demonstration. AJR Am J Roentgenol 156:1189–1190

Gryspeerdt S, Oyen R, Van Hoe L, Baert AL, Boogaerts M (1995) Extramedullary hematopoiesis encasing the pelvicalyceal system: CT findings. Ann Hematol 71:53–56

Guermazi A, Miaux Y, Chiras J (1997) Imaging of spinal cord compression due to thoracic extramedullary haematopoiesis in myelofibrosis. Neuroradiology 39:733–736

Guermazi A, de Kerviler E, Cazals-Hatem D, Zagdanski AM, Frija J (1999) Imaging findings in patients with myelofibrosis. Eur Radiol 9:1366–1375

Harris BK, Ross HA (1974) Hemarthrosis as the presenting manifestation of myeloproliferative disease. Arthritis Rheum 17:969–970

Hasselbalch H (1990) Idiopathic myelofibrosis: a clinical study of 80 patients. Am J Hematol 34:291–300

Heinicke MH, Zarrabi MH, Gorevic PD (1983) Arthritis due to synovial involvement by extramedullary haematopoiesis in myelofibrosis with myeloid metaplasia. Ann Rheum Dis 42:196–200

Hernandez-Boluda JC, Jimenez M, Rosinol L, Cervantes F (2002) Idiopathic myelofibrosis associated with primary biliary cirrhosis. Leuk Lymphoma 43:673–674

Holt SG, Field P, Carmichael P, Mehta A, Jarmulowicz M, Clarke D, Hilson A, Burns A (1995) Extramedullary haematopoiesis in the renal parenchyma as a cause of acute renal failure in myelofibrosis. Nephrol Dial Transplant 10:1438–1440

Humphrey PA, Vollmer RT (1991) Extramedullary hematopoiesis in the prostate. Am J Surg Pathol 15:486–490

Hung SC, Huang ML, Liu SM, Hsu HC (1999) Massive ascites caused by peritoneal extramedullary hematopoiesis as the initial manifestation of myelofibrosis. Am J Med Sci 318:198–200

Jacobs P, Wood L, Robson S (1991) Refractory ascites in the chronic myeloproliferative syndrome: a case report. Am J Hematol 37:128–129

Jones RJ (1992) The role of bone marrow imaging. Radiology 183:321–322

Kaplan KR, Mitchell DG, Steiner RM, Murphy S, Vinitski S, Rao VM, Burk DL, Rifkin MD (1992) Polycythemia vera and myelofibrosis: correlation of MR imaging, clinical, and laboratory findings. Radiology 183:329–334

King BF, Kopecky KK, Baker MK, Clark SA (1987) Extramedullary hematopoiesis in the adrenal glands: CT characteristics. J Comput Assist Tomogr 11:342–343

Kobayashi A, Sugihara M, Kurosaki M, Ishida Y, Takayanagi N, Matsui O, Takashima T (1989) CT characteristics of intrahepatic, periportal, extramedullary hematopoiesis. J Comput Assist Tomogr 13:354–356

Koch BL, Bisset GS, 3rd, Bisset RR, Zimmer MB (1994) Intracranial extramedullary hematopoiesis: MR findings with pathologic correlation. AJR Am J Roentgenol 162:1419–1420

Kosmidis PA, Palacas CG, Axelrod AR (1980) Diffuse purely osteolytic lesions in myelofibrosis. Cancer 46:2263–2265

Kupferschmid JP, Shahian DM, Villanueva AG (1993) Massive hemothorax associated with intrathoracic extramedullary hematopoiesis involving the pleura. Chest 103:974–975

La Fianza A, Alberici E, Torretta L (2001) The irreplaceable image: Rapidly growing extramedullary hematopoiesis in lymph nodes: unusual findings of long-standing idiopathic myelofibrosis. Haematologica 86:784

Lanir A, Aghai E, Simon JS, Lee RG, Clouse ME (1986) MR imaging in myelofibrosis. J Comput Assist Tomogr 10:634–636

Ligumski M, Polliack A, Benbassat J (1978) Myeloid metaplasia of the central nervous system in patients with myelofibrosis and agnogenic myeloid metaplasia. Report of 3 cases and review of the literature. Am J Med Sci 275:99–103

Lund RE, Aldridge NH (1984) Computed tomography of intracranial extramedullary hematopoiesis. J Comput Assist Tomogr 8:788–790

MacKinnon S, McNicol AM, Lee FD, McDonald GA (1986) Myelofibrosis complicated by intestinal extramedullary haemopoiesis and acute small bowel obstruction. J Clin Pathol 39:677–679

Mallouh AA, Sa'di AR (1992) Agnogenic myeloid metaplasia in children. Am J Dis Child 146:965–967

Navarro M, Crespo C, Perez L, Martinez C, Galant J, Gonzalez I (2000) Massive intrahepatic extramedullary hematopoiesis in myelofibrosis. Abdom Imaging 25:184–186

Oesterling JE, Keating JP, Leroy AJ, Earle JD, Farrow GM, McCarthy JT, Silverstein MN (1992) Idiopathic myelofibrosis with myeloid metaplasia involving the renal pelves, ureters and bladder. J Urol 147:1360–1362

Ohtsubo M, Hayashi K, Fukushima T, Chiyoda S, Takahara O (1994) Case report: intracranial extramedullary haematopoiesis in postpolycythemic myelofibrosis. Br J Radiol 67:299–302

Ozsoylu S (1994) Myelofibrosis in children. Pediatr Hematol Oncol 11:339–340, 347

Papavasiliou C, Gouliamos A, Deligiorgi E, Vlahos L, Cambouris T (1990) Masses of myeloadipose tissue: radiological and clinical considerations. Int J Radiat Oncol Biol Phys 19:985–993

Rapezzi D, Racchi O, Ferraris AM (1997) Perirenal extramedullary hematopoiesis in agnogenic myeloid metaplasia: MR imaging findings. AJR Am J Roentgenol 168:1388–1389

Redlin L, Francis RS, Orlando MM (1976) Renal abnormalities in agnogenic myeloid metaplasia. Radiology 121: 605–608

Rozman C, Cervantes F, Rozman M, Mercader JM, Montserrat E (1999) Magnetic resonance imaging in myelofibrosis and essential thrombocythaemia: contribution to differential diagnosis. Br J Haematol 104:574–580

Savader SJ, Otero RR, Savader BL (1988) MR imaging of intrathoracic extramedullary hematopoiesis. J Comput Assist Tomogr 12:878–880

Schnuelle P, Waldherr R, Lehmann KJ, Woenckhaus J, Back W, Niemir Z, van der Woude FJ (1999) Idiopathic myelofibrosis with extramedullary hematopoiesis in the kidneys. Clin Nephrol 52:256–262

Shaldon S, Sherlock S (1962) Portal hypertension in the myeloproliferative syndrome and the reticuloses. Am J Med 32: 758–768

Sharma BK, Pounder RE, Cruse JP, Knowles SM, Lewis AA (1986) Extramedullary haemopoiesis in the small bowel. Gut 27:873–875

Shaver RW, Clore FC (1981) Extramedullary hematopoiesis in myeloid metaplasia. AJR Am J Roentgenol 137:874–876

Siniluoto TM, Hyvarinen SA, Paivansalo MJ, Alavaikko MJ, Suramo IJ (1992) Abdominal ultrasonography in myelofibrosis. Acta Radiol 33:343–346

Solomon D, Goodman H, Jacobs P (1994) Case report: rectal stenosis due to extramedullary haemopoiesis–radiological features. Clin Radiol 49:726–728

Ueda F, Takashima T, Suzuki M, Kadoya M (1994) MR diagnosis of myelofibrosis. Radiat Med 12:135–137

Urman M, O'Sullivan RA, Nugent RA, Lentle BC (1991) Intracranial extramedullary hematopoiesis. CT and bone marrow scan findings. Clin Nucl Med 16:431–434

Warshauer DM, Schiebler ML (1991) Intrahepatic extramedullary hematopoiesis: MR, CT, and sonographic appearance. J Comput Assist Tomogr 15:683–685

Wiener MD, Halvorsen RA, Jr., Vollmer RT, Foster WL, Roberts L, Jr. (1987) Focal intrahepatic extramedullary hematopoiesis mimicking neoplasm. AJR Am J Roentgenol 149:1171–1172

Wright RE (1991) Case report: pararenal extramedullary haematopoietic tissue–an unusual manifestation of myelofibrosis. Clin Radiol 44:210–211

Wyatt SH, Fishman EK (1994) Diffuse pulmonary extramedullary hematopoiesis in a patient with myelofibrosis: CT findings. J Comput Assist Tomogr 18:815–817

Yokoyama T, Saigo K, Maeda N, Hamada Y, Yano Y, Mori T, Tamura M, Tasaka K, Okutani T, Takata M, Maeda Y, Tomofuji Y, Chinzei T (2000) Tumor-like splenic extramedullary hematopoiesis in a patient with myelofibrosis. Intern Med 39:416–418

Yu JS, Greenway G, Resnick D (1994) Myelofibrosis associated with prominent periosteal bone apposition. Report of two cases. Clin Imaging 18:89–92

Yu TF (1965) Secondary gout associated with myeloproliferative diseases. Arthritis Rheum 8:765–771

Zonderland HM, Michiels JJ, ten Kate FJ (1991) Case report: mammographic and sonographic demonstration of extramedullary haematopoiesis of the breast. Clin Radiol 44:64–65

22 Central Nervous System Effects of Therapy in Patients Treated for Hematological Malignancies

ALI GUERMAZI, ELIDA VÁZQUEZ, ELIANE GLUCKMAN, YVES MIAUX

CONTENTS

ALI GUERMAZI, MD
Visiting Associate Professor, Department of Radiology, University of California San Francisco, 350 Parnassus Avenue, Suite 150, San Francisco, CA 94117, USA
ELIDA VÁZQUEZ, MD
Associate Staff, Neuroradiologist, Department of Pediatric Radiology, Hospital Materno-Infantil Vall d'Hebron, Barcelona, Spain, ps. Vall d'Hebron 119–129, 08035 Barcelona, Spain
ELIANE GLUCKMAN, MD
Professor and Chairman, Department of Bone Marrow Transplantation, Saint-Louis University Hospital, AP-HP, 1 Claude Vellefaux Avenue, 75010 Paris, France
YVES MIAUX, MD, MS
Vice President, Department of Reading Services, Synarc Inc., 575 Market Street, 17th Floor, San Francisco, CA 94105, USA

22.1 Introduction

Patients treated for hematological malignancies may develop central nervous system (CNS) complications at some point in the course of the disease. Some complications are caused by the underlying disease itself, while others are treatment-related. The latter include possible toxic side effects of irradiation and/or chemotherapy, infections caused by immunosuppression, thrombocytopenia, nutritional and metabolic stresses, and graft-versus-host disease (GVHD). As a result, CNS effects of therapy may be infectious, vascular, toxic, metabolic, or tumoral. Familiarity with these complications allows early recognition of most problems, and differentiation between CNS complications from the original disease and complications from the treatment. This is of clinical importance as – depending on the cause – patients may require additional or reinforced treatment, or withdrawal from therapy. This chapter presents a range of typical CT and MR imaging appearances of CNS therapeutic abnormalities seen in patients treated for hematological malignancies. Neurological imaging, in combination with electrophysiological studies as well as blood and cerebrospinal fluid investigations, may be helpful for diagnosing most of these complications, as well as in differentiating between the manifestations of the underlying disease and complications of the treatment. The main issues to keep in mind are that certain complications are most likely due to multiple underlying diseases, and that more than one complication can coexist.

22.2 Infectious Side Effects

Infections, including CNS infections, are widely recognized as the most common cause of death among patients treated in hematology (DE MEDEIROS et al. 2000). These patients are severely immunocompromised by both the underlying disease and its treat-ment, especially allogenic bone marrow transplanta-tion (BMT) (GRAUS et al. 1996; MASCHKE et al. 1999). Although the period of neutropenia following BMT has been reduced by the use of growth factor, and the routine use of potent prophylactic antibiotics and antiviral agents has reduced the incidence of infec-tion, unusual or resistant CNS infections continue to arise, often creating difficult treatment choices. The diagnosis is usually made on neurologic imaging and supported by CSF examination and microbiologic studies (ANTONINI et al. 1998). Fungi are the most common causes of brain abscesses in patients after BMT. Post transplant meningitis due to bacterial or viral infections is another cause of CNS morbidity (GALLARDO et al. 1996).

22.2.1
Fungal Infections

Aspergillus species (Fig. 22.1) remains a major prob-lem in BMT patients, with a mortality rate of 95% to 100% (MASCHKE et al. 1999; DE MEDEIROS et al. 2000). Invasive CNS aspergillosis is becoming much more common, largely because of the increased number of immunosuppressed patients. It accounts for 30 to 50% of CNS infections (COLEY et al. 1999; OPENSHAW and SLATKIN 1999; DE MEDEIROS et al. 2000; GUERMAZI et al. 2003). The major cause of inva-sive CNS aspergillosis is BMT, but intensive chemo-therapeutic regimens and the use of corticosteroids also play a role. In most cases, invasive aspergillosis develops in the paranasal sinuses and in the lungs, and secondarily spreads hematogenously to the brain (MIAUX et al. 1995; DELONE et al. 1999).

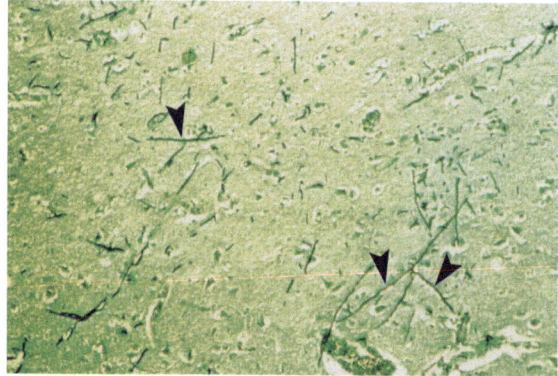

Fig. 22.1. Microscopic view of *Aspergillus fumigatus* (Grocott stain, ×250) shows granulocytes and branched fungal hyphae (*arrowheads*). (With permission from [GUERMAZI et al. 2003])

Imaging of cerebral aspergillosis may present dif-ferent patterns depending on the lesion's age and the immunologic status of the patient (Fig. 22.2) (MIAUX et al. 1994; YUH et al. 1994; MIAUX et al. 1995). The anatomic distribution and radiologic appearance of this vasculopathy-mediated septic infarction is signifi-cantly different from other infarcts and from primary cerebritis or abscess (DELONE et al. 1999). Characteris-tic involvement of the basal nuclei and thalami is fre-quent, indicating that the lenticulostriate and thalamo-perforator arteries are involved (DELONE et al. 1999; GUERMAZI et al. 2003). Corticomedullary involvement is also common, as are neostriatal, thalamic, callosal, or brain stem disease. These lesions present as poorly defined, hypodense lesions with little or no mass effect and faint or no contrast enhancement on CT scans (MIAUX et al. 1995; COLEY et al. 1999). MR imaging detects many more lesions than CT. The additional lesions detected on MR imaging are subcortical and smaller (up to 1 cm diameter) with no enhancement compare to those detected by CT (Fig. 22.3) (MIAUX et al. 1995). On proton density and T2-weighted MR images, lesions present an intermediate signal-inten-sity (isointense to white matter) within a surrounding hyperintense area. As found on autopsies performed shortly after the last MR scans, the intermediate signal intensity center of the lesions could represent areas of coagulative fungal necrosis. These non-enhancing white matter lesions are most conspicuous on proton density and T2-weighted MR images. Fluid-attenu-ated inversion-recovery (FLAIR) MR images are also useful, particularly as fast FLAIR is more sensitive than fast spin-echo T2 for detecting radiologically subtle opportunistic infections. As these lesions are septic infarctions, diffusion-weighted MR images may also be useful for detecting early lesions (DELONE et al. 1999). These lesions are hypointense on T1-weighted MR images (MIAUX et al. 1995). The rare, subtle T1 shortening may represent the petechial hemorrhage often seen in the evolution of an infarct. Absence of contrast enhancement may indicate absence of inflam-matory response related to corticosteroid therapy and to the immunocompromised status (MIAUX et al. 1995; GUERMAZI et al. 2003). Other MR findings correspond to the intravascular enhancement sign and the menin-geal enhancement sign seen in early cerebral infarction. Indications of meningeal enhancement sign are seen only with large infarcts involving a significant portion of a cerebral artery. There is no indication of intravas-cular enhancement in small infarctions restricted to the basal ganglia (MIAUX et al. 1995; DELONE et al. 1999). There is contrast enhancement, as expected in infarc-tion, in less severely immunocompromised patients

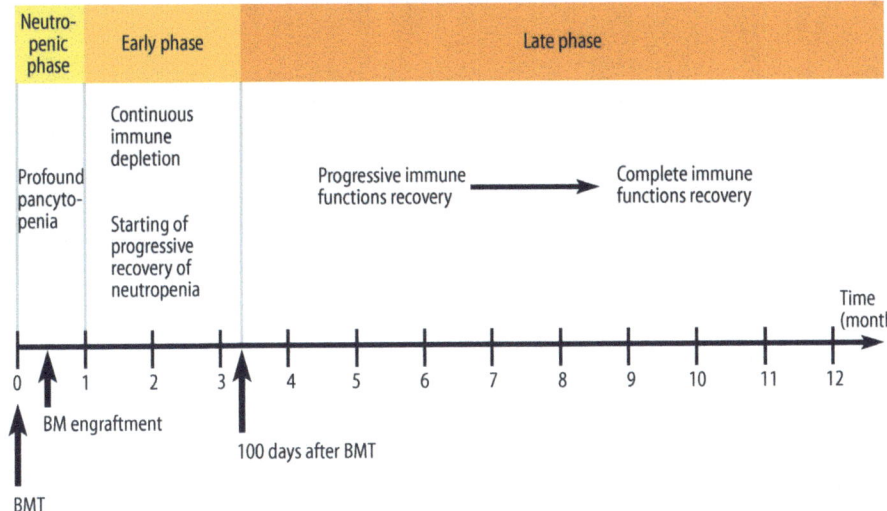

Fig. 22.2. Immune status evolution after bone marrow transplantation. (With permission from [Guermazi et al. 2003])

with prolonged illness who recover. Ring or nodular-enhancing lesions are rare. The presence of true ring or nodular enhancement, consistent with abscess or granuloma formation, indicates that the host defense system is able to isolate or encapsulate the offending organisms, and argues against the aggressive form of cerebral aspergillosis. In a bone marrow transplant recipient who survived, there was progression within several weeks from an infarct to a granuloma (Miaux et al. 1994). The granuloma appeared as a hypointense peripheral rim on T2-weighted MR images that enhances after gadolinium administration (Fig. 22.4) (Miaux et al. 1995). Follow-up imaging studies of long-term survivors indicate that small lesions can be successfully treated, leaving virtually no residual imaging abnormality.

Localized aspergillosis involvement of the spinal cord is exceedingly rare. When Aspergillus involves the spinal cord, hyphae extend into the spinal cord substance, and demyelinating changes and vacuolation are observed. Indeed, blood vessels of the spinal cord are filled with the dichotomously branching Aspergillus with a thrombus-like appearance. MR imaging shows enlargement of the spinal cord that is hypointense on T1-weighted images and hyperintense on long-repetition-time weighted images. Usually, a diffuse intramedullary edema appears as a diffuse hyperintensity within the swelling spinal cord. The MR imaging findings are very similar to those of the typical cerebral lesions and consistent with a medullary infarct. Contrast-enhanced MR imaging shows no enhancement or a mild peripheral contrast enhancement as is usual with medullary infarct (Fig. 22.5) (Guermazi et al. 2002).

CNS infection with Candida albicans is infrequent, occurring in 3% of BMT patients with systemic infection (Openshaw and Slatkin 1999). Patients tend to be clinically asymptomatic and imaging studies are normal (de Medeiros et al. 2000). A case report of Candida encephalitis described multiple intermediate signal intensity lesions within a surrounding hyperintensity on T2-weighted MR images; they were hypointense on T1-weighted MR images, and demonstrated ring enhancement after contrast administration. The lesions were located within the basal ganglia and cerebellum (Maschke et al. 1999). Candida is less likely than Aspergillus to cause fatal compromise of the CNS. Indeed, CNS candidosis as a cause of death is rare (de Medeiros et al. 2000).

Other very rare fungal infections are Cryptococcus neoformans (Gallardo et al. 1996; Openshaw and Slatkin 1999), Pseudallescheria boydii (Fig. 22.6) (Vazquez et al. 2002), Torulopsis glabrata (Gallardo et al. 1996), and Fusarium sp. (Bleggi-Torres et al. 1996). The latter may be confused with Aspergillus in tissue sections, and can only be diagnosed by culture (Bleggi-Torres et al. 1996).

22.2.2
Bacterial Infections

Bacterial abscess and meningitis are unusual since antimicrobial prophylaxis early in the transplant course is effective, and patients usually do not die of CNS problems (Coley et al. 1999; de Medeiros et al. 2000). Organisms responsible for bacterial infections are Staphylococcus aureus, Staphylococcus epidermi-

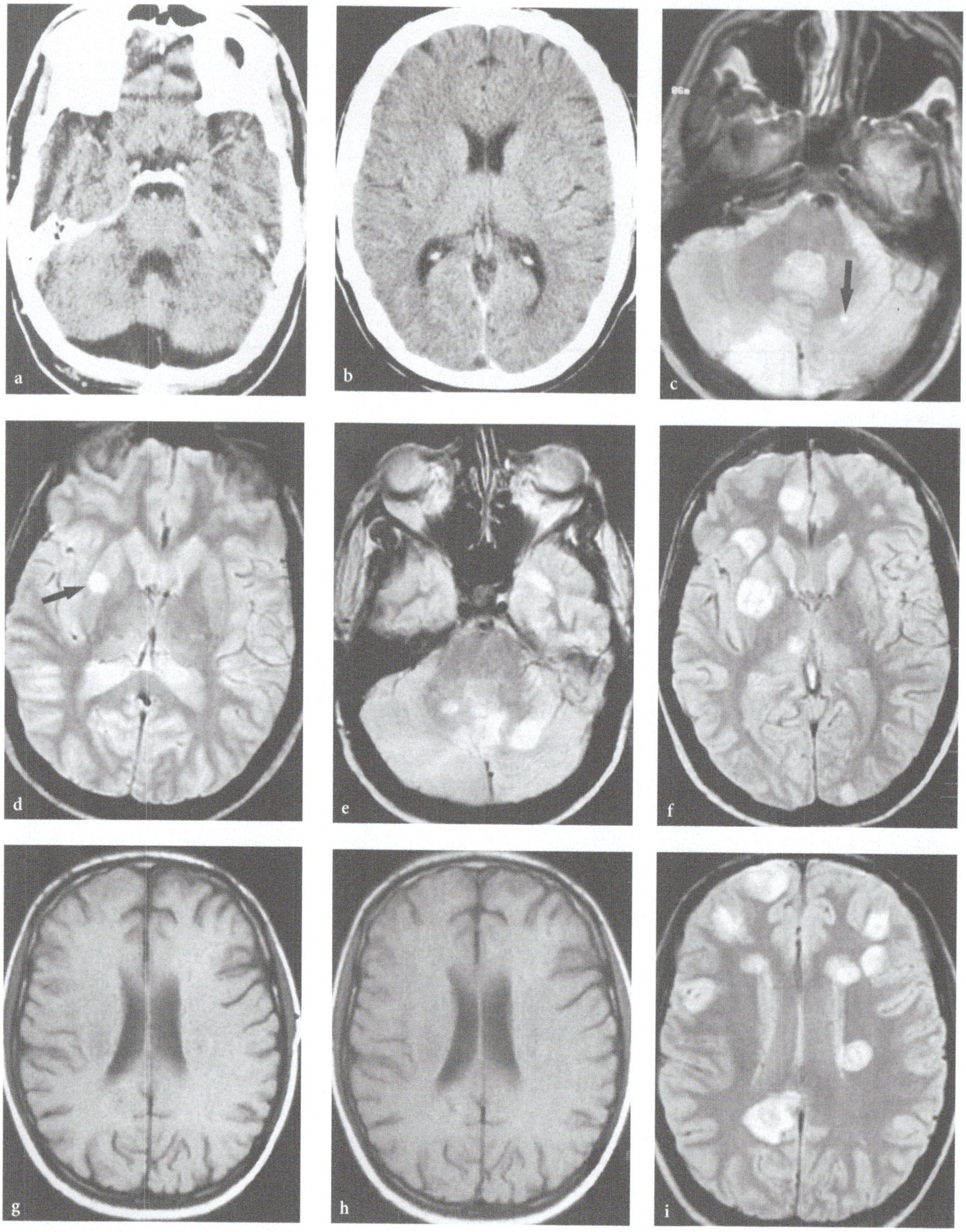

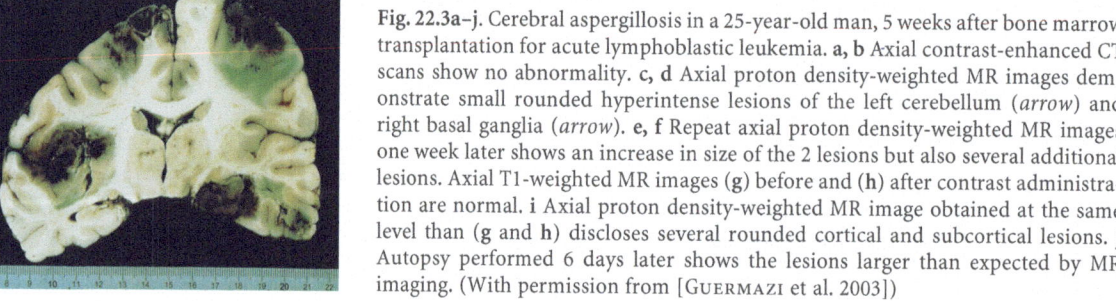

Fig. 22.3a–j. Cerebral aspergillosis in a 25-year-old man, 5 weeks after bone marrow transplantation for acute lymphoblastic leukemia. **a, b** Axial contrast-enhanced CT scans show no abnormality. **c, d** Axial proton density-weighted MR images demonstrate small rounded hyperintense lesions of the left cerebellum (*arrow*) and right basal ganglia (*arrow*). **e, f** Repeat axial proton density-weighted MR images one week later shows an increase in size of the 2 lesions but also several additional lesions. Axial T1-weighted MR images (**g**) before and (**h**) after contrast administration are normal. **i** Axial proton density-weighted MR image obtained at the same level than (**g** and **h**) discloses several rounded cortical and subcortical lesions. **j** Autopsy performed 6 days later shows the lesions larger than expected by MR imaging. (With permission from [Guermazi et al. 2003])

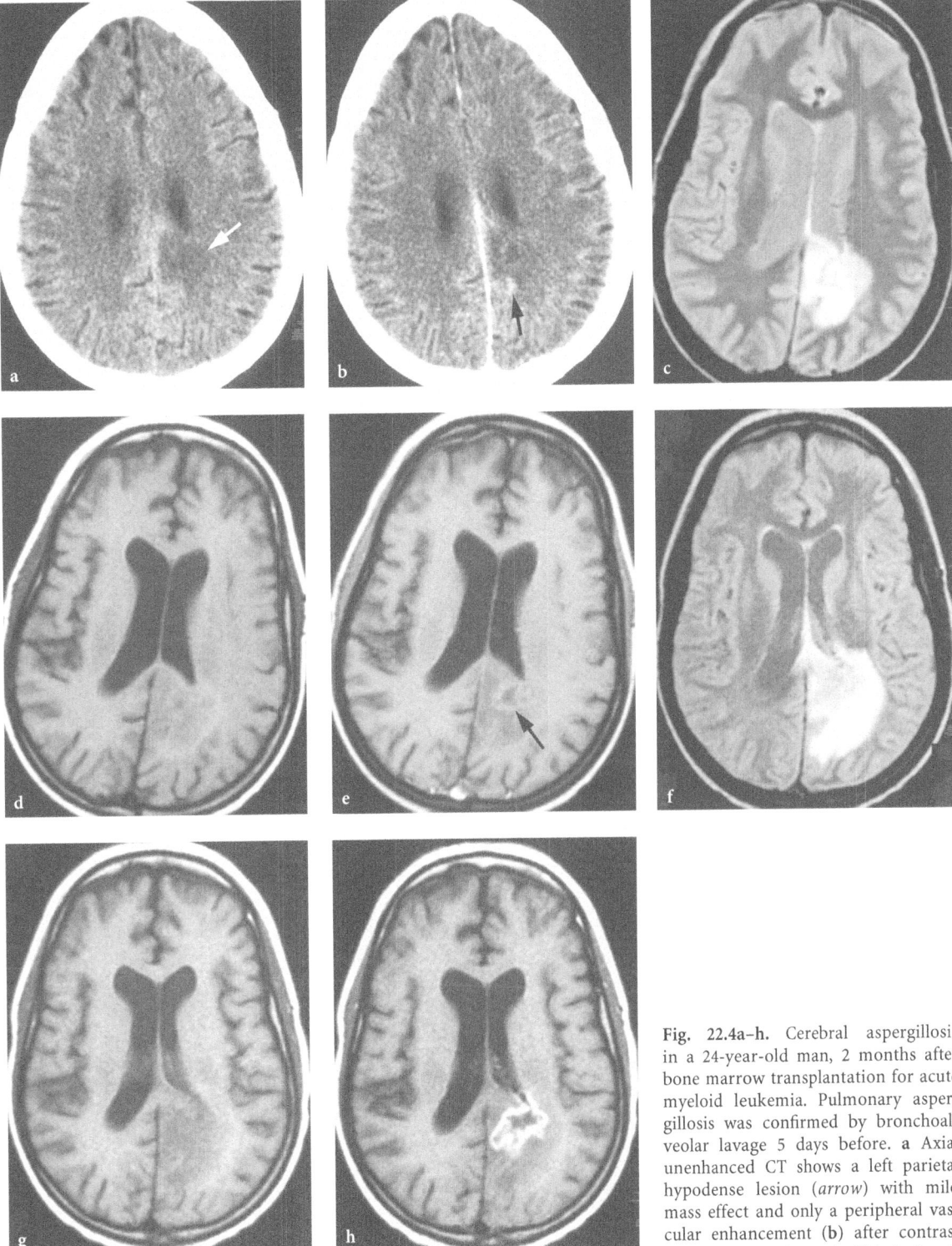

Fig. 22.4a–h. Cerebral aspergillosis in a 24-year-old man, 2 months after bone marrow transplantation for acute myeloid leukemia. Pulmonary aspergillosis was confirmed by bronchoalveolar lavage 5 days before. **a** Axial unenhanced CT shows a left parietal hypodense lesion (*arrow*) with mild mass effect and only a peripheral vascular enhancement (**b**) after contrast administration (*arrow*). This lesion is best seen on (**c**) axial proton density-weighted MR image. **d** Axial unenhanced T1-weighted MR image shows the lesion with poor conspicuity. **e** There is a mild enhancement on axial contrast-enhanced T1-weighted MR image (*arrow*). Patient was receiving antimycotic treatment. Repeat MR imaging 7 weeks later shows an increase in size of the left parietal lesion on axial (**f**) proton density and (**g**) unenhanced T1-weighted MR images. **h** Axial contrast-enhanced axial T1-weighted image shows irregular rim enhancement within the lesion that corresponds to granuloma. (With permission from [GUERMAZI et al. 2003])

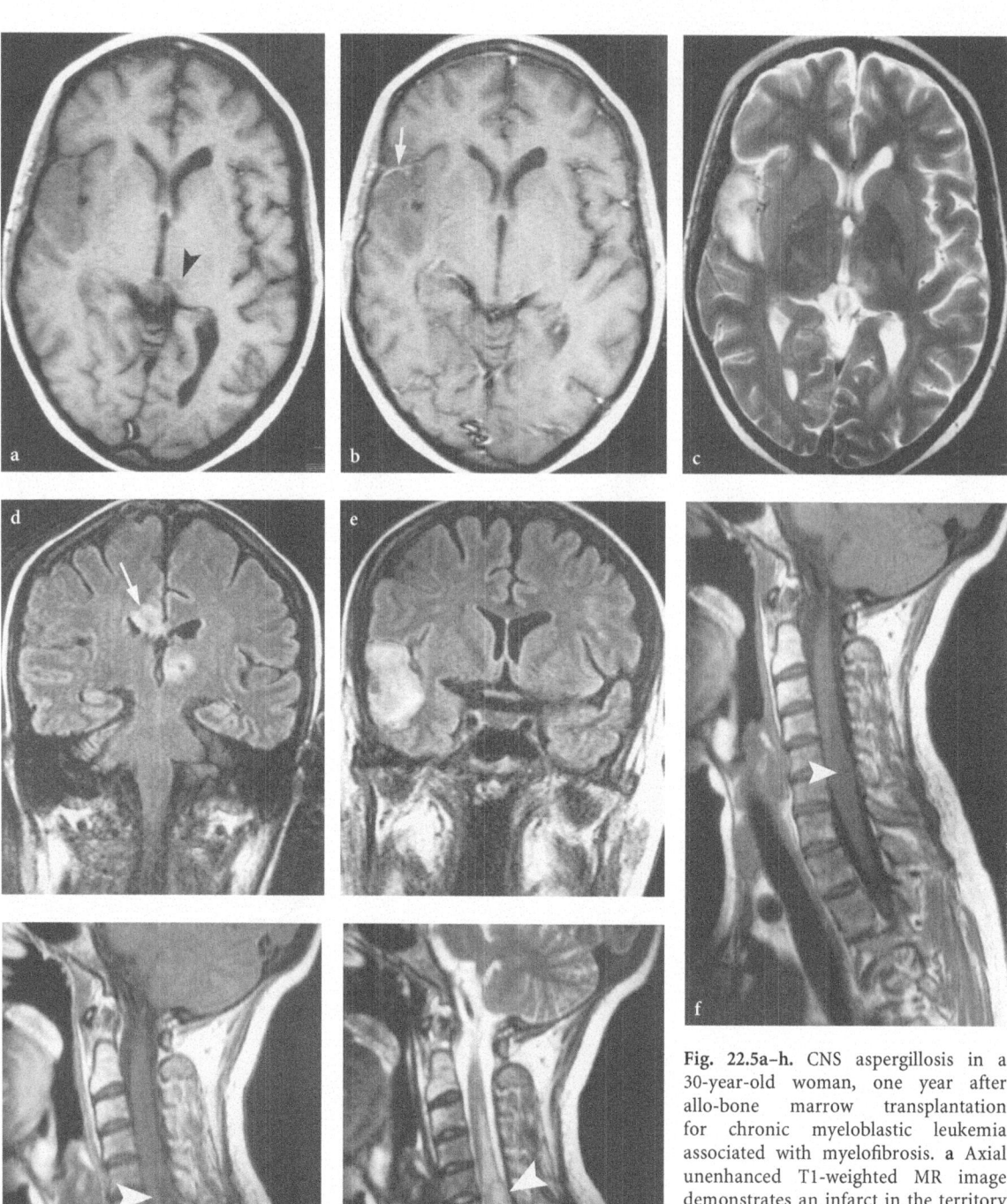

Fig. 22.5a–h. CNS aspergillosis in a 30-year-old woman, one year after allo-bone marrow transplantation for chronic myeloblastic leukemia associated with myelofibrosis. **a** Axial unenhanced T1-weighted MR image demonstrates an infarct in the territory of the right middle cerebral artery. There is also a small hypointense area within the left thalamus (*arrowhead*). **b** There is only a mild contrast enhancement of the adjacent meninges (*arrow*). **c** Axial fast spin-echo T2-weighted MR image shows a mild hyperintensity within the territory of the right middle cerebral artery and also the left thalamus. **d, e** Coronal fluid-attenuated inversion-recovery MR images show better sensitivity for the right middle cerebral artery and the left thalamus infarcts, and also demonstrate another lesion within the genu of the corpus callosum (*arrow*). **f** Sagittal unenhanced T1-weighted MR image of cervical spine shows fusiform enlargement of the cervical cord with an intramedullary hypointense lesion (*arrowhead*). **g** There is a mild peripheral contrast enhancement after contrast administration (*arrowhead*). **h** Sagittal T2-weighted MR image shows the intramedullary lesion to be hyperintense and located posteriorly (*arrowhead*). There is also a diffuse hyperintensity within the swelling spinal cord corresponding to intramedullary edema. (With permission from [GUERMAZI et al. 2002])

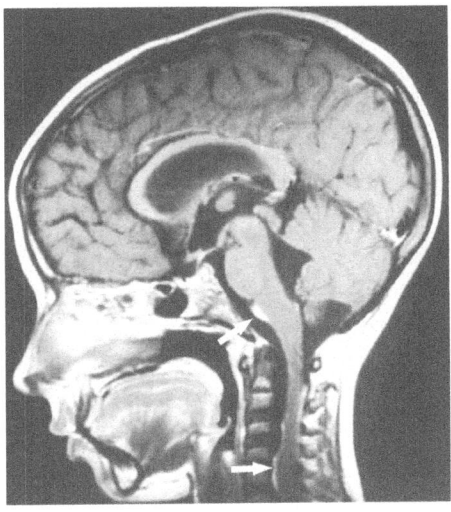
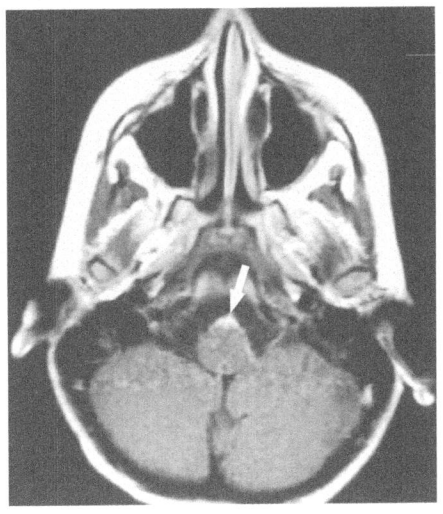

Fig. 22.6a,b. Fungal meningitis due to *Pseudallescheria boydii* in an 8-year-old girl being treated for a cervicothoracic neuroblastoma. She later developed acute myeloid leukemia and during chemotherapy and bone marrow transplantation presented with persistent headaches and fever. **a** Sagittal and (**b**) axial contrast-enhanced TI-weighted MR images show nodular enhancing leptomeningeal lesions along the brainstem and spinal cord (*arrows*). The opportunistic fungus was identified at cerebrospinal fluid culture, and antifungal therapy was intensified with administration via an Ommaya reservoir. However, the patient developed hydrocephalus and eventually died. (With permission from [VAZQUEZ et al. 2002])

dis (OPENSHAW and SLATKIN 1999; DE MEDEIROS et al. 2000), *Listeria monocytogenes* (LONG et al. 1993; COLEY et al. 1999; OPENSHAW and SLATKIN 1999), *Streptococcus pneumoniae* (D'ANTONIO et al. 1992), *Klebsiella pneumoniae* (ABRAHAM et al. 1997), *Diplococcus pneumoniae, Corynebacterium* (MOHRMANN et al. 1990), and *Pseudomonas* (COLEY et al. 1999). Imaging, when performed, may demonstrate brain abscesses and/or purulent meningeal infiltrates (COLEY et al. 1999; BLEGGI-TORRES et al. 2000; DE MEDEIROS et al. 2000).

Stomatococcus mucilaginosus, formerly *Micrococcus mucilaginosus* or *Staphylococcus salivarius*, is a component of the normal oral flora of humans and also may colonize the respiratory tract. It may involve the CNS in the setting of hematologic malignancy accompanied by chemotherapy-induced neutropenia (GUERMAZI et al. 1995; GOLDMAN et al. 1998). *S. mucilaginosus* is recovered from blood prior to discovery of the CNS infection in 62% of cases (GOLDMAN et al. 1998). CT and MR imaging are either normal (GOLDMAN et al. 1998) or demonstrate choroid plexus involvement (GUERMAZI et al. 1995; OPENSHAW and SLATKIN 1999). Indeed, they show abnormal enlargement of the choroid plexus and intense enhancement. There is enhancement of the ependyma with or without periventricular white matter edema adjacent to the involved choroid plexus (Fig. 22.7) (GUERMAZI et al. 1995; GOLDMAN et al. 1998). Although some patients respond to a

regimen of intravenous vancomycin, the addition of intrathecal vancomycin appears to be of benefit in some cases (GOLDMAN et al. 1998).

Mycobacterial infections are relatively uncommon in BMT patients despite their severe immunosuppression (OPENSHAW and SLATKIN 1999). GVHD and T-cell depletion appear to increase the risk of developing these infections (MARTINO et al. 1996). *Mycobacterium tuberculosis* is the cause (MARTINO et al. 1996; OPENSHAW and SLATKIN 1999; CAMPOS et al. 2000). Only a minority of patients with extrapulmonary tuberculosis has coexisting active pulmonary disease. Involvement may be parenchymal (CAMPOS et al. 2000) or meningeal (MARTINO et al. 1996). Imaging of parenchymal abscesses demonstrates contrast-enhanced lesions with surrounding edema (CAMPOS et al. 2000). Specific treatment may be curative even in advanced cases (MARTINO et al. 1996).

22.2.3
Parasitic Infections

Brain infection with *Toxoplasma gondii* following BMT is an uncommon but often fatal complication (MELE et al. 2002). It is usually the result of reactivation of latent infection in patients with positive serology prior to BMT (DEROUIN et al. 1986; DE MEDEIROS et al. 2001) rather than primary infection (MELE et

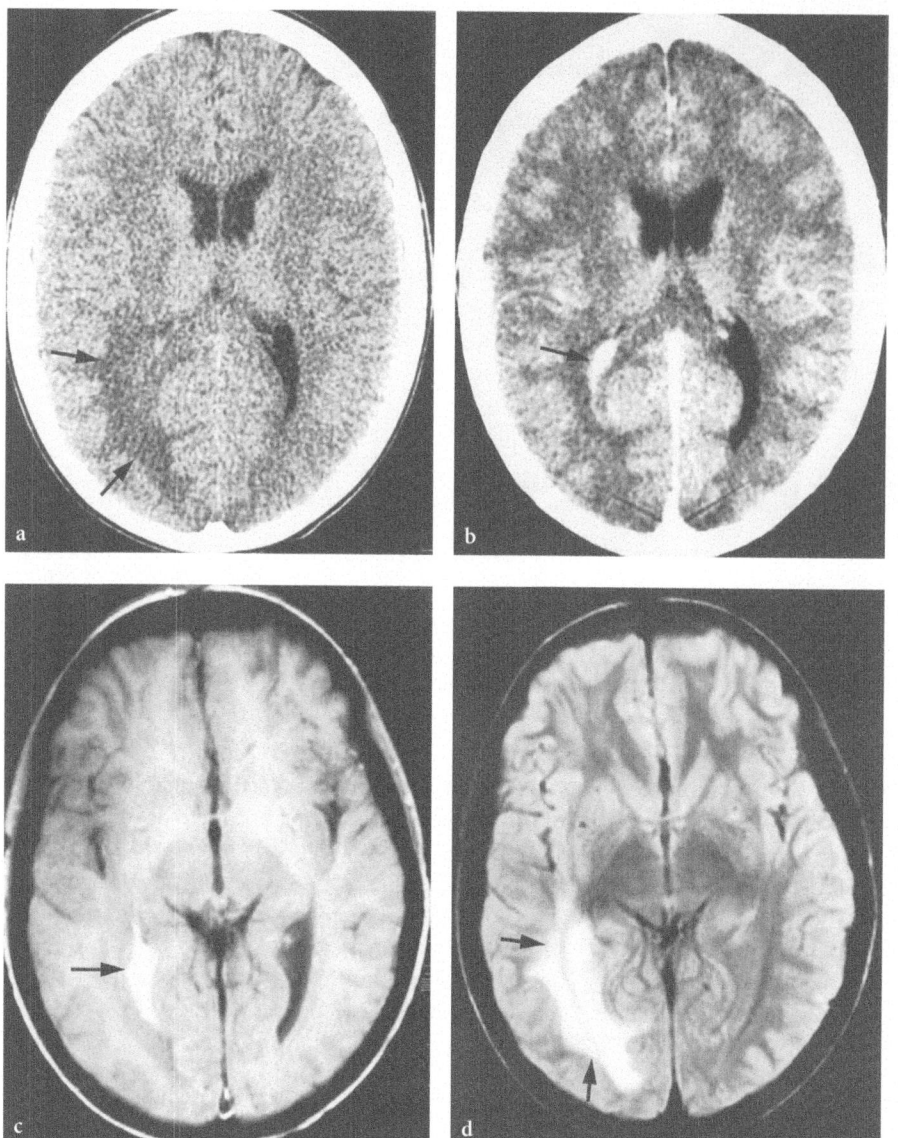

Fig. 22.7a–d. Choroid plexitis due to *Stomatococcus mucilaginosus* in a 14-year-old boy with severe neutropenia after second induction chemotherapy for acute myeloid leukemia. **a** Axial unenhanced CT scan shows right periventricular edema (*arrows*) and asymmetric size of trigones of lateral ventricles attributable to mass effect of edema. Axial contrast-enhanced (**b**) CT scan and (**c**) spin-echo T1-weighted MR image demonstrate marked enhancement of an enlarged right choroid plexus and adjacent parenchyma (*arrow*). **d** Axial proton density-weighted MR image shows hyperintense changes (*arrows*) in the periventricular brain parenchyma attributable to edema. (With permission from [Guermazi et al. 1995])

al. 2002). It is much more amenable to therapy and usually seen during the early post-transplantation period after engraftment (Openshaw and Slatkin 1999). Toxoplasmosis in BMT recipients usually occurs within 6 months of BMT, with the peak at 2–3 months (Derouin et al. 1992). The infection is often disseminated, but isolated cerebral toxoplasmosis have been described (Mele et al. 2002). The radiological appearances of cerebral toxoplasmosis in BMT recipients vary, as does the intensity of contrast enhancement, which has no typical pattern. Indeed, lesions may be unique or multiple, variable in size, and with or without focal hemorrhage (Bleggi-Torres et al. 1999; Dietrich et al.

2000). The most common locations of the lesions are the subcortical white matter, basal ganglia, and cerebellum (Maschke et al. 1999). On T1-weighted MR images, lesions are hypointense, isointense (not visible), or hyperintense indicating hemorrhage (Maschke et al. 1999). After contrast administration, some lesions may not enhance (Brinkman et al. 1998; Maschke et al. 1999; Dietrich et al. 2000), some may enhance while others in the same patient do not (Fig. 22.8) (Picardi et al. 1998), and some may enhance intensively (Tefferi et al. 1998; Dietrich et al. 2000). MR imaging also may show abnormal meningeal and superficial parenchymal enhancement corresponding to meningoencepha-

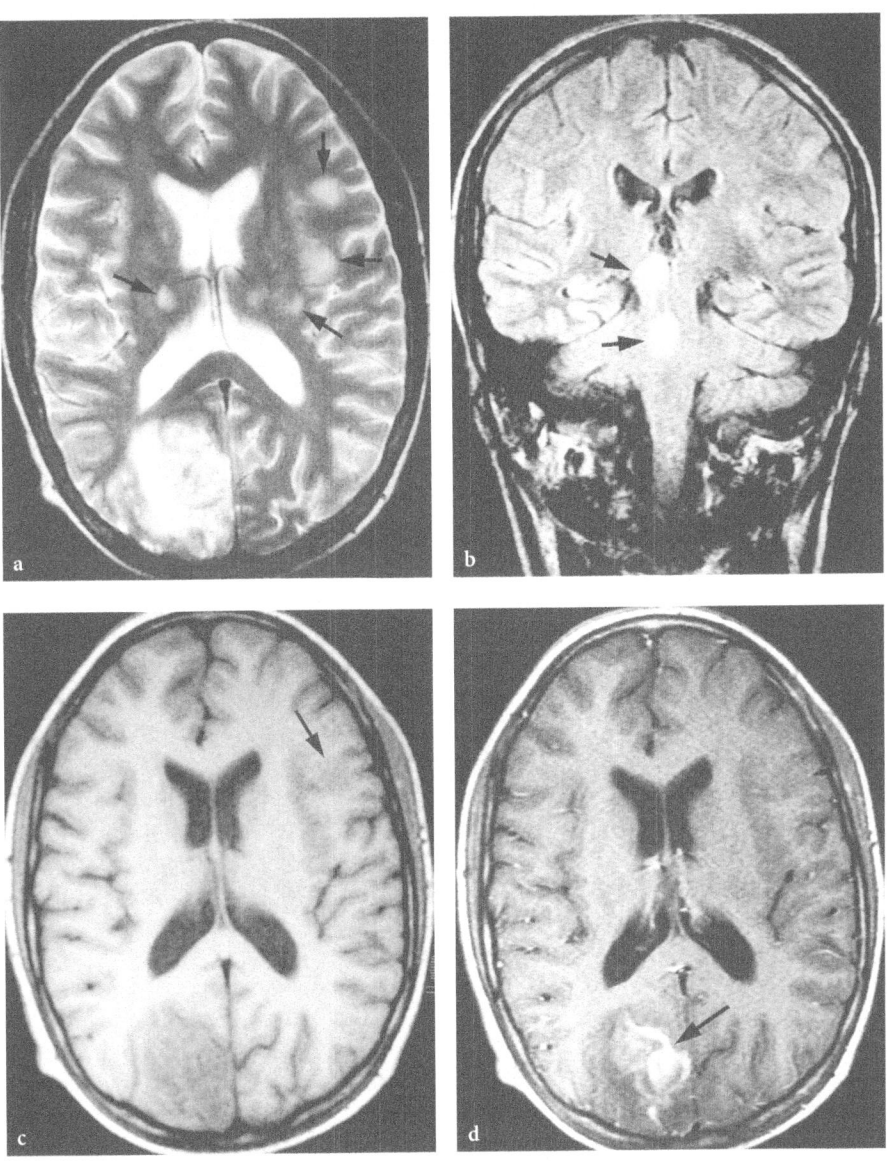

Fig. 22.8a–d. Cerebral toxoplasmosis in an 18-year-old man, eight months after bone marrow transplantation for chronic myeloblastic leukemia. **a** Axial fast spin-echo T2-weighted MR image shows a huge right parietooccipital heterogeneous hyperintense lesion and also several other smaller supratentorial hyperintense lesions (*arrows*). **b** Coronal fluid-attenuated inversion-recovery MR image shows two other lesions within the brain stem (*arrows*). **c** Axial unenhanced T1-weighted MR image shows hypointensities within the right parietooccipital lobe and subcortically within the left frontoparietal lobe (*arrow*). **d** Axial contrast-enhanced spin-echo T1-weighted MR image shows marked enhancement of the right parietooccipital lesion (*arrow*) with adjacent parenchymal edema. There is no enhancement of the other lesions seen on (**a**) T2-weighted and (**b**) fluid-attenuated inversion-recovery MR images. This patient was given a specific treatment and he is still alive 16 months later.

litis (SEONG et al. 1993). Detection and follow-up of hyperintense areas on proton density and T2-weighted MR images may be of value in determining the presence and the activity of brain lesions (DIETRICH et al. 2000). Based on the appearance of the lesions on MR images, Maschke et al (MASCHKE et al. 1999) divided patients with brain toxoplasmosis after BMT into two groups: the first with edema but no contrast enhancement, the second with lesions of typical MR imaging appearance with the exception of frequent hemorrhagic transformation, probably due to reduction in platelet numbers. The first group had a significantly shorter latency between BMT and onset of CNS infection (mean 45 days versus 180

days, P = 0.02) and received a significantly higher daily dose of corticosteroids as treatment for GVHD (P = 0.01). MR imaging is more sensitive for demonstrating lesions undetectable by CT (TEFFERI et al. 1998). Nevertheless, a definite diagnosis of cerebral toxoplasmosis cannot be made from MR imaging alone because other cerebral infections, especially cerebral aspergillosis, may also demonstrate multiple lesions. Biopsy is necessary (TEFFERI et al. 1998; DIETRICH et al. 2000).

Localized toxoplasmosis involvement of the spinal cord is very rare, with only a few case reports in the literature. In one patient with multiple myeloma who underwent autologous peripheral stem-cell transplantation, CNS MR imaging revealed an isolated enlargement of the thoracic spinal cord by a solitary intramedullary lesion localized at the right side of T7 level. The lesion was hyperintense on proton-density and T2-weighted MR images, and enhanced strongly after gadolinium administration (STRAATHOF et al. 2001). Two other patients have been reported with lethal disseminated toxoplasmosis with spinal cord involvement. They were treated for acute-type adult T-cell leukemia/lymphoma: the first had peripheral blood stem-cell transplantation (NAKANE et al. 2000) and the second intravenous and intrathecal chemo-therapy (MACIEL et al. 2000).

22.2.4
Viral Infections

Viral infections are much less common than fungal and bacterial infections, probably because of the widespread use of antiviral drugs (COLEY et al. 1999; OPENSHAW and SLATKIN 1999). After BMT the main pathogens are herpes viruses. They tend to occur in a characteristic temporal sequence: at one week, Herpes simplex virus type 1; 2–3 weeks, Epstein-Barr virus (EBV); 7 weeks, cytomegalovirus (CMV); and 5 months after BMT, Varicella zoster virus (VZV) (COLEY et al. 1999). Although viruses often reactivate with immunosuppression, clinical symptoms rarely occur (OPENSHAW and SLATKIN 1999). CMV infection occurs in approximately 50% of all recipients of allogeneic bone marrow trans-plants and is more frequent in CMV-seropositive patients than in CMV-seronegative patients (SEO et al. 2001). CMV may cause encephalitis with bilateral and symmetrical hypodense areas on CT (CORDONNIER et al. 1983; GRAUS et al. 1996) or ven-triculoencephalitis with progressive hydrocephalus (SEO et al. 2001). VZV infection is frequent following both autologous and allogenic BMT. The CNS infec-tion is considered the most serious infection and it is frequently encountered in seropositive pre-BMT patients (HAN et al. 1994). In a case of a 13-year-old boy with a two-year diagnosis of acute lymphocytic leukemia and who developed VZV leukoencephalitis, brain CT showed subtle white matter changes. MR imaging showed multiple, widespread plaque-like lesions with subtle enhancement, rapid and nearly complete demyelination, and associated hemorrhage (LENTZ et al. 1993). In another case of a 23-year-old patient with BMT for chronic myelogenous leukemia and with a cerebrospinal fluid positive for herpes zoster meningoencephalitis, MR imaging showed bilateral, slightly asymmetrical lesions within the deep gray nuclei and central cerebral white matter (COLEY et al. 1999). Herpes viruses may also involve the spinal cord after BMT. There are two cases in the literature; a 42-year-old man with fatal VZV transverse myelitis after allogenic BMT for chronic myelogenous leukemia (LADRIERE et al. 2001), and a 16-year-old boy with EBV transverse myelitis after unrelated BMT that was successfully treated by ganciclovir and CMV hyperimmune globulin. The same treatment was successful for another case of presumed EBV meningoencephalitis following BMT (DELLEMIJN et al. 1995). In the case of EBV trans-verse myelitis, MR imaging reveals widening of the cervical and thoracic spinal cord with diffuse hyper-intensity on T2-weighted MR images correspond-ing to intramedullary edema. There were several nodular enhancements within the spinal cord after gadolinium administration representing the inflam-matory foci. Follow-up MR imaging 2 months later was normal (GRUHN et al. 1999).

Human herpes virus-6 encephalitis is very rare after BMT. Only two cases have been reported after allogeneic BMT, the first for CML (COLEY et al. 1999) and the second for relapsed Hodgkin disease (DROBYSKI et al. 1994). On MR imaging, the herpetic encephalitis selectively involves the mesial temporal lobe structures, which appear hyperintense on T2-weighted MR images, and spares the reminder of the brain (COLEY et al. 1999).

Before the AIDS epidemic, progressive multifocal leukoencephalopathy caused by polyomavirus JC (DNA virus) was rarely associated among several diseases with chronic lymphocytic leukemia and Hodgkin disease, or after BMT or treatment with fludarabine (SEONG et al. 1996; SAUMOY et al. 2002). Its pathogenesis is still obscure mainly because the route by which the JC virus enters the brain has not been determined (SEONG et al. 1996). Imaging studies are suggestive, showing an asymmetrical distribution of lesions within the white matter, lack of significant mass effect, and incomplete or absent contrast enhancement (SEONG et al. 1996; COLEY et al. 1999). These lesions are hypodense on CT and hyperintense on T2-weighted MR images (SAUMOY et al. 2002).

A case of acute disseminated encephalomyelitis, a parainfectious or postvaccination syndrome, was reported six weeks after para-influenza infection in a 37-year-old patient after BMT for chronic myeloid leukemia. The CT was normal, but MR imaging dem-onstrated demyelination with multifocal hyperin-tense areas on T2-weighted images visible within the pons, centrum semiovale, posterior periventricular and subcortical white matters bilaterally but asymmetrically. These lesions were more obvious on the FLAIR MR images. There were also multiple hyperintense areas on T2-weighted MR images within the thoracic spinal cord. The patient was successfully treated with high-dose corticosteroid and intravenous immunoglobulin (AU et al. 2002).

22.3
Cerebrovascular Side Effects

Cerebrovascular complications may consist of either hemorrhage or thrombosis. They are, with the infections, the most severe complications after BMT (GALLARDO et al. 1996; NEVO and VOGELSANG 2001). They are often multifactorial. Indeed, in addition to abnormal or decreased platelets, multiple coagulopathies are common, with abnormally elevated or decreased coagulation factors. Chemotherapeutic agents may aggravate disease-related coagulopathies, and radiation therapy damages arterial walls. As a result, for a given patient, a particular coagulation imbalance can result in a hypercoagulable state or, alternatively, a bleeding diathesis (GINSBERG and LEEDS 1995).

22.3.1
Hemorrhage

Prolonged thrombocytopenia leads to catastrophic and fatal cerebral hemorrhage (NEVO et al. 1998; COPLIN et al. 2001; NEVO and VOGELSANG 2001; BLEGGI-TORRES et al. 2002). It can be explained by a chemotherapy or radiation-induced decrease in megakaryocytes, or alternatively by immunologic (autoimmune) or drug-induced mechanisms of platelet destruction or dysfunction, particularly L-asparaginase (PRIEST et al. 1980; URBAN and SAGER 1981; PRIEST et al. 1982; MOHRMANN et al. 1990). Coagulopathies may be secondary to disseminated intravascular coagulation or decreased production of coagulation factors (MOHRMANN et al. 1990). Intracranial bleeding has also been reported in children treated with radiation therapy. Patients with the acute promyelocytic leukemia are at particular risk for massive intracerebral hemorrhage, which represents the cause of more than 60% of deaths from that disease (GINSBERG and LEEDS 1995).

Hemorrhage may occur in a variety of locations, i.e., subdural, subarachnoid, and intracerebral (CROSLEY et al. 1978; BLEGGI-TORRES et al. 2002). Almost a fifth of patients have more than one type of hemorrhage.

Usually, CT is more accurate than MR imaging, and shows subarachnoid, intraparenchymal, and/or intraventricular hemorrhage. The lesions range in size from petechiae and focal subarachnoid bleeds, to large, massive, necrotic masses distorting adjacent neural structures (MOHRMANN et al. 1990; BLEGGI-TORRES et al. 2000). Frontal, parietal, and occipital lobes are frequently involved (BLEGGI-TORRES et al. 2002).

The characteristic course of large intraparenchymal bleeding is the abrupt onset of a neurological deficit followed by rapid depression of the sensorium and brainstem signs. Intracerebral hematomas are lethal complications after BMT and appear in about 75% of patients (Fig. 22.9) (POMERANZ et al. 1994).

Subdural hematomas are not rare in patients with leukemia or after BMT (POMERANZ et al. 1994; HENTSCHKE et al. 1999). They are often bilateral, small in size (MOHRMANN et al. 1990; POMERANZ et al. 1994; GRAUS et al. 1996; HENTSCHKE et al. 1999), and symptomatic in only 25% of cases (POMERANZ et al. 1994). The frequency of subdural hematoma after BMT varies. It is surprising that Graus et al found 65% of the CNS hemorrhages to be subdural, most commonly occurring in AML patients receiving autologous BMT. In this series, only platelet refractoriness correlated with the increased risk of subdural hematoma (GRAUS et al. 1996), but pathogenesis is thought to be multifactorial, such as malignancy, thrombocytopenia, heparin treatment, and intrathecal treatment (POMERANZ et al. 1994; HENTSCHKE et al. 1999). Clinically, patients often present with headache (HENTSCHKE et al. 1999). CT scan shows hypodense collection when the subdural hematoma is chronic, hyperdense when hematoma is acute, and isodense when the hematoma is subacute (Fig. 22.10) (POMERANZ et al. 1994). The diagnosis of symptomatic subdural hematoma may be missed initially because CT scans may be normal at the onset of symptoms. MR imaging is more sensitive in detecting small subdural collections. The subdural hematomas may be treated with conservative measures (GRAUS et al. 1996), but surgical drainage is often necessary (HENTSCHKE et al. 1999). The clinical outcome is relatively benign (POMERANZ et al. 1994).

In leukemic patients with coagulopathies, especially thrombocytopenia, diagnostic lumbar punctures may result in spinal subdural or epidural hematoma (GINSBERG and LEEDS 1995; VAZQUEZ et al. 2002).

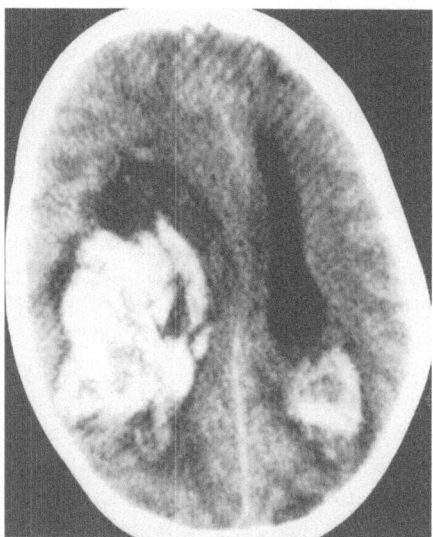

Fig. 22.9. Fatal intracranial hemorrhage in a 6-year-old boy after bone marrow transplantation for acute lymphoblastic leukemia. He presented with rapid sudden headache and was given depression of the sensorium. He has a thrombocytopenia of less than 20,000/mm^3. Axial unenhanced CT scan shows massive bilateral cerebral parenchymal hematomas with surrounding edema. There are signs of pressure on the right lateral ventricle, which is no more visible and side-to-side shift of the midline structures.

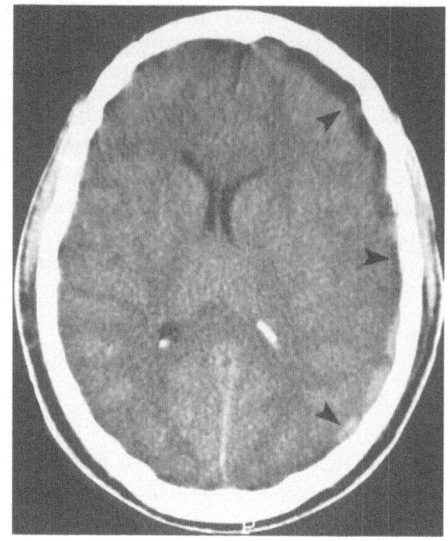

Fig. 22.10. Subdural hematoma in a 35-year-old man with thrombocytopenia (62,000/mm^3) after bone marrow transplantation for non-Hodgkin lymphoma. He had a sudden headache with neurologic deterioration. Axial unenhanced CT scan shows a left-sided hypo and hyperdense subdural collection with marked mass effect, corresponding to mixed chronic and acute subdural hematoma (*arrowheads*).

22.3.2
Thrombosis and Ischemia

Patients with hematological malignancies, and leukemia in particular, are at increased risk for cerebral infarction (GINSBERG and LEEDS 1995). Ischemic strokes in patients treated for hematological malignancies may be embolic from non bacterial thrombotic endocarditis or infective endocarditis, or thrombotic in association with disseminated intravascular coagulation and other hypercoagulable states (MOHRMANN et al. 1990; PATCHELL 1994). The association of high-dose chemotherapy – including high-dose cis-platinum and L-asparaginase – with the hypercoagulable state is known to be related to ischemic strokes (PRIEST et al. 1980; PRIEST et al. 1982). Endarteritis may occur and may be associated with Aspergillus infection, disseminated VZV infection (GRAUS et al. 1996; COPLIN et al. 2001), or with radiation therapy. Infarcts are infrequent in patients undergoing allogeneic and autologous BMT (GALLARDO et al. 1996); nevertheless, a new cause of cerebral infarction, cerebral angiitis after BMT, has recently been reported (TAKATSUKA et al. 2000). This angiitis might be a neurological manifes-

tation of GVHD (PADOVAN et al. 1999) or secondary to CMV infection (TAKATSUKA et al. 2000). The clinical presentation may not be straightforward, and other lesions such as infection or CNS leukemia can present as a stroke like syndrome (GINSBERG and LEEDS 1995). Infarcts vary in size (MOHRMANN et al. 1990). CT may be diagnostic, but MR imaging is more sensitive for diagnosing cerebral infarction. Often more than one area is involved, and infarcts grow contiguously over period of days. This is probably due to the acute onset of cerebrovascular occlusions (COPLIN et al. 2001).

Dural venous thrombosis is more frequently seen in leukemic patients. Besides coagulopathies related to the underlying disease, infiltration of the CNS, and chemotherapeutic drugs particularly L-asparaginase may produce hemostatic effects and favor dural venous sinus thrombosis. Indeed, L-asparaginase is known to produce hypofibrinogenemia, prolonged clotting time, and multiple clotting factor deficiencies (GINSBERG and LEEDS 1995). Vincristine therapy has a well-known venous toxicity at the site of injection, and may play a role in the occurrence of dural venous thrombosis. Coagulopathies have also been reported with prednisone therapy in leukemic patients (GINSBERG and LEEDS 1995). Clinically, dural sinus thrombosis symptoms can mimic CNS infiltration with headache, papilledema, and/or lethargy. Imaging is necessary for diagnosis and differentiation. When patients with hematological malignancy are imaged, especially leukemic patients, the dural sinuses should always be carefully examined. Potential signs of sinus thrombosis on CT are abnormal hyperdensity of a sinus on unenhanced images, abnormal central hypodensity of a sinus on postcontrast images (so-called empty delta-sign), and/or excessive meningeal collaterals. MR imaging is more sensitive than CT and may show abnormal signal intensity or a lack of flow void within the dural sinuses. Venous infarcts may complicate sinus occlusion (Fig. 22.11) (FEINBERG and SWENSON 1988; GINSBERG and LEEDS 1995; GUERMAZI et al. 1997). In equivocal cases, flow sensitive gradient-echo

techniques or MR venography may be necessary (GINSBERG and LEEDS 1995). Conventional cerebral phlebography is no longer performed because of its attendant risks, particularly in such fragile patients.

22.4
Metabolic Side Effects

Metabolic disorders may develop in patients treated for hematological malignancies. The causes of encephalopathy are electrolyte disorders, hypoxia due to pneumonitis, hepatic failure following veno-occlusive disease and/or drug toxicity-related uremia. Imaging is not necessary since the diagnosis is clinical (SNIDER et al. 1994; GRAUS et al. 1996; OPENSHAW and SLATKIN 1999). In a prospective

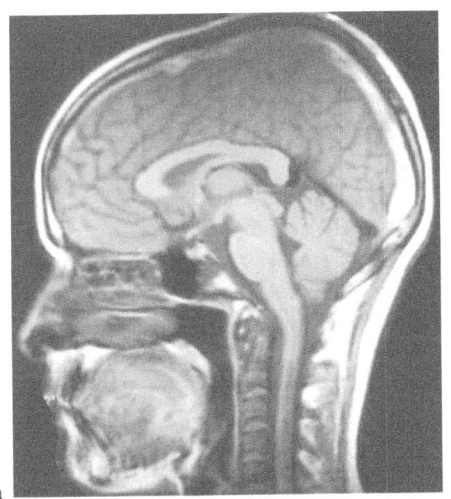

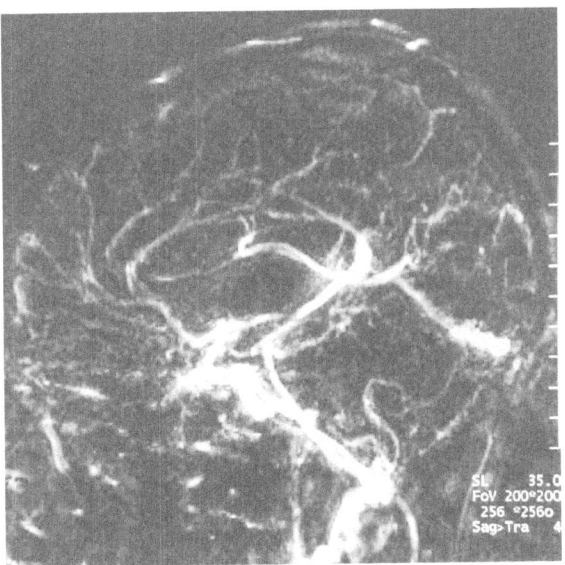

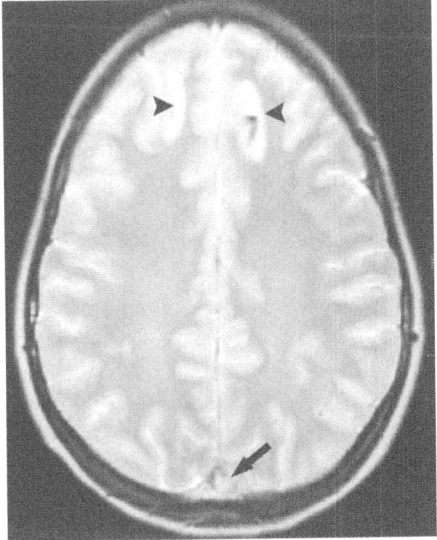

Fig. 22.11a–c. Dural venous thrombosis in a 20-year-old woman treated for acute lymphoblastic leukemia with L-asparaginase. She presented with headaches and seizures. a Sagittal T1-weighted MR image shows hyperintensity along the superior sagittal sinus, a finding suggestive of a subacute thrombus. b Axial T2-weighted MR image shows frontal subcortical hemorrhagic lesions (*arrowheads*) and hyperintensity within the sagittal sinus (*arrow*), which is suggestive of lack of flow. c Sagittal phase-contrast MR venogram shows thrombosis involving the superior sagittal sinus. Anticoagulant therapy was started, and follow-up MR imaging showed resolution of the thrombosis. (With permission from [VAZQUEZ et al. 2002])

study, systematic CT scans were all normal for metabolic encephalopathy (ANTONINI et al. 1998).

On the other hand, imaging, especially MR imaging, is diagnostic for central pontine myelinolysis. This condition is characterized by regions of demyelination throughout the brain that are most prominent in the pons (MILLER et al. 1988). This condition is commonly found in alcoholics (MILLER et al. 1988), and sometimes in both adults and children with leukemia (CROSLEY et al. 1978) and Hodgkin disease (CHINTAGUMPALA et al. 1993).It is also found in other patients with electrolyte abnormalities, most notably hyponatremia that has been corrected rapidly, as it was for a 65-year-old woman with myeloproliferative disorder (MILLER et al. 1988). The pathogenesis of central pontine myelinolysis is still controversial and considered multifactorial, i.e., metabolic, toxic, and/or vascular (CROSLEY et al. 1978; CHINTAGUMPALA et al. 1993). CT sometimes demonstrates hypodensity within the pons, but often the scan is negative. MR imaging is far more sensitive and demonstrates relatively symmetric hypointensity T1-weighted and hyperintensity T2-weighted mostly within the base of the pons; T2-weighted MR images are more sensitive. Lesions have an oval shape on sagittal images, a bat-wing configuration on coronal images, and various shapes on axial images. Indeed, the pons may be triangular, trident (Fig. 22.12),

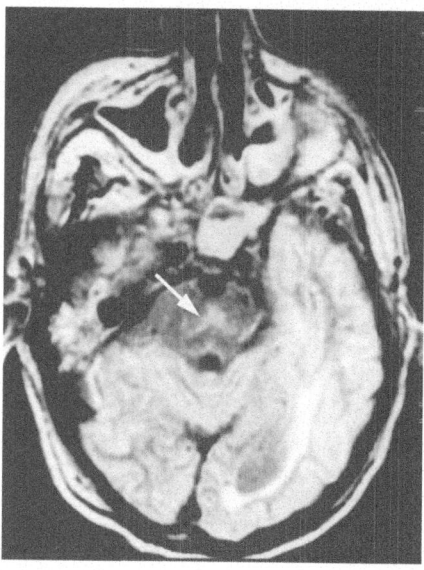

Fig. 22.12. Central pontine myelinolysis in a 34-year-old woman treated for a myeloproliferative disorder. The patient has also a hyponatremia of 94 mEq/l that was corrected to 130 in 45 hours. Axial proton density-weighted MR image shows a hyperintense trident-shaped through the midpons (*arrow*). There is no associated extrapontine abnormality.

trapezoid, round or oval. Associated extrapontine myelinolysis may be visible in the periventricular white matter, basal ganglia, and/or corticomedullary junction bilaterally. The persistence of the pontine lesion as usually seen on MR imaging, particularly if the initial lesion is large, is not correlated with clinical improvement. On the other hand, the lesion may resolve completely, especially if it is very small (MILLER et al. 1988). The imaging findings, especially MR imaging, are not specific and may be encountered in brain stem glioma, after radiation therapy, in multiple sclerosis, after brain stem infarct, and also chemotherapy, namely cyclophosphamide therapy (MILLER et al. 1988).

22.5
Toxic Side Effects

Aggressive treatment of acute leukemia, particularly for preventing or treating CNS relapse, may directly result in neurotoxicity (GINSBERG and LEEDS 1995), as is the case with the more effective classes of immunosuppressants for preventing or treating GVHD. Many chemotherapeutic drugs are known to be associated with neurologic syndromes that may be potentiated by cranial irradiation (GINSBERG and LEEDS 1995). In most cases, neurological disorders and imaging abnormalities are transient, and patients fully recover after treatment is discontinued. In some instances however, neurotoxicity is a significant problem, as a definitive lesions may occur in the white matter, particularly in disseminating necrotizing leukoencephalopathy, with persistent neurological disabilities, limiting the usefulness of potentially effective agents (GINSBERG and LEEDS 1995). It must be stressed that distinguishing chemotherapy-related neurotoxicity from other CNS complications of hematological malignancies could be difficult; therefore, imaging and clinical data must be carefully analyzed prior to discontinuing therapy.

22.5.1
Posterior Reversible Encephalopathy Syndrome

Posterior reversible encephalopathy syndrome (PRES) is a recently proposed clinico-radiological entity with several causes (HINCHEY et al. 1996). There is still some disagreement about the proper name of this syndrome. Different authors use different terms, such as "hypertensive encephalopathy"

(SCHWARTZ 1996), "reversible posterior leukoencephalopathy syndrome" (HINCHEY et al. 1996), or "reversible posterior cerebral edema syndrome" (DILLON and ROWLEY 1998). Since, the syndrome does not represent a true leukoencephalopathy, a better term is "posterior reversible encephalopathy syndrome" (CASEY et al. 2000; PROVENZALE et al. 2001).

The clinical symptoms and neuroradiologic findings are typically indistinguishable among the cases of PRES, regardless of underlying cause (CASEY et al. 2000). Clinically, it is characterized by prodromal headache, visual disturbance or blindness, speech and motor disturbances, altered mental status, and/or seizures (PATCHELL 1994; GINSBERG and LEEDS 1995; CASEY et al. 2000; PROVENZALE et al. 2001). The most common causes of PRES are hypertensive encephalopathy (SCHWARTZ et al. 1992), preeclampsia/eclampsia (CASEY et al. 2000), and also several drugs including cyclosporin A, tacrolimus, and rarely cisplatin and vindesine (HERAN et al. 1990; APPIGNANI et al. 1996; ITO et al. 1998; CASEY et al. 2000; MORI et al. 2000; PROVENZALE et al. 2001). Cyclosporin A and recently tacrolimus (formerly FK 506) therapy is mainly indicated after BMT for chronic maintenance immunosuppression and for the treatment of acute BMT rejection (PATCHELL 1994; MORI et al. 2000). Fifteen to 40% of patients treated with cyclosporine experience neurological side effects (PATCHELL 1994) and 5% cyclosporine encephalopathy (HINCHEY et al. 1996). Cisplatin and vindesine are anticancer drugs used to treat a variety of cancers (ITO et al. 1998), and also used, in association with other antimitotics, for the treatment of lymphomas (HERAN et al. 1990; SEYMOUR et al. 2002). The mechanism of cyclosporin or tacrolimus toxicity is controversial. However, there are clinical and radiographic similarities between cyclosporin or tacrolimus toxicity and eclampsia, a condition of hypertensive encephalopathy. Co-administration of high-dose of methylprednisolone has been reported to be a precipitating factor of cyclosporin/tacrolimus neurotoxicity (MORI et al. 2000).

Imaging studies demonstrate symmetric confluent lesions predominantly within the subcortical white matter that may extend to cortical surface or deep white matter and that typically involve the parietooccipital lobes (Fig. 22.13). An atypical distribution may rarely involve the posterior fossa (Fig. 22.14), corpus callosum, basal ganglia, or frontal/temporal lobes. Unenhanced CT or T1-weighted MR images show decreased density and signal intensity within the parietooccipital regions associated with mild mass effect with sulcal effacement. T2-weighted and, even better, FLAIR MR images show the corresponding foci of hyperintensity, usually involving more than one vascular territory. FLAIR imaging improves the ability to diagnose and detect subcortical and cortical

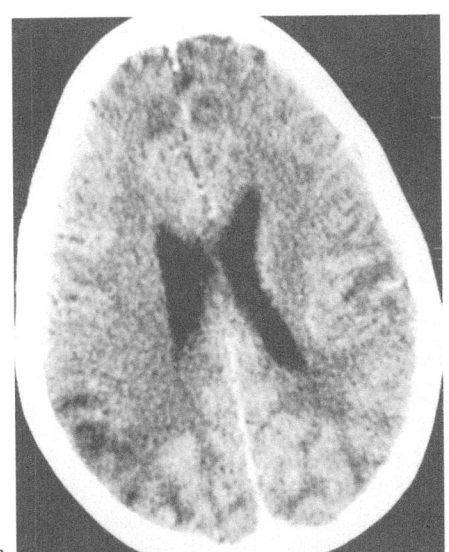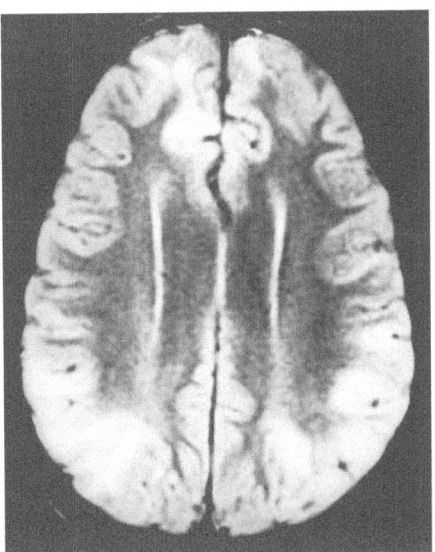

a   b

Fig. 22.13a,b. Cyclosporine neurotoxicity in a 14-year-old boy after bone marrow transplantation for myelodysplasia. He presented with generalized seizures and visual disturbances. **a** Axial contrast-enhanced CT shows multiple subcortical areas of decreased attenuation, predominating in the posterior parietooccipital lobes. **b** Axial proton density-weighted MR image obtained the same day better demonstrates fluffy areas of hyperintensity. MR images returned to normal within one week. Nine years after bone marrow transplantation, the patient is still alive.

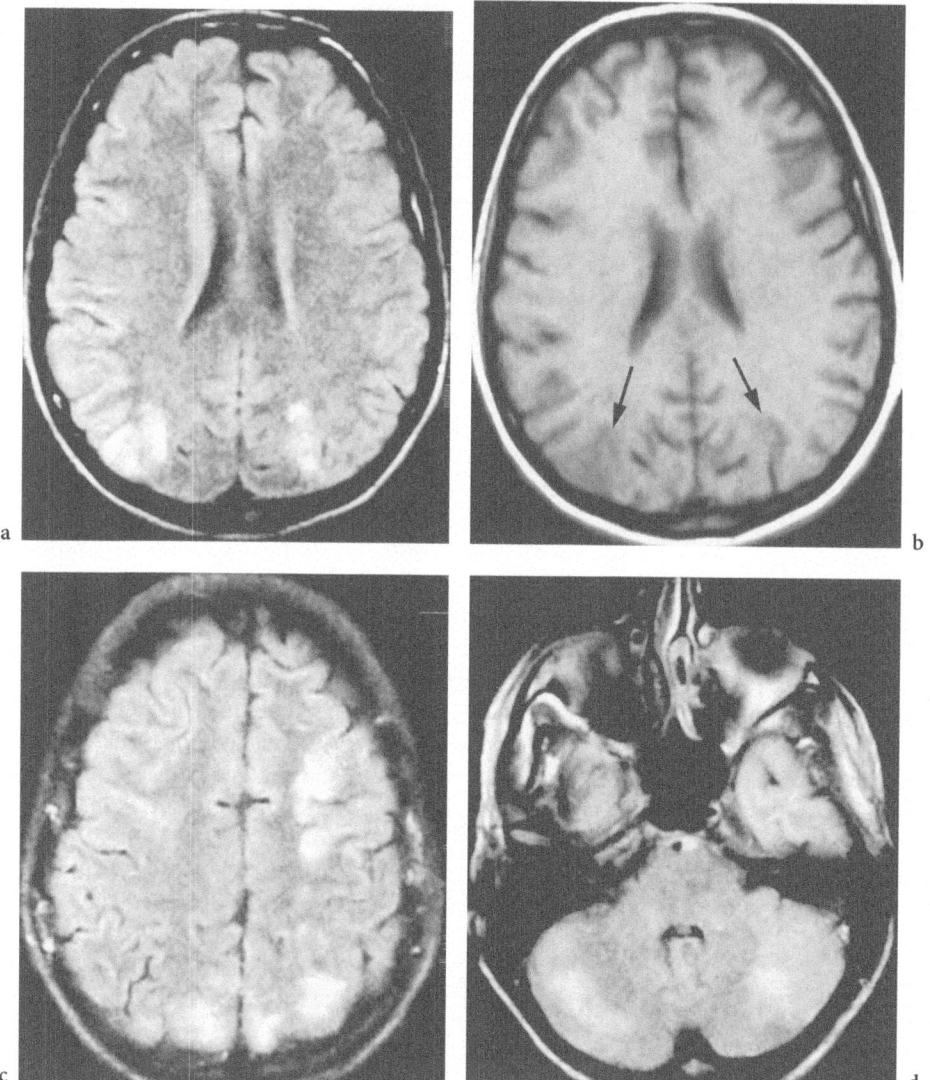

Fig. 22.14a–d. Cisplatin neurotoxicity in a 21-year-old woman treated for acute myeloid leukemia. **a** Axial proton density-weighted MR image shows bilateral hyperintense parietooccipital abnormalities involving the cortex and subcortical white matter, which are more difficult to see as hypointense lesions (*arrows*) on (**b**) axial unenhanced T1-weighted MR image. Axial proton density-weighted MR images at different levels also demonstrate bilateral (**c**) frontal and (**d**) cerebellar hyperintense foci.

lesions (CASEY et al. 2000). After contrast administration, a transient, patchy cortical or leptomeningeal enhancement may rarely be observed, reflecting transient defects in the blood-brain barrier (SCHWARTZ et al. 1992; DILLON and ROWLEY 1998; PROVENZALE et al. 2001). Obviously, MR imaging demonstrates greater extent and conspicuity of lesions than CT. PRES lesions are hypointense or isointense on diffusion-weighted images, indicating that the edema is primarily vasogenic. They are hyperintense on corresponding apparent diffusion coefficient maps, secondary to increased water diffusion (Fig. 22.15)

(SCHWARTZ et al. 1998; PROVENZALE et al. 2001). Transcranial Doppler ultrasound, when performed, shows abnormally elevated cerebral blood flow velocities (SHBAROU et al. 2000).

The pathophysiology of this entity is still incompletely understood and controversial. One early theory suggested that overreaction of brain autoregulation results in reversible vasospasm, which in turn results in potentially reversible ischemia to the brain, especially in vascular border zone areas. Evidence favoring this hypothesis is the large artery vasospasm reported in some cases of preeclampsia and eclampsia. According

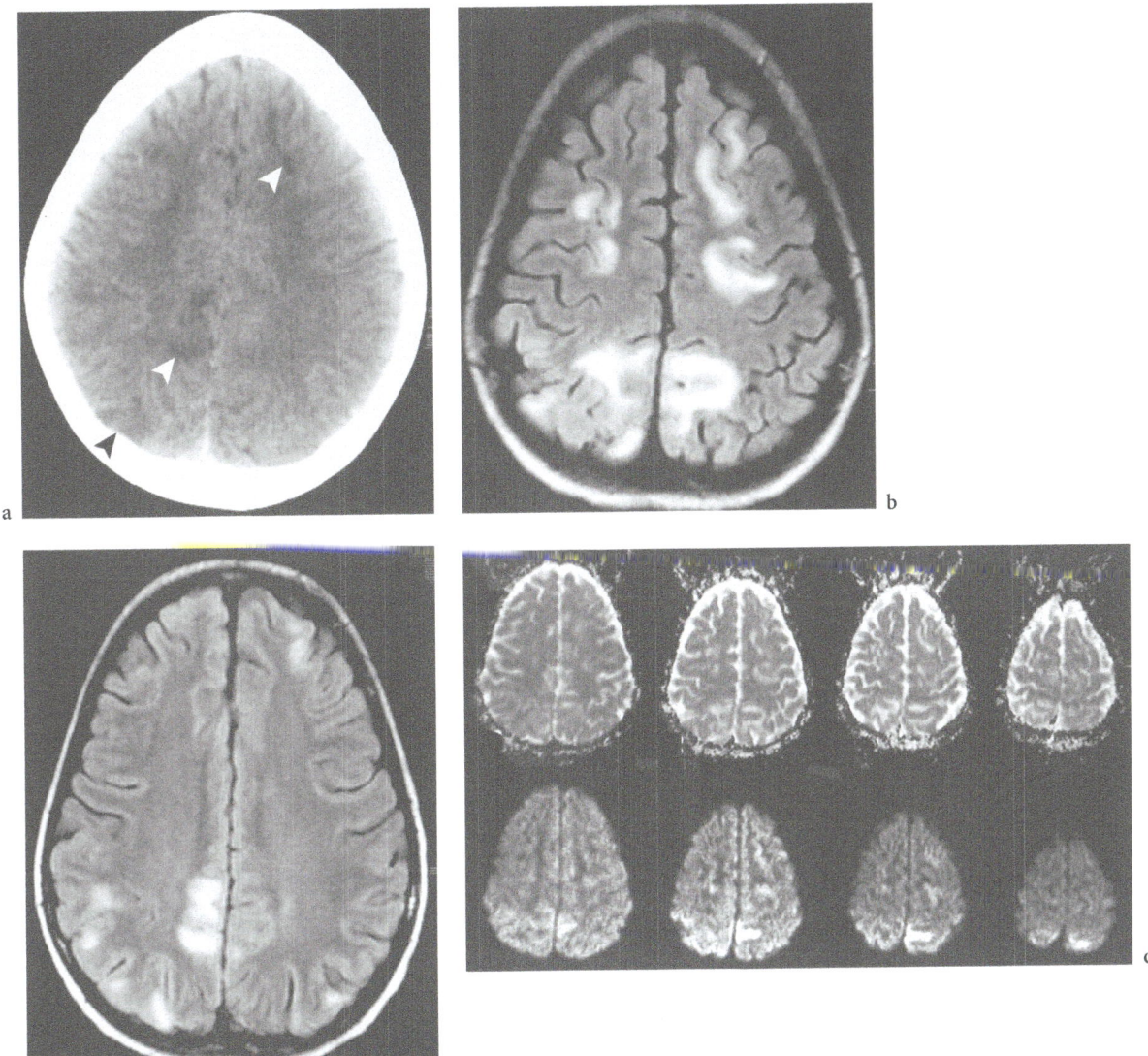

Fig. 22.15a–d. Posterior reversible encephalopathy syndrome in a 12-year-old boy after bone marrow transplantation for acute lymphoblastic leukemia. He presented with a visual disturbances and seizures. The clinical symptoms coincided with arterial hypertension. **a** Axial unenhanced CT scan shows hypodense cortical-subcortical lesions in the frontal and parietal lobes (*arrowheads*). **b, c** Axial fluid-attenuated inversion-recovery MR images show the lesions more clearly. **d** Axial isotropic diffusion-weighted MR images show an elevated apparent diffusion coefficient in regions with the corresponding signal intensity abnormality on T2-weighted MR images. The patient recovered from the neurologic symptoms after blood pressure was controlled, and follow-up MR imaging demonstrated complete resolution of the lesions. (With permission from [VAZQUEZ et al. 2002])

to another hypothesis, favored by most investigators, lesions primarily result from vasogenic edema due to hypertension-induced failure of cerebral autoregulation. Indeed, the brain hyperperfusion is sufficient to overcome the blood-brain barrier, allowing extravasation of fluid, macromolecules, and even red blood cells into the brain parenchyma. Current evidence indicates that both mechanisms are probably associated in PRES, but loss of autoregulation is still considered to be the underlying common pathogenetic mechanism in a number of causes of PRES, including hypertensive encephalopathy and eclampsia (HINCHEY et al. 1996; SCHWARTZ et al. 1998; CASEY et al. 2000; PROVENZALE et al. 2001). Recently, the immune factors were reported to probably play an important etiologic role since the frequency of severe cyclosporin neurotoxicity increases with increasing human leukocyte antigen disparity (ZIMMER et al. 1998).

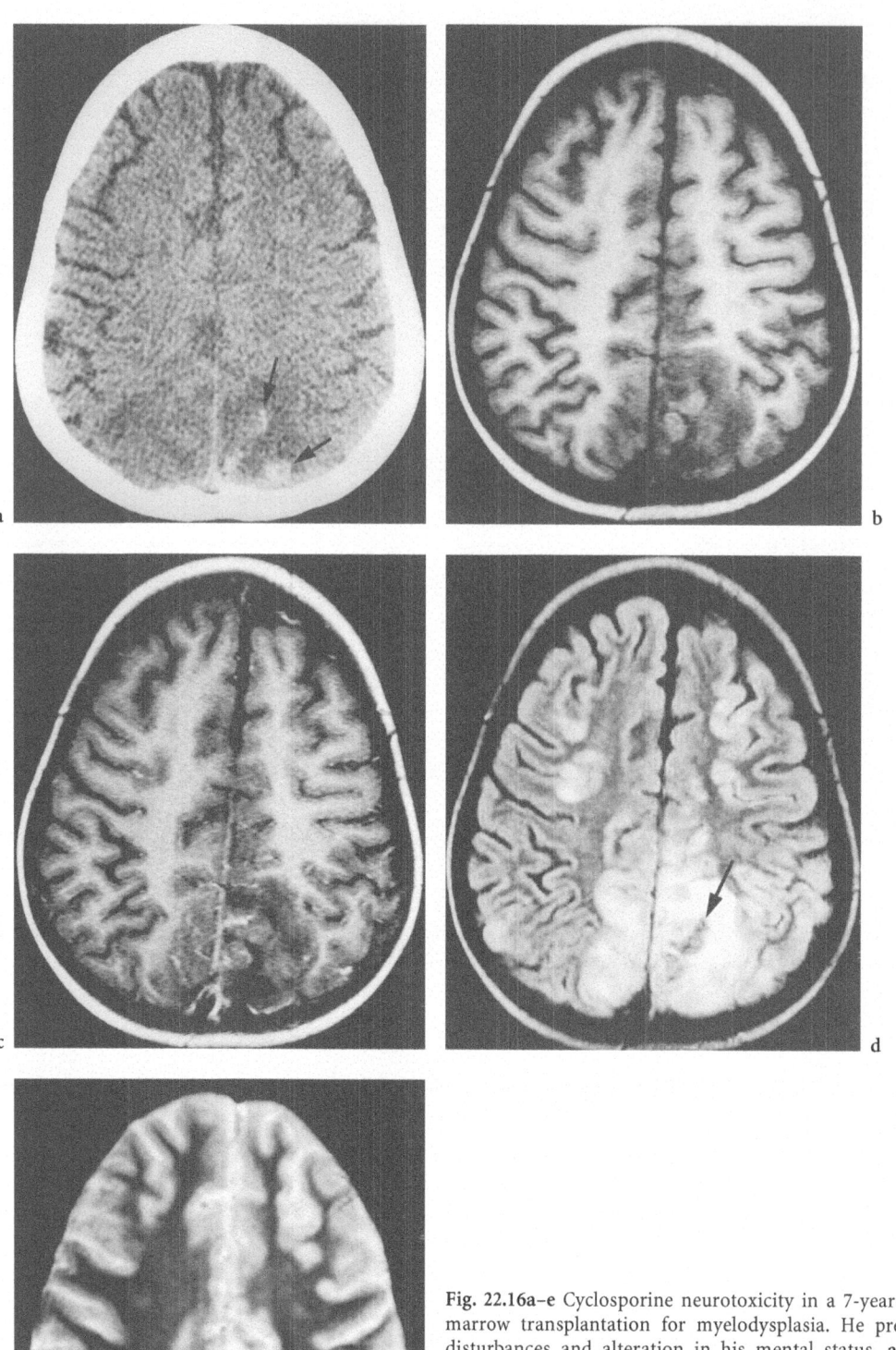

Fig. 22.16a–e Cyclosporine neurotoxicity in a 7-year-old boy after bone marrow transplantation for myelodysplasia. He presented with visual disturbances and alteration in his mental status. **a** Axial unenhanced CT scan shows bilateral parietooccipital hypodensity with hyperdense material within the left lesion (*arrows*). **b** Axial unenhanced T1-weighted MR image shows subtle posterior hypointensity bilaterally, with (**c**) no contrast enhancement. **d** Axial fluid-attenuated inversion-recovery image shows bilateral subcortical areas of hyperintensity in the parietooccipital and also frontal lobes with only minimal cortical involvement. There is a hypointensity (*arrow*) within the left parietooccipital lesion corresponding to an acute hemorrhage and confirmed with (**e**) the gradient-echo T2-weighted MR image.

The treatment for all direct neurotoxic side effects is to decrease the dose or eliminate the drug entirely, if possible. Nearly all of the direct side effects are completely reversible within 1 to 2 weeks as clinical improvement occurs (PATCHELL 1994; GINSBERG and LEEDS 1995; APPIGNANI et al. 1996; ITO et al. 1998; PROVENZALE et al. 2001; TAKAHATA et al. 2001). Nevertheless, occasionally, irreversible findings are seen especially when infarction has occurred (Fig. 22.16). Moreover, some fatal cases of cyclosporin A/tacrolimus encephalopathy have been reported associated with cerebral hemorrhage (SCHWARTZ 1996), transtentorial and tonsillar herniation, and acute or chronic GVHD. In these cases, almost all patients have risk factors of hypertension and become hypertensive, and methylprednisolone was associated with cyclosporin or tacrolimus therapy in all cases (MORI et al. 2000).

22.5.2
Methotrexate

Intrathecal methotrexate is an effective modality for both prophylaxis and treatment of CNS leukemia (GINSBERG and LEEDS 1995; RUBNITZ et al. 1998; KOH et al. 1999), as well as non-Hodgkin lymphoma (ASATO et al. 1992). A variety of neurotoxic effects of methotrexate therapy have been reported and neurotoxicity from intrathecal therapy correlated with CSF concentration of the drug (BLEYER et al. 1973). Low dose intravenous methotrexate causes only occasional and minor neurotoxicity, consisting of headache and dizziness.

Cerebral atrophy is most severe in children treated with intrathecal methotrexate alone or in combination with radiation therapy, in children who are very young at the onset of leukemia, and in children in whom the duration of leukemia is shortest (CROSLEY et al. 1978).

The major progressive and permanent neurological disability usually results from the common combination of intrathecal and intravenous methotrexate, with or without whole brain irradiation (MOHRMANN et al. 1990; KOH et al. 1999). This treatment may lead to progressive encephalopathy (CROSLEY et al. 1978) and finally to a chronic and usually fatal disseminated necrotizing leukoencephalopathy (CROSLEY et al. 1978; GINSBERG and LEEDS 1995) that is variable in size (MOHRMANN et al. 1990). It is characterized by the insidious onset of motor dysfunction, personality changes, lethargy, dementia, and coma (KOH et al. 1999). Risk fac-

tors for developing treatment-related CNS damage include age and meningeal leukemia (PAAKKO et al. 1992). Cases of pure methotrexate encephalopathy have been reported in children with seizures (LOVBLAD et al. 1998). The pathogenesis may result from vasculopathy and/or cerebral edema caused by the treatment (MOHRMANN et al. 1990). Radiation therapy is thought to increase methotrexate toxicity by disrupting the blood-brain barrier (SHALEN et al. 1981). Pathologic changes include multifocal areas of demyelination, coagulative necrosis, glial loss, and axonal swelling in the white matter, mainly centrum semiovale (GINSBERG and LEEDS 1995). The term "disseminated necrotizing leukoencephalopathy" should probably be reserved for the most severe cases since many less severe leukoencephalopathy cases have reversible clinical and radiological findings (ASATO et al. 1992; GINSBERG and LEEDS 1995). CT demonstrates diffuse small foci of decreased attenuation within the periventricular white matter and centrum semiovale that extend by confluence, sometimes with calcifications that may slightly enhance after contrast administration. These calcifications are located subcortically along the U-fibers (SHALEN et al. 1981; LOVBLAD et al. 1998) or within the basal ganglia (GINSBERG and LEEDS 1995). MR imaging is the more sensitive method for early diagnosis (EBNER et al. 1989; ASATO et al. 1992; PAAKKO et al. 1992; SEIDEL et al. 1996) and may show treatment-related leukoencephalopathy changes even before the onset of clinical symptoms (GINSBERG and LEEDS 1995; KOH et al. 1999). It usually reveals multiple symmetric areas within the deep white matter of hypointensity on T1-weighted images, which are best seen as hyperintense on T2-weighted images, and usually without contrast enhancement (Fig. 22.17) (KOH et al. 1999). These lesions, typically with an anterior and posterior periventricular distribution, may rarely enhance after contrast injection (SHALEN et al. 1981; KOH et al. 1999), with a tumor-like pattern in some cases (GINSBERG and LEEDS 1995; KOH et al. 1999). Subcortical white matter, temporal lobes, basal ganglia, thalami, brain stem, and cerebellum are not involved (ASATO et al. 1992). They may or not demonstrate mass effect (SHALEN et al. 1981). With calcifications, susceptibility-sensitive sequences, such as T2-weighted gradient-echo or FLASH sequences might be very helpful (LOVBLAD et al. 1998).

The most emphasized complication is progressive necrotizing myelopathy, also called anterior lumbosacral radiculopathy, which has been reported in patients treated with intrathecal administration of

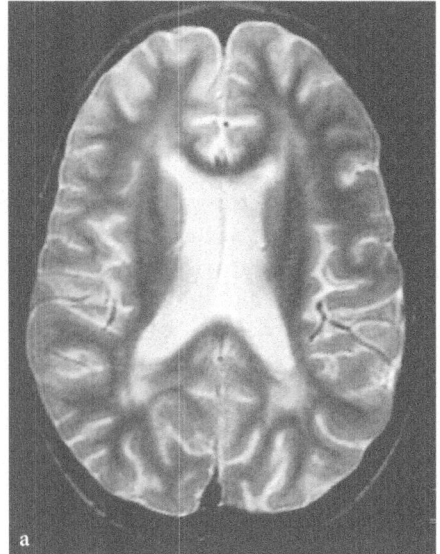 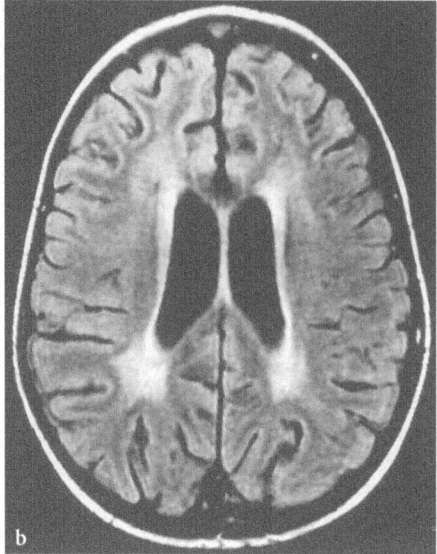

Fig. 22.17a,b. Pure methotrexate leukoencephalopathy in a 6-year-old boy treated for acute lymphoblastic leukemia only with chemotherapy (intravenous and intrathecal methotrexate therapy). He developed progressive neurologic deterioration with motor dysfunction and lethargy. Axial (**a**) T2-weighted and (**b**) fluid-attenuated inversion-recovery MR images show hyperintense symmetrical lesions involving the periventricular white matter. The patient's condition improved, but he was lost to further MR imaging follow-up. (With permission from [Vazquez et al. 2002])

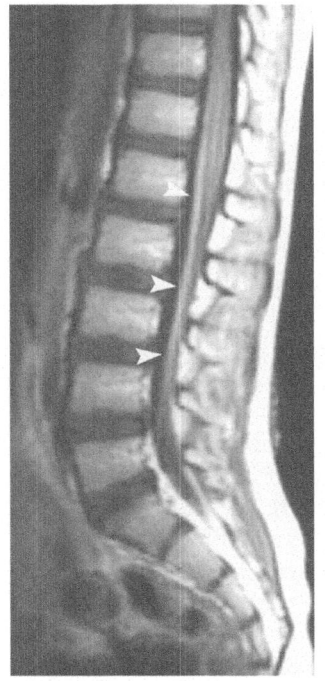

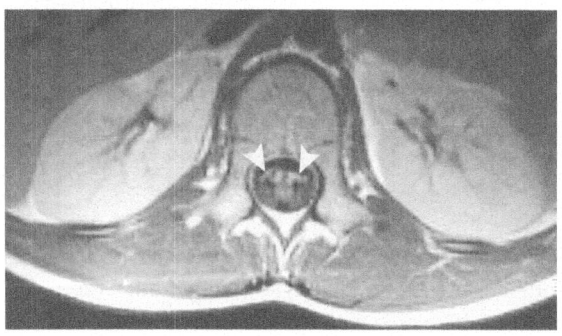

Fig. 22.18a,b. Anterior lumbosacral radiculopathy in a 7-year-old boy with acute lymphoblastic leukemia treated with intrathecal methotrexate. He developed progressive areflexive paraparesis. **a** Sagittal and (**b**) axial contrast-enhanced T1-weighted MR images show selective enhancement of the anterior lumbosacral roots (*arrowheads*). The clinical symptoms improved, and follow-up MR images were normal. (With permission from [Vazquez et al. 2002])

methotrexate (Ginsberg and Leeds 1995; Koh et al. 1999) and/or Ara-C (Koh et al. 1999). Clinically, patients often present with progressive weakness of the legs, incontinence, with or without ascending sensory loss. A rapid progression to complete quadriplegia, brain stem dysfunction, and death can occur in severe cases. MR imaging shows a contrast enhancement of the anterior lumbosacral nerves roots (Fig. 22.18) (Koh et al. 1999; Vazquez et al. 2002). It has been suggested that this finding is related either to a susceptibility of the anterior roots to the toxic effect of methotrexate or to a gravity-dependent increased concentration of the drug around these roots, although a selective autoimmune process cannot be excluded (Koh et al. 1999). Nerve conduction and electromagnetic abnormalities usually correlate with the root enhancement at MR imaging. Spinal MR imaging allows quick differential diagnosis between this anterior toxic radiculopathy and the potential epidural-subdural hematoma occurring after lumbar puncture secondary to thrombocytopenia (Vazquez et al. 2002).

A more common and less explosive neurotoxic reaction to this therapy, aseptic arachnoiditis is a well-recognized and usually transient complication. The symptoms of headache, back pain, meningismus, and fever are seen in 5–40% of patients shortly after intrathecal treatment (Ginsberg and Leeds 1995; Seidel et al. 1996; Koh et al. 1999).

22.5.3
Radiation Therapy

The imaging spectrum of CNS changes after radiation therapy includes leukoencephalopathy of the deep white matter, enhancing radiation necrosis, mineralizing microangiopathy, parenchymal brain volume loss, radiation-induced cryptic vascular malformation, radiation myelitis, and also second neoplasms (Tsuruda et al. 1987; Antunes et al. 2002; Vazquez et al. 2002).

22.5.3.1
White Matter Disease

Radiation injury to the brain has been classified into three categories: acute reactions (1–6 weeks after treatment), early delayed injury (3 weeks to several months after irradiation) and late delayed injury (months to years after treatment) (Tsuruda et al. 1987). Acute reactions usually occur during the therapy and consist of increased capillary permeability and vasodilation leading to vasogenic edema, with hypodense lesions on CT or hyperintense areas on T2-weighted MR images in the periventricular white matter (Fig. 22.19). Acute lesions are in general mild and reversible without clinical or prognostic significance. Early delayed injury includes lesions with vasogenic edema and demyelination that typically present with acute or focal neurologic symptoms. They appear on MR imaging as hyperintense areas on T2-weighted and transient enhancement after contrast administration and often simulate tumor recurrence or progression. They usually improve with steroid therapy, although rare cases of fulminant course and death have been described. Late delayed effects include white matter necrosis, demyelination, astrocytosis and vasculopathy (Ball et al. 1992). Late delayed reactions are irreversible and often fatal, with two imaging patterns of diffuse white matter injury and radiation necrosis. Patients with this latter injury can manifest focal deficits or stupor, but no direct association between mild or moderate changes on imaging studies and clinical symptoms has been found (Edwards-Brown and Jakacki 1999; Parisi et al. 1999). Most, but not all, patients with severe white matter changes have symptoms, particularly neurocognitive deficits (Mulhern et al. 1992). Imaging shows focal or multiple confluent white matter lesions with edema and demyelination which are best seen on MR imaging. The subcortical U-fibers, corpus callosum, posterior fossa, basal ganglia, and internal capsules are relatively unaffected (Tsuruda et al. 1987). Proton MR spectroscopy can demonstrate the neuronal damage remote from the tumor location with reduction of N-acetyl-L-aspartate concentrations (Waldrop et al. 1998).

One of the most severe processes, necrotizing diffuse leukoencephalopathy, which is seen in combined chemotherapy and radiation therapy, is associated with subsequent rapid and progressive clinical deterioration. Extensive areas of white

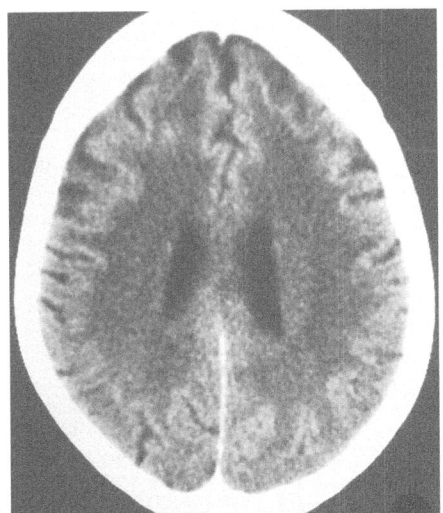 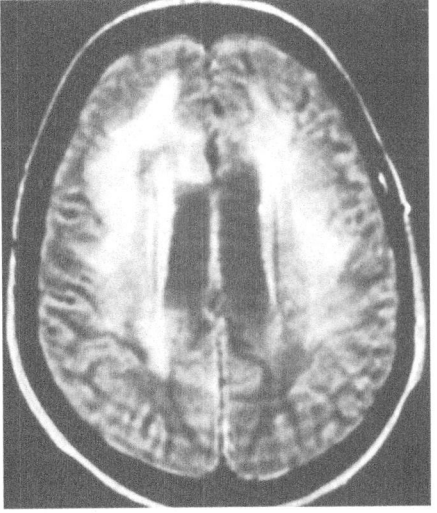

a   b

Fig. 22.19a,b. Radiation therapy-induced acute leukoencephalopathy in mildly symptomatic 45-year-old woman treated for non-Hodgkin lymphoma. **a** Axial contrast-enhanced CT scan shows marked symmetric hypodense non-enhanced periventricular deep white matter. **b** Axial proton density-weighted MR image demonstrates diffuse periventricular deep white matter hyperintensity.

matter necrosis can be seen on neuroimaging, with marked enhancement after contrast administration and a tendency to posterior calcification (Fig. 22.20) (Parisi et al. 1999).

Radiation necrosis may present as late as 10 years after therapy, although most cases occur in the first 2 years. Clinical presentation often mimics primary brain tumor, with increased intracranial pressure, focal deficits, seizures or altered consciousness. The severity of deep white matter changes increases with advancing age. Lesions may partially resolve, stabilize, or progress over several months or several years, leading to widespread, potentially fatal brain destruction. Imaging shows an irregular enhancing and necrotic mass surrounded by vasogenic edema.

This mass is difficult to distinguish from brain tumor and might be biopsy-proved (Tsuruda et al. 1987). Positron emission tomography and MR spectroscopy can be helpful in the differentiation with tumor (Edwards-Brown and Jakacki 1999).

22.5.3.2
Mineralizing Microangiopathy

Radiotherapy produces hyalinization and fibrinoid necrosis of small arteries and arterioles with endothelial proliferation and calcium deposition (Chen et al. 1996; Parker 1997). Dystrophic calcifications in the basal ganglia (putamen) and subcortical white matter were a relatively common finding on cranial

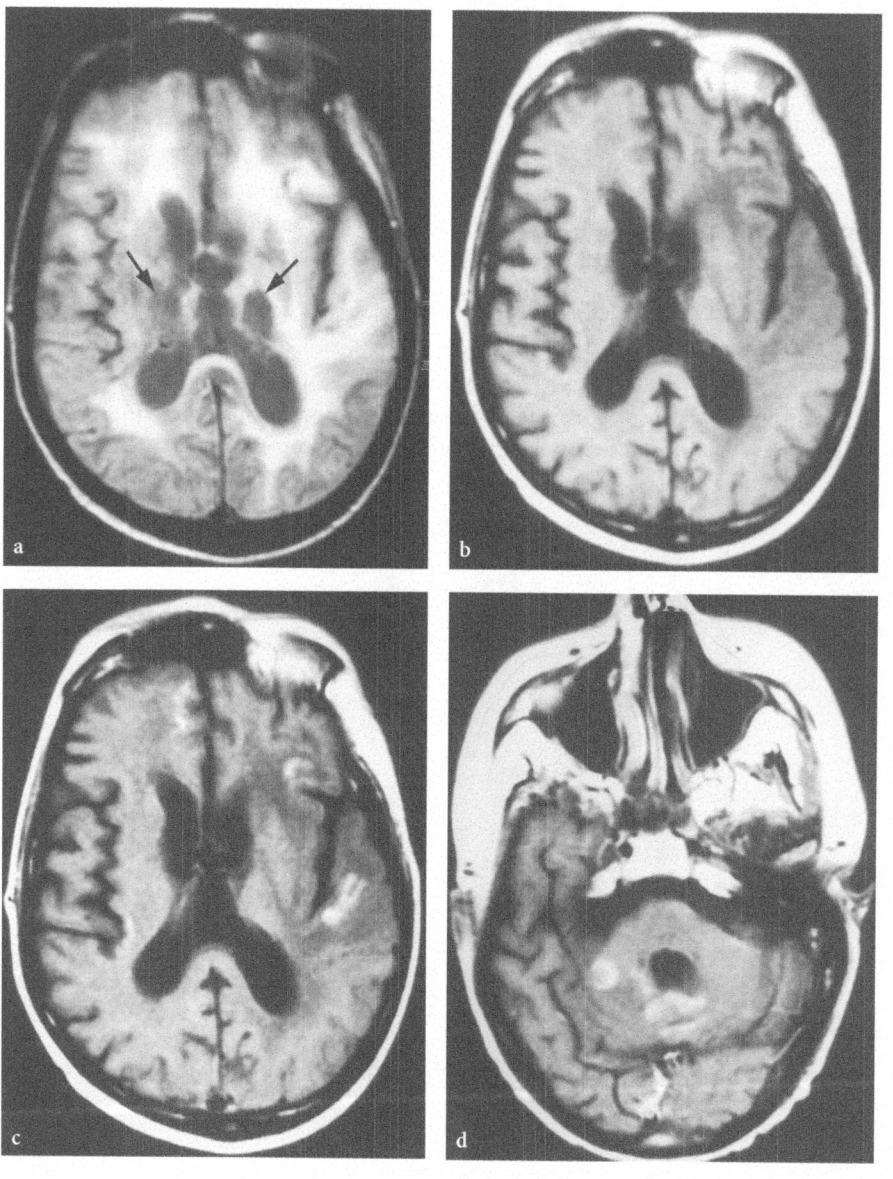

Fig. 22.20a–d. Fatal disseminated necrotizing leukoencephalopathy in a 26-year-man treated for acute lymphoblastic leukemia with high dose intravenous and intrathecal methotrexate in association with brain irradiation. **a** Axial T2-weighted MR image shows marked periventricular hyperintensity. The bilateral dark spots correspond at autopsy to hemosiderin deposition within both thalami (*arrows*). The periventricular changes are hypointense and less obvious on (**b**) axial unenhanced T1-weighted MR image. **c, d** Axial contrast-enhanced T1-weighted MR images demonstrate multiple supra and infratentorial cortical enhancing areas corresponding to radiation therapy necrosis at autopsy. MR images also show cerebral parenchymal volume loss.

CT in children previously treated with radiotherapy and intrathecal methotrexate (Fig. 22.21). Nowadays, with the more conservative protocols, a subtle pattern can be discovered on MR imaging follow-up, with putaminal hyperintensity on T1-weighted images due to a surface-relaxation mechanism, and hypointensity on T2-weighted images (Fig. 22.22). These imaging findings are most common in children receiving both radiation and chemotherapy, particularly intrathecal chemotherapy, but are also seen in children treated with radiation therapy alone. They appear two or more years after therapy and do not clearly correlate with clinical symptoms (BLEYER et al. 1973; SHANLEY 1995).

22.5.3.3
Parenchymal Brain Volume Loss

Patients with leukemia can have reversible enlarged cerebrospinal fluid spaces resulting from therapy, particularly from steroids (WANG et al. 1983). Up to 31% of children with acute lymphoblastic leukemia can have slightly enlarged ventricles before treatment, probably related to communicant hydrocephalus secondary to primary disease (CHEN et al. 1996; PARKER 1997). Nevertheless, when the ventricular and cerebrospinal fluid spaces enlargement does not

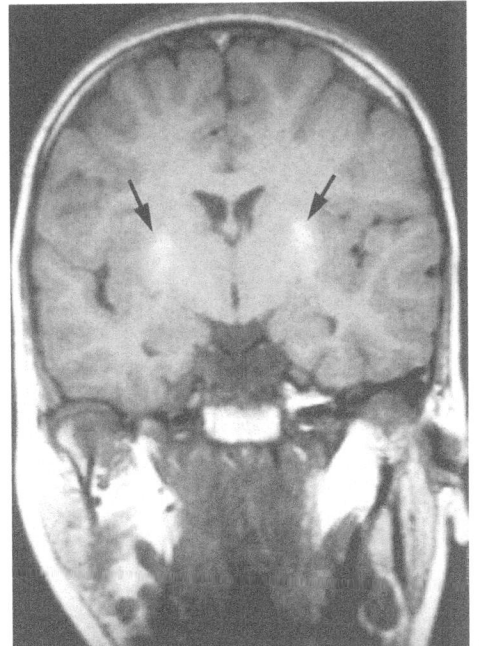

a

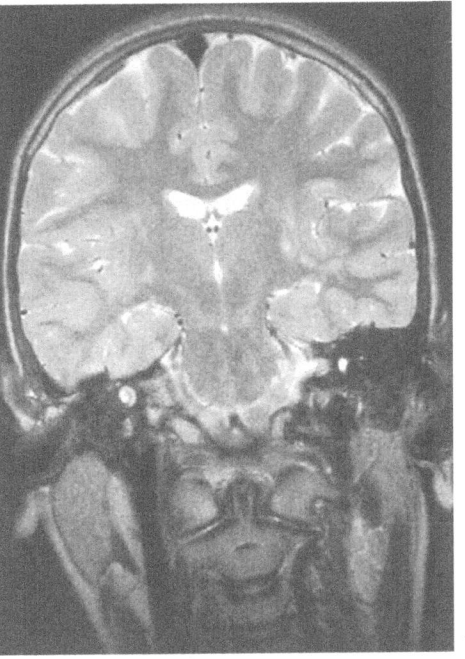

b

Fig. 22.22a,b. Subtle mineralizing microangiopathy in a 10-year-old girl treated for acute lymphoblastic leukemia with radiation therapy and chemotherapy. Follow-up MR imaging was performed 3 years after treatment. **a** Coronal unenhanced T1-weighted MR image shows subtle hyperintense areas (*arrows*) involving the lenticular nuclei. **b** Coronal fast spin-echo T2-weighted MR image shows no clear lesion. The patient was asymptomatic; she did not have liver failure and was not receiving parenteral nutrition, conditions that could also produce hyperintensity of the lenticular nucleus on T1-weighted MR images secondary to manganese deposition. (With permission from [VAZQUEZ et al. 2002])

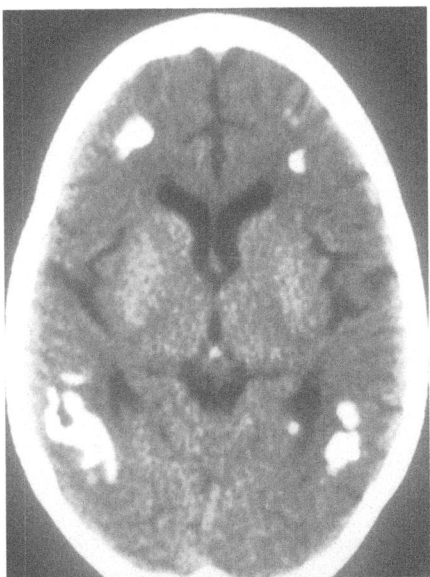

Fig. 22.21. Mineralizing microangiopathy in a 17-year-old boy treated for acute lymphoblastic leukemia with irradiation and intrathecal chemotherapy. Several years after remission, he developed seizures. Axial unenhanced CT scan shows calcifications in the subcortical parenchyma and basal ganglia. (With permission from [VAZQUEZ et al. 2002])

reverse after leukemia remission, but persists or even increases, it is probably related to cranial irradiation (true cerebral atrophy) and is responsible for posterior learning problems in up to 80% of survivors (BERNALDEZ-RIOS et al. 1998).

22.5.3.4
Radiation-Induced Cryptic Vascular Malformations

Patients, especially children, treated with cranial irradiation due to leukemia or CNS primary neoplasms can develop white matter hemorrhagic lesions with heterogeneous signal intensity quite similar to the cryptic malformations or cavernous angiomas on MR images. The interval between therapy and these hem-

orrhagic lesions varies from 1 to 19 years (mean, 8). They mainly appear in cerebral hemispheres, although brain stem and spinal cord involvement have also been described, can be isolated or multiple and can show calcifications on cranial CT. These lesions probably represent capillary telangiectasias secondary to the altered venular endothelium with subsequent venous occlusive disease (GAENSLER et al. 1994; MAEDER et al. 1998). Gradient-echo MR sequences are particularly useful for their identification because of their greater magnetic susceptibility (Fig. 22.23). They should be distinguished from hemorrhage due to leukemia or second or radio-induced tumors. Patients are usually asymptomatic, although some suffer from headaches, seizures or focal signs. These lesions, which appear

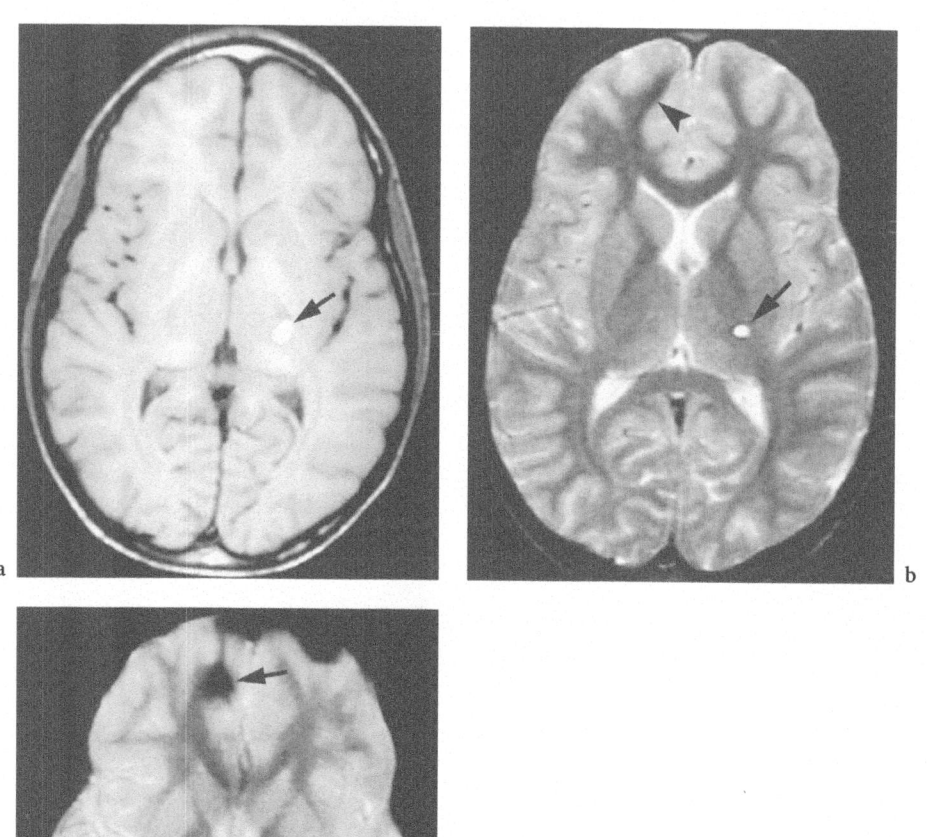

Fig. 22.23a–c. Radiation-induced cryptic vascular malformation in a 15-year-old boy treated for acute lymphoblastic leukemia. The patient presented with headaches. Axial (**a**) T1 and (**b**) T2-weighted MR images show a hyperintense lesion with a hypointense rim in the left thalamic nucleus (*arrow*). A hypointense lesion in the subcortical white matter of the right frontal region is also seen on the T2-weighted image (*arrowhead*). **c** Axial gradient-echo T2-weighted MR image shows both lesions more clearly (*arrows*). These hemorrhagic lesions were unchanged at follow-up MR imaging examinations. (With permission from [VAZQUEZ et al. 2002])

several years after treatment, can have hemorrhagic potential but surgical removal is only justified in cases of symptomatic hemorrhage (POUSSAINT et al. 1995; VAZQUEZ et al. 2002).

22.5.3.5
Radiation Myelitis

Radiation myelitis is an uncommon complication, especially in pediatric age group (ANTUNES et al. 2002). It is secondary to therapeutic radiation exposure to the spinal cord and is characterized by delayed development of paresthesias, sensory changes, and in severe cases, progressive paresis and paralysis (SCHWARTZ et al. 2000). Although accepted radiation therapy tolerance limits for the spinal cord have successfully limited the incidence of this complication (40–45 Gy, in daily 1.8–2 Gy fractions over 4–5 weeks), aggressive systemic therapy may render patients more susceptible to radiation-related neurotoxicity (CHAO et al. 1998; SCHWARTZ et al. 2000). MR imaging of the spinal cord is the exam of choice for the diagnosis of radiation myelitis. It shows intramedullary T2 hyperintensity within the swelling spinal cord, and areas of enhancement on T1-weighted image after contrast administration. These changes always are limited to the radiation field (SCHWARTZ et al. 2000).

22.5.3.6
Radiation-Induced Second Neoplasms

The induction of second neoplasms is a rare but well-documented serious sequela of therapeutic irradiation (GHIM et al. 1993; NISHIO et al. 1998). The initial disease is most frequently acute leukemia (particularly acute lymphoblastic leukemia) and lymphoma (particularly Hodgkin disease). Reported CNS radiation-induced tumors particularly include meningioma and glioma often high-grade glioma. The risk is higher in patients irradiated at an early age, particularly below 5 years of age, with an incidence of 2.6 to 38.8, 6 to 10 times greater than the standard population (MOPPETT et al. 2001). Imperfect repair of the radiation-induced DNA strand breakage in tumor suppressor has been suggested as the genetic basis. The period of latency varies from 8 to 15 years after radiation therapy, and is inversely proportional to irradiation dose, with shorter latencies often seen following higher doses (NISHIO et al. 1998).

Survivors of childhood acute lymphoblastic leukemia form a large population at risk for developing second neoplasms. Brain tumors are one of the most frequently seen, with a drastically different outcome for patients who develop low-grade tumors (primarily meningiomas) (Fig. 22.24) than for those with high-grade tumors (high-grade gliomas). The

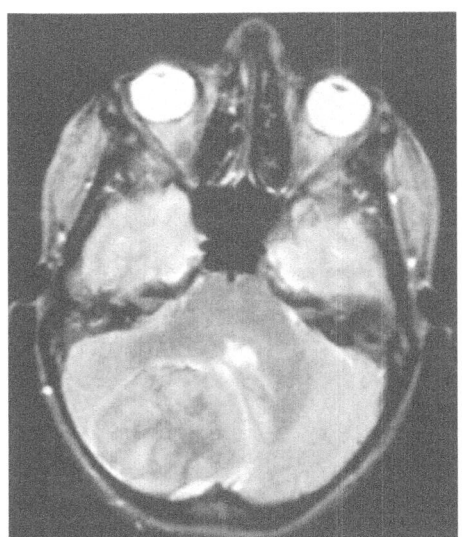
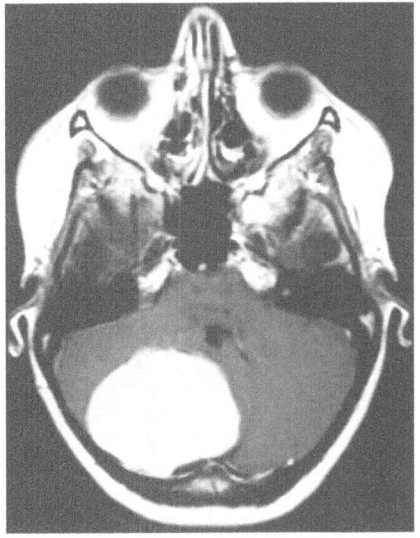

a   b

Fig. 22.24a,b. Secondary meningioma in a 17-year-old girl with occipital headaches who underwent therapy for acute lymphoblastic leukemia (including cranial irradiation) at the age of 2 years. She was treated for papillary carcinoma of the thyroid 2 years earlier. Axial (**a**) T2-weighted and (**b**) contrast-enhanced T1-weighted MR images show an extraaxial mass in the posterior fossa. The mass is slightly hypointense on the T2-weighted image (**a**) and demonstrates homogeneous enhancement on the contrast-enhanced T1-weighted image (**b**). The tumor was resected, and the histopathologic diagnosis was meningioma with anaplastic foci. Follow-up MR imaging examinations did not demonstrate tumor recurrence. (With permission from [VAZQUEZ et al. 2002])

number of second tumors that develop after therapy for acute lymphoblastic leukemia is 62.3 per 100.000 cases annually (WALTER et al. 1998). Cranial irradiation has been particularly implicated, although there are reported cases of a second CNS tumor in survivors of childhood leukemia who had no history of prophylactic irradiation. Other proposed mechanisms have been loss of immune surveillance and genetic factors. The cumulative incidence of both low-grade and high-grade brain neoplasms is related to the presence of CNS leukemic or lymphomatous infiltration at diagnosis, due to the more intensive CNS-directed chemotherapy and irradiation given to these patients (FOREMAN et al. 1995; CHOI and SEEX 2000).

22.5.4
Cytosine Arabinoside

Cytosine arabinoside (Ara-C) has played an important role in the initial intrathecal prevention of disease as well as treatment of CNS acute leukemia and non-Hodgkin lymphoma by both intravenous and intrathecal administration (BAKER et al. 1991; PATEL and RAO 1996; PEASE et al. 2001). Neurotoxicity is an increasingly recognized side effect with patient age (> 60 years) appearing to be the most important risk factor (BAKER et al. 1991). It is also dose-dependent and related to previous CNS toxicities (HERZIG et al. 1987; MILLER et al. 1989; PATEL and RAO 1996; OLAVARRIA et al. 1997), appearing at total dose greater than 18–24 g/m2 per course (PATEL and RAO 1996). Exposure to multiple therapeutic modalities increases the risk of neurotoxicity associated with Ara-C, as is the case with methotrexate (BAKER et al. 1991). High dose Ara-C therapy administrated for acute leukemia causes cerebellar toxicity (ZAWACKI et al. 2000), which is considered the principal side effect of high-dose Ara-C, occurring 10 to 14% of patients (BAKER et al. 1991; PEASE et al. 2001). Complications range from 0 to 16.7% (PATEL and RAO 1996) and are usually transient and mild but may be severe and permanent in rare cases (ZAWACKI et al. 2000) with permanent cerebellar disability in 3% (BAKER et al. 1991). Dysarthria, dysdiadochokinesia, dysmetria, and ataxia are the cardinal manifestation of the cerebellar syndrome (BLEYER et al. 1973; HERZIG et al. 1987). Cerebellar lesions may be seen as one-sided (PATEL and RAO 1996) or bilateral hypodensity at CT (BLEYER et al. 1973) but are much better demonstrated on MR imaging (Fig. 22.25). They consist of areas of hyperintensity on T2-weighted images

within the cerebellum with or without involvement of the pons. Contrast-enhancement of these lesions is rare (PATEL and RAO 1996).

Cerebellar atrophy is rarely reported but is related to Ara-C neurotoxicity. It is seen on noncontrast CT and/or MR imaging performed several months after the onset of symptoms. MR imaging reveals normal parenchymal signal (MILLER et al. 1989; FRIEDMAN and SHETTY 2001).

Disseminated necrotizing leukoencephalopathy, usually observed in patients receiving methotrexate, is also seen in patients receiving high-dose intravenous or intrathecal Ara-C with or without cranial irradiation (BAKER et al. 1991; VAUGHN et al. 1993; GINSBERG and LEEDS 1995). Some other very rare complications may be associated with Ara-C treatment, such as diffuse cerebellar atrophy predominant in midline (ZAWACKI et al. 2000) and acute basal ganglia necrosis (SIRVENT et al. 1998).

Intrathecal Ara-C is also capable of inducing severe transverse myelopathy (HERZIG et al. 1987) with abnormalities of white matter in the spinal cord, severe demyelinization and axonal swellings (BREUER et al. 1977; GRAUS et al. 1996) that are incompletely reversible (BAKER et al. 1991). It also leads to aseptic meningitis, which is usually associated with intrathecal therapy (BAKER et al. 1991) even after low dose (VAN DEN BERG et al. 2001), but very rarely with systemic administration (PEASE et al. 2001). Aseptic meningitis can last up to 8 weeks, and may be prevented with prednisone and H1-receptor antagonist (VAN DEN BERG et al. 2001).

22.5.5
L-Asparaginase

L-asparaginase is an enzymatic inhibitor of protein synthesis used in combination with other chemotherapy drugs in the treatment of acute lymphoblastic leukemia (URBAN and SAGER 1981) and other lymphoid malignancies (FEINBERG and SWENSON 1988). It causes transient deficiencies in plasma proteins important in coagulation and fibrinolysis. L-asparaginase has been linked to hemorrhagic and thrombotic cerebrovascular complications including cortical infarction, capsular infarction, intracerebral hemorrhage, hemorrhagic infarction, and cerebral venous and dural sinus thrombosis (Fig. 22.11) (PRIEST et al. 1980; URBAN and SAGER 1981; PRIEST et al. 1982; FEINBERG and SWENSON 1988). The incidence of the cerebrovascular events in patients treated with L-asparaginase is approximately 1 to 2 %. Clinically, symptoms are similar in the hemorrhagic

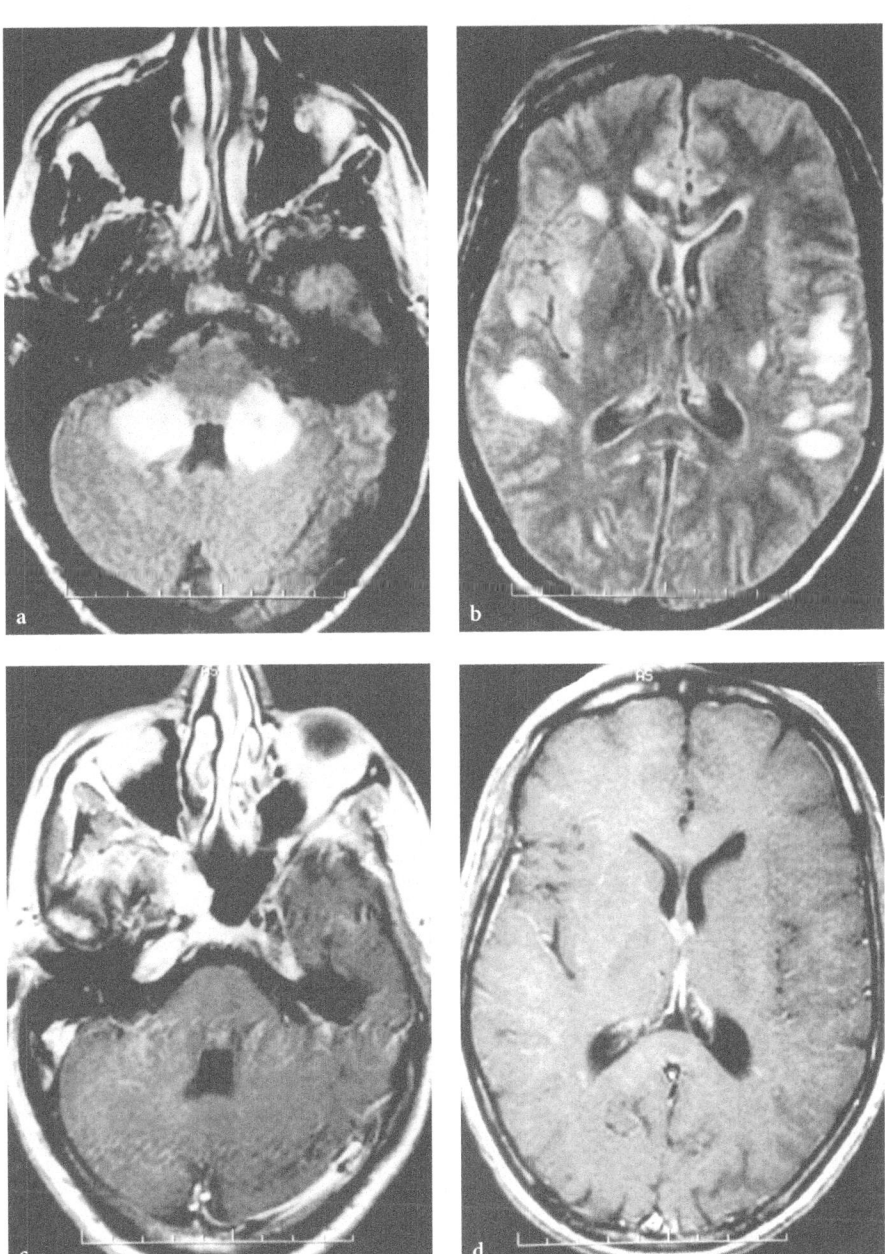

Fig. 22.25a–d. High dose ara-C neurotoxicity in a 26-year-old man presenting with acute cerebellar disability. This patient underwent therapy for acute myeloid leukemia. **a** Axial posterior fossa fluid-attenuated inversion-recovery MR image shows bilateral cerebellar hyperintense abnormalities with mild pressure on the fourth ventricle. **b** Axial supratentorial fluid-attenuated inversion-recovery MR image shows multiple hyperintense lesions of the white matter. **c, d** Enhanced T1-weighted MR images at the same levels show no contrast enhancement of the lesions.

and thrombotic patients with headache the most common initial symptom. Other presenting symptoms are seizures, hemiparesis, altered mental status, and vomiting. The imaging of cerebrovascular complications is presented in the chapter "Cerebrovascular complications". The risk of recurrence with further L-asparaginase therapy is very low, but prophylactic pretreatment with fresh frozen plasma seems to be a prudent therapy (FEINBERG and SWENSON 1988).

22.5.6
Corticosteroids

Corticosteroids as a part of most chemotherapy protocol may induce reversible brain atrophy. Imaging shows reversible ventricular and subarachnoid space enlargement. Pathologic changes consist of gross atrophy without tissue loss or damage (WANG et al. 1983).

Spinal cord or cauda equina compression from epidural lipomatosis caused by corticosteroids in patients treated for hematological malignancies is extremely rare (PENNISI et al. 1985). It usually occurs in patients taking more than the equivalent of 30 mg/day of prednisone. Clinical manifestations include back pain, myelopathy, or radiculopathy (GEORGE et al. 1983). The distribution of epidural lipomatosis through the spinal canal is longitudinal. The mid-thoracic portion of the spine is the most involved, and exclusive lumbar stenosis is not rare. Usually the fat compresses the dural sac from the dorsal epidural compartment. CT reveals the fatty nature of the intraspinal extradural mass. Sagittal T1-weigthed MR images are the best for demonstrating the posterior epidural fatty mass and its longitudinal extent (Fig. 22.26). Moreover, MR imaging with T2-weighted images might be helpful in determining possible structure damage to the myelon (HIERHOLZER et al. 1998). The usual treatment is surgical decompression, although simply stopping the steroid therapy and/or dietary regimen may improve symptoms (GEORGE et al. 1983; HIERHOLZER et al. 1998).

22.6
Treatment-Induced Tumors

As mentioned in the subchapter "Radiation Therapy – Radiation-Induced Second Neoplasms", patients treated for hematological malignancies, especially leukemic children who are long-term survivors, are at risk for second primary tumors, such as gliomablastoma, astrocytoma (GINSBERG and LEEDS 1995; LAITT et al. 1995) or lymphoma (VERSCHUUR et al. 1994). Cranial meningioma, which is a benign tumor, accounts for 70% of all treatment-induced intracranial tumors (Fig. 22.24) (PAAKKO et al. 1994; LAITT et al. 1995; MEIGNIN et al. 1998; VAZQUEZ et al. 2002). Cranial tumors as a late complication are probably secondary to drug therapy and/or radiation therapy (PAAKKO et al. 1994; GINSBERG and LEEDS 1995; LAITT et al. 1995; MEIGNIN et al. 1998). These treatment-induced tumors are more aggressive and highly refractory to therapy (CHOI and SEEX 2000). Secondary meningiomas are also characterized by younger age at presentation, higher male-to-female ratio, and biologically more aggressive variants compared to primary spontaneous meningiomas (VAZQUEZ et al. 2002).

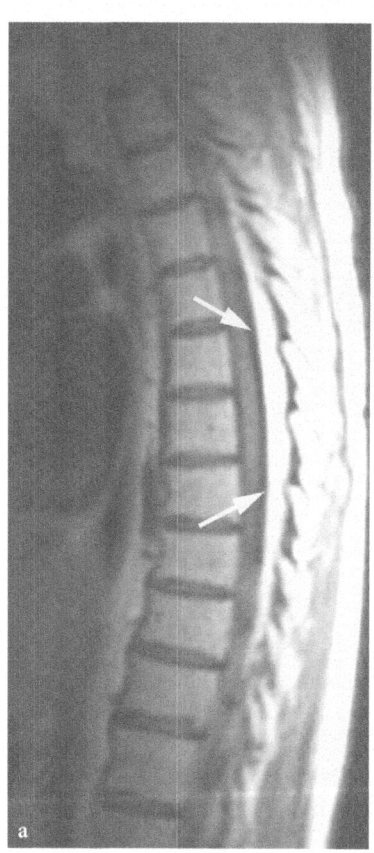
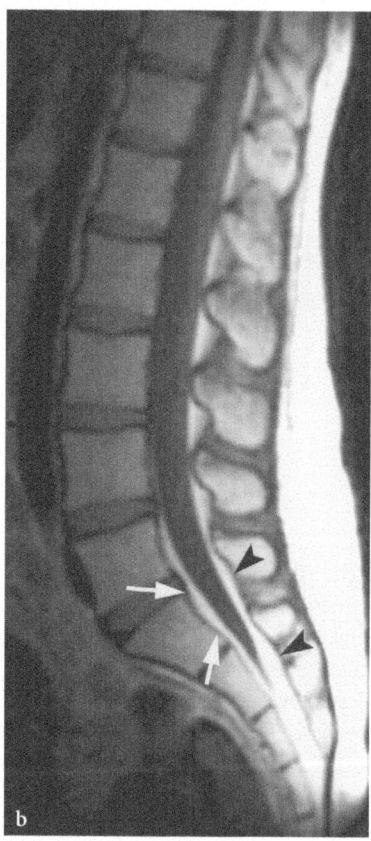

Fig. 22.26a,b. Epidural lipomatosis in a 26-year-woman treated for acute myeloid leukemia with chemotherapy including corticosteroids. The patient had a 1-month history of back pain and proximal muscle weakness. **a** Mid-sagittal unenhanced T1-weighted MR image of the thoracic spine shows extensive posterior mid-thoracic epidural fat overgrowth (*arrows*) with mild cord compression. **b** Mid-sagittal unenhanced T1-weighted MR image of the lumbosacral spine shows accented epidural fat overgrowth leading to a clear dural sac reduction. The anterior epidural space is enlarged by fat accumulation (*arrows*) and the posterior space is recognizable due to increased fat (*arrowheads*).

Also in children, CNS changes in acute leuke-mias include leukemic cellular infiltration of the brain, meninges, and nerve roots. They are more frequent in acute lymphoblastic leukemia (CROSLEY et al. 1978), and reported up to 13% of BMT patients (PATCHELL 1994).

22.7
Conclusion

Patients treated for hematological malignancies are at risk for a variety of CNS complications including among others infections, toxic side effects of high-dose therapy and BMT, and bleeding. Familiarity with these conditions and their imaging appear-ance is essential to determine the correct diagnosis and to avoid a potentially dangerous misdiagnosis. Imaging findings must be considered along with pertinent clinical information, presenting signs and symptoms, and laboratory data so that an accurate evaluation can be made in patients with neurologi-cal signs.

References

Abraham J, Bilgrami S, Dorsky D, et al. (1997) Stomatococ-cus mucilaginosus meningitis in a patient with multiple myeloma following autologous stem cell transplantation. Bone Marrow Transplant 19:639–641

Antonini G, Ceschin V, Morino S, et al. (1998) Early neu-rologic complications following allogeneic bone marrow transplant for leukemia: a prospective study. Neurology 50:1441–1445

Antunes NL, Wolden S, Souweidane MM, Lis E, Rosenblum M, Steinherz PG (2002) Radiation myelitis in a 5-year-old girl. J Child Neurol 17:217–219

Appignani BA, Bhadelia RA, Blacklow SC, Wang AK, Roland SF, Freeman RB Jr (1996) Neuroimaging findings in patients on immunosuppressive therapy: experience with tacrolimus toxicity. AJR Am J Roentgenol 166:683–688

Asato R, Akiyama Y, Ito M, Kubota M, Okumura R, Miki Y, Konishi J, Mikawa H (1992) Nuclear magnetic resonance abnormalities of the cerebral white matter in children with acute lymphoblastic leukemia and malignant lym-phoma during and after central nervous system prophy-lactic treatment with intrathecal methotrexate. Cancer 70:1997–2004

Au WY, Lie AK, Cheung RT, Cheng PW, Ooi CG, Yujenc KY, Kwong YL (2002) Acute disseminated encephalomyelitis after para-influenza infection post bone marrow trans-plantation. Leuk Lymphoma 43:455–457

Baker WJ, Royer GL Jr, Weiss RB (1991) Cytarabine and neu-rologic toxicity. J Clin Oncol 9:679–693

Ball WS, Jr., Prenger EC, Ballard ET (1992) Neurotoxicity of radio/chemotherapy in children: pathologic and MR cor-relation. AJNR Am J Neuroradiol 13:761–776

Bernaldez-Rios R, Villasis-Keever MA, Beltran-Adame G, et al. (1998) Neurological and psychological sequelae in chil-dren with acute lymphoblastic leukemia who had received radiotherapy and intrathecal methotrexate. Gac Med Mex 134:153–159

Bleggi-Torres LF, de Medeiros BC, Neto JZ, Loddo G, Telles FQ, de Medeiros CR, Pasquini R (1996) Disseminated Fusarium sp. infection affecting the brain of a child after bone marrow transplantation.PG – 1013–5. Bone Marrow Transplant 18:1013–1015

Bleggi-Torres LF, de Medeiros BC, Werner B, Pasquini R, de Medeiros CR (1999) Unusual presentation of cerebral toxoplasmosis after BMT. Bone Marrow Transplant 23: 855–856

Bleggi-Torres LF, de Medeiros BC, Werner B, Neto JZ, Loddo G, Pasquini R, de Medeiros CR (2000) Neuropathological findings after bone marrow transplantation: an autopsy study of 180 cases. Bone Marrow Transplant 25:301–307

Bleggi-Torres LF, Werner B, Gasparetto EL, de Medeiros BC, Pasquini R, de Medeiros CR (2002) Intracranial hemor-rhage following bone marrow transplantation: an autopsy study of 58 patients. Bone Marrow Transplant 29:29–32

Bleyer WA, Drake JC, Chabner BA (1973) Neurotoxicity and elevated cerebrospinal-fluid methotrexate concentration in meningeal leukemia. N Engl J Med 289:770–773

Breuer AC, Pitman SW, Dawson DM, Schoene WC (1977) Para-paresis following intrathecal cytosine arabinoside: a case report with neuropathologic findings. Cancer 40:2817–2822

Brinkman K, Debast S, Sauerwein R, Ooyman F, Hiel J, Raemaekers J (1998) Toxoplasma retinitis/encephalitis 9 months after allogeneic bone marrow transplantation. Bone Marrow Transplant 21:635–636

Campos A, Vaz CP, Campilho F, et al. (2000) Central nervous system (CNS) tuberculosis following allogeneic stem cell transplantation. Bone Marrow Transplant 25:567–569

Casey SO, Sampaio RC, Michel E, Truwit CL (2000) Posterior reversible encephalopathy syndrome: utility of fluid-atten-uated inversion recovery MR imaging in the detection of cortical and subcortical lesions. AJNR Am J Neuroradiol 21:1199–1206

Chao MW, Wirth A, Ryan G, MacManus M, Liew KH (1998) Radiation myelopathy following transplantation and radiotherapy for non-Hodgkin's lymphoma. Int J Radiat Oncol Biol Phys 41:1057–1061

Chen CY, Zimmerman RA, Faro S, Bilaniuk LT, Chou TY, Molloy PT (1996) Childhood leukemia: central nervous system abnormalities during and after treatment. AJNR Am J Neuroradiol 17:295–310

Chintagumpala MM, Mahoney DH Jr, McClain K, et al. (1993) Hodgkin's disease associated with central pontine myelin-olysis. Med Pediatr Oncol 21:311–314

Choi D, Seex K (2000) Intracranial meningioma following child-hood irradiation for leukaemia. Br J Haematol 108:665

Coley SC, Jager HR, Szydlo RM, Goldman JM (1999) CT and MRI manifestations of central nervous system infection following allogeneic bone marrow transplantation. Clin Radiol 54:390–397

Coplin WM, Cochran MS, Levine SR, Crawford SW (2001) Stroke after bone marrow transplantation: frequency, aetiology and outcome. Brain 124:1043–1051

Cordonnier C, Feuilhade F, Vernant JP, Marsault C, Rodet M, Rochant H (1983) Cytomegalovirus encephalitis occurring after bone marrow transplantation. Scand J Haematol 31: 248–252

Crosley CJ, Rorke LB, Evans A, Nigro M (1978) Central nervous system lesions in childhood leukemia. Neurology 28: 678–685

D'Antonio D, Di Bartolomeo P, Iacone A, et al. (1992) Meningitis due to penicillin-resistant Streptococcus pneumoniae in patients with chronic graft-versus-host disease. Bone Marrow Transplant 9:299–300

de Medeiros BC, de Medeiros CR, Werner B, Neto JZ, Loddo G, Pasquini R, Bleggi-Torres LF (2000) Central nervous system infections following bone marrow transplantation: an autopsy report of 27 cases. J Hematother Stem Cell Res 9:535–540

de Medeiros BC, de Medeiros CR, Werner B, Loddo G, Pasquini R, Bleggi-Torres LF (2001) Disseminated toxoplasmosis after bone marrow transplantation: report of 9 cases. Transpl Infect Dis 3:24–28

Dellemijn PL, Brandenburg A, Niesters HG, van den Bent MJ, Rothbarth PH, Vlasveld LT (1995) Successful treatment with ganciclovir of presumed Epstein-Barr meningoencephalitis following bone marrow transplant. Bone Marrow Transplant 16:311–312

DeLone DR, Goldstein RA, Petermann G, Salamat MS, Miles JM, Knechtle SJ, Brown WD (1999) Disseminated aspergillosis involving the brain: distribution and imaging characteristics. AJNR Am J Neuroradiol 20:1597–1604

Derouin F, Gluckman E, Beauvais B, Devergie A, Melo R, Monny M, Lariviere M (1986) Toxoplasma infection after human allogeneic bone marrow transplantation: clinical and serological study of 80 patients. Bone Marrow Transplant 1:67–73

Derouin F, Devergie A, Auber P, Gluckman E, Beauvais B, Garin YJ, Lariviere M (1992) Toxoplasmosis in bone marrow-transplant recipients: report of seven cases and review. PG – 267–70. Clin Infect Dis 15:267–270

Dietrich U, Maschke M, Dorfler A, Prumbaum M, Forsting M (2000) MRI of intracranial toxoplasmosis after bone marrow transplantation. Neuroradiology 42:14–18

Dillon WP, Rowley H (1998) The reversible posterior cerebral edema syndrome. AJNR Am J Neuroradiol 19:591

Drobyski WR, Knox KK, Majewski D, Carrigan DR (1994) Brief report: fatal encephalitis due to variant B human herpesvirus-6 infection in a bone marrow-transplant recipient. N Engl J Med 330:1356–1360

Ebner F, Ranner G, Slavc I, Urban C, Kleinert R, Radner H, Einspieler R, Justich E (1989) MR findings in methotrexate-induced CNS abnormalities. AJR Am J Roentgenol 153: 1283–1288

Edwards-Brown MK, Jakacki RI (1999) Imaging the central nervous system effects of radiation and chemotherapy of pediatric tumors. Neuroimaging Clin N Am 9:177–193

Feinberg WM, Swenson MR (1988) Cerebrovascular complications of L-asparaginase therapy. Neurology 38:127–133

Foreman NK, Laitt RD, Chambers EJ, Duncan AW, Cummins BH (1995) Intracranial large vessel vasculopathy and anaplastic meningioma 19 years after cranial irradiation for acute lymphoblastic leukaemia. Med Pediatr Oncol 24: 265–268

Friedman JH, Shetty N (2001) Permanent cerebellar toxicity of cytosine arabinoside (Ara C) in a young woman. Mov Disord 16:575–577

Gaensler EH, Dillon WP, Edwards MS, Larson DA, Rosenau W, Wilson CB (1994) Radiation-induced telangiectasia in the brain simulates cryptic vascular malformations at MR imaging. Radiology 193:629–636

Gallardo D, Ferra C, Berlanga JJ, et al. (1996) Neurologic complications after allogeneic bone marrow transplantation. Bone Marrow Transplant 18:1135–1139

George WE Jr, Wilmot M, Greenhouse A, Hammeke M (1983) Medical management of steroid-induced epidural lipomatosis. N Engl J Med 308:316–319

Ghim TT, Seo JJ, O'Brien M, Meacham L, Crocker I, Krawiecki N (1993) Childhood intracranial meningiomas after high-dose irradiation. Cancer 71:4091–4095

Ginsberg LE, Leeds NE (1995) Neuroradiology of leukemia. AJR Am J Roentgenol 165:525–534

Goldman M, Chaudhary UB, Greist A, Fausel CA (1998) Central nervous system infections due to Stomatococcus mucilaginosus in immunocompromised hosts. Clin Infect Dis 27:1241–1246

Graus F, Saiz A, Sierra J, Arbaiza D, Rovira M, Carreras E, Tolosa E, Rozman C (1996) Neurologic complications of autologous and allogeneic bone marrow transplantation in patients with leukemia: a comparative study. Neurology 46:1004–1009

Gruhn B, Meerbach A, Egerer R, et al. (1999) Successful treatment of Epstein-Barr virus-induced transverse myelitis with ganciclovir and cytomegalovirus hyperimmune globulin following unrelated bone marrow transplantation. Bone Marrow Transplant 24:1355–1358.

Guermazi A, Miaux Y, Laval-Jeantet M (1995) Imaging of choroid plexus infection by Stomatococcus mucilaginosus in neutropenic patients. AJNR Am J Neuroradiol 16: 1331–1334

Guermazi A, Miaux Y, Williams M, Turki C, Frija J (1997) Dural sinus thrombosis: CT and MR imaging of different stages. J Belge Radiol 80:167–169

Guermazi A, Benchaib N, Zagdanski AM, et al. (2002) Cerebral and spinal cord involvement resulting from invasive aspergillosis. Eur Radiol 12:147–150

Guermazi A, Gluckman E, Tabti B, Miaux Y (2003) Invasive central nervous system aspergillosis in bone marrow transplantation recipients: an overview. Eur Radiol 13:377–388

Han CS, Miller W, Haake R, Weisdorf D (1994) Varicella zoster infection after bone marrow transplantation: incidence, risk factors and complications. Bone Marrow Transplant 13:277–283

Hentschke P, Hagglund H, Mattsson J, et al. (1999) Bilateral subdural haematomas following lumbar puncture in three haematopoietic stem cell transplant recipients. Bone Marrow Transplant 24:1033–1035

Heran F, Defer G, Brugieres P, Brenot F, Gaston A, Degos JD (1990) Cortical blindness during chemotherapy: clinical, CT, and MR correlations. J Comput Assist Tomogr 14: 262–266

Herzig RH, Herzig GP, Wolff SN, Hines JD, Fay JW, Phillips GL (1987) Central nervous system effects of high-dose cytosine arabinoside. Semin Oncol 14:21–24

Hierholzer J, Vogl T, Hosten N, Lanksch W, Felix R (1998) Imaging in epidural lipomatosis. Crit Rev Neurosurg 8: 279–281

Hinchey J, Chaves C, Appignani B, et al. (1996) A reversible posterior leukoencephalopathy syndrome. N Engl J Med 334:494–500

Ito Y, Arahata Y, Goto Y, Hirayama M, Nagamutsu M, Yasuda T, Yanagi T, Sobue G (1998) Cisplatin neurotoxicity presenting as reversible posterior leukoencephalopathy syndrome. AJNR Am J Neuroradiol 19:415–417

Koh S, Nelson MD Jr, Kovanlikaya A, Chen LS (1999) Anterior lumbosacral radiculopathy after intrathecal methotrexate treatment. Pediatr Neurol 21:576–578

Ladriere M, Bibes B, Rabaud C, Delaby P, May T, Canton P (2001) Varicella zoster virus infection after bone marrow transplant. Unusual presentation and importance of prevention. Presse Med 30:1151–1154

Laitt RD, Chambers EJ, Goddard PR, Wakeley CJ, Duncan AW, Foreman NK (1995) Magnetic resonance imaging and magnetic resonance angiography in long term survivors of acute lymphoblastic leukemia treated with cranial irradiation. Cancer 76:1846–1852

Lentz D, Jordan JE, Pike GB, Enzmann DR (1993) MRI in varicella-zoster virus leukoencephalitis in the immunocompromised host. J Comput Assist Tomogr 17:313–316

Long SG, Leyland MJ, Milligan DW (1993) Listeria meningitis after bone marrow transplantation. Bone Marrow Transplant 12:537–539

Lovblad K, Kelkar P, Ozdoba C, Ramelli G, Remonda L, Schroth G (1998) Pure methotrexate encephalopathy presenting with seizures: CT and MRI features. Pediatr Radiol 28:86–91

Maciel E, Siqueira I, Queiroz AC, Melo A (2000) Toxoplasma gondii myelitis in a patient with adult T-cell leukemia-lymphoma. Arq Neuropsiquiatr 58:1107–1109

Maeder P, Gudinchet F, Meuli R, de Tribolet N (1998) Development of a cavernous malformation of the brain. AJNR Am J Neuroradiol 19:1141–1143

Martino R, Martinez C, Brunet S, Sureda A, Lopez R, Domingo-Albos A (1996) Tuberculosis in bone marrow transplant recipients: report of two cases and review of the literature. Bone Marrow Transplant 18:809–812

Maschke M, Dietrich U, Prumbaum M, Kastrup O, Turowski B, Schaefer UW, Diener HC (1999) Opportunistic CNS infection after bone marrow transplantation. Bone Marrow Transplant 23:1167–1176

Meignin V, Gluckman E, Gambaraelli D, Devergie A, Ramee MP, Janin A, Socie G (1998) Meningioma in long-term survivors after allogeneic bone marrow transplantation. Bone Marrow Transplant 22:723–724

Mele A, Paterson PJ, Prentice HG, Leoni P, Kibbler CC (2002) Toxoplasmosis in bone marrow transplantation: a report of two cases and systematic review of the literature. Bone Marrow Transplant 29:691–698

Miaux Y, Guermazi A, Bourrier P, Singer B, Leder S (1994) MR of cerebral aspergillosis: different patterns in the same patient. AJNR Am J Neuroradiol 15:1193–1195

Miaux Y, Ribaud P, Williams M, Guermazi A, Gluckman E, Brocheriou C, Laval-Jeantet M (1995) MR of cerebral aspergillosis in patients who have had bone marrow transplantation. AJNR Am J Neuroradiol 16:555–562

Miller GM, Baker HL Jr, Okazaki H, Whisnant JP (1988) Central pontine myelinolysis and its imitators: MR findings. Radiology 168:795–802

Miller L, Link MP, Bologna S, Parker BR (1989) Cerebellar atrophy caused by high-dose cytosine arabinoside: CT and MR findings. AJR Am J Roentgenol 152:343–344

Mohrmann RL, Mah V, Vinters HV (1990) Neuropathologic findings after bone marrow transplantation: an autopsy study. Hum Pathol 21:630–639

Moppett J, Oakhill A, Duncan AW (2001) Second malignancies in children: the usual suspects? Eur J Radiol 37:95–108

Mori A, Tanaka J, Kobayashi S, Hashino S, Yamamoto Y, Ota S, Asaka M, Imamura M (2000) Fatal cerebral hemorrhage associated with cyclosporin-A/FK506-related encephalopathy after allogeneic bone marrow transplantation. Ann Hematol 79:588–592

Mulhern RK, Kovnar E, Langston J, Carter M, Fairclough D, Leigh L, Kun LE (1992) Long-term survivors of leukemia treated in infancy: factors associated with neuropsychologic status. J Clin Oncol 10:1095–1102

Nakane M, Ohashi K, Tominaga J, Akiyama H, Hiruma K, Sakamaki H (2000) Disseminated toxoplasmosis after CD34+-selected autologous peripheral blood stem cell transplantation. Haematologica 85:334–335

Nevo S, Vogelsang GB (2001) Acute bleeding complications in patients after bone marrow transplantation. Curr Opin Hematol 8:319–325

Nevo S, Swan V, Enger C, et al. (1998) Acute bleeding after bone marrow transplantation (BMT)- incidence and effect on survival. A quantitative analysis in 1,402 patients. Blood 91.1469 1177

Nishio S, Morioka T, Inamura T, Takeshita I, Fukui M, Sasaki M, Nakamura K, Wakisaka S (1998) Radiation-induced brain tumours: potential late complications of radiation therapy for brain tumours. Acta Neurochir (Wien) 140: 763–770

Olavarria E, Prieto E, Roman A (1997) Retreatment with low-dose cytarabine in patients with previous central nervous system toxicity. Am J Hematol 54:338

Openshaw H, Slatkin NE (1999) Neurological complications. In: Thomas DE, Blume KG, Forman SJ (eds) Hematopoietic cell transplantation. Blackwell Science, Malden, pp 659–673

Paakko E, Vainionpaa L, Lanning M, Laitinen J, Pyhtinen J (1992) White matter changes in children treated for acute lymphoblastic leukemia. Cancer 70:2728–2733

Paakko E, Talvensaari K, Pyhtinen J, Lanning M (1994) Late cranial MRI after cranial irradiation in survivors of childhood cancer. Neuroradiology 36:652–655

Padovan CS, Bise K, Hahn J, Sostak P, Holler E, Kolb HJ, Straube A (1999) Angiitis of the central nervous system after allogeneic bone marrow transplantation? Stroke 30: 1651–1656

Parisi MT, Fahmy JL, Kaminsky CK, Malogolowkin MH (1999) Complications of cancer therapy in children: a radiologist's guide. Radiographics 19:283–297

Parker BR (1997) Leukemia and lymphoma in childhood. Radiol Clin North Am 35:1495–1516

Patchell RA (1994) Neurological complications of organ transplantation. Ann Neurol 36:688–703

Patel AG, Rao R (1996) Transient Ara-C leukoencephalopathy: MR findings. J Comput Assist Tomogr 20:161–162

Pease CL, Horton TM, McClain KL, Kaplan SL (2001) Aseptic meningitis in a child after systemic treatment with high dose cytarabine. Pediatr Infect Dis J 20:87–89

Pennisi AK, Meisler WJ, Dina TS (1985) Lymphomatous meningitis and steroid-induced epidural lipomatosis: CT evaluation. J Comput Assist Tomogr 9:595–598

Picardi M, De Rosa G, Di Salle F, Pezzullo L, Raiola A, Rotoli B (1998) Post-transplant cerebral toxoplasmosis diagnosed by magnetic resonance imaging. Haematologica 83:570–572

Pomeranz S, Naparstek E, Ashkenazi E, Nagler A, Lossos A, Slavin S, Or R (1994) Intracranial haematomas following bone marrow transplantation. J Neurol 241:252–256

Poussaint TY, Siffert J, Barnes PD, et al. (1995) Hemorrhagic vasculopathy after treatment of central nervous system neoplasia in childhood: diagnosis and follow-up. AJNR Am J Neuroradiol 16:693–699

Priest JR, Ramsay NK, Latchaw RE, et al. (1980) Thrombotic and hemorrhagic strokes complicating early therapy for childhood acute lymphoblastic leukemia. Cancer 46:1548–1554

Priest JR, Ramsay NK, Steinherz PG, et al. (1982) A syndrome of thrombosis and hemorrhage complicating L-asparaginase therapy for childhood acute lymphoblastic leukemia. J Pediatr 100:984–989

Provenzale JM, Petrella JR, Cruz LC Jr, Wong JC, Engelter S, Barboriak DP (2001) Quantitative assessment of diffusion abnormalities in posterior reversible encephalopathy syndrome. AJNR Am J Neuroradiol 22:1455–1461

Rubnitz JE, Relling MV, Harrison PL, et al. (1998) Transient encephalopathy following high-dose methotrexate treatment in childhood acute lymphoblastic leukemia. Leukemia 12:1176–1181

Saumoy M, Castells G, Escoda L, Mares R, Richart C, Ugarriza A (2002) Progressive multifocal leukoencephalopathy in chronic lymphocytic leukemia after treatment with fludarabine. Leuk Lymphoma 43:433–436

Schwartz DL, Schechter GP, Seltzer S, Chauncey TR (2000) Radiation myelitis following allogeneic stem cell transplantation and consolidation radiotherapy for non-Hodgkin's lymphoma. Bone Marrow Transplant 26:1355–1359

Schwartz RB (1996) A reversible posterior leukoencephalopathy syndrome. N Engl J Med 334:1743; discussion 1746

Schwartz RB, Jones KM, Kalina P, Bajakian RL, Mantello MT, Garada B, Holman BL (1992) Hypertensive encephalopathy: findings on CT, MR imaging, and SPECT imaging in 14 cases. AJR Am J Roentgenol 159:379–383

Schwartz RB, Mulkern RV, Gudbjartsson H, Jolesz F (1998) Diffusion-weighted MR imaging in hypertensive encephalopathy: clues to pathogenesis. AJNR Am J Neuroradiol 19:859–862

Seidel H, Nygaard R, Haave I, Moe PJ (1996) Magnetic resonance imaging and neurological evaluation after treatment with high-dose methotrexate for acute lymphocytic leukaemia in young children. Acta Paediatr 85:450–453

Seo SK, Regan A, Cihlar T, Lin DC, Boulad F, George D, Prasad VK, Kiehn TE, Polsky B (2001) Cytomegalovirus ventriculoencephalitis in a bone marrow transplant recipient receiving antiviral maintenance: clinical and molecular evidence of drug resistance. Clin Infect Dis 33:e105–108

Seong D, Bruner JM, Lee KH, et al. (1996) Progressive multifocal leukoencephalopathy after autologous bone marrow transplantation in a patient with chronic myelogenous leukemia. Clin Infect Dis 23:402–403

Seong DC, Przepiorka D, Bruner JM, Van Tassel P, Lo WK, Champlin RE (1993) Leptomeningeal toxoplasmosis after allogeneic marrow transplantation. Case report and review of the literature. Am J Clin Oncol 16:105–108

Seymour JF, Grigg AP, Szer J, Fox RM (2002) Cisplatin, fludarabine, and cytarabine: a novel, pharmacologically designed salvage therapy for patients with refractory, histologically aggressive or mantle cell non-Hodgkin's lymphoma. Cancer 94:585–593

Shalen PR, Ostrow PT, Glass PJ (1981) Enhancement of the white matter following prophylactic therapy of the central nervous system for leukemia: radiation effects and methotrexate leukoencephalopathy. Radiology 140:409–412

Shanley DJ (1995) Mineralizing microangiopathy: CT and MRI. Neuroradiology 37:331–333

Shbarou RM, Chao NJ, Morgenlander JC (2000) Cyclosporin A-related cerebral vasculopathy. Bone Marrow Transplant 26:801–804

Sirvent N, Monpoux F, Benet L, Richelme C, Mariani R, Diaine B (1998) Acute basal ganglia necrosis associated with cytarabine therapy. Med Pediatr Oncol 30:308

Snider S, Bashir R, Bierman P (1994) Neurologic complications after high-dose chemotherapy and autologous bone marrow transplantation for Hodgkin's disease. Neurology 44:681–684

Straathof CS, Kortbeek LM, Roerdink H, Sillevis Smitt PA, van den Bent MJ (2001) A solitary spinal cord toxoplasma lesion after peripheral stem-cell transplantation. J Neurol 248:814–815

Takahata M, Hashino S, Izumiyama K, Chiba K, Suzuki S, Asaka M (2001) Cyclosporin A-induced encephalopathy after allogeneic bone marrow transplantation with prevention of graft-versus-host disease by tacrolimus. Bone Marrow Transplant 28:713–715

Takatsuka H, Okamoto T, Yamada S, et al. (2000) New imaging findings in a patient with central nervous system dysfunction after bone marrow transplantation. Acta Haematol 103:203–205

Tefferi A, O'Neill BP, Inwards DJ (1998) Late-onset cerebral toxoplasmosis after allogeneic bone marrow transplantation. Bone Marrow Transplant 21:1285–1286

Tsuruda JS, Kortman KE, Bradley WG, Wheeler DC, Van Dalsem W, Bradley TP (1987) Radiation effects on cerebral white matter: MR evaluation. AJR Am J Roentgenol 149:165–171

Urban C, Sager WD (1981) Intracranial bleeding during therapy with L-asparaginase in childhood acute lymphocytic leukemia. Eur J Pediatr 137:323–327

van den Berg H, van der Flier M, van de Wetering MD (2001) Cytarabine-induced aseptic meningitis. Leukemia 15:697–699

Vaughn DJ, Jarvik JG, Hackney D, Peters S, Stadtmauer EA (1993) High-dose cytarabine neurotoxicity: MR findings during the acute phase. AJNR Am J Neuroradiol 14:1014–1016

Vazquez E, Lucaya J, Castellote A, et al. (2002) Neuroimaging in pediatric leukemia and lymphoma: differential diagnosis. Radiographics 22:1411–1428

Verschuur A, Brousse N, Raynal B, Brison O, Rohrlich P, Rahimy C, Vilmer E (1994) Donor B cell lymphoma of the brain after allogeneic bone marrow transplantation for acute myeloid leukemia. Bone Marrow Transplant 14:467–470

Waldrop SM, Davis PC, Padgett CA, Shapiro MB, Morris R (1998) Treatment of brain tumors in children is associated with abnormal MR spectroscopic ratios in brain tissue remote from the tumor site. AJNR Am J Neuroradiol 19:963–970

Walter AW, Hancock ML, Pui CH, et al. (1998) Secondary brain tumors in children treated for acute lymphoblastic leukemia at St. Jude Children's Research Hospital. J Clin Oncol 16:3761–3767

Wang AM, Skias DD, Rumbaugh CL, Schoene WC, Zamani

A (1983) Central nervous system changes after radiation therapy and/or chemotherapy: correlation of CT and autopsy findings. AJNR Am J Neuroradiol 4:466–471

Yuh WT, Nguyen HD, Gao F, et al. (1994) Brain parenchymal infection in bone marrow transplantation patients: CT and MR findings. AJR Am J Roentgenol 162:425–430.

Zawacki T, Friedman JH, Grace J, Shetty N (2000) Cerebellar toxicity of cytosine arabinoside: clinical and neuropsychological signs. Neurology 55:1234

Zimmer WE, Hourihane JM, Wang HZ, Schriber JR (1998) The effect of human leukocyte antigen disparity on cyclosporine neurotoxicity after allogeneic bone marrow transplantation. AJNR Am J Neuroradiol 19:601–608; discussion 609–610

23 The Treated Thorax in Patients with Hematological Malignancies

Benoît Mesurolle, Nobuyuki Tanaka, John Kosiuk, François Mignon, Sylvain Choquet

CONTENTS

Benoît Mesurolle, MD
Assistant Professor, McGill University Health Center, Department of Radiology, Royal Victoria Hospital, 687 Pine Avenue West, Montreal PQ, H3A 1A1, Canada
Nobuyuki Tanaka, MD
Assistant Professor, Chest Radiologist, Department of Radiology, Yamaguchi University School of Medicine, 1-1-1 Minamikogushi, Ube, Yamaguchi 755-8505, Japan
John Kosiuk, MD
Assistant Professor, McGill University Health Center, Department of Radiology, Royal Victoria Hospital, 687 Pine Avenue West, Montreal PQ, H3A 1A1, Canada
François Mignon, MD
Assistant Professor, Department of Radiology, Versailles Hospital Center, 177 Rue de Versailles, 78157 Le Chesnay Cedex, France
Sylvain Choquet, MD
Assistant Professor, Department of Hematology, Versailles Hospital Center, 177 Rue de Versailles, 78157 Le Chesnay Cedex, France

23.1 Introduction

Thoracic complications and changes are frequent in patients with hematological malignancies. In those patients with advanced hematological malignancies pulmonary complications, mostly related to chemotherapy, can be a leading cause of death. Tenholder and Hooper found that 98% of leukemic patients showed pulmonary complications at autopsy (Tenholder and Hooper 1980). Of note however, in recent years the frequency of radiation-induced complications has decreased. As the number of survivors increases, several late effects of treatment are becoming evident, some of them – second malignancies, cardiovascular complications – emerging as a major threat to the survival of these patients. To offer the best in patient care, it is imperative to understand the natural history of the disease as well as the treatment related complications and changes. In this chapter, post-therapeutic thoracic changes after chemotherapy and radiation therapy are discussed and illustrated.

23.2
Chest Complications Associated with Chemotherapy

Although chest radiography is an important modality, the findings are often nonspecific or difficult to detect. High-resolution CT (HRCT) is a powerful tool for the detection of early or tiny pulmonary lesions occurring in immunocompromised patients. With progressive improvement in therapy for patients with hematological malignancies, hemopoietic stem cell transplantation (HSCT) has become a standard method for treating aggressive disorders. The frequency of pulmonary complications is different in patients who have undergone HSCT and those who have not. These complications can be divided into two categories: complications not specific to patients treated with HSCT (HSCT non-specific complications) and complications specific to patients treated with HSCT (HSCT specific complications occur in approximately 50% of transplant recipients) (WORTHY et al. 1997a).

Stem cells may be obtained from the patients themselves (autologous HSCT) or from related or unrelated donors (allogeneic HSCT), and may be harvested in the form of bone marrow, peripheral blood stem cells or, less frequently, cord blood (Hows 2001). Autologous HSCT complications are directly related to the conditioning regimen (chemotherapy with or without total body irradiation). Allogeneic HSCT adds the toxicity of the conditioning regimen to a major immunosuppression and, often, graft versus host disease (GVHD). Allogeneic HSCT specific complications occur in a characteristic temporal pattern associated with the period following the procedure (WORTHY et al. 1997a). The period after HSCT is divided into 3 phases: neutropenic, early and late (Fig. 23.1).

23.2.1
HSCT non-Specific Complications

23.2.1.1
Infectious Conditions

Sixty to 75% of reported deaths in leukemia, after HSCT, are due to infectious diseases (HILDEBRAND et al. 1990). Such infectious conditions tend to occur after chemotherapy or in the neutropenic or early phase following HSCT.

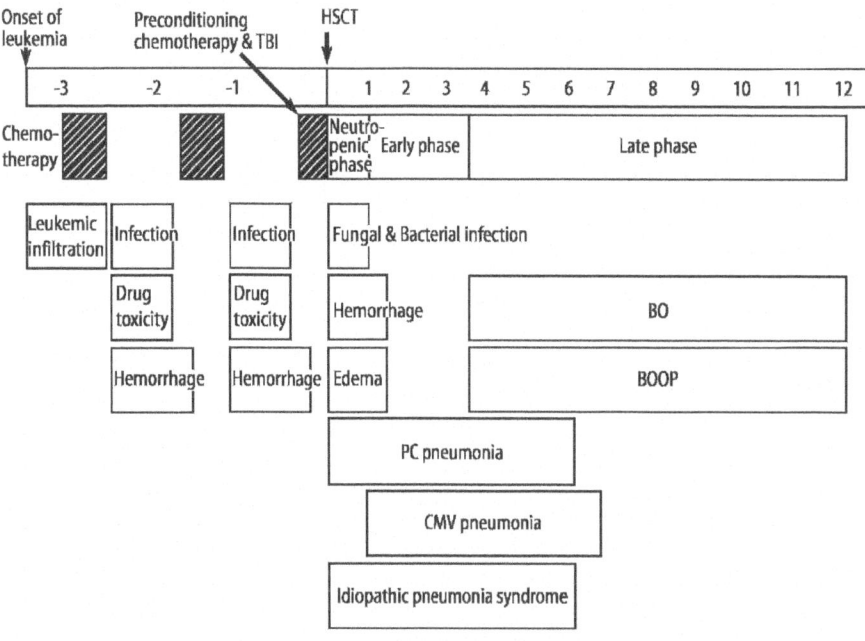

Fig. 23.1. Pulmonary effects of treatment in patients with hematological malignancies. Pulmonary complications often occur in a characteristic temporal pattern associated with hemopoietic stem cell transplantation. (With permission from [TANAKA et al. 2002])

23.2.1.1.1
Bacterial Pneumonia

Granulocytopenia is a major predisposing factor for bacterial infections. This condition occurs after chemotherapy, with or without HSCT. Bacterial pneumonia in HSCT recipients occurs usually in the neutropenic phase, and its incidence is estimated as 20 to 50% (SOUBANI et al. 1996). Gram-negative organisms presumably, from the gastro-intestinal tract or oral mucosa, are classically considered as the predominant group of bacteria, but recent studies show that gram-positive infections represent 60 to 70% of isolated organisms, mainly *Staphylococcus aureus* and coagulase negative *Staphylococcus* (ZINNER 1999). Defective function of the mucociliary system caused by bronchial sicca-like damage from GVHD, impaired production of secretory IgA, abnormal humoral response to pneumococcal polysaccharide antigen, and spleen dysfunction (caused by total body irradiation and/or allogeneic HSCT) are responsible for the increased frequency of these infections.

In bacterial pneumonia, airspace consolidation or ground-glass opacity with centrilobular, acinar, and lobular opacities is observed. Ground-glass opacity seems to occur more frequently in immunocompromised patients than in immunocompetent patients (Fig. 23.2). WINN and CHANDLER (1994) reported that, because the diminution of the inflammatory change in the immunocompromised host was perhaps caused by neutropenia, the radiographic findings were markedly altered by the minimal inflammation. There may be a tendency to produce ground-glass opacity or small opacities like centrilobular opacities on HRCT because the exudative reaction in immunodeficiency states is minimal.

23.2.1.1.2
Pneumocystis carinii Pneumonia

Pneumocystis carinii pneumonia occurs in patients with hematological malignancies who undergo intensive chemotherapy, especially with corticoid and fludarabine, or HSCT. In our institution, it occurs less frequently in HSCT recipients, probably because of the introduction of routine prophylaxis with sulfamethoxazole/trimethoprim. The incidence of *Pneumocystis carinii* pneumonia in HSCT recipients is reported as less than 10% (SOUBANI et al. 1996). Characteristic pathologic findings include intraalveolar histiocytes or a mixture of inflammatory infiltrates with or without associated hemorrhage. The

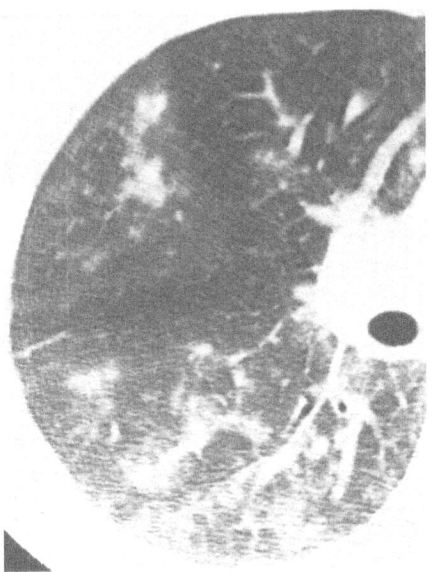

Fig. 23.2. Bacterial pneumonia in a 25-year-old woman with acute lymphocytic leukemia. Axial HRCT scan shows widespread ground-glass opacities and patchy acinar or centrilobular opacities mainly along the bronchovascular bundles.

classic chest radiographic finding of *Pneumocystis carinii* pneumonia is a bilateral perihilar or diffuse symmetric interstitial pattern, which may be finely granular, reticular, or ground-glass in appearance. Chest radiography may have normal or nonspecific findings at the time of initial examination in as many as 40% of cases. In a study of 51 cases with a high clinical suspicion of *Pneumocystis carinii* pneumonia in which chest radiography showed normal, equivocal or non-specific findings by GRUDEN et al. (1997), *Pneumocystis carinii* pneumonia was detected in six of 51 cases. The findings were confirmed by HRCT, which showed abnormal findings in all six cases. It is evident that HRCT is needed for the detection of early lesion of *Pneumocystis carinii* pneumonia when it is strongly suspected in the clinical setting.

On HRCT, widespread ground-glass opacity, which is typically distributed at the perihilar regions, is a frequent and characteristic finding (Fig. 23.3) (WEBB et al. 1996; KUHLMAN et al. 1990). Extensive ground-glass opacity is usually observed with sparing of adjacent secondary pulmonary lobules, called a mosaic or geographic pattern. Occasionally, reticulation or intralobular and interlobular septal thickening within ground-glass opacity may be recognized (crazy-paving appearance), presumably reflecting a combination of fluid and cellular components within the alveolar space as well as thickening of the alveolar septa. Centrilobular opaci-

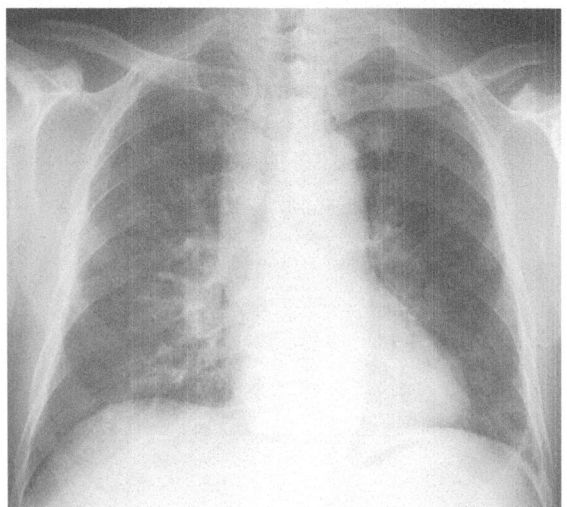

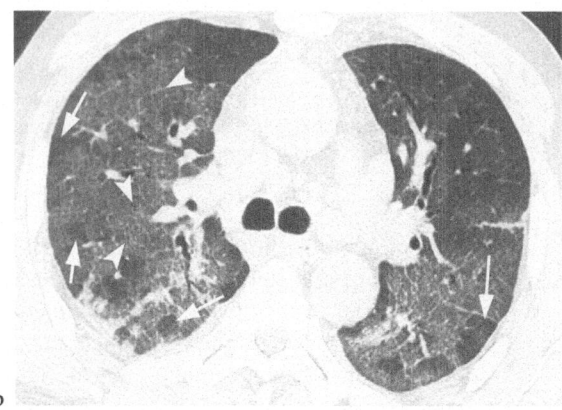

Fig. 23.3a,b. *Pneumocystis carinii* pneumonia in a 60-year-old man with acute lymphocytic leukemia. **a** Posteroanterior chest radiograph shows mixed interstitial and alveolar disease with a right lower lobe predominance. Bilateral hilar and mediastinal lymphadenopathies are also noted. **b** Axial HRCT scan shows widespread ground-glass opacity with sparing of adjacent pulmonary lobules (*arrows*), creating a mosaic pattern. Note the reticular opacities within ground-glass opacity, showing "crazy-paving appearance" (*arrowheads*).

ties or Y-shaped branching structures (tree-in-bud appearance) are sometimes observed, corresponding to bronchiolitis and bronchioles impacted with inflammatory material (WEBB et al. 1996; BOISELLE et al. 1999). In addition to these classical HRCT findings, other atypical findings have been reported in patients with AIDS, such as cystic lesions, upper lobe distribution, lung nodules or masses, lobar consolidation or interstitial fibrosis (BOISELLE et al. 1999). However, we have never encountered such atypical findings in patients with hematological malignancies in our institution.

23.2.1.1.3
Fungal Infections

Fungal infection is a common cause of pneumonia in HSCT recipients. However, it also occurs in patients who do not undergo HSCT. In our series, it occurred more frequently in patients who without HSCT. Granulocytopenia is the most important risk factor (HILDEBRAND et al. 1990). In HSCT recipients, it usually occurs in the neutropenic phase. The pathogens are *Aspergillus*, *Candida*, *Cryptococcus*, and *Mucor*. The most common pathogen in this entity is *Aspergillus*. In general, infection due to *Aspergillus* frequently occurs when the peripheral white blood count decreases to less than $1,000/mm^3$. Invasive pulmonary aspergillosis is the most frequent pattern of infection caused by *Aspergillus* in immunocompromised patients.

Characteristic chest radiographic findings include solitary or multiple focal opacities or consolidation distributed in the peripheral lung. Detection of early lesions of invasive aspergillosis is rather difficult because about one quarter of patients with invasive pulmonary aspergillosis show no abnormal chest radiographic findings. CT is needed in the early diagnosis of invasive pulmonary aspergillosis. Invasive pulmonary aspergillosis includes two types: angio-invasive aspergillosis (angio-invasive pulmonary aspergillosis) and airway-invasive aspergillosis (airway-invasive pulmonary aspergillosis). Usually, invasive pulmonary aspergillosis means angio-invasive pulmonary aspergillosis.

Angio-invasive pulmonary aspergillosis presents two characteristic CT findings: CT-halo sign, an early sign after infection (Fig. 23.4) and the air crescent sign, observed in relatively late phase of infection (KUHLMAN et al. 1988). The CT-halo sign is observed at the period of neutropenia, and represents a hemorrhagic infarction, in which the nodular lesion corresponds to a gray-yellow necrotic center, and the ground-glass opacity to a rim of hemorrhage caused by thrombosis of fungi within pulmonary vessels. This sign was first reported by KUHLMAN et al. (1985) and thought to be characteristic and specific to invasive pulmonary aspergillosis. However, it has been reported in patients with hemorrhagic nodules in the lung, such as candidiasis, CMV infection, Wegener granulomatosis and metastatic angiosarcoma (PRIMACK et al. 1994). The air crescent sign is observed at the period when neutropenia is recovering and represents the cavitation of nodules caused by resorption of necrotic tissue by returning neutrophils (Fig. 23.5) (TANAKA et al. 2002). This sign is usually

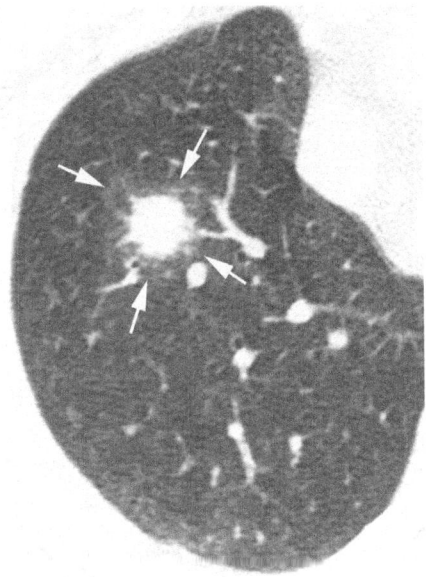

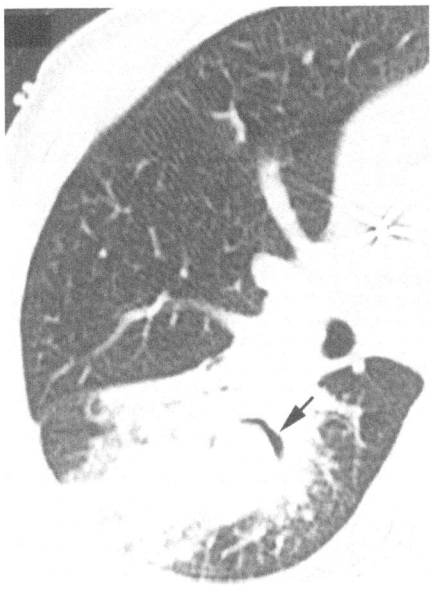

Fig. 23.4. Invasive aspergillosis in a 58-year-old man with chronic myelocytic leukemia. Axial HRCT scan shows a central hyperdense nodule with surrounding halo of ground-glass opacity (CT-halo sign) (*arrow*) in the right upper lobe. (With permission from [TANAKA et al. 2002])

Fig. 23.5. Invasive aspergillosis in a 47-year-old man with acute myelocytic leukemia. Axial HRCT scan shows airspace consolidation with a crescent-like cavity (air crescent sign) (*arrow*) in the right lower lobe.

observed 2–3 weeks after infection. Therefore, it is not useful as an early indication of invasive pulmonary aspergillosis. However, the existence of air crescent sign suggests that the patient is in the recovery phase from infection because it is not seen in patients who do not recover from neutropenia. In a report by GEFTER et al. (1985), the air crescent sign was associated with a good prognosis. We treated a case with extensive ground-glass opacity on CT images induced by the invasion of *Aspergillus* into pulmonary arteries and subsequent pulmonary infarction (Fig. 23.6). The ground-glass opacity was caused by the hemorrhagic changes. It must be noted that extensive pulmonary alveolar hemorrhage can be induced by fungal infection as well as thrombocytopenia or HSCT.

There are few reports concerning airway-invasive pulmonary aspergillosis. It may be seen in 10–30% of patients with invasive pulmonary aspergillosis. Chest radiography shows non-specific findings indicating bronchopneumonia. Pathological findings of airway-invasive pulmonary aspergillosis include bronchiolitis and bronchopneumonia caused by *Aspergillus*. CT findings may show small centrilobular nodules and peribronchial airspace consolidation, which reflect the pathological findings. However, these CT findings are non-specific, and it is difficult to differentiate this entity from other infectious diseases.

Candidiasis frequently occurs concomitantly with bacterial infection, and the characteristic radiographic findings of pulmonary candidiasis are difficult to describe. In the report of a radiographic-pathologic correlative study of candidiasis by DUBOIS et al. (1977), lesions were divided into hematogenous and endobronchial spread. In the former, hemorrhagic nodules are the characteristic pathologic finding. Central areas of necrosis and surrounding hemorrhage are observed. These findings are nearly identical to those of angio-invasive pulmonary aspergillosis (CT-halo sign). Nodules seen in patients with candidiasis are usually smaller than those in invasive pulmonary aspergillosis (Fig. 23.7), therefore, these nodules may be difficult to detect by chest radiography. Miliary nodules may sometimes be seen but in a report of 20 cases of pulmonary candidiasis by BUFF et al. (1982), there were no cases showing a miliary nodular pattern. In the latter type of endobronchial spread, bronchopneumonia is the radiological and pathologic finding.

Cryptococcosis, especially secondary cryptococcosis shows solitary or multiple pulmonary nodules or infiltrative opacities. These lesions may sometimes cavitate. In a CT report of 10 cases with AIDS by SIDER and WESTCOTT (1994), five patients had segmental airspace consolidation with air broncho-

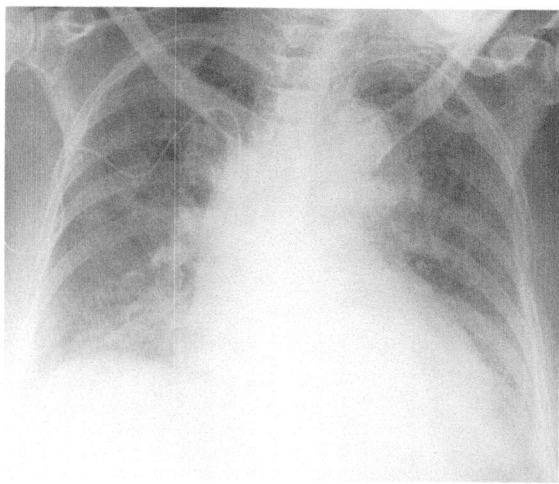

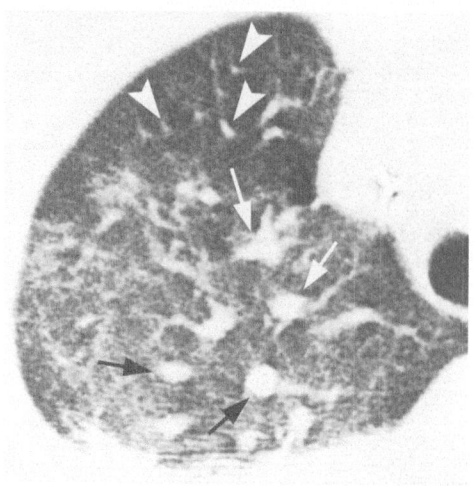

a

b

Fig. 23.6a,b. Mycotic thrombosis in a 70-year-old man with plasma cell leukemia. **a** Posteroanterior chest radiograph shows diffuse bilateral air space disease and cardiomegaly. **b** Axial HRCT scan shows extensive ground-glass opacity with pleural effusion in the right upper lobe. Note that the diameter of pulmonary arteries within the ground-glass opacity became wider (*arrows*) compared with those in the normal lung (*arrowheads*). This patient died after the CT examination. Specimens obtained at autopsy showed extensive hemorrhage and hemorrhagic infarction induced by extensive mycotic (*Aspergillus*) thrombosis within pulmonary arteries.

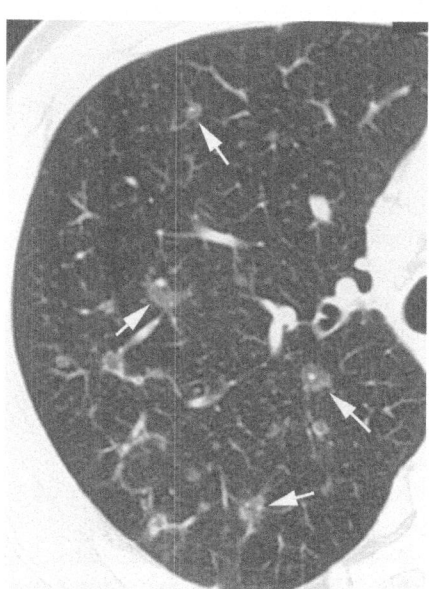

Fig. 23.7. Candidiasis in a 28-year-old man with natural killer-like T-cell leukemia. Axial HRCT scan shows multiple nodules with surrounding ground-glass opacities (*arrows*).

gram, five had ground-glass opacity distributed at the perihilar or lower lung regions, and three had multiple nodules with indistinct borders. It may also be difficult to distinguish cryptococcosis from other infectious conditions based on these reported CT findings.

The CT findings of mucormycosis are indistinguishable from those of invasive pulmonary aspergillosis. Multiple nodules or airspace consolidation are frequent. It should be noted that the CT-halo sign is frequently observed due to hemorrhagic infarction based on the angio-invasive nature of *Mucor* just as with invasive pulmonary aspergillosis (MCADAMS et al. 1997). Cases with pseudoaneurysm or invasive change into the thoracic spine have been reported.

There is an unusual condition induced by the specific nature of fungi including *Aspergillus* and *Mucor*. Hypoxemia without apparent abnormal CT findings may sometimes be observed in patients with fungal infection. This condition seems to be induced by intravascular fungal emboli (Fig. 23.8). The mechanism is the same as that in patients with leukostasis, which is characterized by intravascular leukemic cell emboli due to high leukocyte count (MCKEE et al. 1974).

23.2.1.1.4
Tuberculosis

Pulmonary tuberculosis in immunocompromised patients often has an atypical CT pattern compared with that in immunocompetent patients; it includes non-segmental distribution and multiple small cavities within lesions (IKEZOE et al. 1992). Numerous small nodules with random distribution

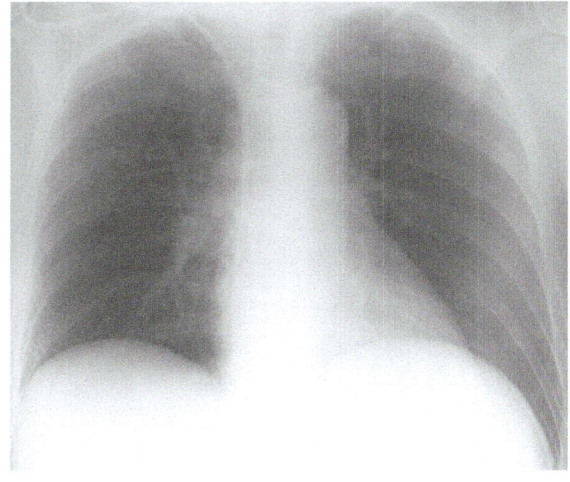

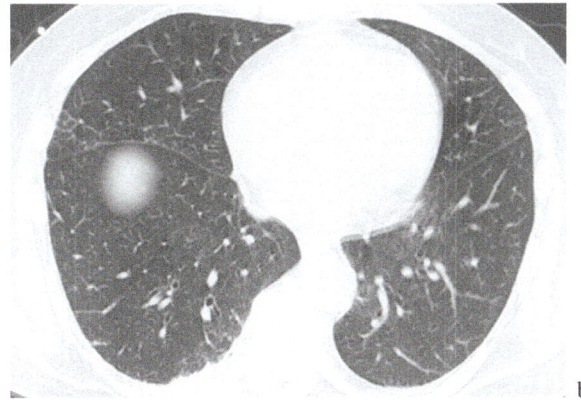

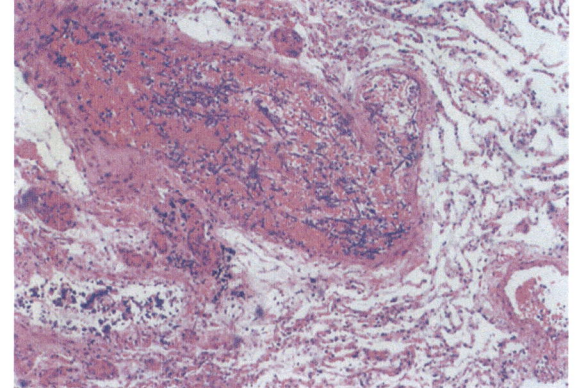

Fig. 23.8a–c. Mycotic thrombosis in a 55-year-old woman with chronic myelocytic leukemia. **a** Posteroanterior chest radiograph shows no abnormal finding. **b** Axial HRCT scan appears almost normal except for linear-reticular opacities in the right lower lobe. This patient showed severe hypoxia and died one week after CT examination. **c** Autopsied specimen shows thrombus with *Candida* filling the pulmonary artery and arterioles.

within secondary pulmonary lobules are a characteristic HRCT finding for miliary tuberculosis (OH et al. 1994). Ground-glass opacity may be present along with nodules (Fig. 23.9) (TANAKA et al. 2002). Ground-glass opacity corresponds pathologically to widespread interstitial granuloma of a size below the limits of resolution on HRCT (OH et al. 1994).

23.2.1.2
Drug Toxicity

Drug-induced lung diseases must always be considered in the differential diagnosis of pulmonary infiltrates in immunocompromised patients who are undergoing chemotherapy, even though the exact incidence is uncertain.

Rossi et al. (2000) reported radiographic findings of drug toxicity based on pathologic findings. As possible pathologic manifestations of pulmonary drug toxicity, they mentioned diffuse alveolar damage, nonspecific interstitial pneumonia, bronchiolitis obliterans organizing pneumonia (BOOP), eosinophilic pneumonia, and others. Diffuse alveolar damage is recognized as a common manifesta-

tion of drug toxicity, and chest radiograph findings include bilateral heterogeneous or homogeneous opacities, often in a mid and lower lung distribution. HRCT shows scattered or diffuse areas of ground-glass opacity. With the progression of lesions, fibrosis, architectural distortion or honeycombing may occur. The concept of nonspecific interstitial pneumonia is relatively new and is thought to be a second most frequent entity among idiopathic interstitial pneumonia. Rossi et al. (2000) found this pattern to be the most frequent in interstitial pneumonia in patients with pulmonary drug toxicity. Nonspecific interstitial pneumonia is characterized pathologically by areas of expansion of the interstitium by mononuclear inflammatory cells and mild interstitial pneumonia with temporal and spatial homogeneity. Interstitial inflammation is typically more cellular than that seen in idiopathic interstitial pneumonia. Chest radiography usually shows diffuse heterogeneous opacities. HRCT shows scattered or diffuse areas of ground-glass opacity. BOOP is a nonspecific pathologic pattern of lung injury that can be a manifestation of pulmonary drug toxicity, characterized by proliferation of immature fibroblas-

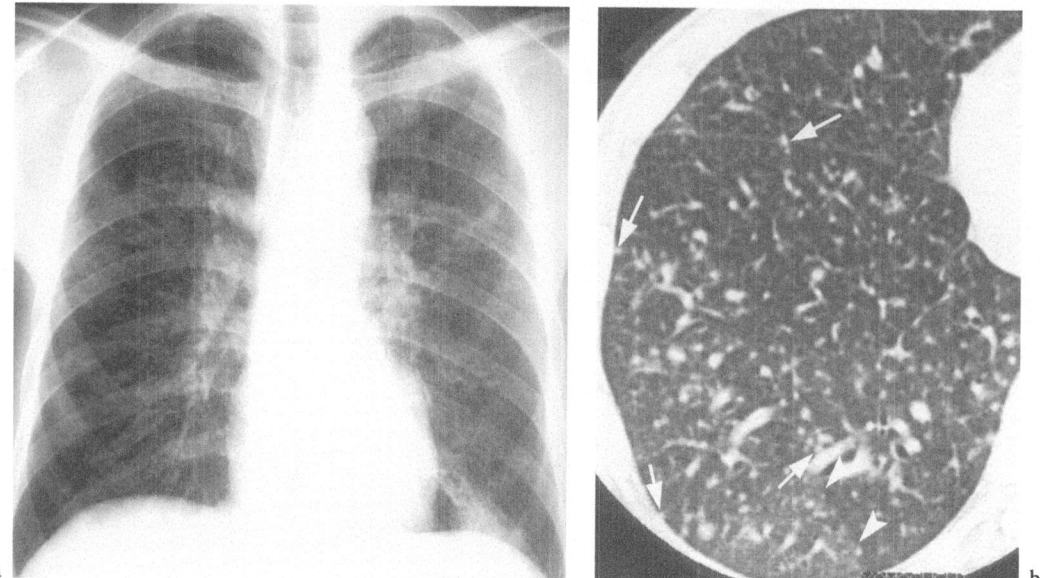

Fig. 23.9a,b. Miliary tuberculosis in a 39-year-old man with acute myelocytic leukemia. **a** Posteroanterior chest radiograph shows diffuse and bilateral pulmonary micronodules with focal consolidations in the left upper and lower lobes. **b** Axial HRCT scan shows numerous miliary nodules throughout both lungs. Some of these nodules are located on the pleural surface or on the pulmonary vessels (*arrows*), showing random distribution of the nodules within the secondary pulmonary lobules. Also note patchy ground-glass opacity in the right lower lobe (*arrowheads*), which probably shows widespread interstitial granuloma of a size below the limits of resolution on HRCT. (With permission from [TANAKA et al. 2002])

tic plugs within the respiratory bronchioles, alveolar ducts, and adjacent alveolar spaces. HRCT shows focal airspace consolidation, poorly-defined masses, or centrilobular nodules. These areas are typically peripheral or peribronchovascular in distribution. Eosinophilic pneumonia is characterized by the accumulation of eosinophils and macrophages in the alveolar spaces or thickened alveolar septa. CT is useful in demonstrating the peripheral nature of the lesions. ROSSI et al. (2000) also mentioned the possibility of pulmonary hemorrhage, bronchiolitis obliterans, pulmonary edema, pulmonary hypertension, or veno-occlusive disease as pathologic features of pulmonary drug toxicity. In a report of 20 patients with drug toxicity who underwent high-dose chemotherapy and autologous HSCT, PATZ et al. (1994) found scattered, predominantly peripheral ground-glass opacity and airspace consolidation in 13 patients (65%). They speculated that a large number of alveoli, alveolar macrophages, type 2 pneumocytes, and a greater density of pulmonary arterioles within the cortical or peripheral region of the lung might be the mechanism of peripheral distribution of lesions. Perfusion differences between the cortical and medullary portions of the lung and longer peripheral blood flow transit times permit

prolonged drug concentration in the cortical lung. The pathologic features of pulmonary drug toxicity are diverse, and the radiographic and CT findings are nonspecific. HRCT findings usually include airspace consolidation, ground-glass opacity and reticulation (Fig. 23.10) (TANAKA et al. 2002). Therefore, it is difficult to diagnose this entity by radiologic findings only. It must be noted that this entity is usually diagnosed by exclusion of alternative diagnoses.

23.2.1.3
Pulmonary Hemorrhage

This entity is associated with complicated thrombocytopenia, infectious disease or HSCT. TENHOLDER and HOOPER (1980) noted that this was the most common cause of non-infectious pulmonary complications in patients with leukemia and BODEY et al. (1996) found it in 54% of 50 autopsied cases of acute leukemia. Diffuse alveolar hemorrhage is also observed in about 20% of HSCT patients (WORTHY et al. 1997a) and occurs especially in the neutropenic phase. The clinical manifestation is acute and nonspecific; it is difficult to diagnose before death since hemoptysis is rare. The mortality rate is high, about 80%. Early diagnosis followed by prompt steroid

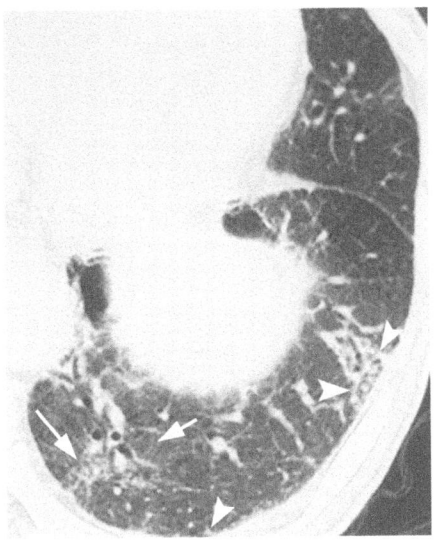

Fig. 23.10. Drug toxicity induced by phosphomycin in a 73-year-old man with chronic myelocytic leukemia. Axial HRCT scan shows patchy ground-glass opacity (*arrows*) and linear-reticular opacities (*arrowheads*) mainly in the subpleural zone.

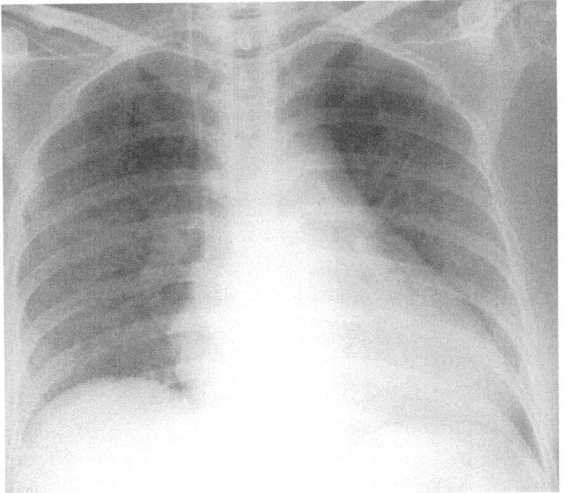

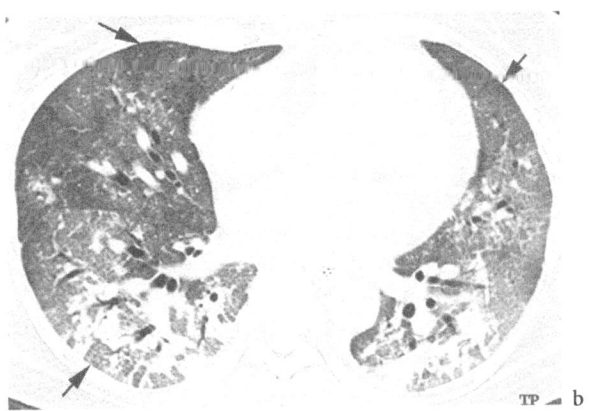

Fig. 23.11a,b. Diffuse pulmonary hemorrhage in a 37-year-old woman with acute lymphocytic leukemia. **a** Posteroanterior chest radiograph shows interstitial changes predominantly distributed in the bilateral lower lung zones. **b** Axial HRCT scan shows extensive ground-glass opacity and airspace consolidation which distribute mainly at the medullary region with the most peripheral zones less involved (*arrows*).

therapy is the only way to improve the survival rate. It is important to perform bronchoalveolar lavage if this entity is suspected because bronchoalveolar lavage can show evidence of hemorrhage by revealing hemosiderin-laden macrophages. The causes of this entity are speculated to be damage to the pulmonary vasculature by GVHD, pre-transplantation chemotherapy or total body irradiation. Whether the process is a distinct entity or whether it represents a part of a spectrum of severe pulmonary edema or idiopathic pneumonia syndrome is not yet known.

The most common, but non-specific CT findings consist of widespread ground-glass opacity or consolidation (Fig. 23.11) (PRIMACK et al. 1995), within which reticulation is often recognized (crazy-paving appearance). Typically, the most peripheral lung zones or subpleural regions are spared.

23.2.2
HSCT Specific Complications

HSCT has made it possible to treat leukemia patients with high-dose chemotherapy and total body irradiation. After HSCT, there is a neutropenic phase, lasting 10 to 12 days with peripheral stem cells, and up to 3 weeks with bone marrow. After the neutropenic phase, an immunosuppressive state continues for about 1 year after allogeneic HSCT. This period is

usually divided into early phase and late phase; the former, by definition, continues for 100 days after HSCT and the latter continues for one year (or more) after HSCT (Fig. 23.1) (HASLETON and DORAN 1996). Chest complications after HSCT are a major problem and occur in 40 to 60% of such patients (KROWKA et al. 1985; WORTHY et al. 1997a).

23.2.2.1.
Infectious Conditions

Although any infectious disorder can occur after HSCT, especially in the neutropenic or early phase, cytomegalovirus pneumonia is the most frequent.

23.2.2.1.1
Cytomegalovirus Pneumonia

Cytomegalovirus (CMV) infection occurs in 70% of allogeneic HSCT recipients, but less than one-third develop CMV pneumonia (WORTHY et al. 1997). It typically occurs in the early phase. The causes of CMV infection include reactivation of endogenous latent virus in profoundly immunosuppressed recipients, or acquisition of exogenous infection from CMV seropositive bone marrow grafts or blood products. Reported mortality rate is up to 85%. Although the detection of early CMV antigen using bronchoalveolar lavage fluid may be a good method in CMV related pneumonia, it should be noted that CMV is sometimes isolated in the absence of active disease. Nowadays, the systematic search for CMV antigens in peripheral leucocytes and early treatment has dramatically decreased the incidence of CMV pneumonia and CMV-related mortality. The basic pathologic finding is an alveolar pattern consisting of alveolar macrophages, fibrin, hyaline membranes, proliferating reactive pneumocytes, and hemorrhagic exudates, consistent with diffuse alveolar damage. Interstitial thickening without airspace disease may sometimes be seen. Interstitial infiltrates consisting of lymphocytes may sometimes result in alveolar wall or interlobular septal thickening.

CMV pneumonia shows various CT findings, including patchy or widespread ground-glass opacity, air-space consolidation, nodules with the CT-halo sign, and centrilobular nodules (Fig. 23.12) (PRIMACK and MÜLLER 1994; WEBB et al. 1996; KANG et al. 1996). In a report of 21 patients with AIDS and CMV pneumonia by McGUINNESS et al. (1994), ground-glass opacity or airspace consolidation were observed in 13 patients and corresponded mainly to an airspace filling process of diffuse alveolar damage. They also reported pulmonary masses and miliary patterns. Nodules with the CT-halo sign correspond to the hemorrhagic nodules. These findings are non-specific, and it is often difficult to differentiate them from those of other entities including *Pneumocystis carinii* pneumonia and pulmonary hemorrhage.

23.2.2.2
Pulmonary Edema

Pulmonary edema is a common complication in the neutropenic phase although the exact incidence is not known. The onset is usually rapid and occurs in the second or third week post transplantation. The causes of this entity are thought to be acute GVHD, cardiac

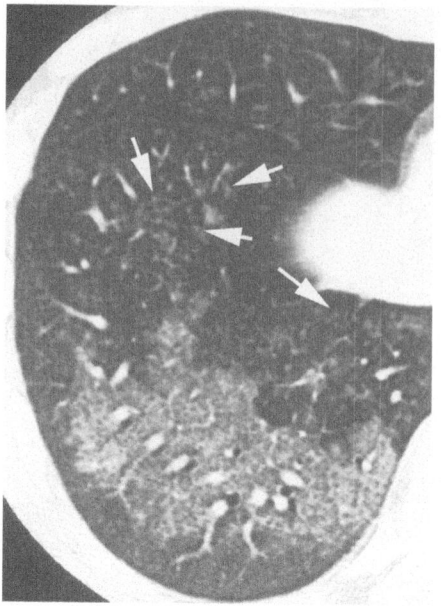

Fig. 23.12. Cytomegalovirus pneumonia in a 35-year-old man with acute myelocytic leukemia. Axial HRCT scan shows extensive ground-glass opacity in the right lower lobe. Note that centrilobular nodules can be seen (*arrows*). It is quite difficult to differentiate this finding from *Pneumocystis carinii* pneumonia.

or renal impairment induced by intensive chemotherapy, the increased permeability of pulmonary vessels induced by total body irradiation, sepsis, cyclosporine A, prophylactic granulocyte transfusions and the infusion of large volumes of fluid to administer drugs (HASLETON and DORAN 1996; WORTHY et al. 1997a). Cardiac dysfunction may be caused by adriamycin, cyclophosphamide or radiation therapy.

Chest radiographic findings include diffusely increased interstitial markings such as Kerley A, B and C lines, peribronchial cuffing, hilar haze, ground-glass appearance and vascular redistribution. Characteristic CT findings include enlargement of pulmonary vessels, ground-glass opacity or air-space consolidation in the hilar or peribronchial regions, thickening of interlobular septa and pleural effusion (Fig. 23.13) (PRIMACK and MÜLLER 1994; WORTHY et al. 1997a).

23.2.2.3
Idiopathic Pneumonia Syndrome

This entity is an early phase complication and occurs in approximately 12% of allogeneic HSCT patients. It is defined as diffuse lung injury occurring after HSCT for which an infectious etiology is not identified (CLARK et

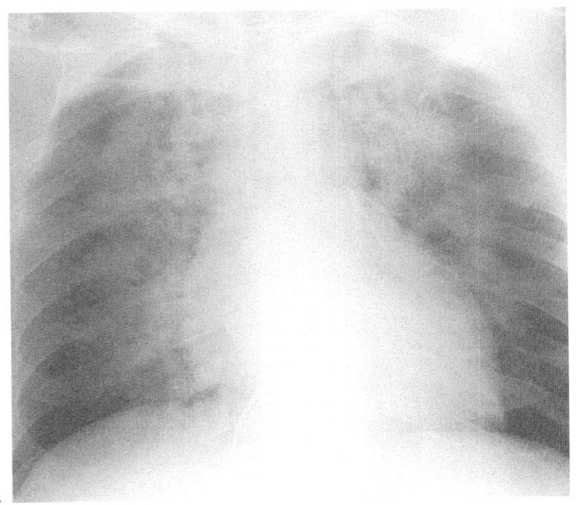

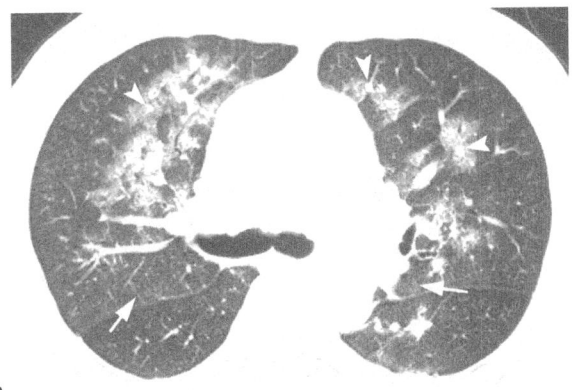

Fig. 23.13a,b. Pulmonary edema in a 58-year-old man with multiple myeloma. a Posteroanterior chest radiograph shows extensive airspace consolidation with air bronchogram distributed mainly in the bilateral hilar regions. Note an associated cardiomegaly. b Axial HRCT scan shows ground-glass opacity and airspace consolidation distributed along the bronchovascular bundles. Thickening of interlobular septa is seen (*arrows*). Note that the pulmonary arteries became greater in diameter (*arrowheads*) than accompanying bronchi.

al. 1993). It is probably caused by toxicity from the pretransplantation chemotherapy and total body irradiation (CLARK et al. 1993; WORTHY et al. 1997a; KROWKA et al. 1985). Mortality rate approaches 80%.

The pathologic feature of idiopathic pneumonia syndrome is diffuse alveolar damage with an interstitial mononuclear cellular infiltrate. Clinically, diffuse alveolar damage is seen in acute interstitial pneumonia or acute respiratory distress syndrome (ARDS). Although it is not clear if idiopathic pneumonia syndrome is the same entity as acute interstitial pneumonia or ARDS, the pathologic feature is the same among these 3 entities. Diffuse alveolar damage is manifested by injury to the alveolar lining and endothelial cells, pulmonary

edema, hyaline membrane formation, and extensive fibroblastic proliferation but little mature collagen deposition. The pathologic appearance of diffuse alveolar damage can be separated into acute exudative, subacute proliferative and chronic fibrotic phases.

HRCT findings of diffuse alveolar damage, focal or diffuse ground-glass opacity were seen in all reported cases. Air-space consolidation is slightly less common, but seen in most cases. Usually, ground-glass opacity and airspace consolidation are denser in attenuation in the dependent lung zone than in the non-dependent lung (Fig. 23.14). ICHIKADO et al. (1997) and PRIMACK et al. (1993) observed areas of ground-glass opacity with focally spared regions that

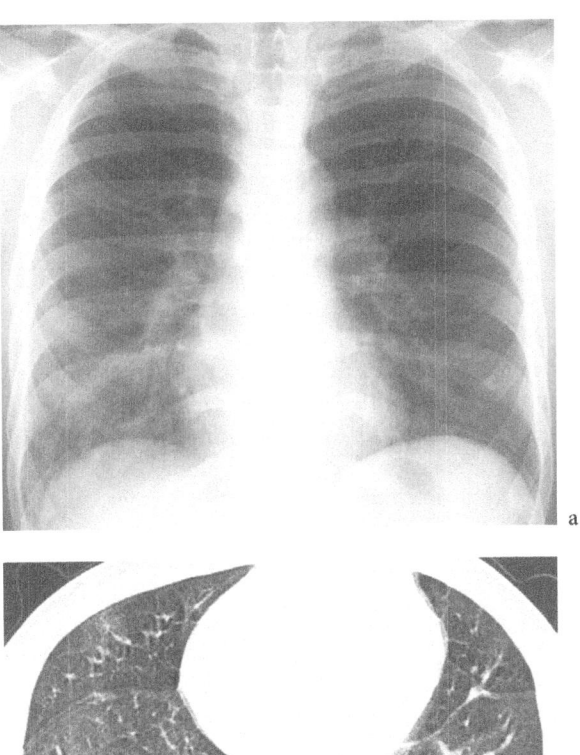

Fig. 23.14a,b. Idiopathic pneumonia syndrome in a 27-year-old man with acute myelocytic leukemia. a Posteroanterior chest radiograph shows bilateral mixed interstitial and alveolar opacities. b Axial HRCT scan shows widespread ground-glass opacity distributed in the bilateral lung field, especially in the dependent lung area, creating a density gradient. Autopsied specimens of this patient showed diffuse alveolar damage. (With permission from [TANAKA et al. 2002])

produced a geographic appearance. In this respect, it might be difficult to distinguish idiopathic pneumonia syndrome from *Pneumocystis carinii* pneumonia. However, a density gradient towards the dependent lung zone may be the key finding of this entity. Traction bronchiectasis and architectural distortion are relatively common findings and probably indicate the proliferative or fibrotic phase. The presence of honeycombing is indicative of the fibrotic phase. It is essentially a diagnosis of exclusion because HRCT findings are non-specific.

23.2.2.4
Bronchiolitis Obliterans

Bronchiolitis obliterans is a late phase complication and occurs in approximately 10% of patients who develop chronic GVHD. Most patients receive an allogeneic HSCT for aplastic anemia or leukemia. It rarely occurs in patients who undergo autologous HSCT. The cause is uncertain, however, it is speculated to be direct damage to the small airways induced by chronic GVHD (HASLETON and DORAN 1996). Risk factors include immunosuppression with methotrexate, pre-HSCT chemotherapy, irradiation, and low serum immunoglobulins after HSCT. This complication usually occurs 6 months after transplantation, with a range of 2–20 months. The mortality rate is high, and the value of treatment is questionable. The pathologic finding of bronchiolitis obliterans is constrictive bronchiolitis; submucosal and peribronchiolar fibrosis, usually irreversible, is present, resulting in extrinsic narrowing and obliteration of the lumen of small bronchi and bronchioles. In the early stages of disease, there is probably a cellular inflammatory and fibroblastic reaction in the bronchiole, but the more typical finding is fibrosis with little active inflammation.

Chest radiography shows hyperinflation with or without focal or diffuse opacities. The diagnosis is based on the clinical findings and the results of pulmonary function tests. Although it can be confirmed histologically by surgical lung biopsy specimen, this is not always necessary. It is possible to diagnose this entity by using the characteristic HRCT findings and the evidence of airflow obstruction shown by pulmonary function tests. HRCT including expiratory technique is essential for the correct diagnosis of this entity. Common HRCT findings consist of patchy or diffuse areas of air trapping (Fig. 23.15), mosaic perfusion, and bronchial dilatation. Centrilobular nodules are sometimes seen. Mosaic perfusion is defined as marked heterogeneity of lung attenuation,

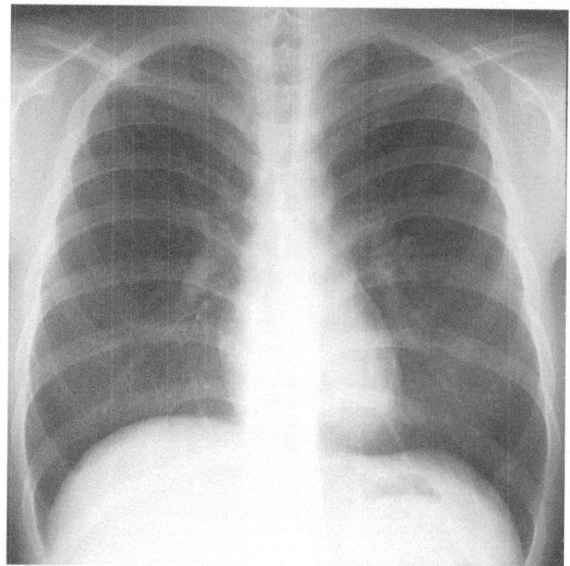

a

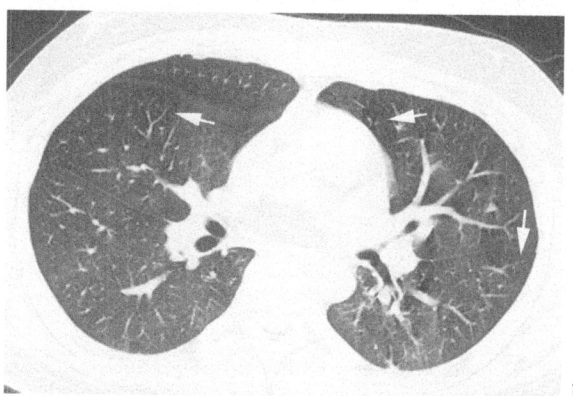

b

Fig. 23.15. Bronchiolitis obliterans in a 15-year-old boy with acute myelocytic leukemia. **a** Posteroanterior chest radiograph shows no abnormal finding except for minimal hyperinflation, which was not previously visible. **b** Expiratory axial thin-section CT scan shows multiple patchy air trapping (*arrows*).

with lobules of increased and decreased lung density that create a striking patchwork pattern. The areas of decreased lung density are presumed to show air trapping, with associated pulmonary oligemia. The areas of increased lung density may be due to redistribution of blood flow to more normal areas of the lung. The pulmonary vessels within the decreased lung attenuation regions may appear smaller in caliber.

Mosaic perfusion is frequently seen in several reports, however, in LAU et al. (1998) study, this finding is not so specific for bronchiolitis obliterans because the control group with normal pulmonary function could represent this finding. In their study, the specificity was 60%. Bronchial dilatation and air trapping are thought to be more reliable findings. In a study by WORTHY et al. (1997b) of 15 patients with bronchiolitis obliterans, the sensitivity of bronchial dilatation and air trapping was 80% for both, and the specificity of bronchial dilatation and air trapping was 78% and 94%, respectively. The combination of bronchial dilatation and air trapping was seen only in patients with bronchiolitis obliterans, in their study. It should be stressed that expiratory CT is needed if bronchiolitis obliterans is suspected in HSCT patients.

23.2.2.5
Bronchiolitis Obliterans Organizing Pneumonia

Bronchiolitis obliterans organizing pneumonia (BOOP) is also a well-recognized late phase complication in HSCT patients. The incidence rate is uncertain. BOOP is characterized pathologically by edematous granulation tissue polyps in the lumina of alveolar ducts and bronchioles in association with a variable degree of interstitial and airspace infiltration by mononuclear cells and foamy macrophages, which can be followed by fibroblast proliferation and collagen deposition. The peribronchial distribution of these changes is a clue to the pathologic diagnosis of BOOP. BOOP is a common pathologic pattern of lung injury, occurring in a variety of diseases. Because of the patchy nature of BOOP, surgical biopsy may be required if transbronchial biopsy is nondiagnostic.

Typical and characteristic CT findings are patchy ground-glass opacity or air-space consolidation often distributed at the peribronchial and subpleural regions (Fig. 23.16). In a study by PREIDLER et al. (1996), all 15 patients showed circumscribed areas of airspace consolidation, almost identical to large nodules. The areas of airspace consolidation were almost always multifocal, and in 14 patients the areas were bilateral and non-segmental, and usually distributed at the lung periphery, and showing lower lung predominance. Although consolidation is more commonly observed in immunocompetent patients, ground-glass opacity or nodules are more frequently observed in immunocompromised patients. Ground-glass opacity, usually random in distribution, is seen in 60% of cases. Nodules are seen in 30% of cases. Centrilobular nodules with branching linear structures mimicking cellular bronchiolitis have been reported. In a study of 8 patients, air-space consolidation and ground-glass opacity were sharply demarcated from each other and from normal lung,

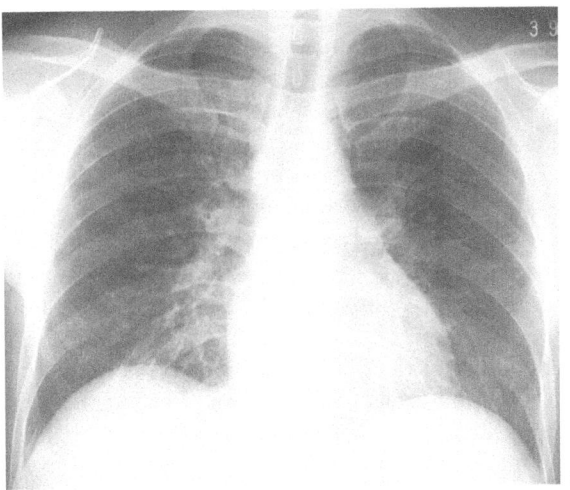

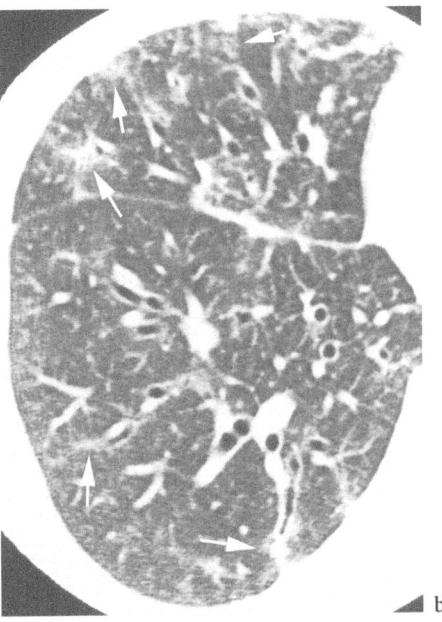

Fig. 23.16. Bronchiolitis obliterans organizing pneumonia in a 36-year-old man with chronic myelocytic leukemia. a Posteroanterior chest radiograph shows minimal patchy subpleural airspace disease. b Axial HRCT scan shows extensive ground-glass opacity and airspace consolidation, which predominantly distribute along the bronchovascular bundles and/or subpleural zones (*arrows*). (With permission from [TANAKA et al. 2002])

exhibiting panlobular or geographic distribution. In that study, air-space consolidation corresponded mostly to organizing pneumonia and ground-glass opacity corresponded to alveolar septal inflammation and alveolar cellular desquamation with a little granulation tissue in the terminal air space (NISHIMURA and ITOH 1992).

23.3
Post Radiation Changes

Patients with intrathoracic lymphoma receive radiation therapy as part of their treatment, or in combination with chemotherapy (BRADY and LEVITT 1998). For these patients, the battle is often won or lost in the thorax. The mantle field used for definitive radiation therapy in patients with Hodgkin or non-Hodgkin lymphomas includes all the major lymph node regions above the diaphragm. The field extends from the inferior portion of the mandible nearly to the level of the insertion of the diaphragm. Lung blocks are designed to conform to patient anatomy and tumor distribution. After radiation therapy, a variety of changes may occur in the thorax. Most patients remain asymptomatic with generally subclinical manifestations of radiation-related changes. Indeed, in recent years, thanks to new modalities of irradiation (decreased intensity, replacement of "mantle field" by "involved field", hyperfractionated irradiation, etc) the frequency of radiation-induced complications has decreased. However, as the number of survivors increases, several late effects of treatment are becoming evident (Table 23.1) (MESUROLLE et al. 2000).

23.3.1
Lung Injuries

23.3.1.1
Radiation Pneumonitis and Fibrosis

Post radiation therapy effects in the lungs are divided into early and late stages (LIBSHITZ 1993; LIBSHITZ and SHUMAN 1984; IKEZOE et al. 1988).

The early stage – radiation pneumonitis – occurs usually about 8–12 weeks after completion of radiation therapy but can occur earlier or much later. It consists of cellular infiltration that is predominantly composed of macrophages. Radiation pneumonitis varies from minimal to extremely marked changes in the paramediastinal areas and in both apices (LIBSHITZ et al. 1973). In case of splenic irradiation (rarely used now), radiation pneumonitis can occur in the left lung base. Radiologically, there is a diffuse haze in the irradiated region with obscuring of vascular outlines (Fig. 23.17). Patchy consolidations appear and then coalesce to form a relatively sharp edge that conforms to treatment portals rather than to anatomic boundaries (Fig. 23.18). CT may reveal radiation changes when the chest X-ray is normal (Fig. 23.19) (IKEZOE et al. 1988). Occasionally, a pleu-

Table 23.1. Post-radiation thoracic injuries. (Modified with permission from [MESUROLLE et al. 2000])

Target Organ	Complication	Time to Onset	Fractionated Dose	Refs
Lung	Pneumonitis	8–12 weeks (acute), 6–24 months (late)	30 Gy	MOSVAS et al. (1997)
	Pneumothorax	16 months	> 30 Gy	PENNIMENT and O'BRIEN (1994)
Lymph nodes	Calcifications	> 12 months	No minimal dose defined	BERETON and Johnson 1974
Esophagus	Stricture	3–18 months	60 Gy	LEPKE and LIBSHITZ (1983)
Vascular tree	Stenosis Occlusion Pseudoaneurysm	10–15 years	Aorta and pulmonary artery, 24–44 Gy; subclavian artery, 40–60 Gy	FAJARDO and BERTHRONG (1983)
Heart	Coronary artery disease	10–15 years	> 30 Gy before 20 years of age	KOPELSON and HERWIG (1978)
	Pericarditis (3 types)	1. During radiation therapy (associated with chemotherapy) 2. Post-therapy, acute effusion 12–18 months 3. Post-therapy, chronic effusion,48 months	40 Gy	APPLEFELD et al. (1981)
	Conduction abnormalities	10 years	40 Gy	COHEN et al. (1981)
Malignancy	Breast carcinoma	15–19 years	> 20 Gy before 35 years of age	BHATIA et al. (1996)
	Sarcoma	> 5 years	No minimal dose defined	LIBSHITZ (1994)

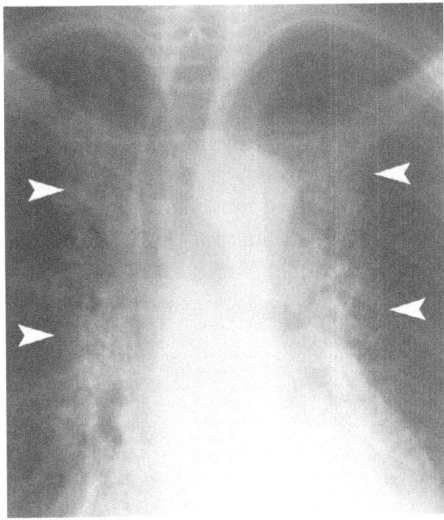

Fig. 23.17. Radiation pneumonitis in a 52-year-old man after radiation therapy for Hodgkin disease. Posteroanterior chest radiograph performed two months after completion of radiation therapy shows typical moderate post-radiation pneumonitis with paramediastinal consolidations (*arrowheads*) obscuring vascular outlines.

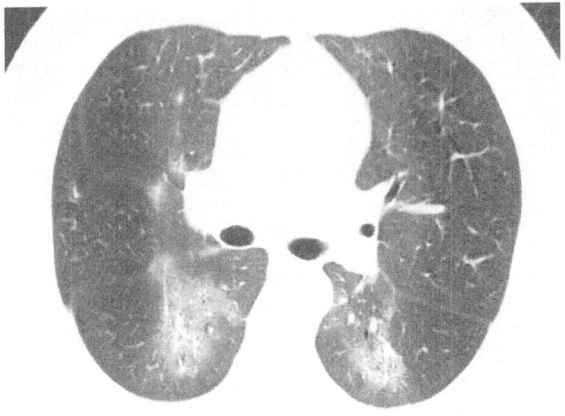

Fig. 23.19. Radiation pneumonitis in a 42-year-old man after radiation therapy for Hodgkin disease. Axial HRCT scan shows mild paramediastinal alveolar and ground glass opacities confined in the radiation port.

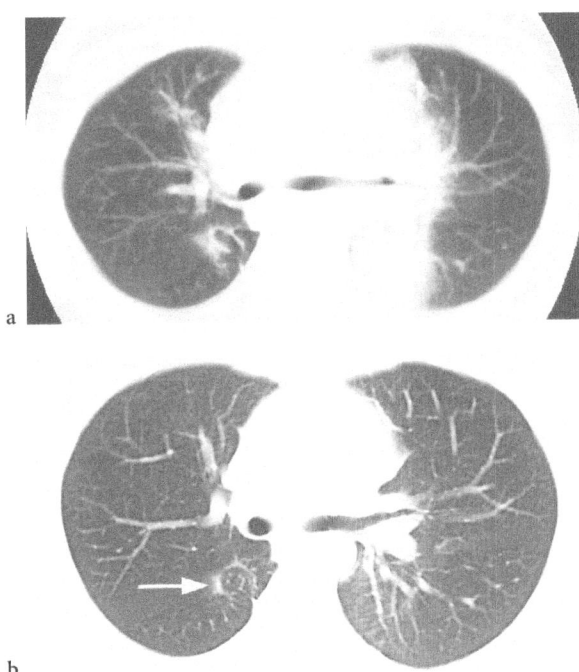

Fig. 23.18a,b. Radiation pneumonitis in a 38-year-old woman after radiation therapy for Hodgkin disease a Axial CT scan performed two months after completion of radiation therapy shows paramediastinal dense consolidation confined to the radiation ports. b Axial CT scan performed eighteen months after completion of irradiation shows no significant injury detected except for slight linear infiltrate (early stage of fibrosis) (*arrow*).

ral effusion develops on the irradiated site. Typically, this effusion is small and is seen with acute radiation pneumonitis (LIBSHITZ 1993).

The late stage is secondary to incompletely resolved radiation pneumonitis. Fibrous changes take 6–24 months to evolve but remain stable after 2 years (LOGAN 1998). These changes are marked by collagen deposition and fibrosis. Volume loss causes coalescence of any linear infiltrates that were present. The borders of the fibrotic area become straight, conforming to the radiation port. Pleural thickening develops in lung apices, and the hilar structures are superomedially retracted (Fig. 23.20). In case of severe changes, marked retraction can induce a narrowing of the cardiomediastinal silhouette (LOYER et al. 2000). CT scans may reveal well-defined areas of atelectasis with parenchymal distortion and traction bronchiectases. These changes are variably present after 30–40 Gy, and universally seen after more than 40 Gy. In hematologic patients, the maximum dose is 40 Gy (MOSVAS et al. 1997). Many factors can alter the risk of developing radiation-related pulmonary damage. These include (a) prior irradiation; (b) chemotherapy (doxorubicin, actinomycin D, busulfan, bleomycin, methotrexate and interferon); (c) a larger target volume, a higher total radiation dose and daily fraction size, and a shorter overall treatment time; and (d) withdrawal of steroid therapy. In addition, radiation to the chest, even when limited to the mediastinum, has been associated with an increased risk of bleomycin-induced pulmonary toxicity (BRICE et al. 1991). The lung target volume irradiated may be the most important factor (RUBIN

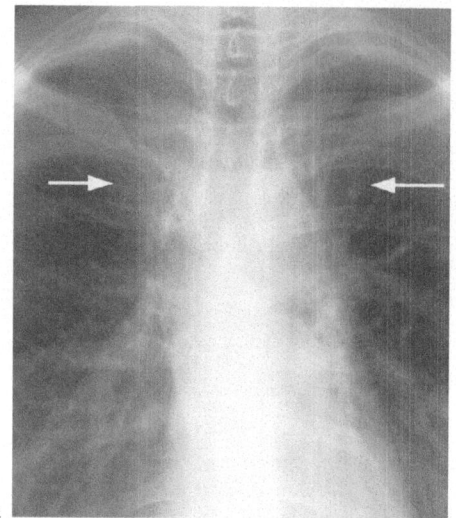

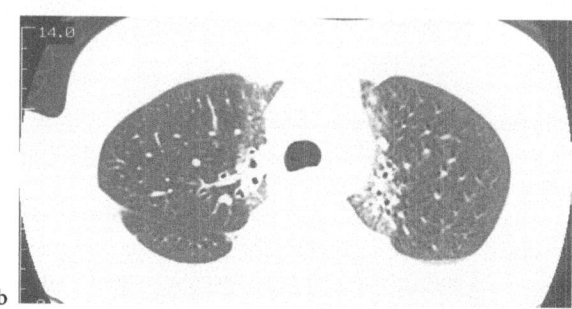

Fig. 23.20a,b. Radiation fibrosis in a 39-year-old woman after radiation therapy for Hodgkin disease. **a** Posteroanterior close-up view chest radiograph demonstrates superomedially retraction of hilar structures associated with moderate post-radiation paramediastinal fibrosis (*arrows*). **b** Axial HRCT scan shows paramediastinal post radiation fibrosis confined to the radiation port. Note traction bronchiectasis, ground glass opacity and sharp demarcation between normal and irradiated lung. These lesions are related to subacute radiation changes.

and CASARETT 1998). A reduction of at least 15–20% of the total dose has been recommended when chemotherapy is administered concurrently (ROSWIT and WHITE 1977) especially with bleomycin, platins or gemcitabine.

23.3.1.2
Spontaneous Pneumothorax

Treatment-related pneumothorax has occasionally been reported in patients who received radiation therapy for a primary malignancy (ROWINSKY et al. 1985). PEZNER et al. (1990) reported a frequency of spontaneous pneumothorax of 2% in patients with Hodgkin disease who were treated with mantle radia-

tion therapy. The patients reported in the literature received more than 30 Gy of radiation (PENNIMENT and O'BRIEN 1994). Pneumothorax can be recurrent, is rarely bilateral, and occurs 1 to 31 months after radiation therapy, with a mean time to onset of 16 months. It usually occurs in patients with radiologic evidence of post-irradiation fibrosis. The volume is usually minimal to moderate, and most cases will reexpand without treatment (ROWINSKY et al. 1985).

23.3.2
Mediastinal Changes

23.3.2.1
Thymic Cysts

Thymic cysts may arise in patients who have undergone irradiation for Hodgkin disease. These cysts are thought to occur either secondarily to treatment of Hodgkin disease of the thymus or exclusively as a result of radiation effects on the thymus (KATZ et al. 1977). They manifest as a stable or progressively enlarging cyst with or without calcified parietal wall (Fig. 23.21) (BARON et al. 1981). The CT and MR imaging appearance is the same as that of a benign cyst. Irregular or thick-walled cysts should be regarded with suspicion and may necessitate biopsy.

23.3.2.2
Calcified Lymph Nodes

Calcifications can arise in lymph nodes after radiation therapy for lymphoma. In Hodgkin disease, calcification of a nonenlarged mass after radiation therapy signifies a favorable response to therapy (KATZ et al. 1977; RIVERO et al. 1984). Calcification generally begins about 1 year after treatment and may become increasingly dense over the years (Fig. 23.22) (BERETON and JOHNSON 1974). Awareness of this condition allows one to avoid confusion with the changes that typify granulomatous infection.

23.3.2.3
Benign Esophageal Injuries

Esophageal dysmotility occurs 4–12 weeks after radiation therapy (LEPKE and LIBSHITZ 1983). Strictures are uncommon but may occur 3–18 months after radiation therapy with a median interval of 6 months. They are usually smooth with tapered margins (Fig. 23.23) but may also have an irregular

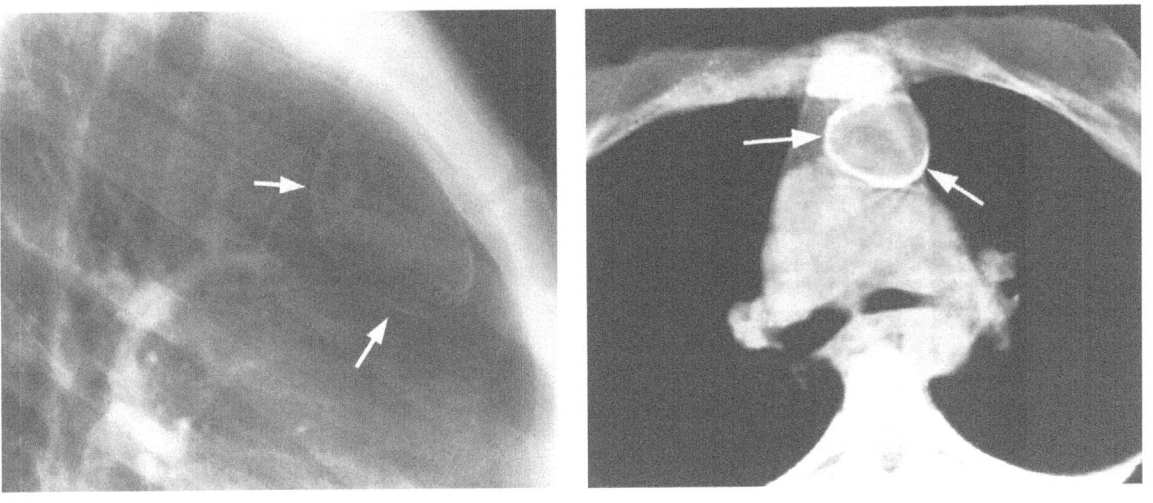

Fig. 23.21a,b. Thymic cyst in a 35-year-old man 10 years after radiation therapy for Hodgkin disease. **a** Lateral chest radiograph shows an ovoid, well defined lesion with a calcified parietal wall located anteriorly in the mediastinum (*arrows*). **b** Axial CT scan shows a thymic cyst with parietal wall calcifications (*arrows*).

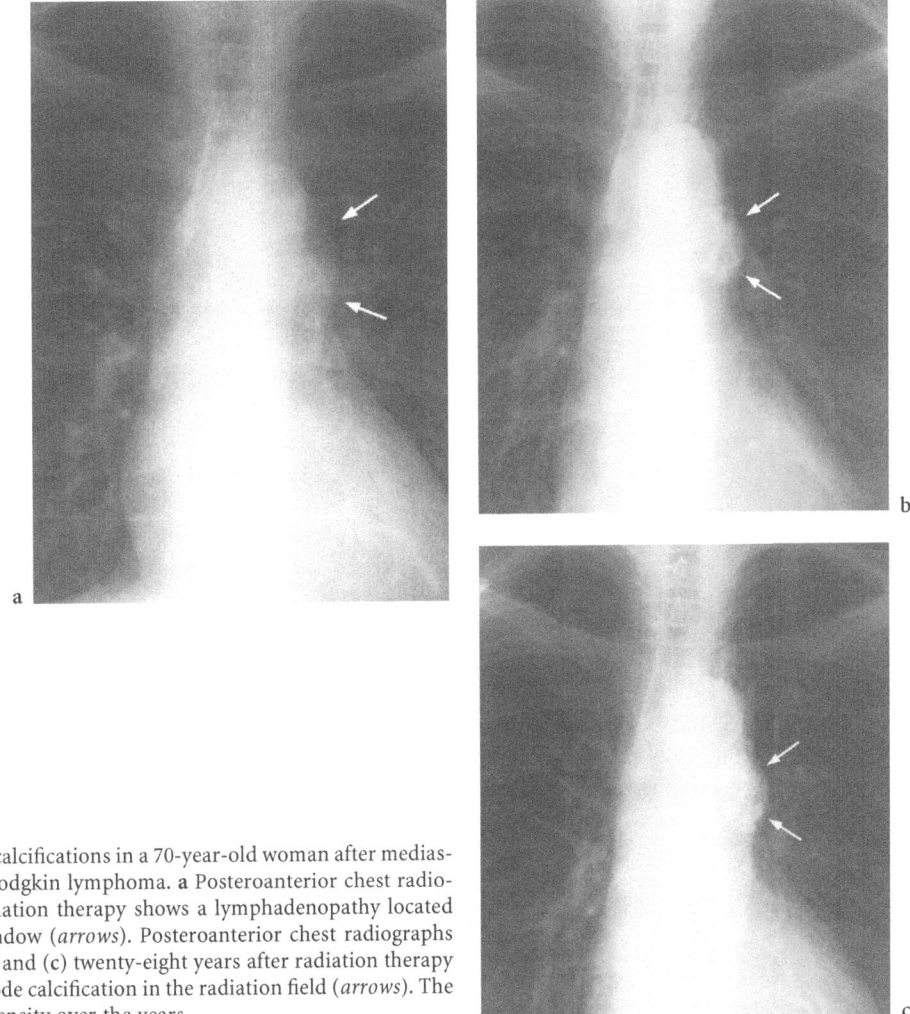

Fig. 23.22a-c. Lymph node calcifications in a 70-year-old woman after mediastinal irradiation for non-Hodgkin lymphoma. **a** Posteroanterior chest radiograph obtained before radiation therapy shows a lymphadenopathy located in the aortopulmonary window (*arrows*). Posteroanterior chest radiographs obtained (**b**) thirteen years and (**c**) twenty-eight years after radiation therapy show mediastinal lymph node calcification in the radiation field (*arrows*). The calcification increased in density over the years.

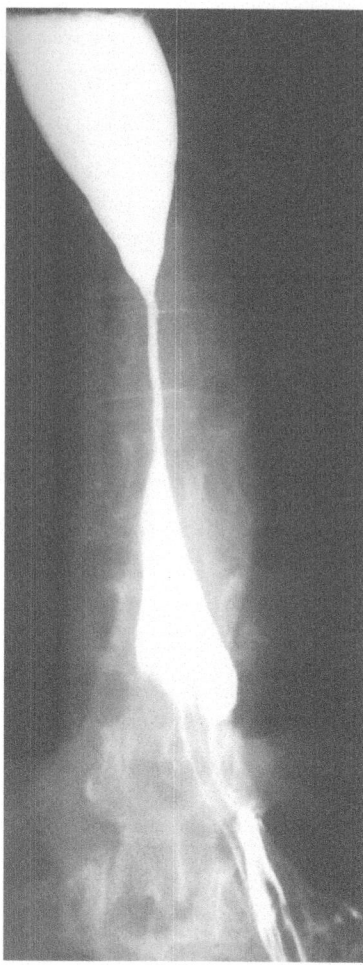

Fig. 23.23. Post radiation esophageal stricture in a 50-year-old woman one and half years after completion of radiation therapy for Hodgkin disease. Barium esophagogram shows marked smooth concentric narrowing of the lower third of the esophagus.

surface. A total dose of 50 Gy or more can lead to stricture formation. The prevalence of symptomatic benign strictures is probably under 2% at doses of 50 Gy or less and may rise to approximately 15% in patients treated with 60 Gy (COIA et al. 1995). However, esophageal strictures can occur even with low-dose radiation therapy when chemotherapy (doxorubicin) is administered (LEPKE and LIBSHITZ 1983).

23.3.3
Cardiovascular Injuries

Cardiovascular complications of radiation therapy are often delayed and insidious. The majority of these complications has been reported in patients previously treated for Hodgkin disease. They are reported to contribute significantly to mortality in long-term survivors of Hodgkin disease, ranking behind only second malignancies and Hodgkin disease itself (LEE et al. 2000; STEWART et al. 1995). The absolute risk of cardiac-related deaths in survivors of Hodgkin disease is estimated between 9.3 and 28 per 10,000 patient years, 2 to 3 times the population risk (AISENBERG 1999; HANCOCK et al. 1993). This risk is higher in younger patients, in patients who received mediastinal doses exceeding 30 Gy (HANCOCK et al. 1993) and in those receiving additive chemotherapy (predominantly MOPP in Hodgkin disease) (GIRINSKY et al. 2000). Such radiation therapy techniques as use of a cobalt beam, preferential weighting of the anterior field, and large daily fractions have been implicated in the development of late cardiac toxic effects (VLACHAKI et al. 1998).

23.3.3.1
Vascular Injuries

Radiation-induced vasculopathy usually occurs after about 10 years. Radiation injuries within the vascular tree most often affect the capillaries, sinusoids, small arteries, veins, and large arteries (FAJARDO and BERTHRONG 1983). When major damage (e.g., thrombosis or rupture) is sustained by an elastic artery, the damage tends to be clinically significant (STEIN and JACOBSON 1993; BENSON 1973). The only differentiating feature from radiation arteritis is that radiation-induced vasculopathy is limited to the radiation field. Stenoses and occlusions are more frequently reported than are perforations and pseudoaneurysms (FAJARDO and LEE 1975). Mediastinal fibrosis produces obliteration of normal fat planes and anatomic landmarks, which is responsible for distortion and stricture of normal vessels (QANADLI et al. 1999).

23.3.3.2
Coronary Artery Disease

The effect of radiation on the coronary arteries continues to fuel debate. Coronary artery stenosis occurs after radiation therapy to the mediastinum, which is usually given for Hodgkin disease. Although some studies indicate that the overall risk of a serious ischemic event in the coronary arteries is not increased in patients who received radiation therapy (BOIVIN and HUTCHISON 1982), more convincing are the reports of young patients with severe coronary artery disease in whom previous irradiation is the only feasible explanation for the development of premature coronary artery stenosis (KOPELSON and HERWIG 1978; TOTTERMAN et al. 1983). Among survivors of Hodgkin disease, two studies found a threefold higher relative risk for coronary artery disease (COSSET et al. 1991; BOIVIN et al. 1992).

Stenosis generally affects the proximal portions of the coronary arteries (Fig. 23.24) (REINDERS et al. 1999). These sites are rarely stenotic in patients who were not treated with radiation therapy, but frequently are stenotic in patients who received radiation therapy to the mediastinum. Post-mortem examinations of young adults treated with radiation therapy for Hodgkin disease have shown marked atherosclerotic disease at the ostia and proximal courses of the coronary arteries, which correspond to the anatomic area exposed to radiation therapy (BROSIUS et al. 1981). Radiation therapy to the heart has also been associated with coronary artery spasm (MILLER et al. 1983; YAHALOM et al. 1983). It is not known whether concurrent use of chemotherapy will increase the risk of coronary artery disease (BOIVIN et al. 1992). The results of treatment appear to be the same in patients who did not undergo adjuvant radiation therapy (STEWART et al. 1995).

23.3.3.3
Calcified Ascending Aorta

Radiation therapy may give rise to calcifications of the ascending aorta after radiation-induced aortitis

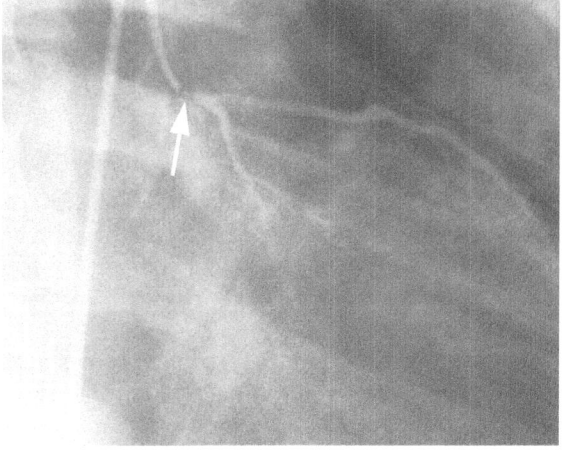

Fig. 23.24. Premature coronary artery stenosis in a non-smoking 27-year-old man fourteen years after radiation therapy for stage IV Hodgkin disease. Selective left coronary arteriogram shows a subocclusive ostial stenosis of the left main coronary artery (arrow). (With permission from [MESUROLLE et al. 2000])

(COBLENTZ et al. 1986). The calcification has a fine, sharp, pencil-like outline. It is due to deposition of calcium salts in tissue as a sequela of a scarred intima or media after aortitis.

23.3.3.4
Pericardial Disease

Historically, the pericardium has been one of the most commonly affected structures of the heart (STEWART and FAJARDO 1984). Previously affecting 20–40% of patients with Hodgkin disease receiving irradiation with older techniques, the prevalence of post–radiation therapy pericarditis is now 2–6% and is very low when the radiation dose is below 40 Gy, anterior and posterior fields are weighted equally, subcarinal blocking is used and daily fraction size is reduced ≤ 2.0 Gy (APPLEFELD et al. 1981). The frequency of pericarditis is significantly greater when a higher radiation dose is delivered per fraction for Hodgkin disease (COSSET et al. 1988). Early acute onset pericarditis is defined as occurring during radiotherapy and is associated with a large tumor contiguous to the heart (STEWART and FAJARDO 1984). This rare form is thought to be a reaction to necrosis of the tumor and has no long-term consequences (STEWART and FAJARDO 1984). Two delayed forms of pericarditis may occur as well. The most common form – pericardial effusion- appears 12–18 months after completion of radiation therapy (delayed acute form) (Fig. 23.25). The second form appears later, usually more than 48 months after radiation therapy, and manifests as chronic pericardial disease (delayed chronic form) (APPLEFELD et al. 1981). Most effusions clear spontaneously, but may take up to 2 years to do so. Constriction is observed in 15–20% of patients with delayed pericarditis (LOYER and DELPASSAND 1993), but it may arise in the absence of a prior adverse pericardial event (STEWART et al. 1995). The normal pericardium is thin, curvilinear, and 1–2 mm thick on CT (BULL et al. 1998). A pericardial thickness of 4 mm on CT or MR imaging is consistent with constriction. CT and MR imaging can provide information about impaired right ventricular diastolic filling when dilatation of the inferior vena cava and right atrium is demonstrated.

23.3.3.5
Valvular Injuries and Conduction Abnormalities

It is not clear whether radiation therapy causes structural alterations in valves (STEWART et al. 1995). These abnormalities are probably related to radiation or due to myocardial fibrosis adjacent to valve rings, resulting

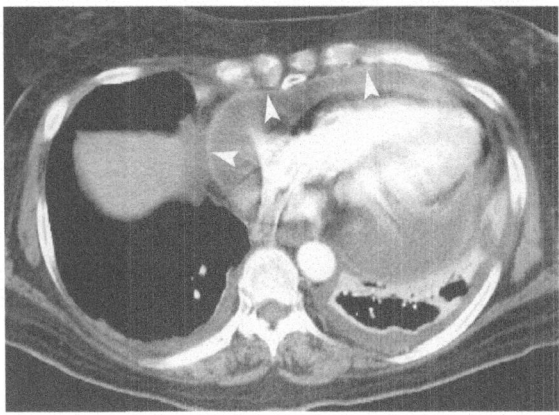

Fig. 23.25. Delayed post radiation pericarditis in a 52-year-old woman after mediastinal radiation therapy for non-Hodgkin lymphoma. Axial CT scan performed eighteen months after completion of radiation therapy shows a large amount of pericardial effusion and a diffuse thickening of the pericardium (*arrowheads*).

in distortion and functional impairment. The mitral, aortic, and tricuspid valves are the most frequently affected. Changes in cardiac rhythm are rarely seen, but the odd event has been attributed to ischemic fibrosis affecting the conduction system. Atrioventricular block, albeit rare, is the most frequent conduction abnormality encountered. It tends to occur about 10 years after treatment (usually after a radiation dose ≥ 40 Gy) and requires insertion of a pacemaker in most cases (COHEN et al. 1981; LOYER and DELPASSAND 1993).

23.3.4
Chest Wall and Nerve Injuries

23.3.4.1
Radiation-Induced Brachial Plexopathy

In patients who undergo radiation therapy to the axillary region, the distinction between recurrent or residual disease and radiation-induced neuropathy can be difficult. Radiation fibrosis may occur generally 5–30 months after the completion of therapy with a peak at 10–20 months and is most likely to occur in patients who have received radiation doses in excess of 60 Gy. Common symptoms include paresthesias, hyperesthesias, pain, and weakness. The utility of MR imaging is in part based on results showing that axillary areas of delayed radiation fibrosis are usually iso- or hypointense relative to muscle on T2-weighted images, thus distinguishing them from tumor infiltration, which is hyperintense (GLAZER et al. 1985). However, patients

with post radiation plexopathy may have hyperintense signal in or near the plexus on T2-weighted images as frequently as patients with tumor infiltration (THYAGARAJAN et al. 1995). Routine administration of gadolinium-based contrast material does not help differentiate radiation fibrosis from metastatic disease, because both may show some degree of enhancement (WOUTER VAN ES et al. 1997). Thus, the morphologic features of the signal abnormalities (absence of a focal mass, and stability of the findings on serial studies) rather than the hyper- or hyposignal, or enhancement, are the key findings that favor a diagnosis of radiation induced plexopathy over recurrent tumor or infection (BOWEN et al. 1996).

23.3.4.2
Left Sided Vocal Cord Paralysis

Anecdotal cases of left-side vocal cord paralysis in patients treated with mediastinal radiotherapy due to mediastinal fibrosis have been reported (ROSANOWSKI 1995). The difference in anatomy of the left and the right recurrent nerve explains the prevalence of left side injuries.

23.3.4.3
Aseptic Necrosis and Osteochondroma

Aseptic necrosis of the humeral heads has been reported after radiation therapy. The humeral heads can usually be blocked when mantle radiation is given (ROSSLEIGH et al. 1986).

Osteochondroma is the only benign bone tumor related to radiation therapy. The prevalence of radiation-induced osteochondromas is about 12% in children whose epiphyses have been irradiated, whereas the prevalence of spontaneous osteochondromas is below 1%. The majority of cases of radiation-induced osteochondromas have been associated with either orthovoltage or megavoltage therapies. The average latent period between radiation and identification of osteochondroma is 8 years (3 –27 years) after radiation (GOROSPE et al. 2002). They tend to be solitary rather than multiple. They do not appear to be premalignant (LIBSHITZ and COHEN 1967). In spinal locations, their detection is difficult on plain radiographs. CT can demonstrate the osseous component of the tumor but fails to show the cartilaginous cap in the majority of cases. MR imaging better evaluates the cartilaginous cap (cartilaginous malignant degeneration should be considered in cartilaginous caps more than 2 cm thick) and the intraspinal involvement (GOROSPE et al. 2002).

23.4
Second Solid Neoplasms

"It is a paradox that radiation can both cure and cause cancer" (ALEXANDER 1957). An increasing number of treatment-associated secondary neoplasms have long been recognized among long-term survivors of Hodgkin disease and non-Hodgkin lymphoma treated either with conventional chemotherapeutic agents or irradiation (BHATIA et al. 1996). However such complications have also been reported after HSCT (BHATIA et al. 2001). Such treatment-induced catastrophes are a consequence of one of the triumphs of cancer management. After HSCT, it is still unclear whether the malignancy is related to pretransplant chemotherapy and radiotherapy, the result of transplant conditioning regimens, or a cumulative effect of all of these factors.

The most commonly reported second malignancies include leukemia and non-Hodgkin lymphoma. Solid cancers have a longer latency period, and they are increasingly being described because of improved survival after treatment. After Hodgkin disease, the actuarial risk of cancer, 25 years after treatment, is 27.7% compared to 4.2% for the general population, at the same age. The relative risk of developing cancer, compared to the population, is estimated at 7 (37.5 for leukemia, 21.5 for lymphoma, 6 for solid tumor) (VAN LEEUWEN et al. 2000).

Solid tumors related to radiation-therapy occur in the irradiated field. Mantle irradiation should be avoided when possible in smokers and young women because of lung and breast cancer risks (AISENBERG 1999).

23.4.1
Mesothelioma, Lung and Esophageal Carcinomas

Radiation-induced mesothelioma and lung carcinoma have been described (HOFMANN et al. 1994; NEUGUT et al. 1994). A two- to eightfold risk of lung carcinoma (compared with the risk in the general population) is observed 5 or more years after Hodgkin disease treatment and persists through the second decade (VAN LEEUWEN et al. 1994). There is general agreement of the excess risk after irradiation and combined regimens of alkylating agents (VAN LEEUWEN et al. 1994) with a direct relationship between lung cancer risk and dose to the previously irradiated lung segments (VAN LEEUWEN et al. 1995). The interval between radiation therapy and the appearance of mesothelioma ranges from 5 to 41 years (median 13.5 years) (HOFMANN et al. 1994).

Radiographic and CT features are non-specific and consist of pleural effusion with or without pleural-based masses (HOFMANN et al. 1994).

Radiation-induced esophageal carcinoma has been described (MICKE et al. 1999; AUDEBERT et al. 2002). The interval between radiation therapy and the appearance of esophageal carcinoma ranges from 5 to 30 years (AUDEBERT et al. 2002). Imaging features are similar to those of other esophageal squamous cell carcinomas (AUDEBERT et al. 2002). These cancers, which are almost all symptomatic, have a poor prognosis.

23.4.2
Breast Carcinoma

Women who undergo thoracic irradiation before age 30 have a high risk of developing a second breast cancer. In the study of BHATIA et al. (1996), women treated for childhood Hodgkin disease had a risk of breast cancer 75 times greater than that of the general population. Breast sensitivity to radiation disappears if the first exposure occurs after 35 years of age. The first breast carcinomas appear at the end of the first decade after Hodgkin disease irradiation. The mean interval between exposure and the development of breast cancer is 15–19 years. Data on the relationship between the radiation field and breast cancer are inconsistent, but the tumor usually appears within or at the edge of treatment fields. YAHALOM et al. (1992) found a higher percentage of breast cancers in the inner quadrants; in the study of DERSHAW et al. (1992), the main site was the upper outer quadrant, with equal distribution between the left and right breasts. Women who undergo thoracic irradiation before the age of 30 years should benefit from screening with mammography earlier than the general population. Any abnormal clinical or mammographic finding should prompt a histologic examination (Fig. 23.26).

23.4.3
Sarcomas

Radiation-induced sarcomas are an infrequent but well-recognized complication of radiation therapy. They were demonstrated in an experimental study conducted by MARIE et al. (1910). The risk of post–radiation therapy sarcoma is very low relative to the beneficial effects of radiation therapy, but they deserve attention because of their often unfavorable

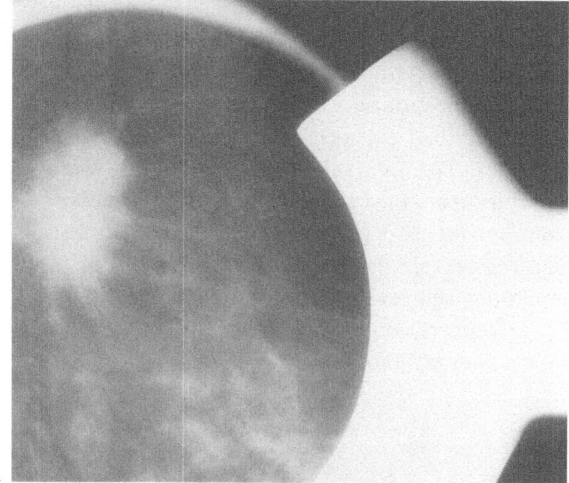

a

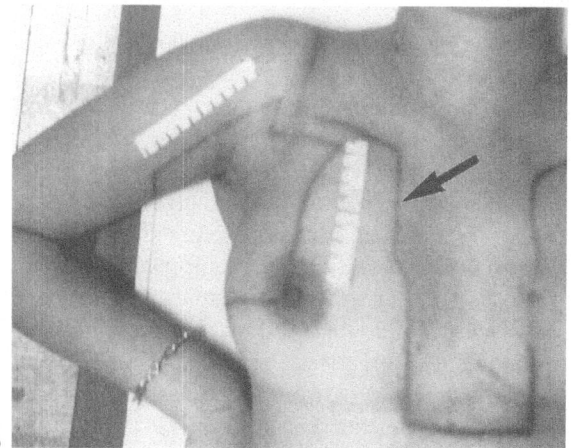

b

Fig. 23.26a,b. Breast cancer in a 47-year-old woman who underwent radiation therapy at the age 23 for Hodgkin disease. At clinical examination, there was a palpable nodule in the right upper inner quadrant, which yielded an infiltrating ductal carcinoma at histology. **a** Lateral mammogram shows a spiculated area of increased opacity. **b** A pretreatment photograph shows the radiation fields for the treatment of Hodgkin disease. The site of the future breast cancer (*arrow*) overlaps the radiation field. (With permission from [MESUROLLE et al. 2000])

outcome when they occur after Hodgkin disease irradiation. The risk of radiation-induced sarcoma is not greater than the risk of death due to surgery or anesthesia (PARKER 1990). Radiation-induced sarcomas occur in approximately 0.1% or fewer of patients who receive radiation therapy and survive 5 years, but constitute a particularly important group of treatment induced neoplasms in the pediatric and adolescent Hodgkin disease population (TUCKER et al. 1987). Such sarcomas can occur 3–30 years after

completion of radiation therapy in either bone or soft tissue. Osteosarcoma is the most frequent variety occurring in bone, and malignant fibrous histiocytoma is the most common cell type arising in soft tissue (LIBSHITZ 1994).

23.4.3.1
Diagnosis of Radiation-Induced Bone Sarcoma

Criteria for diagnosis of a radiation-induced sarcoma arising in bone are: (a) a history of radiation therapy; (b) a neoplasm arising within the irradiated area; (c) a number of years of latency; and (d) histologic proof of sarcoma (CAHAN et al. 1948).

23.4.3.2
Factors Related to Radiation-Induced Sarcomas

A minimal dose, should one exist, has not been defined. Most patients included in earlier studies received orthovoltage radiation therapy. Today, most patients receive megavoltage radiation therapy. The energy attenuation in bone achieved with megavoltage radiation therapy should result in fewer radiation-induced soft-tissue sarcomas. It is not known whether chemotherapy compounds the risk of developing a radiation-induced sarcoma.

23.4.3.3
Imaging Appearance

Radiation-induced sarcomas are aggressive, with a marked tendency toward local recurrence and distant metastasis (Fig. 23.27) (SOUBA et al. 1986). Salvage therapy could be successful in some patients, but early diagnosis is necessary. On radiography, radiation-induced sarcomas of bone do not differ from de novo sarcomas (SMITH 1982), appearing most frequently as an area of bone destruction on conventional radiographs. A radiation-induced sarcoma should be suspected when changes occur in the appearance of previously stable irradiated bone, particularly if an associated soft-tissue mass is present. On CT or MR imaging, a soft-tissue mass and bone destruction are the most common findings (LORIGAN et al. 1989). The differential diagnosis includes metastases, infection, and severe benign changes. Involvement of bone outside the treatment field indicates metastatic disease. Absence of a soft-tissue mass is the most helpful finding in distinguishing extensive benign changes from a radiation-induced sarcoma. Nevertheless, histologic proof is mandatory in all cases.

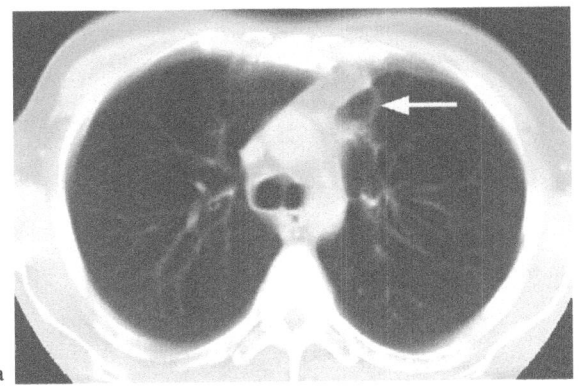

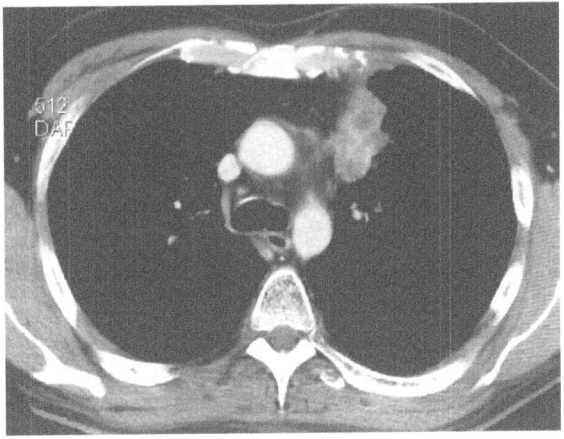

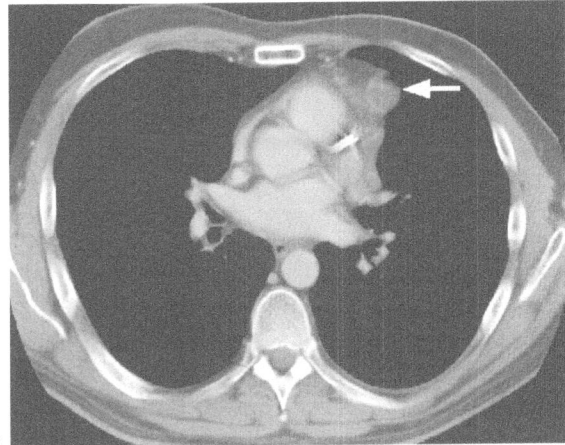

Fig. 23.27a-c. Thoracic sarcoma in a 47-year-old man fifteen years after radiation therapy for Hodgkin disease. a Axial CT scan nine years after completion of radiation therapy showing post radiation changes of the left upper lobe confined to the radiation port with hilar retraction and linear fibrosis (*arrow*). b Axial CT scan thirteen years after completion of radiation therapy demonstrates occurrence of a mass located within the radiation field. Biopsy shows evidence of post-radiation high-grade sarcoma. c More caudal axial CT scan shows extension of the disease along the anterior portion of the pericardium (*arrow*). Note the presence of a coronary stent located within the left anterior descending branch. This coronary stenosis is most likely related to the radiation therapy.

23.5
Residual Masses and Thymic Rebound

23.5.1
Residual Mediastinal Masses

The main therapeutic objective in the treatment of lymphoma is to achieve a complete response, which is associated with a longer disease-free survival and a favorable outcome. Response to treatment is assessed by clinical, imaging and pathological criteria (CHESON et al. 1999). Defining a complete response on CT, however, may be difficult. Residual mediastinal masses are frequently observed (10–20%) on CT scans in patients with mediastinal lymphoma after completed therapy, particularly in patients who initially have bulky masses (TREDANIEL et al. 1992). A residual mass detected on CT after treatment may contain viable tumor cells or, alternatively, may consist of only fibrotic or necrotic tissue. Therefore a common clinical problem arises when a residual abnormality persists on follow-up CT, in spite of the disappearance of clinical symptoms and the reversion of laboratory tests to normal values. The overall

prognosis of patients with residual active disease is poor, and further second-line therapeutic regimens should be initiated as early as possible. In contrast, a benign residual mass is associated with a favorable prognosis and does not warrant any additional treatment (ZINZANI et al. 2001). Apart from calcification of a nonenlarged mass after radiation therapy, which signifies a favorable response to therapy (Fig. 23.28) (KATZ et al. 1977), anatomic imaging with CT does not consistently distinguish between dividing tumor cells and post-therapy fibrosis. Gallium-67 scintigraphy has been shown to be more sensitive for lesions in the chest and to accurately demonstrate active residual disease when there is uptake of Gallium-67 in high-grade non-Hodgkin lymphoma and Hodgkin disease (KOSTAKOGLU et al. 1992; KOSTAKOGLU et al. 2002). However Gallium-67 scintigraphy suffers from the low resolution of the single-photon emission tomography technique in tumors smaller than 2 cm, and false positives have been reported in cases of infection or recent surgery (GASPERINI et al. 1993). MR imaging has been evaluated and compared to Gallium-67 scintigraphy, but it is no better for predicting relapses (HILL et al. 1993). Active tumor foci may be

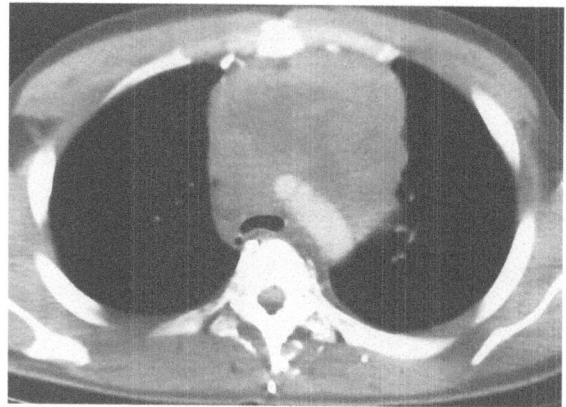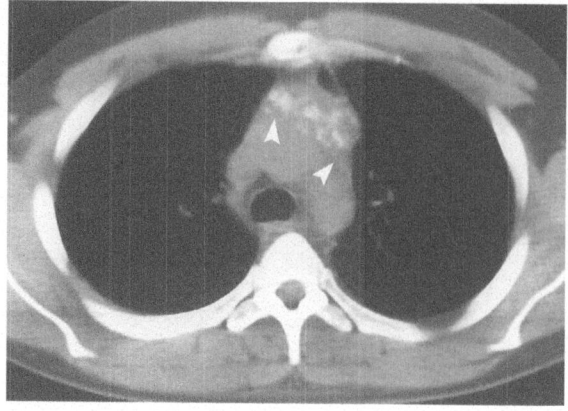

Fig. 23.28a,b. Residual mediastinal mass in a 35-year-old man treated for non Hodgkin lymphoma. **a** Pretreatment axial contrast-enhanced CT scan shows large anterior mediastinal mass. **b** Axial unenhanced CT scan performed eleven months after completion of chemotherapy and radiation therapy shows a residual calcified nonactive mediastinal mass (*arrowheads*).

found within a residual mass with low signal intensity on T2-weighted images. Necrosis, immature fibrotic tissue, edema, and inflammation associated with responding disease can simulate the hyperintensity of a viable tumor, particularly within the first 6 months after therapy. MR imaging evaluation of residual masses requires a pretreatment baseline study for comparison, including both T2-weighting and contrast-enhanced sequences (Rahmouni et al. 2001). 18F-fluorodeoxyglucose (FDG) is a glucose analog known to localize in active lymphoma. Metabolic imaging with FDG positron emission tomography (PET) is gaining in popularity and has proven to have a high sensitivity for the detection of residual tumor and is now a mainstay for treatment evaluation in centers at which this technology is available (Spaepen and Mortelmans 2001; Naumann et al. 2001). It is the most effective means of detecting residual tumor after therapy (Fig. 23.29). Recent studies indicate that the positive predictive value of FDG-PET in lymphoma post therapy is greater than 90%, and that the negative predictive value is slightly lower (De Wit et al. 1997; Jerusalem et al. 1999; Mikhaeel et al. 2000).

23.5.2
Thymic Rebound Hyperplasia

Excessive regrowth of the thymus after chemotherapy, also called thymic rebound hyperplasia (regrowth should be 50% greater than baseline volume) is a rare but well described phenomenon seen in children and young adults (Choyke et al. 1987). The size of the thymus appears to be extremely

sensitive to chemotherapy as the thymus atrophies during the administration of chemotherapy, with regrowth during the recovery phase of chemotherapy (Langer et al. 1992; Choyke et al. 1987). It is generally asymptomatic and detected accidentally as a mediastinal mass on CT scan. There is no reliable non-invasive technique to distinguish thymic rebound hyperplasia from residual or recurrent tumor. It is well known that gallium accumulates in the hyperplastic thymus, inducing false positive Gallium-67 scintigraphy results. The low resolution of Gallium-67 scintigraphy can make it difficult to differentiate homogeneous physiologic uptake of the thymus from irregular uptake seen in mediastinal lymphadenopathy (Peylan-Ramu et al. 1989). A steroid trial has been suggested but should be used cautiously as some lymphomas are steroid-sensitive (Ford et al. 1987). False positive Thallium-201 uptake has been reported as well. In fact, if thymic rebound hyperplasia is suspected because the patient is doing well clinically with no recurrent or residual disease evident in other locations, follow-up imaging is an acceptable method of clarifying the cause of thymic enlargement (Fig. 23.30). Indeed, a gradual reduction in size corroborates the benign cause of the enlargement (Roebuck et al. 1998).

23.6
Transfusion-Related Acute Lung Injury

Transfusion-related acute lung injury (TRALI) is a rare life-threatening complication (fatal in 5–10%

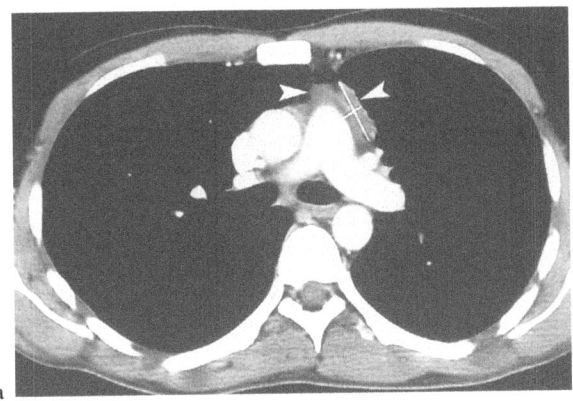

a

Fig. 23.29a,b. Residual mediastinal mass in a 32-year-old man after chemotherapy for Hodgkin disease. **a** Axial CT scan performed at the end of treatment shows a residual anterior mediastinal mass (*arrowheads*). **b** Coronal FDG-PET scan of this patient is negative. Note physiologic uptakes in the cerebral cortex, liver, spleen, and urinary bladder, and also the minimal uptake in the bone marrow. This mass remained stable on follow-up CT examinations.

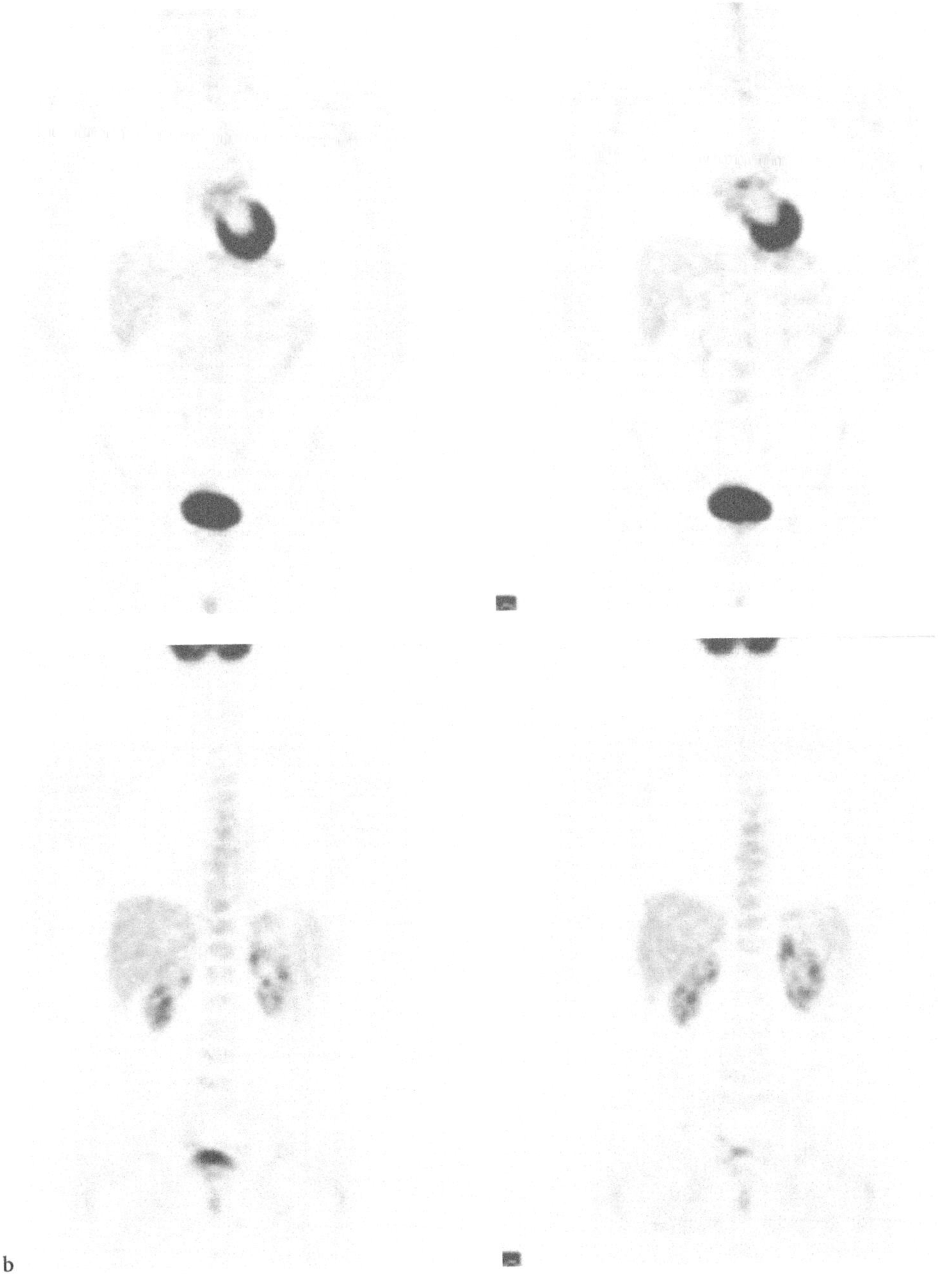

b

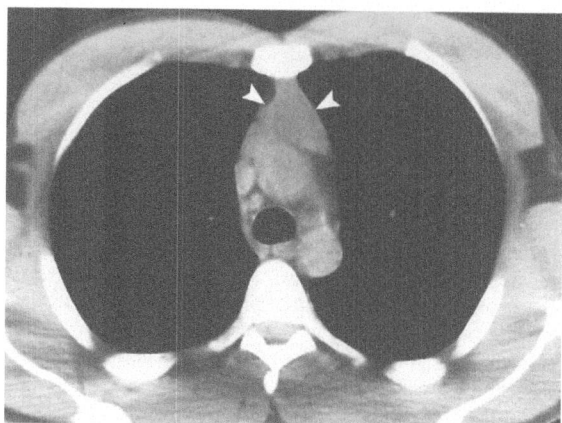
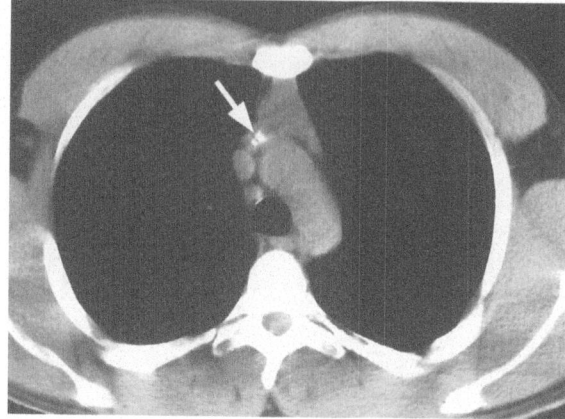

a   b

Fig. 23.30a,b. Thymic rebound in a 25-year-old man treated for non-Hodgkin lymphoma. A CT scan performed three months after completion of treatment showed a small residual mediastinal mass. a Axial unenhanced CT scan performed six months after completion of the treatment shows enlargement of the thymus (*arrowheads*). b Axial unenhanced CT scan performed eighteen months after completion of the treatment shows an unchanged thymic hyperplasia, associated with early stage of calcifications in residual mass (*arrow*).

of cases) occurring within 6 hours of transfusion of a plasma-containing blood product. Patients with underlying hematologic malignancy appear to be at risk (Popovsky and Moore 1985; Silliman et al. 2003). TRALI consists of the insidious onset of pulmonary insufficiency, manifested by severe dyspnea and hypoxia with normal cardiac function. Chest radiographs classically demonstrate pulmonary edema with "white-out" by interstitial and alveolar infiltrates similar to that seen in acute respiratory distress syndrome (Fig. 23.31), but in the first few hours, a patchy pattern may be observed. The key to distinguishing TRALI from other forms of pulmonary edema is recognition that the pulmonary edema is noncardiogenic and that affected patients do not have volume overload (Popovsky 2001).

23.7
Conclusion

Various changes in the thorax can occur in patients with hematological malignancies in relation to the course and/or the phase of therapy. After chemotherapy or/and HSCT, chest CT, especially HRCT, is more sensitive and specific than plain radiography in the assessment of both acute and late complications. Despite the fact that many chest complications show non-specific and overlapping HRCT findings including ground-glass opacity and airspace consolidation, HRCT narrows the differential diagnosis

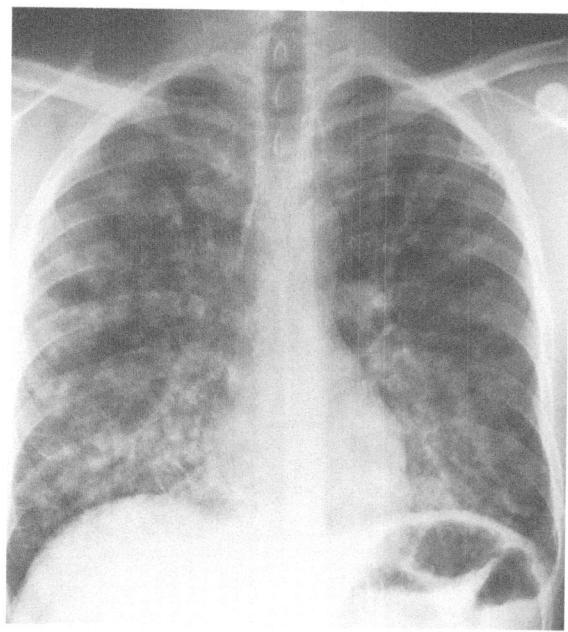

Fig. 23.31. Transfusion-related acute lung injury in a 38-year-old man at the time of induction for an acute B-cell lymphoblastic leukemia. The patient developed a dyspnea two hours after a platelet transfusion. Posteroanterior chest radiograph before transfusion was normal (*not shown*). Posteroanterior chest radiograph performed six hours after transfusion shows extensive and bilateral mixed alveolar and interstitial opacities consistent with a pulmonary edema.

and suggests further diagnostic evaluation such as bronchoalveolar lavage and lung biopsy.

CT scan and Gallium-67 scintigraphy are considered the restaging methods of choice for patients with mediastinal lymphoma. Gallium-67 scintigraphy should be routinely used for early identification of any residual disease after induction so as to allow timely initiation of the appropriate form of second-line treatment. In case of indeterminate lesions on CT scan and Gallium-67 scintigraphy, PET has proven to have a high-sensitivity for the detection of residual tumor.

Large numbers of patients now survive for years following both conventional therapy (chemotherapy and radiation therapy) and HSCT, and several late effects of treatment are now becoming evident. Radiation-induced changes are usually diagnosed on the basis of their characteristic appearance at CT and knowledge of the radiation ports, radiation dose, and interval since therapy. Most importantly, all patients in whom long-term survival is expected should be monitored closely with vigilance regarding potentially lethal iatrogenic complications, such as second cancers and cardiovascular complications, even long after the original disease appears to be cured.

References

Aisenberg AC (1999) Problems in Hodgkin's disease management. Blood 93:761–779

Alexander P (1957) Atomic radiation and life, 1st edn. Penguin Books, Baltimore

Applefeld MM, Cole JF, Pollock SH, et al. (1981) The late appearance of chronic pericardial disease in patients treated by radiotherapy for Hodgkin's disease. Ann Intern Med 94:338–341

Audebert A, Sauvanet A, Mauvais F, et al. (2002) Radiation-induced esophageal carcinoma: report of 11 cases. Ann Chir 127:289–296

Baron RL, Sagel SS, Baglan RJ, et al. (1981) Thymic cysts following radiation therapy for Hodgkin's disease. Radiology 141:593–597

Benson EP (1973) Radiation injury of large arteries: 3 further examples with prolonged asymptomatic intervals. Radiology 106:195–197

Bereton HD, Johnson RE (1974) Calcification in mediastinal lymph nodes after radiation therapy of Hodgkin's disease. Radiology 112:705–707

Bhatia S, Louie AD, Bhatia R, et al. (2001) Solid cancers after bone marrow transplantation. J Clin Oncol 19:464–471

Bhatia S, Robison LL, Oberlin O, et al. (1996) Breast cancer and other second neoplasms after childhood Hodgkin's disease. N Engl J Med 334:745–751

Bodey GP, Powell RD Jr, Hersh EM, et al. (1996) Pulmonary complications of acute leukemia. Cancer 19: 781–793

Boiselle PM, Crans CA, Kaplan MA (1999) The changing face of Pneumocystis carinii pneumonia in AIDS patients. AJR Am J Roentgenol 172:1301–1309

Boivin JF, Hutchison GB (1982) Coronary heart disease mortality after irradiation for Hodgkin's disease. Cancer 49: 2470–2475

Boivin JF, Hutchison GB, Lubin JH, et al. (1992) Coronary artery disease mortality in patients treated for Hodgkin's disease. Cancer 69:1241–1247

Bowen BC, Verma A, Brandon AH, et al. (1996) Radiation-induced brachial plexopathy: MR and clinical findings. AJNR Am J Neuroradiol 17:1932–1936

Brady LW, Levitt SH (1998) Radiation oncology in the 3rd millennium. Radiology 209:593–596

Brice P, Tredaniel J, Monsuez JJ, et al. (1991) Cardiopulmonary toxicity after three courses of ABVD and mediastinal irradiation in favorable Hodgkin's disease. Ann Oncol 2 (suppl 2):73–76

Brosius FC, Waller BF, Roberts WC, et al. (1981) Radiation heart disease. Am J Med 70:519–530

Buff SJ, McLelland R, Gallis HA, et al. (1982) Candida albicans pneumonia: Radiographic appearance. AJR Am J Roentgenol 138: 645–648

Bull RK, Edwards PD, Dixon AK, et al. (1998) CT dimensions of the normal pericardium. Br J Radiol 71:923–925

Cahan WG, Woodard HQ, Hiinbotham NL, et al. (1948) Sarcoma arising in irradiated bone. Cancer 1:3–29

Cheson BD, Horning SJ, Coiffier B, et al. (1999) Report of an international workshop to standardize response criteria for non-Hodgkin's lymphomas. NCI Sponsored International Working Group. J Clin Oncol 17:1244–1253

Choyke PL, Zeman RK, Gootenberg JE, et al. (1987) Thymic atrophy and regrowth in response to chemotherapy: CT evaluation. AJR Am J Roentgenol 149:269–272

Clark JG, Hansen JA, Hertz MI, et al. (1993) Idiopathic pneumonia syndrome after bone marrow transplantation. Am Rev Respir Dis 147:1601–1606

Coblentz C, Martin L, Tuttle R, et al. (1986) Calcification of the ascending aorta after radiation therapy. AJR Am J Roentgenol 147:477–478

Cohen SI, Bharati S, Glass J, et al. (1981) Radiotherapy as a cause of complete atrioventricular block in Hodgkin's disease: an electrophysiological-pathological correlation. Arch Intern Med 141:676–679

Coia LR, Myerson RJ, Tepper JE, et al. (1995) Late effects of radiation therapy on the gastrointestinal tract. Int J Radiat Oncol Biol Phys 30:1213–1236

Cosset JM, Henry-Amar M, Girinski T, et al. (1988) Late toxicity of radiotherapy in Hodgkin's disease: the role of fraction size. Acta Oncol 27:123–129

Cosset JM, Henry-Amar M, Pellae-Cosset B, et al. (1991) Pericarditis and myocardial infarction after Hodgkin's disease therapy. Int J Radiat Oncol Biol Phys 21:447–449

Dershaw DD, Yahalom J, Petrec JA (1992) Breast carcinoma in women previously treated for Hodgkin disease: mammographic evaluation. Radiology 184:421–423

de Wit M, Bumann D, Beyer W, Herbst K, et al. (1997) Whole-body positron emission tomography (PET) for diagnosis of residual mass in patients with lymphoma. Ann Oncol 8 (Suppl 1):57–60

Dubois PJ, Myerowitz RL, Allen CM (1977) Pathoradiologic correlation of pulmonary candidiasis in immunosuppressed patients. Cancer 40:1026–1036

Fajardo LF, Berthrong M (1988) Vascular lesions following radiation. Pathol Annu 23:297–330

Fajardo LF, Lee A (1975) Rupture of major vessels after radiation. Cancer 36:904–913

Ford EG, Lockhart SK, Sullivan MP, et al. (1987) Mediastinal mass following chemotherapeutic treatment of Hodgkin's disease: recurrent tumor or thymic hyperplasia? J Pediatr Surg 22:1155–1159

Gasparini MD, Balzarini L, Castellani MR, et al. (1993) Current role of gallium scan and magnetic resonance imaging in the management of mediastinal Hodgkin lymphoma. Cancer 72:577–582

Gefter WB, Albelda SM, Talbot GH, et al. (1985) Invasive pulmonary aspergillosis and acute leukemia. Limitations in the diagnostic utility of the air crescent sign. Radiology 157:605–610

Girinsky T, Cordova A, Rey A, Cosset JM, et al. (2000) Thallium-201 scintigraphy is not predictive of late cardiac complications in patients with Hodgkin's disease treated with mediastinal radiation. Int J Radiat Oncol Biol Phys 48:1503–1506

Glazer HS, Lee JK, Levitt RG, et al. (1985) Radiation fibrosis: differentiation from recurrent tumor by MR imaging–work in progress. Radiology 156:721–726

Gorospe L, Madrid-Muniz C, Royo A, et al. (2002) Radiation-induced osteochondroma of the T4 vertebra causing spinal cord compression. Eur Radiol 12:844–848

Gruden JF, Huang L, Turner J, et al. (1997) High-resolution CT in the evaluation of clinically suspected pneumocystis carinii pneumonia in AIDS patients with normal, equivocal, or nonspecific radiographic findings. AJR Am J Roentgenol 169:967–975

Hancock SL, Tucker MA, Hoppe RT (1993) Factors affecting late mortality from heart disease after treatment of Hodgkin's disease. JAMA 270:1949–1955

Hasleton PS and Doran HM (1996) Pulmonary changes after transplantation. In: Hasleton PS (ed) Spencer's pathology of the lung. McGraw-Hill, New York, pp 723–765

Hildebrand FL Jr, Rosenow EC 3rd, Habermann TM, et al. (1990) Pulmonary complications of leukemia. Chest 98:1233–1239

Hill M, Cunningham D, MacVicar D, et al. (1993) Role of magnetic resonance imaging in predicting relapse in residual masses after treatment of lymphoma. J Clin Oncol 11:2273–2278

Hofmann J, Mintzer D, Warhol MJ (1994) Malignant mesothelioma following radiation therapy. Am J Med 97:379–382

Hows JM (2001) Status of umbilical cord blood transplantation in the year 2001. J Clin Pathol 54:428–434

Ichikado K, Johkoh T, Ikezoe J, et al. (1997) Acute interstitial pneumonia: high-resolution CT findings correlated with pathology. AJR Am J Roentgenol 168:333–338

Ikezoe J, Takashima S, Morimoto S, et al. (1988) CT appearance of acute radiation-induced injury in the lung. AJR Am J Roentgenol 150:765–770

Ikezoe J, Takeuchi N, Johkoh T, et al. (1992) CT appearance of pulmonary tuberculosis in diabetic and immunocompromised patients: Comparison with patients who had no underlying disease. AJR Am J Roentgenol 159:1175–1179

Jerusalem G, Beguin Y, Fassotte MF, et al. (1999) Whole-body positron emission tomography using 18F-fluorodeoxyglucose for posttreatment evaluation in Hodgkin's disease

and non-Hodgkin's lymphoma has higher diagnostic and prognostic value than classical computed tomography scan imaging. Blood 94:429–433

Kang EY, Patz EF, Müller NL (1996) Cytomegalovirus pneumonia in transplant patients: CT findings. J Comput Assist Tomogr 20:295–299

Katz M, Piekarski JD, Bayle-Weisberger C, et al. (1977) Residual mediastinal mass following radiation therapy for Hodgkin's disease. Ann Radiol 20:667–672

Kopelson G, Herwig KJ (1978) Coronary artery disease in cancer patients. Int J Radiat Oncol Biol Phys 4:895–906

Kostakoglu L, Leonard JP, Kuji I, et al. (2002) Comparison of fluorine-18 fluorodeoxyglucose positron emission tomography and Ga-67 scintigraphy in evaluation of lymphoma. Cancer 94:879–888

Kostakoglu L, Yeh SD, Portlock C, et al. (1992) Validation of gallium-67-citrate single-photon emission computed tomography in biopsy-confirmed residual Hodgkin's disease in the mediastinum. J Nucl Med 33:345–350

Krowka MJ, Rosenow EC, Hoagland HC (1985) Pulmonary complications of bone marrow transplantation. Chest 87:237–245

Kuhlman JE, Fishman EK, Siegelman SS (1985) Invasive pulmonary aspergillosis in acute leukemia: characteristic findings on CT, the CT halo sign, and the role of CT in early diagnosis. Radiology 157:611–614

Kuhlman JE, Fishman EK, Burch PA, et al. (1988) CT of invasive pulmonary aspergillosis. AJR Am J Roentgenol 150:1015–1020

Kuhlman JE, Kavuru M, Fishman EK, et al. (1990) Pneumocystis carinii pneumonia: Spectrum of parenchymal CT findings. Radiology 175:711–714

Langer CJ, Keller SM, Erner SM (1992) Thymic hyperplasia with hemorrhage simulating recurrent Hodgkin's disease after chemotherapy-induced complete remission. Cancer 70:2082–2086

Lau DM, Siegel MJ, Hildebolt CF, et al. (1998) Bronchiolitis obliterans syndrome: Thin-section CT diagnosis of obstructive changes in infants and young children after lung transplantation. Radiology 208:783–788

Lee CK, Aeppli D, Nierengarten ME (2000) The need for long-term surveillance for patients treated with curative radiotherapy for Hodgkin's disease: University of Minnesota experience. Int J Radiat Oncol Biol Phys 48:169–179

Lepke RA, Libshitz HI (1983) Radiation-induced injury of esophagus. Radiology 148:375–378

Libshitz HI (1993) Radiation changes in the lung. Semin Roentgenol 28:303–320

Libshitz HI (1994) Radiation changes in bone. Semin Roentgenol 29:15–37

Libshitz HI, Brosof AB, Southard ME (1973) Radiographic appearance of the chest following extended field radiation therapy for Hodgkin's disease. A consideration of time-dose relationships. Cancer 32:206–215

Libshitz HI, Cohen MA (1967) Radiation-induced osteochondromas. Radiology 142:750–760

Libshitz HI, Shuman LS (1984) Radiation-induced pulmonary change: CT findings. J Comput Assist Tomogr 8:15–19

Logan PM (1998) Thoracic manifestations of external beam radiotherapy. AJR Am J Roentgenol 171:569–577

Lorigan JG, Libshitz HI, Peuchot M (1989) Radiation-induced sarcoma in bone: CT findings in 19 cases. AJR Am J Roentgenol 153:791–794

Loyer EM, Delpassand ES (1993) Radiation-induced heart disease: imaging features. Semin Roentgenol 28:321–332

Loyer E, Fuller L, Libshitz HI, et al. (2000) Radiographic appearance of the chest following therapy for Hodgkin disease. Eur J Radiol 35:136–148

Marie P, Clunet J, Raulot-Lapointe G (1910) Contribution à l'étude du développement des tumeurs malignes sur les ulcères de Roentgen. Bull Assoc France Etude Cancer 3: 404–426

McAdams HP, Rosado de Christenson M, Strollo DC, et al. (1997) Pulmonary mucormycosis: radiologic findings in 32 cases. AJR Am J Roentgenol 168:1541–1548

McGuinness G, Scholes JV, Garay SM, et al. (1994) Cytomegalovirus pneumonitis: spectrum of parenchymal CT findings with pathologic correlation in 21 AIDS patients. Radiology 192:451–459

McKee LC Jr, Collins RD (1974) Intravascular leukocyte thrombi and aggregates as a cause of morbidity and mortality in leukemia. Medicine Baltimore 53:463–478

Mesurolle B, Qanadli SD, Merad M, et al. (2000) Unusual radiologic findings in the thorax after radiation therapy. Radiographics 20:67–81

Micke O, Schafer U, Glashorster M, et al. (1999) Radiation-induced esophageal carcinoma 30 years after mediastinal irradiation: case report and review of the literature. Jpn J Clin Oncol 29:164–170

Mikhaeel NG, Timothy AR, O'Doherty MJ, et al. (2000) 18-FDG-PET as a prognostic indicator in the treatment of aggressive Non-Hodgkin's Lymphoma-comparison with CT. Leuk Lymphoma 39:543–553

Miller DD, Waters DD, Dangoisse V, et al. (1983) Symptomatic coronary artery spasm following radiation for Hodgkin's disease. Chest 83:284–285

Mosvas B, Raffin TA, Epstein AH, et al. (1997) Pulmonary radiation injury. Chest 111:1061–1076

Naumann R, Vaic A, Beuthien-Baumann B, et al. (2001) Prognostic value of positron emission tomography in the evaluation of post-treatment residual mass in patients with Hodgkin's disease and non-Hodgkin's lymphoma. Br J Haematol 115:793–800

Neugut AI, Murray T, Santos J, et al. (1994) Increased risk of lung cancer after breast cancer radiation therapy in cigarette smokers. Cancer 73:1615–1620

Nishimura K, Itoh H (1992) High-resolution computed tomographic features of bronchiolitis obliterans organizing pneumonia. Chest 102:S26-S31

Oh YW, Kim YH, Lee NJ, et al. (1994) High-resolution CT appearance of miliary tuberculosis. J Comput Assist Tomogr 18:862–866

Parker RG (1990) Radiation-induced cancer as a factor in clinical decision making (the 1989 ASTRO Gold Medal address). Int J Radiat Oncol Biol Phys 18:993–1000

Patz EF Jr, Peters WP, Goodman PC (1994) Pulmonary drug toxicity following high-dose chemotherapy with autologous bone marrow transplantation: CT findings in 20 cases. J Thorac Imaging 9:129–134

Penniment MG, O'Brien PC (1994) Pneumothorax following thoracic radiation therapy for Hodgkin's disease. Thorax 49:936–937

Peylan-Ramu N, Haddy TB, Jones E, et al. (1989) High frequency of benign mediastinal uptake of gallium-67 after completion of chemotherapy in children with high-grade non-Hodgkin's lymphoma. J Clin Oncol 12:1800–1806

Pezner RD, Horak DA, Sayegh HO, et al. (1990) Spontaneous pneumothorax in patients irradiated for Hodgkin's disease and other malignant lymphomas. Int J Radiat Oncol Biol Phys 18:193–198

Popovsky MA (2001) Transfusion and lung injury. Transfus Clin Biol 8:272–277

Popovsky MA, Moore SB (1985) Diagnostic and pathogenetic considerations in transfusion-related acute lung injury. Transfusion 25:573–577

Preidler KW, Szolar DM, Moelleken, et al. (1996) Distribution pattern of computed tomography findings in patients with bronchiolitis obliterans organizing pneumonia. Invest Radiol 31:251–255

Primack SL, Hartman TE, Ikezoe J, et al. (1993) Acute interstitial pneumonia: radiographic and CT findings in nine patients. Radiology 188:817–820

Primack SL, Hartman TE, Lee KS, et al. (1994) Pulmonary nodules and the CT halo sign. Radiology 190:513–515

Primack SL, Miller RR, Müller NL, et al. (1995) Diffuse pulmonary hemorrhage: Clinical, pathologic, and imaging features. AJR Am J Roentgenol 164:295–300

Primack SL, Müller NL (1994) High-resolution computed tomography in acute diffuse lung disease in the immunocompromised patient. Radiol Clin North Am 32:731–744

Qanadli SD, El Hajjam M, Mignon F, et al. (1999) Helical CT phlebography of the superior vena cava: diagnosis and evaluation of venous obstruction. AJR Am J Roentgenol 172:1327–1333

Rahmouni A, Divine M, Lepage E, et al. (2001) Mediastinal lymphoma: quantitative changes in gadolinium enhancement at MR imaging after treatment. Radiology 219: 621–628

Reinders JG, Heijmen BJ, Olofsen-van Acht MJ, et al. (1999) Ischemic heart disease after mantlefield irradiation for Hodgkin's disease in long-term follow-up. Radiother Oncol 51:35–42

Rivero H, Gaisie G, Bender TM, et al. (1984) Calcified mediastinal lymph nodes in Hodgkin's disease. Pediatr Radiol 14:11–13

Roebuck DJ, Nicholls WD, Bernard EJ, et al. (1998) Misleading leads. Thallium-201 uptake in rebound thymic hyperplasia. Med Pediatr Oncol 30:297–300

Rosanowski F, Tigges M, Eysholdt U (1995) Esophagomediastinal fistula and recurrent laryngeal nerve paralysis after radiotherapy of Hodgkin's disease. Laryngorhinootologie 74:516–517

Rossi SE, Erasmus JJ, McAdams HP, et al. (2000) Pulmonary drug toxicity: radiologic and pathologic manifestations. Radiographics 20:1245–1259

Rossleigh MA, Smith J, Straus DJ, et al. (1986) Osteonecrosis in patients with malignant lymphoma. A review of 31 cases. Cancer 58:1112–1116

Roswit B, White DC (1977) Severe radiation injuries of the lung. Am J Roentgenol 129:127–136

Rowinsky EK, Abeloff MD, Wharam MD (1985) Spontaneous pneumothorax following thoracic irradiation. Chest 88: 703–708

Rubin P, Casarett GW (1968) Clinical radiation pathology, 1st edn. WB Saunders, Philadelphia, London, Toronto

Sider L, Westcott MA (1994) Pulmonary manifestations of cryptococcosis in patients with AIDS: CT features. J Thorac Imag 9:78–84

Silliman CC, Boshkov LK, Mehdizadehkashi Z, et al. (2003)

Transfusion-related acute lung injury: epidemiology and a prospective analysis of etiologic factors. Blood 101: 454–462

Smith J (1982) Radiation-induced sarcoma of bone: clinical and radiographic findings in 43 patients irradiated for soft tissue neoplasms. Clin Radiol 33:205–221

Souba WW, McKenna RJ Jr, Benjamin R, et al. (1986) Radiation-induced sarcoma of the chest wall. Cancer 57: 610–615

Soubani AO, Miller KB, Hassoun PN (1996) Pulmonary complications of bone marrow transplantation. Chest 109: 1066–1077

Spaepen K, Mortelmans L (2001) Evaluation of treatment response in patients with lymphoma using [18F]FDG-PET: differences between non-Hodgkin's lymphoma and Hodgkin's disease. Q J Nucl Med 45:269–273

Stein JS, Jacobson JH (1993) Axillary-contralateral brachial artery bypass for radiation-induced occlusion of the subclavian artery. Cardiovasc Surg 2:146–148

Stewart JR, Fajardo LF (1984) Radiation-induced heart disease: an update. Prog Cardiovasc Dis 27:173–194

Stewart JR, Fajardo LF, Gillette SM, et al. (1995) Radiation injury to the heart. Int J Radiat Oncol Biol Phys 31: 1205–1211

Tanaka N, Matsumoto T, Miura G, Emoto T, Matsunaga N (2002) HRCT findings of chest complications in patients with leukemia. Eur Radiol 12:1512–1522

Tenholder MF, Hooper RG (1980) Pulmonary infiltrates in leukemia. Chest 78:468–473

Thyagarajan D, Cascino T, Harms G (1995) Magnetic resonance imaging in brachial plexopathy of cancer. Neurology 45:421–427

Totterman KJ, Pesonen E, Siltanen P, et al. (1983) Radiation-induced chronic heart disease. Chest 83:875–878

Tredaniel J, Brice P, Lepage E, et al. (1992) The significance of a residual mediastinal mass following treatment for aggressive non-Hodgkin's lymphomas. Eur Respir J 5:170–173

Tucker MA, D'Angio GJ, Boice JD Jr, et al. (1987) Bone sarcomas linked to radiotherapy and chemotherapy in children. N Engl J Med 317:588–593

Van Leeuwen FE, Klokman WJ, Hagenbeek A, et al. (1994) Second cancer risk following Hodgkin's disease: a 20-year follow-up study. J Clin Oncol 12:312–325

Van Leeuwen FE, Klokman WJ, Stovall M, et al. (1995) Roles of radiotherapy and smoking in lung cancer following Hodgkin's disease. J Natl Cancer Inst 87:1530–1537

Van Leeuwen FE, Klokman WJ, Veer MB, et al. (2000) Long term risk of second malignancy in survivors of Hodgkin's disease treated during adolescence or young adulthood. J Clin Oncol 18:487–497

Vlachaki MT, Ha CS, Hagemeister FB, et al. (1998) Stage I Hodgkin disease: radiation therapy and chemotherapy at the University of Texas M.D. Anderson Cancer Center, 1967–1997. Radiology 208:739–747

Webb WR, Müller NL, Naidich DP (1996) Diseases characterized primarily by parenchymal opacification. In: Webb WR, Müller NL, Naidich DP (eds) High-resolution CT of the lung. Lippincott-Raven, Philadelphia, New York, pp 193–225

Winn WC, Chandler FW (1994) Bacterial infections. In: Dail DH, Hammar SP (eds) Pulmonary pathology. Springer-Verlag, New York, pp 255–330

Worthy SA, Flint JD, Müller NL (1997a) Pulmonary complications after bone marrow transplantation: High-resolution CT and pathologic findings. Radiographics 17:1359–1371

Worthy SA, Park CS, Kim JS, et al. (1997b) Bronchiolitis obliterans after lung transplantation: high-resolution CT findings in 15 patients. AJR Am J Roentgenol 169:673–677

Wouter van Es H, Engelen AM, Witkamp TD, et al. (1997) Radiation-induced brachial plexopathy: MR imaging. Skeletal Radiol 26:284–288

Yahalom J, Hasin Y, Fuks Z, et al. (1983) Acute myocardial infarction with normal coronary angiogram after mantle irradiation therapy for Hodgkin's disease. Cancer 52: 637–641

Yahalom J, Petrec JA, Biddinger PW, et al. (1992) Breast cancer in patients irradiated for Hodgkin disease: a clinical and pathologic analysis of 45 events in 37 patients. J Clin Oncol 10:1674–1681

Zinner SH (1999) Changing epidemiology of infections in patients with neutropenia and cancer: emphasis on gram-positive and resistant bacteria. Clin Infect Dis 29: 490–494

Zinzani PL, Monetti N, Zompatori M, et al. (2001) Importance of gallium scan restaging for curative treatment of mediastinal lymphomas. Haematologica 86:1229–1230

24 Abdominal Effects of Therapy in Patients Treated for Hematological Malignancies

Nobufusa Furukawa and Ali Guermazi

CONTENTS

24.1
Introduction

With the advent of improved diagnostic modalities and aggressive therapy, various gastrointestinal complications of hematological malignancies are becoming more common. Abdominal complications of treated hematological malignancies are no longer a life-threatening event. Early diagnosis and treatment are crucial to improve morbidity of these conditions. However, clinical presentation and plain radiographic manifestations may be non-specific; barium studies may be hard to perform in these patients and carry a risk of bowel perforation. Abdominal US is first choice for patients with abdominal complaints. However, it is entirely operator dependent and significant artifacts caused by bowel gas may be a prob-

Nobufusa Furukawa, MD
Senior Radiologist, Department of Radiology, St. Mary's Hospital, 422 Tusbukuhonmachi, Kurume City, Fukuoka 830-8543, Japan
Ali Guermazi, MD
Visiting Associate Professor, Department of Radiology, University of California, San Francisco, 350 Parnassus Avenue, Suite 150, San Francisco, CA 94117, USA

lem. MR imaging may take a long time and imaging findings of this modality are not yet well reported. CT provides the most comprehensive radiographic evaluation for the detection and characterization of abdominal conditions in such patients. This chapter reviews the important clinical aspects of abdominal complications of treated hematological malignancy and presents mainly CT images.

24.2
General Principles

The etiology of most abdominal complications in treated hematological malignancies is threefold: (1) primary tumor cell invasion; (2) altered immune state from the hematological malignancy itself and from anticancer drugs; and (3) direct and indirect toxic effects of chemotherapeutic agents to abdominal organs (Hunter and Bjelland 1984).

Hematological malignancy not only affects the hematopoietic system directly but also involves many other organs and tissues. The hepatobiliary system and gastrointestinal tract are such areas that often undergo extensive pathological changes produced primarily by the disease process or secondarily by its treatment. The most common sequelae are tumor cell infiltration; mycotic, bacterial, and viral infections; hemorrhagic necrosis; and related surgical and interventional complications (Prolla and Kirsner 1964; Winton et al. 1975; Dewar et al. 1981). Various surgical problems also occur including appendicitis, cecal perforation, liver abscesses, and peritonitis from hemorrhagic proctocolitis (Wall 1992).

BMT or HSCT for treating hematogenous cancer have prevailed as the treatment of choice since the advent of histocompatibility typing (Barrett 1991). Marrow grafting is preceded by intense immunosuppressive, marrow ablative treatment, usually high-dose chemotherapy and whole-body irradiation. Pre-engraftment complications include bacterial, fungal, and viral infections; hepatic veno-occlusive disease; and graft rejection. Postengraftment complications include viral, fungal, and protozonal infections; acute GVHD, and pneumatosis intestinalis (CHAMPLIN and GALE 1984). Delayed complications include chronic GVHD and recurrence of cancer. Recurrent or de novo disease or malignancies may develop, in particular, posttransplantation B-cell NHL may develop in patients who are chronically immunocompromised (SULLIVAN et al. 1984; PATZIK et al. 1991). These malignancies have a high propensity for bowel and brain involvement (SHAPIRO et al. 1988).

24.3
Hepatobiliary System

Hepatic abnormalities can be well delineated with CT (DAY and CARPENTER 1993). Hepatic fungal abscesses are often encountered in immunocompromised patients and patients undergoing aggressive chemotherapy. In one series, all patients with leukemia had candidiasis of the gastrointestinal tract with involvement of the liver in 75% and of the spleen in 94% (MYEROWITZ et al. 1977). CT is probably more sensitive than US and typically shows multiple rounded hypodense areas scattered throughout the liver and/or spleen (Fig. 24.1). Numerous hyperdense areas are seen late in the course of the disease. This finding is considered to be represent calcification. However, negative imaging findings do not rule out the presence of fungal infection, and recurrent tumor

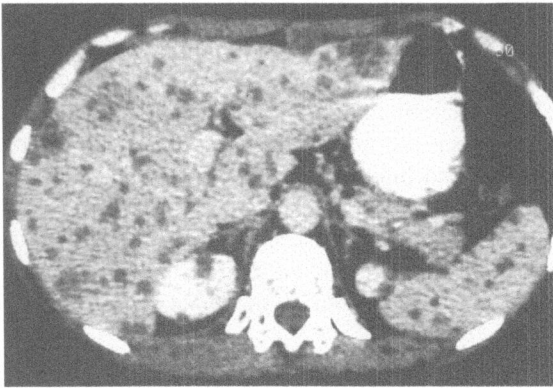

Fig. 24.1. Invasive candidiasis in a 50-year-old woman who underwent bone marrow transplantation for acute myeloid leukemia. Axial contrast-enhanced CT scan of the upper abdomen shows multiple hypodense rounded areas in the liver, spleen, and both kidneys. The patient responded favorably to amphotericin B.

and posttransplantation lymphoma also manifest as focal hypoattenuating liver masses; liver biopsy should be done to confirm the diagnosis (PASTAKIA et al. 1988; SHIRKHODA 1987).

Veno-occlusive disease (VOD) of the liver, clinically characterized by abdominal pain, hepatomegaly, ascites, and jaundice, may be a complication after either autologous or allogenic BMT, usually associated with chemoradiotherapy, particularly myeloblative therapy in combination with BMT. It is a major cause of mortality. This condition is characterized by fibrous obliteration of hepatic venules causing postsinusoidal obstruction and intrahepatic portal hypertension. It may be progressive and fatal (McDONALD et al. 1986). CT findings are hepatomegaly, ascites, thickening of the wall of gallbladder and intestine, and periportal hypodense zones (Fig. 24.2) (BENYA et al. 1993). Hepatofugal or bidirectional portal venous flow on Doppler US can provide the most specific findings, even in the early or subclinical stage (BROWN et al. 1990; HERBETKO et al. 1992).

Gallbladder and biliary tract abnormalities are common in patients treated for hematological malignancies. Hyperalimentation therapy and hepatic GVHD are associated with cholestasis, which contributes to the development of gallbladder sludge and gallstones. Gallbladder or bile duct dilatation may also be seen after BMT. The cause is often obscure, possibly related to infection or GVHD, resolves spontaneously (DAY and CARPENTER 1993).

24.4
Pancreas

In patients with lymphoma or leukemia, acute pancreatitis can be induced by chemotherapy toxic to normal pancreatic cells, by tumor obstruction of the pancreatic duct, or the rapid lysis of tumor metastatic to the pancreas (NICCOLINI et al. 1976; SPIEGEL and MAGRATH 1979; FRANCIS and GLAZER 1982). Although the frequency of acute pancreatitis in these patients is generally low, the disease has substantial morbidity and mortality. It is crucial to identify the cause. Mechanisms suggested for drug induced pancreatitis include pancreatic duct constriction, immuno-supression, cytotoxic, osmotic pressure or metabolic effects, arteriolar thrombosis, direct cellular toxicity, and hepatic involvement. Agents reported to have a definite association with pancreatitis are asparaginase, azathioprine, didanosine, estrogens, furosemide, mercaptopurine,

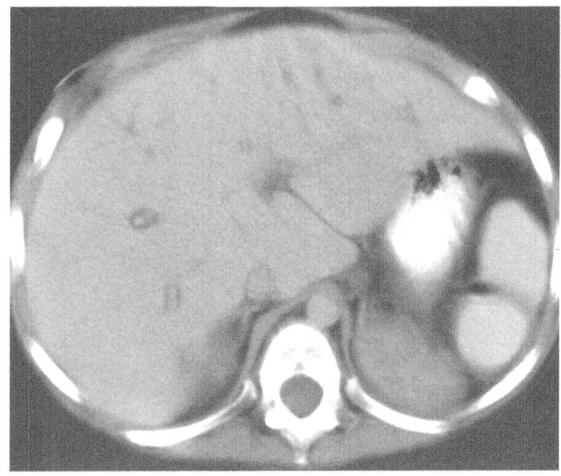
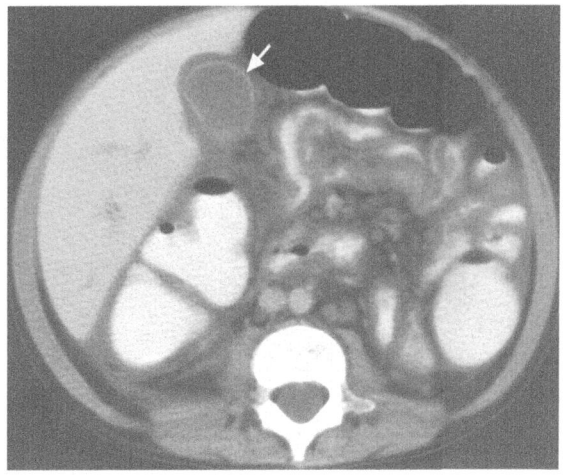

Fig. 24.2a,b. Veno-occlusive disease in a 9-year-old boy who underwent allogenic BMT for non-Hodgkin lymphoma. Axial contrast-enhanced CT scans of the upper abdomen show (**a**) hepatomegaly, hypodense periportal zones of the liver, (**b**) dilatation and thickened bowel, gallbladder wall enhancement (*arrow*), and mesenteric fat obliteration. The diagnosis was confirmed at autopsy.

pentamidine, sulphonamides, sulindac, tetracycline, thiacides, and valproic acid (UNDERWOOD and FRYE 1993). Rapid tumor lysis with effective chemotherapy may produce acute pancreatitis (Fig. 24.3). Radiographs in pancreatitis are often non-specific, but may give some diagnostic clues such as paralytic ileus, focal duodenal dilatation, widening of the duodenal sweep, calcification of the pancreas, and left pleural effusion. Abdominal US is the most frequently performed, reliable imaging modality in patients with suspected acute pancreatitis. Typically US shows a diffusely swollen and hypoechoic pancreas. Ascites and peripancreatic fluid collections are often seen. The main pancreatic duct may be dilated. Contrast-enhanced CT is not usually necessary for diagnosis, but is helpful in evaluating the severity of the pancreatitis and in detecting complications such as abscess or pseudocyst (Fig. 24.4). However, these are not constant findings and the pancreas may appear normal in mild pancreatitis.

24.5
Spleen

Among all splenic complications, splenomegaly is the most common in patients treated for hematological malignancies, especially after BMT. Splenomegaly may be a complication of underlying disease, or it may be associated with posttransplantation infec-

tion or lymphoma (SHIRKHODA 1987). Focal splenic lesions may represent microabscesses (Fig. 24.1), calcified granulomas, or posttransplantation lymphoma, and may be imaged on CT or US. Calcifications may also be seen on plain radiographs. Splenic infarction may occur in BMT recipients and may be focal or diffuse. The cause of this complication remains unclear (DAY and CARPENTER 1993).

24.6
Gastrointestinal Tract

The gastrointestinal tract is frequently affected after chemotherapy, radiation therapy, and BMT. Clinically, affected patients generally complain of severe diarrhea, abdominal pain, and sometimes hemorrhage. Immunosuppressive status also causes various types of gastrointestinal complications.

24.6.1
Typhlitis

Typhlitis is an acute inflammation of the cecum, that may include the terminal ileum; it is also known as the ileocecal syndrome, necrotizing enterocolitis, or neutropenic colitis. It was described initially in children with leukemia and severe neutropenia (WAGNER et al. 1970; MOIR and BALE 1976; DEL FAVA

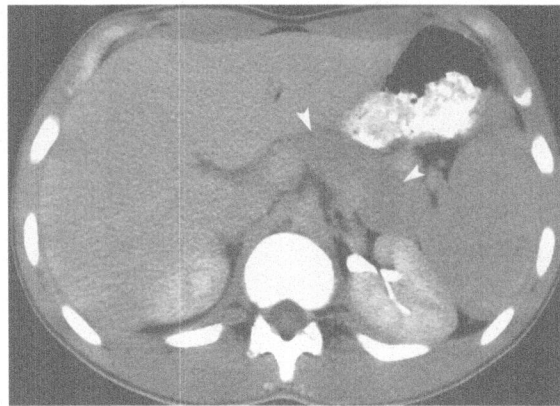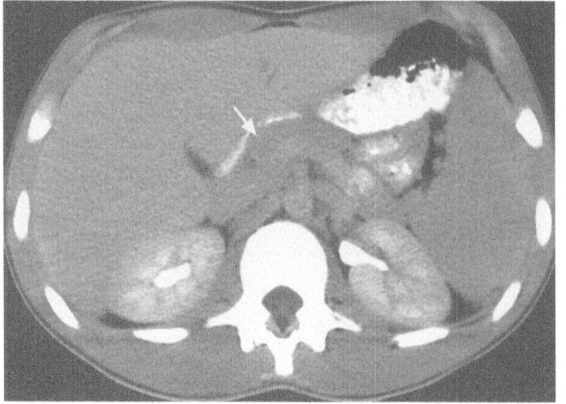

Fig. 24.3a,b. Tumor lysis pancreatitis in a 16-year-old boy with Burkitt lymphoma who developed acute pancreatitis immediately after beginning of chemotherapy. **a** Axial contrast-enhanced CT scan of the upper abdomen reveals focal hypodense enlargement in the body and tail of the pancreas (*arrowheads*). **b** Axial CT scan 10 mm caudate to (**a**) shows the pancreas head appears normal (*arrow*).

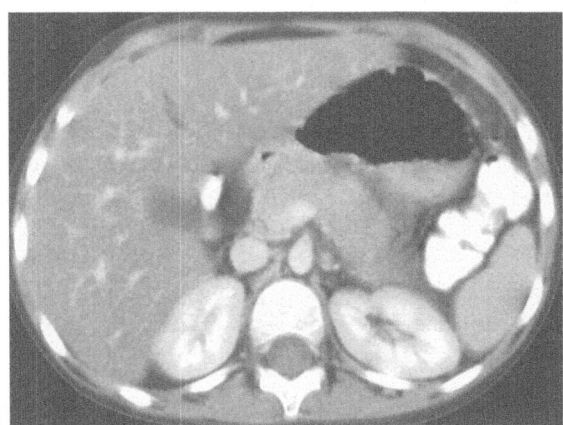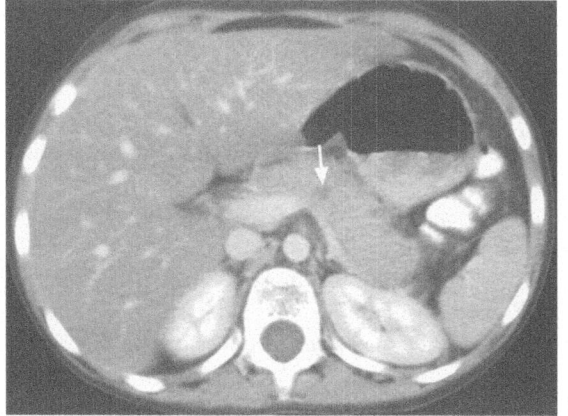

Fig. 24.4a,b. Pancreatitis induced by chemotherapy toxicity in a 7-year-old girl receiving L-asparaginase for acute lymphocytic leukemia. **a, b** Axial contrast-enhanced CT scans of the upper abdomen show diffuse enlargement of the entire pancreas with stranding of the peripancreatic fat. There is focal hypodense area in the body of pancreas (*arrow*) consistent to a pancreatic necrosis.

and CRONIN 1977; DEWAR et al. 1981). However, it is now also recognized in patients with treated hematological malignancies. Pathologically it can be caused by leukemia or lymphoma infiltrates, ischemia, focal pseudomembranous colitis, or infection. The clinical manifestations of typhlitis are non-specific. Colonic diseases such as typhlitis, appendicitis, intussusception, perforation, and intestinal obstruction also may present with symptoms referable to the right lower quadrant of the abdomen.

Plain radiographic findings of typhlitis include a paucity of bowel gas in the right lower quadrant, small bowel ileus, an ill defined soft tissue density in the region of the cecum, ascites, and mechanical obstruction (Fig. 24.5a), although these abnormalities are non

specific. Abdominal ultrasound demonstrates right-side colonic wall thickening with variable echogenecity (Fig. 24.5b) (ALEXANDER et al. 1988). The findings of typhlitis on barium enema usually include a cecal mass, thickened irregular mucosal folds, and thumb printing of the bowel wall. Barium studies are considered a reliable diagnostic tool in typhlitis; however, they carry the risk of bowel perforation in the involved colon.

CT demonstrates not only the thickened colonic wall but also the internal texture and pericolic features. Diffuse right colonic wall thickening is considered a hallmark of typhlitis. Extent of the disease is variable, however the cecum is the most commonly and severely involved (Fig. 24.5). Small bowel involvement is also seen. These findings in neutropenic patients strongly

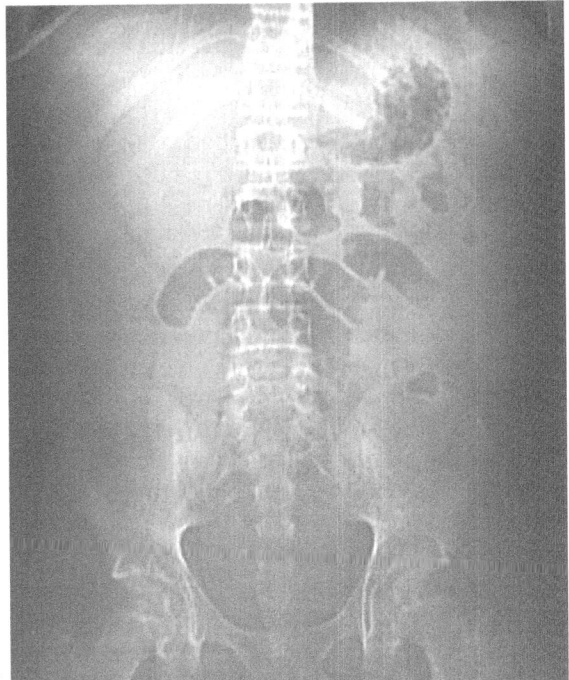

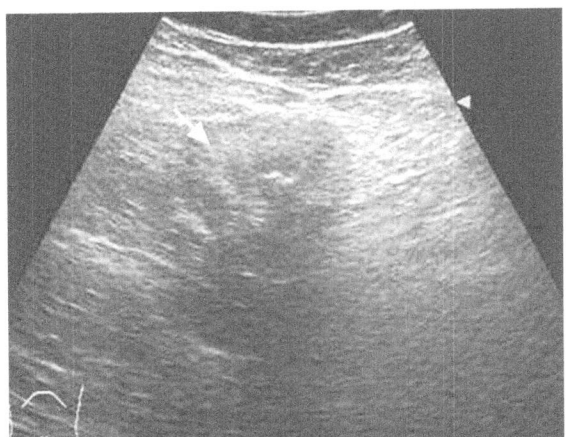

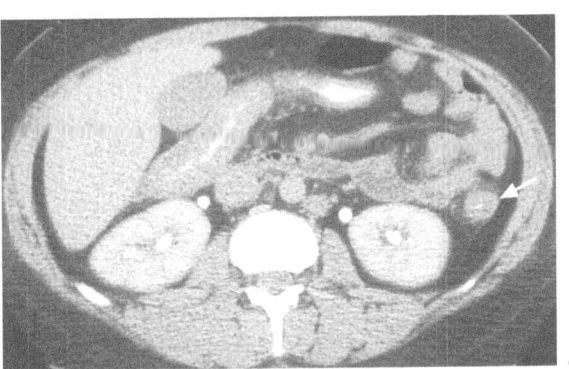

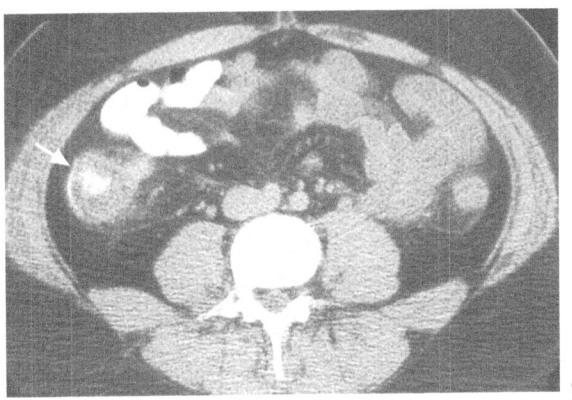

Fig. 24.5a–d. Typhlitis in a 16-year-old boy who underwent chemotherapy for acute lymphocytic leukemia. **a** Antero-posterior plain radiograph of the abdomen demonstrates dilated small bowel loops and paucity of gas in the right lower quadrant. These findings are non-specific, but may suggest typhlitis. **b** Transverse US image of the abdomen shows wall-thickened bowel in the right lower quadrant. The predominate thickening is in the mucosa and submucosa. The increased echogenicity of the thickened submucosa represents hemorrhage (*arrow*). Axial contrast-enhanced CT scans with oral opacification show (**c**) the ascending and descending (*arrow*) colons have thickened walls, most markedly in (**d**) the cecum (*arrow*). Adjacent opaque fat indicates inflammatory change. Small mesenteric lymph nodes are present. These findings correspond to typhlitis, although differentiation of hemorrhagic colitis from other types of infectious colitis may be challenging without clinical information.

indicate typhlitis. Mural attenuation is variable, and is considered to reflect mural edema, hemorrhage or necrosis. Abnormal enhancement is often seen in both mucosa and serosa (Fig. 24.6). Pneumatosis may be a risk for perforation, but does not indicate the need for operation. Pericolic fat obliteration and fluid collection are not constant findings but may indicate the extent of disease (FRICK et al. 1984; ADAMS et al. 1985).

Typhlitis is usually managed conservatively with prophylactic bowel rest, broad spectrum antibiotics, and granulocytic support. Surgical intervention is usually limited to cases with complications such as

perforation, abscess formation, massive gastrointestinal bleeding, uncontrolled sepsis, or obstruction.

24.6.2
Colitis

CMV Colitis

Colitis is the most common gastrointestinal manifestation of the CMV infection. CMV is a herpes-like virus that can be transmitted by contaminated blood, transfusion, urine, bodily secretions, or sexual con-

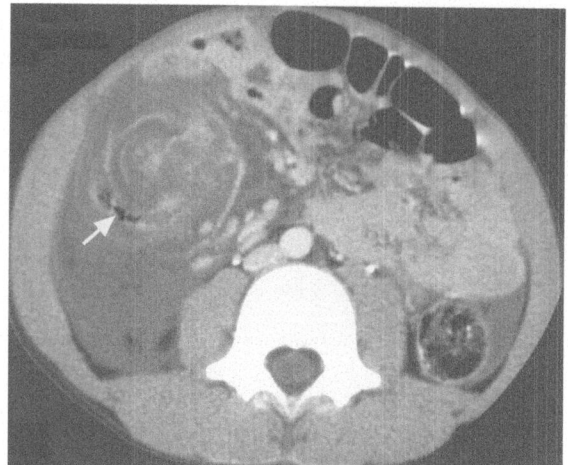

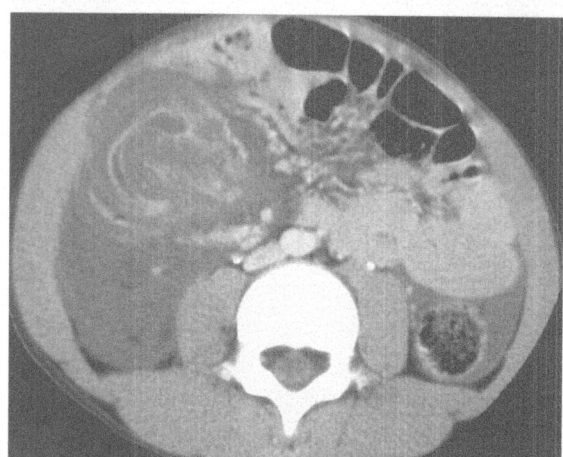

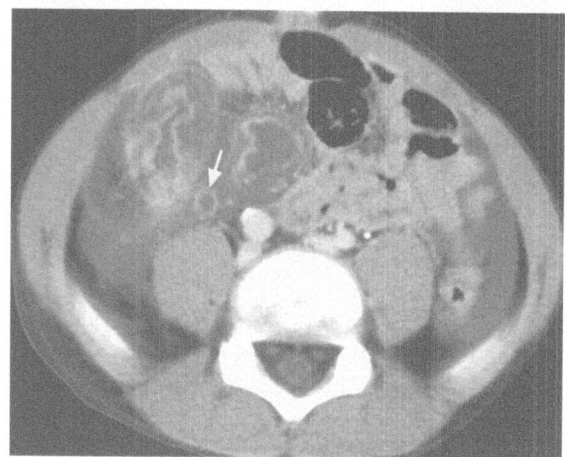

Fig. 24.6a–c. Typhlitis in a 7-year-old boy with acute lymphocytic leukemia who presented abdominal discomfort after chemotherapeutic induction. **a–c** Axial contrast-enhanced CT scans of the abdomen demonstrate marked wall thickening, and abnormal mucosal and serosal enhancement of the cecum, ascending colon, and terminal ileum. CT scans also show (**a–c**) pericolic fluid, (**a**) intramural air in the cecum (*arrow*), (**b**) severe swelling of ileocecal valve, and (**c**) mucosal enhancement of the appendix (*arrow*).

tact. Primary infection is usually asymptomatic, but as with other herpes viruses, CMV remains dormant in the host after infection. With increasing impairment of cell-mediated immunity, particularly with a CD4 lymphocyte count of less than 100 cells/mm³, viral reactivation may occur. CMV involves the colon more frequently than it does the small bowel. In contrast to the often subtle manifestations of CMV in other organ systems, the presenting symptoms of CMV colitis cause significant acute morbidity. Before diagnosis, most patients have persistent diarrhea, fever, weight loss, severe abdominal pain, and hematochezia. Prompt diagnosis and treatment are crucial to avoid future CMV recurrence (DIETERICH et al. 1991).

Since symptoms and radiographic features are nonspecific, total colonoscopy and biopsy are needed for definitive diagnosis (Fig. 24.7a). The diagnosis is suggested when CT shows heterogeneous, eccentric colonic wall thickening with inflammatory stranding in the perirectal and mesenteric fat, particularly if the thickening is associated with mural ulceration. Rectosigmoid colon and right colon are often involved (Fig. 24.7). Pathologically, the most prominent feature of colonic wall thickening is mural edema with ulceration. These changes are thought to be due to CMV invading endothelial cells resulting in severe occlusive vasculitis. This vasculitis may cause tissue edema and necrosis, with ulceration, hemorrhage, and perforation (MURRAY et al. 1995).

Pseudomembranous colitis

Pseudomembranous colitis can develop with use of prophylactic and broad-spectrum antibiotics, and a specific class of immunosuppressive agents, the toxic antibiotics such as actinomycin D. It is due to infection with *Clostridium difficile*, which produces an enterotoxin, and it is treated usually with vancomycin (KELLY et al. 1994). The plain radiographic findings include ileus, thumb printing, and a characteristic" transverse banding"that is due to thickening of the haustral folds. CT findings include diffuse bowel wall thickening, eccentric polypoid wall thickening, prominent haustral folds, pericolic inflammatory changes, and fluid collection (Fig. 24.8). Endoscopy can establish the diagnosis by demonstrating the characteristic adherent yellow plaque, typically in the rectosigmoid colon (Fig. 24.8c) (KAWAMOTO et al. 1999).

24.6.3
Acute GVHD

Acute GVHD is a disease process specific to patients who undergo BMT in which donor T lymphocytes

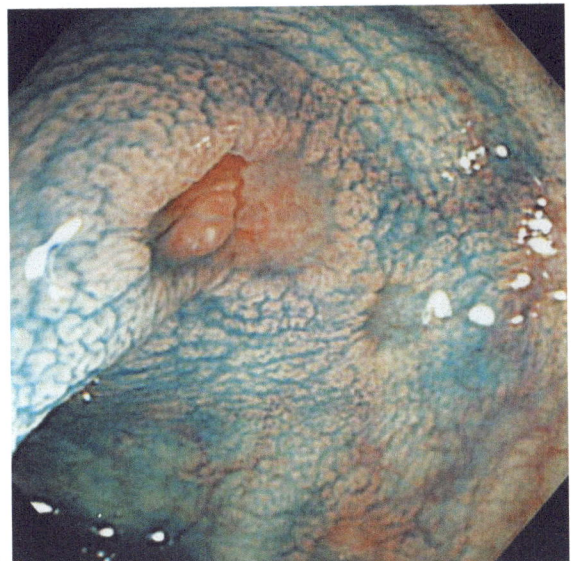

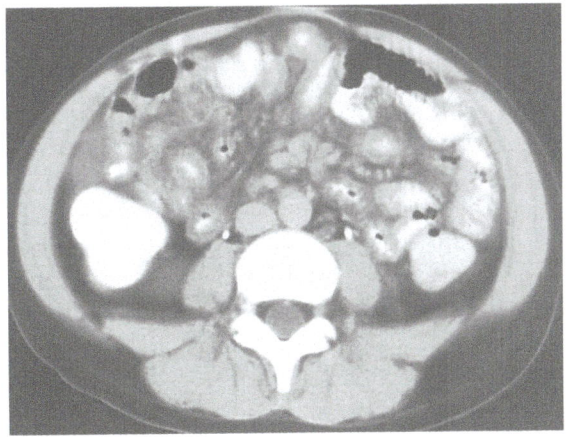

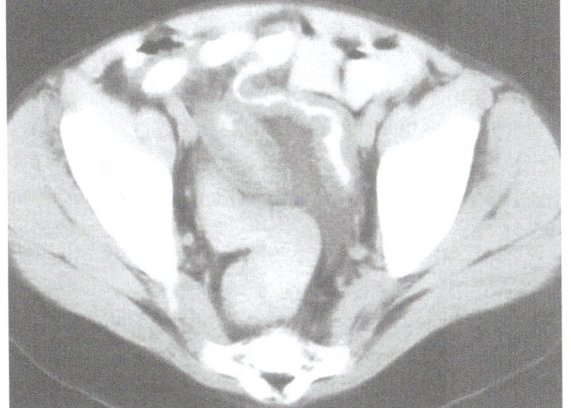

Fig. 24.7a–c. Cytomegalovirus enterocolitis in a 17-year-old boy who underwent chemotherapy for chronic myeloid leukemia. a Endoscopic view demonstrates typical punched-out ulcer indicating Cytomegalovirus colitis. Axial contrast-enhanced CT scans of the (b) abdomen and (c) pelvis demonstrate multiple thick-walled loops of the ileum and sigmoid colon and inflammatory stranding in the mesenteric fat. Ascitic fluid is also seen.

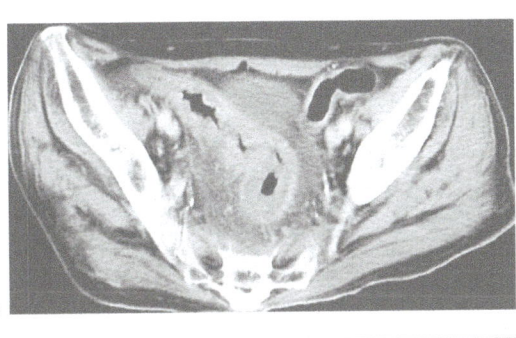

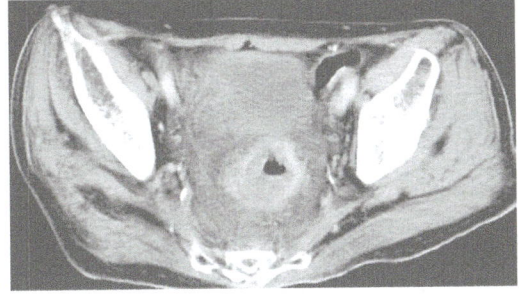

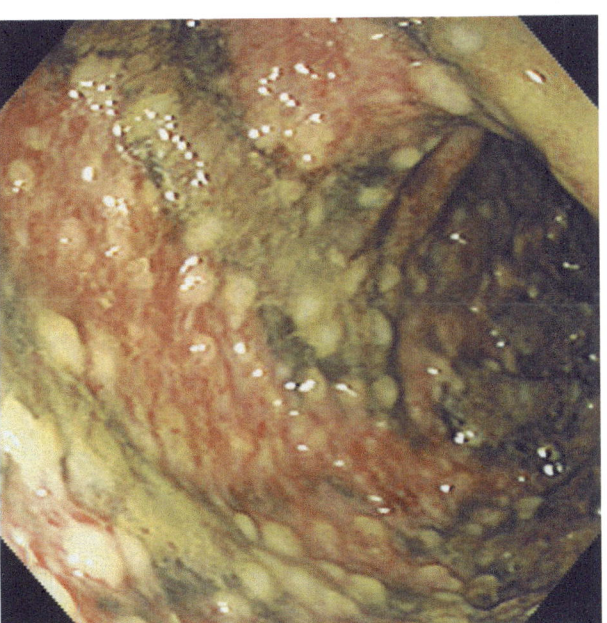

Fig. 24.8a–c. Pseudomembranous colitis following antibiotic therapy in a 68-year-old man with chronic myeloid leukemia. a, b Axial contrast-enhanced CT scans of the pelvis demonstrate circumferential thickening of the edematous wall of the rectosigmoid colon. The enhancement of the luminal surface indicates mucosal hyperemia. Ascites is also seen. c Endoscopic view shows characteristic yellow plaques representing pseudomembranous colitis.

cause selected epithelial damage of recipient target organs. Moderate to severe GVHD occurs in 30–50% of matched allogenic bone marrow recipients. The acute form occurs within the first 100 days after transplantation; the chronic form occurs more than 100 days after transplantation. The organ systems most commonly involved are the skin, liver, and gastrointestinal tract. A maculopapular rash is the most common and often the presenting finding. Hyperbilirubinemia and hepatic dysfunction occur secondary to damaged biliary epithelium. Involvement of the gastrointestinal tract usually appears after the skin rash and, rarely, is the only presenting manifestation. Intestinal symptoms include abdominal pain, diarrhea, anorexia, fever, nausea and vomiting, and, in severe case, intestinal hemorrhage (FERRARA and DEEG 1991). Gastrointestinal involvement has important prognostic and therapeutic implications. Accurate identification of gastrointestinal GVHD on CT scans as the probable source of sepsis obviates further diagnostic tests. Plain radiographic findings are non-specific (Fig. 24.9a). CT provides typical radiographic findings, including multiple, diffuse, fluid-filled, dilated loops of the bowel with a thin, central mucosal layer of bowel wall enhancement. A similar pattern of enhancement may be seen in the walls of the gallbladder and the urinary bladder as well (Fig. 24.9). Abnormal mucosal enhancement corresponds histologically to replacement of destroyed mucosa by a thin layer of highly vascular granulation tissue. Pericolic fat obliteration and ascites are sometimes seen (DONNELLY and MORRIS 1996). Gastric mucosa is usually preserved unless viral infection arises. Bowel wall thickening is sometimes absent. Radiographically such case may be difficult to differentiate from other viral colitis and accurate diagnosis might be obtained with endoscopy (Fig. 24.9e) and mucosal biopsy (JONES et al.1988; CRUZ-CORREA et al. 2002)

24.6.4
Chronic GVHD

Chronic GVHD involves the skin, liver, and gastrointestinal tract and may also produce long-term disability. Radiological findings of this form are reported as bowel stenosis, dilatation, and rupture; surgical resection may sometimes be necessary. No significant mucosal enhancement has been reported (PATZIK et al. 1991).

24.6.5
Other involvements

Other gastrointestinal abnormalities include pneumatosis intestinalis, hemorrhagic colitis (Fig. 24.10), adynamic ileus, and toxic megacolon caused by direct and indirect toxicity of the therapy (ROSENBERG and CARIDI 1983). The gastrointestinal tract is one of the common sites of recurrence or secondary malignancy. Lymphoma is a well known secondary malignancy. Lymphoma may be infiltrative, causing bowel wall thickening, or focal and manifested by mesenteric or bowel-wall mass.

24.7
Urogenital tract

Complications of the urogenital tract may also develop after aggressive chemotherapy and BMT. They include infection of the kidney (Fig. 24.11) and hemorrhagic cystitis. Hemorrhagic cystitis results from after administration of cyclophosphamide (Fig. 24.12) or ifosfamide (DAY and CARPENTER 1993). This adverse effect is related to dose and may occur hours to years after chemotherapy. Viral infection by adenovirus is the second most common cause of hemorrhagic cystitis and is typically seen in patients undergoing allogenic BMT. Abdominal US is considered an accurate investigative tool for this condition and reveals marked bladder wall thickening that represents mucosal edema. Intravesical blood clots from hemorrhagic cystitis can cause bladder outlet or urethral obstruction.

Other common complications include late renal dysfunction, a result of nephrotoxic effects of radiation and chemotherapy and after BMT, papillary necrosis, renal vein thrombosis, nephrolithiasis, and spontaneous subcapsular hematoma of the kidney (KASTE et al. 1999). Late renal dysfunction occurs in up to 20% of survivors of BMT and TBI is considered to be a major risk (COHEN et al. 1995).

Ovarian vein thrombosis (OVT) may develop in patients undergoing high-dose chemotherapy. As OVT is often asymptomatic, and thrombus may resolve without treatment, anticoagulation therapy may not be routinely necessary (JACOBY et al. 1990). Ovarian failure and a small uterus may occur in women who have received radiation therapy for childhood malignancy. Reduction in fertility is a known adverse consequence.

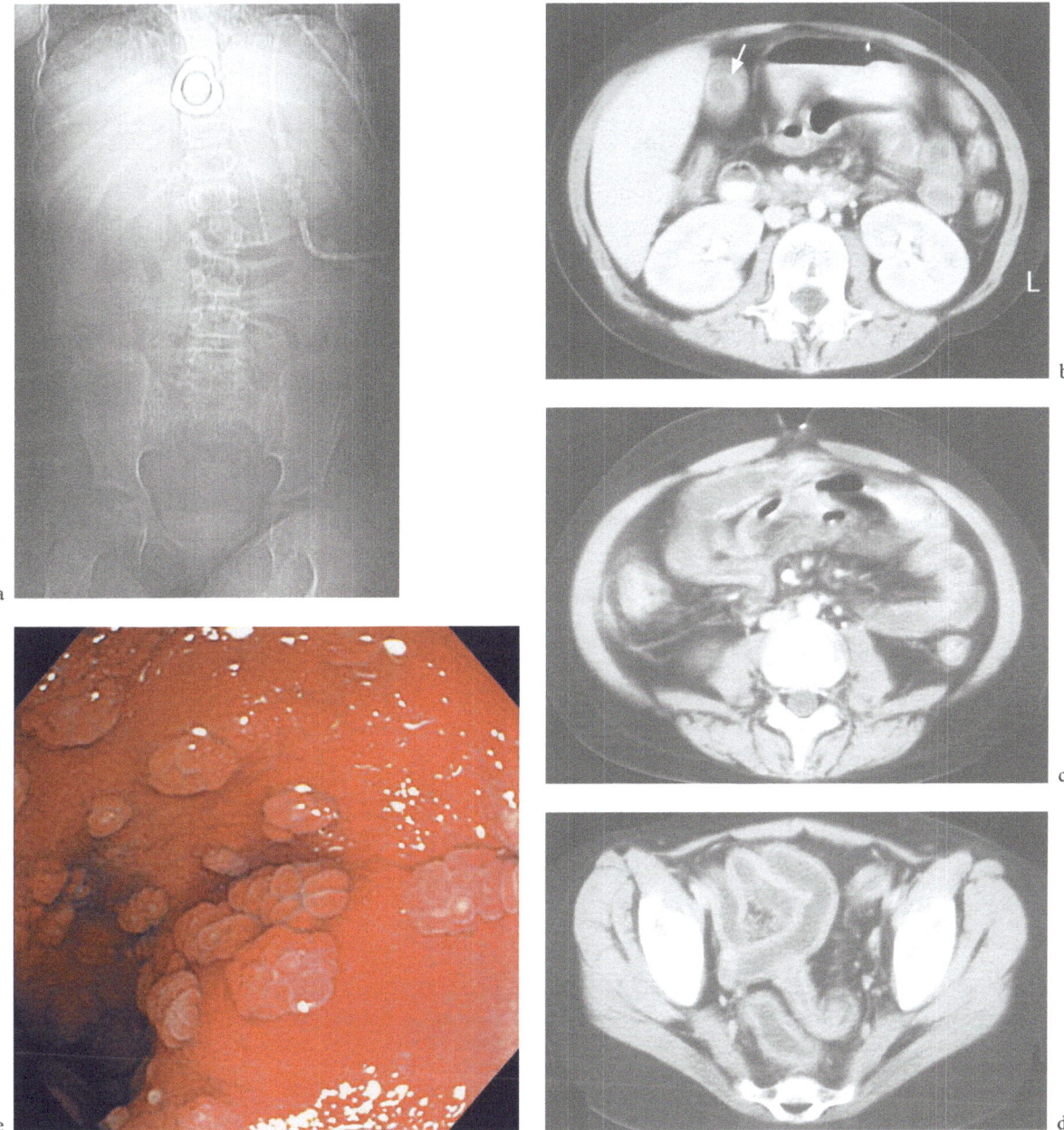

Fig. 24.9a–e. Acute graft-versus-host disease in an 8-year-old girl who underwent allogenic bone marrow transplantation for acute lymphocytic leukemia. **a** Anteroposterior plain radiograph of the abdomen demonstrates dilated small bowel loops in the mid-abdomen indicates non-specific enterocolitis. Axial contrast-enhanced CT scans of the (**b**) upper abdomen, (**c**) lower abdomen, and (**d**) pelvis show diffuse wall thickening, dilated bowel with enhanced thin mucosa from the duodenum to the rectum. The mesentery and pericolic fat are inflamed throughout. The mucosa of gallbladder is also enhanced (*arrow*). **e** Endoscopic view reveals loss of colonic mucosa. Remaining normal mucosa is patchily seen.

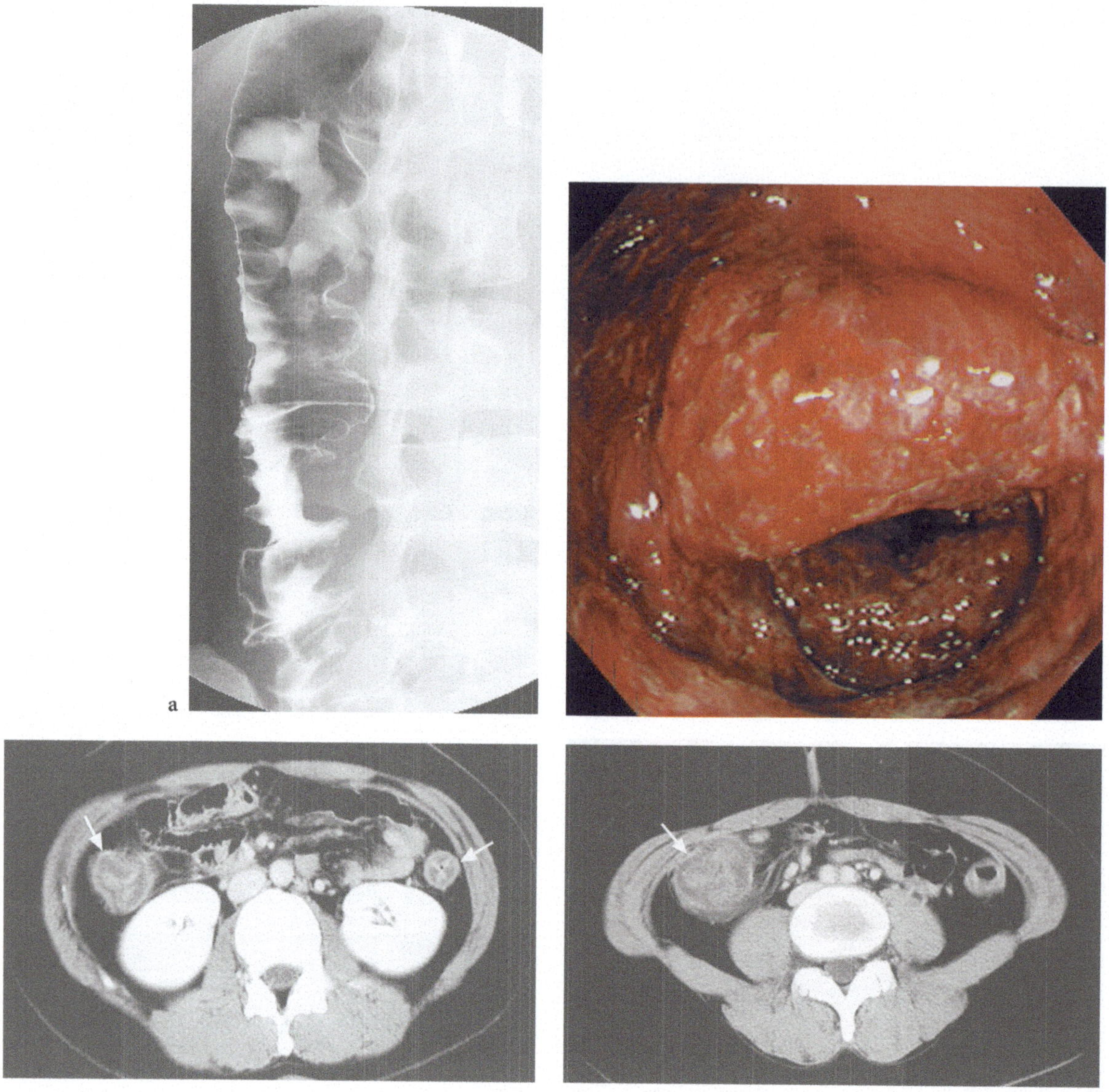

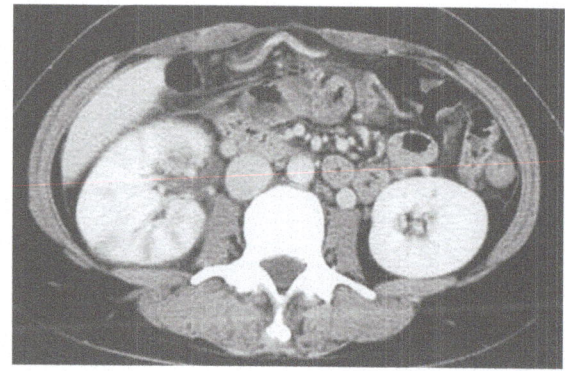

Fig. 24.10a–d. Hemorrhagic colitis in a 24-year-old woman treated with chemotherapy for non-Hodgkin lymphoma. **a** Barium enema view shows massive mucosal edema, the so-called "thumb printing" appearance. **b** Endoscopic view of the ascending colon shows marked edema, erythema, erosion, and facile hemorrhage. Lesions extend over a wide area from cecum to the sigmoid colon and there is no normal mucosal segment between the lesions. Axial contrast-enhanced CT scans of the (**c**) lower abdomen and (**d**) upper pelvis demonstrate massive colonic wall thickening with mucosal serosal enhancement (*arrows*). Ascending colon is predominantly involved. The mucosa of the terminal ileum is normal.

Fig. 24.11. Renal abscesses in a 40-year-old woman treated with chemotherapy for non-Hodgkin lymphoma. Axial contrast-enhanced CT scan of the abdomen shows multiple hypodense lesions within the enlarged right kidney. Causative organism was *Candida albicans*, proved by urine culture.

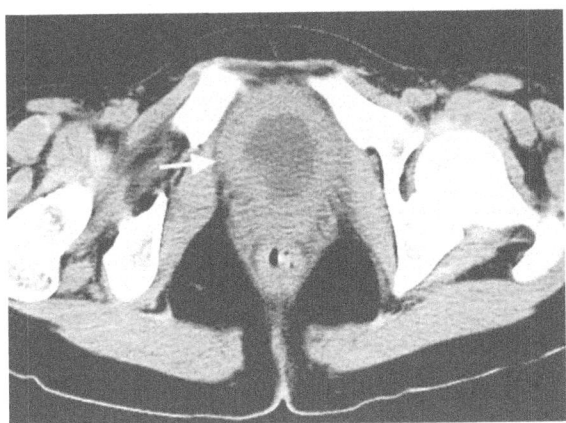

Fig. 24.12. Hemorrhagic cystitis in an 18-year-old girl developed immediately after administration of cyclophosphamide for acute lymphocytic leukemia. Axial unenhanced CT scan of the pelvis shows diffuse thickening of the bladder wall (*arrow*).

24.8
Conclusion

Abdominal effects of therapy in patients treated for hematological malignancies are becoming more common. Radiologists should be familiar with radiographic characteristics of these crucial complications. US is usually the first modality to be implemented, but CT is still considered the most useful for providing information to distinguish these complications from other conditions such as recurrence, and evaluating response to therapy.

References

Adams GW, Rauch RF, Kelvin FM, Silverman PM, Korobkin M (1985) CT detection of typhlitis. J Comput Assist Tomogr 9:363–365

Alexander JE, Williamson SL, Seibert JJ, Golladay ES, Jimenez JF (1988) The ultrasonographic diagnosis of typhlitis (neutropenic colitis). Pediatr Radiol 18:200–204

Barrett J (1991) Worldwide bone marrow transplantation in the last decade: new strategies in bone marrow transplantation. Wiely-Liss, New York, pp 1–6

Benya EC, Sivit CJ, Quinones RR (1993) Abdominal complications after bone marrow transplantation in children: sonographic and CT findings. AJR Am J Roentgenol 161:1023–1027

Brown BP, Abu-Yousef M, Farner R, LaBrecque D, Gingrich R (1990) Doppler sonography: a noninvasive method for evaluation of hepatic venocclusive disease. AJR Am J Roentgenol 154:721–724

Champlin RE, Gale RP (1984) The early complications of bone marrow transplantation. Semin Hematol 21:101–108

Cohen EP, Lawton CA, Moulder JE (1995) Bone marrow transplant nephropathy: radiation nephritis revisited. Nephron 70:217–222

Cruz-Correa M, Poonawala A, Abraham SC, Wu TT, Zahurak M, Vogelsang G, Kalloo AN, Lee LA (2002) Endoscopic findings predict the histologic diagnosis in gastrointestinal graft-versus-host disease. Endoscopy 34:808–813

Day DL, Carpenter BL (1993) Abdominal complications in pediatric bone marrow transplant recipients. Radiographics 13:1101–1112

Del Fava RL, Cronin TG Jr (1977) Typhlitis complicating leukemia in an adult: barium enema findings. AJR Am J Roentgenol 129:347–348

Dewar GJ, Lim CN, Michalyshyn B, Akabutu J (1981) Gastrointestinal complications in patients with acute and chronic leukemia. Can J Surg 24:67–71

Dieterich DT, Rahmin M (1991) Cytomegalovirus colitis in AIDS: presentation in 44 patients and a review of the literature. J Acquir Immune Defic Syndr 4 (Suppl 1):S29–35

Donnelly LF, Morris CL (1996) Acute graft-versus-host disease in children: abdominal CT findings. Radiology 199:265–268

Ferrara JL, Deeg HJ (1991) Graft-versus-host disease. N Engl J Med 324:667–674

Francis IR, Glazer GM (1982) Case report. Burkitt's lymphoma of the pancreas presenting as acute pancreatitis. J Comput Assist Tomogr 6:395–397

Frick MP, Maile CW, Crass JR, Goldberg ME, Delaney JP (1984) Computed tomography of neutropenic colitis. AJR Am J Roentgenol 143:763–765

Herbetko J, Grigg AP, Buckley AR, Phillips GL (1992) Veno-occlusive liver disease after bone marrow transplantation: findings at duplex sonography. AJR Am J Roentgenol 158:1001–1005

Hunter TB, Bjelland JC (1984) Gastrointestinal complications of leukemia and its treatment. AJR Am J Roentgenol 142:513–518

Jacoby WT, Cohan RH, Baker ME, Leder RA, Nadel SN, Dunnick NR (1990) Ovarian vein thrombosis in oncology patients: CT detection and clinical significance. AJR Am J Roentgenol 155:291–294

Jones B, Kramer SS, Saral R, Beschorner WE, Yolken RH, Townsend TR, Yeager AM, Lake A, Tutschka P, Santos GW (1988) Gastrointestinal inflammation after bone marrow transplantation: graft-versus-host disease or opportunistic infection? AJR Am J Roentgenol 150:277–281

Kaste SC, Rodriguez-Galindo C, Furman WL (1999) Imaging pediatric oncologic emergencies of the abdomen. AJR Am J Roentgenol. 173:729–736

Kawamoto S, Horton KM, Fishman EK (1999) Pseudomembranous colitis: spectrum of imaging findings with clinical and pathologic correlation. Radiographics 19:887–897

Kelly CP, Pothoulakis C, LaMont JT (1994) Clostridium difficile colitis. N Engl J Med 330:257–262

McDonald GB, Shulman HM, Sullivan KM, Spencer GD (1986) Intestinal and hepatic complications of human bone marrow transplantation. Part I. Gastroenterology 90:460–477

Moir DH, Bale PM (1976) Necropsy findings in childhood leukaemia, emphasizing neutropenic enterocolitis and cerebral calcification. Pathology 8:247–258

Murray JG, Evans SJ, Jeffrey PB, Halvorsen RA (1995) Cyto-megalovirus colitis in AIDS: CT features. AJR Am J Roent-genol 165:67–71

Myerowitz RL, Pazin GJ, Allen CM (1977) Disseminated can-didiasis. Changes in incidence, underlying diseases, and pathology. Am J Clin Pathol 68:29–38

Niccolini DG, Graham JH, Banks PA (1976) Tumor-induced acute pancreatitis. Gastroenterology 71:142–145

Pastakia B, Shawker TH, Thaler M, O'Leary T, Pizzo PA (1988) Hepatosplenic candidiasis: wheels within wheels. Radiol-ogy 166:417–421

Patzik SB, Smith C, Kubicka RA, Kaizer H (1991) Bone marrow transplantation: clinical and radiologic aspects. Radiographics 11:601–610

Prolla JC, Kirsner JB (1964) The gastrointestinal lesions and complication of the leukemias. Ann Intern Med 61: 1084–1103

Rosenberg RF, Caridi JG (1983) Vincristine-induced megaco-lon. Gastrointest Radiol 8:71–73

Shapiro RS, McClain K, Frizzera G, Gajl-Peczalska KJ, Kersey JH, Blazar BR, Arthur DC, Patton DF, Greenberg JS, Burke B (1988) Epstein-Barr virus associated B cell lymphoprolif-erative disorders following bone marrow transplantation. Blood 71:1234–1243

Shirkhoda A (1987) CT findings in hepatosplenic and renal candidiasis. J Comput Assist Tomogr 11:795–798

Spiegel RJ, Magrath IT (1979) Tumor lysis pancreatitis. Med Pediatr Oncol 7:169–172

Sullivan KM, Deeg HJ, Sanders JE, Shulman HM, Witherspoon RP, Doney K, Appelbaum FR, Schubert MM, Stewart P, Springmeyer S (1984) Late complications after marrow transplantation. Semin Hematol 21:53–63

Underwood TW, Frye CB (1993) Drug-induced pancreatitis. Clin Pharm 12:440–448

Wagner ML, Rosenberg HS, Fernbach DJ, Singleton EB (1970) Typhlitis: a complication of leukemia in childhood. Am J Roentgenol Radium Ther Nucl Med 109:341–350

Wall SD, Jones B (1992) Gastrointestinal tract in the immu-nocompromised host: opportunistic infections and other complications. Radiology 185:327–335

Winton PR, Gwynn AM, Roberts JC, Thomas L (1975) Leuke-mia and the bowel. Med J Aust 131:723–724

25 Musculoskeletal Effects of Therapy in Patients Treated for Hematological Malignancies

Soheil L. Hanna and Barry D. Fletcher

CONTENTS

25.1 Introduction

Considerable progress has been made in therapy for hematological malignancies over the past few decades, particularly for pediatric patients (Bleyer 1990). The increasing number of childhood cancer survivors underscores the need to screen for late adverse effects of therapy that could affect up to one-half of the survivors (Meadows and Hobbie 1986), and the need for radiologists to become familiar with them. The effects of radiation therapy on the musculoskeletal system resulting from interrupted bone growth surface after a latent period are typically permanent and visible radiographically. Musculoskeletal sequelae of chemotherapy, while seemingly less obvious, also exist. Recent studies have dispelled the notion that there are few late effects associated with the prolonged use of anticancer drugs (Fauroux et al. 1996; Gardner 1999; Hockman et al. 1999).

This chapter focuses on the effects of treatment of pediatric and adult hematologic malignancies on bone, bone marrow, and soft tissue with emphasis on plain radiographic and MR imaging findings following radiation therapy, chemotherapy, bone marrow transplantation and biologic response modifiers. Differences in susceptibility between pediatric and adult patients are emphasized.

Soheil L. Hanna, MD
Associate Clinical Professor, Department of Radiology, Musculoskeletal Division, Emory University/The Emory Clinic and Institiue of Orthopedic Imaging, Northside Hospital, 1000 Johnson Ferry Rd, Atlanta, GA 30342, USA
Barry D. Fletcher, MD, CM
Professor of Radiology, Clinical Associate, Department of Radiology, Duke University Medical Center, Box 3808 Med Center, Durham, NC 27710, USA

25.2
Biologic Changes Associated with Therapeutic Modalities

25.2.1
Radiation Therapy

Modern advances in molecular biology have led to improved understanding of the body's response to injury by irradiation. The disclosure that the acute release and up-regulation of several pro-inflammatory cytokines such as interleukin 1 beta (Il1 β) and Il6 contribute to radiation-induced vasculitis and inflammation has provided insight into the mechanism of radiosensitivity of both tumors and normal tissues (FAJARDO et al. 2002; MIZUTANI et al. 2002; RUBIN et al. 1995; VAN DER MEEREN et al. 2001). Also, the release of anti-inflammatory cytokines such as Il4 plays an important regulatory role in post radiation recovery by down-regulating the radiation-induced production of mediators of inflammation (MIZUTANI et al. 2002; VAN DER MEEREN et al. 2001).

Radiation-induced injuries or changes can generally be described as a combination of parenchymal cellular hypoplasia and alterations in the fine vasculature and fibroconnective tissues. Initial recovery at the tissue level is predominantly due to parenchymal cellular repopulation, whereas progressive damage is related to arteriocapillary fibrosis which dominates late irreparable injury and increases the extent of parenchymal cellular depletion (WITHERS and McBRIDE 1998).

Limitations of radiation therapy have been defined according to the tolerance doses for various organs and tissues. The minimal tolerance dose (TD5/5) and the maximal tissue tolerance dose (TD50/5) refer to severe to life-threatening complications occurring in 5 and 50%, respectively, of patients within 5 years of receiving therapeutic radiation. With multimodality treatment, however, additional factors such as chemotherapy or biologic response modifiers have a marked impact on radiosensitivity and toxicity. Thus, the applicability of the previously defined radiation tolerance doses (TD5 and TD50) has changed, and supposedly safe radiation doses can lead to severe late effects. In addition to total dose, irradiated volume, and fractionation including radiation fraction dose, the interval between fractions and the overall duration of therapy are important factors in determining early and late effects (HENDRY et al. 1998), but are well beyond the scope of this chapter.

25.2.2
Chemotherapy

The late effects of chemotherapy are thought to result predominantly from parenchymal cellular depletion with sparing of the microcirculation and fibroconnective tissue stroma (DRYER et al. 2002). Since most chemotherapeutic agents are cell cycle-dependent, the severity of acute toxicities varies according to the proliferation kinetics of individual cell populations. For example, tissues like bone marrow with high cell turnover rates are most susceptible. The least susceptible cells are those that either do not replicate or replicate slowly, such as muscle cells and connective tissue. Exceptions to this correlation include bone injury associated with methotrexate and corticosteroids. Furthermore, injured tissues with low repair potential, such as bone, develop long-lasting or permanent deficits (DRYER et al. 2002). Although children have higher thresholds for acute toxicity enabling them to receive greater doses or dose intensities of most chemotherapeutic agents than adults, growing children are more vulnerable to the delayed adverse musculoskeletal sequelae of cancer therapy.

25.2.3
Combined Radiation and Chemotherapy

Combining radiation and chemotherapy leads to a different clinical-pathological course than either treatment alone. The introduction of chemotherapy in a patient initially treated with radiotherapy can lead to the expression of subclinical damage. Chemotherapy may result in increased morbidity or mortality due to an already apparent post radiation injury. Similar consequences may occur if chemotherapy preceded radiation therapy. Certainly, associated infection or stress can exacerbate the injury (RUBIN et al. 2002).

Chemotherapy acts predominantly on the cellular parenchymal component, whereas radiation acts on the microcirculatory system as well as parenchymal cells of tissues and organs. In rapid renewal systems, where the same stem cell population is affected by both modes, acute toxicity may be reduced by applying chemotherapy and radiation therapy sequentially. In slow renewal tissues, different populations in the same organ system are targeted, which results in an additive effect, particularly when treatments are administered concurrently. The widespread use of drugs is the most common factor altering the tolerance doses of normal tissues (KLEINBERG et al. 1999; TORDIGLIONE et al. 1998). Proliferating tissues are more vulnerable in children than in adults, in whom many normal organs are in a mature steady state with slow cell renewal kinetics (RUBIN et al. 2002).

Clinicians need to be aware of late-effect syndromes secondary to all modes of cancer therapy to avoid confusion with recurrent or metastatic disease. Late-effect syndromes occur within a different time frame from those of tumor progression. Late effect normal tissue (LENT) syndromes at each organ site are predictable events that are expressed in a recognizable biological and temporal fashion (HALL 1994).

25.2.4
Antiangiogenic Agents

Tumor angiogenesis has been increasingly recognized as an important factor in the pathogenesis of hematological malignancies. Recently, thalidomide has been shown to possess antiangiogenic potential in addition to a broad spectrum of properties including immunomodulatory and anti-inflammatory actions. This agent also acts directly on tumor cells and their microenvironment (AMATO 2002; FIEDLER et al. 2001; RAJE and ANDERSON 2002). Thalidomide is being studied for the treatment of hematological cancers including multiple myeloma and myelodysplasia, and solid tumors such as lung, breast, renal, and colon cancer (RAJE and ANDERSON 2002). Recent clinical trials of antiangiogenic therapy with thalidomide demonstrated beneficial activity in a group of patients with relapsed refractory myeloma (RAJE and ANDERSON 2002; RAJKUMAR 2001).

25.2.5
Biologic Response Modifiers

Tumor regression can be achieved by employing prothrombotic response markers to obliterate the tumor vasculature. Thus, these modifiers contribute to antiangiogenesis. Ionizing radiation activates the inflammatory cascade and increases the procoagulative state within blood vessels of both tumors and normal tissues (FAJARDO et al. 2002). Proinflammatory and prothrombotic biological response modifiers given concurrently with ionizing radiation activate homeostatic responses in the endothelium and enhance thrombosis and vasculitis of irradiated

tumor blood vessels. These mechanisms contribute to tumor necrosis by enabling the obliteration of tumor vasculature (HALLAHAN et al. 1999).

Hematopoietic growth factors, such as granulocyte-colony stimulating factor (G-CSF), can stimulate hematopoiesis and marrow recovery in many clinical settings, thus decreasing treatment-related complications and/or allowing the use of more intensive chemotherapy (GROOPMAN et al. 1989; LIESCHKE and BURGESS 1992). G-CSF is typically administered over a period of 10–14 days after each cycle of chemotherapy and is often accompanied by a rapid rise in peripheral neutrophils – sometimes to nearly 10 times their baseline levels (LIESCHKE and BURGESS 1992).

25.2.6
Bone Marrow Transplantation

Bone marrow transplantation is widely used in the treatment of leukemia, recurrent Hodgkin disease and non-Hodgkin lymphoma (ARMITAGE 1994; WEISDORF 1987). The procedure consists of intravenous infusion of hematopoietic progenitor cells from the patient's own stored marrow (autologous transplant) or from donor marrow (allogeneic transplant). Pretransplant treatment involves high-dose, myeloablative chemotherapy and for allogeneic and certain autologous transplants, total body irradiation (TBI), typically 12–15 Gy on a fractionated schedule. The goal of these regimens is to destroy residual malignant cells, provide space for new marrow growth, and prevent rejection of allografts. Marrow repopulation is evaluated by monitoring granulocytes and platelets in the peripheral blood.

25.3
Osseous Effects of Radiation Therapy

25.3.1
Radiation-Induced Abnormalities of Bone Growth

The skeleton is particularly sensitive to radiation effects during the periods of most active growth in early childhood and puberty (PROBERT and PARKER 1975). Therapeutic doses of radiation affect the growing ends of bones by interfering with chondrogenesis and reabsorption of calcified cartilage and bone (RUBIN et al. 1959). Growth retardation was documented in animal experiments performed in the 1940s following doses of at least 600 cGy to the epiphysis whereas, complete cessation of growth ensued following doses of 1200 cGy (NEUHAUSER 1952; RISEBOROUGH 1976). Within a year after therapy, growth arrest lines paralleling the end plates of irradiated vertebrae become apparent and the vertebrae may appear bulbous (BERDON et al. 1965). Later manifestations include decreased height of the irradiated vertebral bodies, with irregular scalloping of the end plates and anterior beaking.

Decreased linear growth is a common problem in children with cancer. While catch-up growth may occur, in some instances short stature is permanent and even progressive. Severe growth retardation, defined as standing height below the fifth percentile, has been observed in 10% to 15% of patients treated with antileukemic regimens (OLIFF et al. 1979; ROBISON et al. 1985). However, comparison of the growth curves of children with ALL treated with various forms of CNS prophylaxis has identified whole brain irradiation as the principal cause of short stature (OLIFF et al. 1979; WELLS et al. 1983).

The mechanism by which cranial irradiation induces short stature is not clear. Doses as low as 2,400 cGy have caused growth hormone deficiency, as suggested by the blunting of spontaneous growth hormone pulses, low plasma insulin-like growth factor-1 (somatomedin C) levels and blunted growth hormone responses to different provocative stimuli (BLATT et al. 1984; DICKINSON et al. 1978; OBERFIELD et al. 1986; ROMSHE et al. 1984; SHALET et al. 1976; SHALET et al. 1979). Early onset of puberty in girls with ALL may contribute to loss of eventual final height. Direct inhibition of vertebral growth by spinal irradiation does contribute to short stature and most commonly follows doses in excess of 3,500 cGy typical of brain tumor patients (BLOOM et al. 1969). Among children who had ALL and received 1,200 cGy of abdominal irradiation in addition to 1,800 to 2,400 cGy of craniospinal irradiation, almost 30% had standing heights less than the fifth percentile (ROBISON et al. 1985). This however, may also have been due to irradiation of the gonads or thyroid and/or scatter radiation of the femoral heads.

As many as 40% of long-term survivors of HD and Wilms tumor who received lower doses of 1,000 to 2,500 cGy, although not necessarily short, have reduced sitting heights (BLOOM et al. 1969; OBERFIELD et al. 1986). Thoracoabdominal preparatory radiation for total lymphoid irradiation also has been associated with short stature. In contrast to radiation, chemotherapy-induced growth retardation is usually temporary, and patients' growth typi-

cally catches up with their peers. Chemotherapeutic agents, such as methotrexate and high-dose corticosteroids, appear to mediate this effect by direct inhibition on bone growth.

Current approaches to pediatric cancer therapy attempt to spare adverse effects on growth. HD protocols for smaller children have successfully limited radiation doses by the addition of chemotherapy. Current leukemia protocols promote the use of intrathecal chemotherapy, high-dose methotrexate, high-dose cytosine arabinoside or other CNS-active systemic chemotherapy in lieu of radiation for CNS prophylaxis. However, craniospinal irradiation may be used in patients at high risk for CNS relapse. Also, the long-term effect on growth of TBI used as a conditioning regimen in BMT appears to decrease with the use of fractionated doses (COHEN et al. 1999).

Scoliosis, a delayed consequence of radiotherapy to a segment of the spinal column, is seen almost exclusively in patients with solid tumors. Scoliosis results from asymmetric vertebral development and decreased height on the irradiated side in addition to muscle atrophy and tissue fibrosis that "act as a bow string across the vertebrae" (Fig. 25.1) (RISEBOROUGH et al. 1976). Patients with hematological malignancies requiring radiation therapy as in total nodal irradiation (TNI) for HD undergo symmetric irradiation of the entire spine, thus limiting the risk of scoliosis. Therapy-induced osteoporosis is another factor that may contribute to scoliosis (MEHLMAN et al. 1999). Kyphosis occurs less frequently and is rare in the absence of scoliosis.

The inclusion of a long bone growth plate in the radiation field results in growth plate abnormalities including metaphyseal fraying and epiphyseal widening resembling rickets (DESMET et al. 1976). These effects are typically observed within one year. If the hip was included in an asymmetric radiation field, underdevelopment will occur and limb length discrepancies may result (IRWIN et al. 1993; MULLEN et al. 1995). Shortening of the clavicles, decrease in interclavicular distance and superior rib hypoplasia are sequelae of mantle irradiation given at a young age for HD.

Slipped femoral capital epiphysis (SFCE), as a sequel to childhood irradiation for malignant tumors including HD, has been documented and results from radiation injury to the proximal femoral growth apparatus combined with weight-bearing stress (DICKERMAN et al. 1979; LIBSHITZ and EDEIKEN 1981; WOLF et al. 1977). The diagnosis is generally made 1–8 years after treatment. SFCE can occur after relatively low radiation doses; we

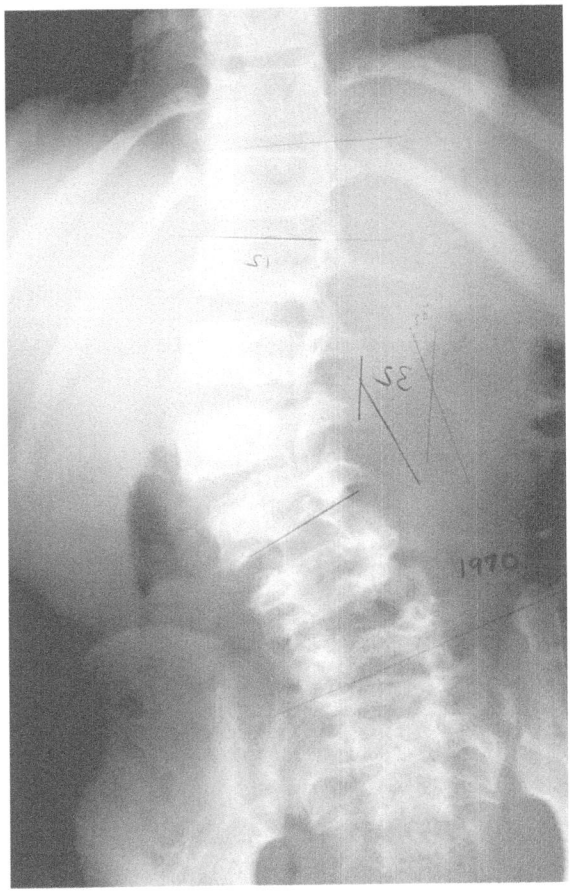

Fig. 25.1. Lumbar scoliosis in an 8-year-old boy who received radiation therapy of the left abdomen. Anteroposterior radiograph of the spine demonstrates lumbar dextroscoliosis as a delayed consequence of prior irradiation of the left abdomen. *(Image courtesy of Dr. T. Hudson)*

mon. Post radiation atrophic changes of bone are the result of combined cellular and vascular damage. Damaged osteoblasts result in decreased matrix production which is manifested radiographically as localized osteopenia (ERGUN and HOWLAND 1980). Osteopenia however, is late in appearing, mainly because of the relative insensitivity of radiographs in detecting demineralization. Osteoporosis and osteopenia, as documented by quantitative computed tomographic scans in survivors of childhood acute lymphoblastic leukemia, may be related more to prior craniospinal irradiation than to the type of chemotherapy (GILSANZ et al. 1990; KASTE et al. 1999; KASTE et al. 2001). Osteopenia may be even severe enough to cause spontaneous fractures in patients who received cranial irradiation in doses less than 2,500 cGy, but may go undetected by plain radiographs. Similarly, post radiation pelvic insufficiency fractures, while infrequent, may be undetected, particularly in post menopausal women (MUMBER et al. 1997). While subsequent delayed healing of post radiation insufficiency fractures is typical, non-union may occasionally ensue (Figs. 25.3, 25.4) (ALTMAN and BAILEY 1996).

observed SFCE in a patient who had undergone TBI with 1,200 cGy 9 years earlier, prior to allogeneic bone marrow transplantation at age 8 months (Fig. 25.2) (FLETCHER et al. 1994; FLETCHER 1997). Radiation-induced slippage of the humeral head has been reported less frequently, possibly because the shoulder is subjected to less stress than the hip (EDEIKEN et al. 1982).

25.3.2
Radiation-Induced Osteopenia

Osteoporosis and osteopenia have been related to radiotherapy and to steroid administration (TEFFT et al. 1976). The primary effect of radiation damage to bone is atrophy while true necrosis of bone is uncom-

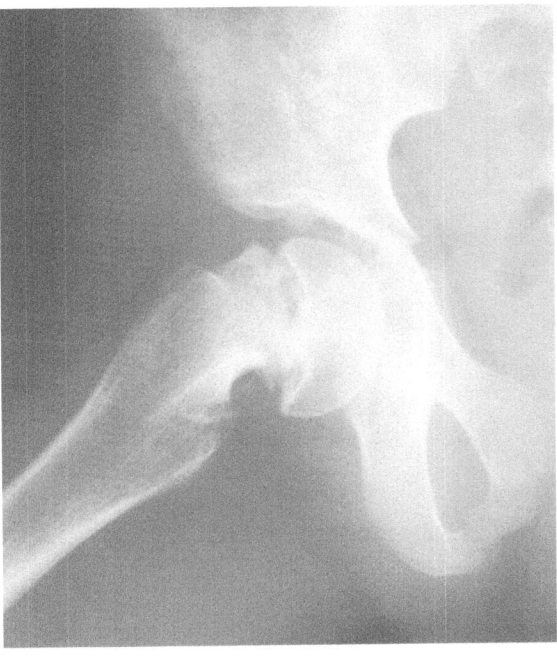

Fig. 25.2. Slipped femoral capital epiphysis in a 9-year-old girl who received 1,200 cGy total body irradiation before allogeneic bone marrow transplantation at the age of 8 months. Anteroposterior radiograph of the right hip shows slipped femoral capital epiphysis. (With permission from [FLETCHER et al. 1994])

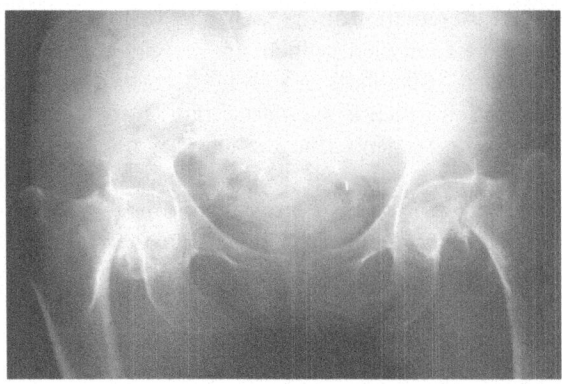

Fig. 25.3. Bilateral femoral neck insufficiency fractures in a 58-year-old man who received 4,500 cGy pelvic irradiation. Anteroposterior radiograph of the pelvis demonstrates bilateral femoral neck insufficiency fractures with non-union.

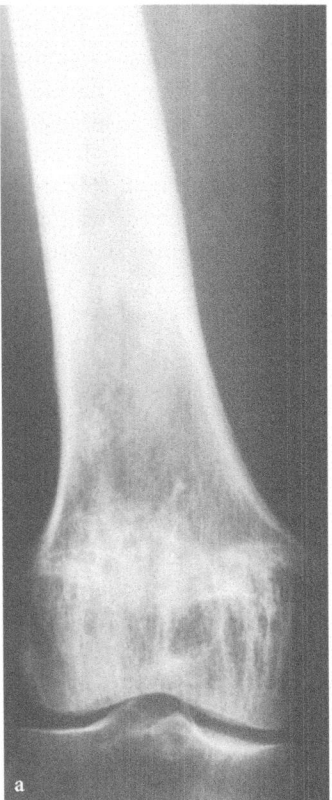
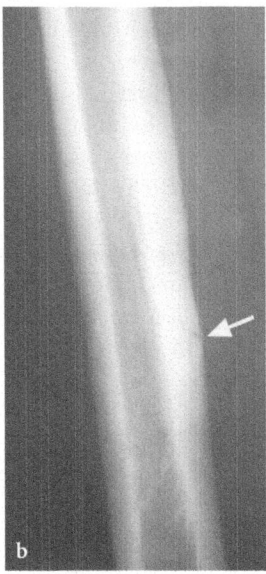
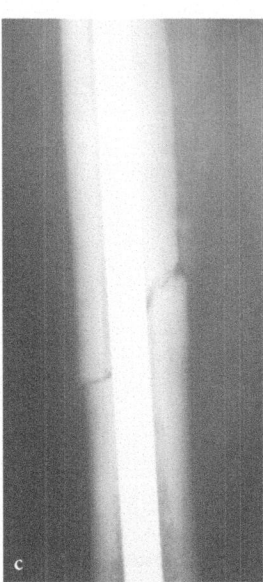

Fig. 25.4a–c. Insufficiency fracture in a 55-year-old man who received radiation therapy for non-Hodgkin lymphoma of the distal femoral shaft. **a** Anteroposterior radiograph of the distal third of the right femoral shaft shows a mottled, predominantly sclerotic process consistent with non-Hodgkin lymphoma. **b** Seven years post irradiation, the femur demonstrates relative osteopenia of the mid femoral shaft with focal, linear medial cortical lucency (*arrow*) consistent with an impending insufficiency fracture. **c** Fifteen months later, there was persistent non-union despite placement of an intramedullary rod. *(Image courtesy of Dr. T. Hudson)*

25.3.3
Radiation-Induced Osteitis

Radiation osteitis is also an atrophic change thought to result from injury to osteoblasts, complicated by late vascular changes, rather than true necrosis (DALINKA and MAZZEO 1985; FLETCHER 1997; HOWLAND et al. 1975). The severity of osteitis appears to be dose-related. On plain radiographs, the involved bone appears osteopenic, with coarse trabeculae and multiple foci of sclerosis (Fig. 25.5).

Pathologic fractures have been reported in more than 20% of these patients (BRAGG et al. 1970). The differential diagnosis in childhood cancer survivors with these radiographic findings includes osteomyelitis, recurrent primary disease, and radiation-induced sarcoma (BRAGG et al. 1970). Radiation osteitis is usually diagnosed within 2–3 years after therapy – very early compared with the latent period of approximately 10 years that precedes most radiation-related second malignancies (LIBSHITZ 1994). Also, unlike tumors, uncomplicated osteitis is not

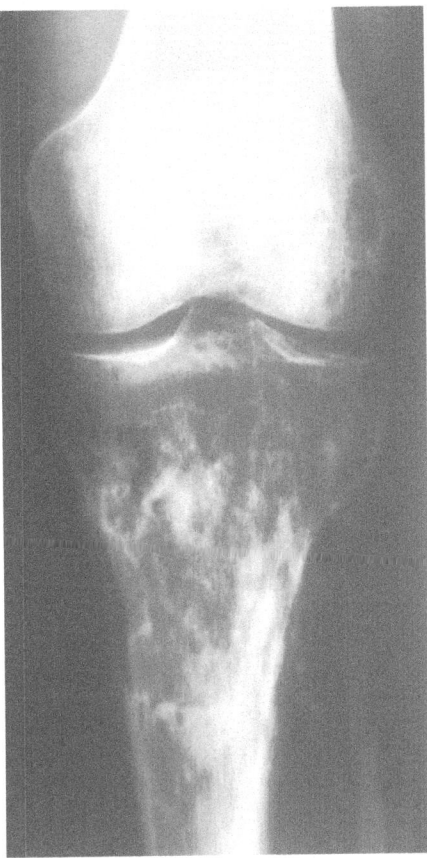

Fig. 25.5. Radiation necrosis in a 66-year-old man 7 months post 4,000 cGy irradiation of a painful solitary plasmacytoma of the tibia. Anteroposterior radiograph of the tibia shows aggressive-appearing mixed lytic/sclerotic process which was histologically confirmed to represent radiation necrosis.

accompanied by a soft tissue mass, a feature that is readily displayed by MR imaging. Subperiosteal abscesses and other features of osteomyelitis are absent. Biopsy should be avoided if possible because of the risk of infection or necrosis (HOWLAND et al. 1975); however, it may be required for definitive diagnosis, especially if imaging studies cannot exclude the possibility of a second malignancy.

25.3.4
Radiation-Induced Osteonecrosis

Clinically significant osteonecrosis presenting as pain has been described in adults and adolescents with HD and NHL, with an incidence of about 3% (TIMOTHY and TUCKER 1978). In the NHL patients, the femoral heads were most commonly affected but osteonecrosis has been described in all locations. It may be multifo-

cal and may be accompanied by SFCE. Osteonecrosis has also been described in patients treated for acute leukemia (BÖMELBURG et al. 1989; FLETCHER 1997; MURPHY and GREENBERG 1990; PIETERS et al. 1987; PRINDULL et al. 1982). It may rarely precede therapy and may be a result of the malignancy itself, presumably due to vascular compromise associated with replacement of normal marrow with leukemic cells (PIETERS et al. 1987). More commonly, it has been attributed to the direct effects of radiotherapy or the systemic effects of corticosteroids administered along with cytotoxic drugs. Cases of both unilateral and bilateral avascular necrosis have been reported 1–13 years after radiation therapy in doses of 30–40 Gy (Fig. 25.6) (LIBSHITZ and EDEIKEN 1981).

The features of osteonecrosis are well recognized by imaging, particularly MR imaging which is a more sensitive diagnostic test than radiography. These include an often asymptomatic infarction of trabecular bone in the medullary cavity and infarction of the subchondral cortex, a painful lesion with significant clinical consequences (MANKIN 1992). The latter process most frequently involves the humeral and femoral heads and distal femoral condyles. Standard MR imaging sequences typically reveal homogeneous regions of decreased signal intensity or well-developed necrotic lesions comprising bands or rings of low signal intensity with higher signal intensity centrally (TOTTY et al. 1984).

25.3.5
Radiation-Induced Osteochondromas

Osteochondromas are common changes after irradiation. Their incidence can be as high as 12% in survivors of childhood cancers treated with irradiation as opposed to 1–2% in the general population (LIBSHITZ and COHEN 1982). Osteochondromas secondary to radiation injury, result from disturbance of orderly chondrogenesis and abnormal endochondral bone growth leading to recapitulation of the physis in an abnormal location and direction (COLE and DARTE 1963). In one study, osteochondromas were seen in 6% of childhood cancer survivors who received 1500 cGy or more of external beam supervoltage radiation therapy between 8 months and 11.5 years of age prior to closure of the epiphysis (Fig. 25.7) (JAFFE et al. 1983). This lesion can occur in almost any irradiated skeletal site and has also been observed in patients who received TBI prior to BMT at a young age (Fig. 25.8) (FLETCHER et al. 1994; FLETCHER 1997).

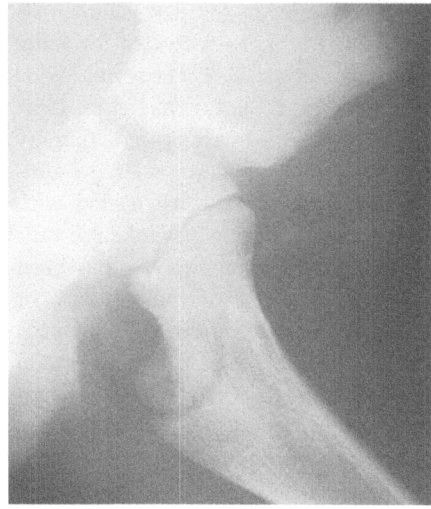
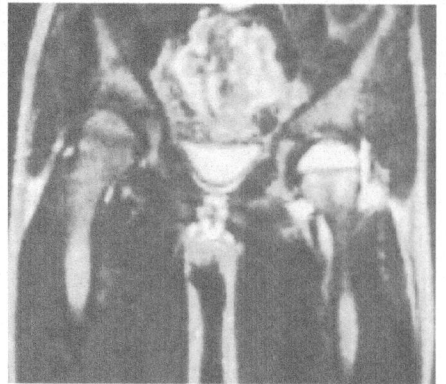
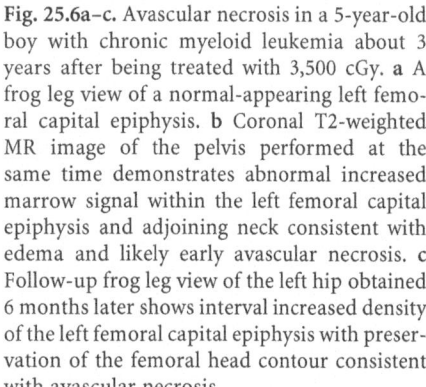

Fig. 25.6a–c. Avascular necrosis in a 5-year-old boy with chronic myeloid leukemia about 3 years after being treated with 3,500 cGy. **a** A frog leg view of a normal-appearing left femoral capital epiphysis. **b** Coronal T2-weighted MR image of the pelvis performed at the same time demonstrates abnormal increased marrow signal within the left femoral capital epiphysis and adjoining neck consistent with edema and likely early avascular necrosis. **c** Follow-up frog leg view of the left hip obtained 6 months later shows interval increased density of the left femoral capital epiphysis with preservation of the femoral head contour consistent with avascular necrosis.

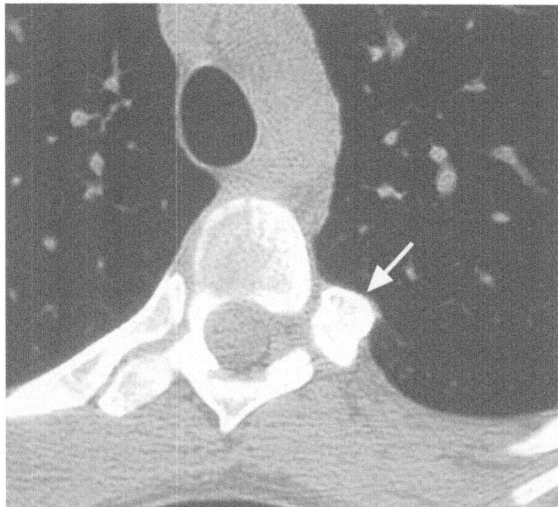
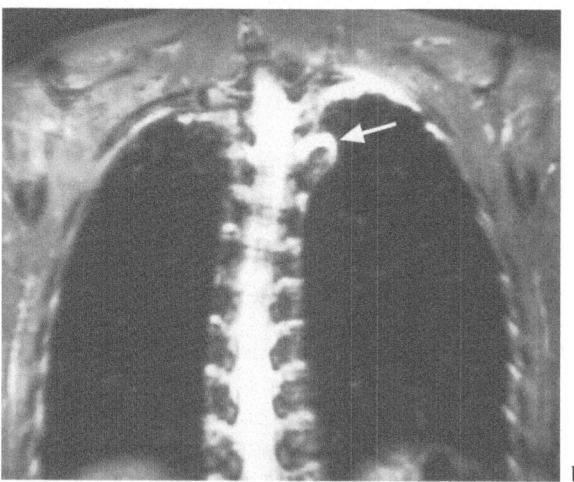

Fig. 25.7a,b. Osteochondroma in a 15-year-old girl with Hodgkin disease treated with mediastinal irradiation 7 years earlier. **a** Axial CT scan and (**b**) coronal T2-weighted MR image of the thorax demonstrate an osteochondroma arising from the most posterior medial aspect of the left third rib (*arrow*). Note intense signal of cartilaginous cap in (**b**).

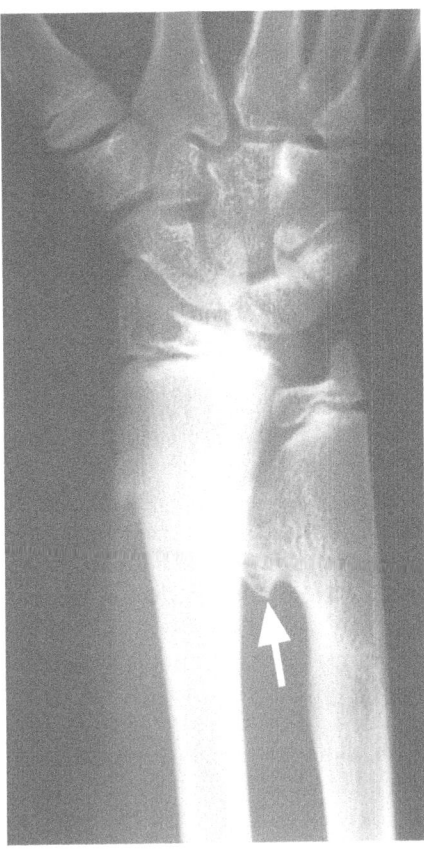

Fig. 25.8. Osteochondroma in an 11-year-old boy treated with total-body irradiation prior to bone marrow transplantation at age 22 months. Posteroanterior radiograph of the wrist shows a large osteochondroma arising from the distal ulnar diametaphysis (*arrow*).

25.4
Osseous Effects of Chemotherapy

25.4.1
Methotrexate-Induced Osteopathy

The routine use of multiple chemotherapeutic agents makes it difficult to accurately determine the adverse effects of cytotoxic drugs. Methotrexate, a folic acid antagonist commonly used to treat a variety of childhood cancers including leukemia, is known to interfere with skeletal growth (O'REGAN et al. 1973; RAGAB et al. 1969; STANISAVLJEVIC and BABCOCK 1977). Using animal models, methotrexate has been shown to decrease cancellous bone volume, cancellous bone formation, and osteoblast activity, while increasing osteoclast activity (TOTTY et al. 1984). Methotrexate-induced bone damage occurs more commonly in the lower extremities, likely due to

weight bearing (ECKLUND et al. 1997; FLETCHER 1997; WHEELER et al. 1995). The radiologic manifestations of skeletal abnormalities associated with long-term methotrexate therapy in patients treated for leukemia include osteoporosis, fractures, evidence of growth disturbance, periosteal reaction, and scurvy-like changes including "ring" epiphysis, and a relative increase in density of the zone of provisional calcification ("white line") and "corner" fractures (Fig. 25.9). The associated bone pain is mostly caused by either occult or frank fractures (FLETCHER 1997; SCHWARTZ and LEONIDAS 1984). While symptoms resolve rapidly with cessation of methotrexate therapy, radiologic improvement occurs over a period of months.

25.4.2
Vincristine and Ifosfamide–Induced Changes

Vincristine, one of the Vinca Alkaloids is used in the treatment of ALL, HD and NHL in addition to various solid tumors. The dose limiting toxicity of the drug

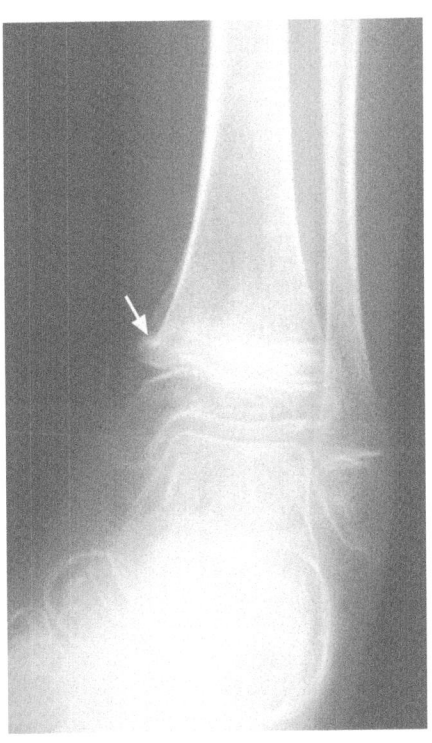

Fig. 25.9. Osteopenia and bone fracture in a 9-year-old boy treated for acute myeloid leukemia with a methotrexate-based regimen. Anteroposterior radiograph of the ankle shows osteoporosis and a subacute non-displaced fracture (*arrow*) of the distal tibial metaphysis. (With permission from [FLETCHER 1997])

is neurotoxicity, rather than myelosuppression as with many other antimetabolites. Among the manifestations of vincristine neurotoxicity are peripheral sensory and motor neuropathy (CAMPBELL et al. 1977; HILDEBRAND et al. 1972; KAUFMAN et al. 1976; TROBAUGH-LOTRARIO et al. 2003). Lack of sensation and suppression of deep tendon reflexes can, rarely, lead to a Charcot-like neuropathic arthropathy with microfractures and reactive bone formation (FLETCHER 1997). In most cases, this complication is avoided by splinting the affected limbs and symptoms can be relieved by discontinuing the drug. However, we have observed its radiologic manifestations in a patient with severe vincristine intoxication (Fig. 25.10).

Ifosfamide, a newer drug related to cyclophosphamide, is being evaluated for treatment of lymphoma as well as a number of solid tumors. Ifosfamide has known nephrotoxicity consisting of renal tubular dysfunction. Diminished phosphate reabsorption results in hypophosphatemic rickets with typical clinical and radiologic manifestations (BURK et al. 1990; RELF and BOAL 1992; ROSSI et al. 1993). This complication is especially prevalent in children with already diminished renal capacity, especially those who have undergone unilateral nephrectomy for Wilms tumor.

25.4.3
Steroid-Induced Osteonecrosis

Osteonecrosis is a significant complication of treatment for various hematological malignancies including acute leukemia, HD and NHL (BÖMELBURG et al. 1989; FLETCHER 1997; MURPHY and GREENBERG 1990; FELIX et al. 1985; PRINDULL et al. 1982; TIMOTHY and TUCKER 1978). While osteonecrosis may develop during therapy, it is detected most commonly after therapy and the latency period can be as long as 13 years (Figs. 25.11, 25.12). Osteonecrosis can also occur after allogeneic BMT in patients who have received steroids for the prevention or treatment of GVHD.

Osteonecrosis secondary to the systemic use of corticosteroids appear to be dose dependent with necrosis reported after cumulative prednisone doses as low as 500 mg. The use of dexamethazone instead of prednisone in pediatric patients during induction, reinduction, or delayed intensification therapy has resulted in a growing number of reports of symptomatic osteonecrosis with high risk for debilitating orthopedic pain that may require eventual joint replacement (FELIX and BLATT 1999; HANIF et al. 1993; MURPHY and GREENBERG 1990; OJALA et al. 1999; STRAUSS et al. 2001).

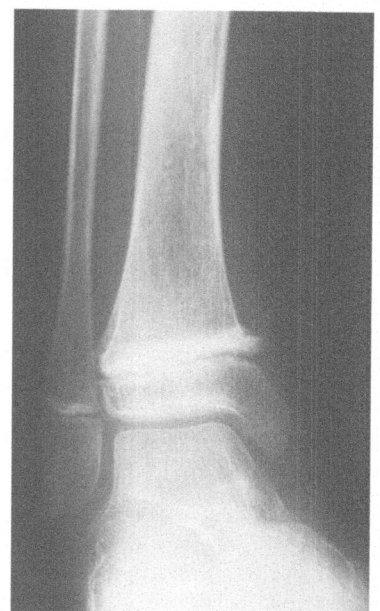
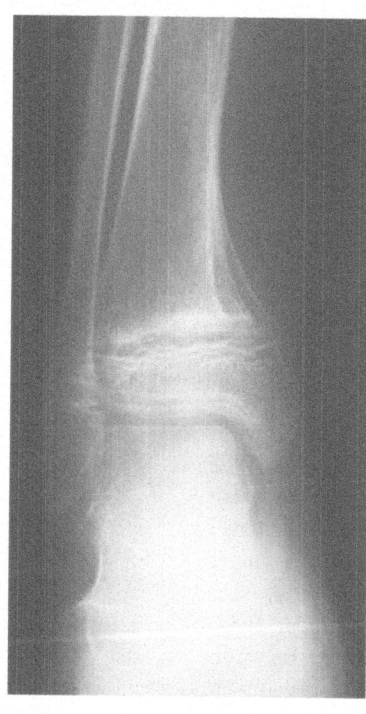

Fig. 25.10a,b. Recurring fracture in a 10-year-old boy treated for acute lymphoblastic leukemia using a vincristin based regimen. a Anteriposterior radiograph of the ankle demonstrates a subacute corner fracture of the distal tibial metaphysis. b Anteriposterior radiograph of the same ankle obtained 18 months later shows interval development of osteopenia with evident reactive new bone formation likely secondary to recurring microfractures resulting from vincristine neurotoxicity.

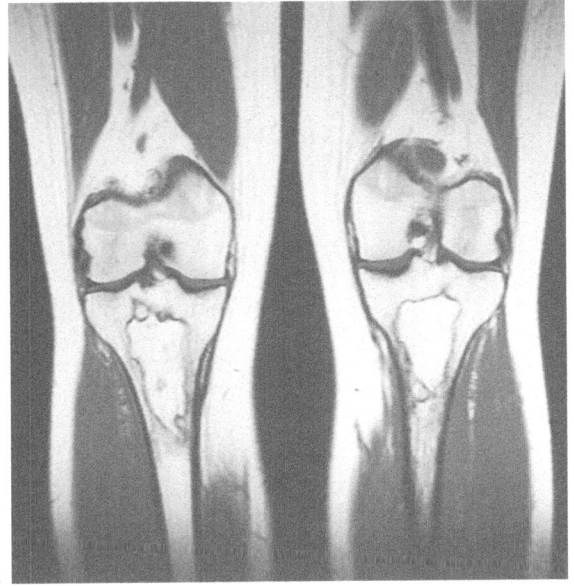
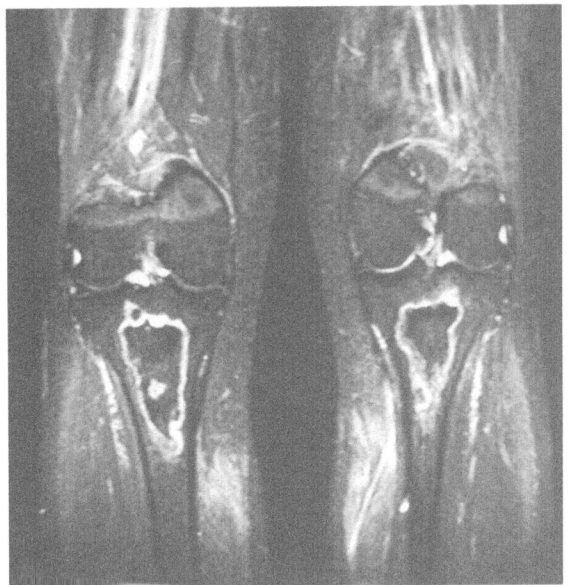

a   b

Fig. 25.11a,b. Intramedullary infarcts in a 19-year-old woman who had received chemotherapy and corticosteroids for 3 years as treatment of acute lymphoblastic leukemia. Coronal (**a**) T1-weighted and (**b**) STIR MR images of the painful knees demonstrate bilateral proximal tibial, well-circumscribed intramedullary serpiginous lines that are hypointense on (**a**) and hyperintense on (**b**) surrounding homogeneous fat-like marrow signal consistent with infarcts. (*Image courtesy of Dr. A. Guermazi*)

25.5
Osseous Effects of Bone Marrow Harvesting

The effect of the multiple needle aspirations used in bone marrow harvesting for later infusion (autologous transplantation) appears on plain radiographs and CT as small round or tubular lytic defects in the ilium and sacrum (ORTIZ et al. 1994). These defects cause foci of increased uptake on bone scintigraphy and focal abnormal MR marrow signal intensities that may mimic metastatic disease.

25.6
Bone Marrow Effects of Therapy

25.6.1
Bone Marrow Imaging

MR evaluation of the marrow changes in patients, particularly children treated for hematological malignancies, is complicated by physiologic age-related changes in the distribution of normal hematopoietic (red) and fatty (yellow) marrow (KRICUN 1985; VOGLER and MURPHY 1988). As previously described by MOORE and DAWSON (1990), physiologic conversion of red to yellow marrow occurs in a centripetal fashion such that by 12–14 years of age, there is macroscopic fat in the mid diaphysis of all long bones. In the femur, red to yellow marrow conversion occurs first in the diaphysis followed by the distal metaphysis. By adulthood, hematopoietic marrow is retained in the femoral neck, intertrochanteric regions and proximal shaft. Adults retain a large proportion of red marrow in the spine, pelvis, ribs and sternum (KRICUN 1985).

While malignant infiltration of yellow marrow results in decreased T1-weighted marrow signal and increased signal intensity on T2-weighted and STIR images (RUZAL-SHAPIRO et al. 1991), these changes are less conspicuous in the still hematopoietic vertebrae of older patients and in the diaphyses of younger children in whom marrow conversion has not yet occurred. Marrow evaluation by MR is further complicated by the rapid reconversion of fatty marrow to hematopoietic marrow when patients are subjected to a variety of stresses associated with cancer treatment.

25.6.2
Radiation-Induced Bone Marrow Changes

The hematopoietic elements of the bone marrow are very sensitive to ionizing radiation, resulting in myeloid depletion after a large volume of marrow is

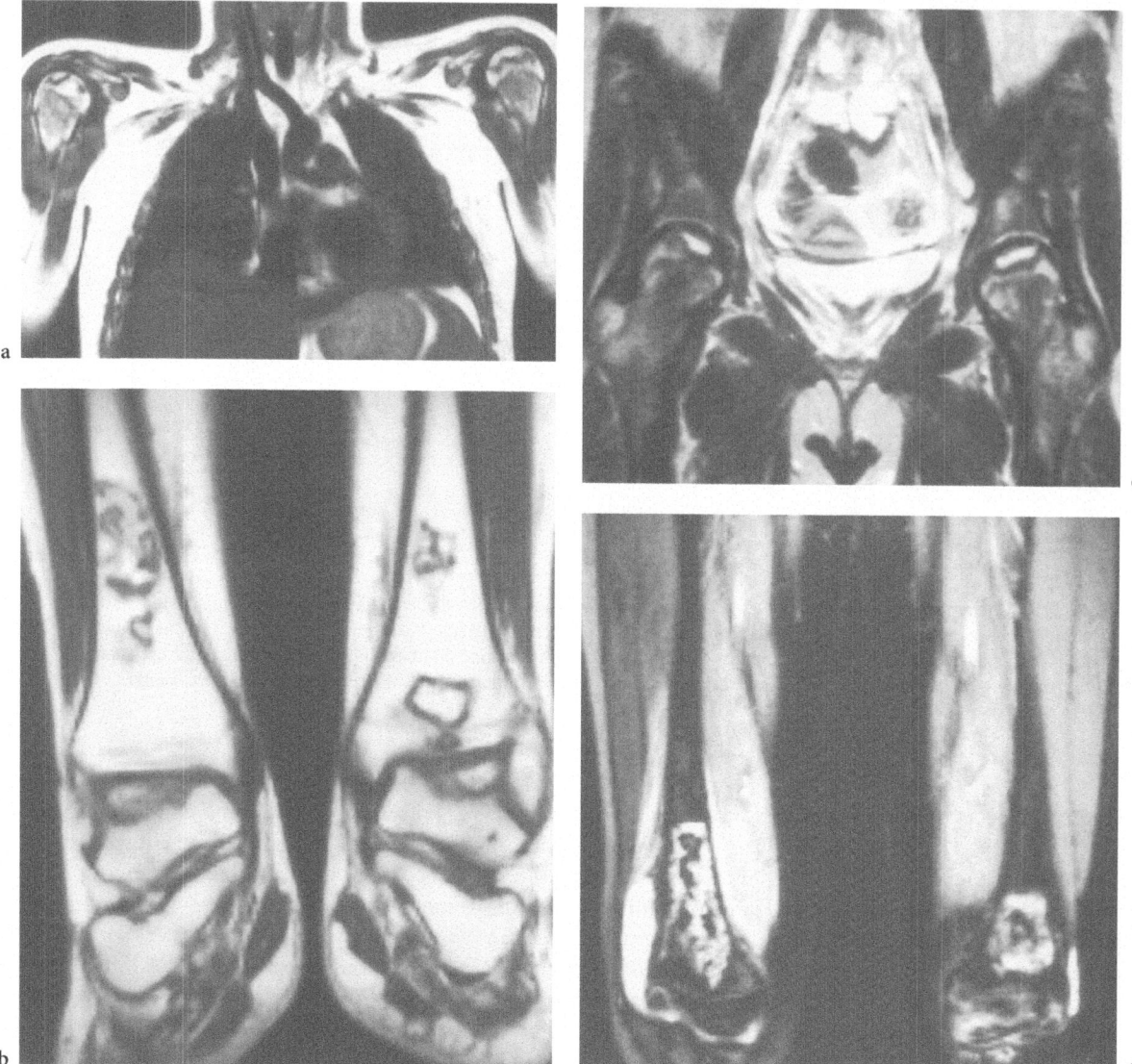

Fig. 25.12a–d. Avascular necrosis in a 13-year-old boy with leukemia treated with chemotherapy and corticosteroids. Coronal T1-weighted MR images of (**a**) the thorax and (**b**) ankles demonstrate avascular necrosis of both humeral heads and talar domes along with bilateral distal tibial medullary infarcts. Coronal (**c**) T2-weighted MR image of the pelvis and (**d**) STIR MR image of the distal femurs also show avascular necrosis of both femoral heads and the left femoral condyle in addition to bilateral distal femoral medullary infarcts.

irradiated. MR imaging confirms findings of marrow depletion previously demonstrated using marrow-seeking radiopharmaceuticals (Rubin and Casarett 1968). The immediate suppression of bone marrow uptake following 30–45 Gy irradiation of the spine or pelvis coincides with early transient post radiation marrow edema, necrosis and hemorrhage. These changes are also shown by increased STIR signal on MR imaging (Stevens et al. 1990b; Sugimura et al. 1994). These early findings are followed by the more enduring replacement of hematopoietic marrow by

adipocytes with a consequent increase in T1-weighted signal intensity (Sugimura et al. 1994). The radiation-induced changes typically conform precisely to the therapy portals and are evident in locations previously occupied by red marrow, particularly the vertebrae and pelvis (Fig. 25.13) (Blomlie et al. 1995; Fletcher 1997; Ramsey and Zacharias 1985).

Radiation tissue injury of the bone marrow is both dose- and time-related. An increase in STIR signal intensity can be seen as early as 1–2 weeks after initiation of radiation therapy (Ramsey and Zacharias

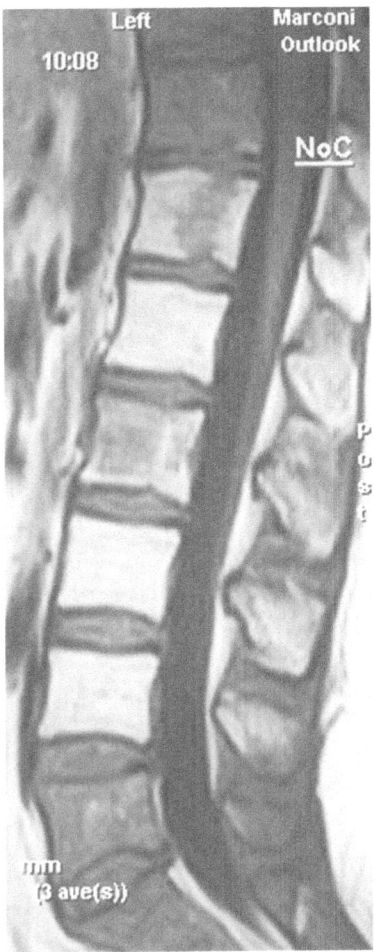

Fig. 25.13. Radiation-induced conversion of hematopoietic to fatty marrow in a 37-year-old woman treated for lymphoma with chemotherapy and irradiation. Sagittal T1-weighted image of the lumbar spine shows the geometrically defined hyperintensity within T12 through L4 vertebral bodies, which conforms to the irradiation field and reflects radiation-induced conversion of hematopoietic to fatty marrow. The noted patchy decreased signal within T12 and L2 raised concern for residual/recurrent disease. Subsequent percutaneous CT-guided biopsy of L2 revealed no viable tumor.

1985; YANKELEVITZ et al. 1991); whereas complete conversion to fatty marrow has been observed after 6–8 weeks (RAMSEY and ZACHARIAS 1985). Fatty marrow replacement with increased T1-weighted marrow signal may occur more slowly after lower doses of radiation (REMEDIOS et al. 1988). Recovery of bone marrow following radiation therapy is also dose dependent and correlates with the length of time since completion of therapy. Recovery after a dose below 30 Gy is likely, whereas marrow damage following doses exceeding 50 Gy appear to be irreversible (CASAMASSIMA et al.

1989). A progressive decrease in T1-weighted marrow signal indicates vertebral marrow recovery and has been documented in pediatric patients 11–30 months after receiving 20–40 Gy spinal radiation (CAVENAGH et al. 1995). Similar findings were documented in the marrow of long bone metaphyses after radiation. SACKS et al. (1978) found that marrow of patients under 18 years of age had increased capacity to regenerate but regeneration of marrow irradiated with more than 40 Gy was infrequent.

25.6.3
Chemotherapy-Induced Bone Marrow Changes

While antineoplastic drugs can induce long-term damage to the hematopoietic system, the precise mechanism of drug-induced myelosuppression is not well defined. Both acute and long term effects have been documented, with changes similar to those that occur after radiation found in the cellular marrow within 48 hours (MAUCH et al. 1995). Alterations in peripheral blood counts are not apparent for 1–3 weeks, reflecting the kinetics of cell maturation and the life span of mature peripheral blood cells (1 to 2 days for granulocytes, 10 to 20 days for platelets, and 120 days for erythrocytes).

On MR imaging, acute bone marrow response to chemotherapy appears similar to that after irradiation. Within a few days, tissue edema leads to a decrease in T1-weighted marrow signal followed by an increase in T1-weighted signal due to gradual fatty replacement. Contrary to local radiation injury, chemotherapy-induced alterations in bone marrow signal are diffuse in nature, less conspicuous and lack the sharp delineation caused by conformation to therapy portals. Bone marrow changes after chemotherapy are also temporary with hematopoietic marrow reseeding commencing after 3 to 4 weeks and leading to eventual marrow signal recovery (HUSBAND and REZNEK 1998).

25.6.4
Combined Radiation and Chemotherapy-Induced Bone Marrow Changes

The temporal sequence of treatment affects patients' tolerance to therapy. Irradiated bone marrow has less tolerance to chemotherapy because of the ablation of radiated marrow segments and because of compensatory increased sensitivity of hyperactive, unexposed marrow segments. Lack of marrow reserve following chemotherapy can also render the subsequent delivery of full courses of radiation difficult. MOPP therapy for example, is well tolerated following TNI, whereas the poor tolerance of TNI after MOPP for patients with advanced HD requires lowering the radiation dose. The simultaneous administration of chemotherapy and radiotherapy may, in some instances, be better tolerated than sequential courses that trigger compensatory mechanisms (KROGER et al. 1998).

25.6.5
Hematopoietic Growth Factors-Induced Bone Marrow Changes

Hematopoietic growth factors, such as granulocyte-colony stimulating factor (G-CSF), aim to stimulate hematopoiesis and marrow recovery thus decreasing treatment-related complications and allowing the use

of more intensive chemotherapy for hematologic and solid malignancies (GROOPMAN et al. 1989; LIESCHKE and BURGESS 1992). Bone marrow MR imaging signal alterations compatible with reconversion of yellow to red marrow often accompany a rise in peripheral neutrophil counts associated with proliferation of mature and immature myeloid elements and numerous granulocytes within the marrow (Fig. 25.14) (FLETCHER et al. 1993; SALGIA et al. 1994).

On MR imaging, G-CSF-induced marrow reconversion causes diminished T1-weighted marrow signal and mildly increased signal on T2-weighted and STIR images (FLETCHER et al. 1993; RYAN et al. 1995). Signal changes may be diffuse or patchy, affecting the entire marrow cavity of long bones, or predominantly and asymmetrically affecting the metaphyses (Fig. 25.15) (MULLEN et al. 1995; RYAN et al. 1995). While marrow MR imaging signal changes may be observed incidentally on studies performed

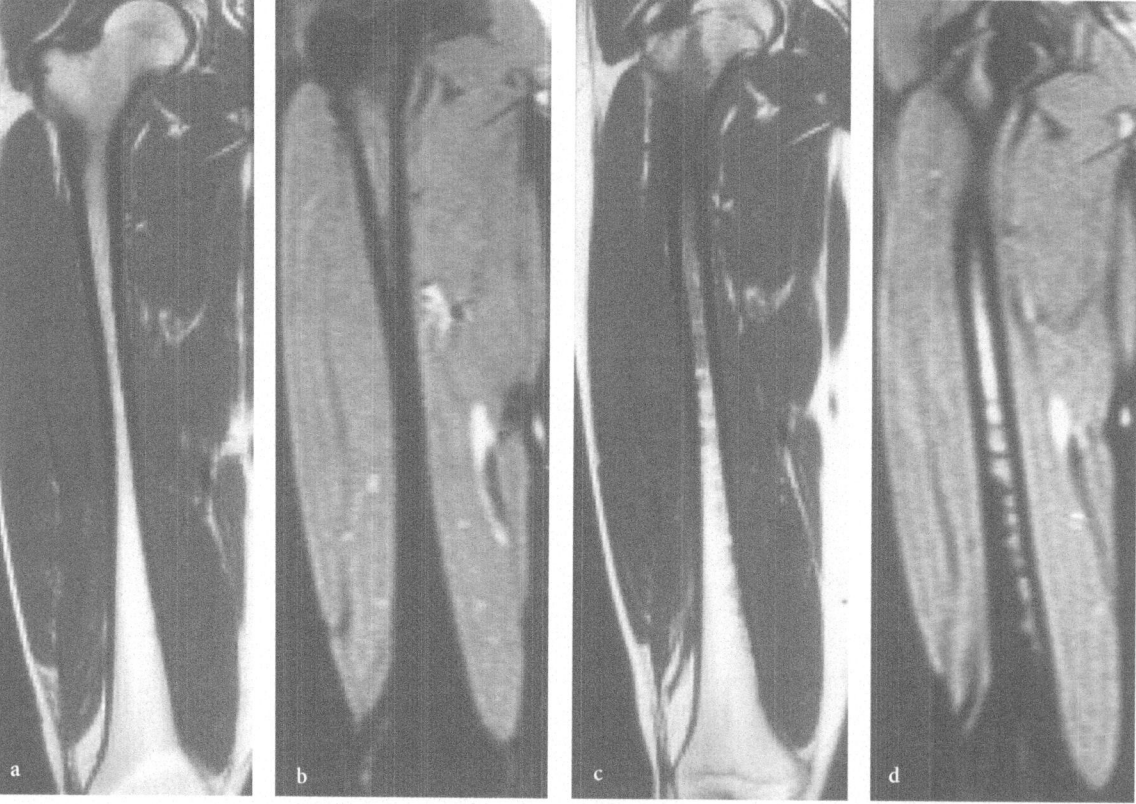

Fig. 25.14a–d. Red marrow stimulation in a 19-year-old woman treated with chemotherapy and granulocyte-colony stimulating factor (G-CSF). Coronal (**a**) T1-weighted and (**b**) STIR MR images of the femur obtained before administration of chemotherapy and granulocyte-colony stimulating factor (G-CSF) show normal medullary signal reflecting predominantly yellow marrow. Coronal (**c**) T1-weighted and (**d**) STIR MR images obtained 4 days after two 14-day courses of G-CSF show interval development of focal and diffuse changes in marrow signal intensity attributed to red marrow stimulation. (With permission from [FLETCHER et al. 1993])

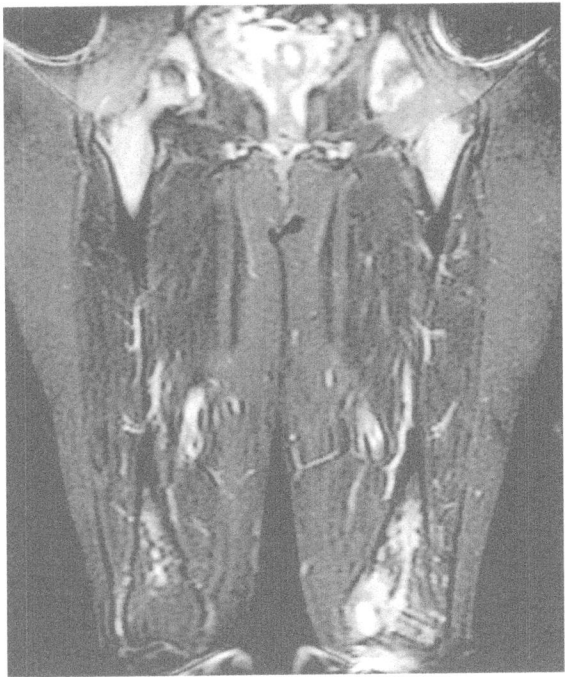
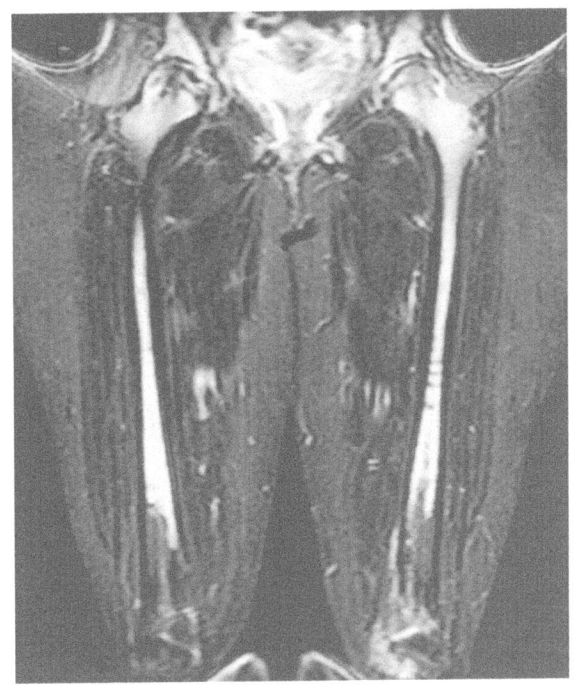

a   b

Fig. 25.15a,b. Red marrow stimulation in a 21-year-old woman following the completion of three cycles of chemotherapy and granulocyte-colony stimulating factor (G-CSF). **a, b** Coronal STIR MR images of the femurs demonstrate extensive bilateral femoral diffuse marrow signal hyperintensity attributed to red marrow stimulation.

for other purposes, the MR studies may be prompted by bone pain accompanying G-CSF administration. Diminished T1-weighted vertebral marrow signal with moderate Gadolinium-DTPA uptake has also been reported in adults treated with G-CSF (UNGER et al. 1990). Such findings may mimic metastatic disease, particularly in patients with G-CSF-related increased activity on bone and gallium scintigraphy (ITOH et al. 1995; SALGIA et al. 1994).

25.6.6
Bone Marrow Transplantation-Induced
Bone Marrow Changes

Post-BMT MR imaging marrow signal changes are variable. STEVENS et al. (1990a) noted a slight decrease in T1-weighted lumbar vertebral marrow signal along with increased STIR signal following a pre-transplant regimen of chemotherapy with or without fractionated TBI. Within three months after transplantation, they detected a "band" pattern consisting of a peripheral zone of intermediate signal intensity surrounded by a central zone of high intensity in the vertebrae of most patients (Fig. 25.16). This pattern apparently reflects earlier peripheral than central reconstitution of hemat-

opoietic marrow within the vertebral body (FLETCHER 1997; STEVENS et al. 1990a). LIEN et al. (1997) noted a more heterogeneous marrow pattern following bone marrow transplantation of lymphoma patients. Sharply defined focal T1-weighted low signal intensity areas were noted in 5 of 22 patients who were in complete remission after transplantation, particularly in those aged 40–45 years. Other groups however, noted little or no difference on T1 weighted images between successfully transplanted patients and volunteers (KAUCZOR et al. 1993; SMITH et al. 1989).

Early studies using quantitative MR techniques such as T1 relaxation (STEVENS et al. 1990a), T1 mapping (SMITH et al. 1991; TANNER et al. 1996) and chemical shift imaging (KAUCZOR et al. 1993) suggest that these techniques may be sensitive indicators of marrow repopulation. In one study, changes in the T1 relaxation rate corresponded temporally with recovery of peripheral neutrophils and platelet counts (SMITH et al. 1989). Using T1 mapping, TANNER et al. (1996) showed that pixels with low T1 values consistent with fat tended to occur mainly in the center of the vertebral body around the basivertebral vein. In another study employing chemical shift imaging in patients 2–6 years after autologous BMT, the relative lumbar and pelvic fat marrow signal was

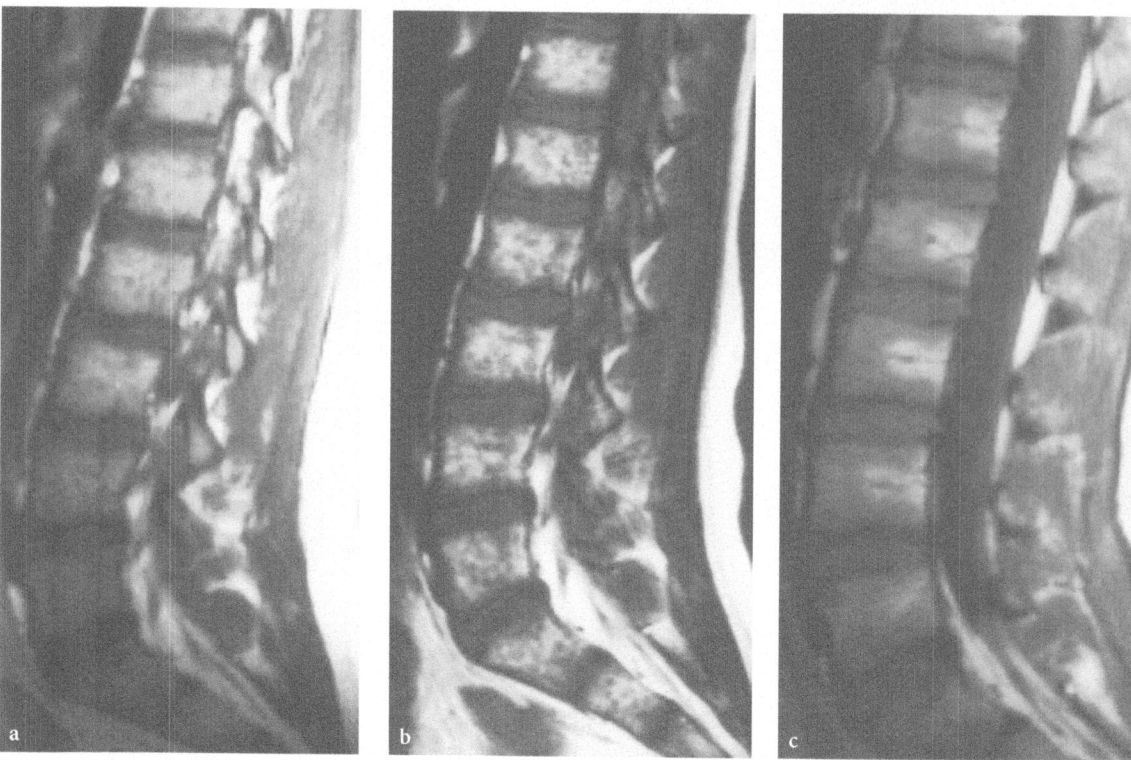

Fig. 25.16a–c. Normal bone marrow repopulation in a 14-year-old patient with Hodgkin disease after autologous bone marrow transplantation. The spine was not irradiated. **a** Sagittal T1-weighted MR image of the spine obtained before the bone marrow transplantation demonstrates a homogeneous intermediate vertebral body signal intensity. Sagittal T1-weighted MR images of the spine obtained (**b**) 6 weeks, and (**c**) one year after bone marrow transplantation show the change to a mottled pattern (**b**) and a "band" pattern (**c**) of central hyperintensity and peripheral intermediate signal intensity. (With permission from [FLETCHER 1997])

higher in the transplanted patients than age-matched volunteers. However, no significant differences between the marrow of patients and controls were detected on T1-weighted imaging (KAUCZOR et al. 1993). Using MR imaging and spectroscopic techniques, SCHICK et al. (1996) detected considerable increase in the amount of paramagnetic hemosiderin following transplantation. This result is likely related to iron overload which commonly accompanies BMT (KORNREICH et al. 1997). Such findings suggest a potential value of quantitative MR imaging in screening for residual marrow disease and monitoring bone marrow recovery following transplantation.

25.6.7
Bone Marrow Necrosis

Bone marrow necrosis is a distinct pathologic entity associated with a variety of diseases (BROWN 1972; KIRALY and WHEBY 1976; NOGARD et al. 1979; PUI et al. 1985). Extensive bone marrow necrosis is neverthe-

less, rarely encountered in living patients and is seen predominately in malignant infiltration of the bone marrow as in ALL and lymphoma. Various risk factors including chemotherapy and radiotherapy have been implicated in bone marrow necrosis (BROWN 1972; KIRALY and WHEBY 1976; MASON et al. 1978). Patients usually present with fever and excruciating and diffuse bone pain, accompanied by a precipitous drop in peripheral blood counts. Diagnosis is established pathologically using multiple bone marrow aspirates and biopsies showing necrotic marrow cells in a background of amorphous eosinophilic material (BROWN 1972; KIRALY and WHEBY 1976).

Previously reported MR features of bone marrow necrosis range from a pattern similar to periarticular osteonecrosis or bone infarctions occurring diffusely in the pelvis and spine (CHIM et al. 1998), to multifocal fluid-filled foci (WEISSMAN et al. 1992). In one patient with relapsing ALL who developed bone marrow necrosis 2 months after allogeneic BMT, CHIM et al. (1998) described multiple, well marginated foci of marrow signal abnormality with a double-line sign on T2-weighted MR images. Other less frequent findings were enhancing lesions showing increased T1 and T2-weighted signal characteristics consistent with MR imaging features of blood or proteinaceous material. However, they noted no fluid necrotic lesions and postulated that the degree of marrow necrosis in their patient may not have yet reached the final fluid-filled stage described by WEISSMAN et al. (1992). CHIM et al. (1998) also indicated that the histologically confirmed foci of bone marrow necrosis enhanced marginally as opposed to the homogenous enhancement of the foci of malignant infiltration. The potential ability to differentiate viable tumor from necrosis highlights the utility of MR imaging in non-invasive bone marrow evaluation and for the selection of potential biopsy sites.

25.7
Soft Tissue Effects of Therapy

25.7.1
Post-Irradiation Soft Tissue Inflammation

Even though striated muscle is relatively resistant to radiation, an inflammatory response may occur that is characterized by edema of the muscles and subcutaneous tissues. Vascular damage with eventual muscle atrophy typically ensues (BLOMLIE et al. 1996; RUBIN and CASARETT 1968). In a retrospective study, we documented increased T2-weighted and STIR signal intensity in irradiated muscle along with evidence of Gd-DTPA enhancement as early as the sixth week after treatment with doses of 59.5–65 Gy (FLETCHER et al. 1990). The findings were visible up to 69 weeks post radiation. The area of signal abnormality conforms to the irradiated volume often associated with clinical evidence of skin, soft tissue and epithelial radiation effects (Fig. 25.17) (FLETCHER 1997; FLETCHER et al. 1990; SOVIK et al. 1993).

The MR findings of increased signal on T2-weighted, STIR and Gd-DTPA enhanced T1-weighted images of irradiated tissues typically reflect minor, usually subclinical, tissue damage with edema and inflammation. These signal changes are consistent with an increase in total water content and extracellular fluid volume of the affected tissues (HERFKENS et al. 1983). The reduced fiber size of grossly atrophic muscles and the consequent expansion of extracellular fluid space likely contributes to the MR signal abnormality (POLAK et al. 1988). Clinically apparent soft tissue changes during and immediately after irra-

diation include epithelial reactions, often associated with subcutaneous and submucosal edema. Subacute soft tissue changes, clinically apparent as "cellulitis-like" events, have been described anecdotally. Clinical effects of radiation on normal tissues are well documented (BLOOMER and HELLMAN 1975).

25.7.2
Treatment-Related Increased Propensity to Infections

Therapy of patients with hematological malignancies may result in long-term sequelae which include compromised immune function and decreased bone marrow reserve. Impairment of cell-mediated immunity, as noted by decreased numbers of peripheral T cells and absolute lymphocyte counts, and inversion of CD4/CD8 ratios, has followed TNI in patients with HD (WATANABE et al. 1997), TBI (VEDA et al. 1984), and dose-intensive multiagent regimens (MACKALL et al. 1997).

The impaired humoral immunity that follows splenectomy is well documented and is typically associated with overall decrease in serum levels of immunoglobulin M and immunoglobulin A (HANCOCK et al. 1976). In one study, 8% of the patients with HD who had undergone splenectomy as part of a staging laparotomy developed fulminant infections, generally with encapsulated organisms. Some of these patients developed infection 3 years after splenectomy, which indicates a long-term risk for sepsis (LANZKOWSKY et al. 1976). This underscores the necessity of pneumococcal vaccination and the use of prophylactic penicillin for indefinite periods in splenectomized survivors of HD (HAYS et al. 1984).

Splenic atrophy with consequences similar to those of splenectomy has also been reported after splenic irradiation (approximately 4 Gy) of patients with HD and NHL (DAILEY et al. 1980). Total nodal irradiation, in the absence of a splenic port, does not impair antibody production on a long-term basis. The current tendency to avoid staging laparotomy, the use of partial rather than total splenectomy, and the reduced reliance on larger doses of extensive radiation help to avoid these problems.

25.7.3
Treatment-Related Increased Propensity to Bleeding Diathesis

The degree of marrow damage and subsequent clinical consequences depends on the volume irradiated and

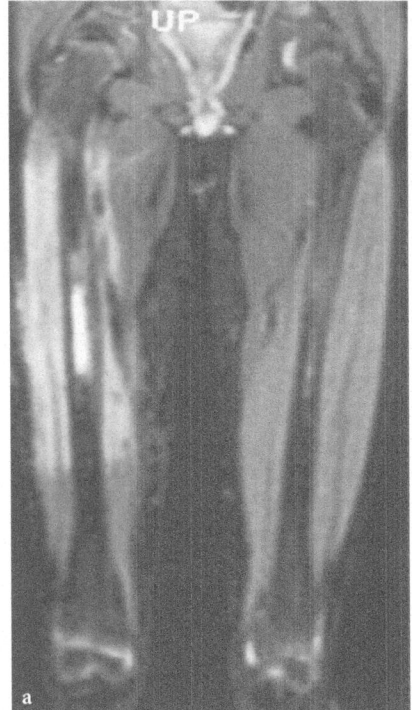

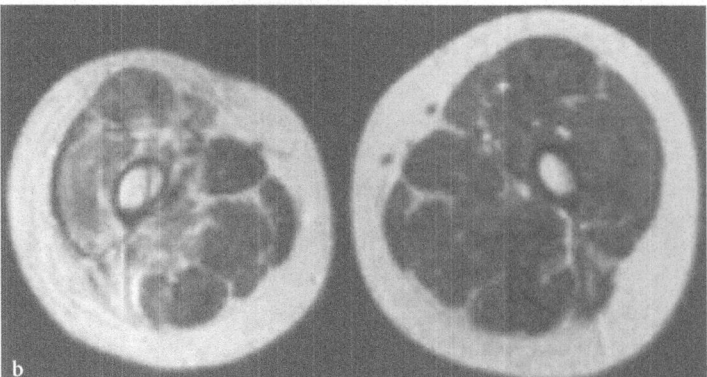

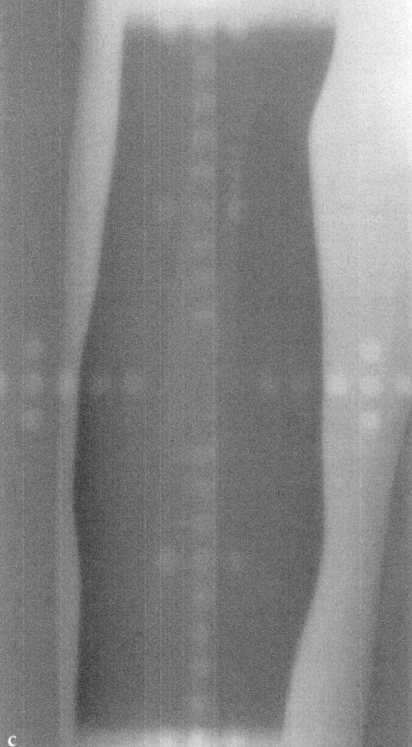

Fig. 25.17a–c. Soft-tissue inflammation in an 11-year-old boy at 28-weeks post radiation therapy using 6,000 cGy. **a** Coronal STIR and (**b**) axial T2-weighted MR images of the right thigh demonstrate geometric distribution of the hyperintensity in the muscles and subcutaneous fat that conform to (**c**) the radiation port. Note also that there is relative atrophy of the right thigh muscles. (With permission from [FLETCHER et al. 1990])

the dosage used. Following 850 to 1,000 cGy of single-dose TBI and marrow transplantation for various hematological abnormalities, about 25% of patients have platelet counts of fewer than 100,000 per cubic millimeter after 4 months (FIRST et al. 1985). Concomitant chemotherapy may increase the degree of radiation-induced marrow damage. Despite the well documented short-term effects of chemotherapy on bone marrow function, the long-term effects have not been adequately evaluated. However, methotrexate given as much as 18 months after craniospinal irradiation in patients with ALL (MACLENNAN et al. 1975), or chemotherapy instituted as long as 3 years after irradiation in patients with HD (CURRAN and JOHNSON 1970), may result in long-term excessive myelosuppression. This in turn increases the propensity to bleeding diathesis (Figs. 25.18, 25.19) and infection, including osteomyelitis.

25.8
Second Malignant Neoplasms

Survivors of childhood malignancies are at risk for significant late effects, the most devastating of which

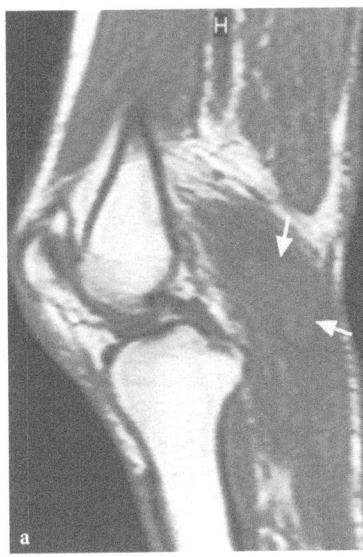
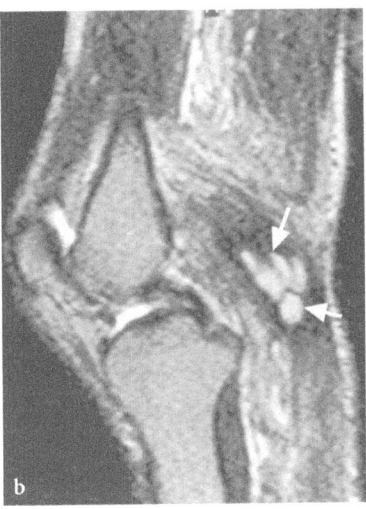
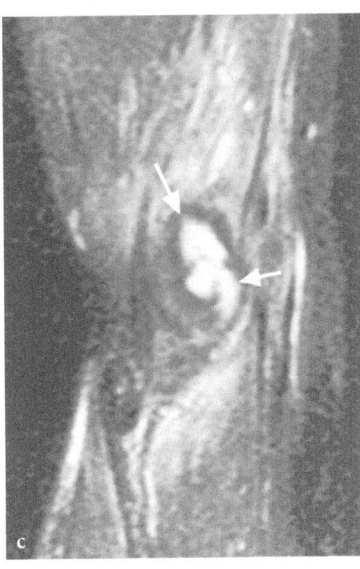

Fig. 25.18a–c. Intramuscular hematoma in a 55-year-old man receiving chemotherapy for leukemia. **a** Sagittal T1-weighted, and (**b**) sagittal and (**c**) coronal T2-weighted MR images of the knee obtained after the patient complained of recent upper calf pain demonstrate evidence of subacute intramuscular hematoma manifested by a localized area of subtle T1-weighted hyperintensity (*arrows*) and corresponding T2-weighted hyperintensity within the medial head of the gastrocnemius muscle. The hematoma is surrounded by a hypointense hemosiderin ring and mild muscle edema.

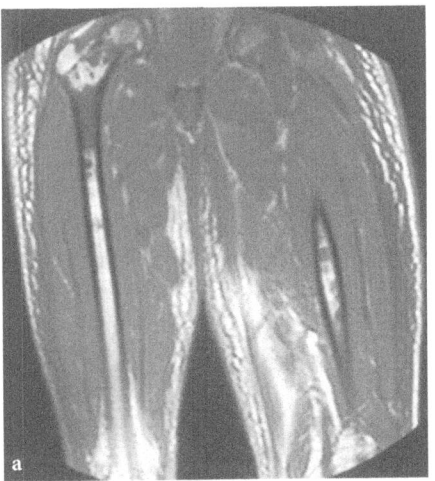
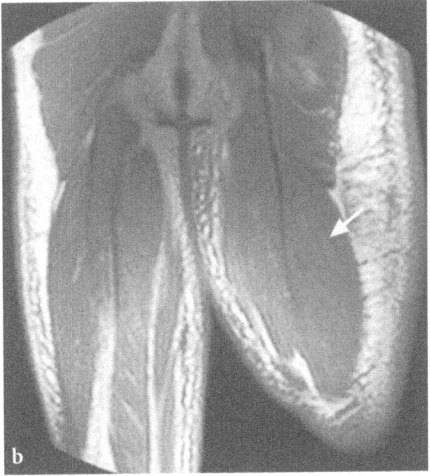

Fig. 25.19a–d. Intramuscular hemorrhage in a 39-year-old man treated with chemotherapy for relapsing acute myeloid leukemia. **a, b** Coronal T1-weighted MR images of the thighs show multiple foci of bone marrow signal abnormality within both femoral shafts consistent with leukemic marrow deposits in addition to a subtle hyperintense area within the left biceps femoris muscle (*arrow*). **c** Coronal and (**d**) axial T2-weighted MR images demonstrate a large fusiform-shaped hyperintense area with a hemosiderin ring and marked surrounding edema within the left biceps femoris muscle consistent with subacute hemorrhage.

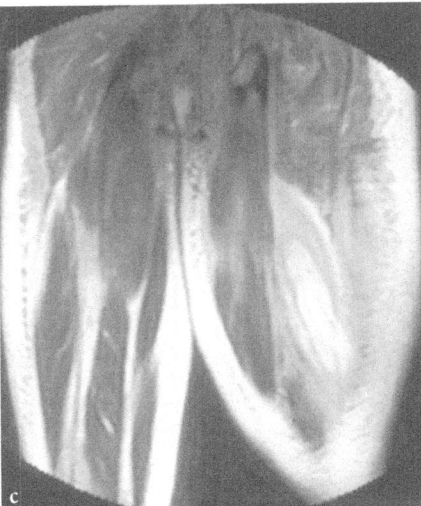
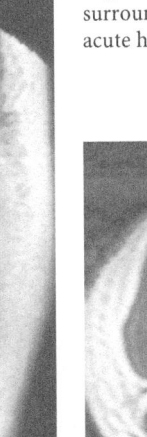
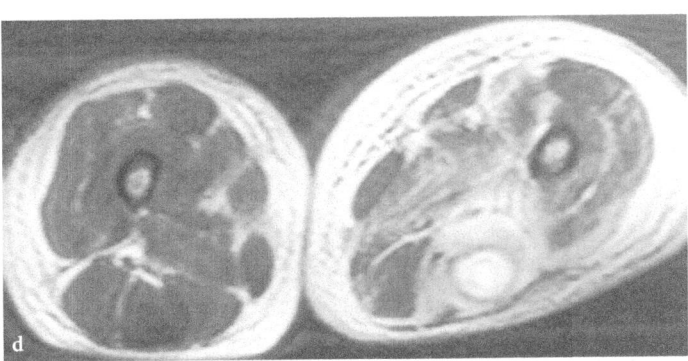

is a second malignant neoplasm (SMN). The lifetime risk of a SMN in such patients has been estimated to be 10 to 20 times that of age-matched controls (NEGLIA et al. 2001). The incidence of SMN within the first 20 years after the initial diagnosis ranges from 3% to 12% (NEGLIA et al. 2001; TUCKER et al. 1988) and SMN is the most common cause of death in long-term survivors after the recurrence of the primary cancer (MERTENS et al. 2001; NICHOLSON et al. 1994). The risk and type of SMN depend on several variables, including the initial diagnosis, patient age, nature and intensity of prior therapy, the presence of genetic predisposition and the time lapsed since original diagnosis and therapy. Childhood cancer survivors are at particularly high risk if their primary diagnosis was HD, retinoblastoma, or the genetic form of Wilms tumor.

The low incidence of SMN in ALL patients treated with conventional therapy is worthwhile noting since that group comprises the largest cohort of childhood cancer survivors. MIKE et al. (1982) estimated the risk to be 62 per 100,000 patients per year, while the risk of SMN in HD survivors is 280 per 100,000 patients per year at 15 years from diagnosis (NEGLIA et al. 1991). The most common SMN in ALL survivors is other forms of leukemia and NHL (MIKE et al. 1982) followed by an increased incidence of brain tumors (ROSSO et al. 1994; SOCIE et al. 2000). High risk factors include therapy with at least 2,400 cGy of cranial irradiation or TBI at an age younger than 5 years.

Acute nonlymphoblastic leukemia (ANLL), including myelodysplasia, is the most common hematopoietic SMN and has been reported in 10% to 20 % of patients

(NEGLIA et al. 2001; TUCKER et al. 1988). Causation in survivors of childhood and adolescent HD has been linked to mechlorethamine and cyclophosphamide, two alkylating agents commonly used in the MOPP multiagent chemotherapeutic regimen (ARSENEAU et al. 1972; BEATTY et al. 1995; COLEMAN 1986; COLTMAN and DIXON 1982; TUCKER et al. 1988; VALAGUSSA et al. 1986; VAN LEEUWEN et al. 1994). The role of nodal radiotherapy in the development of secondary leukemia is inconclusive (COLTMAN and DIXON 1982). In fact, some series suggest that MOPP alone carries the same risk as MOPP plus radiation (ARSENEAU et al. 1972; BEATTY et al. 1995). The risk of secondary ANLL appears to plateau by 10 years from initial diagnosis (BLAYNEY et al. 1987; NEGLIA et al. 1991). Secondary leukemias after treatment of HD with alkylating agents have a mean latency of 5 to 7 years (FELIX 1998). Secondary ANLL following leukemia has been ascribed to epipodophylotoxin etoposide (VP-16) and has a brief latent period, less than 2 years from initial diagnosis (FELIX 1998; FELIX and BLATT 1999; HEYN et al. 1994; KUSHNER et al. 1998; PUI et al. 1989).

In contrast to leukemias, solid tumors have been attributed to radiation therapy with most radiation-induced tumors occurring within or adjacent to the directly irradiated tissues and radiation ports (BLATT et al. 1992; BRESLOW et al. 1988; FLETCHER 1997; HANCOCK et al. 1993; HASELOW et al. 1978; HAWKINS et al. 1996; HEYN et al. 1993; KOVALIC et al. 1991; NEGLIA et al. 2001; SOCIE et al. 2000; TUCKER et al. 1988; TUCKER et al. 1987). Bone and soft tissue sarcomas, breast carcinomas and carcinomas of the

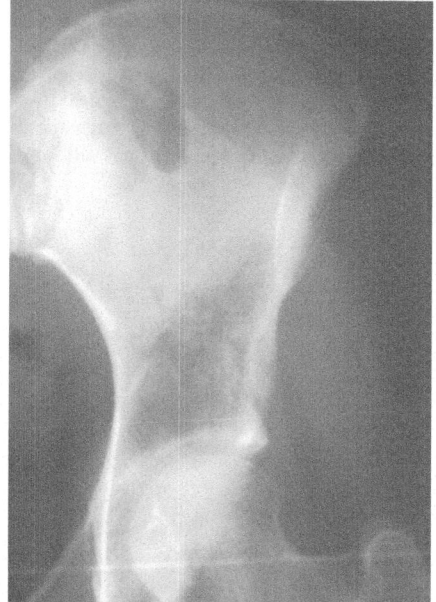
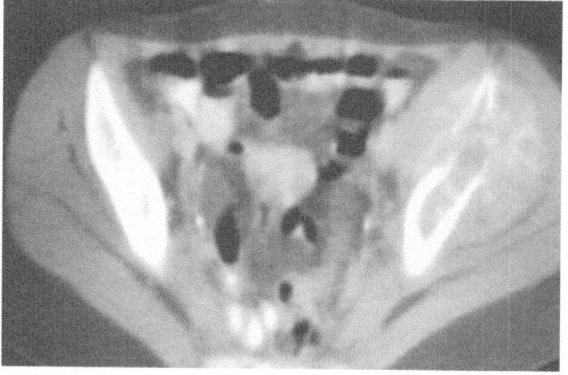

Fig. 25.20a,b. Post-radiation sarcoma in a 35-year-old Hodgkin disease survivor treated 15-years earlier with chemotherapy and irradiation to the chest, abdomen and pelvis. Patient presented with lingering pain and limited ability to walk. **a** Anteroposterior radiograph and (**b**) axial CT scan of the left iliac bone demonstrate an aggressive lytic destructive lesion with malignant periosteal reaction and soft tissue component involving the left iliac bone. Findings were consistent with post radiation sarcoma. (*Image courtesy of Dr. T. Hudson*)

skin and thyroid are the most common solid tumors (Fig. 25.20) (BECHLER et al. 1992; HAWKINS et al. 1996; NEWTON et al. 1991; SMITH et al. 1993; TUCKER et al. 1987). The risk appears to rise with increasing levels of radiation exposure (HEYN et al. 1993), as well as with time since initial therapy (mean latency about 10 years) (TUCKER et al. 1987). HANCOCK et al. (1993) reported that 25 of 885 women with HD who were treated with radiation developed invasive breast carcinoma and an additional patient developed multi focal carcinoma in situ. They concluded that treatment with mantle therapy before age 30 years is a risk factor for breast cancer that raises the relative risk to 14-fold that of the general female population. The relative risk was especially high for those irradiated between the ages of 10 and 15 years (HANCOCK et al. 1993). Thyroid cancer, which occurs after HD at an incidence of approximately 18-fold that of the general population may also occur after low doses of radiation (BLAYNEY et al. 1987).

The risk of a malignant bone tumor following BMT appears to be low (DEEG 1984). Osteosarcoma, the most common type of musculoskeletal second malignancy (SMITH et al. 1993; TUCKER et al. 1987), is particularly prevalent following treatment of retinoblastoma and Ewing sarcoma (BECHLER et al. 1992; HAWKINS et al. 1996) and has a dismal prognosis. Other musculoskeletal second malignancies include Ewing sarcoma, malignant fibrous histiocytoma and malignant mesenchymoma (HAWKINS et al. 1996; SMITH et al. 1993; TUCKER et al. 1987). Most secondary bone tumors occur in patients who have received radiation therapy for their primary malignancy (NEWTON et al. 1991); however, chemotherapy with alkylating agents has also been implicated (HAWKINS et al. 1996).

25.9
Conclusion

Remarkable progress in the management of hematological malignancies, particularly childhood hematological malignancies, during the past two decades has resulted in greatly improved rates of long-term survival and cure. Consequently, there is an increasing need to monitor the health of these patients, and diagnostic imaging plays a central and major role in these efforts. Radiologists should be able to recognize the various therapy-related effects or complications and to differentiate them from recurrent or concomitant disease.

References

Altman K, Bailey BM (1996) Non-union of mandibulotomy sites following irradiation for squamous cell carcinoma of the oral cavity. Br J Oral Maxillofac Surg 34:62–65

Amato RJ (2002) Thalidomide: an antineoplastic agent. Curr Oncol Rep 4:56–62

Armitage JO (1994) Bone marrow transplantation. N Engl J Med 330:827–838

Arseneau JC, Sponzo RW, Levin DL et al (1972) Nonlymphomatous malignant tumors complicating Hodgkin's disease. Possible association with intensive therapy. N Engl J Med 287:1119–1122

Beatty O, Hudson MM, Greenwald C et al (1995) Subsequent malignancies in children and adolescents after treatment for Hodgkin's disease. J Clin Oncol 13:603–609

Bechler JR, Robertson WW, Meadows AT et al (1992) Osteosarcoma as a second malignant neoplasm in children. J Bone Joint Surg [Am] 74:1079–1083

Berdon WE, Baker DH, Boyer J (1965) Unusual benign and malignant sequelae to childhood radiation therapy. AJR Am J Roentgenol 93:545–556

Blatt J, Bercu BB, Gillin JC et al (1984) Reduced pulsatile growth hormone secretion in children after therapy for acute lymphoblastic leukemia. J Pediatr 104:182–186

Blatt J, Olshan A, Gula MJ et al (1992) Second malignancies in very long-term survivors of childhood cancer. Am J Med 93:57–60

Blayney DW, Longo DL, Young RC et al (1987) Decreasing risk of leukemia with prolonged follow-up after chemotherapy and radiotherapy for Hodgkin's disease. N Engl J Med 316:710–714

Bleyer WA (1990) The impact of childhood cancer on the United States and the world. CA Cancer J Clin 40:355–367

Blomlie V, Rofstad EK, Skjonsberg A et al (1995) Female pelvic bone marrow: serial MR imaging before, during and after radiation therapy. Radiology 194:537–543

Blomlie V, Rofstad EK, Tvera K et al (1996) Noncritical soft tissues of the female pelvis: serial MR imaging before, during and after radiation therapy. Radiology 199:461–468

Bloom HJ, Wallace EN, Henk JM (1969) The treatment and prognosis of medulloblastoma in children: a study of 82 verified cases. AJR Am J Roentgenol 105:43–62

Bloomer WD, Hellman S (1975) Normal tissue responses to radiation therapy. N Eng J Med 29:80–83

Bömelburg T, von Legerke H-J, Ritter J (1989) Aseptic osteonecrosis in the treatment of childhood acute leukaemias. Eur J Pediatr 149:20–23

Bragg DG, Shidnia H, Chu FCH et al (1970) The clinical and radiographic aspects of radiation osteitis. Radiology 97:103–111

Breslow NE, Norkool PA, Olshan A et al (1988) Second malignant neoplasms in survivors of Wilms' tumors: a report from the National Wilms' Tumor Study. J Natl Cancer Inst 80:592–595

Brown CH (1972) Bone marrow necrosis. A study of seventy cases. Johns Hopkins Med J 131:189–203

Burk CD, Restaino I, Kaplan BS et al (1990) Ifosfamide-induced renal tubular dysfunction and rickets in children with Wilms tumor. J Pediatr 177:331–335

Campbell RH, Marshall WC, Chessels JM (1977) Neurological complications of childhood leukemia. Arch Dis Child 52:850–858

Casamassima F, Ruggiero C, Caramella D et al (1989) Hemato-poietic bone marrow recovery after radiation therapy: MRI evaluation. Blood 73:1677–1681

Cavenagh EC, Weinberger E, Shaw DWW et al (1995) Hematopoietic marrow regeneration in pediatric patients undergoing spinal irradiation: MR depiction. AJNR Am J Neuroradiol 16:461–467

Chim CS, Ooi C, Ma SK et al (1998) Bone marrow necrosis in bone marrow transplantation: the role of MR imaging. Bone Marrow Transplant 22:1125–1128

Cohen A, Duell T, Socie G et al (1999) Nutritional status and growth after bone marrow transplantation (BMT) during childhood: EBMT late-effects working party retrospective data. European group for blood and marrow transplantation. Bone Marrow Transplant 23:1043–1047

Cole ARC, Darte JMM (1963) Osteochondromata following irradiation in children. Pediatrics 32:285–288

Coleman CN (1986) Secondary malignancies after treatment of Hodgkin's disease: an evolving picture. J Clin Oncol 4:821–824

Coltman CA, Dixon DO (1982) Second malignancies complicating Hodgkin's disease: a Southwest Oncology Group 10-year follow-up. Cancer Treat Rep 66:1023–1033

Copelan EA (1992) Conditioning regimens for allogeneic bone marrow transplantation. Blood Reviews 6:234–242

Curran RE, Johnson RE (1970) Tolerance to chemotherapy after prior irradiation for Hodgkin's disease. Ann Intern Med 72:505–509

Dailey MO, Coleman CN, Kaplan HS (1980) Radiation-induced splenic atrophy in patients with Hodgkin's disease and non-Hodgkin's lymphomas. N Engl J Med 302:215–217

Dalinka MK, Mazzeo VP (1985) Complications of radiation therapy. Crit Rev Diagn Imaging 23:235–267

Deeg HJ (1984) Bone marrow transplantation: a review of delayed complications. Br J Haemat 57:185–208

DeSmet AA, Kuhns LR, Fayos JV et al (1976) Effects of radiation therapy on growing long bones. AJR Am J Roentgenol 127:935–939

Dickerman JD, Newbert AH, Moreland MD (1979) Slipped capital femoral epiphysis (SCFE) following pelvic irradiation for rhabdomyosarcoma. Cancer 44:480–482

Dickinson WP, Bezzy H, Dickinson L et al (1978) Differential effects of cranial radiation on growth hormone response to arginine and insulin infusion. J Pediatr 92:754–757

Dryer ZE, Blah J, Bleyer A (2002) Late effects of childhood cancer and its treatment. In: Pizzo PA, Poplack DG (eds) Principles and practice of pediatric oncology. Lippincott Williams & Wilkins, Philadelphia, pp 1431–1461

Ecklund K, Laor T, Goorin AM et al (1997) Methotrexate osteopathy in patients with osteosarcoma. Radiology 202:543–547

Edeiken BS, Libshitz HJ, Cohen MA (1982) Slipped proximal humeral epiphysis: a complication of radiotherapy to the shoulder in children. Skeletal Radiol 9:123–125

Ergun H, Howland WJ (1980) Postradiation atrophy of mature bone. CRC Crit Rev Diagn Imaging 12:225–243

Fajardo L-G LF, Prionas SD, Kaluza GL et al (2002) Acute vasculitis after endovascular brachytherapy. Int J Radiat Oncol Biol Phys 53:714–719

Fauroux B, Clement A, Tournier G (1996) Pulmonary toxicity of drugs and thoracic irradiation in children. Rev Mal Respir 13:235–242

Felix C (1998) Secondary leukemias induced by topoisomerase targeted drugs. Biochim Biophys Acta 1400:233–255

Felix C, Blatt J, Goodman MA et al (1985) Avascular necrosis of bone following combination chemotherapy for acute lumphocytic leukemia. Med Pediatr Oncol 13:269–272

Felix CA, Blatt J (1999) Etoposide and Langerhans cell histiocytosis: second malignancies, a second look. Pediatr Hematol Oncol 16:183–185

Fiedler W, Staib P, Kuse R et al (2001) Role of angiogenesis inhibitors in acute myeloid leukemia. Cancer J 3:129–133

First LR, Smith BR, Lipton J et al (1985) Isolated thrombocytopenia after allogeneic bone marrow transplantation: existence of transient or chronic thrombocytopenia syndromes. Blood 65:368–374

Fletcher BD (1997) Effects of pediatric cancer therapy on the musculoskeletal system. Pediatr Radiol 27:623–636

Fletcher BD, Crom DB, Krance RA et al (1994) Radiation-induced bone abnormalities after bone marrow transplantation for childhood leukemia. Radiology 191:231–235

Fletcher BD, Hanna SL, Kun LE (1990) Changes in MR signal intensity and contrast enhancement of therapeutically irradiated soft tissue. Magn Reson Imaging 8:771–777

Fletcher BD, Wall JE, Hanna SL (1993) Effect of hematopoietic growth factors on MR images of bone marrow in children undergoing chemotherapy. Radiology 189:745–751.

Gardner RV (1999) Long term hematopoietic damage after chemotherapy and cytokine. Front Biosci 4:47–57

Gilsanz V. Carlson ME, Roe TF et al (1990) Osteoporosis after cranial irradiation for acute lymphoblastic leukemia. J Pediatr 117:238–244

Groopman JE, Molina JM, Scadden DT (1989) Hematopoietic growth factors. Biology and clinical applications. N Engl J Med 321:1449–1459

Hall EJ (1994) Radiobiology for the radiologist, 4th edn. JB Lippincott, Philadelphia

Hallahan DE, Chen AY, Teng M et al (1999) Drug-radiation interactions in tumor blood vessels. Oncology (huntingt) 13:71–77

Hancock BW, Bruce L, Ward AM et al (1976) Changes in immune status in patients undergoing splenectomy for the staging of Hodgkin's disease. Br Med J 1:313–315

Hancock SL, Tucker MA, Hoppe RT (1993) Breast cancer after treatment of Hodgkin's disease. J Natl Cancer Inst 85:25–31

Hanif I, Mahmoud H, Pui C-H (1993) Avascular femoral head necrosis in pediatric cancer patients. Med Pediatr Oncol 21:655–660

Haselow RE, Nesbit M, Dehner LP et al (1978) Second neoplasms following megavoltage radiation in a pediatric population. Cancer 42:1185–1191

Hawkins MM, Wilson LMK, Burton HS et al (1996) Radiotherapy, alkylating agents, and risk of bone cancer after childhood cancer. J Natl Cancer Inst 88:270–278

Hays DM, Ternberg JL, Chen TT et al (1984) Complications related to 234 staging laparotomies performed in the Intergroup Hodgkin's disease in childhood study. Surgery 96:471–478

Hendry JH, Mackay RI, Roberts SA et al (1998) Outstanding issues in radiation dose-fractionation studies. Int J Radiat Biol 73:383–394

Herfkens RJ, Sievers R, Kaufman L et al (1983) Nuclear magnetic resonance imaging of the infracted muscle: A rat model. Radiology 147:761–764

Heyn R, Haeberlen V, Newton WA et al (1993) Second malignant neoplasms in patients treated for rhabdomyosarcoma. J Clin Oncol 11:262–270

Heyn R, Khan F, Ensign L et al (1994) Acute myeloid leukemia in patients treated for rhabdomyosarcoma with cyclophosphamide and low dose etoposide on Intergroup Rhabdomyosarcoma study III: an interim report. Med Pediatr Oncol 23:99–106

Hildebrand J, Kenis Y, Mubashir BA et al (1972) Vincristine neurotoxicity. N Eng J Med 287:517

Hockman K, Van der Vijgh WJ, Vermorken JB (1999) Clinical and preclinical modulation of chemotherapy-induced toxicity in patients with cancer. Drugs 57:133–155

Howland WJ, Loeffler RK, Starchman DE et al (1975) Postirradiation atrophic changes of bone and related complications. Radiology 117:677–685

Husband JE, Reznek RH (1998) Imaging in oncology, 1st ed. Isis Medical Media, Oxford

Irwin CJR, Thomson E, Plowman PN (1993) Case report: paediatric radiotherapy—the avoidance of late radiation damage to the growing hip. Br J Radiol 66:369–374

Itoh K, Kanegae K, Kato C (1995) Increased symmetric bone uptake during treatment with granulocyte colony stimulating factor and erythropoietin. Clin Nuclear Med 20:932

Jaffe N, Ried HL, Cohen M et al (1983) Radiation induced osteochondroma in long-term survivors of childhood cancer. Int J Radiation Oncology Biol Phys 9:665–670

Kaste SC, Chesney RW, Hudson MM et al (1999) Bone mineral status during and after therapy of childhood cancer: an increasing population with multiple risk factors for impaired bone health. J Bone Miner Res 14:2010–2014

Kaste SC, Jones-Wallace D, Rose SR et al (2001) Bone mineral decrements in survivors of childhood acute lymphoblastic leukemia: frequency of occurrence and risk factors for their development. Leukemia 15:728–734

Kauczor H-U, Brix G, Dietl B et al (1993) Bone marrow after autologous blood stem cell transplantation and total body irradiation: magnetic resonance and chemical shift imaging. Magn Reson Imaging 11:965–975

Kaufman IA, Kung FH, Koenig HM et al (1976) Overdosage with vincristine. J Pediatr 89:671–674

Kiraly JF, Wheby MS (1976) Bone marrow necrosis. Am J Med 60:361–368

Kleinberg L, Grossman S, Piantadosi S (1999) The effects of sequential versus concurrent chemotherapy and radiotherapy on survival and toxicity in patients with newly diagnosed high-grade astrocytoma. Int J Radiat Biol Phys 44:535–543

Kornreich L. Horev G, Yaniv I et al (1997) Iron overload following bone marrow transplantation in children: MR findings. Pediatr Radiol 27:869–872

Kovalic JJ, Thomas PR, Beckwith JB et al (1991) Hepatocellular carcinoma as second malignant neoplasms in successfully treated Wilms' tumor patients. Cancer 67:342–344

Kricun ME (1985) Red-yellow marrow conversion: its effect on the location of some solitary bone lesions. Skeletal Radiol 14:10–19

Kroger N, Hoffknecht M, Hanel M (1998) Busulfan, cyclophosphamide and etoposide as high-dose conditioning therapy in patients with malignant lymphoma and prior dose-limiting radiation therapy. Bone marrow transplant 21:1171–1175

Kushner BH, Cheung NK, Kramer K et al (1998) Neuroblastoma and treatment-related myelodysplasia/leukemia: the memorial Sloan-Kettering experience and a literature review. J Clin Oncol 16:3880–3889

Lanzkowsky P, Shende A, Karayalcin G et al (1976) Staging laparotomy and splenectomy: treatment and complications of Hodgkin's disease in children. Am J Hematol 1: 393–404

Libshitz HI (1994) Radiation changes in bone. Semin Roentgenol 29:15–37

Libshitz HI, Cohen MA (1982) Radiation-induced osteochondromas. Radiology 142:643–647

Libshitz HI, Edeiken BS (1981) Radiotherapy changes of the pediatric hip. AJR Am J Roentgenol 137:585–588

Lien HH, Blomlie V, Blystad AK et al (1997) Bone-marrow MR imaging before and after autologous marrow transplantation in lymphoma patients with known bone-marrow involvement. Acta Radiol 38:896–902

Lieschke GJ, Burgess AW (1992) Granulocyte colony stimulating factor and granulocyte-macrophage colony stimulating factor. N Engl J Med 327:28–35

Mackall CL, Fleicher TA, Brown MR et al (1997) Distinctions between CD8+ and CD4+ T cell regenerative pathways result in prolonged T cell subset imbalance after intensive chemotherapy. Blood 89:3700–3707

MacLennan IC, Kay HE, Festenstein M et al (1975) Analysis of treatments in childhood leukemia. I. Predisposition to methotrexate-induced neutropenia after craniospinal irradiation. Report to the Medical Research Council of the Working Party on Leukaemia in Childhood. BMJ 1: 563–567

Mankin HJ (1992) Nontraumatic necrosis of bone (osteonecrosis). N Engl J Med 22:1473–1479

Mason BA, Klug PP, Cohen SP (1978) Bone marrow necrosis during chemotherapy for lymphoma. JAMA 239: 1158–1162

Mauch P, Constine L, Greenberger J (1995) Hematopoietic stem cell compartment: acute and late effects of radiation therapy and chemotherapy. Int J Radiat Oncol Biol Phys 31:1319–1339

Meadows AT, Hobbie WL (1986) The medical consequences of cure. Cancer 58:524–528

Mehlman CT, Crawford AH, McMath JA (1999) Pediatric vertebral and spinal cord tumors: a retrospective study of musculoskeletal aspects of presentation, treatment and complications. Orthopedics 22:49–55

Mertens AC, Yasui Y, Neglia JP et al (2001) Late mortality experience in five-year survivors of childhood and adolescent cancer: the childhood cancer survivor study. J Clin Oncol 19:3163–3172

Mike V, Meadows AT, D'Angio GJ (1982) Incidence of second malignant neoplasms in children: results of an international study. Lancet 2:1326–1331

Mizutani N, Fujikura Y, Wang YH et al (2002) Inflammatory and anti-inflammatory cytokines regulate the recovery from sublethal x irradiation in rat thymus. Radiat Res 157:281–289

Moore SG, Dawson KL (1990) Red and yellow marrow in the femur: age-related changes in appearance at MR imaging. Radiology 175:219–223

Mullen LA, Berdon WE, Ruzal-Shapiro C et al (1995) Soft-tissue sarcomas: MR imaging findings after treatment in three pediatric patients. Radiology 195:413–417

Mumber MP, Greven KM, Haygood TM (1997) Pelvic insufficiency fractures associated with radiation atrophy: clinical recognition and diagnostic evaluation. Skeletal Radiol 26: 94–99

Murphy RG, Greenberg ML (1990) Osteonecrosis in pediatric patients with acute lymphoblastic leukemia. Cancer 65: 1717–1721

Neglia JP, Friedman DL, Yasui Y et al (2001) Second malignant neoplasms in five-year survivors of childhood cancer: childhood cancer survivor study. J Natl Cancer Inst 93: 618–629

Neglia JP, Meadows AT, Robison LL et al (1991) Second neoplasms after acute lymphoblastic leukemia in childhood. N Engl J Med 325:1330–1336

Neuhauser EBD, Wittenborg MH, Berman CZ et al (1952) Irradiation effects of roentgen therapy on the growing spine. Radiology 59:637–650

Newton WA, Meadows AT, Shimada H et al (1991) Bone sarcomas as second malignant neoplasms following childhood cancer. Cancer 67:193–201

Nicholson HS, Fears TR, Byrne J (1994) Death during adulthood in survivors of childhood and adolescent cancer. Cancer 73:3094–3102

Nogard MJ, Carpenter JT, Conrad ME (1979) Bone marrow necrosis and degeneration. Arch Intern Med 139:905–911

O'Regan S, Melhorn DK, Newman AJ (1973) Methotrexate-induced bone pain in childhood leukemia. Am J Dis Child 126:489–490

Oberfield SE, Allen JC, Pollack J et al (1986) Long-term endocrine sequelae after treatment of medulloblastoma: prospective study of growth and thyroid function. J Pediatr 108:219–223

Ojala AE, Paakko E, Lanning FP et al (1999) Osteonecrosis during the treatment of childhood acute lymphoblastic leukemia – a prospective MRI study. Med Pediatr Oncol 32:11–17

Oliff A, Bode V, Bercu BB et al (1979) Hypothalamic pituitary dysfunction following CNS prophylaxis in acute lymphocytic leukemia: correlation with CT scan abnormalities. Med Pediatr Oncol 7:141–151

Ortiz SS, Miller JH, Villablanca JG et al (1994) Bone abnormalities detected with skeletal scintigraphy after bone marrow harvest in patients with childhood neuroblastoma. Radiology 192:755–758

Pieters R, van Brenk AI, Veerman AJP et al (1987) Bone marrow magnetic resonance studies in childhood leukemia. Cancer 60:2994–3000

Polak JF, Jolesz FA, Adams DF (1988) Magnetic resonance imaging of skeletal muscle prolongation of T1 and T2 subsequent to denervation. Invest Radiol 23:365–369

Prindull G, Weigel W, Jentsch E et al (1982) Aseptic osteonecrosis in children treated for acute lymphoblastic leukemia and aplastic anemia. Eur J Pediatr 139:48–51

Probert JC, Parker BR (1975) The effects of radiation therapy on bone growth. Radiology 114:155–162

Pui C, Behm SG, Raimondi SC et al (1989) Secondary acute myeloid leukemia in children treated for acute lymphoid leukemia. N Engl J Med 321:136–142

Pui CH, Stass S, Green A (1985) Bone marrow necrosis in children with malignant disease. Cancer 56:1522–1525

Ragab AH, Frech RS, Vietti TJ (1969) Osteoporotic fractures secondary to methotrexate therapy of acute leukemia in remission. Cancer 25:580–585

Raje N, Anderson KC (2002) Thalidomide and immuno-modu-latory drugs as cancer therapy. Curr Opin Oncol 14:635–640

Rajkumar SV (2001) Current status of thalidomide in the treatment of cancer. Oncology (Huntingt) 15:867–874

Ramsey RG, Zacharias CE (1985) MR imaging of the spine after radiation therapy: easily recognizable effects. AJR Am J Roentgenol 144:1131–1135

Relf M. Boal DKB (1992) Rickets – a complication of ifosfamide chemotherapy for Wilms tumor. Pediatr Radiol 22:209–210

Remedios PA, Colletti PM, Raval JK et al (1988) Magnetic resonance imaging of bone after radiation. Magn Reson Imaging 6:301–304

Riseborough EJ, Grabias SL, Burton RI et al (1976) Skeletal alterations following irradiation for Wilms' tumor. J Bone Joint Surg (Am) 58:526–536

Robison LL, Nesbit ME, Sather HN et al (1985) Height of children successfully treated for acute lymphoblastic leukemia: a report from the Late effects study committee of children's cancer study group. Med Pediatr Oncol 13:14–21

Romshe CA, Zipf WB, Miser A et al (1984) Evaluation of growth hormone release and human growth hormone treatment in children with cranial irradiation – associated short stature. J Pediatr 104:177–181

Rossi R, Kleinebrand A, Gödde A et al (1993) Increased risk of ifosfamide-induced renal Fanconi's syndrome after unilateral nephrectomy. Lancet 341:755

Rosso P, Terracini B, Fears TR et al (1994) Second malignant tumors after elective end of therapy for a first cancer in childhood: a multicenter study in Italy. Int J Cancer 59: 451–456

Rubin P, Andrews JR, Swarm JR et al (1959) Radiation induced dysplasia of bone. Am J Roentgenol 82:206–216

Rubin P, Casarett GW (1968) Muscle. In: Rubin P, Casarett GW (eds) Clinical radiation pathology. WB Saunders, Philadelphia, pp 768–777

Rubin P, Johnston CJ, Williams JP et al (1995) A perpetual cascade of cytokines postirradiation leads to pulmonary fibrosis. Int J Radiat Oncol Biol Phys 33:99–109

Rubin P, Landman S, Mayer E et al (1973) Bone marrow regeneration and extension after extended field irradiation in Hodgkin's disease. Cancer 32:699–711

Rubin P, Wefer A, Hricak H et al (2002) Late effects. In: Bragg DG, Rubin P, Hricak H (eds) Oncologic imaging. WB Saunders, Philadelphia, pp 895–939

Ruzal-Shapiro C. Berdon WE, Cohen MD et al (1991) MR imaging of diffuse bone marrow replacement in patients with cancer. Radiology 181:587–589

Ryan SP, Weinberger E, White KS et al (1995) MR imaging of bone marrow in children with osteosarcoma: effect of granulocyte colony-stimulating factor. AJR Am J Roentgenol 165:915–920

Sacks EL, Goris ML, Glatstein E et al (1978) Bone marrow regeneration following large field radiation. Cancer 42: 1057–1065

Salgia R, Demetri GD, Kaplan WD (1994) Changes in Tc99m radionuclide bone scan images and peripheralization of marrow hematopoietic activity associated with the administration of granulocyte colony stimulating factor as an adjunct to dose-intensified chemotherapy for breast cancer. A case report. Cancer 74:1887–1890

Schick F, Einsele H, Weiss B et al (1996) Assessment of the composition of bone marrow prior to and following autologous BMT and PBSCT by magnetic resonance. Ann Hematol 72:361–370

Schwartz AM, Leonidas JC (1984) Methotrexate osteopathy. Skeletal Radiol 11:13–16

Shalet SM, Beardwell CG, Jones PH et al (1976) Growth hormone deficiency after treatment of acute leukemia in children. Arch Dis Child 51:489–493

Shalet SM, Price DA, Beardwell CG et al (1979) Normal growth despite abnormalities of growth hormone secretion in children treated for acute leukemia. J Pediatr 94:719–722

Smith MB, Xue H, Strong S, Takahashi H et al (1993) Forty-year experience with second malignancies after treatment of childhood cancer: analysis of outcome following the development of the second malignancy. J Pediatr Surg 28:1342–1348

Smith SR, Roberts N, Edwards RHT (1991) Marrow repopulation after bone marrow transplantation. Radiology 178:581

Smith, SR, Williams CE, Edwards RHT et al (1989) Quantitative magnetic resonance imaging in autologous bone marrow transplantation for Hodgkin's disease. Br J Cancer 60: 961–965

Socie G, Curtis RE, Deeg HJ et al (2000) New malignant diseases after allogeneic marrow transplantation for childhood acute leukemia. J Clin Oncol 18:348–357

Sovik E, Lein HH, Tveit KM (1993) Postirradiation changes in the pelvic wall. Findings on MR. Acta Radiol 34:573–576

Stanisavljevic S, Babcock AL (1977) Fractures in children treated with methotrexate for leukemia. Clin Orthop 125:139–144

Stevens SK, Moore SG, Amylon MD (1990a) Repopulation of marrow after transplantation: MR imaging with pathologic correlation. Radiology 175:213–218

Stevens SK, Moore SG, Kaplan ID (1990b) Early and late bone-marrow changes after irradiation: MR evaluation. AJR Am J Roentgenol 154: 745–750

Strauss AJ, Su JT, Dalton VM et al (2001) Bone morbidity in children treated for acute lymphoblastic leukemia. J Clin Oncol 19:3066–3072

Sugimura H, Kisanuki A, Tamura S et al (1994) Magnetic resonance imaging of bone marrow changes after irradiation. Invest Radiology 29:35–41

Tanner SF, Clarke J, Leach MO et al (1996) MRI in the evaluation of late bone marrow changes following bone marrow transplantation. Br J Radiol 69:1145–1151

Tefft M, Lattin PB, Jereb et al (1976) Acute and late effects on normal tissue following combined chemo – and radiotherapy for childhood rhabdomyosarcoma and Ewing's sarcoma. Cancer 37:1201–1207

Timothy AR, Tucker AK (1978) Osteonecrosis in Hodgkin's disease. Br J Radiol 51:328

Tordiglione M, Kalli M, Vavassori V et al (1998) Combined modality treatment for esophageal cancer. Tumors 84:252–258

Totty WG, Murphy WA, Ganz WI et al (1984) Magnetic resonance imaging of the normal and ischemic femoral head. AJR Am J Roentgenol 143:1273–1280

Trobaugh-Lotrario AD, Smith AA, Odom LF (2003) Vincristine neurotoxicity in the presence of hereditary neuropathy. Med Pediatr Oncol 40:39–43

Tucker MA, Coleman CN, Cox RS et al (1988) Risk of second cancers after treatment for Hodgkin's disease. N Eng J Med 318:76–81

Tucker MA, D'Angio GJ, Boice JD Jr et al (1987) Bone sarcomas linked to radiotherapy and chemotherapy in children. N Engl J Med 317:588–593

Unger HR, Ryan KP, Shelton DK et al (1990) False positive MRI for malignancy involving vertebral marrow of patients treated with neupogen. Presented at ASNR 30th Annual Meeting, St. Louis, MO, 31 May-June 5

Valagussa P, Santoro A, Fossati-Bellani F et al (1986) Second acute leukemia and other malignancies following treatment for Hodgkin's disease. J Clin Oncol 4:830–837

Van der Meeren A, Monti P, Lebaron-Jacobs L et al (2001) Characterization of the acute inflammatory response after irradiation in mice and its regulation by interleukin 4 (Il4). Radiat Res 155:858–865

van Leeuwen FE, Chorus AM, van den Belt-Dusebout AW et al (1994) Leukemia risk following Hodgkin's disease: relation to cumulative dose of alkylating agents, treatment with teniposide combinations, number of episodes of chemotherapy and bone marrow damage. J Clin Oncol 12:1063–1073

Veda M. Harada M, Shiobara S et al (1984) T lymphocyte reconstitution in long-erm survivors after allogeneic and autologous marrow transplantation. Transplantation 37:552–556

Vogler JB, Murphy WA (1988) Bone marrow imaging. Radiology 168:679–693

Watanabe N, DeRosa SC, Cmelak A et al (1997) Long-term depletion of naive T cells in patients treated for Hodgkin's disease. Blood 90:3662–3672

Weisdorf DJ (1987) Bone marrow transplantation for acute leukemia. Invest Radiol 22:839–846.

Weissman DE, Negendank WG, Al-Katib AM et al (1992) Bone marrow necrosis in lymphoma studied by magnetic resonance imaging. Am J Hematol 40:42–46

Wells RJ, Foster MB, D'Ercole AJ et al (1983) The impact of cranial irradiation on the growth of children with acute lymphocytic leukemia. Am J Dis Child 137:37–39

Wheeler DL, Vander Griend RA, Wronski TJ et al (1995) The short- and long-term effects of methotrexate on the rat skeleton. Bone 16:215–221

Withers HR, McBride WH (1998) Biologic basis of radiation therapy. In: Perez CA, Brady LW (eds) Principles and practice of radiation oncology. Lippincott-Raven, Philadelphia, pp 79–118

Wolf EL, Berdon WE, Cassady JR et al (1977) Slipped femoral capital epiphysis as a sequela to childhood irradiation for malignant tumors. Radiology 125:781–784

Yankelevitz DF, Henschke CI, Knapp PH et al (1991) Effect of radiation therapy on thoracic and lumbar bone marrow: evaluation with MR imaging. AJR Am J Roentgenol 157:87–92

26 Percutaneous Image-Guided Lymph Node Needle Biopsy

Ali Guermazi and Gerald D. Dodd III

CONTENTS

26.1
Introduction

Open surgical biopsy has long been considered the conventional gold standard for obtaining thoracic and abdominal lymph node samples in patients with lymphoma, especially for the original diagnosis. However, this procedure can have significant complications. With advances in cytopathologic diagnostic techniques, percutaneous image-guided needle biopsy with its high overall accuracy has become the procedure of choice, and is taking a prominent place in the management of lymphoma in both adults and children. It is now considered a relatively painless, quick, safe, low cost, and valuable tool for patients with suspected or recurrent lymphomas. A well-planned and executed biopsy provides an accurate diagnosis and facilitates treatment. CT is a widely available imaging modality and allows image-guided needle biopsy in a large majority of

Ali Guermazi, MD
Visiting Associate Professor, Department of Radiology, University of California San Francisco, 350 Parnassus Avenue, Suite 150, San Francisco, CA 94117, USA
Gerald D. Dodd III, MD
Professor and Chairman, Department of Radiology, University of Texas Health Science Center at San Antonio, 7703 Floyd Curl Drive, San Antonio, TX 78284, USA

patients. US-guided biopsy is an alternative method of guidance and at some institutions is the guidance technique of choice. In this chapter, we will describe the technique and give some alternatives for when the procedure tends to be difficult, especially in posterior and/or deep-seated lymph nodes.

26.2
Background

Among all diseases that can be diagnosed by image-guided needle biopsy, lymphomas are probably the greatest challenge for the pathologist. Indeed, tissue sampling should allow not only diagnosis but also accurate subtyping of the disease prior to initiation of therapy. Moreover, it is sometimes difficult to differentiate lymphomas from other lymphoproliferative diseases, benign hyperplasia, primary tumors or metastases, or even infectious processes. Therefore, for many years patients with suspected lymphomas have undergone excisional lymph node biopsy rather than a needle biopsy. Because of progress in tissue sampling and immunochemistry studies, image-guided needle biopsy has been advocated as the method of choice to obtain an accurate pathologic diagnosis (Silverman et al. 1994; Demharter et al. 2001).

26.3
Prebiopsy Procedures

In the absence of peripheral lymph nodes in patients with lymphoma, image-guided needle biopsy should be used judiciously and preferably as part of a multidisciplinary team discussion. Consultation with the referring physician should always be employed to clarify objectives, approach, and to identify potential risks of the procedure. Often, the consultation may lead to a change in the initial management plan or the proposed diagnostic procedure. For instance, the imaging findings might suggest a significantly different diagnosis than that being considered by the referring physician, or indicate a more plausible biopsy site over that originally chosen. This multidisciplinary approach also allows the identification of and potential resolution of contraindications for percutaneous biopsy under local anesthesia, such as patients with uncontrollable movements, or coagulopathies (platelets < 50,000/mm³, anemia < 8 g/dl, prothrombin time < 50%, INR > 2) (DEMHARTER et al. 2001).

The procedure should be explained to the patient and informed consent obtained. In children, informed consent should be obtained from their parents (SKLAIR-LEVY et al. 2001). Informed consent should include a review of the proposed procedure, the reason for choosing to perform a biopsy, the potential risks and benefits of the procedure, and alternative diagnostic techniques. In preparation an intravenous catheter should be placed for vascular access. It can be used for administration of anesthetics if necessary, and is absolutely essential for the treatment of potential complications such as a vasovagal reflex, anaphalaxic reaction, coronary arrest, or severe hemorrhage. This low cost procedure is typically performed on an outpatient basis and rarely requires hospitalization (DEMHARTER et al. 2001).

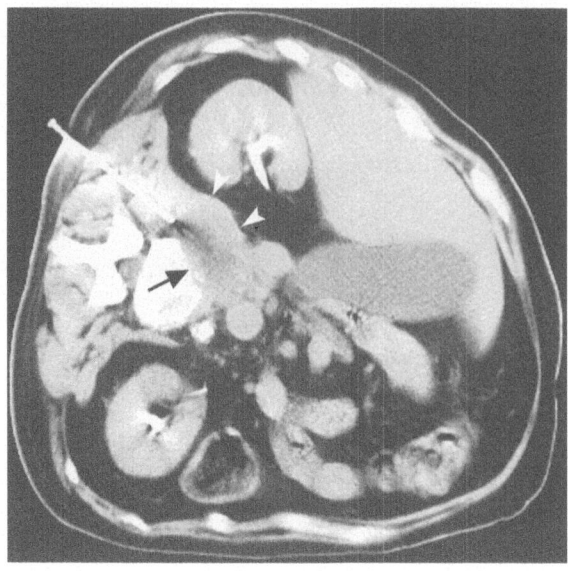

Fig. 26.1. Lateral decubitus positioning in a 56-year-old man who underwent CT-guided biopsy for paravertebral lymph node mass. The patient had undergone treatment for Hodgkin disease with complete remission. Axial contrast-enhanced CT scan of the abdomen shows the biopsy is performed in a lateral approach. The 16-Gauge needle is inserted into the right paraspinous muscle with its tip touching the proximal edge of the retroperitoneal paravertebral mass (*arrowheads*). There is associated erosion by the lymph node mass of the anterior border of the vertebrae (*arrow*). Histologic examination revealed recurrent Hodgkin disease.

26.4
Biopsy Technique

Proper positioning is important for the comfort of the patient and for the success of the procedure. The patient may be supine or prone, or even in the lateral decubitus position (Fig. 26.1) depending on lesion location. The vertical and horizontal approaches are preferable when using CT scanning to guide the procedure, although, oblique approaches (Fig. 26.2), while more challenging, can be used. With US guidance, complex angulation is less problematic with the approach typically dictated by intervening anatomy and adequate visualization of the biopsy site.

After disinfecting and sterilely draping the skin of the patient, local anesthesia is given. For children, general anesthesia may sometimes be required (SKLAIR-LEVY et al. 2001). When US guidance is to be used, the transducer should be sterilized or covered with a sterile sheath. For both CT and US guidance, limited scanning is performed to localize the lesion and determine its margins, to determine the entry

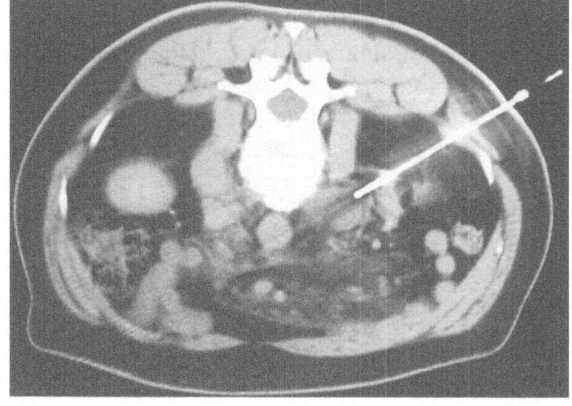

Fig. 26.2. Oblique approach in a 60-year-old man who underwent CT-guided biopsy for paraaortic mass. Axial CT scan of the abdomen obtained with the patient in the prone position shows the 16-Gauge needle inserted coaxially through a 17-Gauge needle and entering the paraaortic lymph node mass. Histologic examination revealed follicular mixed non-Hodgkin lymphoma.

site of the needle and to document needle progression to the depth of the target. Needle advancement is performed while respiration is suspended. If inadequate, the needle placement is readjusted, and the patient is scanned again until satisfactory needle positioning is achieved. US-guided biopsy has had the advantage of a real time procedure; recently a new method has been reported using real-time CT fluoroscopy, which provides effective real-time reconstruction and display of CT images (KATADA et al. 1996). Although it is a useful targeting technique, significant radiation exposure may result in spite of the possible use of needle holders (KATO et al. 1996). Thus, it is indicated mainly for guiding external compression and needle placement into lesions that may be considered difficult with standard CT assistance (SCHWEIGER et al. 2000). Other advantages of US over CT are the possibility of reducing the skin-to-lesion distance by transducer compression, multiplanar capability, lack of ionizing radiation, and mobility of the equipment (FISHER et al. 1997).

At the time of the biopsy, the physician should avoid blood vessels to avoid the risk of hemorrhage (Fig. 26.3). When performing the procedure using CT guidance, this may be achievable by the administration of intravenous contrast material (HUSSAIN et al. 2001).

This also may help to visualize necrosis in the lymph node mass (Fig. 26.4) and so avoid histological negative results by sampling viable tissue (SKLAIR-LEVY et al. 2000). Indeed, most biopsies should be directed such that the outer margin of the lesion is sampled, as it is the area least likely to be necrotic. When performing a biopsy using US guidance, color Doppler should be used to identify and avoid blood vessels within the anticipated path of the biopsy needle (Fig. 26.5). Image guided biopsy should also avoid targeting nerves because of pain, and the large bowel to avoid perforation and subsequent infection. Although it is preferable to avoid transgressing the small bowel, in practice narrow gauge needles can be passed through it with little risk of complications. Both large and small bowel are easily identified by CT after the administration of oral contrast material; however, visualization of the bowel by US is more difficult and often requires close anatomic correlation with a previous CT scan. No biopsy should be performed without confirmation of the precise location of the tip of the biopsy needle. When using an automated biopsy "gun", care must be exercised to assure that an adequate amount of tissue is present to accommodate the full excursion of the needle; failure to do so may result in unintentional injury to vital structures adjacent to the nodal mass.

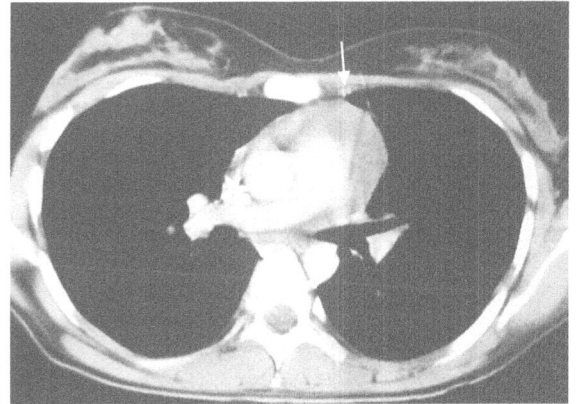

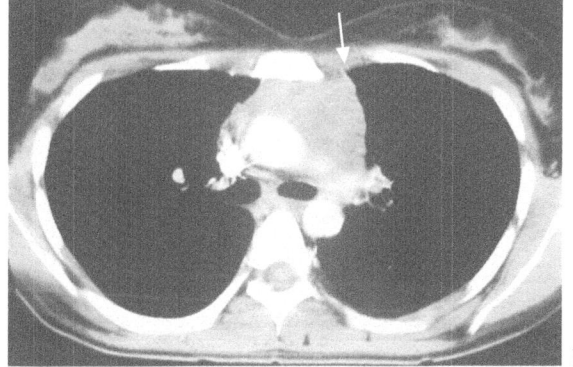

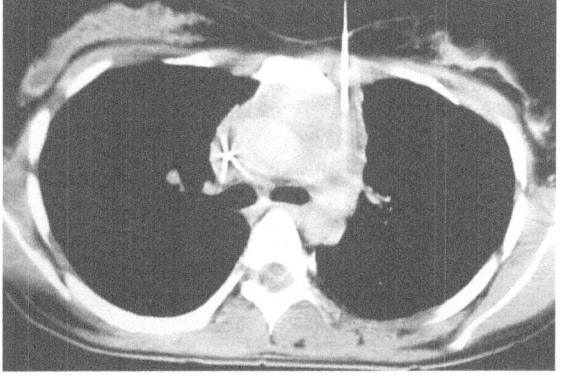

Fig. 26.3a–c. Anterior thoracic approach in a 25-year-old woman who underwent CT-guided biopsy for anterior mediastinal mass. a, b Axial contrast-enhanced CT scans of the thorax before the procedure clearly delineate the anterior mediastinal mass and identify the left internal mammary (*arrow*) as well as the mediastinal vessels. They also allow choosing the best entry site for the biopsy. c At the time of biopsy, the 14-Gauge needle is placed in the mass, avoiding the vessels. Histologic examination revealed Hodgkin disease.

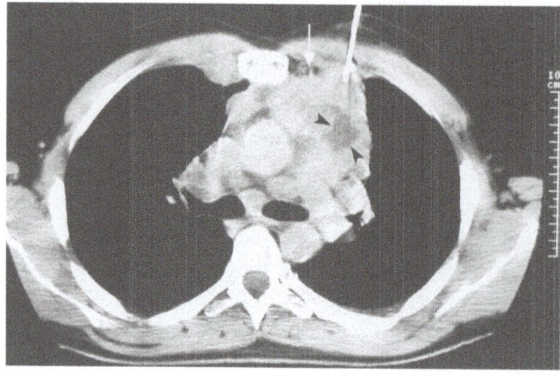

Fig. 26.4. Anterior thoracic approach in a 32-year-old man who underwent CT-guided biopsy for anterior mediastinal mass. Axial contrast-enhanced CT scan of the thorax at the time of biopsy clearly shows the necrosis (*arrowheads*) in the anterior mediastinal mass and identifies the left internal mammary vessels (*arrow*) as well as the mediastinal vessels. The 14-Gauge needle is placed in the outer margin of the lesion, away from the necrosis. Histologic examination revealed Hodgkin disease.

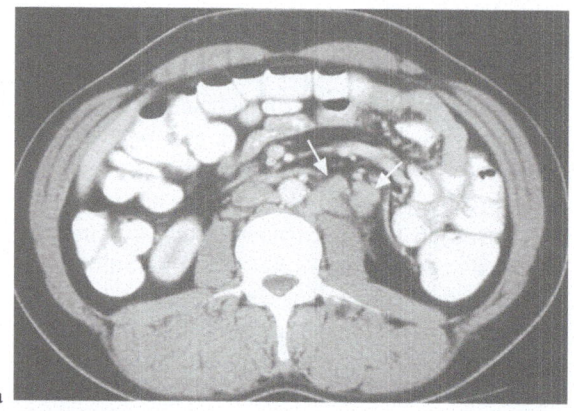

a

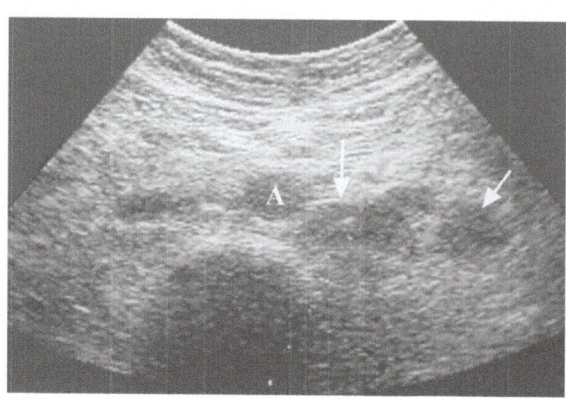

b

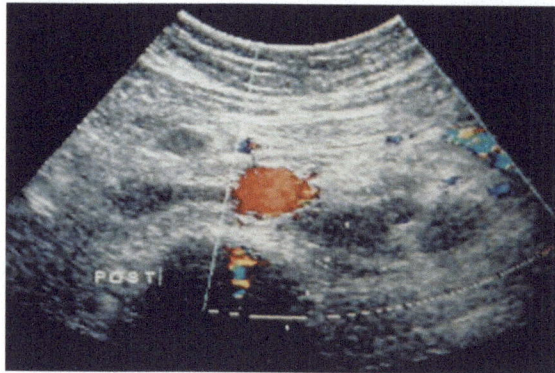

c

Fig. 26.5a–c. Anterior abdominal approach in a 23-year-old man who underwent US-guided biopsy for deep paraaortic lymph node. a Axial contrast-enhanced CT scan through mid-abdomen shows left paraaortic lymph node (*arrows*). b Transverse US image shows biopsy guide track projected over lymph node (*arrows*) to left of aorta (*A*). c Transverse color Doppler US image confirms no flow in the paraaortic lymph node and also avoids blood vessels within the path of the biopsy needle. Histologic examination revealed non-Hodgkin lymphoma.

Unlike fine-needle aspiration biopsy which yields a pathologic diagnosis in only two-thirds of cases, larger gauge percutaneous cutting needles or core needle biopsy needles yield large specimens that are amenable to histologic analysis and subtyping (Zinzani et al. 1998; Demharter et al. 2001; Sklair-Levy et al. 2001). The simplified coaxial technique is now widely performed in thoracic, abdominal and pelvic approaches. Its main advantage is its ability to sample several core specimens with a single biopsy tract (Moulton and Moore 1993), allowing an accurate and reproducible insertion of flexible needles especially for deep biopsy of small lymph nodes (Fig. 26.6) (Jeffrey 1988). The biopsy sample should be large enough to enable the pathologic diagnosis and to grade specimens. This goal is usually best reached with a 16 gauge biopsy needle (de Kerviler et al. 2000; Demharter et al. 2001); but an 18 or 20 gauge needle is also efficient (Ben-Yehuda et al. 1996). An automated-gun biopsy device is now recommended (Protopapas and Westcott 2000) and the number of passes is determined according to the amount of biopsy material obtained.

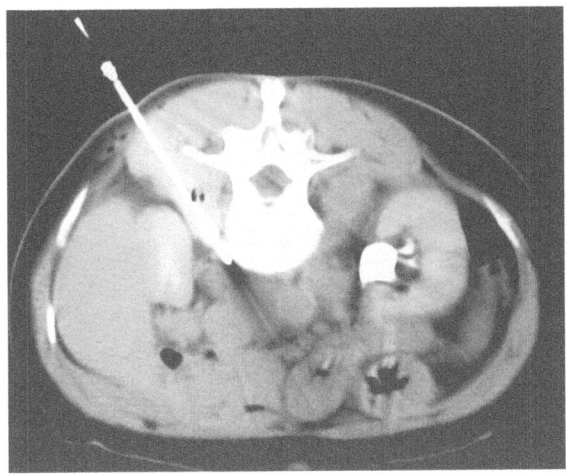

Fig. 26.6. Prone positioning in a 59-year-old woman who underwent CT-guided biopsy for deep retrocaval lymph node mass. Axial contrast-enhanced CT scan through the mid-abdomen shows the oblique approach of the 16-Gauge biopsy needle inserted coaxially through a 17-Gauge needle and entering the retrocaval lymph node mass. This allows getting 4 core specimens with a single biopsy tract. Histologic examination revealed non-Hodgkin lymphoma.

26.4.1
Thoracic Biopsy

The histologic diagnosis of mediastinal lymphoma has always been problematic. Imaging guidance should enable an individualized approach to mediastinal lymph nodes to avoid penetration of the visceral pleura, large blood vessels, and the bronchial tree. Fluoroscopy guided biopsy has been employed in the past with much success. This widely available technique is usually performed in large anterior mediastinal masses > 4 cm, and located at maximum 3 cm from the chest wall (ZINZANI et al. 1999). US-guided biopsy allows for real time cross-sectional monitoring during the biopsy, but requires an adequate sonographic window. It is mainly used for biopsy of mediastinal masses that extend to the anterior chest wall (PROTOPAPAS and WESTCOTT 2000). It may also be used for large mediastinal masses in children (GARRETT et al. 2002). The development of new guidance techniques for percutaneous biopsy under CT control has changed the approach to the routine diagnosis of mediastinal lymphoma (SKLAIR-LEVY et al. 2000). Indeed, CT is now the preferred method, allowing biopsy of small and deep mediastinal lesions. CT is also useful with large lesions close to the chest wall to avoid extensive necrotic areas (ZINZANI et al. 1999). Contrast-enhanced CT is usually needed to determine the relationship of the lesion to adjacent cardiovascular structures (Fig. 26.7).

For staging lymphomas, biopsy specimens should be placed in formalin so that monoclonal antibody analysis (LCA, CD 3, CD 20, CD 30, CD 35, CD 68, CD 79 a, bcl-2), can be performed to determine cell lineage and histologic subtypes. An additional specimen should be frozen for subsequent immunochemistry, cytogenetic and molecular analyses (CARRASCO et al. 1990; BEN-YEHUDA et al. 1996; PAPPA et al. 1996).

US or CT scanning is performed routinely immediately after the procedure to detect possible complications. Patients should than be monitored in the adjacent nursing area for 2–4 hours, and discharged only if there are no signs or symptoms suggestive of complication. Patients are told to call the physician in the event of a complication or unexpected symptoms (SKLAIR-LEVY et al. 2000).

Several authors stress the importance of performing a repeat image-guided needle biopsy when the results of the first biopsy are either negative or insufficient for a confident diagnosis (WITTICH et al. 1992; SILVERMAN et al. 1994; BEN-YEHUDA et al. 1996; PAPPA et al. 1996; PROTOPAPAS and WESTCOTT 1997; SKLAIR-LEVY et al. 2000). The radiologist should bear in mind how the first biopsy was performed so that the technique might be altered as necessary to yield diagnostic tissue.

An anterior parasternal approach is preferred for most anterior mediastinal masses, whereas a posterior paravertebral approach is used for posterior mediastinal masses (Fig. 26.8) (PROTOPAPAS and WESTCOTT 2000). Care must be taken during the anterior approach to avoid the internal mammary vessels (Figs. 26.7, 26.9) (MOULTON 1993). Anterior and middle mediastinal masses superior to the heart have different approaches according to their location. Right-sided masses located anterior to the superior vena cava can undergo biopsy using an anterior approach, whereas right paratracheal and retrotracheal masses usually require a right posterior paravertebral approach. Although this approach is deep, it avoids puncture of the superior vena cava (PROTOPAPAS and WESTCOTT 2000). Nevertheless, traversing the vena cava with an anterior approach for biopsy of juxtatracheal lymphadenopathy has been reported without complications (PROTOPAPAS and WESTCOTT 1997). Midline (retrosternal) masses can undergo biopsy by a trans-sternal approach if they are not easily accessible parasternally (HAGBERG et al. 2000). Aortopulmonary lymph nodes are reached using a left anterior parasternal approach. Subcarinal

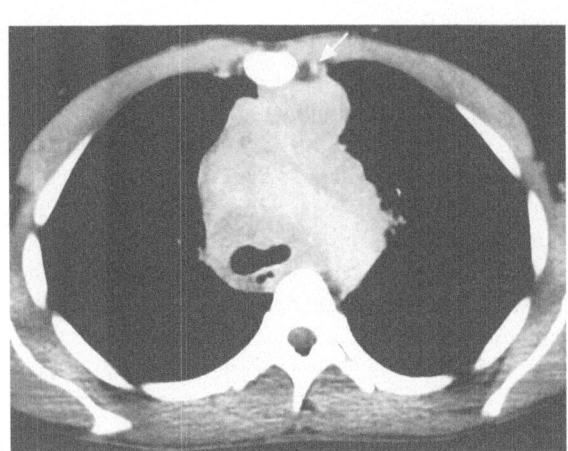
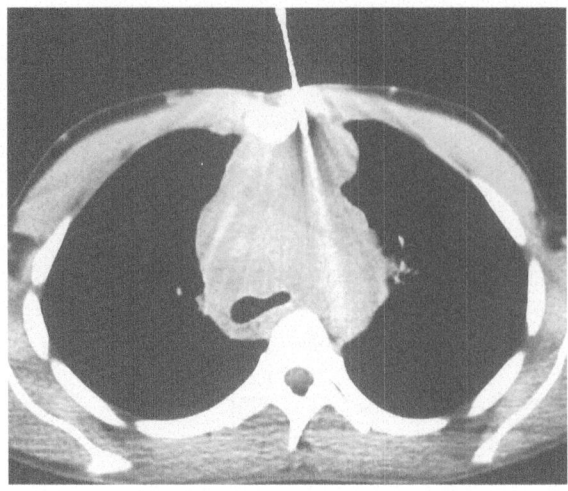

Fig. 26.7a,b. Left parasternal approach in a 27-year-old man who underwent CT-guided biopsy for anterior mediastinal mass. **a** Axial contrast-enhanced CT scan of the chest before the procedure clearly delineates the anterior mediastinal mass and identifies the left internal mammary (*arrow*) as well as the mediastinal vessels. **b** Axial CT scan at the time of biopsy shows the 14-Gauge needle is placed parasternally in the outer margin of the lesion. Histologic examination revealed B-cell non-Hodgkin lymphoma.

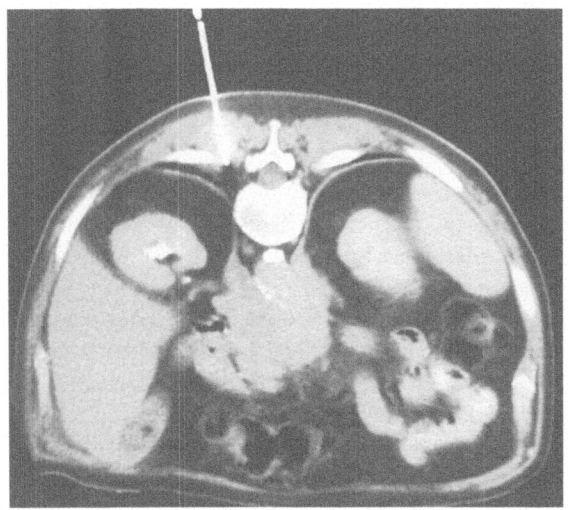
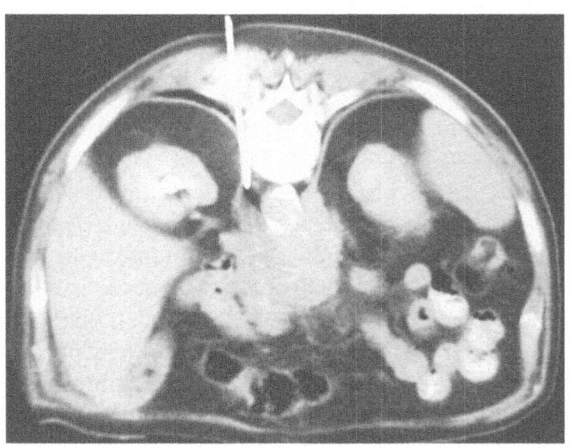

Fig. 26.8a,b. Right posterior paravertebral approach in a 72-year-old man who underwent CT-guided biopsy for posterior inferior mediastinal and upper abdominal lymph node mass. **a** Axial contrast-enhanced CT scan of the upper abdomen obtained with the patient in the prone position shows the 16-Gauge needle is placed medially to the very distal part of the right pleural sulcus. **b** Final localizing axial CT scan shows the needle is placed in the lymph node mass after entering the posterior inferior mediastinum via the connective tissue space between the descending aorta and spine. Histologic examination revealed non-Hodgkin lymphoma.

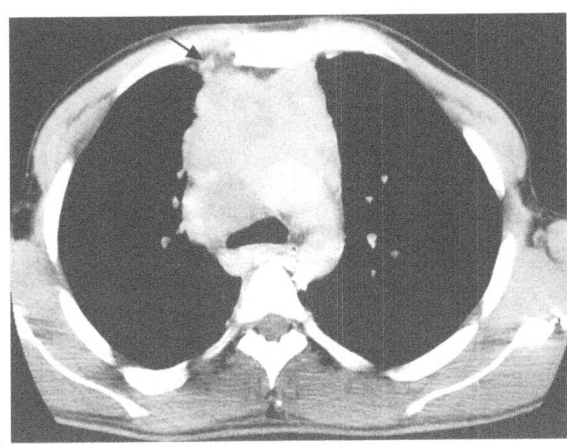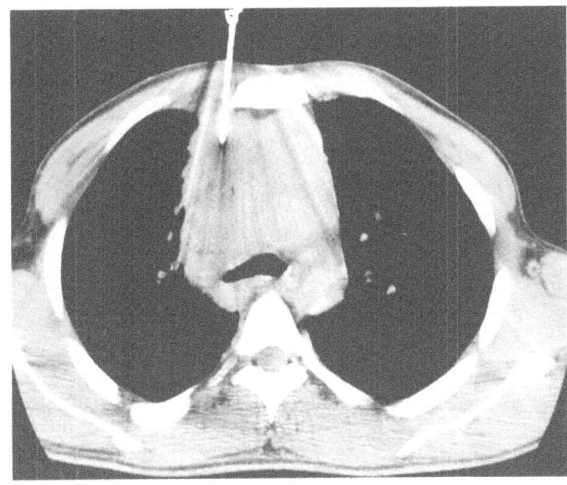

a
b

Fig. 26.9a,b. Right parasternal approach in a 30-year-old man who underwent CT-guided biopsy for anterior mediastinal mass. a Axial contrast-enhanced CT scan of the thorax obtained before the procedure delineates clearly the anterior mediastinal mass and identifies the right internal mammary (*arrow*) as well as the mediastinal vessels. b Axial CT scan at the time of biopsy shows the 14-Gauge needle is placed parasternally in the outer margin of the lesion. Histologic examination revealed Hodgkin disease.

masses are usually accessed using a right posterior paravertebral approach by entering the mediastinum via the connective tissue space between the descending aorta and spine, but occasionally they may be reached with a left parasternal approach. Hilar masses may be accessed by an anterior, posterior, or lateral approach depending on the relationship of the mass to the hilar vessels (PROTOPAPAS and WESTCOTT 2000).

Whenever possible, a direct mediastinal approach is preferable to a transpulmonary one, to avoid risk of pneumothorax. A simple way to improve the approach to the mediastinal lymph nodes is to change the patient's position. Placing the patient in the lateral decubitus or oblique position may put an unreachable anterior mass sufficiently in contact with the anterior parasternal chest wall to allow a direct mediastinal approach (BRESSLER and KIRKHAM 1994). The injection of 60 to 180 mL of normal saline solution, mixed or not with 1–2 mL of contrast material, into the paravertebral or substernal extrapleural space may also be useful for creating or expanding an extrapleural window for a direct mediastinal approach (Fig. 26.10). No pneumothoraces or bleeding complications occurred, and only mild discomfort was reported during creation of the posterior pathway (MOULTON 1993).

An artificial pleural window for mediastinal biopsy has been described. The pleural space leading to the lesion is widened by an existing effusion or expanded by creation of an iatrogenic pneumothorax to avoid puncturing the visceral pleura. After

positioning maneuvers, a pleural effusion ipsilateral to the mediastinal mass may interpose between the skin entry site and the lesion, providing a pleural window that avoids traversing lung parenchyma (BRESSLER and KIRKHAM 1994).

A suprasternal approach under CT or US guidance has been reported for large anterior and right paratracheal masses. The patient is imaged in a semicoronal position allowing for direct visualization of the needle path (BRESSLER and KIRKHAM 1994; DODD et al. 1996; ESOLA et al. 1997).

26.4.2
Abdominal Biopsy

CT is generally considered the guidance technique of choice for biopsy of abdominal, pelvic and retroperitoneal lymph nodes. US has been reserved traditionally for biopsy of masses in superficial locations. However, at some centers it has become the guidance technique of choice for deep nodes as small as 1 cm in diameter (Fig. 26.11). It is a technique that requires specific training but once learned has the advantages of real-time guidance, speed, direct compression of the abdominal wall, and low cost. The use of US for this application may be limited by lack of visualization of the biopsy site and intervening bowel (MEMEL et al. 1996; FISHER et al. 1997).

In abdominal image-guided needle biopsy, the needle should progress through the peritoneal and

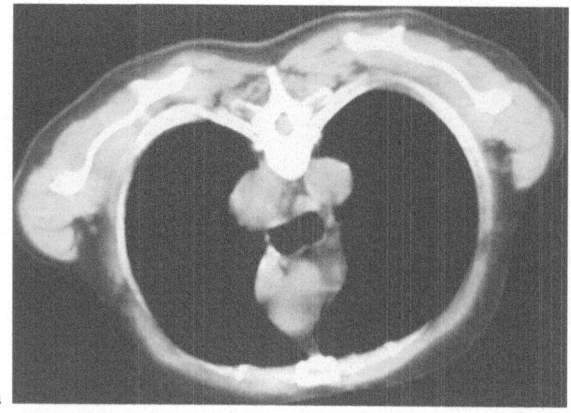

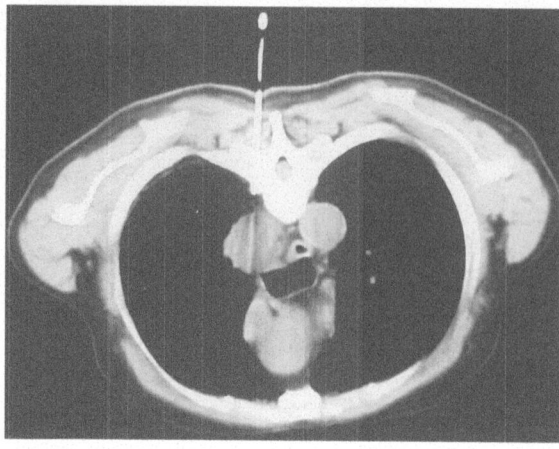

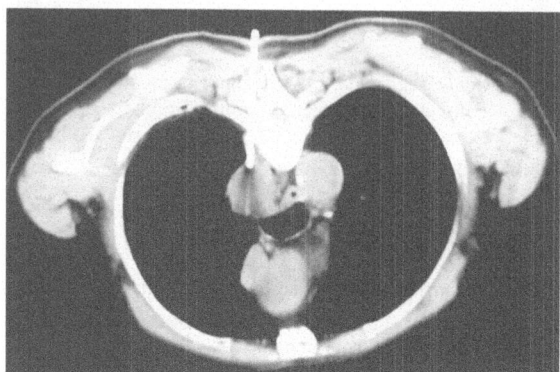

Fig. 26.10a–c. Prone positioning in a 64-year-old man who underwent CT-guided biopsy for deep subcarinal lymph nodes mass. **a** Axial CT scan of the thorax before the procedure shows subcarinal lymph node mass. **b** Axial CT scan at the time of biopsy shows the vertical approach of the 18-Gauge biopsy needle entering the mediastinum via the connective tissue space between the paravertebral parietal pleura and spine. **c** Final localizing axial CT scan shows the lymph node mass is easily reached through a direct mediastinal tract after injecting 40 mL of normal saline solution into paravertebral space resulting into an expansion of the extrapleural window. Histologic examination revealed non-Hodgkin lymphoma.

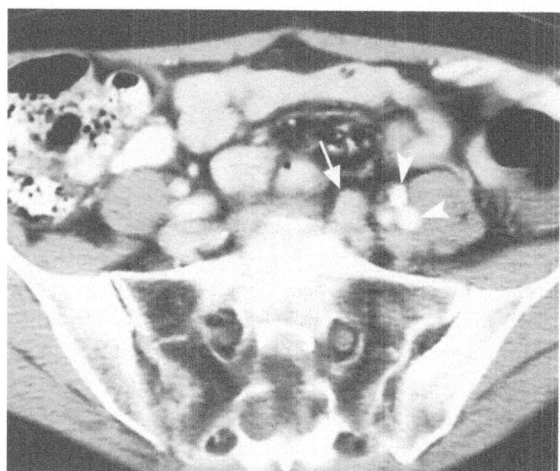

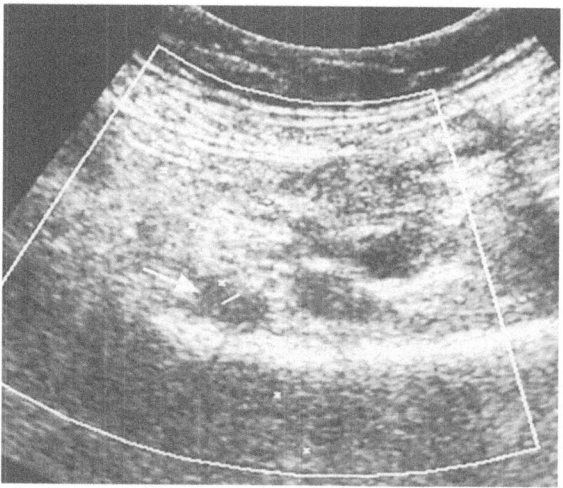

Fig. 26.11a,b. Anterior pelvic approach in a 48-year-old woman who underwent US-guided biopsy for deep left common iliac lymph node. **a** Axial contrast-enhanced CT scan of the pelvis shows a lymph node (*arrow*) medial to the left common iliac vessels (*arrowheads*) and resting on the sacrum. **b** Transverse US image shows biopsy guide track projected over hypoechoic iliac lymph node (*arrow*). The route to the lymph node is safe, without intervening vascular structures. Histologic examination revealed non-Hodgkin lymphoma.

retroperitoneal fat, and avoid traversing digestive structures, kidneys, pancreas and spleen. It may traverse the hepatic parenchyma safely if needed (Fig. 26.12).

When needed, a gantry angulation may be implemented in upper abdomen CT-guided percutaneous biopsy to avoid vital structures such as pleura (HUSSAIN 1996). This safe method was first used for percutaneous biopsy but may also be implemented for lymph node biopsy. In the same way, profound expiration may be useful in diminishing the depth of the posterior pleural sulcus, thereby avoiding the pneumothorax during a dorsal or lateral approach of the upper abdominal lymph node (Fig. 26. 13) (DE KERVILER et al. 1998).

For the biopsy of retroperitoneal lymph nodes using CT guidance, a dorsal approach is ordinarily implemented with the patient prone. If there is no intervening transverse process it is possible to insert the needle directly vertically into the paraspinous muscle, thus avoiding any angulation (Figs. 26.14–26.16) (JEFFREY 1988). For the deep retroperitoneal lymph nodes and especially those located in the midline retroperitoneum or of small size, bowel loops can still block the projected pathway of the needle (DE KERVILER et al. 1996). The large bowel should be avoided to prevent leaking bacteria into the peritoneal cavity and the possibility of peritoni-

tis. Traversing the colon may be a rare factor in the development of postbiopsy pancreatitis (DACHMAN 1998). There are some very effective techniques for active displacement of anatomic structures from the needle pathway. Among them, abdominal compression (Fig. 26.17) is now probably the most efficient and easy to implement, allowing the displacement of bowel during retroperitoneal biopsies. The patient is placed in the supine position and the entry site of the needle is chosen adjacent to the outer surface of bowel. To move the bowel from the preferred trajec-

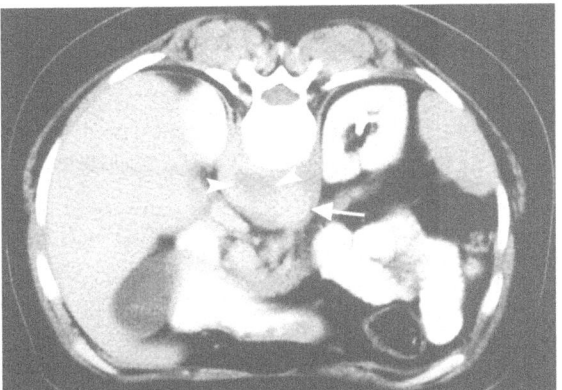

a

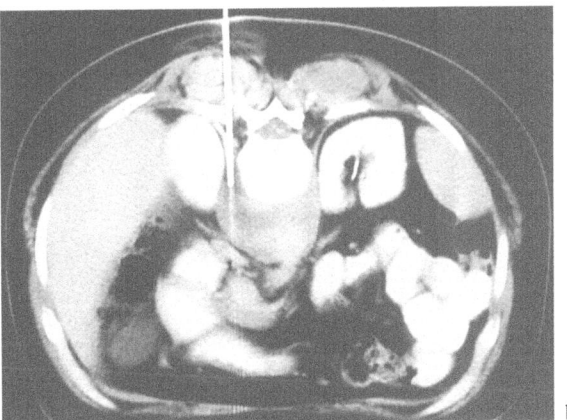

b

Fig. 26.13a,b. Right posterior paravertebral approach in a 51-year-old woman who underwent CT-guided biopsy for posterior inferior mediastinal and upper abdominal lymph node mass. a Axial contrast-enhanced CT scan of the upper abdomen obtained before the procedure and with the patient in the prone position and during suspended respiration shows a paravertebral mass encasing the aorta (*arrow*) with hypodense area corresponding to necrosis (*arrowheads*). The very distal part of the right pleural sulcus is still visible. b Final localizing axial CT scan obtained at the same level as (a) and after profound expiration shows the 16-Gauge needle is placed in the lymph node mass and the right pleural sulcus is no longer visible. The tip of the needle is placed away from the necrosis. The histologic examination revealed small cleaved cell follicular non-Hodgkin lymphoma.

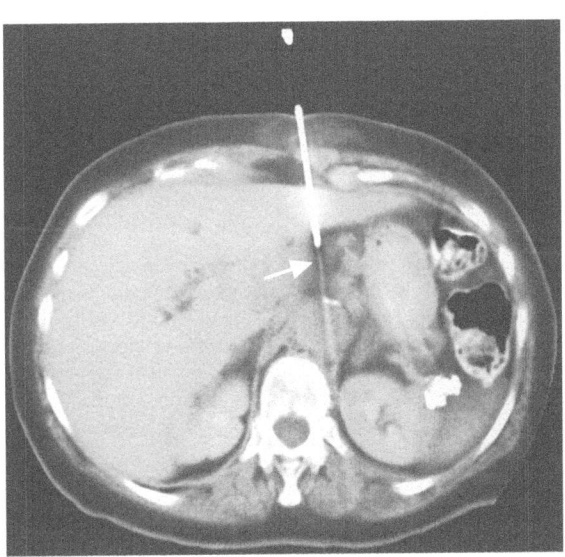

Fig. 26.12. Transhepatic approach in an 80-year-old woman who underwent CT-guided biopsy for small hepatic hilar lymph node. Axial CT scan of the upper abdomen shows the 18-Gauge needle is traversing the left liver lobe and is placed in the lymph node (*arrow*). Histologic examination revealed non-Hodgkin lymphoma.

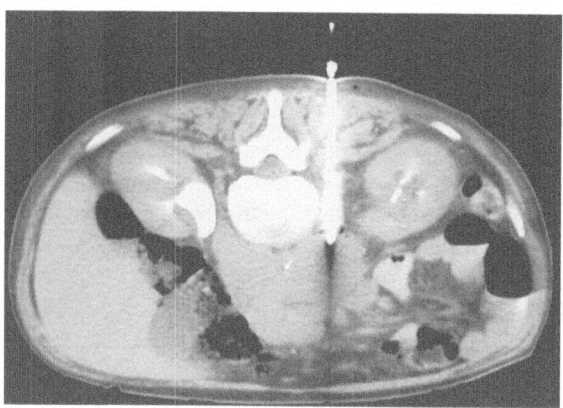

Fig. 26.14. Prone positioning in a 59-year-old man who underwent CT-guided biopsy for paraaortic lymph node mass. The patient had undergone treatment for Waldenström macroglobulinemia with complete remission. Axial CT scan through the mid-abdomen shows the vertical approach of the 16-Gauge needle which is inserted into the left paraspinous muscle with its tip touching the proximal edge of the paraaortic mass. Note that there is no intervening transverse process. Histologic examination revealed relapsed lymph node Waldenström macroglobulinemia.

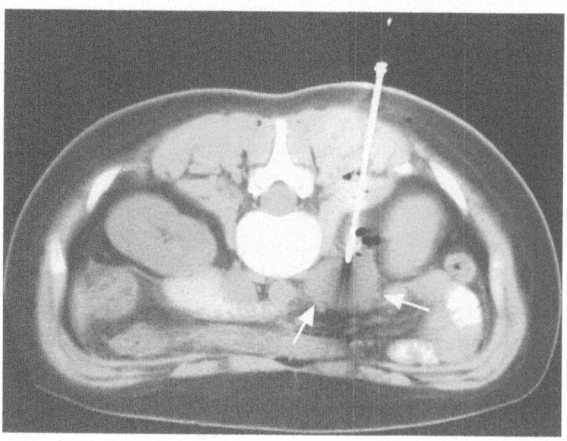

Fig. 26.15. Prone positioning in a 17-year-old girl who underwent CT-guided biopsy for deep paraaortic residual lymph node mass. The patient had undergone treatment for stage III Hodgkin disease. Axial unenhanced CT scan through the mid-abdomen shows the vertical approach of the 16-Gauge needle which is inserted into the left paraspinous muscle with its tip touching the residual mass (*arrows*). Histologic examination revealed residual nonactive mass.

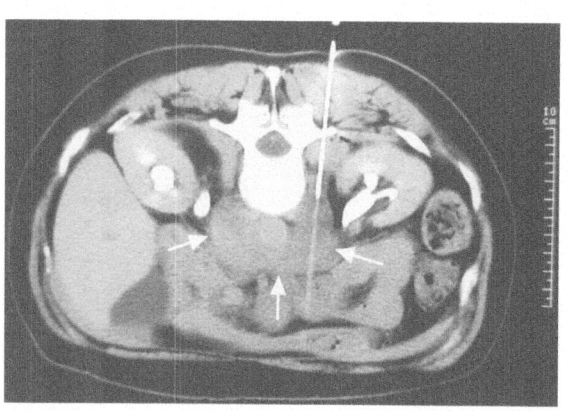

Fig. 26.16. Prone positioning in a 54-year-old woman who underwent CT-guided biopsy for deep retroperitoneal lymph node mass. Axial contrast-enhanced CT scan through the mid-abdomen shows the vertical approach of the 16-Gauge needle which is inserted into the left paraspinous muscle with its tip touching the proximal edge of the retroperitoneal mass (*arrows*). Histologic examination revealed non-Hodgkin lymphoma.

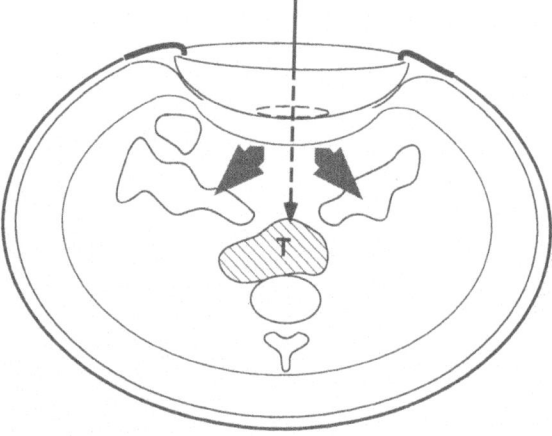

Fig. 26.17. View of the abdominal compression device. Plastic bowl with perforated bottom is applied to abdominal wall. Adjustable strap encompassing patient's abdomen is fixed at edges of bowl by two removable hooks. Compression displaces bowel loops (*arrows*) and shortens distance between skin and tumor (*T*). (With permission from [DE KERVILER et al. 1996])

tory, the device is placed on the patient by compressing its edge to the skin, pressing down, and "milking" the skin upward to deviate the bowel cephalad (DE KERVILER et al. 1996; DACHMAN 1998). A similar approach can be used for US, MR imaging, or fluoroscopically guided procedures (DACHMAN 1998; MEMEL et al. 1996). This abdominal compression allows the displacement of the colon (Fig. 26.18), small bowel (Figs. 26.19–26.21), stomach or bladder away from the needle and also reduces the distance between the skin and the retroperitoneal lesions by 15–54% (DACHMAN 1998; DE KERVILER et al. 1998). Also the anterior approach permits patients to remain supine for the entire procedure (DE KERVILER et al. 1996). Patients usually tolerate the procedure

well with minimal pain reported. The procedure is relatively safe with only minor complications such as periduodenal or abdominal wall hematomas reported. The contraindications for this procedure include recent abdominal surgery and abdominal aorta aneurysms (DE KERVILER et al. 1998).

Artificial displacement of the kidneys (Fig. 26.22), spleen, and colon by CT-guided paravertebral injection of physiologic saline fluid and/or CO_2 as an aid to percutaneous procedures has also been described and found very effective in gaining an access route to the retroperitoneum especially for large needle

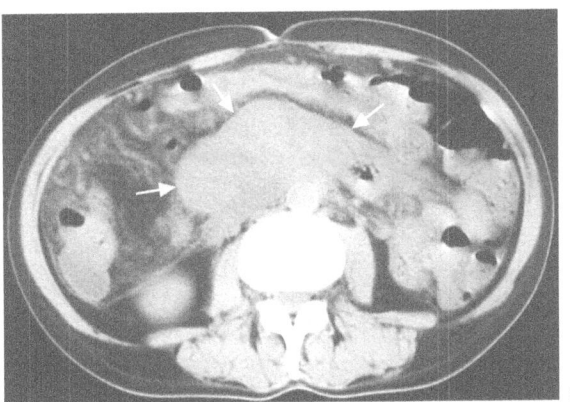

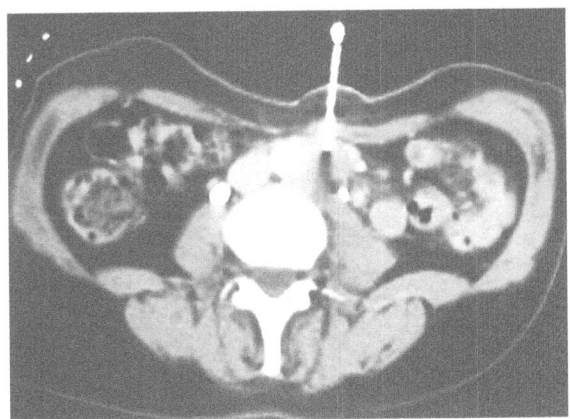

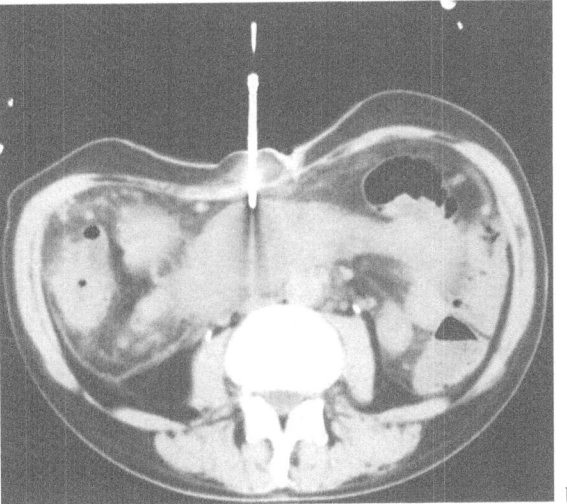

Fig. 26.18a,b. Abdominal compression in a 53-year-old woman who underwent CT-guided biopsy for deep paraaortic lymph node mass. a Axial contrast-enhanced CT scan through the mid-abdomen shows the deep paraaortic mass (*arrows*) and colon intervening in expected needle pathway. b Axial CT scan with abdominal compression obtained at the same level as (a) shows colon is displaced away from the 16-Gauge needle pathway while skin-to-mass distance is reduced by 56%. The lesion now sits right under the abdominal wall and is easily sampled. Histologic examination revealed non-Hodgkin lymphoma.

Fig. 26.19a,b. Abdominal compression in a 56-year-old woman who underwent CT-guided biopsy for mesenteric lymph node mass. a Axial contrast-enhanced CT scan through the mid-abdomen shows the mesenteric mass (*arrows*) and bowel loops intervening in expected needle pathway. b Axial CT scan with abdominal compression obtained at the same level as (a) shows bowel loops are displaced away from the 16-Gauge needle pathway while skin-to-mass distance is reduced by 42%. The lesion now sits right under the abdominal wall and is easily sampled. Histologic examination revealed B-cell non-Hodgkin lymphoma.

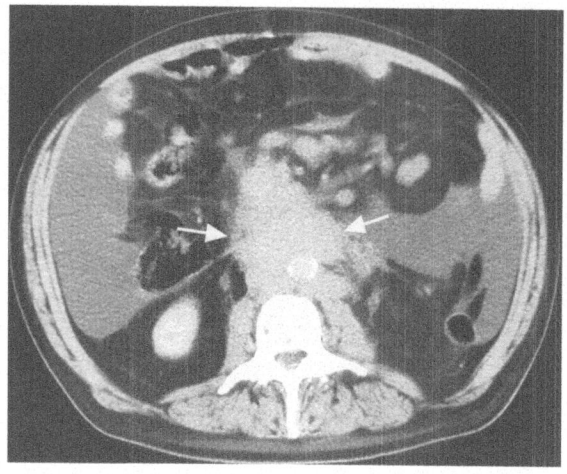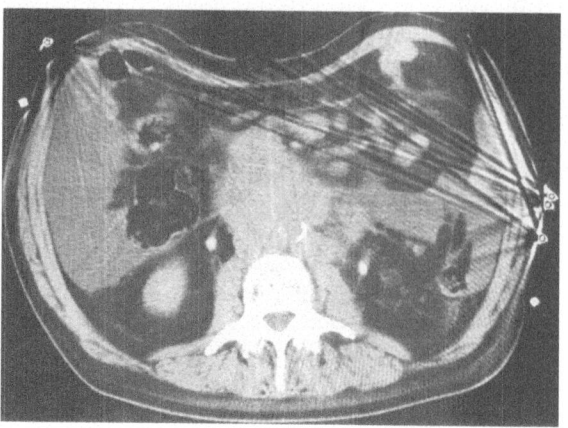

Fig. 26.20a,b. Abdominal compression in a 53-year-old man who underwent CT-guided biopsy for deep retroperitoneal mass. **a** Axial contrast-enhanced CT scan through the mid-abdomen shows the retroperitoneal mass (arrows) and bowel loops intervening in the expected needle pathway. **b** Axial CT scan with abdominal compression obtained at the same level as (**a**) shows bowel loops are displaced away from the needle pathway while skin-to-mass distance is reduced by 52%. Artifacts result from metallic buckle of trap of compression device. Histologic examination revealed non-Hodgkin lymphoma. (With permission from [DE KERVILER et al. 1996])

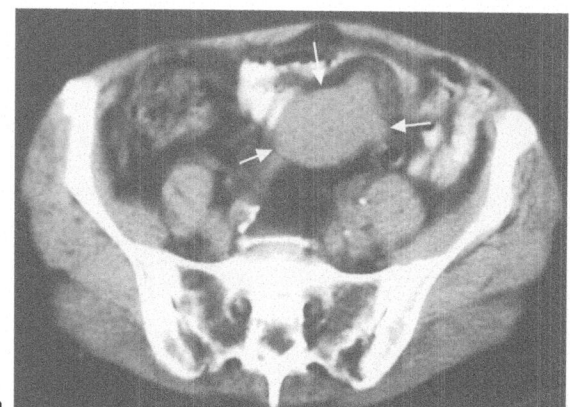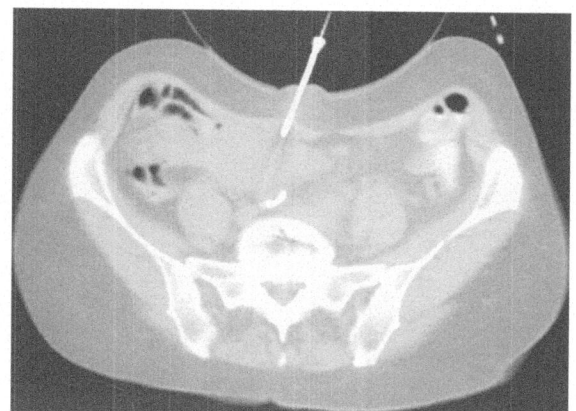

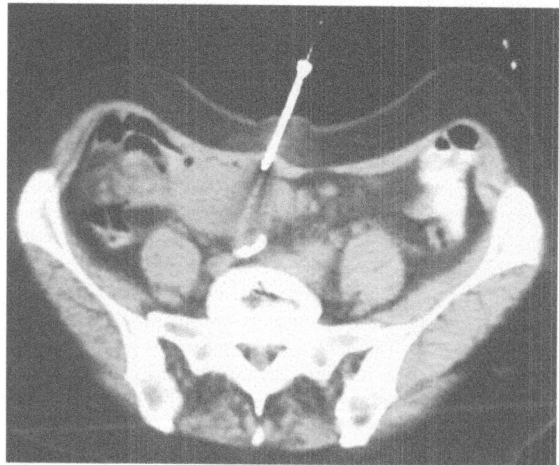

Fig. 26.21a–c. Pelvic compression in a 70-year-old woman who underwent CT-guided biopsy for pelvic lymph node mass. The patient had undergone treatment for non-Hodgkin lymphoma with complete remission. **a** Axial CT scan through the pelvis shows the pelvic mass (*arrows*) and opacified bowel loops intervening in the expected needle pathway. **b** Axial CT scan with pelvic compression shows bowel loops are displaced away from the 16-Gauge needle pathway while skin-to-mass distance is reduced by 32%. The lesion now sits right under the abdominal wall and is easily sampled. **c** Bone windowing of (**b**) shows clearly the device used for the pelvic compression. Histologic examination revealed relapsed non-Hodgkin lymphoma.

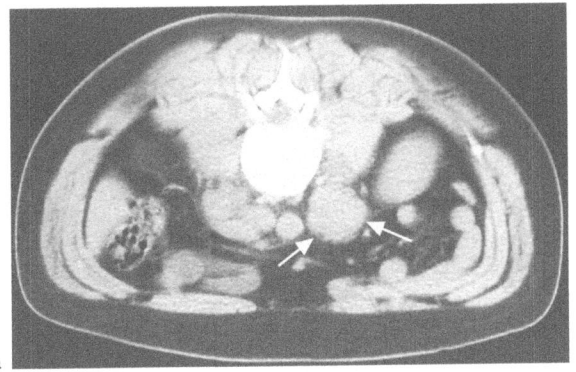
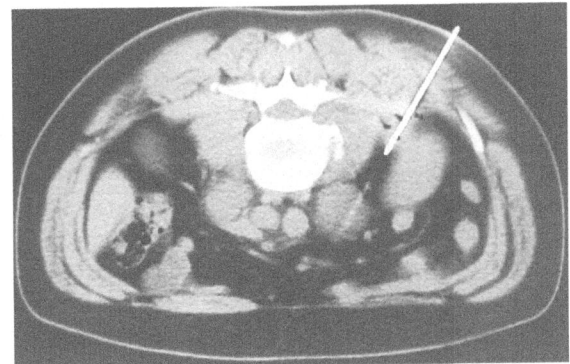
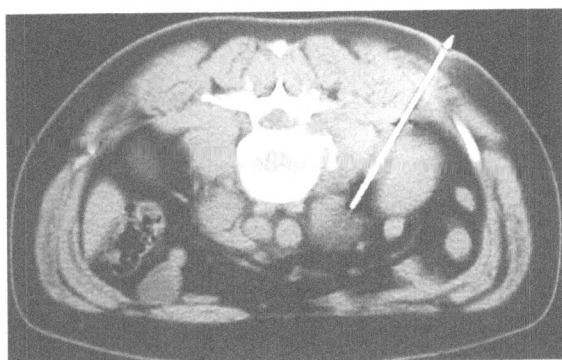

Fig. 26.22a–c. Prone positioning in a 32-year-old man who underwent CT-guided biopsy for paraaortic lymph node mass. **a** Axial unenhanced CT scan through the mid-abdomen obtained before the procedure shows the paraaortic mass (*arrows*). **b** Axial CT scan at the time of biopsy shows the oblique approach of the 16-Gauge biopsy needle entering the pathway between the psoas muscle and left kidney. The latter is being displaced after the injection of 40 mL of normal saline solution. **c** Final localizing axial CT scan shows the mass is easily reached through the psoas-left kidney pathway after a total injection of 75 mL of normal saline solution resulting in an expansion of the pathway window. Histologic examination revealed non-Hodgkin lymphoma.

biopsy (LANGEN et al. 1995). By injecting as small a quantity as 50 ml of blood quickly absorbed CO_2 through the needle, it is possible to move the bladder or bowel from the intended pathway. This procedure, which requires special equipment for CO_2 injection, works well for the retroperitoneum and the pelvis, but is not effective for the midabdomen, paraspinal regions and mediastinum; also it is ineffective for displacing solid organs such as the kidneys and the spleen (HAAGA and BEALE 1986).

26.5
Complications

Minor complications after lymph node biopsy may occur in 7–8% of cases. They include perilesional hematomas, mild hemoptysis, small pneumothorax or hemothorax, and mild hemoperitoneum (AGID et al. 2003; WITTICH et al. 1992; ZINZANI et al. 1999; SKLAIR-LEVY et al. 2000; DEMHARTER et al. 2001). The complication rate increases as the needle size increases and as the bowel is traversed (DE KERVILER et al. 1996). Most complications usually remain asymptomatic and rarely require specific treatment (WITTICH et al. 1992; DEMHARTER et al. 2001). Major

or catastrophic complications are rare. In fact, some studies have reported no complications (ZINZANI et al. 1998; SKLAIR-LEVY et al. 2001).

26.6
Efficacy

In their series of image-guided needle biopsy in patients with suspected or recurrent lymphomas, DE KERVILER et al. (2000) obtained total success in 88% providing a diagnosis of lymphoma with subtyping, partial success in 11% providing a diagnosis of lymphoma without subtyping, and failure in 1%. Treatment of lymphoma was initiated on the basis of image-guided needle biopsy findings in 72% (SILVERMAN et al. 1994; SKLAIR-LEVY et al. 2000), 81% (ZINZANI et al. 1999), 83% (AGID et al. 2003; PAPPA et al. 1996), 84% (QUINN et al. 1995), 86% (BEN-YEHUDA et al. 1996), 91% (MOULTON and MOORE 1993), 93% (DE KERVILER et al. 2000), 96% of cases (ZINZANI et al. 1998).

The diagnosis of recurrent disease was achieved in 77% (PAPPA et al. 1996) to 82% (DE KERVILER et al. 2000), and progression in 82% (DE KERVILER et al. 2000) to 88% (PAPPA et al. 1996) of cases.

In series including nodal and also extranodal biopsies, the authors found no significant statistical difference between nodal or extranodal involvement, the site of the lesion, nor the age of patients (PAPPA et al. 1996; de KERVILER et al. 2000). There was also no difference between fine versus large needle biopsies in tumor grade determination (SILVERMAN et al. 1994; PAPPA et al. 1996; ZINZANI et al. 1998; DE KERVILER et al. 2000). Nevertheless, large needles may be necessary to distinguish between some low-grade lymphomas and intermediate-grade lymphomas (SILVERMAN et al. 1994). Large needles also are recommended in children with suspected Hodgkin disease (GARRETT et al. 2002). The image-guided needle biopsy is equally successful in the primary diagnosis of lymphoma and in the diagnosis of relapse or progression. Also the rate of success is similar in the diagnosis of non-Hodgkin lymphomas and Hodgkin disease (PAPPA et al. 1996; ZINZANI et al. 1998; DE KERVILER et al. 2000; SKLAIR-LEVY et al. 2000; DEMHARTER et al. 2001). The technique is effective for both intraabdominal and intrathoracic structures (PAPPA et al. 1996). The ability to obtain a definitive subclassified diagnosis of malignant lymphoma is not affected by image guidance modality (SILVERMAN et al. 1994).

Among the causes of failure, small size of the sample or inappropriate tissue sampled are the most frequent (ZINZANI et al. 1999; DEMHARTER et al. 2001; HUSSAIN et al. 2001). In fact, sampling errors are secondary to either missed pathologic area in a heterogeneously involved lymph node, or tissue obtained from a normal lymph node adjacent to the lymph node involved with the disease (PROTOPAPAS and WESTCOTT 2000; DEMHARTER et al. 2001). Occasionally, it can be difficult to differentiate reactive changes of lymph node from a low-grade non-Hodgkin lymphoma on the core-biopsy specimen. Furthermore, the percutaneous biopsy can miss the transformation of a known low-grade non-Hodgkin lymphoma to a high-grade non-Hodgkin lymphoma if the specimen does not encompass the transformed portion of the lymphoma (DEMHARTER et al. 2001).

26.7
Conclusion

Percutaneous image-guided needle biopsy, as a minimally invasive procedure, is an effective alternative to surgical biopsy in the original diagnosis, recurrence or progression of lymphomas. It is also safe, quick, accurate and cost-efficient. It should be the first procedure performed in the diagnosis of lymphoma, except at easily accessible superficial neck, inguinal, and axillary nodal sites. It provides sufficient information for the diagnosis of and subsequent therapeutic decision to treat most cases of lymphoma. Importantly, it should be performed as part of a multidisciplinary team approach. A surgical approach to the thoracic or abdominal lymph nodes should be avoided as a first diagnostic procedure in patients with suspected or recurrent lymphoma, unless a previous percutaneous biopsy has failed or is contraindicated, or there is a high suspicion of Hodgkin disease. In such cases, video-assisted surgery should be implemented because of its high diagnostic yield and its low morbidity (cf next chapter). For the same reasons and because of its potential morbidity, open surgery should nowadays be banished as a diagnostic procedure in patients with lymphomas.

References

Agid R, Sklair-Levy M, Bloom AI, Lieberman S, Polliack A, Ben-Yehuda D, Sherman Y, Libson E (2003) CT-guided biopsy with cutting-edge needle for the diagnosis of malignant lymphoma: experience of 267 biopsies. Clin Radiol 58: 143–147

Ben-Yehuda D, Polliack A, Okon E, Sherman Y, Fields S, Lebenshart P, Lotan H, Libson E (1996) Image-guided core-needle biopsy in malignant lymphoma: experience with 100 patients that suggests the technique is reliable. J Clin Oncol 14:2431–2434

Bressler EL, Kirkham JA (1994) Mediastinal masses: alternative approaches to CT-guided needle biopsy. Radiology 191:391–396

Carrasco CH, Richli WR, Lawrence D, Katz RL, Wallace S (1990) Fine needle aspiration biopsy in lymphoma. Radiol Clin North Am 28:879–883

Dachman AH (1998) A biopsy compression device for use in cross-sectional or fluoroscopic imaging. AJR Am J Roentgenol 171:703–705

de Kerviler E, Guermazi A, Cazals-Hatem D, Frija J (1996) Use of abdominal compression as an aid to CT-guided retroperitoneal biopsies. AJR Am J Roentgenol 167:1346–1347

de Kerviler E, Guermazi A, Gossot D, Cazals-Hatem D, Zagdanski AM, Mariette X, Brice P, Frija J (1998) Use of an abdominal compression device for CT-guided biopsy of enlarged abdominal or pelvic lymph nodes. J Vasc Interv Radiol 9:353–357

de Kerviler E, Guermazi A, Zagdanski AM, Meignin V, Gossot D, Oksenhendler E, Mariette X, Brice P, Frija J (2000) Image-guided core-needle biopsy in patients with suspected or recurrent lymphomas. Cancer 89:647–652

Demharter J, Muller P, Wagner T, Schlimok G, Haude K, Bohndorf K (2001) Percutaneous core-needle biopsy of enlarged lymph nodes in the diagnosis and subclassification of malignant lymphomas. Eur Radiol 11:276–283

Dodd GD 3rd, Esola CC, Memel DS, Ghiatas AA, Chintapalli KN, Paulson EK, Nelson RC, Ferris JV, Baron RL (1996) Sonography: the undiscovered jewel of interventional radiology. Radiographics 16:1271–1288

Esola CC, Chopra S, Dodd GD (1997) Sonographic guidance in biopsies and drainages: techniques and applications. Semin Intervent Rad 14:343–369

Fisher AJ, Paulson EK, Sheafor DH, Simmons CM, Nelson RC (1997) Small lymph nodes of the abdomen, pelvis, and retroperitoneum: usefulness of sonographically guided biopsy. Radiology 205:185–190

Garrett KM, Hoffer FA, Behm FG, Gow KW, Hudson MM, Sandlund JT (2002) Interventional radiology techniques for the diagnosis of lymphoma or leukemia. Pediatr Radiol 32:653–662

Haaga JR, Beale SM (1986) Use of CO2 to move structures as an aid to percutaneous procedures. Radiology 161:829–830

Hagberg H, Ahlstrom HK, Magnusson A, Sundstrom C, Astrom GK (2000) Value of transsternal core biopsy in patients with a newly diagnosed mediastinal mass. Acta Oncol 39:195–198

Hussain HK, Kingston JE, Domizio P, Norton AJ, Reznek RH (2001) Imaging-guided core biopsy for the diagnosis of malignant tumors in pediatric patients. AJR Am J Roentgenol 176:43–47

Hussain S (1996) Gantry angulation in CT-guided percutaneous adrenal biopsy. AJR Am J Roentgenol 166:537–539

Jeffrey RB, Jr. (1988) Coaxial technique for CT-guided biopsy of deep retroperitoneal lymph nodes. Gastrointest Radiol 13:271–272

Katada K, Kato R, Anno H, Ogura Y, Koga S, Ida Y, Sato M, Nonomura K (1996) Guidance with real-time CT fluoroscopy: early clinical experience. Radiology 200:851–856

Kato R, Katada K, Anno H, Suzuki S, Ida Y, Koga S (1996) Radiation dosimetry at CT fluoroscopy: physician's hand dose and development of needle holders. Radiology 201:576–578

Langen HJ, Jochims M, Gunther RW (1995) Artificial displacement of kidneys, spleen, and colon by injection of physiologic saline and CO2 as an aid to percutaneous procedures: experimental results. J Vasc Interv Radiol 6:411–416

Memel DS, Dodd GD, 3rd, Esola CC (1996) Efficacy of sonography as a guidance technique for biopsy of abdominal, pelvic, and retroperitoneal lymph nodes. AJR Am J Roentgenol 167:957–962

Moulton JS (1993) Artificial extrapleural window for mediastinal biopsy. J Vasc Interv Radiol 4:825–829

Moulton JS, Moore PT (1993) Coaxial percutaneous biopsy technique with automated biopsy devices: value in improving accuracy and negative predictive value. Radiology 186:515–522

Pappa VI, Hussain HK, Reznek RH, Whelan J, Norton AJ, Wilson AM, Love S, Lister TA, Rohatiner AZ (1996) Role of image-guided core-needle biopsy in the management of patients with lymphoma. J Clin Oncol 14:2427–2430

Protopapas Z, Westcott JL (1997) Transthoracic hilar and mediastinal biopsy. J Thorac Imaging 12:250–258

Protopapas Z, Westcott JL (2000) Transthoracic hilar and mediastinal biopsy. Radiol Clin North Am 38:281–291

Quinn SF, Sheley RC, Nelson HA, Demlow TA, Wienstein RE, Dunkley BL (1995) The role of percutaneous needle biopsies in the original diagnosis of lymphoma: a prospective evaluation. J Vasc Interv Radiol 6:947–952

Schweiger GD, Yip VY, Brown BP (2000) CT fluoroscopic guidance for percutaneous needle placement into abdominopelvic lesions with difficult access routes. Abdom Imaging 25:633–637

Silverman SG, Lee BY, Mueller PR, Cibas ES, Seltzer SE (1994) Impact of positive findings at image-guided biopsy of lymphoma on patient care: evaluation of clinical history, needle size, and pathologic findings on biopsy performance. Radiology 190:759–764

Sklair-Levy M, Polliack A, Shaham D, Applbaum YH, Gillis S, Ben-Yehuda D, Sherman Y, Libson E (2000) CT-guided core-needle biopsy in the diagnosis of mediastinal lymphoma. Eur Radiol 10:714–718

Sklair-Levy M, Lebensart PD, Applbaum YH, Ramu N, Freeman A, Gozal D, Gross E, Sherman Y, Bar-Ziv J, Libson E (2001) Percutaneous image-guided needle biopsy in children–summary of our experience with 57 children. Pediatr Radiol 31:732–736

Wittich GR, Nowels KW, Korn RL, Walter RM, Lucas DE, Dake MD, Jeffrey RB (1992) Coaxial transthoracic fine-needle biopsy in patients with a history of malignant lymphoma. Radiology 183:175–178

Zinzani PL, Corneli G, Cancellieri A, Magagnoli M, Lacava N, Gherlinzoni F, Bendandi M, Albertini P, Baruzzi G, Tura S, Boaron M (1999) Core needle biopsy is effective in the initial diagnosis of mediastinal lymphoma. Haematologica 84:600–603

Zinzani PL, Colecchia A, Festi D, Magagnoli M, Larocca A, Ascani S, Bendandi M, Orcioni GF, Gherlinzoni F, Albertini P, Pileri SA, Roda E, Tura S (1998) Ultrasound-guided core-needle biopsy is effective in the initial diagnosis of lymphoma patients. Haematologica 83:989–992

27 Surgical Endoscopic Techniques in Patients with Lymphoma

Dominique Gossot and Domenico Galetta

CONTENTS

27.1
Introduction

As described in the previous chapter, the diagnostic yield of image-guided needle biopsies (IGNB) is high, as much as 85% (BEN-YEHUDA et al. 1996; PAPPA et al. 1996; SILVERMAN et al. 1994), so that surgery is now seldom indicated in these patients. However, there is still a place for surgical techniques when large specimens are required for specialized studies such as immunophenotyping or cytogenetic analysis, or when IGNB fails, or when size and/or location of the target make it difficult to reach.

Until recently, it was common to use laparotomy or thoracotomy for diagnostic purposes. In most cases, a surgical approach may now be employed using a minimally invasive technique (CHILDERS et al. 1993; CHILDERS and SURWIT 1994; CONLON et al.

DOMINIQUE GOSSOT, MD
Senior Surgeon, Department of Thoracic Surgery, Institut Mutualiste Montsouris, 42 Jourdan Boulevard, 75015 Paris, France
DOMENICO GALETTA, MD
Associate Surgeon, Department of Thoracic Surgery, Institut Mutualiste Montsouris, 42 Jourdan Boulevard, 75015 Paris, France

1996; D'EMILIA et al. 1996). In this chapter we will describe the surgical endoscopic techniques used as an alternative to IGNB in patients with lymphoma.

27.2
Techniques

All surgical techniques described here require general anesthesia.

27.2.1
Laparoscopy

The procedure is performed using peritoneal insufflation at 12 mmHg and a 3 or 4-port technique, depending on how difficult it is to reach the target. A 0° or a 30°–10 mm telescope is used, usually inserted at the umbilicus level. The procedure is performed with the patient supine, when the targets are celiac or hepatic lymph nodes (Fig. 27.1). For retroperitoneal tumors and/or lateroaortic lymph nodes lateral positioning is preferable since it allows the intestine to drop by gravity, thus facilitating the approach to the large retroperitoneal vessels. All biopsies – tumor, lymph nodes, liver – are extracted through one of the trocar after having been placed in an endoscopic specimen retrieval bag. Patients can be discharged one or two days after surgery.

27.2.2
Thoracoscopy

The procedure is performed under double-lumen tracheal intubation in all cases, except those patients who present with either a narrowing of the trachea related to the lymphoma or a poor respiratory function contraindicating split ventilation (GOSSOT et al, 1996a). Thoracoscopy provides an excellent view of the mediastinum (Figs. 27.2,

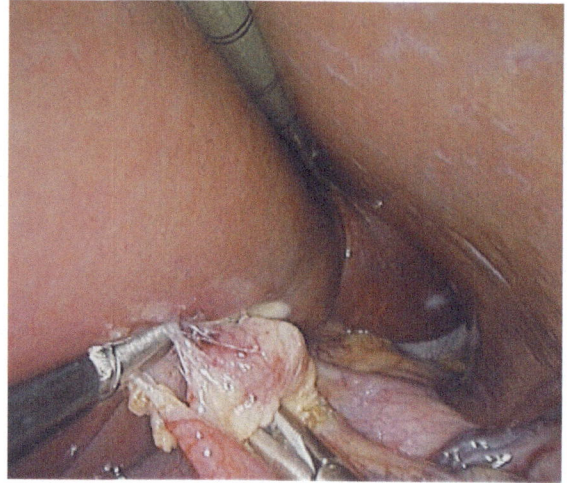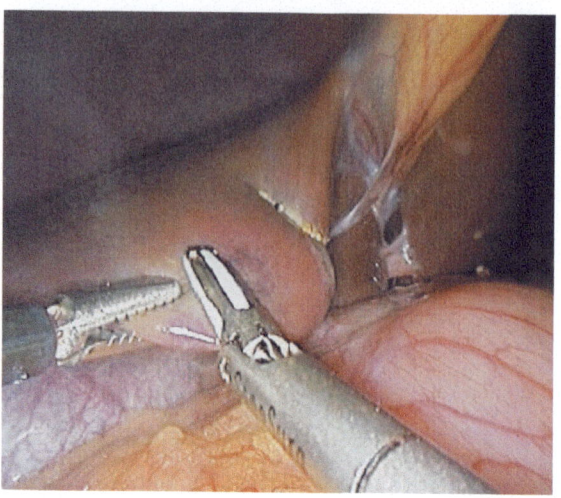

Fig. 27.1a,b. High suspicion of lymphoma in a 30-year-old man. **a** Laparoscopy view shows celiac lymph nodes. **b** Laparoscopic hepatic biopsy is performed during the same procedure, looking for hepatic localization of the lymphoma. Pathology yielded non-Hodgkin lymphoma.

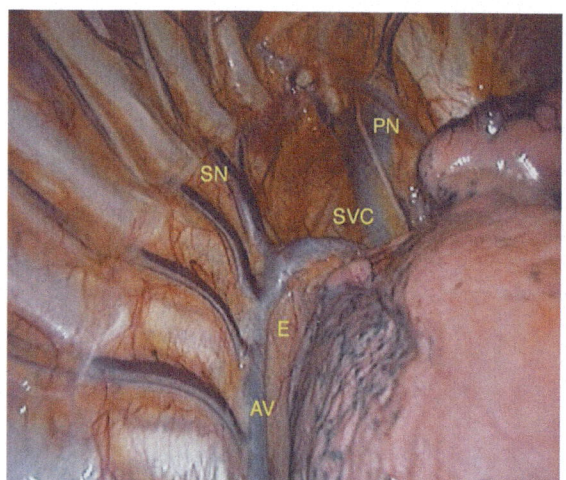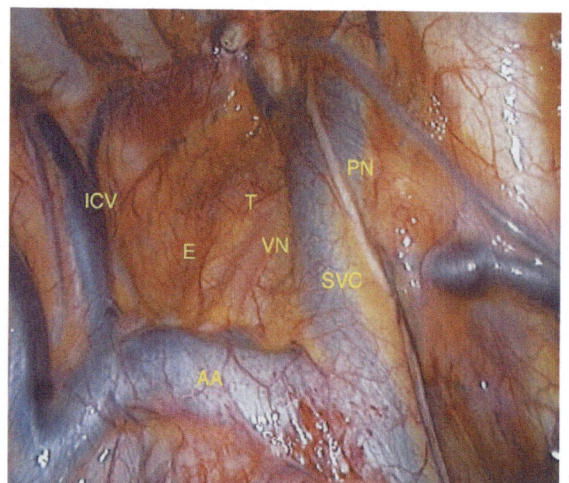

Fig. 27.2a,b. Thoracoscopic approach of normal mediastinum. **a** Thoracoscopic view of normal right middle mediastinum (*SVC* = superior vena cava, *E* = esophagus, *SN* = sympathetic nerve, *PN* = phrenic nerve, *AV* = azygos vein). **b** Close-up view of normal right paratracheal region (*SVC* = superior vena cava, *T* = trachea, *E* = esophagus, *VN* = vagus nerve, *PN* = phrenic nerve, *AA* = azygos arch, *ICV* = intercostal vein).

27.3) and allows complete removal of lymph nodes (Figs. 27.4, 27.5). A 0° or a 30° telescope is used, usually inserted in the 5th intercostal space (ICS) and 2 additional ports. A fourth port is rarely required, except when an examination of the subcarinal area or of the aorto-pulmonary window is necessary. In patients operated on for a small-sized lung nodule, a preoperative CT-guided localization using a hookwire or methylene blue labeling or both may be used (Fig. 27.6) (GOSSOT et al 1994). Pleural effusions of unknown origin are frequently encountered in these patients. Thoracoscopy helps differentiate non-specific pleural lesions (Fig. 27.7) from true recurrences (Fig. 27.8).

At the end of the procedure a single 24-French chest tube is placed. It is usually removed the day after surgery, after checking the chest X-ray, and the patient is discharged on the same day or one day later. Considering that the procedure is minor with a short period of drainage, no postoperative analgesia is given, as we usually do for other major thoracoscopic procedures.

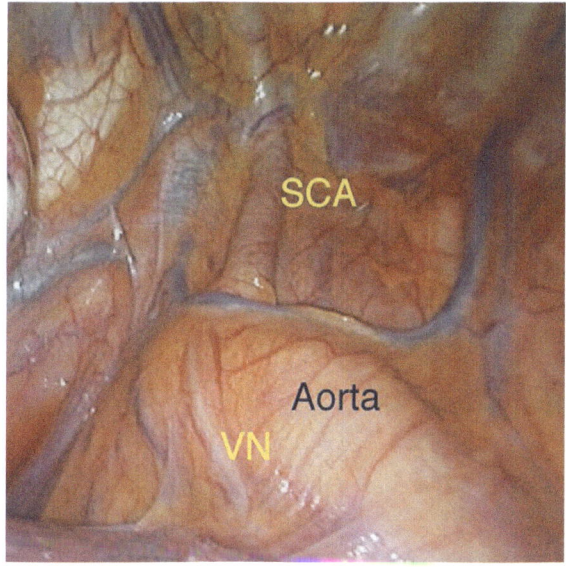

Fig. 27.3. Thoracoscopic view of normal left middle mediastinum *(SCA = subclavian artery, VN = vagus nerve)*.

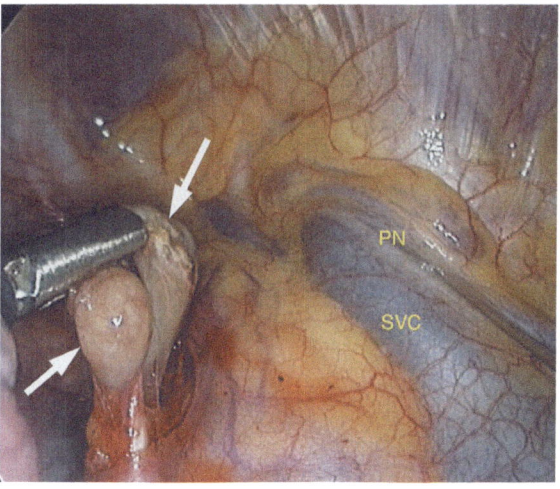

Fig. 27.4. Right paratracheal lymph nodes in a 28-year old man with high suspicion of lymphoma. Thoracoscopic view shows the right paratracheal lymph nodes *(arrows)* *(SVC = superior vena cava, PN = phrenic nerve)*. Histology of the thoracoscopic tissue samples yielded non-Hodgkin lymphoma.

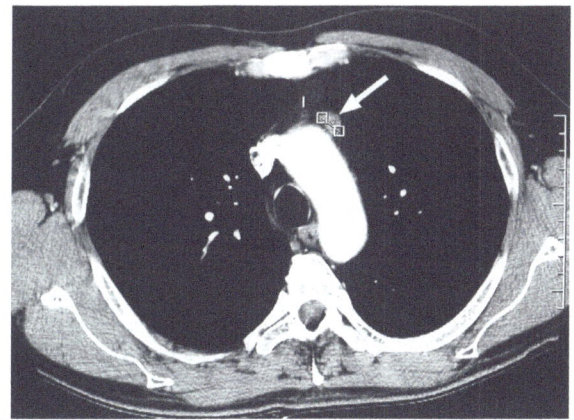
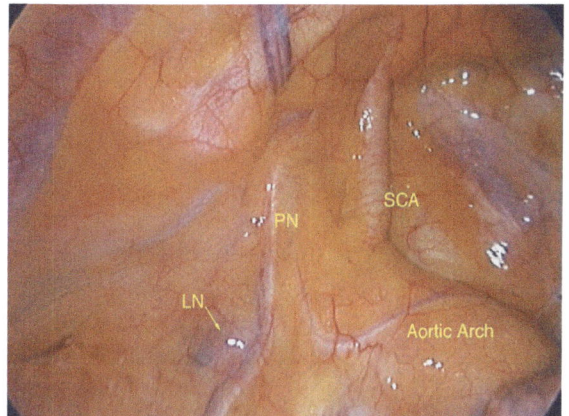

a   b

Fig. 27.5a,b. Non-Hodgkin lymphoma in a 56-year-old man who was considered in remission after treatment. **a** Axial contrast-enhanced thoracic routine follow-up CT scan shows an isolated small anterior mediastinal lymph node *(arrow)*. **b** This lymph node was picked via left thoracoscopy *(SCA = subclavian artery, PN = phrenic nerve, LN = lymph node)*. Pathological examination yielded recurrence.

27.2.3
Mediastinoscopy

A video-mediastinoscope is inserted through a mini-transversal cervicotomy. Whenever possible we try to dissect and take out at least a whole lymph node, rather than performing multiple small size biopsies (Fig. 27.9) which may make pathological examination more difficult. The skin is closed with a resorbable subcutaneous suture and a small suction drain is kept in place for a few hours. Mediastinoscopy is performed as an out-patient procedure, or during a one day hospitalization.

In the case of mediastinal tumors or lymph nodes enlargement, the indication for using either mediastinoscopy or thoracoscopy is mainly based on anatomical considerations. For instance, tumors or lymph nodes of the anterior or posterior and/or inferior mediastinum are reachable only through the thoracoscope. On the other hand, paratracheal lymph nodes are usually approached through mediastinoscopy. However, even for lesions of the upper

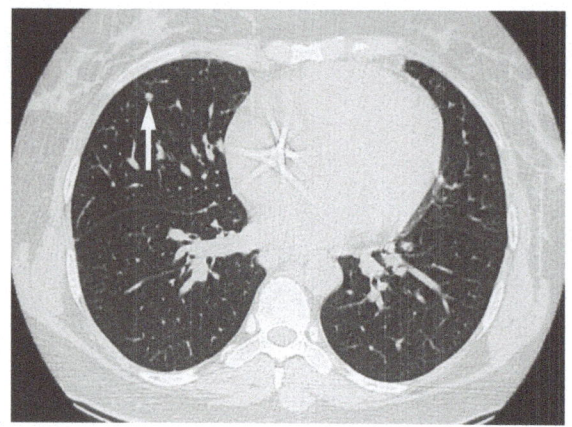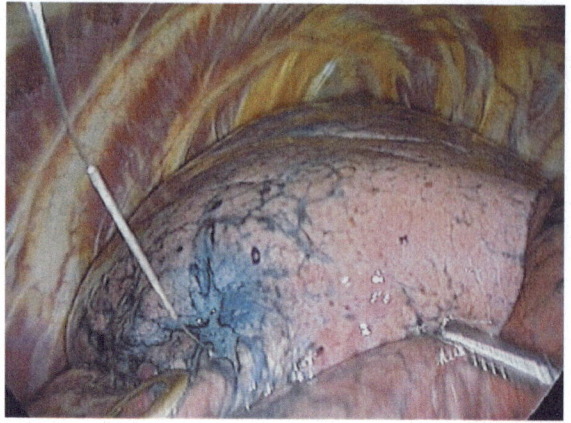

Fig. 27.6a,b. Non-Hodgkin lymphoma in a 26-year-old woman with pulmonary localization. **a** Axial CT scan of the chest shows a right small lung nodule persisting at the end of treatment (*arrow*). **b** Thoracoscopic view after preoperative methylene blue labeling and placement of a hook-wire within the nodule under CT-guidance. Pathology yielded fibrotic non-malignant lesion.

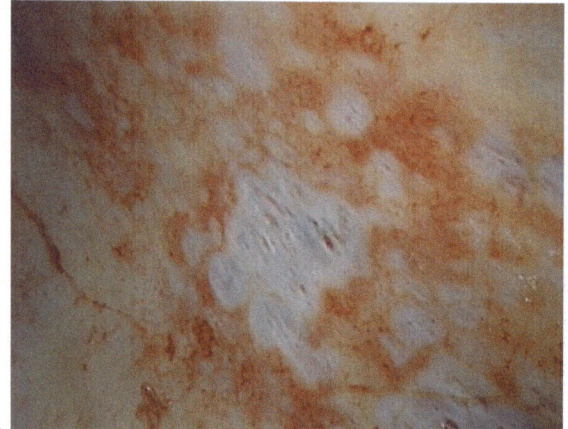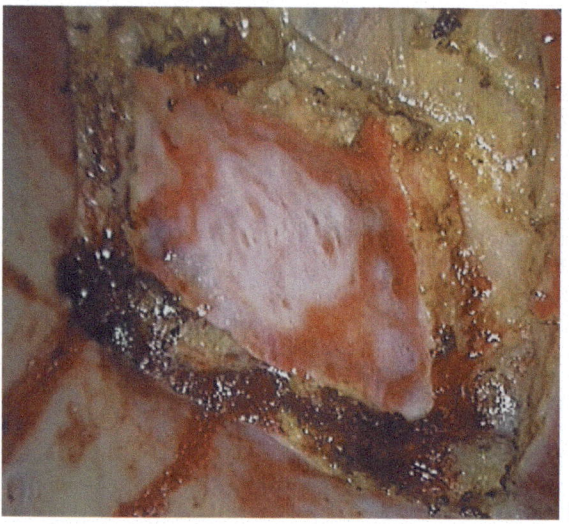

Fig. 27.7a,b. Hodgkin disease in a 31-year-old man who presented with left pleural effusion 6 months after treatment. **a** Thoracoscopic view shows an inflammatory and thickened pleura without nodule. **b** A large pleural flap is removed. Pathological examination revealed nonspecific fibrotic pleura, most likely secondary to radiation therapy.

third of the middle mediastinum, some criteria may indicate thoracoscopy rather than mediastinoscopy: (1) when multiple biopsies are required, such as for restaging of non-Hodgkin lymphoma or Hodgkin disease, thoracoscopy is preferred; (2) same as for patients for whom biopsy of other organs – e.g. lung – is needed; (3) some cosmetic reasons in young women may influence the choice of thoracoscopy, since 2 or 3 lateral punctures are usually less unesthetic than a cervical scare.

27.3
Results

In 1998, we reported on 92 patients presenting with suspected or confirmed lymphoma (GOSSOT et al. 1998). They were referred to the surgeon for a surgical biopsy of a deeply located intrathoracic or intraabdominal mass or lymph node. None of these patients had peripheral lymph nodes. Only the 86 patients operated on through a surgical endoscopic technique

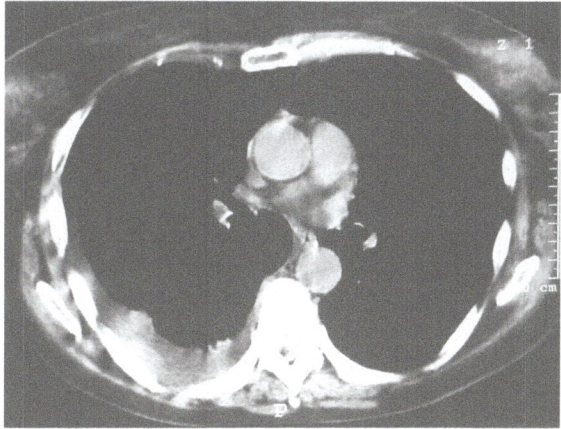

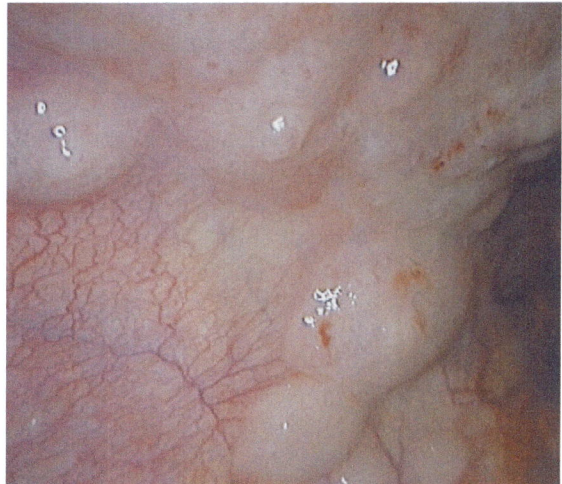

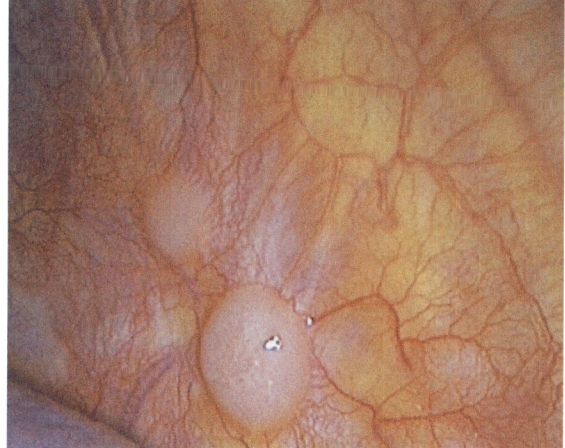

Fig.27.8a–c. Non-Hodgkin lymphoma in a 45-year-old man who presented with right pleural disease 5 years after treatment. **a** Axial contrast-enhanced CT scan of the chest shows a right pleural effusion and thick irregular pleura. **b** Right thoracoscopic view shows confluent large pleural nodules. **c** Right thoracoscopic view also shows small pleural nodules. Biopsy of both lesions confirmed recurrence.

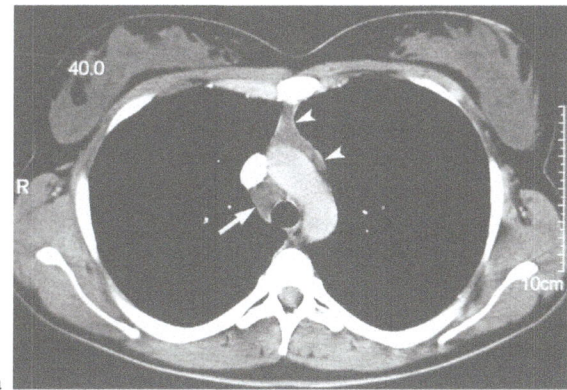

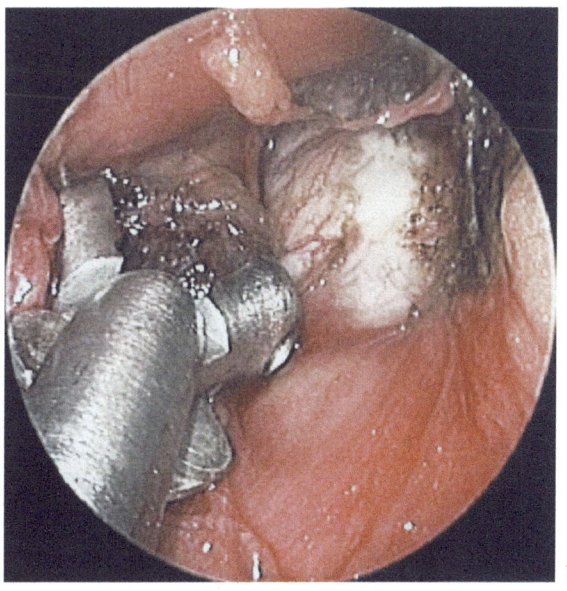

Fig. 27.9a,b. Mild mediastinal enlargement in an 18-year-old man. **a** Axial contrast-enhanced CT scan of the chest shows anterior mediastinal (*arrowheads*) and right paratracheal (*arrow*) lymph nodes. **b** Mediastinoscopic view during the biopsy of the right paratracheal lymph node. Pathology yielded Hodgkin disease.

were included in this study. Most were selected directly for surgery while 5 were operated on after failure of an IGNB. During the same period, 82 IGNB were performed. The different techniques used in this study are summarized in Table 27.1. Only 5 patients underwent conventional open surgery. Surgical biopsies were indicated in 3 different situations: (1) at presentation of the disease in patients with suspected but unproved lymphoma (48 cases); (2) at progression of the lymphoma, e.g. in case of histological modification or outset of another localization of the disease (23 cases); or (3) because of the need for restaging at completion of medical treatment. In patients with residual mass, the main concern was to determine its nature, i.e. fibrosis or persistent disease (15 cases) (Table 27.2).

The study comprised 86 patients in whom 89 endoscopic procedures were performed. A procedure was considered successful when it provided sufficient information for the pathologist and the physician thus allowing treatment. A small size biopsy that allowed for obtaining a pathological diagnosis, i.e. Hodgkin disease or non-Hodgkin lymphoma, but which did not permit subtyping was considered a semi-failure. A biopsy that did not permit any diagnosis was considered a complete failure.

Table 27.1. Surgical techniques used in 86 patients (89 procedures) with suspected or confirmed lymphoma.

Procedure	Number
Surgical endoscopic technique	
Laparoscopy	15
Thoracoscopy	61
Mediastinoscopy	13
Conventional open technique	
Laparotomy	2
Thoracotomy	0
Sternotomy	0
Mediastinotomy	3

Table 27.2. Final pathological diagnosis after thoracoscopy in 15 patients presenting with residual thoracic mass.

Diagnosis	Number
Success	14
Hodgkin disease	4
Non-Hodgkin lymphoma	1
Fibrosis	4
Necrotic tissue	1
Tuberculosis	2
Normal enlarged thymus	2
Failure	1

There were no deaths in this series. One intra-operative complication occurred in the thoracoscopic group (1.1%): a pulmonary hemorrhage during a lung biopsy could not be controlled thoracoscopically and required a thoracotomy whose post-operative course was uneventful. Two post-operative complications were noticed (2.2%): one pleural effusion which did not necessitate chest drainage and which faded after physiotherapy and one intraabdominal abscess in the laparoscopy group. The later required a laparotomy that failed to determine a cause. However, it was assumed that a pancreatic injury during the laparoscopic biopsy of a peripancreatic lymph nodes might have provoked a pancreatic fistula leading to an abscess. Indeed pancreatic tissue was found with the lymph nodes sample by the pathologist.

Three patients required conversion to open surgery (3.4%). As mentioned above, one patient had a thoracotomy for pulmonary hemorrhage. A second had a mediastinotomy because of inefficient lung collapse that did not permit a safe thoracoscopic examination. Finally, in the laparoscopic group, a technical problem led to a laparotomy. In these 3 patients, a pathological diagnosis was obtained. The average post-operative stay was 1.1 days in the mediastinoscopy group (range: 1–2 days), 2.8 days in the thoracoscopy group (range 1–10 days) and 3.1 days in the laparoscopy group (range: 2–14 days).

The global success rate of surgical endoscopic procedures was 86.5%. All but one mediastinoscopy were successful (93.3%). The patient whose mediastinoscopy was not contributory was reoperated on one month later via thoracoscopy. In the thoracoscopic group, the success rate was 93.4%. It was only 60% in the laparoscopic group. In the later, we had 3 complete failures and 3 partial failures. These were due to inadequate size of the lymph nodes biopsies. The reasons will be discussed below. In total, 4 patients had a difficult phenotyping (partial failure). In two no further surgery was carried out, while in the 2 others, a repeat endoscopic procedure was performed successfully.

27.4
Which Technique for Diagnosis of Lymphomas?

Despite the rapid development of surgical endoscopy which is now established in many fields, the use of laparoscopy and/or thoracoscopy as diagnostic and staging tools has not yet become routine in the management of lymphomas (Tables 27.3–27.5). In our institution, it is still not uncommon to manage second-hand patients

Table 27.3. Major experiences in diagnosis and staging of abdominal lymphomas by laparoscopy.

Authors	Year	Number of patients	Complica- tions (%)	Diagnostic Yield (%)
SALKY et al.	1988	12	0	83
CONLON et al.	1996	55*	1.8	100
FERZLI et al.	1997	6	0	100
GOSSOT et al.	1998	14	7	60
BACCARANI et al.	1998	15	20	100
STRICKER et al.	1998	51	NR	47
SILECCHIA et al.	1999	66*	3	94
COWLES and YAHANDA	2000	18	11	78
LEV-CHELOUCHE et al.	2001	15	0	93

NR = Not reported
* Operative procedures

Table 27.4. Major experiences in diagnosis and staging of intrathoracic lymphomas by thoracoscopy.

Authors	Year	Number of patients	Complica- tions (%)	Diagnostic Yield (%)
CELIKOGLU et al.	1992	9	0	78
RIEGER et al.	1996	9	0	89
DMITRIEV and SIGAL	1996	8	0	100
GOSSOT et al.	1998	61	3	92
SOLAINI et al.	1998	10	0	100
CIRINO et al.	2000	17	6	100
ROVIARO et al.	2000	42	0	100

Table 27.5. Major experiences in diagnosis and staging of mediastinal lymphomas by mediastinoscopy.

Authors	Year	Number of patients	Complica- tions (%)	Diagnostic Yield (%)
ELIA et al.	1992	46	NR	80
RENDINA et al.	1994	18	0	89
VENUTA et al.	1997	50	4	100
GOSSOT et al.	1998	13	0	92
MINEO et al.	1999	17	0	100
RENDINA et al.	2002	34	0	100

NR = Not reported

whose diagnosis of lymphoma was established using a large abdominal or thoracic incision. Performing a laparotomy, a thoracotomy or a sternotomy, leads to the inherent and well-known morbidity of these incisions. In a series of 133 laparotomies for Hodgkin disease, JOCKOVITCH et al. (1994) reported a 9.8% rate of small

bowel obstruction, requiring repeat laparotomy in most cases. Considering the advantages of minimally invasive surgery, using those disabling and unesthetic incisions just to pick a node or a tumor sample – moreover in patients who are usually young and whose prognosis is most often good – appears questionable.

This may explain the rise of ultrasound (US) and computed tomography (CT)-guided biopsies. In recent years, both safety and accuracy of these techniques have improved. Radiologically-guided biopsies were previously performed using fine needle aspiration. Pathological diagnoses were obtained in only 64% of the patients (ZORNOZA et al. 1981). With core-needle biopsies, the diagnostic accuracy is around 80% in many recent series, especially when several samples can be obtained using a coaxial technique (BEN-YEHUDA et al. 1996; PAPPA et al. 1996). In the series of BEN-YEHUDA et al. (1996), 86% of the patients received therapy on the basis of the core-needle biopsy without need for subsequent open biopsy. In the series of PAPPA et al. (1996), the rate was similar (83%). In the latter study, the size of the samples was sufficient for phenotyping in all cases. The authors point out that they did not encounter the problem of missing large follicles, a theoretical limitation of IGNB for assessment of follicularity (CARRASCO et al. 1990). All failures of IGNB reported have then required an open surgical biopsy (BEN-YEHUDA et al. 1996; CARRASCO et al. 1990).

Since 1991, we have used a surgical endoscopic technique rather than open surgery whenever possible. This policy has resulted in an indisputable advantage for those patients whose biopsy was successful, because of the limited cosmetic harm and short hospital stay. The 93% success rates of thoracoscopy and mediastinoscopy found in our series is close to the rates reported in other studies dealing with the use of these techniques for mediastinal masses and/or lymph nodes (LANDRENEAU et al. 1993; RENDINA et al. 1994; RIEGER et al. 1996). With regard to the use of laparoscopy for biopsy of lymphomas, few studies are available. Most of them are case reports (CHILDERS et al. 1993; CHILDERS and SURWIT 1994; D'EMILIA et al. 1996) or limited series (CONLON et al. 1996). In our series, laparoscopy yielded less than thoracoscopy or mediastinoscopy, since its accuracy was only 60%. Overlooking positive lymph nodes during laparoscopy has already been mentioned as a limitation of the method in other studies (HEMMING et al. 1995; SALKY et al. 1988). Conversely, in a series of 55 laparoscopies performed in 52 patients with suspected lymphoma, CONLON et al. (1996) reported a diagnostic accuracy of 98.2%. We attribute the high failure rate in our series to the following causes: (1) At our institution, most abdominal masses or lymph nodes are referred to the radiologist, given the high success rate of percutaneous biopsies for abdominal masses (SILVERMAN et al. 1994). Only those patients not selected for IGBN undergo surgery. This means they have either a small-sized lesion which may be difficult to reach laparoscopically, especially in overweight patients, or a high suspicion of Hodgkin disease or low-grade non-Hodgkin lymphoma. In the latter situation, examination of a whole lymph node is usually essential. We have found that dissecting and removing a whole lymph node located in the retroperitoneum was sometimes difficult. Oozing and proximity of large vessels and/or pancreas may prompt excessive prudence thus leading to small size and non-contributory biopsies. (2) The second reason for failure during laparoscopy may be inexperience. In the later cases, we have found that adapting the patient's positioning to the procedure was helpful in exposing the target and made the operation easier and safer, allowing for a better diagnostic yield.

Eventually, the following management may be proposed:

- All abdominal masses or lymph nodes, provided that their size is suitable for percutaneous biopsy should be primarily approached through IGNB (DE KERVILER et al. 1996). However, when there is a high suspicion of Hodgkin disease, the need to examine a complete lymph nodes may make surgery preferable. Indeed, in both series of SILVERMAN et al. (1994) and ZORNOZA et al. (1981), only two thirds of the patients with Hodgkin disease could be treated on the basis of IGNB. In nodular sclerosing Hodgkin disease, as in follicular low-grade lymphomas or in residual masses in general, extensive sclerosis makes cellular samples difficult to obtain.

- For patients presenting with lymph nodes of the middle mediastinum, mediastinoscopy is the procedure of choice because of its high diagnostic yield as well as its low morbidity and short post-operative stay (CYBULSKY and BENNET 1994; GOSSOT et al. 1996b; PATTISON et al. 1989). Patients presenting with lung nodules or other mediastinal masses are better managed by thoracoscopy (GOSSOT et al. 1996b; LANDRENEAU et al. 1993; RIEGER et al. 1996). CT-guided biopsies are however indicated for those masses that are close to the chest wall and/or in patients in poor respiratory condition (WITTICH et al. 1992). Minimally invasive approaches such as image-guided biopsies and surgical endoscopic techniques have become two methods of choice in the management of patients with lymphoma at presentation. From a practical standpoint, we recommend image-guided biopsies as a first step when non-Hodgkin lymphoma is suspected, provided that the target can be reached safely. In the remaining cases, i.e. suspicion of Hodgkin disease and small B-cell lymphoma or deep mediastinal masses or lymph nodes, or in case of failure of previous IGNB, surgical endoscopic techniques are the method of choice for obtaining tissue samples (SUTCLIFFE et al. 1982; GOODMAN et al. 1982).

27.5
How Should Residual Masses Be Approached?

An intrathoracic residual mass is present in more than 20% of patients after treatment of Hodgkin disease or a non-Hodgkin lymphoma (BRICE et al. 1993). Eighteen percent of these patients experience a relapse at the level of the residual mass (CANELLOS 1988). Theoretically, only a complete surgical resection of the residual mass could assert that the patient is disease-free. A second-look surgery has been advocated as the method of choice by some authors (GOODMAN et al. 1982; SUTCLIFFE et al. 1982). This attitude is questionable because (1) complete removal of tumoral and fibrotic tissues requires large incisions in patients who have often undergone previous surgery, (2) morbidity is high, and (3) less than 20% of mediastinal residual mass lead to relapse (RADFORD et al. 1988).

Thus, the use of noninvasive methods such as CT or Gallium scan (GS) or positron emission tomography (PET) scan seems preferable. However, there is no consensus on the method of choice. CT alone does not allow discrimination between residual tumor and fibrosis or necrosis. According to most recent studies, CT has a poor sensitivity with respect to the diagnosis of residual disease. In a retrospective review of Hodgkin disease and non-Hodgkin lymphoma, Stumpe et al. have found the specificity of CT to be only 41% for Hodgkin disease and 67% for non-Hodgkin lymphoma (STUMPE et al. 1998). MR imaging has been shown to be slightly more reliable with respect to the diagnosis of fibrosis (DEVIZZI et al. 1997). The GS is much more reliable than CT and MR imaging since gallium uptake is proportional to the amount of residual cells (FRONT et al. 1992). A recent study demonstrated that GS has a high specificity (91%) and a positive predictive value of 81% in 53 patients with residual mass after treatment of Hodgkin disease (IONESCU et al. 2000). Other authors have found similar results for aggressive diffuse non-Hodgkin lymphoma. However, for follicular non-Hodgkin lymphoma, results appear to be less reliable (GALLAMINI et al. 1997). The specificity of GS is not optimal because of numerous causes of false positives, such as tuberculosis, sarcoidosis, bronchitis, or thymic hyperplasia (BARTHOLD et al. 1997). The later is a commonplace cause of mediastinal enlargement after chemotherapy. It is known as "rebound" thymic hyperplasia (Fig. 27.10) (KISSIN et al. 1987). It may occur up to 14 months after completion of chemotherapy and is found in more than 11% of patients. Although thymic enlargement usually appears as a homogeneous mass of the anterior mediastinum, doubt may remain in some cases. Furthermore, most thymic rebounds are cause for ^{67}Ga uptake (PEYLAN-RAMU et al. 1989). In addition, GS must not be performed near the end of chemotherapy to avoid false negative results. Partially necrotic or small sized tumors may also lead to false negatives of GS.

PET seems to reach higher specificity. In a series of 44 residual mass with positive CT, ZINANI et al. (1999) found 100% relapse among the 13 patients with positive PET and only 1 relapse (4%) among the 24 patients with negative PET. STUMPE et al. (1998) have found CT and PET to have similar sensitivities but PET is significantly more specific than CT. Its specificity for residual mass is 96% after Hodgkin disease and 100% after non-Hodgkin lymphoma. However, although the predictive positive value of PET is 100%, it seems than PET mainly predicts for early progression but cannot exclude the presence of minimal residual disease (JERUSALEM et al. 1999). Indeed, in the series of JERUSALEM et al. (1999), clinical relapses were observed more frequently in patients with than without residual mass. These data and the limited follow-up do not allow definite conclusion about the accuracy of PET.

Thus, there are still circumstances where doubt remains and where a pathological proof is required. Due to their minimal invasiveness, CT-guided biopsies are often seen as the method of choice. However, our data indicate its limitations when dealing with residual mass. In these residual mass, performing multiple biopsies is essential since residual disease usually coexists with fibrotic and/or necrotic tissue or thymic hyperplasia (Figs. 27.11, 27.12) (GOSSOT et al. 2001).

27.6
Conclusion

Despite the increasing use of gallium and positron emission tomography scans, there are still cases where certainty is wanted i.e. where a biopsy is required. Only surgery allows for multiple biopsies at different sites (benign and malignant lesions may coexist), thus avoiding the risk of missing malignant cells. In these patients submitted to invasive therapeutic programs, open conventional surgery should be avoided for two reasons. First, satisfactory specimens can be obtained by endoscopic surgical techniques; and second, open surgery makes an eventual secondary thoracoscopy more difficult and less profitable.

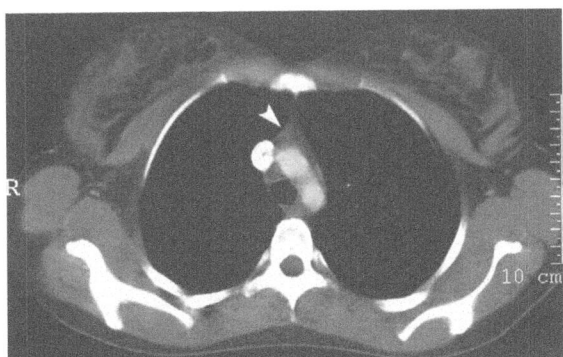 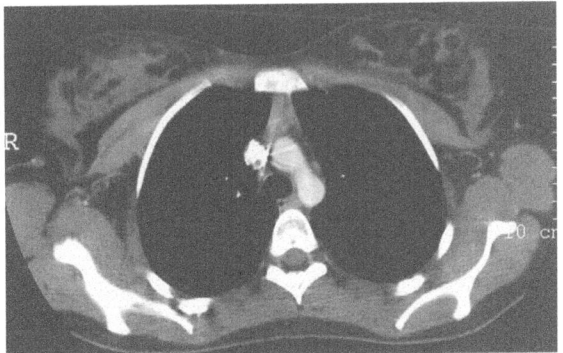

Fig. 27.10a,b. Hodgkin disease in a 15-year-old-girl with rebound thymic hyperplasia. **a** Axial contrast-enhanced thoracic CT scan at the end of treatment shows small residual anterior mediastinal lymph node mass (*arrowhead*) which increased in size on (**b**) axial contrast-enhanced thoracic CT scan 6 months later. Pathology allowed the diagnosis of rebound thymic hyperplasia with no sign of disease recurrence.

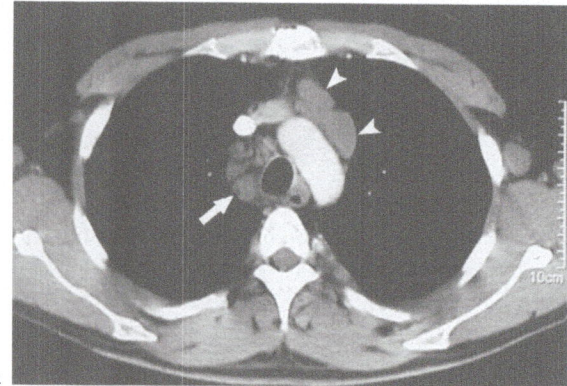

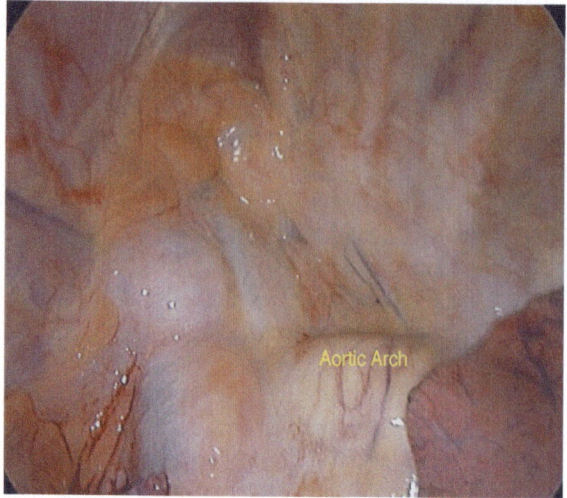

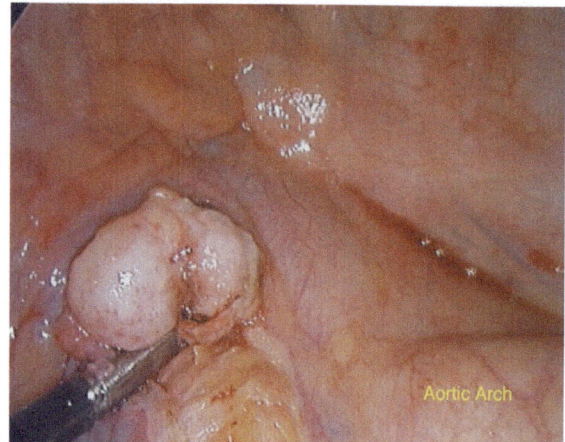

Fig. 27.11a–c. Hodgkin disease in a17-year-old girl with a residual mass. **a** Axial contrast-enhanced CT scan of the chest at the end of chemotherapy shows residual right paratracheal lymph node (*arrow*) and anterior mediastinal mass (*arrowheads*). Left thoracoscopic views show the mass (**b**) before and (**c**) while removing a large sample. Pathology yielded presence of Sternberg cells, and thus confirmed the active nature of this residual mass.

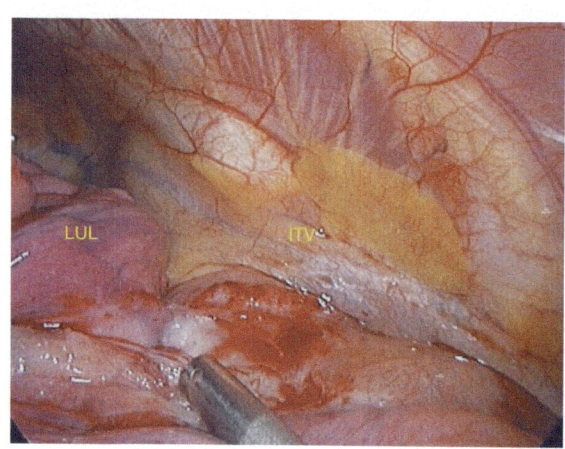

Fig. 27.12. Non-Hodgkin lymphoma in a 31-year-old man with anterior mediastinal residual mass at completion of treatment. Thoracoscopic view shows the anterior mediastinal mass (*LUL* = left upper lobe, *ITV* = internal thoracic vessels). Biopsy during thoracoscopy yielded residual active lymphoma within fibrotic tissue.

References

Baccarani U, Carroll B, Hiatt J et al (1998) Comparison of laparoscopic and open staging in Hodgkin disease. Arch Surg 133:517–522

Barthold S, Donohoe K, Fletcher J (1997) Procedures guideline for Gallium scintigraphy in the evaluation of malignant disease. J Nucl Med 38:990–994

Ben-Yehuda D, Pollicak A, Okon E et al (1996) Image-guided core-needle biopsy in malignant lymphoma: experience with 100 patients that suggests the technique is reliable. J Clin Oncol 14:2431–2434

Brice P, Rain JD, Miaux Y et al (1993) Residual mediastinal mass in malignant lymphoma: value of magnetic resonance imaging and gallium scan. Nouv Rev Fr Hematol 35:457–461

Canellos GP (1988) Residual mass in Lymphoma may not be residual disease. J Clin Oncol 6:931–933

Carrasco C, Richli W, Lawrence D, Katz R, Wallace S (1990) Fine needle aspiration biopsy in lymphoma. Radiol Clin North Am 28:879–883

Celikoglu F, Teirstein A, Krellenstein D, Strauchen J (1992) Pleural effusion in non-Hodgkin's lymphoma. Chest 101: 1357–1360

Childers J, Balserack J, Kent T, Surwit E (1993) Laparoscopic staging of Hodgkin's lymphoma. J Laproendosc Surg 3: 495–499

Childers J, Surwit E (1994) Laparoscopic para-aortic lymph node biopsy for diagnosis of a non-Hodgkin's lymphoma. Surg Laparosc Endosc 2:139–142

Cirino LM, Milanez de Campos JR, Fernandez A et al (2000) Diagnosis and treatment of mediastnal tumors by thoracoscopy. Chest 117:1787–1792

Conlon K, Zelentez A, LaQuaglia M, Dougherty E (1996) Laparoscopy: redefining the role of the surgeon in abdominal lymphoma (Abstr). Surg Endosc 10:179

Cowles R, Yahanda A (2000) Laparoscopic biopsy of abdominal retroperitoneal lymphadenopahy for the diagnosis of lymphoma. J Am Coll Surg 191:108–113

Cybulsky I, Bennet F (1994) Mediastinoscopy as a routine outpatient procedure. Ann Thorac Surg 58:176–178

D'Emilia J, Neff P, DeMaria E (1996) Laparoscopic staging for Hodgkin's disease (abstr). Surg Endosc 10:203

de Kerviler E, Guermazi A, Cazals-Hatem D, Frija J (1996) Use of abdominal compression as an aid to CT-guided retroperitoneal biopsies. AJR Am J Roentgenol 167: 1346–1347

Devizzi L, Maffioli L, Bonfante V et al (1997) Comparison of gallium scan, computed tomography, and magnetic resonance in patients with mediastinal Hodgkin's disease. Ann Oncol 8:53–56

Dmitriev EG, Sigal EI (1996) Thoracoscopic surgery in the management of mediastinal masses. Indications, complications, limitations. Surg Endosc 10:718–720

Elia S, Cecere C, Giampaglia E, Ferrante G (1992) Mediastinoscopy vs anterior mediastinoscopy in the diagnosis of mediastinal lymphoma: a randomized trial. Eur J Cardiothorac Surg 6:361–365

Ferzli G, Fiorillo M, Solis R et al (1997) Laparoscopic stagig of Hodgkin's disease. J Laparoendosc Adv Surg Tech A 7: 353–355

Front D, Ben-Haim S, Israel O et al (1992) Lymphoma: predictive value of Ga-67 scintigraphy after treatment. Radiology 182:359–363

Gallamini A, Biggi A, Fruttero A et al (1997) Revisiting the prognostic role of gallium scintigraphy in low-grade Non-Hdgkin's lymphoma. Eur J Nucl Med 24:1499–1506

Goodman G, Jones S, Villar H (1982) Surgical restaging of Hodgkin's disease. Cancer Treat Rep 66:751–757

Gossot D, Miaux Y, Guermazi A, Frija J, Celerier M (1994) The hook-wire technique for localisation of pulmonary nodules during thoracoscoic resection. Chest 105:1467–1469

Gossot D, Toledo L, Celerier M (1996a) The thoracoscope as diagnostic tool for solid mediastinal masses. Surg Endosc 10:504–507

Gossot D, Toledo L, Fritsch S, Celerier M (1996b) Mediastinoscopy vs Thoracoscopy for mediastinal biopsy. Results of a prospective non-randomized trial. Chest 110:1328–1331

Gossot D, de Kerviler E, Brice P (1998) Surgical endoscopic techniques in the diagnosis and follow-up of patients with lymphoma. Br J Surg 85:1107–1110

Gossot D, Girard P, de Kerviler E et al (2001) Thoracoscopy or CT-guided biopsy for residual intrathoracic masses after treatment of lymphoma. Chest 120:289–294

Hemming A, Nagy A, Scudamore C, Edelmann K (1995) Laparoscopic staging of intraabdominal malignancy. Surg Endosc 9:325–328

Ionescu I, Brice P, Simon D et al (2000) Restaging with Gallium scan identifies chemosensitive patients and predicts survival of poor-prognosis mediastinal Hodgkin's disease patients. Med Oncol 17:127–134

Jerusalem G, Beguin Y, Najjar F, Paulus P, Rigo P, Fillet G (1999) Whole-body positron emission tomography using fluorodeoxyglucose for posttreatment evaluation in Hodgkin's disease and non-Hodgkin's lymphoma has higher diagnostic and pronostic value than classical computed tomography scan imaging. Blood 94:429–433

Jockovitch M, Mendenhall N, Sombeck M, Talbert J, Copeland E, Bland K (1994) Long-term complications of laparotomy in Hodkin's disease. Ann Surg 219:615–621

Kissin CM, Husband JE, Nicholas D, Eversman W (1987) Bening thymic enlargement in adults after chemotherapy: CT demonstration. Radiology 163:67–70

Landreneau R, Hazelrigg S, Mack M et al (1993) Thoracoscopic mediastinal lymph node node sampling: useful for mediastinal lymphn node stations inacessible by cervical mediastinoscopy. J Thoracic Cardiovasc Surg 106:554–558

Lev-Chelouche D, Margal D, Klausner JM, Szold A (2001) Diagnostic laparoscopy: a useful tool in abdominal lymphoma. Harefuah 140:103–105

Mineo T, Ambrogi V, Anfroni I, Pistolese C (1999) Mediastinoscopy in superior vena cava obstruction: analysis of 80 consecutive patients. Ann Thorac Surg 68:223–226

Pappa V, Hussain H, Reznezk R et al (1996) Role of image-guided core-needle biopsy in the management of patients with lymphoma. J Clin Oncol 14:2427–2430

Pattison C, Westaby S, Wetter A, Townsend E (1989) Mediastinoscopy in the investigation of primary mediastinal lymphadenopathy. Scand J Thor Cardiovasc Surg 23: 177–179

Peylan-Ramu N, Haddy TB, Jones E, Horvath K, Adde MA, Magrath IT (1989) High frequency of benign mediastinal uptake of Gallium-67 after completion of chemotherapy in children with high-grade non-Hodgkin's lymphoma. J Clin Oncol 7:1800–1806

Radford J, Cowan R, Flanagan M (1988) The significance of residual mediastinal abnormality on the chest radiograph following treatment for Hodgkin's disease. J Clin Oncol 6: 940–946

Rendina E, Venuta F, DeGiacomo T et al (2002) Biopsy of anterior mediastinal masses under local anesthesia. Ann Thorac Surg 74:1720–1723

Rendina E, Venuta F, DeGiacomo T et al (1994) Comparative merits of thoracoscopy, mediastinoscopy and mediastinotomy for mediastinal biopsy. Ann Thorac Surg 57:992–995

Rieger R, Schrenck P, Woisetschläger R, Wayand W (1996) Videothoracoscopy for the management of mediastinal mass lesions. Surg Endosc 10:715–717

Roviaro G, Varoli F, Nucca O, Vergani C, Maciocci M, Scalambra S (2000) Videothoracoscopic approach to medistinal pathology. Chest 117:1179–1183

Salky B, bauer J, Gelernt I (1988) The use of laparoscopy in retroperitoneal pathology. Gastrointest Endosc 34:227–230

Silecchia G, Fantini A, Raparelli L et al (1999) Management of abdominal lymphoproliferative diseases in the era of laparoscopy. Am J Surg 177:325–330

Silverman S, Lee B, Mueller P (1994) Impact of positive findings at image-guided biopsy of lymphoma on patient care: evaluation of clinical history, needle size and pathologic findings on biopsy performance. Radiology 190:759–764

Solaini L, Bagioni P, Campanini A, Poddie B (1998) Diagnostic role of videothoracoscopy in mediastinal diseases. Eur J Cardio-Thoracic Surg 13:491–493

Stricker J, Donohue J, Porter L, Habermann T (1998) Laparoscopic biopsy for suspected abdominal lymphoma. Mod Pathol 11:831–836

Stumpe K, Urbinelli M, Steinert H, Glanzmann C, Buck A, von Schulthess G (1998) Whole-body positron emission tomography using fluorodeoxyglucose for staging of lymphoma: effectiveness and comparison with computed tomography. Eur J Nucl Med 25:721–728

Sutcliffe S, Wrigley P, Timothy A (1982) Post-treatment laparotomy as a guide to management in patients with Hodgkin's disease. Cancer Treat Rep 66:759–765

Venuta F, Rendina E, Pescarmona E et al (1997) Ambulatory mediastinal biopsy for hematoogic malignancies. Eur J Cardio-Thoracic Surg 11:218–221

Wittich G, Nowels K, Korn R et al (1992) Coaxial transthoracic fine-needle biopsy in patients with a history of malignant lymphoma. Radiology 183:175–178

Zinani P, Magagnoli M, Chierichetti F et al (1999) The role of positron emission tomography (PET) in the management of lymphoma patients. Ann Oncol 10:1181–1184

Zornoza J, Cabanillas F, Altof T (1981) Percutaneous needle biopsy in abdominal lymphoma. AJR Am J Roentgenol 135:97–103

28 Imaging-guided Therapeutic Percutaneous Procedures

Afshin Gangi, Stéphane Guth, Ali Guermazi

CONTENTS

28.1
Introduction

Patients treated for hematological malignancies almost always suffer from pain and disability late in the course of their disease. Over the past few years, imaging-guided percutaneous procedures have become useful for providing short, and sometimes long-term, pain relief, as well as bone strengthening. Patient selection is essential to the success of these techniques. Thus, the interventional radiologist should play an active central role in minimally invasive management of pain in patients treated for hematological malignancies, and should be part of an interdisciplinary team that determines the appropriate therapy (Gangi et al. 1998). Indeed, the choice between a therapeutic percutaneous procedure and alternative methods of treatment depends on several factors: the location of the lesion, the local and general extent of the disease, the pain and functional disability experienced by the patient, and the patient's state of health and life expectancy (Cotten et al. 1999). In this chapter, we will primarily, and most importantly, focus on the cementoplasty technique and give secondarily some details about ethanol injection in bone osteolytic lesions.

28.2
Cementoplasty

Afshin Gangi, MD, Ph D
Professor, Department of Radiology B, University Hospital of Strasbourg, Pavillon Clovis Vincent BP 426, 67091 Strasbourg, France
Stéphane Guth, MD
Senior Radiologist, Department of Radiology B, University Hospital of Strasbourg, Pavillon Clovis Vincent BP 426, 67091 Strasbourg, France
Ali Guermazi, MD
Visiting Associate Professor, Department of Radiology, University of California, San Francisco, 350 Parnassus Avenue, Suite 150, San Francisco, CA 94117, USA

Percutaneous injection of polymethylmethacrylate (PMMA), also referred to a bone cement, provides notable pain relief and bone strengthening in patients with malignant vertebral and acetabular osteolyses. Multiple myeloma involving vertebral bodies and the weight-bearing part of the acetabulum (i.e., the acetabular roof) is therefore a classical indication for cementoplasty (Cotten et al. 1999; Gangi et al. 2003). It should be stressed that performing this procedure requires excellent radiological skills and special training.

28.2.1
Mechanism

Percutaneous injection of PMMA reduces pain and strengthens bone. PMMA, which hardens as polymerization occurs, also provides bone strengthening with stabilization of microfractures and reduction of mechanical forces. Consequently, injection of PMMA is indicated when the object is to improve mobility in patients with osteolysis involving the weight-bearing part of the vertebral body and acetabulum) (COTTEN et al. 1999). The pain-reducing effect of cement cannot be explained by consolidation of the pathologic bone alone. In fact, good pain relief occurs after injection of only 2 ml of cement in a myeloma.

PMMA injection may be performed prior to radiation therapy, which complements its action due to similar but delayed effects on pain; alternatively, it may be performed after radiation therapy that has failed to relieve pain or in cases of local recurrence. Patients do not begin to experience pain relief until 10–14 days after start of radiation therapy. More importantly, radiation therapy results in minimal, 2–4 months delay in bone strengthening, which is usually more effective in patients with myeloma. However, this delay in bone strengthening increases the risk of vertebral collapse and subsequently of neural compression. Therefore, vertebroplasty can be used to provide pain relief and to produce bone strengthening and vertebral stabilization when the lesion threatens the stability of the spine (COTTEN et al. 1998). Likewise, injection of PMMA in lesions of the acetabular roof prior to radiation therapy is recommended to decrease the risk of pathologic fracture of the acetabulum and to improve walking (COTTEN et al. 1999).

28.2.2
Vertebroplasty

Percutaneous vertebroplasty with acrylic cement consists of injecting PMMA into vertebral bodies destabilized by osseous lesions. The aim is to obtain an analgesic effect by reinforcing lesions of spine (COTTEN et al. 1998; DERAMOND et al. 1998). Developed in France in the late 1980's, minimally invasive vertebroplasty was first used to treat aggressive or painful vertebral hemangiomas (GALIBERT et al. 1987) and was quickly applied to other lesions that weaken the vertebral body, including osteolytic metastases or multiple myeloma (COTTEN et al. 1996; CALLANDER and ROODMAN 2001; JENSEN and KALLMES 2002)

and osteoporotic vertebral body collapse (BARR et al. 2000; KALLMES et al. 2002; EVANS et al. 2003). Rarely, vertebral lymphoma (COTTEN et al. 1998; BARR et al. 2000; JENSEN and KALLMES 2002; FOURNEY et al. 2003) and intravertebral pseudoarthrosis caused by avascular necrosis (JANG et al. 2003) can also be an indication for vertebroplasty. Although injection of PMMA does not, commonly, significantly reexpand a collapsed vertebra, it does reinforce and stabilize the vertebra, which seems to alleviate pain (BARR et al. 2000; FOURNEY et al. 2003) before radiation therapy or chemotherapy alone or in combination with surgical osteosynthesis. It also can be useful in recurrent pain after chemotherapy and/or radiation therapy (COTTEN et al. 1996; CHIRAS et al. 1997).

28.2.2.1
Equipment

Materials used for vertebroplasty include (Fig. 28.1):
- 15-gauge needle for cervical spine, and 10 cm or 15 cm 10-gauge vertebroplasty beveled needle for thoracic and lumbar spine, respectively
- Surgical hammer
- PMMA cement mixed with 3g of tantalum or tungsten to increase the radiopacity of the acrylic glue.
- Pressure syringe to facilitate the injection of this viscous glue.
- Sterile drapes and towels.
- 22-gauge needle for anesthesia.
- Scalpel.
- Iodine.
- 1% lidocaine.

28.2.2.2
Imaging Guidance

The procedure is performed under guidance of CT and/or fluoroscopy. For either method, the injection of the acrylic cement should be controlled by real-time fluoroscopic guidance to avoid major complications.

28.2.2.2.1
Dual Guidance

For skeletal, minimally invasive procedures, the best and safest guidance technique seems to be combined CT and fluoroscopy (GANGI et al. 1994b). This combination allows precise needle placement, reduces complications and increases the comfort of the operator. The dual guidance technique using CT and C-arm fluoroscopy is particularly interesting in per-

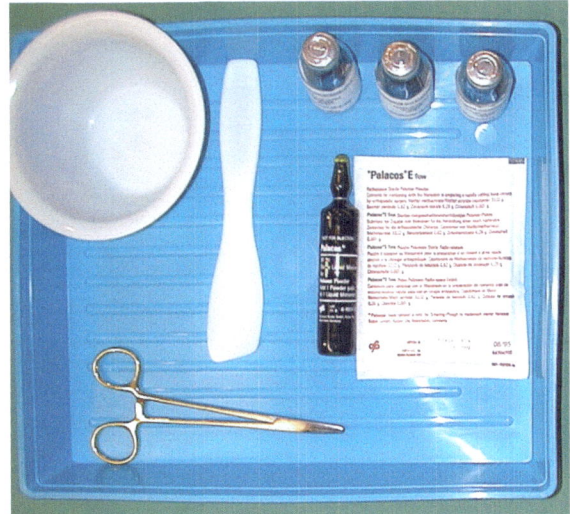
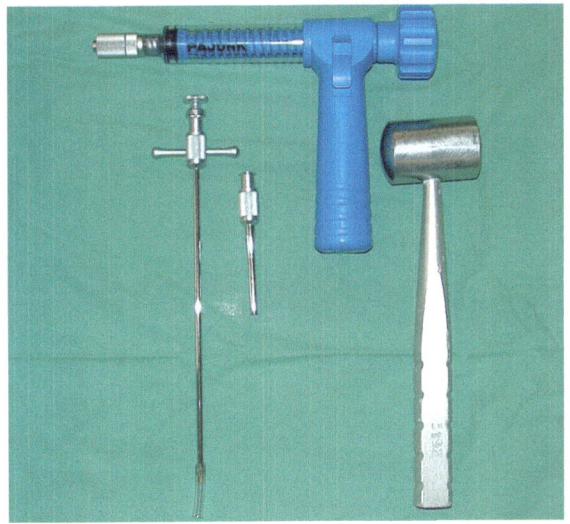

a

b

Fig. 28.1a,b. Photographs show materials used for vertebroplasty.

cutaneous cementoplasty (GANGI et al. 1994b; GANGI et al. 2003). However, fluoroscopy and biplane fluoroscopy can be used for percutaneous vertebroplasty by a well-trained radiologist if access to the CT room is difficult (COTTEN et al. 1996).

For fluoroscopy, a mobile C-arm is used, positioned in front of the CT-gantry (Fig. 28.2). By using a rotating fluoroscope and CT, the structure to be punctured can be visualized three dimensionally and with exact differentiation of anatomic structures, which in many cases is not possible with fluoroscopy alone. Two mobile monitors are placed in front of the physician, displaying the last stored image and the fluoroscopic image. The operator can switch from CT to fluoroscopy and vice versa at any time. In percutaneous vertebroplasty, the intervention begins with CT and is followed by fluoroscopy. The needle is placed precisely and safely under CT guidance (Fig. 28.3). The injection of the PMMA requires real-time imaging and is therefore performed under fluoroscopic control (Fig. 28.4). This combination has many advantages. The possibilities of the simultaneous combination of the two imaging methods are almost unlimited and other applications in interventional radiology are possible (GANGI et al. 2003).

28.2.2.2.2
Fluoroscopic Guidance

Puncture can be done under fluoroscopic guidance (Fig. 28.5). It is, however, more difficult under fluoroscopy alone than with dual guidance.

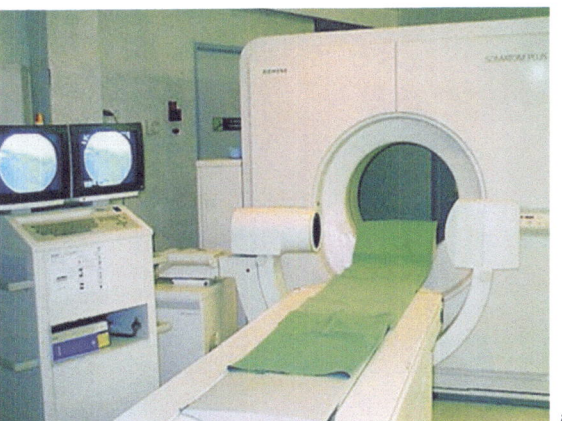

a

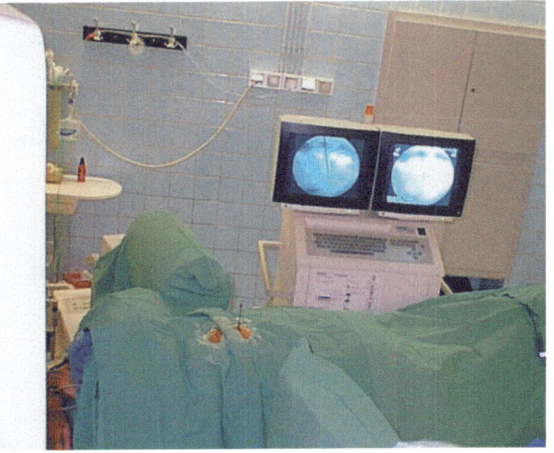

b

Fig. 28.2a,b. Dual guidance CT and fluoroscopy. **a** View before the procedure of the mobile C-arm positioned in front of the CT gantry. Two mobile monitors face the operator. **b** View of dual guidance during the procedure.

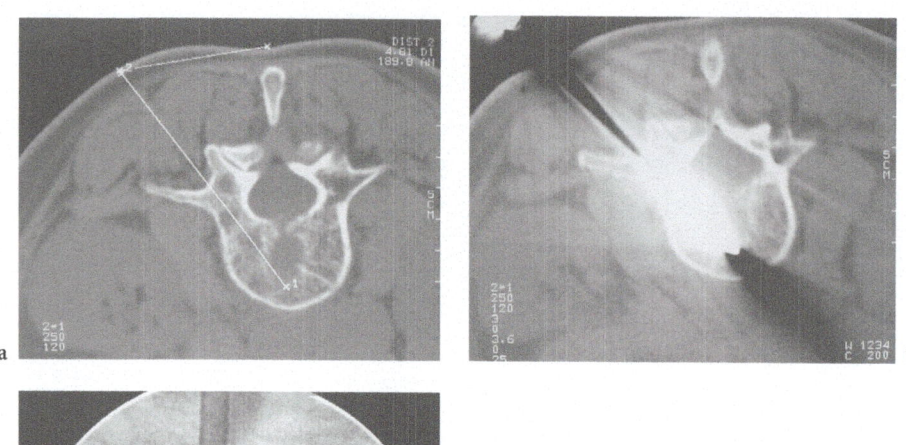

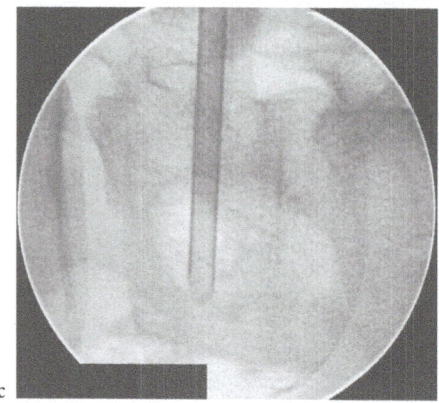

Fig. 28.3a–c. CT-guided needle placement during vertebroplasty in a 68-year-old woman with multiple myeloma. a Axial CT scan of L4 shows the expected needle placement in the anterior portion of the vertebral body. b Axial control CT scan and (c) view from fluoroscopic control show the needle placed in the optimal position which is the anterior portion of the vertebral body.

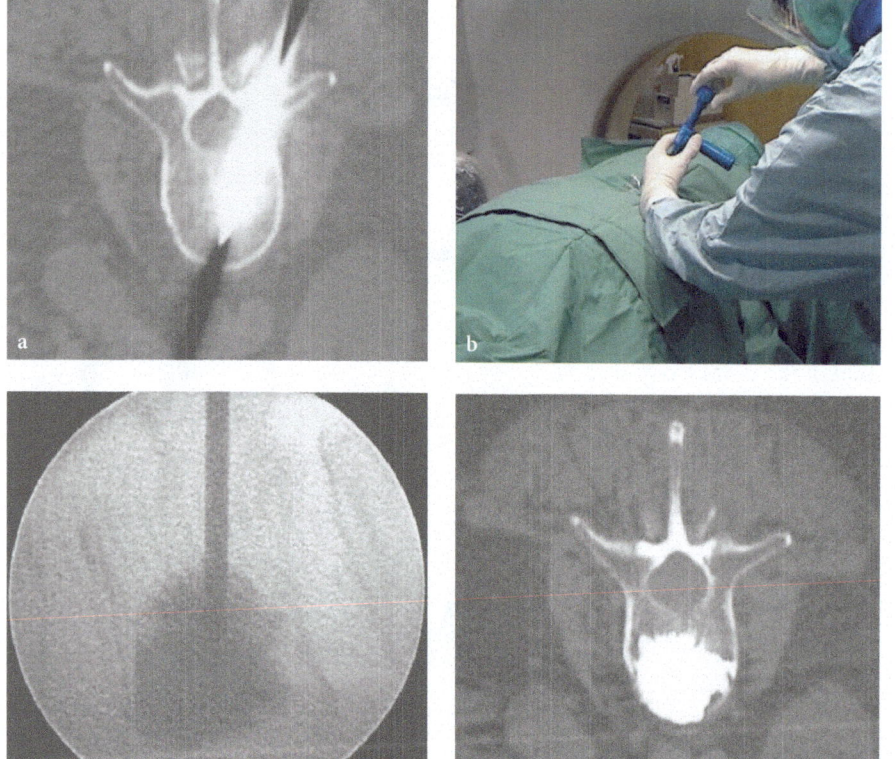

Fig. 28.4a–d. Cement injection under fluoroscopic control in a 59-year-old man with multiple myeloma. a View from video of control CT scan of the optimal needle placement in anterior aspect of L3 vertebral body. b View of the physician during the cement injection. c View of cement injection in L3 under fluoroscopic control, the patient in prone position. d View from video of control CT scan of the satisfactory filling of L3 vertebral body without complications.

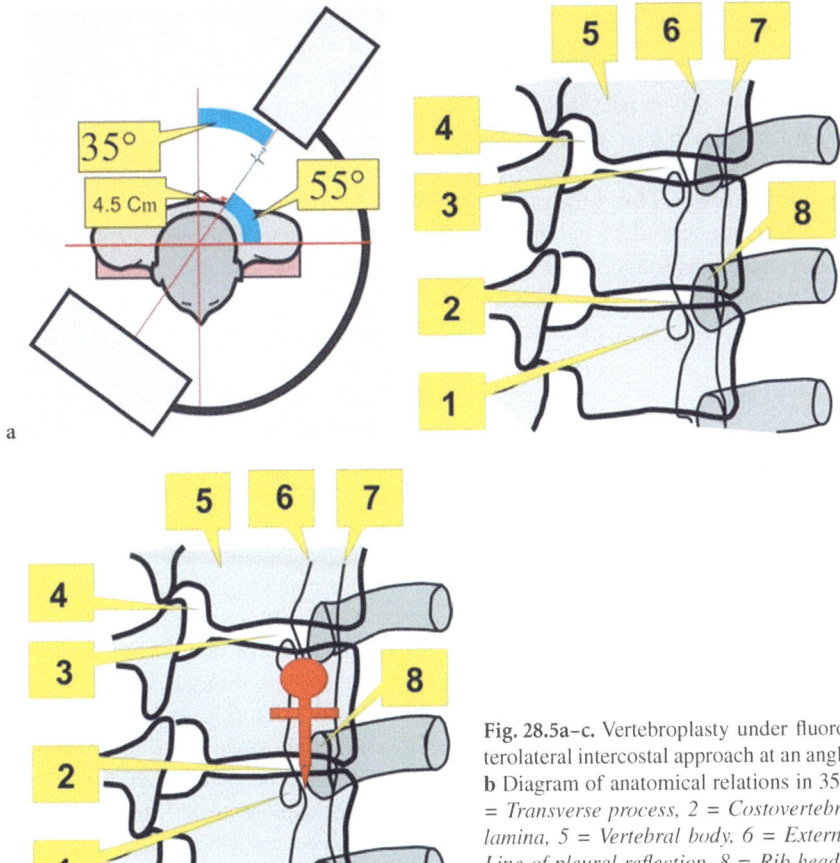

Fig. 28.5a–c. Vertebroplasty under fluoroscopic guidance. a View of the posterolateral intercostal approach at an angle 35° from the patient's sagittal plane. b Diagram of anatomical relations in 35° oblique procubitus position (left) *(1 = Transverse process, 2 = Costovertebral joint, 3 = Disk, 4 = Contralateral lamina, 5 = Vertebral body, 6 = External edge of the articular process, 7 = Line of pleural reflection, 8 = Rib head)*. c Puncture shown in red represents the vertebroplasty needle under fluoroscopy control.

The patient is placed in prone position. The appropriate radiographic profile for a pedicular approach is a straight anteroposterior view, with 5° to 10° angulation. The pedicle, with an oval shape, is localized with fluoroscopy. The needle is advanced into the pedicle under fluoroscopic control. For an optimal approach, the entry point and its distance from the midline (spinous process) can be measured on the axial CT scan or MR imaging film of the patient. The needle tip is positioned in the anterior part of the vertebral body. With this technique, the needle is placed in the ipsilateral half of the vertebra, although a bipediculate approach is often necessary for an optimal filling of the vertebral body. However, placement of the needle in the opposite pedicle prolongs the procedure and increases the risk of extravasation (KIM et al. 2002; GANGI et al. 2003).

For the unipediculate approach, the fluoroscopy tube is angled more laterally in the lumbar region until the oval appearance of the pedicle is transformed into the "Scotty dog" appearance over the pedicle. This typically requires a 30° angulation of the anteroposterior fluoroscopy tube. In the thoracic region, the tube is empirically angled to approximately 20°. This angulation projects a thin oval appearance of the pedicle. The needle is advanced until it approaches the anterolateral wall of the contralateral half of the vertebra (GANGI et al. 2003).

28.2.2.3
Patient Selection

Vertebroplasty is usually indicated when osteolysis involves the weight-bearing part of the vertebra, i.e., the vertebral body. This osteolysis should be symptomatic and also refractory to medical therapy (CORTET et al. 1997; McGRAW et al. 2003). Because multiple myeloma and rarely lymphoma of the vertebral body frequently cause severe pain and functional disability, they are excellent indications for vertebroplasty (GANGI et al. 2003).

PMMA injection is contraindicated in patients with coagulation disorders due to the large diameter of the needles used, and in case of infection (COTTEN et al. 1998; GANGI et al. 2003).

Extensive vertebral destruction and significant vertebral collapse (i.e., vertebra reduced to less than 1/3 of its original height) may lead to a technically difficult vertebroplasty procedure and may constitute a relative contraindication. Neurologic symptoms related to compression by vertebral body lesion or epidural tumoral extension require careful injection to prevent epidural overflow that could increase the compression. However, such symptoms do not constitute an absolute contraindication for the procedure (COTTEN et al. 1998).

28.2.2.4
Technique

Radiography and CT, and/or MR imaging, must be performed in the days preceding therapeutic percutaneous injection to assess the location and extent of the lytic process, the visibility and degree of involvement of the pedicles, the presence of epidural or foraminal stenosis caused by tumor extension or bone fragment retropulsion, the presence of cortical destruction or fracture especially of the vertebral posterior wall, and the presence of soft-tissue involvement (COTTEN et al. 1998; GANGI et al. 2003).

The procedure is performed under local anesthesia, usually combined with neuroleptanalgesia to control pain. The arterial blood pressure and oxygen saturation are monitored during the procedure.

After positioning the patient, a 10 or 15-gauge trocar needle is introduced into the lytic part of the tumor. Different approach routes can be selected for the vertebral body and depend on the experience of the radiologist. For the cervical spine, the anterolateral route is used (Fig. 28.6) (COTTEN et al. 1998; DUFRESNE et al. 1998; GANGI et al. 2003). The fingers are placed in such a way as to push the large vessels laterally, and the needle is advanced between the vessels and the pharyngolarynx. For the upper cervical spine, the route ascends markedly because the needle has to be introduced below the mandible (COTTEN et al. 1998; TONG et al. 2000). This approach is relatively difficult at the C2 level. A transoral approach to the C2 vertebral body has been described in a patient with myeloma, with benefits including precise needle placement and decreased risk to adjacent neurovascular structures (TONG et al. 2000). It should be stressed that this is a very difficult, high-risk approach. A transpedicular or intercostovertebral (Fig. 28.7) route is used for the thoracic level, and a posterolateral or transpedicular (Fig. 28.8) route for the lumbar level (GANGI et al. 2003). Use of the transpedicular route avoids spinal segmental nerve injury and decreases the risk of leakage of PMMA into the paravertebral tissue. Such access is not possible when

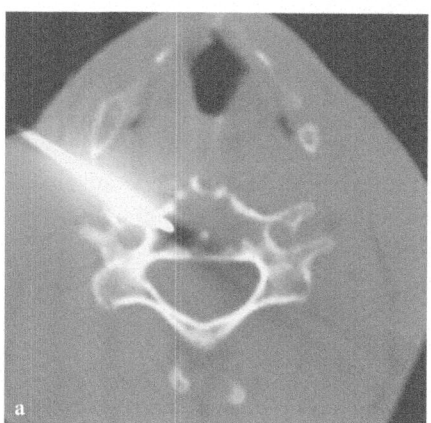
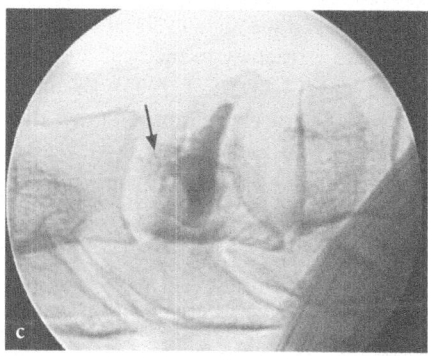
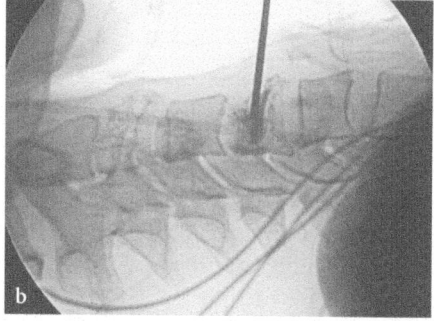
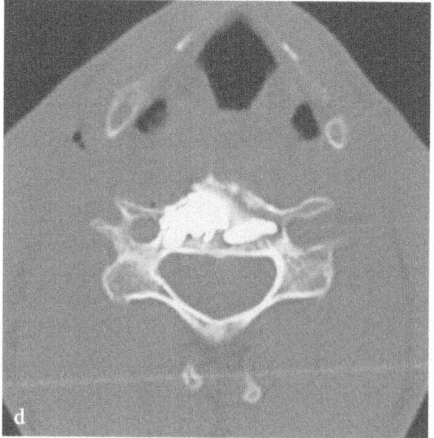

Fig. 28.6a–d. Cervical vertebroplasty under CT and fluoroscopic guidance in a 45-year-old man with multiple myeloma. **a** Axial control CT and (**b**) lateral fluoroscopic control of the cervical spine show right anterior route of the needle in C5. **c** Lateral fluoroscopic control and (**d**) axial CT scan after the procedure show good filling of C4 with PMMA. There is a small discal leak (*arrow*), only seen on (**c**). The patient was pain free 48 hours after the intervention.

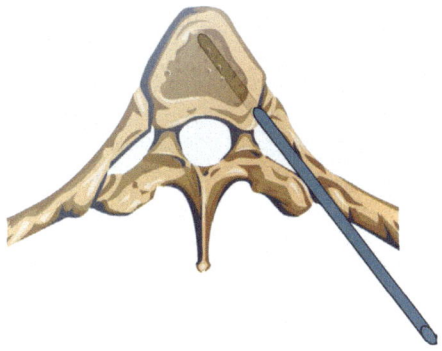

Fig. 28.7.
tebral route for thoracic vertebroplasty in axial view.

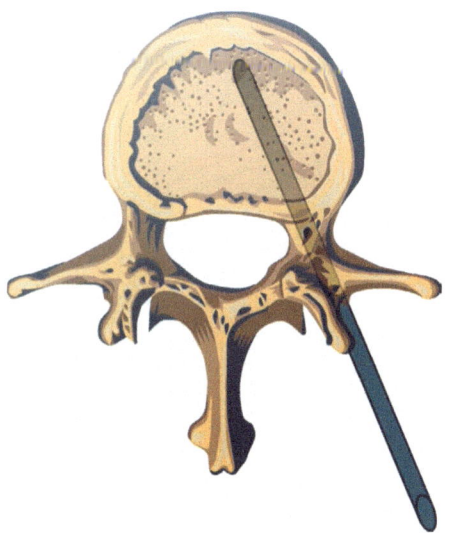

Fig. 28.8. Artist's rendering of the ideal needle transpedicular route for lumbar vertebroplasty in axial view.

osteolysis involves the pedicles or when there is surgical osteosynthesis. In such cases, the posterolateral route is easy to use for the lumbar spine but is more difficult for the thoracic spine due to risk of pneumothorax (CHIRAS et al. 1997; COTTEN et al. 1998).

The needle is introduced through a small dermatotomy and advanced to the posterior aspect of each pedicle along its superolateral cortex. Cortical perforation requires the aid of a surgical hammer. The bevel of the needle is directed so that the tip is pointed laterally, to avoid penetration of the spinal canal. The needle is directed anteriorly, medially, and caudally through the pedicle to reach a point within the anterior third of the vertebral body, near the midline in the sagittal plane (Fig. 28.9) (FOURNEY et al. 2003). The needle is safely guided under CT and the bevel of the needle must be oriented to facilitate injection of the cement in the desired direction. When the needle is in the optimal position, the imaging mode is switched to fluoroscopy. The cement is prepared by using 30 g of methacrylate powder and 12 g of barium sulfate. This powdered mixture is vigorously mixed. Approximately 10 ml is removed and combined with approximately 6 ml of methacrylate liquid monomer. The resultant PMMA with the consistency of paste (Fig. 28.10) is then injected until resistance is met or until the cement reaches the borders of the osteolytic lesion. This phase of the procedure is guided with fluoroscopy (Figs. 28.11, 28.12). The average volume of PMMA injected is 2.8 ml, ranging from 1.8 ml to 6.5 ml. If filling does not occur across the midline, then contralateral transpedicular injection is performed. The contralateral pedicle is approached in a manner similar to that described above (KIM et al. 2002; GANGI et al. 2003).

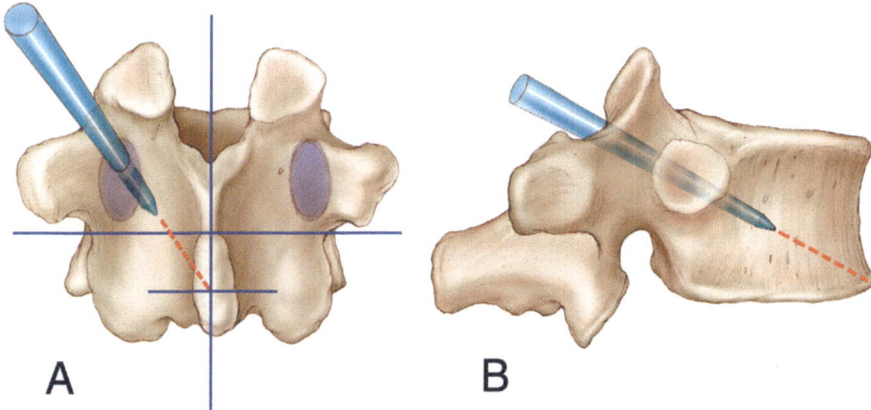

Fig. 28.9. Artist's rendering of the ideal needle trajectory for the vertebroplasty in anteroposterior (left) and lateral (right) views. The optimal position of the needle tip is also shown. (With permission from [Fourney et al. 2003])

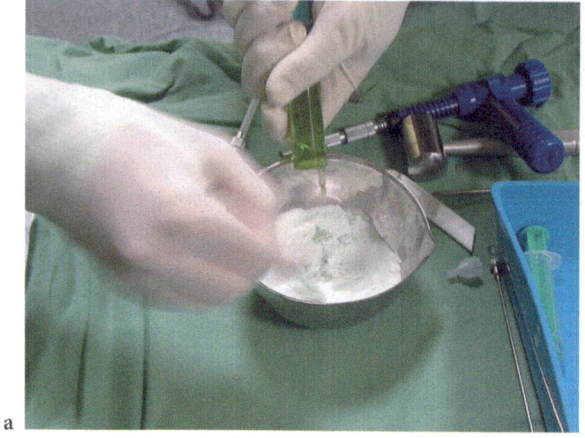
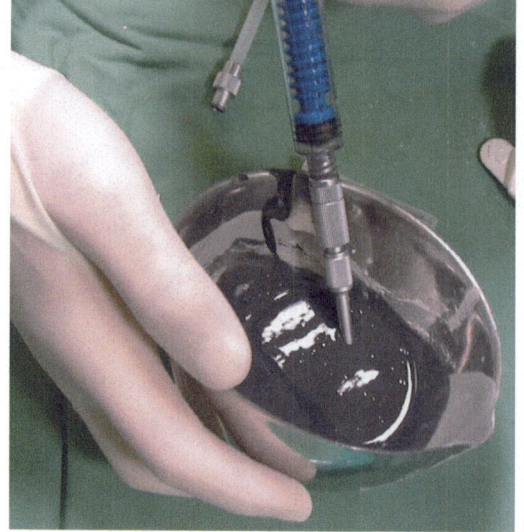

Fig. 28.10a,b. Views of (**a**) the methacrylate powder and (**b**) the PMMA cement before injection.

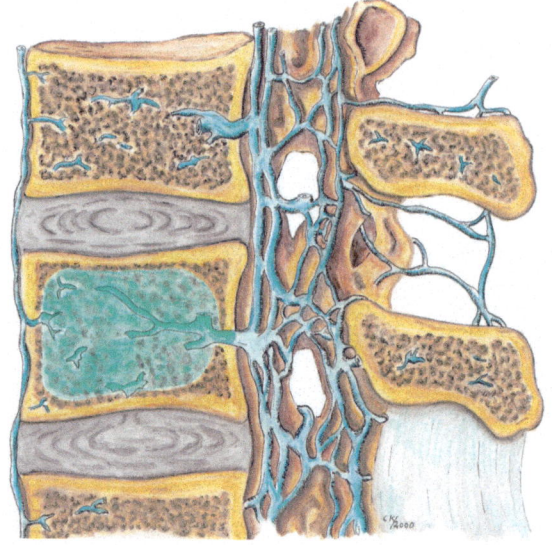
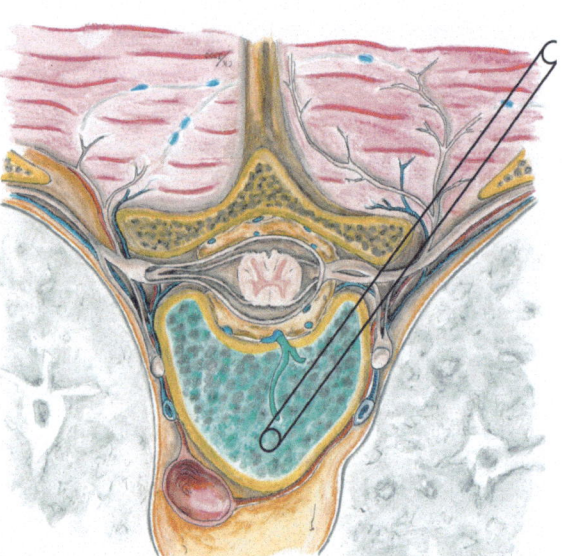

Fig. 28.11a,b. Artist's rendering of the ideal vertebral body filling with cement in (**a**) sagittal and (**b**) axial views.

Use of a unipediculate approach in percutaneous vertebroplasty (Fig. 28.13) allows filling of both vertebral halves from a single puncture site with no statistically significant difference in clinical outcome from that of bipediculate vertebroplasty. In this case, the tip of the needle is placed in the contralateral half of the vertebra. Filling across the midline was achieved in 96% of unipediculate injections, with a mean filling of 77% in both vertebral halves (KIM et al. 2002).

Injection is immediately stopped if epidural, foraminal, or venous leakage of cement is detected. One or more injections may be performed depend-ing on the distribution of cement in the vertebral body as demonstrated by radiographs and CT scan. The degree of lesion filling varies with myelomatous lesions, probably because of the different texture of this lesion (COTTEN et al. 1998). The procedure usually lasts from 1 to 2 hours unless cement is injected into 2 or more vertebral bodies. It is highly recommended that CT, which allows assessment of lesion filling (Fig. 28.14) as well as detection of PMMA leakage, be performed immediately after cement injection (COTTEN et al. 1998; KIM et al. 2002; GANGI et al. 2003).

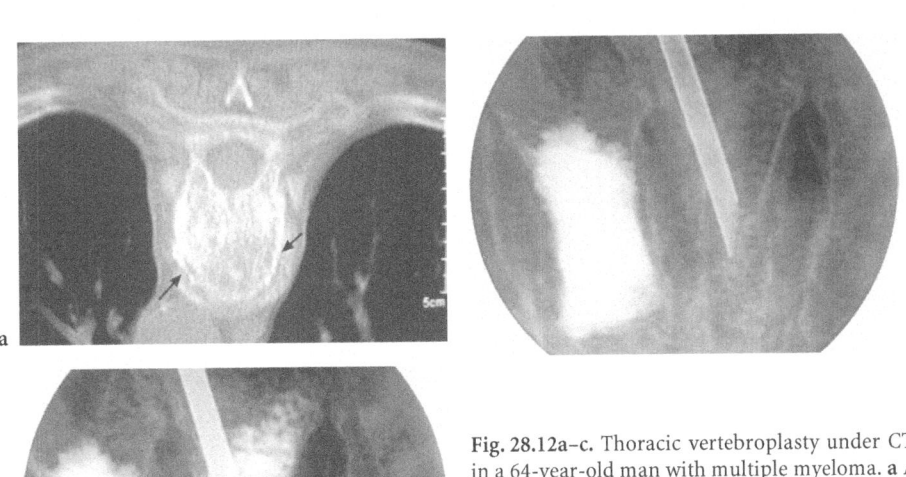

Fig. 28.12a–c. Thoracic vertebroplasty under CT and fluoroscopic guidance in a 64-year-old man with multiple myeloma. **a** Axial CT scan of the thoracic spine before the procedure shows heterogeneous involvement of T8 vertebral body with anterior pathologic fracture (*arrows*). Lateral fluoroscopic controls of the thoracic spine during the procedure show (**b**) the needle placed in the optimal position within the anterior aspect of the T8 vertebral body, and (**c**) satisfactory cement filling of the vertebral body without visible leakage. Note previous vertebroplasty of vertebra T7. Good pain relief was obtained 48 hours after the procedure.

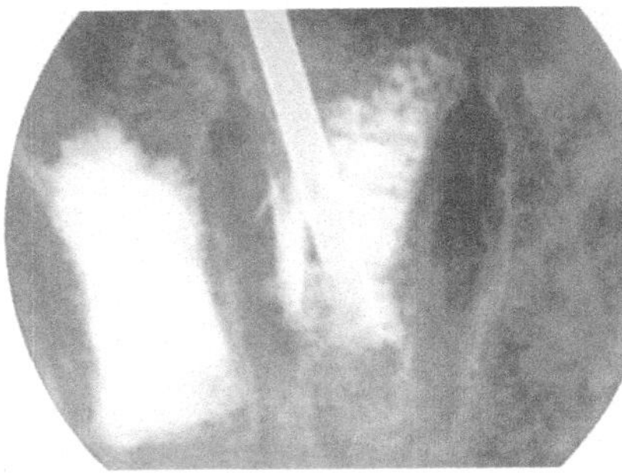

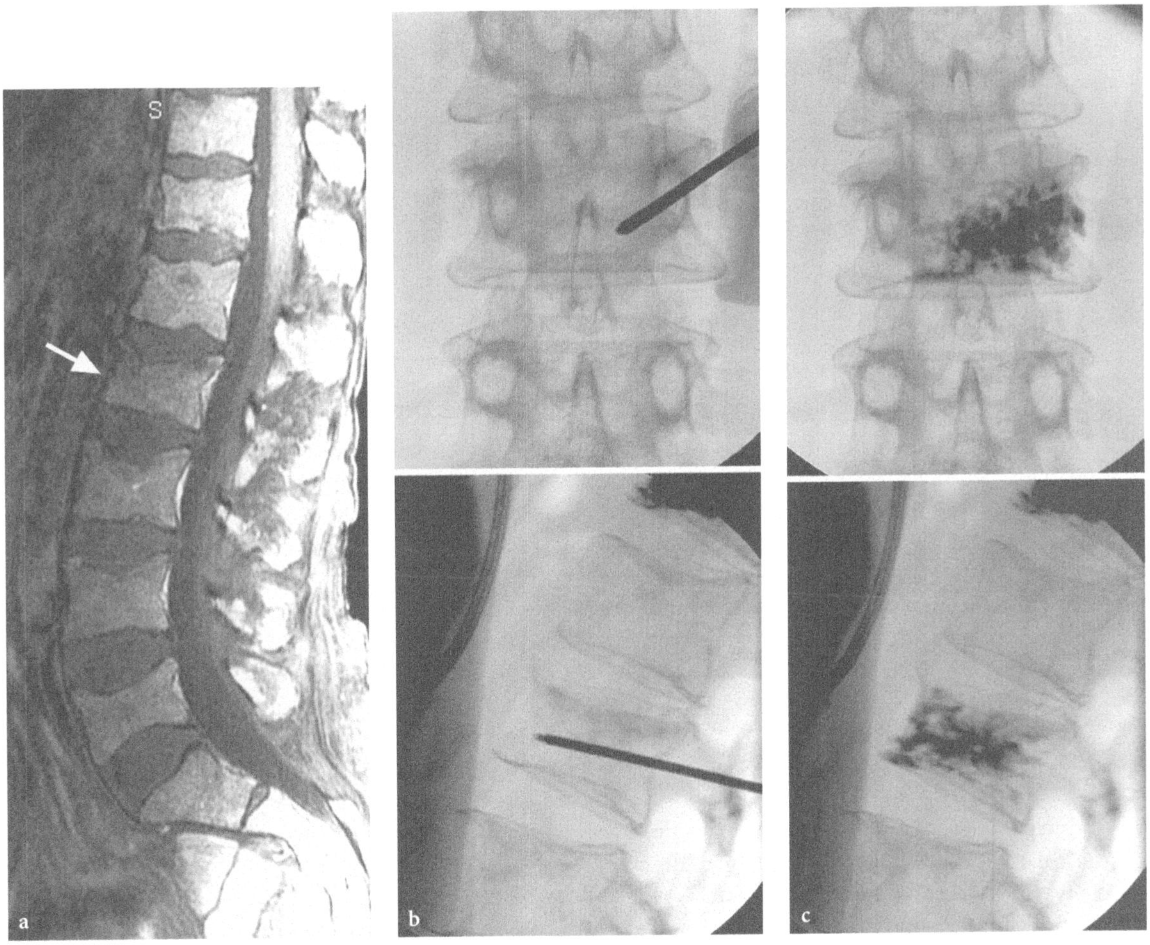

Fig. 28.13a–c. Lumbar unipedicular vertebroplasty under fluoroscopic guidance in a patient with multiple myeloma. **a** Preoperative sagittal T1-weighted MR image of the lumbar spine shows abnormal hypointensity of L2 with osteolytic compression fracture (*arrow*). L3 is also involved, but less importantly. Anteroposterior (*upper*) and lateral (*lower*) fluoroscopic images obtained during the procedure, demonstrate (**b**) the needle trajectory with the tip ideally positioned and (**c**) final PMMA casting. (With permission from [FOURNEY et al. 2003])

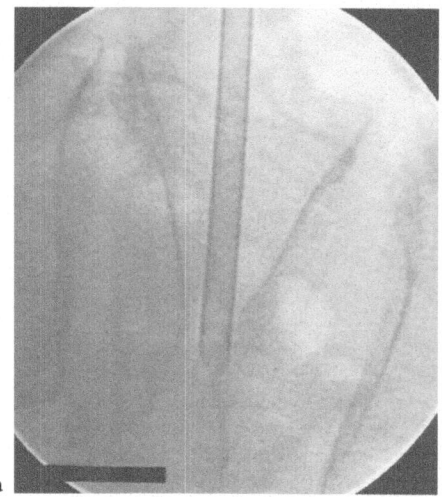
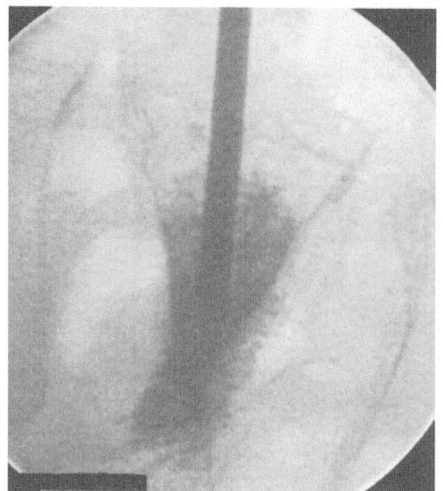
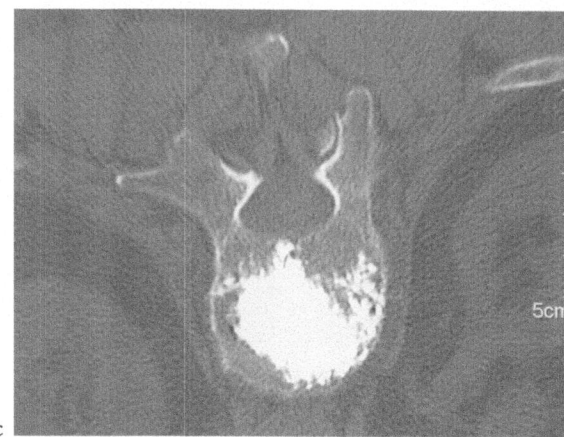

Fig. 28.14a–c. Lumbar vertebroplasty under CT and fluoroscopic guidance in a 72-year-old man with multiple myeloma. Fluoroscopic images obtained during the procedure show (a) the needle was placed in the optimal position which is the anterior portion of the compressed L2 vertebral body, and (b) satisfactory filling of the lesion. c Axial CT scan performed after the procedure demonstrates good packing of the vertebral body, and the absence of cement leakage. The patient was pain free 24 hours after the intervention.

In patients without a history of tumor who are suspected of having neoplastic vertebral collapse, or those with a known tumor who have vertebral lesions not typical of malignant collapse, a vertebral body biopsy is needed. In such cases, it can be performed at the same time as the vertebroplasty. The procedure is performed under fluoroscopic guidance via a coaxial bitranspedicular approach used for vertebroplasty (Fig. 29. 15) (MINART et al. 2001).

28.2.2.5
Patient Outcome

The principal effect of percutaneous injection of PMMA is early – and frequently striking – pain relief, especially when there is considerable pain initially. Marked or complete pain relief has been demonstrated in 70–83% of patients with vertebral myeloma. Pain relief has been reported within a few hours to 4 days (mean, 24 hours) after PMMA injection (COTTEN et al. 1998; GANGI et al. 2003). This pain relief is probably attributable to tumor necrosis and destruction of sensitive nerve endings in surrounding tissue by vascular, chemical, thermal, or mechanical effects (COTTEN et al. 1998; DERAMOND et al. 1998). The pain relief obtained with this technique is not correlated with the volume of PMMA injected; in tumoral bone for example, as little as 1.5 ml of cement is usually enough to reduce considerably the patient's pain (COTTEN et al. 1996; CORTET et al. 1997; GANGI et al. 2003).

The rapidity of clinical improvement allows most patients to stand upright the next day. Consequently, hospitalization time is short (mean, 4 days) which is especially beneficial to elderly patients and patients with a short life expectancy (COTTEN et al. 1998).

28.2.2.6
Side Effects and Complications

Fever and transitory worsening of pain may occur secondary to inflammatory reaction in the hours following injection. These side effects resolve spon-

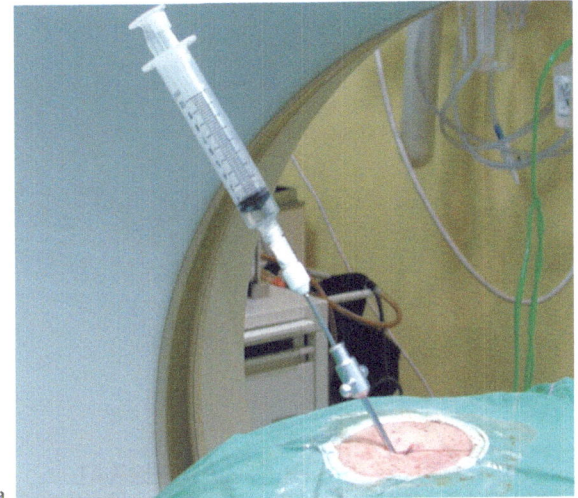

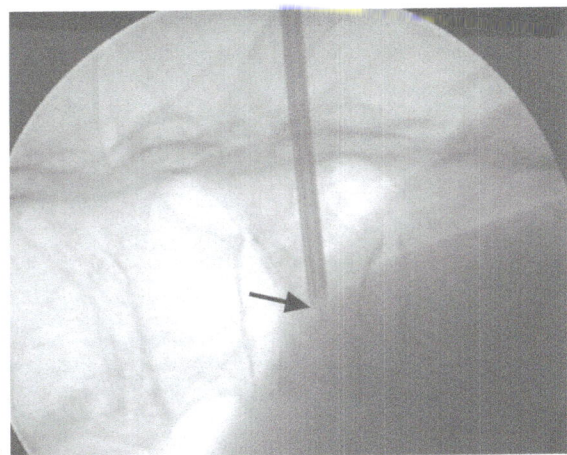

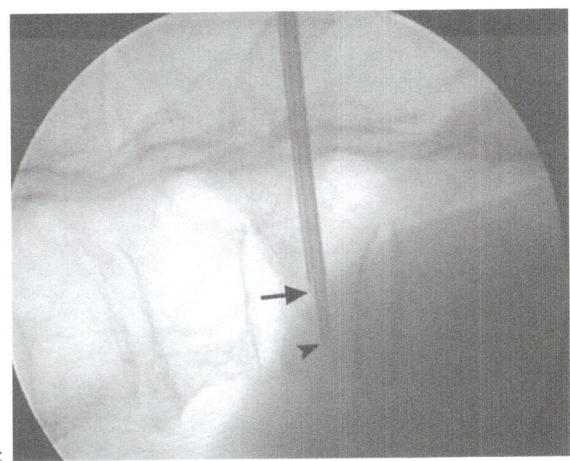

Fig. 28.15a–c. Coaxial transpedicular vertebral biopsy during vertebroplasty in a 63-year-old man with multiple myeloma. **a** View of the needle in place for L2 vertebral body biopsy during vertebroplasty. **b** Lateral fluoroscopic control shows the tip of the 10-gauge vertebroplasty needle (*arrow*) is within the central portion of the vertebral body, and (**c**) the 14-gauge biopsy needle (*arrowhead*) is introduced coaxially and is advanced into the vertebral body to extract a core biopsy sample.

taneously within days (mean, 1–3 days) following the procedure (GANGI et al. 2003). To minimize these side effects, steroidal or nonsteroidal anti-inflammatory drugs may be administered for 2–4 days (COTTEN et al. 1998).

Complications are minor and infrequent (BARR et al. 2000; JANG et al. 2002). Leakage of bone cement represents the principal risk associated with PMMA injection, a risk that increases when there is rupture of the posterior wall of the vertebral body, and the cement is too fluid. Cement can leak toward the epidural veins, epidural space and neural foramina, as well as the intervertebral disk, perivertebral veins and paravertebral soft tissue (Fig. 28.16). In patients with malignant tumors, the complication rate is increased due to the destruction of the vertebral body by the primary tumor (CHIRAS et al. 1997; MATHIS et al. 2001). Nevertheless, the risk can be minimized by monitoring the bone filling with a high-quality fluoroscopy unit, and by adequate radiopacity (tantalum) of acrylic glue (GANGI et al. 2003).

The major complication during injection is epidural overflow of PMMA (Fig. 28.17) with spinal cord compression (Fig. 28.18). The risk is greater when there is posterior cortical destruction and associated epidural tumor extension (COTTEN et al. 1996). Spinal cord compression may necessitate emergency decompressive surgery; orthopedic or neurosurgical support should be available (COTTEN et al. 1998; GANGI et al. 2003). However, this neurological complication is uncommon (CHIRAS et al. 1997; COTTEN et al. 1998).

Radiculopathy is the major risk with neural foramina leaks. Intercostal neuralgia occurs immediately after cementoplasty if there is filling of epidural veins and neural foramina. This complication can be successfully treated with a series of intercostal steroid infiltrations (GANGI et al. 2003) or by surgery (COTTEN et al. 1996; CORTET et al. 1997). Epidural veins (vertebral plexus) filling alone does not systematically cause neuralgia (GANGI et al. 2003). In fact, the major technical drawback of percutaneous vertebroplasty is the potential for neural compromise from leakage of PMMA toward epidural or perivertebral veins. Recently, a combined intrathecal injection of contrast medium with vertebroplasty has been reported to be very useful for better delineating spinal canal encroachment during injection when the posterior vertebral wall is compromised by myeloma (SARZIER and EVANS 2003).

Cement leakage into perivertebral veins (Fig. 28.19) can lead to pulmonary cement embolism, which is usually asymptomatic. It may lead to pulmonary

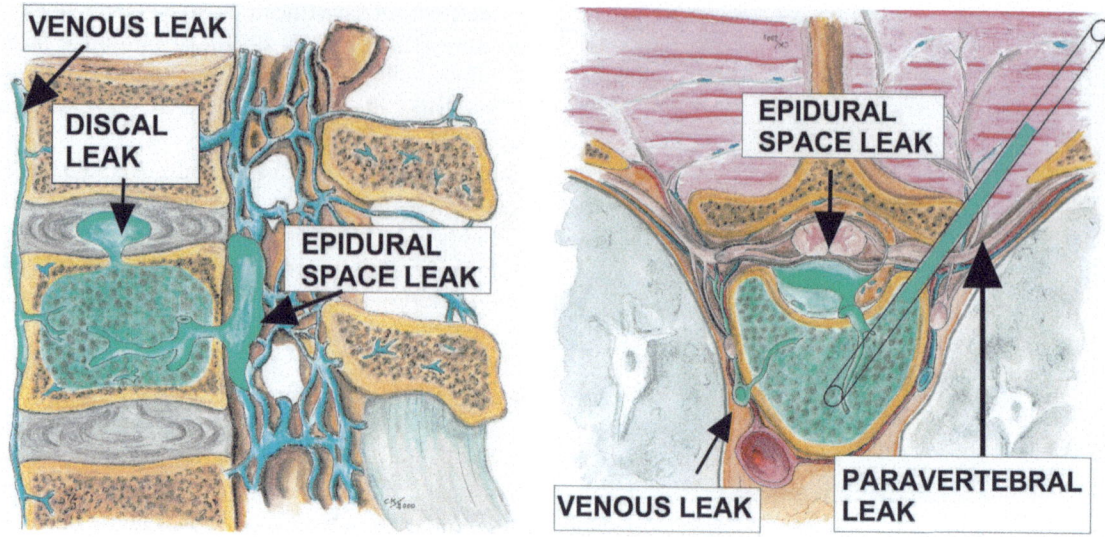

Fig. 28.16a,b. Artist's rendering of the potential leaks as complications from cement injection in (**a**) sagittal and (**b**) axial views.

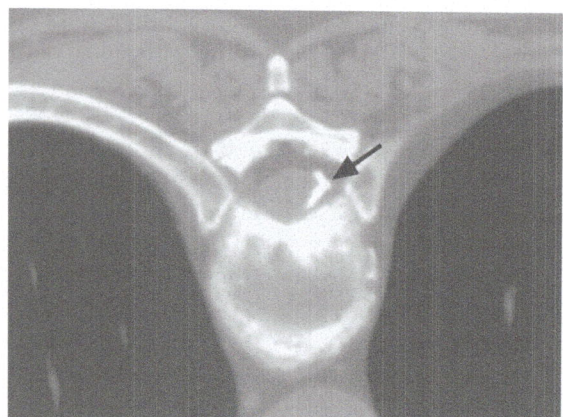

Fig. 28.17. Epidural cement leak during vertebroplasty in a 62-year-old man with multiple myeloma. The patient was clinically asymptomatic. Axial CT scan of the thoracic spine performed right after the procedure shows a small amount of cement (*arrow*) in the epidural space around the spinal cord.

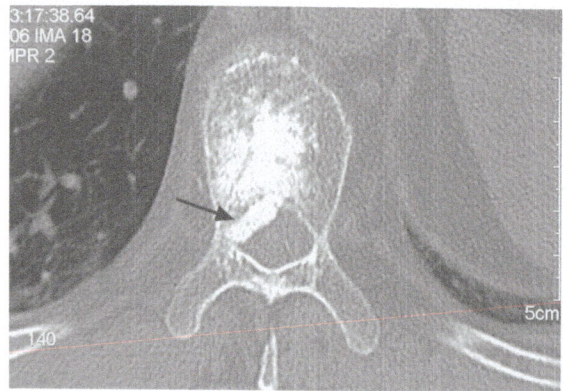
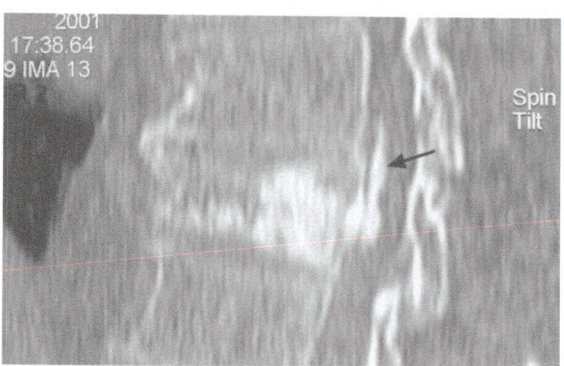

Fig. 28.18a,b. Epidural cement leak during vertebroplasty in a 65-year-old woman with multiple myeloma. Clinically, the patient was suspected of spinal cord compression. **a** Axial CT scan of the thoracic spine performed immediately after the procedure shows right anterolateral epidural leak of the cement (*arrow*) with compression of the spinal cord, best demonstrated on (**b**) 2D sagittal reconstruction of the thoracic spine. The patient underwent successful neurosurgical decompression.

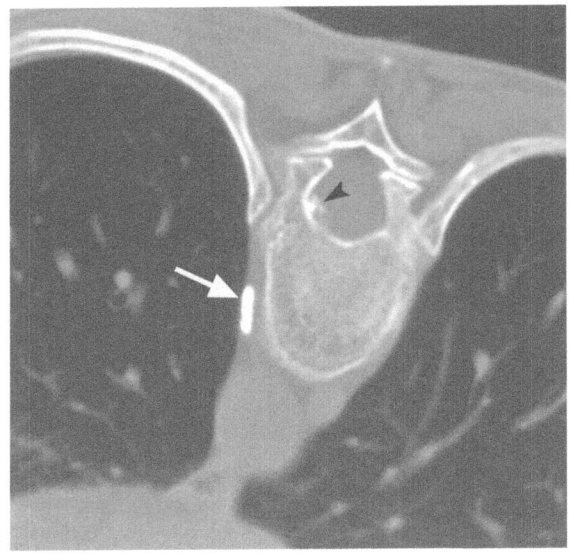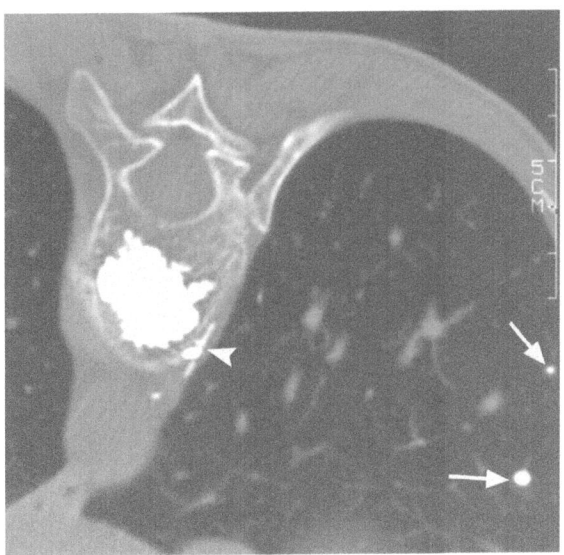

a   b

Fig. 28.19a,b. Perivertebral veins leak during vertebroplasty in a 71-year-old man with multiple myeloma. The patient was clinically asymptomatic. **a** Axial CT scan of the thoracic spine shows right perivertebral veins filled by the cement (*arrow*). There is also a small amount of cement in the right anterior epidural space (*arrowhead*). **b** Axial CT scan at the level of T10 and caudad to (**a**) shows cement also filling the left vertebral veins (*arrowhead*) and hyperdense intra-luminal cement embols within the intrapulmonary arteries (*arrows*). It also shows final casting of T10 vertebral body.

infarction involving necrosis of the lung parenchyma, due to interference with the blood supply (JANG et al. 2002). In case of pulmonary embolism of PMMA, perivertebral venous opacification is observed. To avoid major pulmonary infarction, the glue should be injected slowly during its pasty polymerization phase under fluoroscopic control, and the injection should be stopped immediately if a venous leak is observed (COTTEN et al. 1996; PADOVANI et al. 1999; GANGI et al. 2003). There is a higher risk of pulmonary embolism in multilevel than in single-level vertebroplasty. Therefore, greater caution should be taken during the multilevel procedure (JANG et al. 2002).

Cement leakage towards the disk (Fig. 28.20) associated with cortical fracture or osteolysis of the vertebral end plates is usually without clinical consequence (COTTEN et al. 1996). However, this leak may increase the risk of adjacent vertebrae collapse (GANGI et al. 2003) and secondary degenerative changes (COTTEN et al. 1996).

Cement leaks into paravertebral soft tissues are the most frequent complication and have no clinical significance (COTTEN et al. 1996). They can occur in relation with the path of the needle (Fig. 28.21) or with cortical rupture (CHIRAS et al. 1997; GANGI et al. 2003).

In only one reported case, the control CT scan showed an asymptomatic leak of acrylic cement into an intercostal artery (GANGI et al. 2003).

The risk of infection is under 5% and should be minimized with careful sterilization of the skin and aseptic procedure (CHIRAS et al. 1997; COTTEN et al. 1998).

Since the PMMA mixture is prepared at the time of the procedure, the patient and medical staff can be exposed to PMMA vapor, which, in high concentrations, can have toxic effects. A recent study demonstrated that the PMMA vapor levels to which patient and medical staff are exposed during percutaneous vertebroplasty are well below the level typically considered hazardous. However, it is important to note that some individuals may experience adverse effects, such as asthma, coughing, nausea, and decreased appetite, when exposed to levels typically considered to be within acceptable limits (CLOFT et al. 1999).

28.2.3
Kyphoplasty

Percutaneous balloon kyphoplasty, a recent modification of vertebroplasty, involves inflation of a balloon within a collapsed vertebral body to restore height and reduce kyphotic deformity, prior to stabilization with PMMA. The risk of cement extravasation is theoretically reduced because inflation of the balloon creates a void within the vertebral body into which cement can be injected under relatively low pressure (FOURNEY et

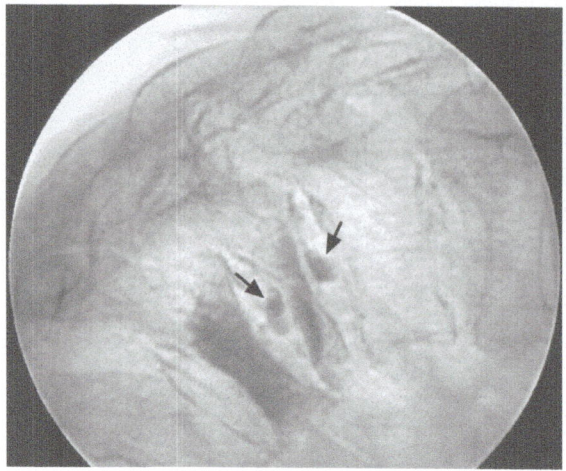

Fig. 28.20. Discal leak during vertebroplasty in a 70-year-old man with multiple myeloma. The patient was clinically asymptomatic. Lateral fluoroscopic control of the thoracic spine shows cement leaks towards both superior and inferior disks (*arrows*). Note previous vertebroplasty of above T8 vertebra.

al. 2003). However, this technique is still under evaluation, and a full understanding of its risks and benefits will require randomized clinical trials.

28.2.3.1
Patient Selection

Kyphoplasty is favored over vertebroplasty in the presence of (1) kyphosis that is deemed to contribute significantly to morbidity (that is, deformity > 20°), and (2) disruption of the posterior vertebral cortex, where more controlled delivery of bone cement is desired. In patients with significant vertebral collapse (vertebra plana), kyphoplasty is preferred to restore height; although vertebroplasty is necessary when the collapse is too severe to permit insertion of the balloon device. Finally, vertebroplasty is performed if the patient can not tolerate general anesthesia or the relatively longer procedure time required for kyphoplasty (FOURNEY et al. 2003).

28.2.3.2
Technique

Kyphoplasty is always performed with the patient in prone position after induction of general anesthesia. Bilateral access to the vertebral body is preferred. The needle is advanced as for vertebroplasty. However, the endpoint is within the posterior one third of the vertebral body. A series of instruments are used to create two working channels (Fig. 28.22). A

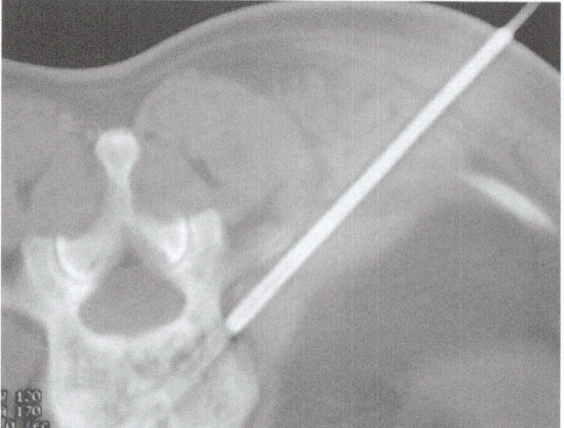

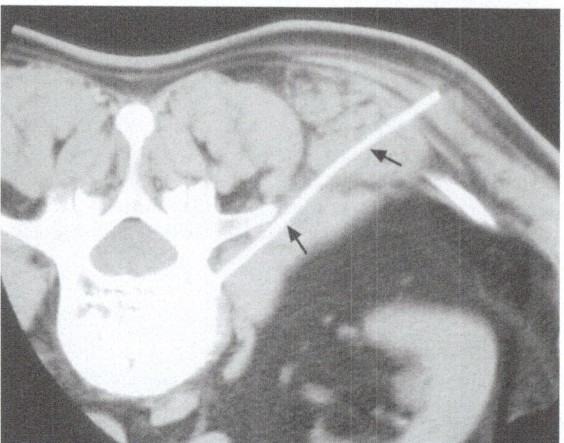

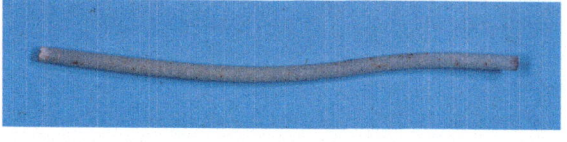

Fig. 28.21a–c. Paravertebral soft tissue leak in a 62-year-old woman with multiple myeloma. The patient was clinically asymptomatic. **a** Axial CT scan during the procedure shows the needle is filled with compact cement. **b** Axial control CT scan shows the cement (*arrows*) is filling the hole produced by the needle after its removal. **c** View of the cement after its removal from the path of the needle.

hand-mounted drill is used to create bilateral channels within the anterior aspect of the vertebral body for placement of the inflatable bone tamp.

The inflatable bone tamp is a high-pressure balloon designed to restore the vertebral body to its original height by creating a cavity that is subsequently filled with PMMA (Fig. 28.23). Its length varies depending on the anteroposterior diameter of the vertebral body. There are two radiopaque markers that identify the balloon for accurate placement

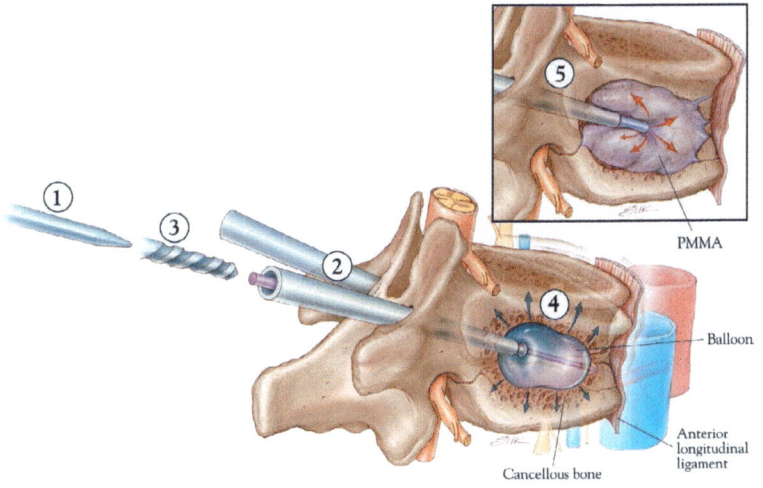

Fig. 28.22. Artist's rendering of the kyphoplasty technique. Using a bilateral transpedicular approach, bone biopsy needles are directed into the posterior third of the vertebral body. Guide pins (K-wires) are used to exchange the biopsy needles for blunt cannulated obturators (1). Working cannulas (2) are then advanced, and the obturators and K-wires are removed. A hand-mounted drill (3) creates bilateral channels within the anterior aspect of the vertebral body for the placement of the inflatable bone tamps (4). Balloon inflation allows restoration of vertebral height. Inset: The inflatable bone tamps are removed and the osseous void is filled with PMMA displaced from bone cement cannulae (5). (With permission from [Fourney et al. 2003])

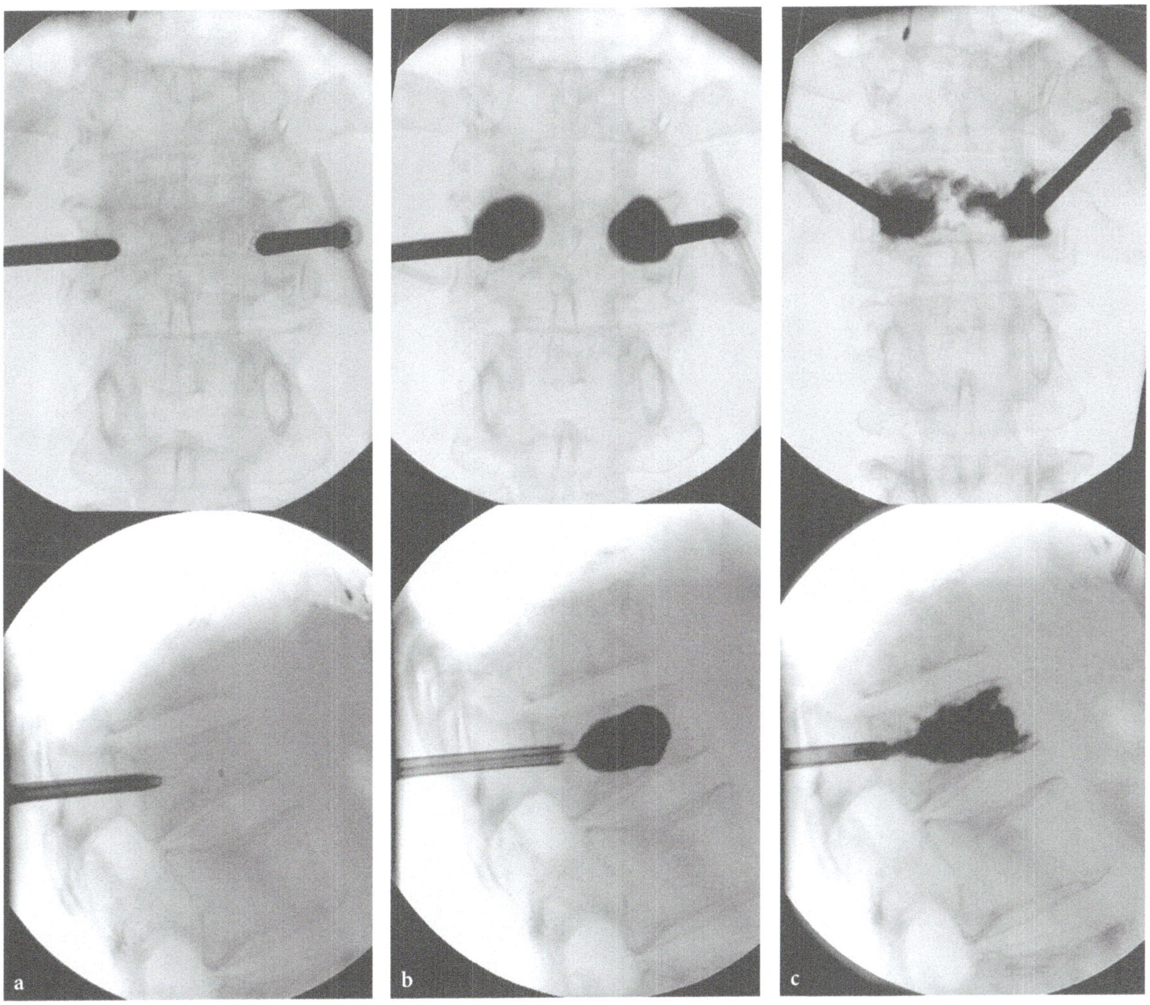

Fig. 28.23a–c. Thoracic kyphoplasty in a patient with multiple myeloma. Sequentially anteroposterior (upper) and lateral (below) fluoroscopic images obtained during the procedure demonstrate (**a**) transpedicular placement of the working cannulas in T12 vertebral body, (**b**) inflation of the inflatable bone tamps, and (**c**) filling of the bone voids with PMMA. (With permission from [Fourney et al. 2003])

(Fig. 28.24). The balloon is inflated under strict lateral fluoroscopic control, with the inflation pressure monitored via an in-line pressure gauge. Inflation endpoints are: (1) fracture reduction, (2) contact of the balloon with any cortical surfaces, or (3) attaining the maximum inflation pressure of 220 psi.

Specialized bone cement cannulas are filled with the PMMA preparation. The inflatable bone tamps are deflated and exchanged for the cement cannulas. A stylet, which acts as a plunger, displaces the cement into the vertebral body. Filling is stopped once the void left by the inflatable bone tamp is filled and the PMMA is observed to extend out into the trabecular spaces (FOURNEY et al. 2003).

28.2.3.3
Patient Outcome

Besides the improvement or complete pain relief, restored vertebral body height and kyphosis correction are seen after kyphoplasty.

For the assessment of restored vertebral body height, the vertical height (endplate to endplate) at the center of the vertebral body on the lateral radiographs is measured before and after kyphoplasty. The vertebra above the fracture is also measured as an estimate of prefracture height (LIEBERMAN et al. 2001). The mean vertebral height lost prior to kyphoplasty is 9.7 +/- 5.1 mm and the mean height

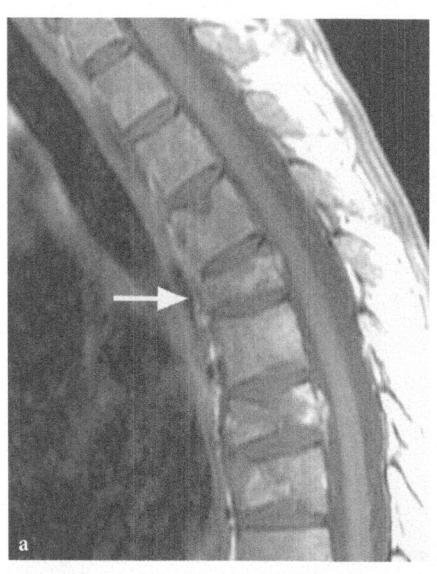
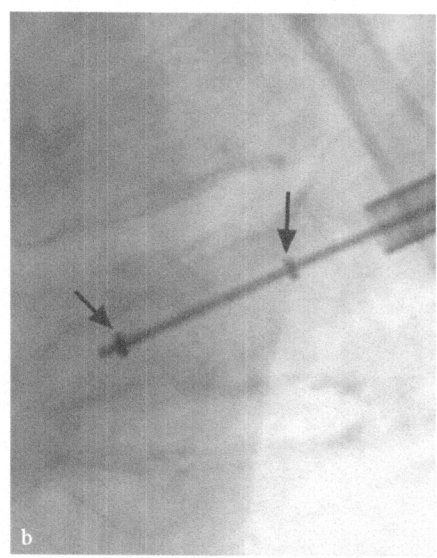
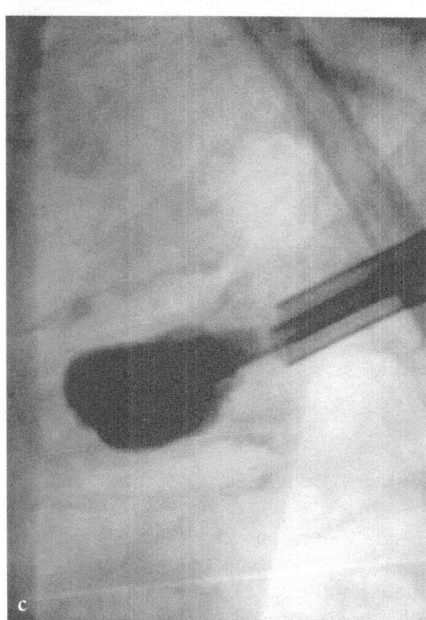
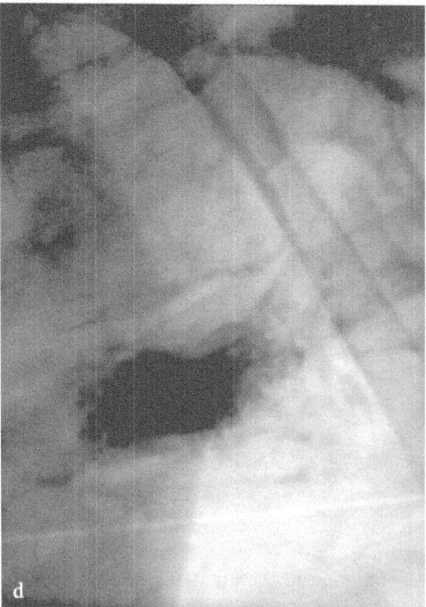

Fig. 28.24a–d. Thoracic kyphoplasty under fluoroscopic guidance in a patient with multiple myeloma. a Preoperative sagittal T1-weighted MR image reveals T6 osteolytic compression fracture (*arrow*). Sequentially lateral fluoroscopic images obtained during the procedure demonstrate (b) the trajectory of the inflatable bone tamps, (c) inflation of the balloons, and (d) filling of the bone voids with polymethylmethacrylate. Two markers identify the balloon position for accurate placement (b, *arrows*). (With permission from [Fourney et al. 2003])

regained by the procedure is 4.5 +/- 3.6 mm. The mean percentage of vertebral height lost restored by kyphoplasty is 42 +/- 21% (FOURNEY et al. 2003).

Local kyphosis is assessed on the lateral radiographs by measuring the angle obtained by a line parallel to the inferior endplate of the fractured vertebra and that of the vertebra on level above (Fig. 28.25) (LIEBERMAN et al. 2001). The mean local kyphosis measured during kyphoplasty is 25.7 +/- 9.7° and 20.5 +/- 8.7° after the procedure. Man improvement in local kyphosis is 4.1 +/- 3.7° (FOURNEY et al. 2003).

28.2.3.4
Side Effects and Complications

The side effects and complications are the same as with vertebroplasty. However, kyphoplasty appears to be associated with fewer instances of bone cement extravasation (FOURNEY et al. 2003).

28.2.4
Acetabular Cement Injection

Therapeutic percutaneous injection of PMMA for malignant acetabular osteolysis is a palliative procedure that should be offered only to patients who are unable to tolerate surgery (COTTEN et al. 1999).

28.2.4.1
Patient Selection

PMMA injection is contraindicated in patients with coagulation disorders due to the large diameter of the needles used. Fracture or destruction of the articular cortex of the acetabulum is not a contraindication for injection of cement but should prompt extreme caution during the procedure to prevent leakage into the joint space. In contrast, associated osteolysis of the acetabular fossa, which increases the risk of traumatic acetabular protrusion when the patient stands, may be a relative contraindication for the injection of bone cement; the mechanical improvement and relief of pain may encourage such patients to stand and walk, actually increasing the risk of traumatic protrusion (COTTEN et al. 1999).

28.2.4.2
Technique

Radiography and CT including contiguous thin-section acquisition must be performed preceding therapeutic percutaneous injection to assess the location and extent of the lytic process, the presence of cortical destruction or fracture (especially of the acetabular roof and acetabular fossa), and the presence of soft-tissue involvement. The procedure is performed with the patient under neuroleptanalgesia (COTTEN et al. 1999).

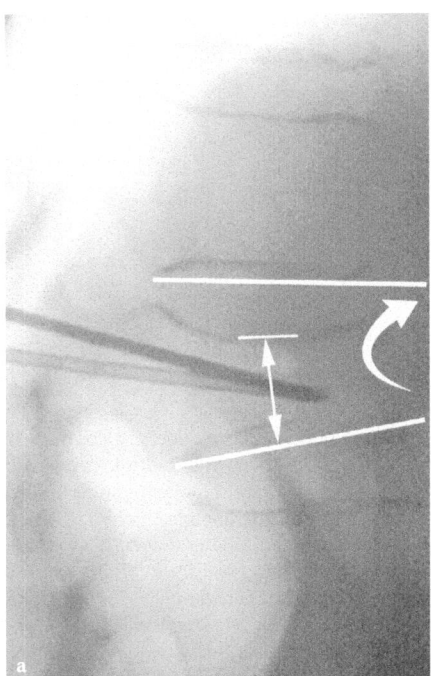
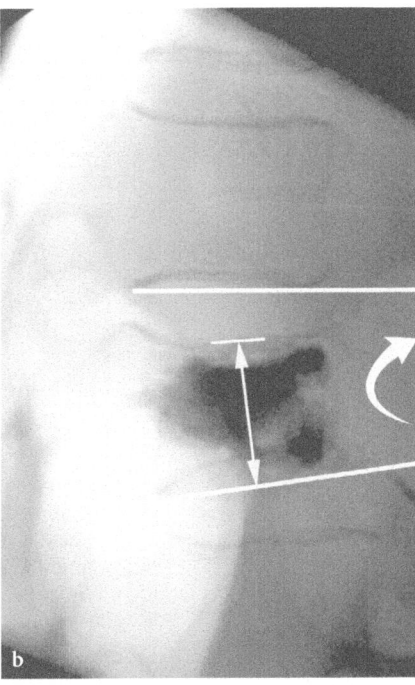

Fig. 28.25a,b. Correction of central vertebral height and local kyphosis angles after kyphoplasty. Lateral radiograph of the lumbar spine (a) before and (b) after kyphoplasty show regaining of central vertebral body height (*double arrowheads*) and improvement of local kyphosis angles (*curved arrows*). (With permission from [FOURNEY et al. 2003])

Injection is usually performed under anteropos-terior and lateral fluoroscopic guidance, but CT may be used for needle positioning. A 10-gauge needle is inserted into the osteolytic lesion via a posterior or posterolateral (Fig. 28.26) access route with the bevel oriented to spread the cement in the desired direction (COTTEN et al. 1999; GANGI et al. 1996). PMMA with the consistency of paste is then injected until resistance is met or until the cement reaches the borders of the osteolytic lesion. Additional injections may be performed depending on the distribution of the cement. A total of 7–25 ml (mean, 16 ml) of bone cement is usually injected. Injection stops if leakage of bone cement into the joint space or soft tissue is detected. It is highly recommended that CT, which allows assessment of lesion filling as well as detection of PMMA leakage, be performed in the hours following cement injection (COTTEN et al. 1999).

28.2.4.3
Patient Outcome

The principal effect of percutaneous injection of PMMA or ethanol is early – and frequently striking – pain relief, especially when there is considerable pain initially. Pain relief has been reported within hours to 4 days (mean, 24 hours) after PMMA injection. This pain relief is probably attributable to tumor necrosis and destruction of sensitive nerve endings in surrounding tissue by vascular, chemical, thermal, or mechanical effects (COTTEN et al. 1999).

PMMA injection of the weight-bearing parts of the acetabulum may also allow improved walking. is the effects are usually seen within 1–5 days (mean, 3 days) of bone cement injection, especially in previously bedridden patients. This improvement in walking is not necessarily synchronous with pain relief and does not appear to be proportional to the quality of lesion filling. Indeed, excellent clinical and functional results can be obtained in some patients despite what appears to be insufficient lesion filling (COTTEN et al. 1999; GANGI et al. 1996).

28.2.4.4
Side Effects and Complications

Fever and transitory worsening in pain may occur secondary to inflammatory reaction in the hours following injection; however, these side effects usually resolve spontaneously within 1–3 days (COTTEN

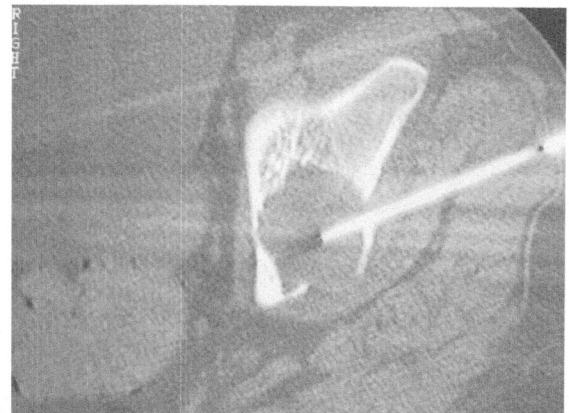

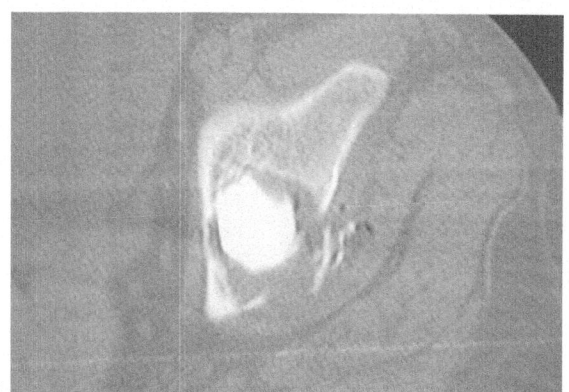

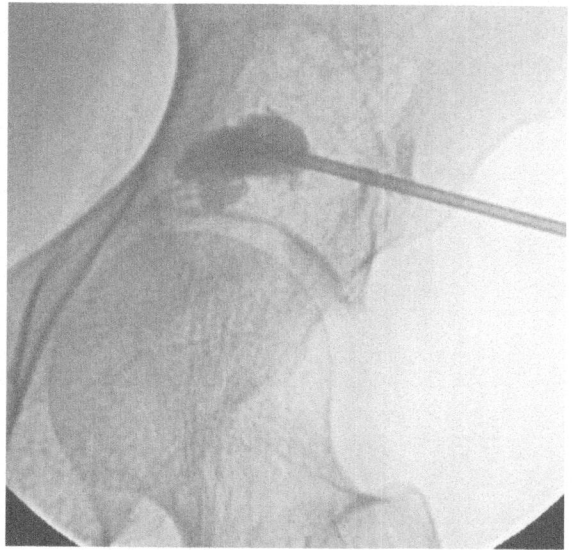

Fig. 28.26a–c. Acetabular cementoplasty under CT and fluoro-scopic guidance in a 58-year-old man with multiple myeloma. **a** Axial CT scan during the procedure shows a 10-gauge needle positioned in the center of the lytic bone lesion by means of a posterolateral approach. Note the lateral cortical destruction of the left acetabulum. **b** View from fluoroscopic control shows subsequent injection of the cement in the left acetabular lesion. **c** Axial control CT scan after the procedure shows satisfactory filling of the myeloma lesion with 4 ml of PMMA. Good pain relief was obtained 48 hours after the procedure.

et al. 1995; GANGI et al. 1996). To minimize these side effects, nonsteroidal anti-inflammatory drugs may be administered during this time (COTTEN et al. 1999).

Transitory renal insufficiency has been reported after PMMA injection in one patient with myeloma and may have been related to the disease (COTTEN et al. 1995).

Leakage of bone cement represents the principal risk associated with PMMA injection, a risk that increases when there is destruction of the cortex of the acetabular roof and too fluid cement injection (COTTEN et al. 1995; GANGI et al. 1996). As soon as a leak is detected, the injection should be stopped and the hip mobilized to flatten the cement while it still has the consistency of paste. Leaks are associated with a striking transitory increase in pain but they do not prevent either secondary pain relief or improved walking. Small leaks of PMMA into the acetabular fossa are without clinical significance at follow-up. Small cement leaks into soft tissue due to cortical osteolysis or puncture holes are detected in about half of patients but are also without clinical significance at follow-up (COTTEN et al. 1995; GANGI et al. 1996).

Other potential complications include vascular injury, nerve injury, and infection (COTTEN et al. 1995).

28.3
Bone Lesion Alcoholization

Percutaneous alcoholization of tumoral bone is indicated in patients with painful, severe, osteolytic bone lesion if conventional anticancer therapy is ineffective and high doses of opiates are necessary to control pain and rapid pain relief is necessary (GANGI et al. 1994a; GANGI et al. 1996). Particularly, ethanol injection in the acetabulum is preferred to PMMA whenever the acetabular roof is not involved (COTTEN et al. 1999). Ethanol and PMMA injections may be performed together if both weight-bearing and non weight-bearing parts of the acetabulum are involved or extensive soft-tissue involvement is present. Moreover, these injections may be performed prior to radiation therapy, which complements their action due to similar although delayed effects on pain, or after radiation therapy that has failed to relieve pain, or in cases of local recurrence (COTTEN et al. 1999).

There are no reported contraindications for ethanol injection in tumoral bone. Indeed, the thin

needles used allow injections to be performed, albeit cautiously, in these patients (COTTEN et al. 1999). Nevertheless, radiologists must be aware of the major risk of ethanol diffusing into vital structures (GANGI et al. 1996), such as nerves and vascular structures adjacent to the tumor (GANGI et al. 1994a).

Radiography and CT must be performed before the percutaneous injection to assess the location and extent of the lytic process, the presence of cortical destruction or fracture, and the presence of soft-tissue involvement. Contrast-enhanced CT is usually performed to determine the necrotic part of the tumor (GANGI et al. 1996). The procedure must be performed with the patient under neuroleptanalesia to palliate the painful alcohol injection (GANGI et al. 1996).

CT is usually used for both needle positioning and the injection of the ethanol itself. A thin (20–22-gauge) needle is inserted into the lesion, and a mixture of lidocaine (1%) and contrast material is injected first to assess the expected distribution of ethanol and decrease the pain produced by the ethanol injection (Fig. 28.27) (COTTEN et al. 1999). If leakage of contrast material is detected, especially into the joint space, the needle is repositioned and a second test injection is performed. If no contrast material is visualized,

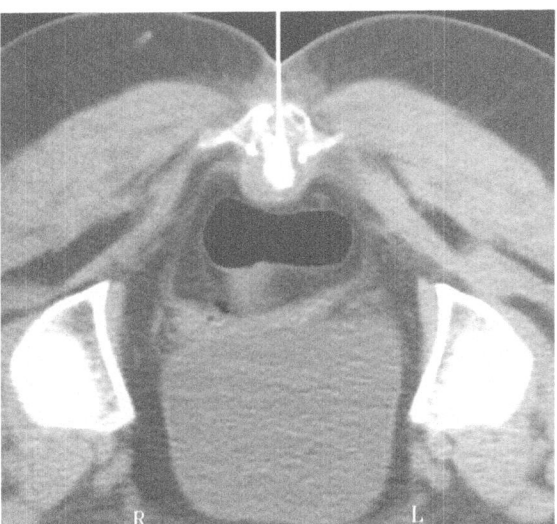

Fig. 28.27. Ethanol percutaneous injection in a sacral osteo-lytic bone lesion with soft tissue mass in a 56-year-old woman with multiple myeloma. The patient underwent local radiation therapy with insufficient pain relief and was unable to tolerate additional therapy. Axial CT scan of the pelvis on prone position shows a 22-gauge needle inserted into the center of the osteolytic lesion of the sacrum. It also shows injection of a mixture of lidocaine (1%), contrast material and 2 ml of a solution of 95% ethanol. Good pain relief was obtained after 36 hours and analgesia lasted until the death of the patient 3 weeks after the procedure.

the needle has been positioned intravascularly and needs to be repositioned (GANGI et al. 1996). Then, a solution of 96% ethanol is injected slowly. Injection volume depends on lesion size and diffusion of contrast material. A volume of 1–4 ml is usually sufficient for osteolytic lesions, but in patients with extensive soft-tissue involvement, the volume can reach 20–30 ml (GANGI et al. 1994a; COTTEN et al. 1999). In these large tumors, alcohol is selectively injected into regions considered to be responsible for pain. One or more injections may be performed at different sites on the same day, especially in bulky lesions. With bulky lesions, repeat injections performed over the ensuing weeks may improve pain relief and decrease tumor size (GANGI et al. 1996).

As with PMMA injection, the principal effect of percutaneous injection of ethanol is early and frequently striking pain relief (GANGI et al. 1994a).

Ethanol injection usually does not lead to serious complications. As with PMMA injection, a fever and transitory worsening in pain may occur secondarily to inflammatory reaction in the hours following injection. These side effects resolve spontaneously within days (mean, 1–3 days) following the procedure. Other rare possible complications of the procedure are neurolysis and massive tumor necrosis with fever and hyperuricemia (GANGI et al. 1994a; GANGI et al. 1996). No intraarticular leaks of ethanol have been reported (COTTEN et al. 1995).

28.4
Conclusion

Therapeutic percutaneous procedures are palliative imaging-guided techniques that may be helpful in patients treated for hematological malignancies, especially multiple myeloma, by providing rapid and frequently striking pain relief and sometimes improved walking. The decision to use these procedures should be made by a multidisciplinary team because the choice between therapeutic percutaneous procedure and surgery, radiation therapy, medical treatment, or a combination of these alternative methods depends on several factors. These factors include the location of the lesion, the local and general extent of the disease, the pain and functional disability experienced by the patient, and the patient's state of health and life expectancy. Interventional radiologists using an efficient imaging-guided technique can increase the precision of the analgesic procedures, improving the results and significantly reducing complications.

Acknowledgments
We thank Professor Ziya L. Gokaslan for providing the excellent images to illustrate this chapter.

References

Barr JD, Barr MS, Lemley TJ, McCann RM (2000) Percutaneous vertebroplasty for pain relief and spinal stabilization. Spine 25:923–928
Callander NS, Roodman GD (2001) Myeloma bone disease. Semin Hematol 38:276–285
Chiras J, Depriester C, Weill A, Sola-Martinez MT, Deramond H (1997) Percutaneous vertebral surgery. Technics and indications. J Neuroradiol 24:45–59
Cloft HJ, Easton DN, Jensen ME, Kallmes DF, Dion JE (1999) Exposure of medical personnel to methylmethacrylate vapor during percutaneous vertebroplasty. AJNR Am J Neuroradiol 20:352–353
Cortet B, Cotten A, Boutry N, Dewatre F, Flipo RM, Duquesnoy B, Chastanet P, Delcambre B (1997) Percutaneous vertebroplasty in patients with osteolytic metastases or multiple myeloma. Rev Rhum Engl Ed 64:177–183
Cotten A, Deprez X, Migaud H, Chabanne B, Duquesnoy B, Chastanet P (1995) Malignant acetabular osteolyses: percutaneous injection of acrylic bone cement. Radiology 197:307–310
Cotten A, Dewatre F, Cortet B, Assaker R, Leblond D, Duquesnoy B, Chastanet P, Clarisse J (1996) Percutaneous vertebroplasty for osteolytic metastases and myeloma: effects of the percentage of lesion filling and the leakage of methyl methacrylate at clinical follow-up. Radiology 200:525–530
Cotten A, Boutry N, Cortet B, Assaker R, Demondion X, Leblond D, Chastanet P, Duquesnoy B, Deramond H (1998) Percutaneous vertebroplasty: state of the art. Radiographics 18:311–320; discussion 320–313
Cotten A, Demondion X, Boutry N, Cortet B, Chastanet P, Duquesnoy B, Leblond D (1999) Therapeutic percutaneous injections in the treatment of malignant acetabular osteolyses. Radiographics 19:647–653
Deramond H, Depriester C, Galibert P, Le Gars D (1998) Percutaneous vertebroplasty with polymethylmethacrylate. Technique, indications, and results. Radiol Clin North Am 36:533–546
Dufresne AC, Brunet E, Sola-Martinez MT, Rose M, Chiras J (1998) Percutaneous vertebroplasty of the cervico-thoracic junction using an anterior route. Technique and results. Report of nine cases. J Neuroradiol 25:123–128
Evans AJ, Jensen ME, Kip KE, DeNardo AJ, Lawler GJ, Negin GA, Remley KB, Boutin SM, Dunnagan SA (2003) Vertebral compression fractures: pain reduction and improvement in functional mobility after percutaneous polymethylmethacrylate vertebroplasty retrospective report of 245 cases. Radiology 226:366–372
Fourney DR, Schomer DF, Nader R, Chlan-Fourney J, Suki D, Ahrar K, Rhines LD, Gokaslan ZL (2003) Percutaneous vertebroplasty and kyphoplasty for painful vertebral body fractures in cancer patients. J Neurosurg 98:21–30
Galibert P, Deramond H, Rosat P, Le Gars D (1987) Preliminary note on the treatment of vertebral angioma by percutaneous acrylic vertebroplasty. Neurochirurgie 33:166–168

Gangi A, Kastler B, Klinkert A, Dietemann JL (1994a) Injection of alcohol into bone metastases under CT guidance. J Comput Assist Tomogr 18:932–935

Gangi A, Kastler BA, Dietemann JL (1994b) Percutaneous vertebroplasty guided by a combination of CT and fluoroscopy. AJNR Am J Neuroradiol 15:83–86

Gangi A, Dietemann JL, Schultz A, Mortazavi R, Jeung MY, Roy C (1996) Interventional radiologic procedures with CT guidance in cancer pain management. Radiographics 16:1289–1304; discussion 1304–1286

Gangi A, Dietemann JL, Mortazavi R, Pfleger D, Kauff C, Roy C (1998) CT-guided interventional procedures for pain management in the lumbosacral spine. Radiographics 18: 621–633

Gangi A, Guth S, Imbert JP, Marin H, Dietemann JL (2003) Percutaneous vertebroplasty: indications, technique, and results. Radiographics 23:e10

Jang JS, Lee SH, Jung SK (2002) Pulmonary embolism of polymethylmethacrylate after percutaneous vertebroplasty: a report of three cases. Spine 27:E416–418

Jang JS, Kim DY, Lee SH (2003) Efficacy of percutaneous vertebroplasty in the treatment of intravertebral pseudarthrosis associated with noninfected avascular necrosis of the vertebral body. Spine 28:1588–1592

Jensen ME, Kallmes DE (2002) Percutaneous vertebroplasty in the treatment of malignant spine disease. Cancer J 8: 194–206

Kallmes DF, Schweickert PA, Marx WF, Jensen ME (2002) Vertebroplasty in the mid- and upper thoracic spine. AJNR Am J Neuroradiol 23:1117–1120

Kim AK, Jensen ME, Dion JE, Schweickert PA, Kaufmann TJ, Kallmes DF (2002) Unilateral transpedicular percutaneous vertebroplasty: initial experience. Radiology 222:737–741

Lieberman IH, Dudeney S, Reinhardt MK, Bell G (2001) Initial outcome and efficacy of "kyphoplasty" in the treatment of painful osteoporotic vertebral compression fractures. Spine 26:1631–1638

Mathis JM, Barr JD, Belkoff SM, Barr MS, Jensen ME, Deramond H (2001) Percutaneous vertebroplasty: a developing standard of care for vertebral compression fractures. AJNR Am J Neuroradiol 22:373–381

McGraw JK, Cardella J, Barr JD, Mathis JM, Sanchez O, Schwartzberg MS, Swan TL, Sacks D (2003) Society of Interventional Radiology quality improvement guidelines for percutaneous vertebroplasty. J Vasc Interv Radiol 14: 827–831

Minart D, Vallee JN, Cormier E, Chiras J (2001) Percutaneous coaxial transpedicular biopsy of vertebral body lesions during vertebroplasty. Neuroradiology 43:409–412

Padovani B, Kasriel O, Brunner P, Peretti-Viton P (1999) Pulmonary embolism caused by acrylic cement: a rare complication of percutaneous vertebroplasty. AJNR Am J Neuroradiol 20:375–377

Sarzier JS, Evans AJ (2003) Intrathecal injection of contrast medium to prevent polymethylmethacrylate leakage during percutaneous vertebroplasty. AJNR Am J Neuroradiol 24:1001–1002

Tong FC, Cloft HJ, Joseph GJ, Rodts GR, Dion JE (2000) Transoral approach to cervical vertebroplasty for multiple myeloma. AJR Am J Roentgenol 175:1322–1324

Subject Index

List of Contributors

IBRAHIM FIKRY ABDELWAHAB, MD
Clinical Professor of Radiology
Weill Medical College, Cornell University of New York
Adjunct Clinical Professor of Pathology
Mount Sinai School of Medicine
104-60 Queens Blvd #16A
Forest Hills, NY 11375
USA

CARMEN ADEM, MD
Senior Neuroradiologist
Department of Neuroradiology
Val de Grâce Military Hospital
74 Boulevard du Port-Royal
75005 Paris
France

YASUO AMANO, MD
Assistant Professor
Department of Radiology
Nippon Medical School
1-1-5 Sendagi, Bunkyo-ku
Tokyo 113-8603
Japan

TSUTOMU ARAKI, MD
Professor and Chairman
Department of Radiology
University of Yamanashi School of Medicine
1110 Shimokatou, Tamaho-chou Nakakoma-gn
Yamanashi 409-3938
Japan

JAQUES CHIRAS, MD
Professor and Chairman
Department of Neuroradiology
La Salpêtrière University Hospital, AP-HP
47-83 Boulevard de l'Hôpital
75013 Paris
France

BYUNG IHN CHOI, MD
Professor
Department of Radiology
Seoul National University College of Medicine
28 Yongon-dong, Chongno-Gu
Seoul 110-744
Korea

SYLVAIN CHOQUET, MD
Assistant Professor
Department of Hematology
Versailles Hospital Center
177 Rue de Versailles
78157 Le Chesnay Cedex
France

KATHERINE B. M. COLQUHOUN, MD
Specialist Registrar Radiologist
Department of Clinical Radiology
C Level, Centre Block
Southampton General Hospitals Trust
Tremona Road
Southampton S016 6YD
UK

PHILIP COSTELLO, MD
Professor of Radiology
Harvard Medical School
Director of Thoracic Imaging
Brigham and Women's Hospital
75 Francis Street
Boston, MA 02114
USA

AGNÉS COULON, MD
Clinical Fellow
Department of Radiology
Croix-Rousse Hospital
Grande Rue de la Croix-Rousse
69004 Lyon
France

KAZUO DAN, MD
Professor
Department of the 3rd Internal Medicine
Nippon Medical School
1-1-5 Sendagi, Bunkyo-ku
Tokyo 113-8603
Japan

MELETIOS A. DIMOPOULOS, MD
Professor
Department of Medical Oncology
Alexandra Hospital
University of Athens Medical School
80 Vas. Sophias Avenue and Lourou Street
11528 Athens
Greece

ELISABETH DION, MD
Associate Professor
Department of Radiology
Pitié-Salpêtrière University Hospital, AP-HP
83 Boulevard de l'Hôpital
75013 Paris
France

PAMELA J. DiPIRO, MD
Assistant Professor of Radiology
Harvard Medical School
Clinical Director of CT
Dana Farber Cancer Institute
44 Binney Street
Boston, MA 02115
USA

GERALD D. DODD III, MD
Professor and Chairman
Department of Radiology
University of Texas Health Science Center at San Antonio
7703 Floyd Curl Drive
San Antonio, TX 78284
USA

ELLIOT K. FISHMAN, MD, FACR
Professor of Radiology and Oncology
Johns Hopkins University School of Medicine
Director, Diagnostic Radiology and Body CT
Department of Radiology
Johns Hopkins Hospital
600 North Caroline Street, JHOC 3254
Baltimore, MD 21287
USA

BARRY D. FLETCHER, MD
Professor of Radiology
Clinical Associate
Department of Radiology
Duke University Medical Center
Box 3808 Med Center
Durham, NC 27710
USA

MATAKAZU FURUKAWA, MD
Clinical Attending, Neuroradiologist
Department of Radiology
Yamaguchi University School of Medicine
1-1-1 Minamikogushi, Ube
Yamaguchi 755-8505
Japan

NOBUFUSA FURUKAWA, MD
Senior Radiologist
Department of Radiology
St. Mary's Hospital
422 Tusbukuhonmachi, Kurume City
National Kyushu Medical Center
Fukuoka 830-8543
Japan

DOMENICO GALETTA, MD
Associate Surgeon
Department of Thoracic Surgery
Institut Mutualiste Montsouris
42 Boulevard Jourdan
75014 Paris
France

AFSHIN GANGI, MD, PhD
Professor
Department of Radiology B
University Hospital of Strasbourg
Pavillon Clovis Vincent BP 426
67091 Strasbourg
France

HARRY K. GENANT, MD
Professor of Radiology and Orthopaedics
Department of Radiology
Chef Executive Officer
Osteoporosis & Arthritis Research Group
University of California, San Francisco
350 Parnassus Avenue, Suite 150
San Francisco, CA 94117
USA

ELIANE GLUCKMAN, MD
Professor and Chairman
Department of Bone Marrow Transplantation
Saint-Louis University Hospital, AP-HP
1 Avenue Claude Vellefaux
75010 Paris
France

DOMINIQUE GOSSOT, MD
Senior Surgeon
Department of Thoracic Surgery
Institut Mutualiste Montsouris
42 Boulevard Jourdan
75014 Paris
France

ALI GUERMAZI, MD
Visiting Associate Professor
Department of Radiology
Director, Radiographic Laboratory
Osteoporosis & Arthritis Research Group
University of California, San Francisco
350 Parnassus Avenue, Suite 150
San Francisco, CA 94117
USA

R. PAUL GUILLERMAN, MD
Assistant Professor of Radiology
Baylor College of Medicine
Department of Diagnostic Imaging
Texas Children's Hospital
6621 Fannin Street, MC 2-2521
Houston, TX 77030
USA

Stéphane Guth, MD
Senior Radiologist
Department of Radiology B
University Hospital of Strasbourg
Pavillon Clovis Vincent BP 426
67091 Strasbourg
France

Joon Koo Han, MD
Associate Professor
Department of Radiology
Seoul National University Hospital
28 Yongon-dong, Chongno-gu
Seoul 110-744
Korea

Soheil L. Hanna, MD
Associate Clinical Professor
Department of Radiology, Musculoskeletal Division
Emory University, The Emory Clinic
Northside Hospital, 1000 Johnson Ferry Rd
Atlanta, GA 30342
USA

George Hermann, MD, FACR
Professor of Radiology
Department of Radiology
Mount Sinai School of Medicine
One Gustave L. Levy Place
New York, NY 10029-6574
USA

Matthew C. Hull, MD
Radiation Oncologist
Department of Radiation Oncology
University of Florida College of Medicine
2000 SW Archer Road, PO Box 100385
Gainesville, FL 32610-0385
USA

Ah-Young Kim, MD
Assistant Professor
Department of Radiology
Asan Medical Center
University of Ulsan College of Medicine
388-1 Poongnapdong Songpagu
Seoul 138-736
Korea

Michael J. Klein, MD
Professor of Pathology
Head, Section of Surgical Pathology
Department of Pathology
University of Alabama at Birmingham School of Medicine
1922 Seventh Avenue – Room 506
Birmingham, AL 35233
USA

John Kosiuk, MD
Assistant Professor
McGill University Health Center
Department of Radiology
Royal Victoria Hospital
687 Pine Avenue West
Montreal PQ, H3A 1A1
Canada

Tatsuo Kumazaki, MD
Professor
Department of Radiology
Nippon Medical School
1-1-5 Sendagi, Bunkyo-ku
Tokyo 113-8603
Japan

François Lafitte, MD
Senior Radiologist
Department of Radiology
Adolphe de Rothschild Foundation
25-29 Rue Manin
75019 Paris
France

Frédéric E. Lecouvet, MD, PhD
Assistant Professor
Department of Radiology and Medical Imaging
Saint Luc University Hospital
Université Catholique de Louvain
10 Avenue Hippocrate
1200 Brussels
Belgium

Hyun Ju Lee, MD
Instructor of Diagnostic Radiology
Department of Radiology
Seoul National University College of Medicine
28 Yongon-dong, Chongno-Gu
Seoul 110-744
Korea

Baudouin E. Maldague MD
Professor
Department of Radiology and Medical Imaging
Saint Luc University Hospital
Université Catholique de Louvain
10 Avenue Hippocrate
1200 Brussels
Belgium

Jaques Malghem, MD
Professor
Department of Radiology and Medical Imaging
Saint Luc University Hospital
Université Catholique de Louvain
10 Avenue Hippocrate
1200 Brussels
Belgium

Stephen I. Marglin, MD, FACR
Director of Radiology
Seattle Cancer Care Alliance
Associate Professor
Department of Radiology
University of Washington School of Medicine
825 Eastlake Avenue, E.
Seattle, WA 09109-1023
USA

Tsuneo Matsumoto, MD
Associate Professor, Chest Radiologist
Department of Radiology
Yamaguchi University School of Medicine
1-1-1 Minamikogushi, Ube
Yamaguchi 755-8505
Japan

Nancy Price Mendenhall, MD
Professor and Chairman
Department of Radiation Oncology
University of Florida College of Medicine
2000 SW Archer Road, PO Box 100385
Gainesville, FL 32610-0385
USA

Benoît Mesurolle, MD
Assistant Professor
McGill University Health Center
Department of Radiology
Royal Victoria Hospital
687 Pine Avenue West
Montreal PQ, H3A 1A1
Canada

Yves Miaux, MD, MS
Vice President
Department of Reading Services
Synarc Inc.
575 Market Street, 17th Floor
San Francisco, CA 94105
USA

François Mignon, MD
Assistant Professor
Department of Radiology
Versailles Hospital Center
177 Rue de Versailles
78157 Le Chesnay Cedex
France

Shuichi Monzawa, MD
Staff Radiologist
Department of Radiology
Hyogo Medical Center for Adults
Kitaohji 13-70, Akashi City
Hyogo 673-8558
Japan

Lia A. Moulopoulos, MD
Assistant Adjunct Professor
MD Anderson Cancer Center
Assistant Professor
Department of Radiology
Areteion Hospital
University of Athens Medical School
76 Vas. Sophias Avenue
11528 Athens
Greece

Clara G.C. Ooi, MD
Associate Professor and Honorary Consultant
Department of Radiology
University of Hong Kong
Queen Mary Hospital
Pokfulam Road, Room 405, Block K
Pokfulam
Hong Kong SAR
China

Noboru Oriuchi, MD
Associate Professor
Department of Nuclear Medicine
Gumma University School of Medicine
3-39-22 Showa-machi, Maebashi-shi
Gumma 371-8511
Japan

Bruce R. Parker, MD
Professor of Radiology
Baylor College of Medicine
Chief, Department of Diagnostic Imaging
Texas Children's Hospital
6621 Fannin Street, MC 2-2521
Houston, TX 77030
USA

Ilona M. Schmalfuss, MD
Assistant Professor
Department of Radiology
University of Florida College of Medicine
2000 SW Archer Road
Gainesville, FL 32610-0385
USA

Sheila Sheth, MD
Associate Professor of Radiology
Johns Hopkins University School of Medicine
Director of Biopsy Service
Department of Radiology
Johns Hopkins Hospital
600 North Wolfe Street
Baltimore, MD 21287
USA

Susumu Sugai, MD
Professor
Department of Internal Medicine
Division of Hematology and Immunology
Kanazawa Medical University
Daigaku 1-1, Uchinada, Kahoku
Ishikawa 920-0293
Japan

Kenji Tajika, MD
Assistant Professor
Division of Hematology
Department of the 3rd Internal Medicine
Nippon Medical School
1-1-5 Sendagi, Bunkyo-ku
Tokyo 113-8603
Japan

Nobuyuki Tanaka, MD
Assistant Professor, Chest Radiologist
Department of Radiology
Yamaguchi University School of Medicine
1-1-1 Minamikogushi, Ube
Yamaguchi 755-8505
Japan

Bachir Taouli, MD
Assistant Professor
Department of Radiology
New York University Medical Center
560 First Avenue, TCH-HW 202
New York, NY10016-6497
USA

Osamu Tokuda, MD
Clinical Attending, Muscloskeletal Radiologist
Department of Radiology
Yamaguchi University School of Medicine
1-1-1 Minamikogushi, Ube
Yamaguchi 755-8505
Japan

Hisao Tonami, MD
Professor
Department of Radiology
Kanazawa Medical University
Daigaku 1-1, Uchinada, Kahoku,
Ishikawa 920-0293
Japan

Ken Tung, MD
Consultant Radiologist
Department of Clinical Radiology
C Level, Centre Block
Southampton General Hospitals Trust
Tremona Road
Southampton S016 6YD
UK

Bruno C. Vande Berg, MD, PhD
Associate Professor
Department of Radiology and Medical Imaging
Saint Luc University Hospital
Université Catholique de Louvain
10 Avenue Hippocrate
1200 Brussels
Belgium

Elida Vázquez, MD
Associate Staff, Neuroradiologist
Department of Pediatric Radiology
Hospital Materno-Infantil Vall d'Hebron
Ps. Vall d'Hebron 119-129
08035 Barcelona
Spain

Itaru Yamamoto, MD
Professor
Department of Radiology
Kanazawa Medical University
Daigaku 1-1, Uchinada, Kahoku,
Ishikawa 920-0293
Japan

MEDICAL RADIOLOGY Diagnostic Imaging and Radiation Oncology

Titles in the series already published

DIAGNOSTIC IMAGING

Innovations in Diagnostic Imaging
Edited by J. H. Anderson

Radiology of the Upper Urinary Tract
Edited by E. K. Lang

The Thymus – Diagnostic Imaging, Functions, and Pathologic Anatomy
Edited by E. Walter, E. Willich, and W. R. Webb

Interventional Neuroradiology
Edited by A. Valavanis

Radiology of the Pancreas
Edited by A. L. Baert, co-edited by G. Delorme

Radiology of the Lower Urinary Tract
Edited by E. K. Lang

Magnetic Resonance Angiography
Edited by I. P. Arlart, G. M. Bongartz, and G. Marchal

Contrast-Enhanced MRI of the Breast
S. Heywang-Köbrunner and R. Beck

Spiral CT of the Chest
Edited by M. Rémy-Jardin and J. Rémy

Radiological Diagnosis of Breast Diseases
Edited by M. Friedrich and E.A. Sickles

Radiology of the Trauma
Edited by M. Heller and A. Fink

Biliary Tract Radiology
Edited by P. Rossi

Radiological Imaging of Sports Injuries
Edited by C. Masciocchi

Modern Imaging of the Alimentary Tube
Edited by A. R. Margulis

Diagnosis and Therapy of Spinal Tumors
Edited by P. R. Algra, J. Valk, and J. J. Heimans

Interventional Magnetic Resonance Imaging
Edited by J. F. Debatin and G. Adam

Abdominal and Pelvic MRI
Edited by A. Heuck and M. Reiser

Orthopedic Imaging Techniques and Applications
Edited by A. M. Davies and H. Pettersson

Radiology of the Female Pelvic Organs
Edited by E. K.Lang

Magnetic Resonance of the Heart and Great Vessels Clinical Applications
Edited by J. Bogaert, A.J. Duerinckx, and F. E. Rademakers

Modern Head and Neck Imaging
Edited by S. K. Mukherji and J. A. Castelijns

Radiological Imaging of Endocrine Diseases
Edited by J. N. Bruneton in collaboration with B. Padovani and M.-Y. Mourou

Trends in Contrast Media
Edited by H. S. Thomsen, R. N. Muller, and R. F. Mattrey

Functional MRI
Edited by C. T. W. Moonen and P. A. Bandettini

Radiology of the Pancreas
2nd Revised Edition
Edited by A. L. Baert
Co-edited by G. Delorme and L. Van Hoe

Emergency Pediatric Radiology
Edited by H. Carty

Spiral CT of the Abdomen
Edited by F. Terrier, M. Grossholz,and C. D. Becker

Liver Malignancies Diagnostic and Interventional Radiology
Edited by C. Bartolozzi and R. Lencioni

Medical Imaging of the Spleen
Edited by A. M. De Schepper and F. Vanhoenacker

Radiology of Peripheral Vascular Diseases
Edited by E. Zeitler

Diagnostic Nuclear Medicine
Edited by C. Schiepers

Radiology of Blunt Trauma of the Chest
P. Schnyder and M. Wintermark

Portal Hypertension Diagnostic Imaging-Guided Therapy
Edited by P. Rossi
Co-edited by P. Ricci and L. Broglia

Recent Advances in Diagnostic Neuroradiology
Edited by Ph. Demaerel

Virtual Endoscopy and Related 3D Techniques
Edited by P. Rogalla, J. Terwisscha Van Scheltinga, and B. Hamm

Multislice CT
Edited by M. F. Reiser, M. Takahashi, M. Modic, and R. Bruening

Pediatric Uroradiology
Edited by R. Fotter

Transfontanellar Doppler Imaging in Neonates
A. Couture and C. Veyrac

Radiology of AIDS A Practical Approach
Edited by J.W.A.J. Reeders and P.C. Goodman

CT of the Peritoneum
Armando Rossi and Giorgio Rossi

Magnetic Resonance Angiography
2nd Revised Edition
Edited by I. P. Arlart, G. M. Bongratz,and G. Marchal

Pediatric Chest Imaging
Edited by Javier Lucaya and Janet L. Strife

Applications of Sonography in Head and Neck Pathology
Edited by J. N. Bruneton in collaboration with C. Raffaelli and O. Dassonville

Imaging of the Larynx
Edited by R. Hermans

3D Image Processing Techniques and Clinical Applications
Edited by D. Caramella and C. Bartolozzi

Imaging of Orbital and Visual Pathway Pathology
Edited by W. S. Müller-Forell

Pediatric ENT Radiology
Edited by S. J. King and A. E. Boothroyd

Radiological Imaging of the Small Intestine
Edited by N. C. Gourtsoyiannis

Imaging of the Knee Techniques and Applications
Edited by A. M. Davies and V. N. Cassar-Pullicino

Perinatal Imaging From Ultrasound to MR Imaging
Edited by Fred E. Avni

Radiological Imaging of the Neonatal Chest
Edited by V. Donoghue

Diagnostic and Interventional Radiology in Liver Transplantation
Edited by E. Bücheler, V. Nicolas, C. E. Broelsch, X. Rogiers, and G. Krupski

Radiology of Osteoporosis
Edited by S. Grampp

Imaging Pelvic Floor Disorders
Edited by C. I. Bartram and J. O. L. DeLancey
Associate Editors: S. Halligan, F. M. Kelvin, and J. Stoker

Imaging of the Pancreas Cystic and Rare Tumors
Edited by C. Procassi and A. J. Megibow

High Resolution Sonography of the Peripheral Nervous System
Edited by S. Peer and G. Bodner

Imaging of the Foot and Ankle Techniques and Applications
Edited by A. M. Davies, R. W. Whitehouse, and J. P. R. Jenkins

Radiology Imaging of the Ureter
Edited by F. Joffre, Ph. Otal, and M. Soulie

Imaging of the Shoulder Techniques and Applications
Edited by A. M. Davies and J. Hodler

Radiology of the Petrous Bone
Edited by M. Lemmerling and S. S. Kollias

Interventional Radiology in Cancer
Edited by A. Adam, R. F. Dondelinger, and P. R. Mueller

Duplex and Color Doppler Imaging of the Venous System
Edited by G. H. Mostbeck

Multidetector-Row CT of the Thorax
Edited by U. J. Schoepf

Functional Imaging of the Chest
Edited by H.-U. Kauczor

Radiology of the Pharynx and the Esophagus
Edited by O. Ekberg

Radiological Imaging in Hematological Malignancies
Edited by A. Guermazi

Imaging and Intervention in Abdominal Trauma
Edited by R. F. Dondelinger

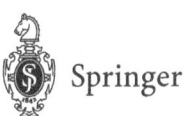

Springer

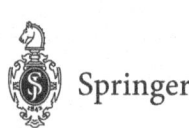 Springer

The manufacturer's authorised representative in the EU is Springer
Nature Customer Service Centre GmbH, Europaplatz 3, 69115 Heidelberg,
Germany. If you have any concerns regarding our products, please
contact ProductSafety@springernature.com

Printed and bound by CPI Group (UK) Ltd, Croydon, CR0 4YY
29/04/2026
02099553-0006